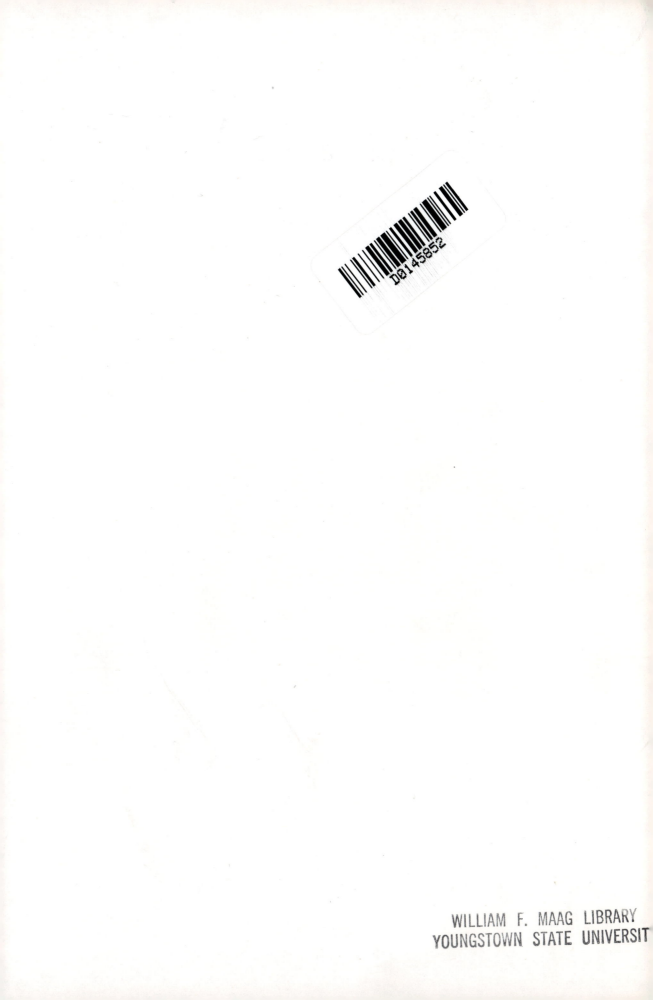

Geriatric Medicine

Volume I

Medical, Psychiatric and
Pharmacological Topics

Geriatric Medicine

Volume I

Medical, Psychiatric and Pharmacological Topics

Edited by
Christine K. Cassel
John R. Walsh

With 136 Figures

Springer-Verlag
New York Berlin Heidelberg Tokyo

Christine K. Cassel, M.D.
Department of Geriatrics
Mt. Sinai Medical Center
1 Gustave Levy Place
New York, New York 10029
U.S.A.

John R. Walsh, M.D.
Section of Geriatric Medicine
Veterans Administration Medical
 Center
Portland, Oregon 97201
U.S.A.

Principal Illustrator:
Kate Simon
Beaverton, Oregon 97007
U.S.A.

Library of Congress Cataloging in Publication Data
Main entry under title:
Geriatric medicine.
   Bibliography: p.
   Includes indexes.
   Contents: v. 1. Medical, psychiatric and pharmacolog-
ical topics—v. 2. Fundamentals of geriatric care.
   Bibliography: p.
   Includes indexes.
   1. Geriatrics.   I. Cassel, Christine K., 1945–   II. Walsh,
John R. (John Richard), 1926–   . [DNLM: 1. Geriatrics.
WT 100 G36635]
RC952.G393   1984   618.97   84-1332

Typeset by Bi-Comp, Incorporated, York, Pennsylvania.
Printed and bound by Halliday Lithograph Corporation, West Hanover,
   Massachusetts.
Printed in the United States of America.

9 8 7 6 5 4 3 2 1

Volume I
ISBN 0-387-90944-3   Springer-Verlag   New York   Berlin   Heidelberg   Tokyo
ISBN 3-540-90944-3   Springer-Verlag   Berlin   Heidelberg   New York   Tokyo
Volume II
ISBN 0-387-90958-3   Springer-Verlag   New York   Berlin   Heidelberg   Tokyo
ISBN 3-540-90958-3   Springer-Verlag   Berlin   Heidelberg   New York   Tokyo
Volumes I and II (as a set)
ISBN 0-387-96023-6   Springer-Verlag   New York   Berlin   Heidelberg   Tokyo
ISBN 3-540-96023-6   Springer-Verlag   Berlin   Heidelberg   New York   Tokyo

To our parents and grandparents

Contents of Volume I

Contents of Volume II

Foreword

With the appearance of a textbook as comprehensive as this one, it is clear that the field of geriatrics is coming of age. The broad scope of these volumes shapes a substantial answer to the question, "What is geriatrics and why should we be interested in it?" As I see it, there are at least five reasons.

First, the scientific or intellectual reason: gerontology is the study of aging from the biologic, psychological, and social perspectives. There is increasing interest in the fascinating insights into the biologic mechanisms of aging, errors in protein synthesis, DNA repair mechanisms, alterations of the neuroendocrine system, changes in the immune system, genetic controls, and somatic mutations.

Second, the demographic reason: this is the century of old age. There has been a 26-year gain in the average life expectancy. This gain compares with that acquired from 3,000 years B.C. (the Bronze Age) to the year 1900, which was about 29 years. Therefore, in one century, there has been a gain in the average life expectancy almost equal to 5,000 previous years of human history.

In 1830, one of three newborn infants survived beyond 60 years of age. Today 8 of 10 newborn babies are expected to live a full life. In 1870, only 44 of 100 women who did not die of scarlet fever, diphtheria, chicken pox, or other diseases, and who survived to 15 years of age, enjoyed what we take for granted as the natural course of human life today. In 1920, a 10-year-old person had about a 40% chance of having two of his or her four grandparents alive. At present, that probability is over 80%. From birth, women today will outlive men by nearly 8 years. This is a mixed blessing, because many of the problems of age are the special problems of women.

Third, the epidemiologic reason: the high incidence and prevalence of disease and disabilities with age is striking. Certain diseases pose "silent epidemics," which rise with the aging population. One, senile dementia of the Alzheimer's type, probably is the fourth leading cause of death; yet, it only has received significant attention recently. Another, osteoporosis, is unknown to 80% of the public according to one survey, but it is one of the main causes of disability. Along with senile dementia of the Alzheimer's type, osteoporosis is one of the true scourges of old age. These are only two examples of the kinds of medical disorders that affect great numbers of people of advanced age and that, nonetheless, have, until recently, attracted little research attention. These are frontiers of scientific knowledge that are now responding to inquiry and experimentation.

Fourth, the health costs: In 1982, about 10% of the gross national product, or $320 billion, was spent on health care; $83 billion was spent for Medicare and Medicaid, largely but not exclusively for elderly persons. Of all health costs, 30% are associated with persons over 65 years of age; 40% of all Medicaid funds go to nursing homes. There are about 20,000 nursing homes in the United States, in which about 1.5 million people reside; 1.4 million are over 65 years of age. On any given day, there are more patients in nursing homes than there are in hospitals. Attempts to contain costs often focus on the elderly population. Considerations of health care policy are a critical part of effective, prudent, and humane geriatric practice.

Fifth, attitude: negativism toward old age. In my medical school days, I was offended by the use of the word "crock" and other insensitive epithets. These attitudes are deep, widespread, and compel us to rethink our approach to the evident resistance to the development of geriatrics in our institutions of health care. Changing these negative attitudes requires more than exhortation. It requires developing a sense of competence in handling the clinical problems of elderly persons, a working knowledge of the social, economic, and institutional barriers to respectful treatment and how to change them, and the intellectual background to meet ethical issues with both analytic and humanistic skills.

Geriatrics clearly is a topic of great complexity and breadth. Some 40–50% of the time of most internists, family practitioners, gynecologists, neurologists, and others already is devoted to the diagnosis, treatment, and care of older persons. The field of geriatrics demands more than attention to one's body. It requires a greater appreciation of the social and psychological forces that operate within us. In medical education, we emphasize the search for a single explanation in the diagnostic evaluation of a patient. We refer to a medieval philosopher, William Occam, and his "razor." He is said to have propounded the principle of searching for a single explanation to any complex group of symptoms. This has been a cardinal principle of differential diagnosis. Yet, the multiplicity of illnesses, their complexity, associated polypharmacy, the disguise of one disease by another, and the effect of the age of the host in altering the presentation and the course of diseases all must change our reasoning. Multiple interacting disorders more likely explain the problems of elderly persons. The same factors also may change the character of treatment response.

The future of medicine is coupled with the "graying of America" and "the triumph of survivorship." We will have 55 million people over 65 years of age in the range of the years 2020–2030. We see corporate medicine expanding rapidly. Some 20% of all voluntary hospitals are now owned or managed by private corporations. It is possible that physicians will take a distant third place to business and government in the conduct of health delivery. Thus, understanding the social, political, and economic realities of health care systems is essential to a geriatrician.

In geriatrics, we stress the team, the egalitarian collaboration of a nurse, social worker, and other professionals with physicians. We stress the importance of assessing function and, even more importantly, maintaining and improving function. We can no longer depend on brief, mechanistic, overly economical, and, therefore, superficial forms of assessment. Older patients in contemporary hospitals deteriorate because they often are neglected after their acute episode has been taken care of. There frequently are no efforts toward continuing function, even ambulation. There should be signals that herald discharge planning at the very moment of admission. Hospitals and physicians should be prepared to respond on an urgent basis with rehabilitative and other restorative efforts when a high-risk older person is in a medical crisis.

Charcot, the great French physician, one century ago said, "The importance of a special study of the diseases of old age would not be contested at the present time." However, it has taken time. An American physician, Ignatz Nascher, introduced the term "geriatrics" just after the turn of the century. In Great Britain in the late 1930s, a unique physician, Marjorie Warren, took leadership in the development of geriatrics. In 1976, the National Institute of Aging inaugurated a Geriatric Medicine Academic Award. It also sponsored the Institute of Medicine, of the National Academy of Sciences, special task force under the leadership of Paul B. Beeson to study "aging and medical education." This report concurs with most leaders in geriatrics in not promoting a primary care practice specialty to which patients would be referred at some arbitrary age. However, most leaders in geriatrics do favor the creation of an academic specialty to insure that there will be new ideas and innovations in diagnosis and treatment, as well as critical leadership in research and education. This specialty must represent a broad range of knowledge rather than a focused one, which is characteristic of other kinds of specialties.

Not long ago, there were those who objected that geriatrics did not possess a distinct body of knowledge. If ever a book demonstrates the falseness of that statement, it is this two-volume work concerning the fundamentals of geriatric care, biomedicine, and psychiatry. It highlights the fact that geriatrics is distinct in the breadth of its concern rather than being a more narrow definition of a specialty. The goal of this unique book is to integrate biomedical and psychosocial information with the perspectives of ethics and social policy. These volumes provide the basic information that most medical textbooks do not have, for example, on such topics as law and the role of the environment in health. All of these perspectives and data bases are necessary to achieve excellence in clinical practice and to foster the further evolution of this expanding field.

Robert N. Butler, M.D.

Preface

"Old age ain't for sissies"*

In the last decade, two developments have changed the practice of medicine: the aging of the population and the dominance of medical technology. Both medical education and medical practice have responded to these events. Aging, chronic illness, and long-term care now are frequently written about in medical journals. Advances in diagnostic and therapeutic technologies have out-stripped our ability to evaluate or to pay for the new services. The field of geriatric medicine is a response to the first development and a reaction to the second.

The medical response to the demographic imperative of aging has been to codify a field of medical specialization that is relevant and useful to the increasing numbers of elderly persons. The reaction is to emphasize a broadly comprehensive, humane, and personal approach to patient care. There no longer is any doubt that there exists a body of scientific knowledge, which characterizes the field of geriatrics. In addition to a distinct body of knowledge, most geriatricians also will describe a special approach and philosophy that characterizes the practice of geriatrics. There is a growing awareness in academic medicine that special knowledge, skills, and attitudes are needed to deal effectively with elderly patients, particularly very old or frail patients. However, many physicians in primary care specialties such as internal medicine, family practice, and general surgery claim (and accurately so) that they function as geriatricians because many of their patients are elderly. In fact, in many instances, clinical practices of these generalists predominantly consist of elderly patients. Even with the advent of full-time geriatricians, the proportion of elderly persons in general practice populations will increase within the next 2 decades.

Both viewpoints are correct. Geriatrics is a specialty and also an essential component of almost any clinical practice. It is true that many physicians, especially those in primary care settings, will have a large proportion of elderly patients in their practice and (to a certain extent) will be practicing geriatrics. Until recently, most graduate training programs in medicine, family practice, or psychiatry did not include special consideration of

---

* Moore, H: Sayings, in Alvarez J, Oldham P (eds): *Old Age Ain't For Sissies.*

geriatrics. Many physicians have learned some of the practical information of their own; however, the body of knowledge referred to in the recent Institute of Medicine report and the theoretic and scientific progress in this field has not been generally accessible.† It also is true that we have, in the last 5 years in the United States, codified a specialty of geriatrics that includes training programs in geriatric medicine at the fellowship level. Many of the graduates of these programs will assume academic roles and bring the content of geriatrics to all relevant areas of health care education.

In these volumes, we have tried to assemble the material in a way that is useful for both practicing clinicians and physicians-in-training, especially those who have selected training in geriatrics. In addition, this text is meant to be a comprehensive resource for a practitioner who needs information for the clinical demands of the moment. For a research scientist or physician in advanced training, there is an introduction to the theoretical basis of each subject and a substantial bibliography. We hope that, in this way, these volumes also will provide access to the new areas of research and the new understandings that are now emerging.

Because we attempt to bring together in one place the full content of geriatric medicine, this work is deliberately compendious. Geriatrics has a broad basis; it includes clinical medicine, humanities, and the social sciences. Also, *Geriatric Medicine* accordingly has several sections organized into two volumes. The division into two volumes is primarily in the interest of the reader's convenience and, thus, inevitably somewhat arbitrary. Nonetheless, our underlying concept is that the biological, the psychosocial, and the philosophical are essential parts of a single whole. We have called on a large number of contributors, in many different fields, to assure that the subject matter is treated authoritatively.

Aging is an important and exciting area of biomedical research, which is represented largely in Volume I. The diseases that are the greatest scourges of old age are principally the chronic and degenerative disorders such as osteoporosis, parkinsonism, stroke, Alzheimer's disease, osteoarthritis, and peripheral vascular disease. Until recently, the level of research activity into the causes and treatments of these disorders has been markedly inadequate when measured against the numbers of people who are afflicted and the costs—both financial and humanitarian—to our society. However, there are areas of knowledge and research outside of biomedicine that also are critical to progress in geriatrics. These include disciplines that are based in social sciences and humanities, rather than in biology and medicine. Health services research and bioethics are especially important to geriatrics. A geriatrician may need to emulate the Renaissance scholar. The body of knowledge is broad and its relevance is undeniable.

Geriatrics is unique as a medical specialty, because it is broader, rather than narrower, than the parent disciplines. An effective clinician must have some grasp of social gerontology, architectural design, law, psychology and psychiatry, spiritual counseling, health policy and health care economics, interprofessional sociology, epidemiology, and philosophical ethics to claim a firm competence in the care of elderly persons. For this reason, much of Volume II is devoted to chapters that are written by

---

† Institute of Medicine: *Aging and Medical Education.* National Academy of Sciences, Washington, DC, 1978.

experts in these fields. These authors provide information that is both practical and relevant to clinicians, and that also may encourage a deeper exploration of this field.

The breadth of subjects covered in these two volumes is a demonstration of the need for interdisciplinary practice in geriatrics and gerontology. No one person can be an expert in each of these areas. Yet, each subject will be relevant to the needs of an elderly patient at one time or another. It is important for a geriatrician to be able to work effectively with other health care providers as well as with social scientists and policymakers, and to know where his or her own limits have been surpassed and where consultation is necessary. For appropriate and effective consultation, one must have a basic understanding of the sphere of knowledge of consultants.

The theoretical and clinical basis of geriatrics is a rich tapestry of different disciplines. In weaving this tapestry, it was inevitable that there would be overlappings and crossings of one discipline into another. The reader occasionally may find material that is apparently redundant from one chapter to another. We feel that such duplication is appropriate in a comprehensive resource text such as this. In most cases, the areas of overlap will provide a different perspective on the same topic and will enrich the understanding of the reader in the process. We hope that the indexing and cross-referencing will provide guidance to those who are specifically seeking these different perspectives.

For a project of this magnitude, it is impossible to adequately acknowledge all those who helped. It has been a project of many rewards, both in the content and meaning of the work itself and in the expanding community of scholarship and advocacy. From inception to completion, this project has taken 3 years. During this time, innumerable persons have contributed significant support. The staff of Springer-Verlag has given us stimulating concepts and good ideas, in addition to steadfast sensible guidance. The details of organizing, phone-calling, letter-writing, library research, and manuscript preparation cannot be overemphasized in a work of this size and complexity. Special acknowledgment in these areas is due to Pamela Beere Briggs and Carol Saatzer. We also acknowledge the generous support of the Henry J. Kaiser Family Foundation.

We are aware that we have joined the beginning of a very important process. The profession of medicine is at a turning point; it is caught between the successes of scientific and technologic progress and concerns about the rising costs of care and the depersonalization of its delivery. Patients—disaffected, frustrated, and often in real need—are caught in between these unresolved issues. The moral center of the profession is at risk in the policy debates. An understanding of geriatrics requires competent familiarity with the capabilities of the latest in medical technology, a discerning sense of judgment about when and when not to use such interventions, and the courage and energy to take seriously the social role of advocate for a patient. The complexity, richness, and mystery of aging cannot be described better than it has been by T.S. Eliot in *East Coker:*

> Home is where one starts from. As we grow older
> The world becomes stranger, the pattern more complicated
> Of dead and living. Not the intense moment
> Isolated, with no before and after,
> But a lifetime burning in every moment
> And not the lifetime of one man only
> But of old stones that cannot be deciphered.

We choose to view the challenge posed by the geriatric imperative not as a burden, but as an opportunity for medicine to restructure its priorities and to respond to the real needs of modern society. Geriatrics can be a vehicle for returning the values of compassion, moderation, and moral judgment to both medicine and scientific progress. These volumes, in themselves, will not create the complete clinician, but they can provide the groundwork for the excellence that is possible in geriatrics. That excellence not only is possible, but it is a duty we owe to our patients, our profession, our society, and—in the final analysis—to ourselves.

Christine K. Cassel, M.D.
John R. Walsh, M.D.

Contributors

Itamar B. Abrass, M.D., *Geriatric Research Education and Clinical Center, Veterans Administration Medical Center, Sepulveda, CA 91343 and University of California, Los Angeles School of Medicine, Multicampus Division of Geriatric Medicine, Los Angeles, CA 90024, U.S.A.*

James S. Bennett, D.M.D., M.S., *Director, General Dental Residency Program, Oregon Health Sciences University, Portland, OR 97201, U.S.A.*

Christine K. Cassel, M.D., *Department of Geriatrics, Mt. Sinai Medical Center, New York, NY 10029, U.S.A.*

Thomas G. Cooney, M.D., *Medical Director Hospital Based Home Care, Ambulatory Care Service, Veterans Administration Medical Center, and Division of General Medicine, Oregon Health Sciences University, Portland, OR 97201, U.S.A.*

Bruce M. Coull, M.D., *Department of Neurology, Director, Comprehensive Stroke Center of Oregon, Oregon Health Sciences University, Portland, OR 97201, U.S.A.*

Howard R. Creamer, Ph.D., *School of Dentistry, Oregon Health Sciences University, Portland, OR 97201, U.S.A.*

Kent Crossley, M.D., *Department of Medicine, University of Minnesota Medical School, Minneapolis, MN 55455 and St. Paul Ramsey Medical Center, St. Paul, MN 55101, U.S.A.*

Henry DeMots, M.D., *Chief, Cardiology Section, Veterans Administration Medical Center, and Division of Cardiology, Oregon Health Sciences University, Portland, OR 97201, U.S.A.*

Eugene F. Fuchs, M.D., *Division of Urology, Oregon Health Sciences University, Portland, OR 97201, U.S.A.*

David P. Gardner, M.D., Ph.D., *Department of Neurology, Oregon Health Sciences University, Portland, OR 97201, U.S.A.*

Ralph Goldman, M.D., *Associate Chief of Staff for Education, Los Angeles Veterans Administration Medical Center, and Department of Medicine, UCLA School of Medicine, Los Angeles, CA 90073, U.S.A.*

Thomas A. Golper, M.D., *Division of Nephrology, Oregon Health Sciences University, Portland, OR 97201, U.S.A.*

James S. Goodwin, M.D., *Chief, Division of Gerontology, University of New Mexico School of Medicine, Albuquerque, NM 87131, U.S.A.*

John P. Hammerstad, M.D., *Department of Neurology, Oregon Health Sciences University, Portland, OR 97201, U.S.A.*

William R. Hazzard, M.D., *Department of Medicine, Johns Hopkins Hospital, Baltimore, MD 26205, U.S.A.*

Louis A. Healey, M.D., *Department of Medicine, University of Washington, Virginia Mason Medical Center, Seattle, WA 98101, U.S.A.*

Patrick Irvine, M.D., *Director, Program of Geriatric Medicine, University of Minnesota Medical School, Minneapolis, MN 55455 and St. Paul Ramsey Medical Center, St. Paul, MN 55101, U.S.A.*

E. Paul Kirk, M.D., *Department of Gynecology and Obstetrics, Oregon Health Sciences University, Portland, OR 97201, U.S.A.*

Stanley G. Korenman, M.D., *Chairman, Department of Medicine, UCLA, San Fernando Valley Program, Veterans Administration Medical Center, Sepulveda, CA 91343, U.S.A.*

Michael R. McClung, M.D., *Chief, Endocrinology Section, Veterans Administration Medical Center, and Division of Endocrinology, Oregon Health Sciences University, Portland, OR 97201, U.S.A.*

Walter J. McDonald, M.D., *Chief, Medical Service, Veterans Administration Medical Center, and Department of Medicine, Oregon Health Sciences University, Portland, OR 97201, U.S.A.*

Diane E. Meier, M.D., *Department of Geriatrics and Adult Development, Mt. Sinai Medical Center, New York, NY 10029, U.S.A.*

James F. Morris, M.D., *Chief, Pulmonary Disease Section, Veterans Administration Medical Center, and Pulmonary Disease Division, Oregon Health Sciences University, Portland, OR 97201, U.S.A.*

Edward S. Murphy, M.D., *Cardiology Section, Veterans Administration Medical Center, and Division of Cardiology, Oregon Health Sciences University, Portland, OR 97201, U.S.A.*

Michael Myers, R.Ph., *Pharmacy Department, Bess Kaiser Medical Center, Portland, OR 97217, U.S.A.*

John G. Nutt, M.D., *Department of Neurology, Oregon Health Sciences University, Portland, OR 97201, U.S.A.*

Eric Orwoll, M.D., *Endocrinology Section, Veterans Administration Medical Center, and Division of Endocrinology, Oregon Health Sciences University, Portland, OR 97201, U.S.A.*

Robert M. Palmer, M.D., *Division of Nephrology, Oregon Health Sciences University, Portland, OR 97201, U.S.A.*

Frank Parker, M.D., *Chairman, Department of Dermatology, Oregon Health Sciences University, Portland, OR 97201, U.S.A.*

B. Z. Rappaport, Ph.D., *Audiology Service, Veterans Administration Medical Center, and Division of Gerontology, Oregon Health Sciences University, Portland, OR 97201, U.S.A.*

James B. Reuler, M.D., *Chief, General Medicine Section, Veterans Administration Medical Center, and Division of General Medicine, Oregon Health Sciences University, Portland, OR 97201, U.S.A.*

Larry F. Rich, M.S., M.D., *Department of Ophthalmology, Oregon Health Sciences University, Portland, OR 97201, U.S.A.*

Matthew C. Riddle, M.D., *Head, Division of Metabolism, Oregon Health Sciences University, Portland, OR 97201, U.S.A.*

Frederic W. Smith, M.D., *Chief, Gastroenterology Section, Veterans Administration Medical Center, and Division of Gastroenterology, Oregon Health Sciences University, Portland, OR 97201, U.S.A.*

Elmer E. Specht, M.D., *Chairman, Department of Rehabilitation, Ralph K. Davies Medical Center, San Francisco, CA 94114, U.S.A.*

Michael Spilane, M.D., *St. Paul Ramsey Medical Center, St. Paul, and Chief, Section of General Internal Medicine, University of Minnesota, Minneapolis, MN 55101*

Susan Stanik, M.D., *UCLA-San Fernando Valley Program, Veterans Administration Medical Center, Sepulveda, California, Olive View Medical Center, Van Nuys, CA 91343*

Jane E. Stilwell, M.D., *Geriatric Medicine Section, Veterans Administration Medical Center, and Division of Gerontology, Oregon Health Sciences University, Portland, OR 97201, U.S.A.*

Richard C. U'Ren, M.D., *Department of Psychiatry, Oregon Health Sciences University, Portland, OR 97201, U.S.A.*

John R. Walsh, M.D., *Chief, Geriatric Medicine Section, Veterans Administration Medical Center, and Head, Division of Gerontology, Oregon Health Sciences University, Portland, OR 97201, U.S.A.*

Geriatric Medicine

Volume I

Medical, Psychiatric and Pharmacological Topics

PART I
Fundamentals

CHAPTER 1

The Cell Biology of Aging

DIANE E. MEIER, M.D.

No one can doubt that, as preventive medicine improves and food and housing become healthier, as a way of life is established that develops our physical powers by exercise without ruining them by excess, as the two most virulent causes of deterioration, misery and excessive wealth, are eliminated, the average length of human life will be increased and a better health and a stronger physical constitution will be ensured. The improvement of medical practice, which will become more efficacious with the progress of reason and of the social order, will mean the end of infectious and hereditary diseases and illnesses brought on by climate, food, or working conditions. It is reasonable to hope that all other diseases may likewise disappear as their causes are discovered. Would it be absurd then to suppose that this perfection of the human species might be capable of indefinite progress; that the day will come when death will be due only to extraordinary accidents or to the decay of the vital forces, and that ultimately the average span between birth and decay will have no assignable value? So, in the example under consideration, we are bound to believe that the average length of human life will forever increase . . .

Condorcet on the Progress of the Human Spirit, 1793

The study of the cellular biology of aging has long been spurred by the quest for immortality. Although current methods are more scientific than they once were, the aims of aging research are still often directed at slowing or halting the process of senescence. Shedding light on some basic cellular and molecular mechanisms of aging may, at the very least, offer hope of ameliorating some of the disabilities that all too often accompany chronological aging. This chapter will define the terms, list the verifiable observations, and describe the more popular theories invoked to explain the biology of aging.

Aging may be defined as follows: First, aging is universal in a species. It is distinguished from disease and pathology, which are sometimes reversible and are, at least, not observed equally in all subjects. Second, it is a deleterious process, leading to loss of function. It is distin-guished from development, whereby an organism achieves maturation of function. Third, it is progressive. Fourth, aging is intrinsic; that is, not due to modifiable environmental factors.[1] The aging process is measured in terms of numbers surviving over time in a given population. Wild animals and Stone Age men in hostile environments die randomly at all ages, and the survival curve shows an exponential decay. In more protected populations, the curve "rectangularizes" as death tends to occur more frequently among the older members of the population (*see* Volume I, Chapter 2). It is important to note that although the mean human life expectancy has increased over the last 2,000 years, the maximum life span has remained fixed at about 110 years. As our ability to prevent and treat disease and to ameliorate hostile environmental factors has improved, the curve has become more rectangular, with most people living to old age in good health and dying in a cluster around the age of 80 (*see* Figure 2-1).[2]

Verifiable Observations

The following verifiable observations have contributed to the development of current theories of aging (*see* Table 1-1). First, mammalian species, which emerged only about 30–40 million years ago, have variable and predictable mean life spans (e.g., rats live about 3 years, cows 30 years, and humans 73 years). This period of time is too short for an evolutionary mutational process leading to life span differences, and it lends support to a genetic basis for life span variability.[3] Second, longevity is a hereditary function. For example, short-lived people come from short-lived families, and vice versa. This also lends support to a genetic locus controlling the life span, with some families having a longer "genetic tape" than others. The fact that monozygotic twins have a more equal life span than dizygotic twins or siblings is further evidence for genetic control over longevity. In support of this, certain major histocompatibility loci have been associated with life span.[4] Third, the average number of potential offspring per year in different species is inversely proportional to their life span. Species that require a long period of time to bear and rear their young require a suitably prolonged life span in which to achieve perpetuation of their line.[5] Fourth, rats that are calorie deprived prior to sexual maturation live longer than rats allowed to feed freely. Teleologically, it is not in the species' best in-

TABLE 1-1   Cell Biology of Aging: Verifiable Observations

Variable life spans among mammals
Longevity as a hereditary function
Number offspring per year inversely related to species life span
Caloric deprivation prematuration increases life span
Linear decline in organ physiologic functioning with age
Cells and organs die as a part of normal growth and development, as well as aging
Cellular function declines with age
Disease models of premature aging: Progeria, Werner's syndrome, diabetes mellitus, Down's syndrome
Finite dividing potential of human cells in culture

terest to reproduce under adverse conditions of scarcity. This is evidence for the plasticity of aging and against a pre-set genetic tape, and it may indicate that life span is amenable to interventions aimed at prolonging it.[6] Fifth, the physiologic functioning of many human organ systems declines predictably with age at a linear rate after age 30 (*see* Figure 1-1).[5] An increase in the chance of death occurs simultaneously; risk increases exponentially until the 9th and 10th decades, when the curve flattens. The oldest part of the population represents a selected robust group with a longer genetic tape and an unusual resistance to disease and environmental insults.[5]

These observations have led to the concept of the "aging hot spot" organ, such as the heart, central nervous system, and immune system. These postmitotic organs must repair or replace cellular components and enzymes regularly to prevent breakdown, because the cells cannot divide and replace themselves after maturity. Eventually, these critical organs simply wear out and the organism dies.[7] The immune system is believed by many investigators to be the biological clock that controls aging.

The sixth verifiable observation is that the organism normally loses some tissues, such as the pro- and mesonephron and the placenta, as a part of embryonic development. Just as cells and organs die as a normal developmental process, individuals may be seen to die as a normal part of the evolutionary development of the species.

Seventh, cellular function declines with age. For example, oxidative phosphorylation, cellular synthesis of RNA (ribonucleic acid) and DNA (deoxyribonucleic acid), and incorporation of radiolabelled amino acids, measurably decrease in older organisms. Receptor number and affinity (e.g., cellular beta-adrenergic receptors) are reduced with age.[1] Lipid and protein breakdown products called lipofuscin accumulate with age in many organs, particularly in postmitotic organs such as the heart, skeletal muscle, and central nervous system. Labelling studies have shown that endoplasmic reticulum and golgi apparatus are incorporated into lipofuscin. Although lipofuscin has been invoked as the cause of gradual cellular, organ, and individual deterioration in function, the harmfulness of this pigmented accumulation has not been documented.[1] Organelles undergo changes

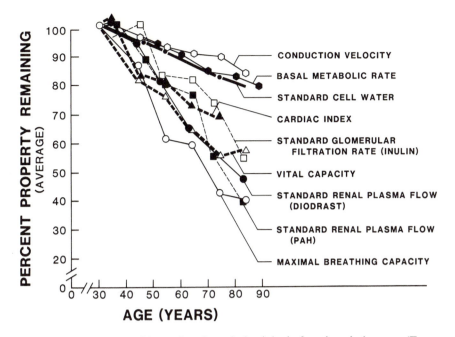

FIGURE 1-1   Decline with age in selected physiologic functions in humans (From Shock, 1960).

in morphology and function with age as well. For example, aged mitochondria show impaired viability after a hypoxic stimulus, lipoprotein membrane components undergo oxidative polymerization and become cross-linked, enzymes may decrease or increase in measurable level and activity, and a longer time is required to induce enzyme synthesis. This lag time has a linear correlation with the chronological age of the organism.[6]

Eighth, there are disease models demonstrating premature aging. These include progeria, Werner's syndrome, diabetes mellitus, and Down's syndrome. Progeria is a human disease leading to severe growth deceleration, characterized by generalized atherosclerosis that usually causes death in the 2nd decade. Werner's syndrome is similar to progeria although the life span approximates 5 decades and the clinical picture includes an increased incidence of neoplasm, predisposition to diabetes mellitus, osteoporosis, cataracts, and hair loss.[8,9] The clinical relevance of these diseases to normal human aging is not known; however, cell cultures from individuals with these diseases demonstrate doubling and morphological characteristics similar to cultures of normal aged human cells. Persons with trisomy 21 (Down's syndrome) die at a younger age than other retarded people; they

evidence a progressive dementia that overlaps their retardation and has both a clinical and a pathological resemblance to Alzheimer's disease. Epidemiologic observations of families with Alzheimer's disease have revealed an increased incidence of Down's syndrome and carcinoma. Further evidence supporting Down's syndrome as a model of accelerated aging is found in the immune system. There is an increased incidence of infection, and certain immunologic dysfunctions are found in both normal elderly individuals and in those with Down's syndrome.[3]

Ninth, Leonard Hayflick's observations on the finite dividing potential of human cells in culture provides further empiric support for genetic control of longevity; this will be discussed in detail later in this chapter.

This listing of empiric data supports many different theories of aging. It is likely that aging is a multifactorial process, and that there is no unitary explanation for the observed phenomena that precede death. The following discussion of current theory should be read with this in mind.

The two major theories of aging are the "wear and tear" theory and the genetic program theory. The "wear and tear" theory assumes that aging is due to progressive damage to the organism from its internal and external environment. Processes occurring before the reproductive age are thought to be under the control of genetic information arrived at through natural selection. Once the germ cell line has been replicated, the finite life span of somatic cells is determined by the quality of the structures built by the developmental program (strong or weak) and its interactions with the environment over time.[5] An example frequently used is that of the car sitting in the garage, rarely used, protected from the elements, lasting far longer than the one driven 50,000 miles per year and parked on the street. The theories subsumed under the "wear and tear" concept include the error-catastrophe, free radical, somatic mutation, lipofuscin accumulation, and collagen cross-linkage theories.[10,11]

The genetic program theory suggests that growth, maturation, and senescence are genetically controlled through codon restriction. Senescence is caused by a switching off of the capacity to translate messages whose products are necessary for cellular function. Mechanisms permitting successive repressions and derepressions, which normally occur in code word groups to produce needed proteins, are somehow terminated. Each organism is thought to have its own "genetic tape" that begins playing at conception and then comes to an end at some predetermined moment, thus causing death. Disease and a hostile environment might cause the organism to die before the tape reaches its conclusion; however, even a totally protected

healthy animal will eventually surrender to its genetically determined life span. The "organ hot spot theory" postulates that the genetic program in certain critical organs runs out first and initiates aging within the organism. The immune senescence and endocrine theories of aging, therefore, are classified with the genetic program concept of aging (see Table 1-2).[11]

Wear and Tear Theories

Free Radicals

Free radicals are chemicals with an unpaired electron (O, O_3^*, O^*-OH, $H_2O_2^*$), which are highly reactive with the unsaturated lipids, nucleic acids, proteins, and polysaccharides that comprise living organisms. They are formed from exogenous (radiation) and endogenous (enzymatic degradation) stimuli and cause disruption of chemical bonds and membranes. This leads to polymerization, accumulation of debris, loss of membrane and enzymatic integrity, and cell death.[6,10] Several mechanisms exist in vivo that afford protection from free radicals. First, antioxidants are found in living organisms, including Vitamin E, selenium, and superoxide dismutase. Second, the structural integrity of cells protects vulnerable unsaturated lipids and genetic material by burying them so that they are inaccessible to free radicals. Third, oxygen tension is lower in vivo and, thus, fewer free radicals are formed. Fourth, highly charged metals (such as iron and copper) are bound and chelated in vivo, thus preventing production of free radicals.[4] Attempts to prolong life by decreasing ingestion of unsaturated fatty acids or increasing ingestion of antioxidants have proven only minimally effective in laboratory animals. Mice of differing life spans show no difference in superoxide dismutase antoxidant levels, nor do these levels alter with age in rat brains.[6] Radiation exposure, known to induce free radicals, can be shown to decrease the life span of mammalian white blood cells. Resistance of white blood cells of different species to radiation is directly proportional to the median life span. However, human studies, to date, have not shown a correlation between radiation exposure and shortened life expectancy.[10]

TABLE 1-2   Cell Biology of Aging: Theories

Wear and tear theories
  Free radical (Harman)
  Lipofuscin accumulation (Strehler, Mann and
    Yates, Bjorkerud)
  Macromolecular cross-linking (Bjorksten, Kohn)
  Somatic mutation (Szilard, Maynard-Smith,
    Curtis, Martin)
  Error-catastrophe (Orgel, Martin, Holiday, Tarrant)

Genetic program theories
  Finite doubling potential (Hayflick)
  Codon Restriction (Strehler)
  Immune senescence (Weksler, Walford,
    Goodwin)
  Endocrine pacemaker (Timiras, Finch)

Lipofuscin Accumulation

Lipofuscin is thought both to consist of breakdown products of mitochondria, lysosomal debris, and golgi apparatus, and to accumulate as a result of decreased exocytic function. It increases in amount with age, particularly in post-mitotic organs. It can be induced experimentally by a Vitamin E-deficient diet, leading to the postulate that auto-oxidation causes its accumulation.[12] Lipofuscin has not been clearly linked to cellular dysfunction, although a rough correlation exists between the amount of lipofuscin in the brain and the degree of dementia in Alzheimer's disease.[13,14] Some researchers claim that meclofenoxate, a lipofuscin-removing chemical, can decrease confusion and cognitive dysfunction in demented patients.[4]

Macromolecular Cross-Linking

Build up of cross-linked collagen also has been proposed as an aging mechanism leading to abnormal mechanical properties and altered permeability in cells. Both free radicals and aldehydes (products of metabolism toxic to cells) have been invoked as etiologic agents in macromolecular cross-linking; however, to date, little evidence is available to support this process as a primary event in aging.[4,5,10]

Somatic Mutations

This theory proposes that life span is determined by the rate of somatic mutation. In other words, enough errors of DNA replication that are not accurately repaired will lead to aging and death.[3,4,16] In support of this theory, the efficiency of DNA repair is directly proportional to life span among animal species. The major argument against somatic mutation as the cause of senescence is the fact that mutations occur randomly, and aging is clearly a nonrandom process. Differences in gene regulation, not in gene structural mutation, have led to phenotypic changes in the life span that occur over time in hominid-human precursors. The relatively rapid evolution of hominids with both larger head sizes and associated increases in longevity occurred over millions of years. This could not have been due to the slower evolutionary process of random mutation through

structural amino acid substitutions that require billions of years. For example, the DNA and protein in chimpanzees is identical to that in humans and, therefore, it must be gene regulation and expression that is responsible for the observed phenotypic differences between the ape and man, including the life span.[3,16,17]

Error-Catastrophe Theory

A related theory postulates a random error in translation or transcription, which leads to an abnormal protein. This abnormal protein is itself needed to make other proteins (e.g., RNA polymerase). The accumulation of abnormal end-products leads to a negative feedback loop to the genome with an increasing production of the original abnormal protein. This leads to catastrophe and cell death.[3,7,16–18] The theory requires both random accumulation of somatic mutations and kinetics of accumulation appropriate to the varying life spans of mammalian species. Evidence for this proposal is the redundancy of the genetic message, with extra sequences normally repressed and then derepressed if the active gene is damaged. The theory assumes that when all repetition has been completed catastrophe and death occurs. The degree of gene redundancy among species is directly proportional to their life span. Another argument in support of the error-catastrophe theory observes that evolutionary change and genetic diversity require occasional somatic errors; that is, there is an optimal error rate in order for natural selection to occur.[7] Although germ cells are highly stable in their translation to insure continuity of information to the next generation, somatic cells may be less protected from error. Accuracy in error regulation, both in surveillance and repair, requires energy. Accordingly, the organism may need to permit some somatic error to balance energy needed for growth and reproduction. This theory views aging as an organism's eventual inability to maintain energy for error surveillance and repair. Arguments against this construct point out that although cellular enzymatic function decreases with age, it does not occur in the exponential or random manner predicted by the theory. Furthermore, a viral genome added to young and old cells undergoes no loss of fidelity of viral replication in the older cells. Chromosomal abnormalities are a constant feature of neoplastic cells, which are immortal, despite their theoretic vulnerability to error-catastrophe due to aneuploidy. Finally, animals fed amino acid analogues, which should theoretically increase the risk of an error-catastrophe, demonstrate no alterations in life span. Rather, the abnormal proteins are simply turned over faster.[3,16–18] This theory is an area of active controversy and research.

Genetic Programming Theories

Finite Doubling Potential

Genetic theory places control of aging in the nucleus of the cell, which is thought to be programmed in a finite manner. Age changes are normal genetic signals in a series whose ultimate purpose is to bring the organism to and through the reproductive phases. The work of Leonard Hayflick is at the foundation of this theory, and it supports the genetic predetermination of life span.[2,8,9,15,21,22] Using cell culture techniques, Hayflick found that the number of human fibroblast divisions is fixed at about 50 doublings, in vitro. This cellular senescence cannot be overcome by placing an old cell into the protected environment of a young animal, which supports the thesis that it is a process within the cell itself—and not a lack of some environmental requirement—that is responsible for cellular aging. Similarly, transplantation of an old cell nucleus into a young cytoplast results in a hybrid cell with the life span of the transplanted nucleus. Alterations in nutrients of the culture medium will not alter the number of doublings. If cells are allowed to double 20 times, are frozen, and then thawed, they will continue to double 30 times for a total of 50 divisions, which is indicative of the constancy of cell division. Cells from donors of varied ages display growth potentials inversely related to the age of the donor; cells from species of varied life spans display growth potentials directly proportional to the donor species' life span.

Evidence of cellular aging in the later divisions has been observed and measured by decreases in nutrient uptake, decreased repair of chromosomal damage, changes in enzyme synthesis, and organelle morphologic abnormalities. Both in vivo and in vitro aged cells demonstrate lobed and irregular nuclei, pleomorphic vacuolated mitochondria, dilated and vesicular golgi apparatus, increased number of lysosomes, decreased rough endoplasmic reticulum, and an increase in lipofuscin. The time required to complete a division is greater in older cells, thus demonstrating functional as well as morphologic decline during the later doublings. Significant clonal variation exists between and within cell cultures; some cells do not divide at all, others go through all 50 divisions. Cells from individuals with progeria, Werner's syndrome, or diabetes mellitus, model diseases of premature human aging, demonstrate a striking decrease in their in vitro cell-doubling potential. Finally, normal cells may be transformed into immortal cells via incorporation of the cancer-causing viral genome SV40, which provides further evidence for genetic control of the cellular life span. Bacterial cultures are also immortal, although individual bacteria die with a fixed life span. Similarly, the infinite capacity of human germ cells to divide is responsible for the propagation of the species.[2,8,9,15,21,22]

Hayflick's cell culture technique has been criticized on several counts. First, the in vitro medium is an artificial environment that may not approximate the normal biologic needs of a cell. The experiments showing that old cells have a finite number of divisions, even when transplanted into young hosts, begins to counter this criticism; however, the relevance of the in vitro experiment to the in vivo cellular milieu remains at issue. Structuring of cells into units and organs may affect their longevity through cell-to-cell interactions that cannot be observed using cell culture techniques. Finally, highly differentiated postmitotic cells, where critical aging changes take place, cannot be maintained in cell culture; an overgrowth of fibroblasts occurs through cell selection.[1,4,23,24] There are three categories of somatic cells: 1) Continuously dividing cells, such as bone marrow stem cells, skin, and the lining of the gastrointestinal tract; 2) Intermittently dividing cells with slow doubling and a preserved capacity to repair injury through regeneration, such as hepatocytes and fibroblasts; and 3) postmitotic cells, which do not divide after maturity and cannot regenerate after cell death, such as nerve and muscle cells.

The division and regenerative capacity of the first two types of cells remains fairly intact in aged humans; thus, a simple cellular inability to divide does not seem to be responsible for aging. In fact, the Hayflick limit for dividing cells is probably never reached during a normal human life time. Instead, aging is probably the result of functional changes at the postmitotic cellular level that leads to loss of organ function. In other words, even if it is acknowledged that human cells have a finite replicative capacity, the primary aging process does not necessarily result from reaching that limit. It may occur for other reasons, usually deterioration in function of highly differentiated non-dividing cells of the heart, brain, or immune system.[2]

The primary event of senescence may be the chance deterioration of long-lived macromolecules and postmitotic cells whose synthesis and division stops early in life. The development of these stable cellular components, without repair or replacement capability, is thought to lead to some selective advantage for the species. A finite intrinsic error rate is advantageous because it allows for natural selection. The existence of highly differentiated non-dividing cells increases adaptability and insures propagation of the germ cell line.[7] Thus, the loss of ability of parts of an organism to divide and repair errors is exchanged for the protective function of specialized postmitotic organs. The continued existence of the species is insured at the expense of individual immortality.[4,7]

What is the relevance of the Hayflick limit to the aging of organs made up of specialized postmitotic cells? Many of the observed cellular, morphologic, and enzymatic changes that occur during the later divisions of fibroblasts are identical to those that occur in aging cells of the heart or central nervous system. An understanding of why normal fibroblasts lose their ability to divide may provide insight into other age-related losses of function.[2] The observed inverse correlation of age to the remaining number of cell divisions, the decreased dividing potential in cells from individuals with diseases characterized by premature aging, and the positive correlation of species life span to the maximum number of divisions in cell culture, are evidence of the relation of the Hayflick limit to the processes underlying aging.[2,8,9,15,19–21]

These conclusions remain controversial.

Some authors have postulated that it is artifactual overgrowth of cells committed to senescence that hides the existence of uncommitted immortal cells in culture.[22,23] Other investigators have interpreted the loss of ability to divide as evidence of differentiation to new functions, rather than evidence of senescence. In other words, the cessation of cell doubling is not necessarily preliminary to cell death, which is exemplified by postmitotic cells such as nerve and muscle that live and function for years after they have stopped dividing.[22,23]

Although changes in cell morphology and function occurring in tissue culture may not be directly applicable to aging, in vivo, Hayflick's work does focus attention on intrinsic cellular and molecular processes that are controlled by genetic information.

Codon Restriction Theory

This theory postulates that there is a continuously operating program in chromosomes, which begins with embryonic development, continues with growth and differentiation, and terminates with senescence. The primary aging event is thought to be the switching off of the capacities to translate messages whose products are required for mitosis or other cell functions. The successive repressions and derepressions needed to produce required proteins throughout the life span would include the senescent repression of genes coding for proteins that may be vital to cellular functioning.[24,25] The result of this cessation of mitosis, and of synthesis of needed proteins, is cellular degeneration and death.

Immune Senescence Theory

This theory proposes that aging results from variations in antigens and antibodies that determine the recognition of self. Loss of tolerance to self leads to autoimmune phenomena, degenerative changes, aging, and death. Implicit in this construct is that the decline of immune function is a genetically determined primary event, with the thymus playing the role of an "organ clock" that reaches the end of its genetic information first, thus determining longevity.[25–28] Evidence in favor of this theory includes the observation that parameters increasing the life span, such as prepubertal malnutrition and hypothermia, also lead to improved immune function. By age 50, the thymic mass is less than 15% of its maximum. T-cell proliferative capacity steadily declines with age. Skin test reactivity can be shown to decrease with age, and the decline is correlated with an increased mortality.[25-28] Increases in antithyroglobulin, antinative DNA and antiIgG antibodies, immune complexes, monoclonal gammopathies, rheumatoid factors, and amyloid deposition can be shown with age. In addition, an increase in the number of B cells with a specific antibody to self, a decreased avidity (speed and intensity) of immune reaction, an increase in blocking antibodies (binds to antigenic site, but without efficacy), and an increased macrophage elaboration of prostaglandin E can be demonstrated in aging humans.[24] Despite this increase in measurable evidence of autoimmunity, there is no associated increase in the incidence of autoimmune disease in the elderly.[26] However, incidence of neoplasm and infection does increase with age.

Investigators have observed multiple, and occasionally contradictory, changes in B and T cell function with age.[24-26] Normally, B cells originate in bone marrow and form antibodies. Some are T-cell dependent and some T-independent. Helper T cells stimulate, and suppressor T cells inhibit, B cell differentiation to plasma cells. Sensitized T lymphocytes and antigens produce migration inhibitory factors and chemotactic factors, and they mediate delayed hypersensitivity. Cytolytic T lymphocytes cause cell lysis and cell-mediated immunity. Aging leads to thymic involution and decreases in secretion of, and response to, humoral regulatory factors, delayed hypersensitivity, cytotoxic T cell generation, graft rejection, quantitative and qualitative antibody response, and phytohemagglutinin response. This suggests that age-related, T-cell functional alterations are occurring at a number of different loci.

Intrinsic B cell function is said by some researchers to remain normal, and by others to decline with age.[25-28] The importance of thymic hormones in immunity is supported by studies showing that old T cells transplanted into young thymectomized and irradiated animals do not improve functionally, and that an infusion of thymic hormones into an older animal subject will improve T cell function.[25] A decrease in helper T cell function that causes a lowered response to exogenous antigens may lead to the increased incidence of infection that is seen with age.[25,26] Likewise, a decrease in suppressor T cell function that causes a lowered tolerance of self may lead to the observed increase in serologic markers of autoimmunity.[25,26] Other researchers propose that a decrease in self-tolerance may permit development of clonal, autoreactive B cells, with a secondary compensatory increase in the numbers of suppressor T cells. This might lead to some modulation of clinical manifestations of autoimmunity, but it could cause a non-specific T suppression of B cells that respond to exogenous infectious agents and endogenous neoplastic antigens.[25,26] Yet, a third theory postulates a primary decrease in intrinsic B cell function with age, which leads to compensatory increases in helper T cells and decreases in suppressor T cells.[27,28] This might lead to increased autoimmunity via diminished T-cell suppressor function; the increased rate of infection might be due to the inadequacy of the compensatory increase in helper T cells. Older subjects have been shown to have increased sensitivity to prostaglandin E-mediated inhibition of suppressor T cells, with a resultant relative increase in helper T cell-B cell production of autoantibodies. Indomethacin, a prostaglandin synthetase inhibitor, has been shown to increase skin test reactivity in the elderly, presumably by restoring the balance of T helper and suppressor function.[27,28]

Attempts to slow the aging process through the manipulation of T and B cell function may lend credence to the theory that the immune system is the organ clock or "hot spot" of senescence (see Figure 1-2).

Endocrine Pacemaker Theory

An organ hot spot theory similar to the immune senescence theory postulates that the endocrine system contains the aging pacemaker through its failing hypothalamic neuroendocrine control over end-organ function.[29]

The study of the cell biology of aging raises basic questions that the preceding discussion of current theory attempts to answer. Why do we age? What prevents eternal life? Can aging be

FIGURE 1-2 Theoretical mechanisms of immune senescence (From Goodwin, 1982).

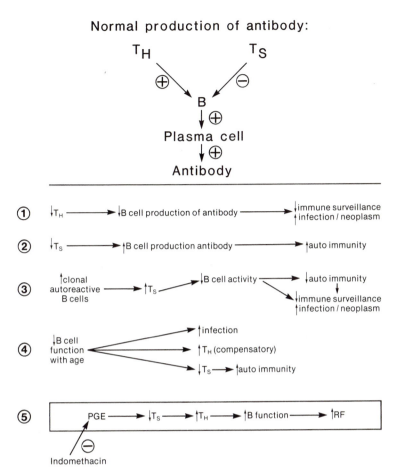

prevented or delayed? Should it be? The growing number of verifiable observations about senescence await a unifying explanatory theory.

References

1. Rowlatt C, Franks LM: Aging in tissues and cells, in Brocklehurst JC (ed). *Geriatric Medicine and Gerontology.* ed. 2, New York, Churchill Livingstone, 1978, pp 3–17.
2. Fries JF, Crapo LM: *Vitality and Aging.* San Francisco, WH Freeman & Co, 1981, pp 25–40.
3. Martin G: Genetic and evolutionary aspects of aging. *Fed Proc,* 38:6, May 1979, pp 1962–1967.
4. Schofield JD, Davies I: Theories of aging, in Brocklehurst JC: *Geriatric Medicine and Gerontology.* ed. 2, New York, Churchill Livingstone, 1978, pp 38–70.
5. Comfort A: *The Biology of Senescence.* ed. 3, Elsevier Press, 1964.
6. Scoggins CH: The cellular basis of aging. *West J Med* 135:521–525, December 1981.
7. Latham KR, Johnson LK: Aging at the cellular level, in Rossman I: *Clinical Geriatrics.* ed. 2, Philadelphia, Lippincott, 1979, pp 60–81.
8. Hayflick L: Cell aging. Annual review of gerontology and geriatrics. vol. 1, New York, Springer, 1980, pp 26–67.
9. Hayflick L: The biology of human aging. *Am J Med Sci* 265(1):432–445, June 1973.
10. Harman D: The aging process. *Proc Natl Acad Sci USA* 78:7124–7128, 1981.
11. Scoggin CH: The cellular, biochemical and genetic basis of aging, in Shrier RW (ed): *Clinical Internal Medicine in the Aged.* Philadelphia, WB Saunders & Co, 1982, pp 24–28.
12. Sanadi DR: Metabolic changes and their significance in aging, in Finch CE, Hayflick L (eds): *Handbook of the Biology of Aging.* New York, Van Nostrand Reinhold Co, 1977, pp 73–93.
13. Finch CE: Neuroendocrine and autonomic aspects of aging, in Finch CE, Hayflick L (eds): *Handbook of the Biology of Aging,* New York, Van Nostrand Reinhold Co, 1977, chap 11, pp 262–274.

14. Brody H, Vijayashankar N: Anatomical changes in the nervous system, in Finch CE, Hayflick L (eds): *Handbook of the Biology of Aging.* New York, Van Nostrand Reinhold Co, 1977, chap 10, pp 241–256.

15. Hayflick L: Cell biology of aging. *Bio Science* 25:629–636, 1975.

16. Martin GM: Genotropic theories of aging: An overview, in Finch CE, Hayflick L (eds): *Handbook of the Biology of Aging.* New York, Van Nostrand Reinhold Co, 1977, chap 1, pp 5–20.

17. Martin GM: Evidence against somatic mutation as a mechanism of clonal senescence. *Adv Exp Med Biol* 129:139–145, 1980.

18. Orgel LE: The maintenance of the accuracy of protein synthesis in its relevance to aging. *Proc Natl Acad Sci USA* 49:517–521, 1963.

19. Hayflick L: Cell biology of human aging. *Sci Am,* 242:58–65, 1980.

20. Hayflick L: Current theories of biological aging. *Fed Proc* 34:9–13, 1975.

21. Hayflick L: The longevity of cultured human cells. *J Am Geri Soc* 22:1–12, 1974.

22. Holliday R, Huschtcha LI, Tarrant GM, et al: Testing the commitment theory of fibroblast aging. *Science* 198:366–372, 1979.

23. Kirkwood TBL: Evolution of aging. *Nature* 270:301–304, 1977.

24. Strehler BL, Hirsch G, Gusseck D: Codon restriction theory of aging and development. *J Theor Biol* 33:429–474, 1971.

25. Weksler ME: The senescence of the immune system. *Hosp Pract,* pp 53–63, October 1981.

26. Walford RL: *The Immunologic Theory of Aging.* Fed Proc 33:2020–2027, 1974.

27. Goodwin JS: *Suppressor Cells in Human Disease.* New York, Marcel Dekker, 1981, pp 99–135.

28. Goodwin JS, Searles RP, Tung KSH: Immunological responses of a healthy elderly population. *Clin Exp Immunol* 48:403–410, 1982.

29. Timiras PS: Biological perspectives on aging. *Amer Sci* 66:605–613, 1978.

CHAPTER 2

Normal Human Aging: A Theoretical Context

RALPH GOLDMAN, M.D.

The striking prolongation in life expectancy has greatly increased the proportion of older individuals in the population. After many years of disinterest, medical attention is now necessarily focused on geriatrics. As would be expected, the approach is one that has been successful in the resolution of all previous problems in medicine. However, there are reasons to suspect that these methods may not be relevant, since the problems may be based on an entirely different set of conditions.

There is an oft-quoted cliché that nobody ever died of old age. Physicians are oriented to the concept of disease and, as a corollary, that all diseases are potentially reversible and eventually preventable. Since death comes in many guises, and natural death should appear in but one, this concept is believed to be valid. It may not be.

What will be presented is the concept that life is intrinsically limited, that natural death need not be stereotyped, that many of what are now considered chronic diseases may be the natural, age-related, systematic manifestations of aging, and that an impressive body of evidence has been developed to support these views.[1–5]

Survival

Until recently, death usually has been considered to be an accidental and environmentally induced event. The accident may be overtly physical, but it can also be due to famine, infection, or less obvious causes. In any essentially unchanging environment, the risks are relatively constant; survival should follow that of curve 1B (*see* Figure 2-1), in which a 50% risk of death occurs in an identifiable period of time. Progressive reduction of extrinsic risks should lengthen this period and produce the shallower curves 1C and 1D. If all risks could be eliminated and all deaths were environmentally induced, there should be no deaths and individuals would be immortal, as exemplified by curve 1A (*see* Figure 2-1).

Obviously, this is an oversimplification. Old age has been clearly identified with characteristic bodily changes and an associated increase in vulnerability to death. A fundamental question that must be resolved is whether aging changes are inherent in an organism or are the result of cumulative, extrinsic sublethal trauma. If there is an intrinsic biologic limit, survival of a cohort should follow pattern 1E in the absence of accidents or, more probably, pattern 1F, if allowance is made for individual variation and a normal distribution of risk. Although the concept of such patterns tends to be rejected initially, these patterns are not uncommon in nature. Annual plants do not survive beyond a season, adult mayflies have no mouth parts and can reproduce although not feed, and salmon die after spawning. An intrinsically controlled life span can be the result of a specific genetic program (*see* Volume I, Chapter 1), or the result of program exhaustion after the function of assuring species survival has been accomplished.

The foregoing paradigms assume a constant vulnerability to risk; however, if a newborn infant has a greater vulnerability, the early death

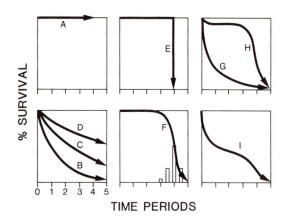

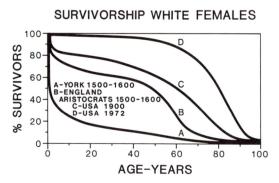

FIGURE 2-1 Theoretical patterns of cohort survival. (A) Infinite survival in the absence of environmental hazards. (B) Death due to a constant rate of environmental hazard. (C,D) Deaths due to reduced, but constant, levels of environmental hazard. (E) Death due to a precisely timed intrinsic mechanism. (F) Death due to an intrinsic mechanism, but with a distribution of time among individuals. (G) Death due to environmental hazards, but with a greater risk in infancy and childhood. (H) Early deaths due to faulty development, late deaths due to intrinsic mechanisms. (I) Deaths within a cohort due to all of the above. (From Goldman R: The aging process and the gerontologist, in Haley NB, Kennan PA (eds): *Health and Health Care of the Aging.* Charlottesville, University Press of Virginia, 1981, used by permission.)

FIGURE 2-2 Actual patterns of survival. (A) Females in the city of York, England (compare with curve 1G). (B) English aristocrats, Sixteenth Century. (C) White females, United States, 1900 (compare B and C with curve 1I). (D) White females, United States, 1972 (compare with curve 1H). (Curves A and B adapted from Cowgill in *Sci Amer, 1970,* and curves C and D from *Statistical Abstracts of the United States, 1975.* From Goldman R: Aging and geriatric medicine, in Beeson PB, McDermott W, Wyngaarden JB (eds): *Cecil Textbook of Medicine.* Philadelphia, WB Saunders & Co, 1979, p 34 used by permission.)

rate would be greater at any risk level and curve 1G would apply. In this case, the accelerated risk occurs early and, at some point in maturation, the risk stabilizes as shown in curve 1B. Example 1H demonstrates a pattern in which there is abnormal development; death occurs shortly after birth, following the withdrawal of maternal support and despite a risk-free environment. Finally, pattern 1I synthesizes all these possible factors, including lethal maldevelopment, reduced early resistance to stress, environmental risk, and (finally) ultimate-intrinsic life limitation.

With these possibilities in mind, it is interesting and instructive to examine actual human experience. Figure 2-2 exemplifies this experience and is representative of a large body of data. Curve 2A is the experience of females in the city of York, England, during the Sixteenth Century. There was a 45% survival rate the first year, 18% to age 20, 11% to age 40, and 3–4% to age 65.[6] This curve strongly resembles 1G (*see* Figure 2-2), in which a stressful environ-

ment causes excessive infantile and juvenile mortality, then reaches a constant one-half survival time of approximately 20 years. This pattern would have resulted in the depopulation of York were it not for the constant influx of residents from the countryside. Curve 2B is the concurrent example for the aristocracy and resembles curve 1I.[6] This curve is the one most frequently observed in nature, and it is probable that the contemporary populace of the countryside resembled this pattern more than it did pattern 2A. It is of interest that through the Middle Ages and Renaissance, the total population growth was extremely slow; a very small decrease in reproductive success would have led to a population decline. Curve 2C represents the survival of white females in the United States at the onset of the Twentieth Century.[7] It closely resembles curve 2B, although there has been significant improvement. Finally, curve 2D resembles curve 1H. There has been both a striking improvement in survival and a significant alteration in the pattern. Survival is now 96.7% at age 40, 83.9% at age 65, and 36.6% at age 85. There is little evidence of accidental death and most deaths occur within a relatively small age range. Gerontologists refer to this as "squaring" of the survival curve (see Table 2-1).

TABLE 2-1   Percent Survival at Various Ages: 1900 and 1978

| | White | | | | All Other | | | |
| | Male | | Female | | Male | | Female | |
Age	1900	1978	1900	1978	1900	1978	1900	1978
1	86.7	98.7	88.9	98.9	74.7	97.7	78.5	98.1
20	76.4	97.3	79.0	98.2	56.7	96.1	59.0	97.2
40	65.0	93.7	67.9	96.7	43.0	88.7	46.1	94.1
65	39.2	71.1	43.8	83.9	19.0	56.4	22.0	73.4
85	5.2	16.8	7.1	36.6	2.0	13.8	3.6	27.9

SOURCE: *Vital Statistics of the United States.* Washington, DC, Government Printing Office, 1980.

There have been at least two obvious results of this change. The progressive increase in female survival through the reproductive period, at extremes from 11–96%, has reduced the number of births needed to sustain a population level. With the delay in adaptation to a lower birth rate, it has caused a massive surge in population growth. In addition, this is the first time any animal species has achieved survival to old age as the norm, rather than the exception.

Death Rates

It is usually accepted that the risk of death is greatest at the extremes of life, but the data have not been generalized for clinical use. Figure 2-3A shows such data for United States females for 1978.[7] As expected, there is a relatively high infant mortality, then a rapid decrease in the first few years, reaching a nadir at puberty. In adolescence and early maturity, there is an excessive mortality followed by a consistently accelerating death rate with increasing age. When the log of the age-specific death rate is plotted on the ordinate (*see* Figure 2-3B), it appears to be a straight line after early maturity. This phenomenon was first recognized by a British actuary, Benjamin Gompertz, in 1825; it has been identified since with his name as Gompertz's Law.[8] Presumably, it has been used by the insurance industry since that time, but it was not until more than one century later that it began to appear in biological literature. The equation is:

$$Y_x = Y_o e^{ax},$$

where Y_o is the risk of death at age o, Y_x is the risk at age x, e is the natural logarithm, and a is a constant.

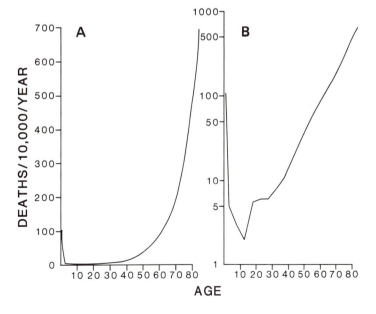

FIGURE 2-3   Risk of death at various ages in the United States, females, 1978. In Figure 2-3A, the risk is plotted on a rectangular scale; in Figure 2-3B, the risk is plotted on a logarithmic scale. Age is plotted on the abscissa and the risk of death at a specific age, the age-specific death rate, is shown on the ordinate.

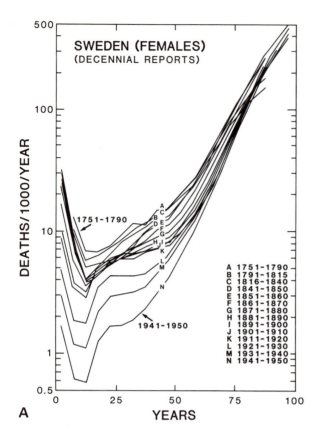

FIGURE 2-4A   Age-specific death rates for females in Sweden, 1751–1950. (From Jones HB: The relation of human health to age, place, and time, in Birren JE (ed): *Handbook of Aging and the Individual: Psychological and Biological Aspects*. Chicago, University of Chicago Press, 1959, used by permission.)

The implication of Gompertz's Law is that the risk of death is directly related to age, regardless of cause. This implies a fixation of risk and raises questions as to the goals and evaluation of medical intervention. Figure 2-4A shows the changes in mortal risk of Swedish women from 1750–1950[9] and Figure 2-4B shows the changes in the actual risk curve in the United States at intervals between 1900–1978.[7] The sequence of curves demonstrates a decreasing infantile and juvenile mortality. The adolescent-young adult anomaly progressively decreases,

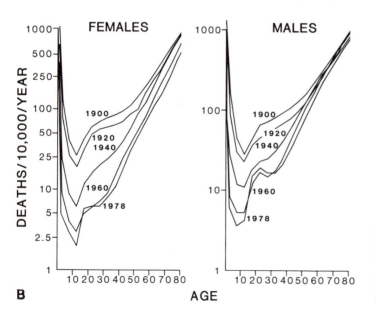

FIGURE 2-4B Age-specific death rates of females and males in the United States, 1900–1978. (From *Vital Statistics of the United States*, Washington, DC, Government Printing Office, 1980.)

the straight portion of the curve starts at a lower level and at an earlier age, and its slope increases. These changes have been observed in all mortality risk curves and must be reconciled with Gompertz's concept. Another British actuary, Makeham,[10] made such an adjustment in 1867 by combining the Gompertz formula with the concept of accidental death, which is represented by a constant risk, k:

$$Y_x = Y_o e^{ax} + k$$

In high-risk environments, k is large and dominates the total risk factor in early life. It then approaches the Gompertz line with advancing age until the latter component, increasing geometrically, assumes major importance. As the environmental risk decreases, the incremental straight-line portion of the curve becomes steeper and approaches the asymptote defined by the Gompertz component of the equation at an earlier age (*see* Figure 2-5).

This approximation is much closer to observed phenomena, but further conceptual modifications are necessary. It is improbable that there has been a significant reduction in major developmental defects, although recent therapeutic methods, mainly surgical, may have

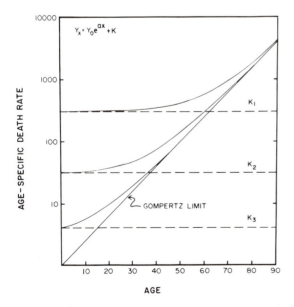

FIGURE 2-5   Theoretic age-specific death rates combining a constant, extrinsic age-independent risk (K_1, K_2, K_3) with the increasing intrinsic, age-dependent (Gompertz) risk. Note that as each curve approaches the asymptote it appears virtually straight, with a slope that increases as K decreases.

caused a significant reduction in mortality. Most early deaths in the past were associated with infection, trauma, and the fetal and maternal risks of childbirth. Although exposure to infection may have been constant in the past, first exposure always carried the greatest and often the only risk. For example, exposure to diphtheria resulted either in death or the subsequent, immunity-based total absence of risk on recovery. Public health measures, immunizations, and antibiotics have largely eliminated infection as a cause of premature death.

Risk of maternal mortality has not only been reduced per episode, but the reduction in the number of needed pregnancies has further reduced the risk per individual. Inexperience and the recklessness of youth exacerbate the risks of accidents among adolescents and young adults, particularly males. The better management of trauma, education, seat belts, and crash helmets may have reduced these deaths as well. The reductions in age-related environmental causes of death undoubtedly are reflected in the reduced excessive mortality within this age group; the recent increase in mortality rates for the 15–30-year-old group may reflect the violence of the period.

Having once recognized the Gompertz-Makeham phenomenon, it can be easily identified in clinical statistics. Figure 2-6 shows the mortality rates for pneumonia in three eras.[11] In 1900, there was no specific therapy, and the mortality was about 30%. There was little improvement by 1930, although diagnosis was more precise, hospitalization and nursing care may have improved, and oxygen was available. Then, in rapid succession, specific pneumococcus antisera, the sulfonamides and penicillin, were introduced between 1934–1943. The mortality dropped impressively. Yet, the greatest gains were among adolescents, with decreased improvement at the extremes of age; the curves, except for the lesser risks of death, resemble those of Figure 2-4. Since pneumonia is an acute disease, the evidence suggests that the ability to cope with this specific acute stress is age related. Many other examples strengthen this presumption of the relationship between age and the ability to cope with acute stress in general.

The virtual elimination of acute diseases has drawn attention to chronic diseases and their

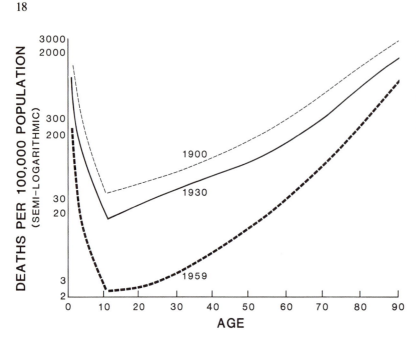

FIGURE 2-6 Age and mortality rates from pneumonia. (From Reimann HA: Prevention and treatment of pneumonias in the older person. *Geriatrics,* 1963, used by permission.)

acute complications. It is of interest that the frequency of death due to these causes also increases geometrically. The risks for the four most frequent causes of death, which account for 75% of the total, are plotted in Figure 2-7.[7] Ischemic heart disease and cerebral vascular disease show a linear increase on the semilogarithmic plot, while age-specific cancer mortality increases at the same rate until advanced age, then seems to decrease. It may be that cancer-susceptible individuals with a specific genetic predisposition or exposure to carcinogens have approached numeric exhaustion and their fraction of the remaining population at risk has declined. However, deaths from vascular disease are age related and comprise the largest fraction defined by the total mortality. The deaths due to accidents follow a remarkably pure Gompertz-Makeham model, as would be expected. This risk remains essentially constant from age 25–65, then gradually increases to approach the slope of the others as the intrinsic vulnerability achieves dominant proportions. The pattern closely resembles k_1 of Figure 2-5. The frequency of most generally non-lethal, chronic diseases increases on this same slope; it includes such diverse disorders as arthritis, diabetes mellitus, chronic obstructive pulmonary disease, fracture of the hip, cataracts, prostatic hypertrophy, and Alzheimer-like dementia. The consistency of the data suggests that these

changes may be manifestations of the aging process, rather than diseases in the usual sense.

All available data show that as early deaths decrease, the straight portion of the mortality risk curve gets steeper. This indicates that although at any age the risk has decreased, the rate of risk acceleration has increased approaching (as a limit) the fixed slope of the Gompertz component.

The concept that aging is due to extrinsic trauma carries certain implications. Sublethal trauma should increase vulnerability in proportion to the amount of trauma sustained, both per episode and cumulatively. It seems improbable that in an environment where the risks of lethal episodes decrease, the frequency of non-lethal episodes should increase. Thus, a reduction in environmental risk should reduce the steepness of the Gompertz slope if it is the product of environmental stress. The reverse has been the case up to the present time. There is no evidence that with a reduction in lethal environmental risks the acceleration of the Gompertz component has decreased, with one possible exception to be noted later.

Thus, in addition to the questionable assumption that it is possible to decrease lethal risks without, at the same time, decreasing sublethal injury, the data suggest an environmental independence of the asymptote. The 1963 *Report of the Surgeon General* on the risks of

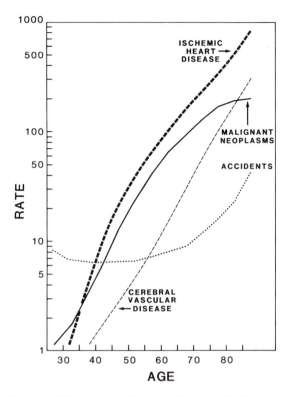

FIGURE 2-7 Age-specific mortality rates for the four most common causes of death plotted per 10,000 males, United States, 1974. (From *Vital Statistics of the United States,* 1975.)

DEATH RATE (logarithmic scale)
PLOTTED AGAINST AGE, PROSPECTIVE STUDY
OF MORTALITY IN U.S. VETERANS

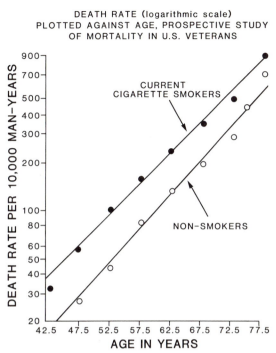

FIGURE 2-8 Comparison of age-specific mortality rates of smokers and non-smokers. Note that with increasing age, the risk differential decreases, despite a longer history of exposure. (From the *Report of the Surgeon General on Smoking and Health,* 1963.)

smoking offer an interesting example (*see* Figure 2-8). If smoking is a cumulative risk factor, then the longer the history of smoking the greater the risk should be. The curves suggest, however, that 1) there are degrees of vulnerability that are inversely related to survival, and that 2) some individuals who normally are limited in ultimate survival only by old age are immune to life-long smoking.

Some years ago, Benjamin[12] presented the idea that there was a fixed, average, normal life span with a normal distribution. This idea has been revived by Fries and Crapo,[2] who propose the average natural life span to be 85 years, with a standard deviation of 4 years. Current projections indicate that almost two thirds of white females in the United States will die between 75–95 years of age. However, a precise projection based on the Gompertz-Makeham equation should show an asymmetric curve with increasing deaths until the remaining individuals become so reduced that, even with the increasing risk, the number of deaths declines rapidly. It

may be reasonable to allow a small terminal splay for individual variation in natural vitality. The data appear to be approaching the latter form. Whichever one of these concepts is correct, it is interesting that as life expectation has increased, there has been little shift in the mode of this curve (*see* Figure 2-9).

Risk Factors

The most perplexing problem in gerontology is the separation of normal aging phenomena from disease and injury. Growth and development are associated with preponderantly incremental processes, whereas during maturity and senescence injury and loss exceed the reparative processes. In all individuals, postmitotic cells of nerve and muscle tissue, which are incapable of reproduction, are gradually lost, mitotic cells are now known to have a limited reproductive capability, and the macromolecules of the intercellular matrix cross-link and lose their earlier

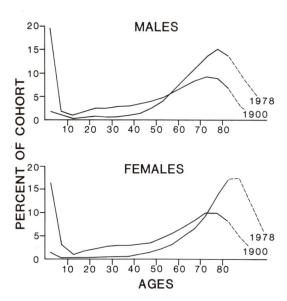

FIGURE 2-9   The fraction of deaths occurring during 5-year intervals, 1900 and 1978. Although the terminal mode shifts slightly toward the higher ages, this is due to reduced deaths at earlier ages. (From *Vital Statistics of the United States,* Washington, DC, Government Printing Office, 1980.)

functional characteristics. Other progressive changes also are noted in almost all intracellular organelles and in the organs and tissues. The universality and variety of change implies that these multiple processes are so diverse that they are unlikely to be the result of any one mechanism, type of injury, or disease.

There are certain biologic parameters that vary from one individual to another. A prototype could be blood pressure. Blood pressure elevation is secondary to specific and identifiable abnormalities in a small proportion of individuals. However, an examination of the remaining population as a whole shows an essentially normal distribution of pressures, with an entirely arbitrary dividing point between normotension and hypertension. Not only is there no evident discontinuity, but the point at which hypertension is stated to be present is well within two standard deviations from the mean. The etiology of such hypertension has not been found, and it may not be. It may represent only a graded and continuous set of vascular, neuronal, and hormonal interactions. There is much evidence that hereditary factors determine the relationship to the normal range; however, there also is good evidence

TABLE 2-2   Relative Risk of Death Related to Blood Pressure Levels (BP)

Systolic BP	Mortality Ratio	Diastolic BP	Mortality Ratio
88– 97	0.78	48– 67	0.83
98–127	0.88	68– 82	0.97
128–137	1.18	83– 87	1.29
138–147	1.55	88– 92	1.50
148–157	1.94	93– 97	1.88
158–167	2.44	98–102	2.34
168–177	2.42	103–112	2.62

From a 1959 Blood Pressure Study, (males, policy issue ages 15–69), Society of Actuaries. The mortality ratio is the ratio of subset mortality to that of the entire group at risk.

that pressure can be modified by environmental manipulation and drugs (*see* Volume I, Chapter 32).

If one examines the effect of blood pressure (either diastolic or systolic) on life expectation, there are striking data that indicate a continuum in which the higher the pressure, the shorter the life expectation (*see* Table 2-2). While this increased risk is modest at low pressure levels, it accelerates rapidly and without any discontinuity as the pressure rises. A graphic representation is presented in Figure 2-10.

Since there is no conclusive evidence that there is more than one population, and there is a normal distribution of the risk factor, it is difficult to attribute the increased risk to disease. Moreover, it is apparent that the normal distribution of this factor is highly correlated with mortal risk throughout the range.

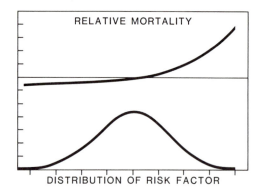

FIGURE 2-10   The relationship of individual risk factor status to mortal risk. (From Goldman R: The aging process and the gerontologist, in Haley HB, Keenan PA (eds): *Health and Health Care of the Aging.* Charlottesville, University Press of Virginia, 1981, used by permission.)

Collagen macromolecules cross-link and form dense bundles, which become more rigid with age. Elastin becomes fragmented and loses its elasticity. These two changes contribute to the age-related dilatation and rigidity of the elastic arteries. It is possible that the traumatic effects of increasingly high pressures on the elastic arteries lead to an acceleration of these changes, with earlier atherosclerosis and its resulting complications. Coronary occlusion and stroke are acute episodes; however, they require vascular alteration, which develops over time.

Although intrinsic factors may govern the blood pressure range in an individual, this range also can be modified by environmental factors. There are now many therapeutic methods by which this range can be altered. Ultimate vascular damage may be inevitable, but blood pressure control may delay its course. A number of other risk factors have been identified, including glucose tolerance and the blood levels of uric acid, cholesterol, blood lipids, and blood lipoproteins. There should be many others, and a systematic search is warranted. If these intrinsic risk factors can be favorably modified by environmental factors, there should be a measurable reduction in the Gompertz slope. This is a phenomenon that did not occur as a result of reduction in environmental trauma, but which may be measurable in the recently observed improved risks of heart disease and stroke. It may be that the apparent failure of the 1960 and 1978 curves of females and the 1978 curves of males in Figure 2-4B to converge on the earlier curves is real; it may be a reflection of risk factor control via diet, exercise, and other possibly unidentified life style changes.

Evidence has also been developed showing that the effectiveness of the immune mechanisms decreases with age (*see* Volume I, Chapter 20). Burnet had proposed that there is a relationship between immunocompetence and the appearance of cancer.[13] Figure 2-7 suggests that 1) only a limited segment of the population may be susceptible to cancer and 2) the age-specific frequency of cancer increases, perhaps as immunocompetence decreases, until the entire population at risk has succumbed.

While these examples present data that fit the concept, the relationships are not conclusive. However, the close association of age and the incidence of principal remaining causes of disability and death cannot be overlooked. The possibility that this relationship may be the result of quantitative differences in normal processes, rather than of extrinsic factors, is supported strongly by extensive available data. There is evidence that modification of these processes, even if they are intrinsic in origin, can delay the onset of overt changes. The data and concepts presented rationalize both the differential character of aging complications and the precise patterns of survival and morbid risk.

Implications

If these concepts are acceptable, there is an implication that some of our traditional procedural concepts should be revised; if they are proven, it is our responsibility to react appropriately.

First, the striking and continued increase in longevity means that there has been a consistent improvement in the environment; increasing stress is not compatible with increased longevity. This stands in contrast to the generally negative view so popular today. This is not to say that constant vigilance and improvement are not necessary; however, there is a special danger that an attitude of defeatism may be self-fulfilling because of a resultant decline in the willingness to sustain legitimate protective standards. In addition, it seems a tragedy that instead of rejoicing at the saving of younger lives, and enjoying the bonus of longevity, we deplore the increased numbers of aged and the fact they are at risk.

As physicians, we are still bound to prolong life by preventing premature death, within the context just outlined. The concept of inevitable limits is not a justification for failing to diagnose and treat entities that are reversible or whose progression can be favorably influenced.

One of the oft-quoted anxieties is that life prolongation will result in longer periods of incapacity. While it is true that there are more elderly people, with their attendant chronic disabilities, one implication of the increasing steepness of the Gompertz curve is that terminal disease or disability should be of a shorter duration. A reasonable goal is the shortest possible period of disability and decline following the longest possible healthy and competent survival.

On the other hand, we must be aware of prolonging the process of dying. We must improve our basic knowledge and our clinical skills so that we can recognize inappropriate therapeutic goals. If there is evidence of age-related and irreversible decremental change, it is inhumane to manage the patient as if reversal were possible. In order to achieve a social consensus, we must develop objective criteria, as we have with brain death. If we persist in the belief that all disorders of aging are due to disease and are preventable, our treatment will be unkind to our patients and profligate of our resources.

Clearly, prolongation of the natural life span will not be achievable using the concepts of disease prevention and treatment. It will be necessary to elucidate the basic mechanisms of aging and to devise methods to slow or change them. This must be accomplished without altering the quality of life. Thus, instead of seeking the abnormal and converting it to the normal, we must find the normal and make it favorably abnormal. And, despite attempts to identify a single basic mechanism, it seems more probable that there are multiple aging changes, many of which will require modification.

Ultimately, we are faced with a dilemma. If life can be prolonged, it will be. But is there a moral imperative to do so? If immortality were achievable, what would be gained? If nobody died on so crowded an earth, where would we place the newborn? How would humanity be renewed? Even if there is life prolongation without immortality, what have we gained? Why is it better to die at age 150 than at age 85? Will we be less anxious, less afraid? It is argued that wisdom comes with age, and that if effective productivity were spread over a longer period, it would achieve higher levels. Would youth be required to wait longer, perhaps generations, for its chance at maturity? These are important questions for those who would seek a cure for the "disease of aging." In the mean-

time, a full and healthy life, within the present parameters, with survival to see our children and possibly our grandchildren mature, followed by a rapid, painless decline, is a worthy, reasonable, achievable, and morally justifiable goal.

References

1. Comfort A: *The Biology of Senescence,* ed 3. New York, Elsevier Press, 1979.
2. Fries JF, Crapo LM: *Vitality and Aging.* San Francisco, WH Freeman & Co, 1981.
3. Goldman R: Aging and geriatric medicine, in Wyngaarden JB, Smith LH, Jr, (eds): *Cecil Textbook of Medicine,* ed 16. Philadelphia, WB Saunders & Co, 1979, pp 34–39.
4. Goldman R: The aging process and the gerontologist, in Haley HB, Keenan PA (eds): *Health and Health Care of the Aging.* Charlottesville, University Press of Virginia, 1981, pp 20–32.
5. Strehler BL: *Time, Cells, and Aging,* ed 2. New York, Academic Press, 1977.
6. Cowgill UM: The people of York: 1538–1812. *Sci Am* 222:104–112, 1970.
7. *Vital Statistics of the United States.* Washington, DC, Government Printing Office, 1980.
8. Gompertz B: On the nature of the function expressive of the law of human mortality and on a new mode of determining the value of life contingencies. *Philos Trans R Soc Lond (Biol)* 115:513–585, 1825.
9. Jones HB: The relation of human health to age, place and time, in Birren JE (ed): *Handbook of Aging and the Individual.* Chicago, University of Chicago Press, 1959, pp 336–363.
10. Makeham WM: On the law of mortality. *J Inst Actuaries* 13:325–358, 1867.
11. Reimann HA: Prevention and treatment of pneumonias in the older person. *Geriatrics* 18:423–432, 1963.
12. Benjamin B: Actuarial aspects of human life spans, in Wolstenholme GEW, O'Connor M (eds): *Ciba Foundation Colloquium on Aging,* 5. Boston, Little Brown & Co, 1959, pp 2–20.
13. Burnet M: *Immunology, Aging and Cancer.* San Francisco, WH Freeman & Co, 1976.

PART II

Medical Disorders in the Geriatric Patient

CHAPTER 3

Cerebrovascular Disease

BRUCE M. COULL, M.D.

In the adult population of the United States and Canada, stroke is the third most common cause of death and a major cause of disability and invalidism. Although no age group is spared, stroke primarily is a disease of the elderly. A recent survey of over 4,000 cases showed the average age of acute stroke victims to be 72 years, with women being slightly older than men.[1] About 50% of hospitalized stroke patients are discharged to their homes, 20% die during hospitalization, and 30% require long-term or institutional care. Thus, in addition to considerable human suffering, the monetary cost of this disease is staggering, with estimates measured in billions of dollars.[2]

The term "stroke" implies the sudden onset of focal neurologic dysfunction that is due to an interference of blood flow within a region of the brain or spinal cord. The concept of a regional disturbance in cerebral blood flow that causes focal brain ischemia serves to separate stroke from more global insults to the brain, which occur in cardiac arrest, anoxic encephalopathy or prolonged and severe hypoglycemia. Although certain mechanisms of brain injury may differ, any distinction between focal and global cerebral insults is (in part) arbitrary since cerebral infarctions resulting from large arterial occlusions may cause massive brain injury, whereas relatively small and quite focal infarctions can follow cardiac arrest or anoxic-metabolic encephalopathy. The clinician's task is to recognize the symptoms of focal cerebral ischemia, to identify the vascular territory involved, the underlying cause, and to direct appropriate therapy.

Epidemiology

Epidemiologic studies show that the incidence of stroke is declining, and that it has been doing so for approximately 3 decades.[3,4] There is approximately a 25% decline in the overall incidence of stroke since 1945.[3] Although a decline in all age groups was found, persons over 70 years of age seemed to benefit most. This important advance in stroke prevention is ascribed primarily to early and better risk-factor recognition and reduction.[5] Despite the decline in incidence, the actual number of persons suffering from stroke may increase during the next decade as the number of elderly within the population rises. Moreover, age remains a major risk factor for stroke. Compared to persons 55–59 years of age, stroke incidence is 5-fold greater for persons 70–74 years of age and 10-fold greater for persons over age 75.[4]

Types of Stroke

There are many causes of stroke; hence, stroke is a syndrome not a diagnosis. From the standpoint of management, the underlying cause of stroke should be identified. The major categories of stroke include: 1) Cerebral infarction due to atherosclerotic cerebrovascular disease; 2) Cardioembolic cerebral infarction; 3) Intracerebral hemorrhage; 4) Subarachnoid hemorrhage; and 5) A miscellaneous group that includes infarction due to cerebral vasculitis, venous thrombosis, and hyperviscosity or hypercoagulable states. The emphasis in our discussion will

TABLE 3-1   Frequency of Major Categories of Stroke

Cerebral infarction	72%
Atherosclerotic-thromboembolic*	22%
Lacunar	7%
Cardioembolic	28%
Infarction type unknown	15%
Intracerebral hemorrhage	5%
Subarachnoid hemorrhage	5%
Other causes†	7%
Stroke NOS††	11%

* Atherosclerotic-thromboembolic infarction is attributed to arteriosclerosis of carotid or vertebrobasilar arteries (see text for details).
† Vasculitis, hypercoagulable or hyperviscous states, arteriovenous malformation, and so on.
†† Stroke NOS—not otherwise specified.

be on the more common causes of stroke in elderly persons. The frequency of the major types of stroke seen in a university medical center is shown in Table 3-1. The vast majority of strokes, especially in the aged, are due to cerebral infarctions related to cerebrovascular atherosclerosis. Because of the coexistence of significant cardiovascular and cerebrovascular diseases, it is sometimes difficult to distinguish a definitive cause of infarction. As shown in Table 3-1, and in accordance with data from the Harvard Cooperative Stroke Registry compared to earlier studies of causes of stroke, cerebral embolism is becoming an increasingly frequent cause of stroke.[6,7,8]

Cerebral Infarction

As the most common cause of stroke in aged adults, cerebral infarction occurs following an acute occlusion of a cerebral artery or arteriole. Infarction also can follow cerebral vein thrombosis, but compared to arterial causes such an occurrence is rare. In elderly persons, most cerebral infarctions are related to underlying disseminated atherosclerosis. In atherothromboembolic infarction degenerative changes within an atheromatous lesion, typically at the carotid bifurcation or involving the vertebral or basilar arteries, can encourage the formation of a friable thrombus made up of a meshwork containing platelet-fibrin and red blood cell aggregates. Portions of this clot or the atheroma itself can embolize distally into the cerebral circulation, thus causing vascular occlusions and a re-

sultant cerebral infarction. Particularly when the atheromatous lesion at the carotid bifurcation is advanced, thrombus formation may completely occlude the internal carotid artery. Although such a lesion may be asymptomatic, in many cases massive cerebral infarction ensues in the territory of both the ipsilateral middle and anterior cerebral arteries. If the process occurs in the vertebrobasilar circulation, symptomatic distal embolization of a thrombus is less frequent. Most strokes are caused by a thrombosis within the vertebral or basilar arteries themselves, or from propagation into the basilar artery of a clot that formed within a small penetrating branch artery of the vertebral or basilar vessels.[9]

As a general rule, atherothromboembolic infarctions are large and have a dramatic clinical signature. In the carotid territory, the middle cerebral artery and its branches are involved most often so that the clinical presentation is one of profound weakness, sensory disturbances, and (with dominant hemisphere infarction) various forms of aphasia. The less common infarction in the distribution of the anterior cerebral artery can produce a most profound paresis in the contralateral lower extremity, which is accompanied by alterations in affect and loss of initiative. With massive hemispheric infarctions, alterations in consciousness and Cheyne-Stokes pattern breathing may be observed. Such patients frequently exhibit complete hemiplegia, hemianesthesia, hemianopsia, and bilateral Babinski signs. In this setting, a poor recovery and high mortality is common. Brainstem and cerebellar infarctions of the atherothromboembolic type are no less dramatic. Cerebellar infarctions with an accompanying edema and pressure on the brainstem tegmental structures can be life threatening if not promptly treated by surgical decompression. Large infarctions within the brainstem, depending upon location, produce a variety of cranial nerve abnormalities, ataxia, abnormalities in eye movements, bulbar palsy, and bilateral abnormalities in motor or sensory function over the trunk and extremities. Alterations in consciousness, including profound coma, are frequent. Massive brainstem infarctions that cause coma have a poor prognosis, whereas other brainstem infarction syndromes, such as Wallenberg's syndrome or the lateral medullary

TABLE 3-2 The Wallenberg Syndrome: Infarction in the Distribution of the Posterior Inferior Cerebellar Artery

Symptoms	Signs
Dizziness, vertigo	Ipsilateral
Nausea, vomiting	Cranial nerves V, IX, X, XI
Ataxia, hiccup	Horner's sign
Dysphagia	Cerebellar ataxia
Ipsilateral numbness of face and arm	Contralateral
	Loss of pain and temperature
	Gaze-evoked nystagmus

plate infarction syndrome, have a relatively good prognosis. Infarction in the distribution of the posterior inferior cerebellar artery (PICA), termed Wallenberg's syndrome, often is caused by an occlusion of the distal vertebral artery (see Table 3-2).

Lacunar Infarction

Lacunar infarction, for the most part, results from a disease of the small, deep-penetrating arterioles located at both the base of the brain and along the basilar artery within the pons and midbrain. Lacunar infarction accounts for up to one in five of all cerebral infarctions, but the prevalence of clinically silent lacunar infarctions is probably much higher.[6] From the French meaning "small hole," the term "lacune" was first used by Durant-Fardel. It now connotes small infarctions usually of 2–15 mm in diameter within the basal ganglia, internal capsule, thalamus, and pons.[10] They occur frequently in multiples and need not be confined

entirely to any single vascular territory or to subcortical structures. The nature of the vascular injury that gives rise to lacunar infarction remains controversial. It has been proposed that arteriolar damage results from poorly controlled hypertension.[11] This change, termed lipohyalinosis, is seen in arterioles measuring 40–200 μm in diameter, and it is characterized by a thickened arterial wall with a reduction in luminal diameter. The vascular tissue contains segmental areas of necrosis, which sometimes give rise to small aneurysmal dilatations termed Charcot-Bouchard aneurysms. In some vessels microatheroma appear. In the setting of extremely high blood pressure that is sufficient to produce hypertensive encephalopathy, a third pathology occurs, termed fibrinoid necrosis. Ongoing debates still argue whether lipohyalinosis, fibrinoid necrosis, and microatheroma represent a spectrum of a common underlying mechanism.[12] The predilection for this to occur within the deep vascular beds, but not in the cortical microvascular territory, remains controversial. The clinical features of the common lacunar syndromes are summarized in Table 3-3. Pure motor hemiparesis by far is the most common syndrome and presents as hemiplegia or paresis of the face, arm, and leg. All of these need not be affected; the syndrome can present as monoparesis of the arm or leg. Lacunes that produce this syndrome are commonly situated within the internal capsule, where they disrupt descending motor pathways. Pure motor syndromes may follow strokes occurring within the midbrain and ventral pons. In contradistinction to the pure motor stroke, pure sensory syndromes occur with lacunar infarctions within the thalamus. In such cases only contralateral hemisensory symptoms

TABLE 3-3 Lacunar Syndromes

Designation	Symptoms	Location of Infarction
Pure motor hemiparesis	Paresis of face, arm, and leg	Contralateral internal capsule, contralateral basis pontis
Pure sensory stroke	Paresthesias of arm, leg, and face	Contralateral thalamus
Ataxic hemiparesis	Hemiparesis, ipsilateral ataxia	Contralateral basis pontis, contralateral internal capsule
Dysarthria, clumsy hand	Dysarthria, hemiataxia	Contralateral basis pontis, contralateral internal capsule

SOURCE: Miller VT: Lacunar Stroke: A Reassessment. *Arch Neurol* 40:129–134, 1983.

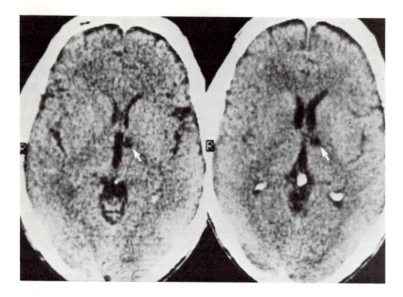

FIGURE 3-1 Two closely spaced CT-scan cuts showing lacunar infarction within the right thalamus (arrows).

occur, which include paresthesias that are sometimes painful. Pure sensory strokes, compared to pure motor strokes, are rare, and neurologic findings may be minimal and difficult to document. With ataxic hemiparesis, patients complain of incoordination and gait difficulties accompanied at times by sensory disturbances. This syndrome is caused most often by lacunar infarction within the regions of the thalamus and internal capsule. Lacunar infarctions in the basis pontis seem to account for the "dysarthria-clumsy hand syndrome," although neither the location nor the cause is exclusive for this common presentation of stroke.[10]

The patient with lacunar stroke is recognized not only by the syndrome presentation, but by the lack of accompanying disturbances in the level of consciousness, preservation of language function, and absence of large visual field abnormality. The computed tomography (CT scan) of the brain is frequently normal or may show (*see* Figure 3-1) the corresponding, well-circumscribed small lucency within the basal ganglia or deep white matter structures. Cerebral angiography reveals markedly atherosclerotic involvement in only one third of all cases. About 75% of all persons with lacunar stroke are hypertensive and roughly 20% are diabetic. Thus, although most lacunar syndromes are caused by intracranial vasculopathy, occasional atherothromboembolic or cardioembolic sources may contribute.

Cerebral Embolism

Embolism to the brain of a thrombus or other friable material arising from within the heart is another common cause of stroke. Recent studies suggest that the incidence of cardioembolic stoke is rising.[6–8] Cardioembolic infarction is the main cause of stroke in persons under 45 years of age and is the probable cause in the majority of postoperative strokes among all age groups.[13] The clinical presentation has a usually abrupt onset—a "bolt from the blue"; however, this apoplectic presentation is not universal and symptoms may evolve slowly or include stuttering. Most emboli lodge within the territory of the middle cerebral artery, but no vascular distribution, including vertebrobasilar, is spared. Pathologic studies suggest that embolic infarctions often have a hemorrhagic component, but a recent clinical study using CT scanning has not confirmed this observation.[14] This issue needs to be resolved since persons with embolic stroke are frequently considered candidates for therapeutic anticoagulation to prevent a recurrence of emboli. A diagnosis of embolic infarction is established by clinical evidence that suggests multiple systemic or cerebral emboli in the presence of a recognized cardiac source of emboli.

As shown in Table 3-4, rheumatic and atherosclerotic heart disease are the underlying causes in most cases of cerebral embolism.[15] In

TABLE 3-4 Major Causes of Cardiogenic Cerebral Embolism

Non-valvular atrial fibrillation	50%
Coronary heart disease	
Myocardial infarction	20%
Rheumatic heart disease	
Mitral stenosis ± atrial fibrillation	15%
Prosthetic cardiac valves	10%
Other	5%
Cardiomyopathy	
Cardiac tumors	
Septic endocarditis	
Non-bacterial thrombotic endocarditis	
(marantic)	
Congenital heart disease	
Venous clots/intracardiac shunt (paradoxic	
emboli)	
Mitral annulus calcification*	
Calcific aortic stenosis*	
Mitral valve prolapse*	

* Uncertain significance in an individual patient, but statistically linked to stroke.

the appropriate setting, less common causes such as atrial myxoma, right-to-left shunts, and congenital heart disease should be considered. Once a diagnosis of embolic infarction is established, and evidence for intracerebral hemorrhage is excluded, several therapeutic questions need attention: What are the risks of early re-embolization compared to the risks of immediate anticoagulation? Also, what are the long-term risks of re-embolization as opposed to the long-term risks of chronic anticoagulation therapy? Depending upon the underlying form of heart disease, these questions can be answered only in part. Experience with CT scanning of acute infarctions confirms that this procedure is very selective in excluding intracerebral blood clots; at present no better method exists for excluding hemorrhagic infarction.[16] A word of caution, however, is necessary. A CT scan early in the course of a large infarction may not show any abnormality or only mild swelling and edema, whereas spontaneous hemorrhage may appear several days later in the absence of anticoagulation. The predilection for ''spontaneous'' hemorrhage seems to be associated with larger cerebral infarctions. With this caution, recent data suggest that early short-term anticoagulation therapy (i.e., anticoagulation for 2 weeks to 3 months) can be safely performed in non-hemorrhagic embolic strokes due to non-

infectious causes.[17–19] Although these studies suggest that immediate anticoagulation may be beneficial, it remains to be proven that this intervention reduces the 10–20% rate of early re-embolization. The commitment to long-term anticoagulation therapy lasting months to years presents a dilemma since this therapy, particularly in persons over 65 years of age, has a high morbidity and mortality.[20] Unless a disabling illness dictates otherwise, persons who experience emboli in association with rheumatic heart disease should receive long-term anticoagulation therapy. In this setting, this therapy reduces the recurrence of emboli from roughly 50% to the 2–25% range. Anticoagulation therapy in the presence of chronic atrial fibrillation alone, without valvular or rheumatic heart disease, has not been adequately evaluated. It would appear that persons with symptoms of systemic or cerebral emboli who are younger than 65 years of age may benefit from long-term anticoagulation therapy, whereas in those 65 years old or older antiaggregate treatment with aspirin or other similar agents may be a safer albeit less effective treatment.

Hemorrhagic Stroke

Subarachnoid Hemorrhage (SAH)

The two main types of hemorrhagic stroke are subarachnoid hemorrhage (SAH) and intracerebral hemorrhage (ICH). The principal cause of SAH is a ruptured berry aneurysm. Berry aneurysms distribute around the arteries at the base of the brain. They occur most frequently at the first portion of the posterior communicating artery near the internal carotid artery, the origin of the middle cerebral artery, the anterior communicating artery, and the distal internal carotid artery. The vertebral basilar arteries may be involved. The aneurysms may be single or multiple and can vary in size from a few millimeters to giant aneurysms many centimeters in diameter. Aneurysmal rupture occurs often in aneurysms of 1–2 cm in diameter and is rare in those less than 7 mm in diameter.[21] Giant aneurysms produce symptoms by mass effect and rupture, per se, occurs infrequently. Symptoms of aneurysmal rupture are a severe and sudden headache, often described as explosive, accompanied by collapse. Loss of consciousness may be brief; a deep coma resulting in death can rapidly develop. Focal neurologic signs are often absent in mild cases, but weakness in the lower extremities, even if brief, suggests an anterior communicating artery aneurysm. Lateralized weakness indicates a middle cerebral artery aneurysm. Complete third cranial nerve palsy suggests a posterior communicating artery aneurysm. Most aneurysms are asymptomatic before rupture, but they occasionally give rise to distal emboli producing transient or completed infarctions. Besides headache, alterations in consciousness, and focal neurologic signs, subarachnoid blood produces meningeal irritation manifested by nuchal rigidity. Hemorrhage often can be seen within the retina at the inner limiting membrane. These circular hemorrhages are referred to as subhyoid hemorrhages and are a helpful confirmatory sign in SAH. The CT scan may show blood in the subarachnoid space and it sometimes visualizes the aneurysm itself, but in 50% of all cases the CT scan is within the normal range.[22] Cerebral angiography remains the best tool for defining the location and anatomy of an aneurysm. Of those who suffer SAH, 50% will die of the initial or repeat hemorrhage, about 15% will have disability, and the remainder will recover.[23]

The management of SAH during the initial posthemorrhage period requires the coordinated efforts of skilled neurosurgical, neurological, and critical care personnel. Definitive therapy entails the surgical correction of the aneurysm. Medical management is directed at stabilizing the patient to prevent re-bleeding and to assure an optimal chance for a good surgical result. In particular, blood pressure regulation to prevent dangerously high ranges is necessary. In this regard, bowel function must be maintained in such a way that the patient does not strain. For the same reason, agitation needs to be controlled with suitable drugs.

When an excessive clot exists within the subarachnoid space at the basal meninges, cerebrovasospasm may complicate the management late in the first week after the SAH or during the second week. Recent evidence suggests that calcium channel antagonists may help prevent vasospasm if instituted early in the course of the illness.[24] Basilar collections of blood also can lead to obstruction of cerebrospinal fluid (CSF) flow with resultant hydrocephalus. Thus, patients with SAH may deteriorate further within 5–20 days because of a variety of mechanisms that include re-bleeding of the aneurysm, vasospasm producing frank infarction, and the production of hydrocephalus. To successfully manage SAH, it is necessary to anticipate these and other potential complications and to begin treatment early after the first onset of symptoms.

Intracerebral Hemorrhage

The incidence of intracerebral hemorrhage (ICH) is declining; however, nonetheless, this remains (along with SAH) one of the more lethal forms of stroke. Whereas 15–20% of persons with cerebral infarctions die during the initial hospitalization period, 35–40% of those hospitalized with ICH die.[1] Most often, ICH occurs in a setting of poorly controlled hypertension, the treatment of which has contributed to the declining incidence of ICH. In persons under 40 years of age, arteriovenous malformations (AVM) contribute to a substantial portion of brain hematomas, while in very elderly persons amyloid angiopathy has recently been recognized as an important cause of ICH.[25] For ICH associated with hypertension, the distribution of hematomas is similar to the location of most lacunar infarctions: in the basal ganglia, deep white matter, thalamus, pons, and cerebellum. It is possible that hypertensive ICH and lacunar infarction represent two ends of the spectrum of the same vasculopathy—possibly arteriolosclerosis.

Hematomas vary in size, but those sufficiently large enough to produce mass effect or rupture of blood into the ventricular system are often life threatening if not promptly treated. As with cerebellar infarction, cerebellar hematoma can produce an irreversible coma because of the compression of vital structures within the pons. An early indication of pontine compression is the presence of very small, equal in size, and reactive pupils. Large hematomas within the thalamus cause tonic deviation of the eyes downward so that the patient appears to be looking at his nose. When they are massive, hematomas produce headache, alterations in consciousness, and elevated intracranial pressure with its attendant findings. There is no better way to diagnose ICH than with CT scanning.[16] Once diagnosed, patients should be investigated for abnormalities in blood clotting and, if present, these should be corrected. Hypertension should be controlled, but overaggressive measures that produce hypotension can cause clinical worsening. If increased intracranial pressure is present, corticosteroids or other edema-reducing agents should be employed. It is frequently helpful to monitor intracranial pressure during the acute stages since uncontrolled elevations in pressure constitutes an indication for either surgical evacuation of the clot or decompression to control brain swelling. Whenever possible, it is best to manage the patient without surgical intervention since evacuation of the clot seldom lessens neurologic deficit. The exception to this rule as, already mentioned above, is that of threatened brainstem compression. Despite combined medical and surgical efforts, ICH remains a morbid form of stroke.

Transient Ischemic Attacks

Transient ischemic attacks (TIAs) of the brain are characterized by the sudden onset of focal neurologic dysfunction. Symptoms correspond to the neuroanatomic vascular territory of the compromised blood vessel. Most TIAs are 5 minutes or less in duration, and the vast majority are resolved in less than 1 hour from onset. By generally accepted criteria, however, any focal ischemic-neurologic deficit that clears within 24 hours may be considered a TIA. When a transient arteriolar occlusion occurs within the retinal circulation, the monocular blindness ensues, termed amaurosis fugax. These events are sometimes designated separately as transient monocular blindness (TMB). TIAs and TMB are considered together since blood supply to the retina and most of the cerebral hemispheres derive from the internal carotid circulation.

The importance of TIA stems from the fact that it is a harbinger of stroke. Although the literature varies, 20–30% of all stroke patients will experience a prior TIA.[1,26,27] Perhaps two thirds or more of all individuals in whom stroke arises from atherosclerosis within the carotid or vertebral basilar arteries will experience a prior TIA. In the carotid territory, the majority of individuals experience only one or two TIAs

before a stroke, whereas multiple TIAs prior to a stroke within the vertebrobasilar circulation are the rule.[28,29] In round figures, the rate of stroke after TIA is 5–7% per year although considerable extremes are present in several series reported in the literature.[30,31] Persons with a single TIA or only a few tightly grouped TIAs are at a particularly high risk for several weeks to several months after the onset of symptoms. Such patients require immediate attention to determine the cause of the TIAs so that they may receive proper treatment to reduce the risk of a completed stroke.

Typical symptoms of TIAs are shown in Table 3-5. It is helpful to characterize the vascular territory in which symptoms arise since this may provide insight into the pathogenesis, and because it has important therapeutic implications. When certain symptoms such as vertigo, dizziness, and syncope occur in the absence of additional focal neurologic symptoms, a diagnosis of TIA is suspect and other causes such as cardiac arrhythmia or vestibular dysfunction should be sought.

TABLE 3-5 Symptoms of TIA

Carotid System TIA
Unilateral weakness—usually hemiparesis
Unilateral sensory complaints—numbness, paresthesia
Aphasia—language comprehension, output or both
Monocular visual loss (amaurosis fugax)

Vertebrobasilar System TIA
Motor deficit—especially if bilateral
Sensory complaints—especially if bilateral
Simultaneous, bilateral visual complaints
Diplopia
Vertigo
Dysarthria*   only in combination,
Ataxia without   not as isolated symptoms
   weakness
Dysphagia

Either Carotid or Vertebral TIA
Severe dysarthria*
Homonymous visual complaints

Isolated Symptoms Rarely Due to TIA
Vertigo, dizziness
Diplopia
Loss of consciousness
Confusion
Bilateral leg weakness, falling spells

* Often difficult to distinguish from non-fluent aphasia on the basis of history.

Evaluation and Management

Since persons with a completed stroke are at risk for another stroke, they require the same scrutiny that patients with TIA undergo. Certainly, any patient with a cerebral infarction who makes a good recovery and returns to the premorbid level of function should not be dismissed without a thorough investigation into the course of the infarction. Once identified, all treatable causes, including contributing risk factors, should receive proper therapy and management. The differential diagnosis of the stroke patient is identical to that of the patient with TIAs. History, physical examination, and usual routine laboratory investigation will provide clues to the presence of systemic illness that produces cerebrovascular symptoms. In order to establish specific diagnosis, a CT scan of the brain is necessary. This procedure can rule in or out many non-vascular causes of stroke-like syndromes, and it is extremely helpful in the diagnosis of intracranial hemorrhage. In certain debilitated, severely ill patients, exhaustive investigation may not be carried out regardless of the diagnosis because of the absence of therapeutic options. There are relatively few patients, however, in whom a CT scan could provide no potential therapeutic information.

Invasive angiography, is reserved for patients in whom a vascular lesion, such as an internal carotid stenosis at the bifurcation of the common carotid artery, will lead to surgical endarterectomy. At present, invasive angiography remains the standard for imaging the carotid bifurcation and intracranial vasculature. However, in experienced hands, it carries a morbidity of major complications of about 1% and a mortality of under 0.3%.[32] Various non-invasive procedures have shown promise as a way of providing a safe and accurate means of evaluating carotid arterial pathology; but their clinical utility as a replacement for angiography remains to be proven.[2,33] All patients who undergo cerebral angiography or CT scanning with contrast administration should be well hydrated to avoid potential renal complications.

If cerebral embolism is suspect, holter monitoring (for cardiac arrhythmias) and echocardiography can provide evidence of cardiac pathology that gives rise to emboli. These studies are reserved for the setting in which a cardiac source of emboli is suspect since they provide low yield as a routine screening procedure in stroke.[34,35]

Depending upon the type of stroke or cause of the TIA, a variety of therapies are available. Medical therapy may take the form of general risk-factor reduction or be directed at the specific pathogenesis of the vascular symptoms. Accepted surgical therapy is directed at atherosclerosis and the complications thereof, which occur at the carotid bifurcation. Recently, various microvascular procedures have been advocated as a means of "revascularizing" or bypassing totally occluded precerebral arteries, especially the internal carotid artery. The efficacy of this procedure remains to be proven.

Cerebrovascular disease, as with other forms of vascular disease (especially heart disease), is common in elderly persons. Its presence alone does not assure that both symptoms will be present or that stroke will occur. These facts must be kept in mind when confronted with the patient who is found to have an asymptomatic bruit or asymptomatic carotid stenosis. A carotid bruit can be found in as many as 20% of all persons with symptomatic cardiovascular symptoms, and it occurs with increasing frequency after the 4th decade.[36] Large population studies confirm that men and women with asymptomatic bruits are two to seven times at risk for stroke compared to age-matched controls.[37,38] The location of the bruit does not, however, predict the location of the subsequent stroke. Prophylactic endarterectomy in an elderly person with asymptomatic bruit has not proved beneficial in reducing the incidence of subsequent stroke when compared to the risk of morbidity and mortality from endarterectomy.[39] Persons with asymptomatic cerebrovascular disease benefit most from both education about the symptoms of TIA and the recognition and reduction of risk factors for stroke. Whether or not treatment with antiaggregates serves to reduce risk of stroke in this group remains speculative.

The role of surgical and medical therapy is better defined in persons with symptomatic cerebrovascular atherosclerosis. Carotid endarterectomy is recommended for patients with symptoms appropriate for an artery in which either surgically accessible atherosclerosis sufficient to produce 50% or greater obstruction or large ulceration within the atheromatous plaque is present. For a good outcome, patients should be able to undergo general anesthesia, have a life expectancy of 5 years, and have a surgical risk of less than 3–4% for mortality and major morbidity. Not all patients, medical centers, or medical communities achieve this acceptable level of health and skill.[40,41] Under these circumstances, patients should be referred elsewhere or receive only medical therapy. It is important to keep in mind that the risk for stroke after endarterectomy does not fall to 0, but remains elevated at 2–4% per year, albeit reduced from 5–7% per year.[42,43]

Medical management is directed both at risk-factor reduction and, if possible, at the underlying cause of symptoms. Medical and surgical therapies are by no means exclusive; all patients who receive carotid endarterectomy, for example, will benefit from risk-factor reduction and potentially from antiaggregate therapy. In a well-designed clinical trial, the benefits of aspirin in reducing stroke and death by 50% in males were shown.[44] These beneficial results in males as well as in females has been confirmed in one large study, whereas a smaller study showed no benefit.[45,46] The weight of evidence supports the position that aspirin is a useful drug in the treatment of patients with TIAs. Clinical experience suggests that this protection is only partial and incomplete. Presumably, aspirin and other antiaggregating agents influence the reactivity of circulating platelets so as to reduce the chance of arterial thrombus formation. These events, in part, are mediated by various prostaglandins of which prostacyclin (PGI_2) and thromboxane (TXA_2) play a pivotal role.[47] PGI_2 is a potent vasodilator and has platelet disaggregating effects, whereas TXA_2 causes vasoconstriction and promotes platelet aggregation and thrombosis. The exact role of these and other prostaglandins in the genesis of stroke, particularly cerebral infarction, remains to be determined.

Risk Factors

Risk factors play an important role in the genesis of stroke. How they do so has not been fully determined. Risk factors include hereditary makeup such as sex and family history of premature atherosclerosis, cardiac disease and stroke, age, hypertension, heart disease, diabetes, TIAs, and prior stroke. Various combinations of risk factors can increase the risk of stroke 2–12-fold.[48,14] At present, the roles of obesity, a sedentary life style, stress, smoking, and elevated blood lipids in producing stroke needs further clarification. Since these factors are contributory to atherosclerosis and heart disease, despite a lack of epidemiologic significance, it is prudent to consider them as potential risk factors for stroke. Hypertension is the most important treatable risk factor for stroke. Data from the Framingham Study show 1) a striking increase in the incidence of atherothrombotic cerebral infarction with increasing age and degree of hypertension; 2) Gender having less of an effect in reducing risk in post-menopausal females with borderline elevations in blood pressure.[4] A similar relationship was found for intracerebral hemorrhage.

Cardiac diseases of all types contribute to stroke of all types. Relative risk depends upon both the type of heart disease and the type of stroke. For example, persons with non-rheumatic, but chronic, atrial fibrillation have a 5–6-fold increase in risk for embolic stroke; those with rheumatic heart disease and atrial fibrillation have 17 times the risk for stroke compared to non-affected age-matched persons.[15,49] Overt diabetes mellitus was found in 22% of acute stroke cases in a recent survey of nearly 4,000 strokes.[1] This figure is in agreement with the findings of Lavy and is about 4-fold greater than the figure found in the general age-matched population.[50] The exact role of any one risk factor or combination thereof in the pathogenesis of stroke requires further investigation. Nevertheless, there is no doubt that a reduction in risk factors, especially the treatment of hypertension, has led to a decline in the incidence of stroke. Furthermore, the early recognition and treatment of risk factors for stroke remains the most beneficial and cost-effective therapy available.

References

1. Yatsu FM, Coull BM, Toole JF, et al: Regional stroke survey: Demography and outcome. *Stroke* 13:124–128, 1982.
2. Yatsu FM, Coull BM: Stroke, in Appel AH (ed):

Current Neurology. New York, John Wiley & Sons, 1981, chap 7, pp 159–203.

3. Garraway WM, Whisnant JP, Furlan AJ, et al: The declining incidence of stroke. *N Engl J Med* 300:449–452, 1979.

4. Wolf PA, Kannel WB, Dawber TR: Prospective investigations: The Framingham study and the epidemiology of stroke. *Adv Neurol* 19:107–120, 1978.

5. Soltero I, Liu K, Cooper R, et al: Trends in mortality from cerebrovascular diseases in the United States, 1960 to 1975. *Stroke* 9:549–558, 1978.

6. Mohr JP, Caplan LH, Melski JW, et al: The Harvard Cooperative Stroke Registry: a prospective registry. *Neurology (NY)* 28:754–762, 1978.

7. Hart RG, Miller VT: Cerebral infarction in young adults: a practical approach. *Stroke* 14:110–114, 1983.

8. Caplan LR, Hier DB, D'Cruz I: Cerebral Embolism in the Michael Reese Stroke Registry: a prospective registry. *Neurology (NY)* 28:754–762, 1978.

9. Kubik CS, Adams RD: Occlusion of the basilar artery—a clinical and pathological study. *Brain* 69:6–121, 1946.

10. Miller VT: Lacunar stroke—a reassessment. *Arch Neurol* 40:129–134, 1983.

11. Fisher CM: The arterial lesions underlying lacunes. *Acta Neuropathol (Berl)* 12:1–15, 1969.

12. Mohr JP: Lacunes. *Stroke* 12:3–11, 1982.

13. Hart R, Hindman B: Mechanisms of perioperative cerebral infarction. *Stroke* 13:733–766, 1982.

14. Hart RG, Coull BM, Hart PD: Early recurrent emboli associated with non-valvular atrial fibrillation. *Stroke* 14:(in press), 1983.

15. Easton JD, Sherman DG: Management of cerebral embolism of cardiac origin. *Stroke* 11:433–442, 1980.

16. Weisberg LA: Computerized tomography in intracranial hemorrhage. *Arch Neurol* 36:422–426, 1979.

17. Furlan AJ, Cavalier SJ, Hobbs RE, et al: Hemorrhage and anticoagulation after nonseptic emboli brain infarction. *Neurology (NY)* 32:280–282, 1982.

18. Koller RL: Recurrent emboli cerebral infarction and anticoagulation. *Neurology (NY)* 32:283–285, 1982.

19. Cerebral Embolism Study Group: Immediate anticoagulation in emboli stroke. Part I: A prospective study. Stroke 14:(in press), 1983.

20. Conneally PM, Oyken ML, Futty DE, et al: Co-operative study of hospital frequency and character of transient ischemic attacks VIII. Risk Factors. *JAMA* 240:742–746, 1978.

21. Wiebers DO, Whisnant JP, O'Fallon WM: The natural history of unruptured intracranial aneurysms. *N Engl J Med* 304:696–698, 1981.

22. Weisberg LA: Computed tomography in the diagnosis and management of patients with subarachnoid hemorrhage and intracranial aneurysms. *Neurology (NY)* 29:802–808, 1979.

23. McKissock W, Paine KW, Walsh LS: An analysis of the results of treatment of ruptured intracranial aneurysms: A report of 722 consecutive cases. *J Neurosurg* 17:762–776, 1960.

24. Allen GS, Ahn HS, Preziosi TJ, et al: Cerebral Arterial Spasm—A controlled trial of nimodipine in patients with subarachnoid hemorrhage. *N Engl J Med* 308:619–624, 1983.

25. Okazaki IH, Reagan TJ, Campbell RJ: Clinicopathologic studies of primary central amyloid angiopathy. *Mayo Clin Proc* 54:22–31, 1979.

26. Boust JCM: Transient ischemic attacks: natural history and anticoagulation. *Neurology (NY)* 27:701–707, 1977.

27. Joint Committee for Stroke Facilities: Transient focal cerebral ischemia: epidemiological and clinical aspects. *Stroke* 5:277–287, 1974.

28. Cartlidge NEF, Whisnant JP, Elveback LR: Carotid and vertebral-basilar transient cerebral ischemic attacks. *Mayo Clin Proc* 52:117–120, 1977.

29. Ziegler DK, Hassanein RS: Prognosis in patients with transient ischemic attacks. *Stroke* 4:666–673, 1973.

30. Millikan C: The transient ischemic attack, in Goldstein M, et al: *Advances in Neurology*. New York, Raven Press, 1979, chap 25, pp 135–140.

31. Toole JF: Management of TIAs and acute cerebral infarction, in Thompson RA, Green JR (eds): *Advances in Neurology*. New York, Raven Press, 1977, chap 15, pp 71–80.

32. Eisenberg RL, Bank WO, Hedycock MW: Neurologic complications of angiography in patients with critical stenosis of the carotid artery. *Neurology (NY)* 30:892–895, 1980.

33. Ackerman RH: A perspective on noninvasive diagnosis of carotid disease. *Neurology (NY)* 29:615–622, 1979.

34. Knopman DS, Anderson DC, Asinger RW, et al: Indications for echocardiography in patients with ischemic stroke. *Neurology (NY)* 32:1005–1011, 1982.

35. Lovett JR, Sandok BA, Guiliani ER, et al: Two-dimensional echocardiography in patients with focal cerebral ischemia. *Ann Int Med* 95:1–4, 1981.

36. Barnes R, Marszalek P: A symptomatic carotid disease in the cardiovascular surgical patient: is prophylactic end arterectomy necessary? *Stroke* 12:497–500, 1981.

37. Heyman A, Wilkerson WE, Heyden S, et al: Risk of stroke in asymptomatic persons with cervical bruits. *N Engl J Med* 302:838–841, 1980.

38. Wolf PA, Kannel WB, Sorlie P, et al: Asymptomatic carotid bruit and risk of stroke: The Franklin Study. *JAMA* 245:1442–1445, 1981.

39. Jaird H, Ostermiller WE, Hengesh JW, et al: Carotid end arterectomy for asymptomatic patients. *Arch Surg* 102:389–391, 1971.

40. Whisnant JP, Sandok BA, Sundt TM: Carotid end arterectomy for unilateral carotid system transient cerebral ischemia. *Mayo Clin Proc* 58:171–175, 1983.

41. Easton JD, Sherman DG: Stroke and mortality rate in carotid endarterectomy: 228 consecutive operations. *Stroke* 8:565–568, 1977.

42. Toole JF, Yuson CP, Janeway R, et al: Transient ischemic attacks: a prospective study of 225 patients. *Neurology (NY)* 28:746–753, 1978.

43. Allen GS, Preziosi TJ: Carotid endarterectomy: a prospective study of its efficacy and safety. *Medicine* 60:298–309, 1981.

44. Barnett HJM, Gent M, Sackett DL, et al: A randomized trial of aspirin and sulfinpyrazone in threatened stroke: the Canadian Cooperative Study Group. *N Engl J Med* 299:53–59, 1978.

45. Bousser MG, Eschwege E, Haguenau M, et al: "AICLA" controlled trial of aspirin and dipyridamole in the secondary prevention of atherothrombotic cerebral ischemia. *Stroke* 14:5–14, 1983.

46. Sorensen PS, Pedersen H, Marquardsen J, et al: Acetylsalicylic acid in the prevention of stroke in patients with reversible cerebral ischemic attacks. A Danish cooperative study. *Stroke* 14:15–22, 1983.

47. Moncada A, Vane JR: Arachadonic acid metabolites and the interactions between platelets and blood-vessel walls. *N Engl J Med* 300:1142–1147, 1979.

48. Kannel WB, Wolf PA, Verker J, et al: Epidemiological assessment of the role of blood pressure in stroke: The Framingham Study. *JAMA* 214:301–310, 1970.

49. Wolf PA, Dawber TR, Thomas HE, et al: Epidemiologic assessment of chronic atrial fibrillation and risk of stroke: The Framingham Study. *Neurology (NY)* 28:973–977, 1978.

50. Lavy S: Medical risk factors in stroke. *Adv Neurol* 25:127–133, 1979.

CHAPTER 4

Neurologic Aspects of Dementia

BRUCE M. COULL, M.D.

The Royal College of Physicians Committee on Geriatrics defines dementia as

. . . the global impairment of higher cortical functions including memory, the capacity to solve the problems of day-to-day living, the performance of learned perceptuo-motor skills, the correct use of social skills and control of emotional reactions, in the absence of gross clouding of consciousness. The condition is often irreversible and progressive.[1]

Dementia has no single cause; it may result either from a disease limited to the brain, such as Alzheimer's disease, or as a result of widespread systemic involvement, such as in hypothyroidism. Dementia is the end result of greatly varied pathologic processes, and it may be static, progressive, reversible, or irreversible. The clinician must have a commanding knowledge of both the subtleties of the clinical presentation of this syndrome and the nuances of evaluation to properly evaluate, diagnose, and manage the patient with dementia. The early detection of dementia and a specific causal diagnosis can present a considerable diagnostic challenge.

Epidemiology

The exact incidence rate is unknown, but it is estimated that as many as one individual in six over 65 years of age suffers from dementia.[2,3] The prevalence in the United States is estimated at 550 per 100,000 persons. The prevalence increases with age, becoming as high as 20% in those over 80 years of age.[4,5] These figures suggest that there are at least 2 million persons in the United States with dementia, but the actual figure may be as high as 5 million. Among elderly persons, dementia or disease relating to it accounts for 75% of all first admissions to hospitals and between 70,000–110,000 deaths per year in the United States.

Disturbances in Cognitive Function: The Dementia Syndromes

Disturbances in cognitive function may accompany many disease processes and, thereby, produce a syndrome of dementia (see Volume I, Chapter 35). Not all strictly fulfill the requirements of the definition of dementia as advanced above. Such dementia syndromes can be broadly classified into three general categories: 1) Psychological disturbances; 2) Disordered cognition accompanying focal neurologic dysfunction; and 3) Dementia in association with global disturbance in neurologic function.[6] Disease in groups 1 and 2 are sometimes referred to as pseudodementia, while those in group 3 comprise the "true" dementias. This distinction of pseudodementia from dementia is of uncertain value, except insofar as such terminology serves to emphasize differential diagnosis and the need to establish the definitive causes underlying impaired cognition. Of the psychological disturbances, psychoses, hysteria, and malingering may all present as apparent dementia; however, the most common psychological disturbance constituting a dementia syndrome is that of depression.[7,8] Depression masquerading as dementia is a form of treatable and potentially reversible dementia (*see* Volume I, Chapter 36). One long-term study of persons initially diagnosed as having presenile dementia suggests that depression may be causal in roughly 20%.[9] The clinician should suspect depression as a cause for dementia if the patient's daily behaviors and activities are carried out with better performance than would be predicted by the performance in mental status testing. As opposed to the individual with a loss of intellectual function who may be oblivious, the depressed individual often complains bitterly of memory loss. Usually, mood and affect are markedly altered, and anxiety level is high, and there may exist a tendency to ruminate on a past life event. Psychometric testing often shows widely scattered and "inconsistent" results, but no single psychometric test or clinical study is sufficient to diagnose depression that mimics dementia. Rather, the syndrome is diagnosed after thorough evaluation fails to reveal any organic brain dysfunction, there is no evident progression over the follow-up period, and improvement follows the administration of antidepressant or other therapy. It is important, however, to keep in mind that depression may coexist with organic dementia.

The dementia syndromes that accompany focal neurologic dysfunction usually reflect lesions affecting three main brain regions: the frontal, temporal (or "limbic"), and parietal lobes (*see* Table 4-1).[6,10] In each of these types, preservation of intellect is the rule. Memory function is usually little affected in the frontal and parietal syndromes, while in "limbic" lesions an amnestic syndrome appears to be characterized by an almost pure loss of memory function and a preservation of other higher cortical modalities. Perhaps the most common and best example of this is the memory impairment seen in the Wernicke-Korsakoff syndrome of chronic alcoholism caused by thiamine deficiency. The clinical features of acute Wernicke encephalopathy encompass more than a disturbance of memory function and include abnormalities in extraocular motility, which include ophthalmoplegia and nystagmus, ataxia (especially of the trunk and lower extremities), and global confusion. Peripheral neuropathy is present in the majority of cases.

When chronic, the syndrome is termed Korsakoff's psychosis, characterized by an anterograde amnesia and, to a variable degree, a disturbance of past memory. When severe, persons may be incapable of learning even the simplest of new facts, despite excellent retention of language and many other aspects of intellectual function. A similar selective loss of anterograde memory function may, however, accompany head trauma, encephalitis, diencephalic tumors or, rarely, vertebrobasilar stroke.[11,12]

TABLE 4-1 Focal Deficits in Higher Mental Function

Type	Nature of Deficits	Other Signs	Common Causes
Frontal lobe syndrome	Social disintegration Emotional disinhibition Personal neglect Loss of judgment	Incontinence Adversive seizures Anosmia Grasp reflex Word finding difficulty Broca's aphasia	Space occupying lesion Frontal meningioma Chronic abscess, other primary or metastatic tumors Normal pressure hydrocephalus Head trauma
Amnestic syndrome (bitemporal or "limbic" lobes)	Loss of recent memory Inability to learn new material Confabulation	Hemianopsia Temporal lobe seizures Wernicke's aphasia	Thiamine deficiency (Korsakoff's) Herpes encephalitis or paraneoplastic "limbic" encephalitis Cerebral infarction Head trauma
Parietal lobe syndromes	Loss of visuo-spatial recognition Unawareness for contralateral body and illness	Cortical sensory loss Hemianopsia	Cerebral infarction Space occupying lesions, brain tumor, abscess, and so on

A common form of selective brief amnesia in elderly persons is the syndrome of transient global amnesia (TGA). In TGA, memory impairment is caused by ischemia to the hippocampus and mesial temporal structures, probably because of circulation disturbances in arterial branches of the posterior cerebral arteries although ischemia in the anterior choroidal artery also has been proposed.[13,14] In TGA, memory impairment is profound, lasts less than 24 hours, clears completely and does not recur.[14] During the amnestic episode personal identity is retained, the patients are usually agitated, but without any accompanying functional limitations and no focal neurologic abnormalities. Although this syndrome is presumed to be caused by focal vascular insufficiency, it remains controversial. It is important to recognize the syndrome, however, since it is both common and usually benign.

Another source of diagnostic confusion accompanies lesions (usually vascular) of the dominant hemisphere temporal lobe, which produce fluent aphasia of the Wernicke's type. With Wernicke's aphasia patients often seem confused, language shows normal fluency, but it contains meaningless jargon, termed neologisms, and paraphasic errors.[15] Language comprehension, reading, and writing are usually affected equally. Verbal discourse is, thus, so disrupted that patients may mistakenly be diagnosed as being psychotic or delirious. A history of apoplectic onset and careful attention to the character of language errors allows a recognition of this focal cortical disturbance.

Dementia with global impairment in neurologic function must be distinguished from delirium, in which global impairment in higher cortical function exists but in concert with decreased consciousness. The major causes of dementia and delirium are listed in Volume I, Chapter 35. Delirium presents clinically with an abrupt decrease in consciousness, usually in the setting of an already impaired cerebral cortex. Thus, pneumonia, fever or drug intoxication are important causes of delirium in elderly persons. Episodic delerium, which accompanies nocturnal sensory deprivation common in hospital and nursing home settings, is termed "sun downing." This is caused by environmental sensory deprivation, which follows the removal of orienting cues. Delirium may last hours or days,

but it is rarely prolonged for weeks or months (e.g., chronic intoxication) and clears with proper treatment. Depending on the cause, the return to the previous level of neurologic function may be gradual and incomplete.

A common misconception that cerebrovascular atherosclerosis is a cause of dementia because of chronic global cerebral ischemia is not supported by investigations of cerebral blood flow and metabolism.[16] Although amyloidosis of the intracerebral vasculature has been implicated in dementia, the only confirmed atherosclerotic cause of dementia is that accompanying multiple cerebral infarctions. Cardioembolic or cerebrovascular atherosclerosis thus produce dementia secondary to recurrent cerebral infarctions that are characterized by the sudden onset of focal neurologic deficits, which include hemiparesis, hemiplegia, aphasia, bulbar palsy, hemianopsia, or monoclear amaurosis.[17] A direct correlation between the presence of dementia and the amount of brain tissue infarcted has been shown.[18] Clinical skill is needed not only in recognizing the syndrome, but also in diagnosing the underlying cause of the vascular pathology.

Hydrocephalus

A potentially reversible form of dementia is that accompanying hydrocephalus (see Table 4-2). Any intracranial lesion that obstructs the outflow of cerebrospinal fluid (CSF) from the intracerebral ventricular system can produce obstructive hydrocephalus. The clinical presentation of acute obstructive hydrocephalus includes headache, nausea, vomiting, obtundation, and hyperactive reflexes. Papilledema and focal neurologic findings are frequent. CSF pressure is elevated, and because of shifts of brain tissue within the intracranial compartment lumbar puncture may be contraindicated. In contradistinction, communicating hydrocephalus occurs when the flow of CSF is obstructed in the subarachnoid space, usually within the meninges or at the site of CSF absorption in arachnoid villi at the sagittal sinus. Dementia that follows the onset of hydrocephalus, particularly when the obstruction to CSF flow is incomplete and chronic, may resolve with relief to the obstruction. Besides de-

TABLE 4-2 Common Causes of Hydrocephalus

Type	Mechanism	Common Causes
Obstructive hydrocephalus	Obstruction of CSF flow within the cerebral ventricles	Parenchymal tumors, mostly posterior fossa Intraventricular tumors (i.e., colloid cyst of third ventricle) Aqueductal stenosis Ventriculitis
Communicating hydrocephalus	Obstruction of CSF flow in subarachnoid space or impairment of CSF resorption	Subarachnoid hemorrhage Chronic meningitis Head injury Idiopathic (i.e., normal pressure hydrocephalus)
Hydrocephalus ex vacuo	Diffuse cerebral atrophy with replacement of brain parenchyma by CSF	Alzheimer's disease Alcoholic dementia Multiinfarct dementia

mentia, additional prominent clinical features of communicating hydrocephalus include the early appearance of urinary and, at times, bowel incontinence and apraxia of gait.[19] Papilledema and elevated CSF pressure with lumbar puncture are uncommon, but some patients improve clinically after removal of 15–20 cc of CSF. Additional clues that suggest a clinical diagnosis include an antecedent history of head trauma, meningitis, or subarachnoid hemorrhage. A computed tomography (CT) scan of the brain is useful in excluding an intracranial tumor and may suggest aqueductal stenosis, communicating hydrocephalus, or diffuse cerebral atrophy (hydrocephalus exvacuo).[20,21] The role of radiolabelled serum albumin (RISA) in studying the flow of CSF when communicating hydrocephalus is suspected is controversial, since several studies report conflicting or inconsistent responses in patients with dementias of various causes.[22]

Intracranial Mass Lesions

Intracranial mass lesions usually produce headache and focal neurologic symptoms before causing global impairment of higher cortical functions. Rarely, tumors of the brain and subdural hematomas (SDH) present with alterations in behaviors or mentation. The elderly are at risk for SDH because they are more prone to falling and because age-related cerebral atrophy places bridging cerebrodural veins at particular

risk for rupture after a head injury. The classic presentation of SDH is that of head trauma followed by a lucid interval before headache, stupor, and focal neurologic signs appear. Once symptomatic, and particularly if consciousness is disturbed, the mortality approaches 60% despite surgical evacuation.[23,24] SDH in elderly persons may follow trivial trauma of may even arise without antecedent trauma thus producing "spontaneous" SDH. The lesion is bilateral in about 15% of all cases or it may be confined to the posterior fossa. If chronic, SDH is often accompanied by changes in mentation and behavior alone, or only with headache as the clinical presentation. Acute neurologic deterioration can terminate the course of chronic SDH. Frequently, the diagnosis of chronic SDH is missed in a patient with coincidental metabolic abnormalities. Accordingly, SDH should be considered whenever mental function does not clear with correction of metabolic abnormalities or when focal neurologic findings, such as hemiparesis, exist.

Both primary brain malignancies and metastatic tumors of the brain are a cause of deterioration in behavior, mentation, and neurologic function in elderly persons.[25–27] Headache, lateralized weakness or clumsiness, visual complaints, and seizures (often with focal motor components) are common early symptoms. In roughly 20% of all cases intellectual decline is prominent early in the course of illness.[25,26] Symptoms usually are gradually progressive, but apoplectic onset of symptoms can occur.

Besides focal neurologic findings, the presence of papilledema confirms the clinical suspicion of an intracranial mass lesion. The CT scan should be performed with and without contrast, since some tumors are "isodense" with normal brain tissue. The presence of multiple round (spherical) densities suggests a metastatic tumor of the brain. It is sometimes difficult to distinguish the CT picture of a brain abscess and other infectious or parasitic diseases from that of a neoplasm. An elevated white blood cell count, fever, and symptoms of systemic or focal infection elsewhere in the body point to the diagnosis; however, in debilitated elderly persons these are not always present.

Infections of the Brain

Infectious disease of the brain and its surroundings causes alterations in mentation, behavior, and the level of consciousness. Other symptoms, which include a fever, stiff neck, nausea and vomiting, and a variety of focal neurologic findings, usually suggest the diagnosis of infection; however, when insidious, a nervous system infection can cause a diagnostic difficulty. Although uncommon, a brain abscess may arise without a history of antecedent infection and remain quiescent for weeks or months before presenting as a focal mass lesion.[28] With a chronic brain abscess, frequent headache, deterioration in behavior, and intellect are recalled as the initial manifestation only after focal seizures or other focal symptoms appear. Since brain abscesses, whether single or multiple, are intracranial "mass" lesions, caution in performing lumbar puncture is advised.

Chronic Basilar Meningitis

The chronic meningitides encountered most often are listed in Table 4-3. Besides changes in mentation, these are usually associated with one or more cranial nerve abnormalities and other focal neurologic signs. Neurosyphilis is the "classic" chronic meningeal and brain infection producing both tabes dorsalis and dementia.[29] Although less common than they once were, these infections still occur. Behcet's syndrome and sarcoidosis are accompanied by cutaneous lesions, uveitis, and systemic symp-

TABLE 4-3   Chronic Meningitis

"Common" Meningitis	"Rare" Uveo-Meningeal Syndromes
Tuberculous	Behcet's disease
Fungal	Vogt-Koyanagi-Harada
Neurosyphilis	Cogan's syndrome
Sarcoidosis	

toms.[30–32] Examination of the CSF usually provides clues to a diagnosis with protein elevation of moderate degree and a predominant lymphocytic pleocytosis. In fungal and tuberculosis infections of the nervous system, initial CSF examination with india ink preparations and stains such as acid fast may be negative.[33–35] Cultures sometimes take weeks or longer periods to grow out. If the overall clinical picture is strongly suggestive, negative culture and stain results should not dissuade an early institution of appropriate therapy, since this may be lifesaving. "Opportunistic" infectious agents, including progressive multifocal leukoencephalopathy (PML), toxoplasmosis, cytomegalovirus, cryptococcus, and a variety of fungi present a special problem for diagnosis in the immune suppressed host. Isolated cerebral vasculitis (granulomatous angiitis), systemic vasculitidies, or vasculitis in association with chronic nervous system infections can account for changes in higher cortical function.[36]

Slow Virus Infection

Although several important slow viral infections of humans are identified, Creutzfeldt-Jacob disease (CJD) is the most important in relation to dementia. CJD is a rare disease (incidence rate approximately equals a prevalence of 1 case per 1 million persons), but it is of considerable importance to all health professionals who evaluate or treat demented persons. Kuru, a disease similar if not identical to CJD, is caused by a transmissible agent referred to as a slow or "unconventional" virus.[37,38] The term prions describe small, proteinaceous infectious particles.[39] Although not fully characterized, prions are small in size (i.e., less than 50,000 daltons), have no capsule, contain no nucleic acids, and produce no known host immune response. They have a long incubation period (several months to 2 or more years), but transmission of CJD from man-to-animal and man-to-man via contaminated tissues or instruments has occurred.[40,41] Once symptoms are manifest, there is a rapid progression with dementia, myoclonic jerks, severe ataxia, gait instability, and visual symptoms as prominent features. Death follows in most cases within 9 months to 1 year from onset of symptoms. Because CJD is transmissible, great care must be used when handling tissues from patients in whom CJD is suspect. Furthermore, the CJD prion is not inactivated by some routine methods of sterilization or formalin fixation. Established guidelines should be followed in this regard.[42] Since the cause of many forms of dementia remains unknown, precautionary measures are warranted whenever handling tissues from patients with dementia.

Systemic Diseases and Intoxications

Chronic encephalopathy with apparent dementia is sometimes a major symptom of several metabolic, nutritional, and toxic states. The aging brain, because of impaired compensatory mechanisms, is particularly sensitive to the adverse metabolic effects brought about by systemic disease.[43] A small decrement in cardiac or pulmonary function, in the setting of underlying chronic cardiopulmonary failure, may cause a sudden decompensation in higher cerebral function because of brain hypoperfusion and hypoxia, which follows already compromised cerebral blood flow autoregulation.[44–46] Similarly, hepatic, renal, and endocrine dysfunction can produce derangements in electrolyte, glucose, or thyroid hormone levels that result in apparent dementia and/or delirium.[47–49] Hepatic and renal failure are accompanied by accumulations of circulating toxic metabolic products that impair brain function.[50–61] Major organ failure also impairs or prolongs the metabolism and excretion of many drugs, thereby resulting in dangerous levels that may be toxic to the brain.[62] It is not uncommon in large medical centers to encounter patients with encephalopathy in whom multiple organs systems have failed and complicated multi-drug therapies have made identifying the single cause of brain dysfunction almost impossible.

The frequently encountered forms of organ system failure that produce encephalopathy are shown in Table 4-4. Encephalopathy in this setting always is attended by additional systemic symptoms and signs, which suggest a diagnosis. In elderly persons this is more difficult, since encephalopathy can follow subtle metabolic changes which in a younger individual would not lead to decompensation. The problem of distinguishing between intrinsic brain disease and disease caused by underlying systemic illness such as congestive heart failure in elderly persons has been emphasized.[43] Sound advice under such circumstances is to treat the systemic illness with the expectation that brain function will improve. Return of higher cortical function often occurs gradually, sometimes over weeks or even months despite prompt correction of offending metabolic abnormalities.

Intoxicants

The common intoxicants that cause confusion in elderly persons are listed in Table 4-5. Pharmaceutical drugs and ethyl alcohol are most often the offending agents. Alcoholism is not confined to any particular age group and can arise later in life (see Volume II, Chapter 17). Elderly persons with several disease processes may require multiple medicines, which with delayed metabolism and clearance can lead to drug accumulation up to toxic levels. Combinations of medicines are particularly prone to causing adverse side effects because of competition for binding sites and metabolic pathways. Confused or demented patients sometimes complicate the problem further by taking more of a drug than directed, or doing so in a haphazard fashion. As a general rule, the clinician should consider all drugs as suspect when dealing with recently onset encephalopathy. Drug regimens in elderly persons, or those with intellectual impairment, should be simplified to the least number of medicines in the lowest possible dosages given at regular intervals.[62] To design effective drug regimens and to avoid these pitfalls, a working knowledge of pharmacokinetics is necessary. For example, some soporific drugs, such as flurazepam, although given only once per night for sleep, may gradually accumulate to levels producing adverse effects on mental function because of its very long elimination half-life of 1–4 days.[62]

TABLE 4-4 Organ System Failure Causing Encephalopathy

Organ System	Clinical Symptoms and Signs	Laboratory Findings	References
Cardiopulmonary failure	Headache, confusion, stupor	$\downarrow$ PaO$_2$, $\uparrow$ CO$_2$, elevated CSF pressure	44–46
Hepatic failure	Asterixis, papilledema, myoclonic jerks	Synchronous "tri-phasic" slowing on EEG, $\uparrow$ blood NH$_3$, low serum copper, low ceruloplasmin, high urinary copper	47,48
	Confusion, stupor or coma; focal or generalized seizures		49,50
	Asterixis, signs of chronic liver disease		
Renal failure	Apathy, fatigue, confusion, stupor, generalized seizures, "dialysis dementia," "disequilibrium syndrome"	Elevated CSF* pressure and protein, elevated BUN† and creatinine, electrolyte abnormalities, paroxysmal "epileptiform" bursts on EEG‡	51–53
	Myoclonic jerks, asterixis, hypertension, peripheral polyneuropathy		54,55
Endocrine			
Glucose	Focal neurologic signs, hemiparesis, peripheral polyneuropathy, diabetic retinopathy	Elevated or low blood glucose, large sudden drop in blood glucose, elevated serum osmolality, ketoacidosis, electrolyte abnormalities	56–58
Hypoglycemia			
Hyperglycemia	Episodic headaches, sweats, seizures, confusion, coma		
Thyroid			
Hypothyroidism	Delayed reflex relaxation, hypothermia, cerebellar ataxia	Elevated thyroid stimulating hormone, low T$_3$ and T$_4$ in hypothyroidism (B$_4$), elevated T$_3$ in "T$_3$ toxicosis," EEG slowing	59–61
Hyperthyroidism (apathetic)	Apathy, psychosis, coma		
Hypophysioadrenal axis	Increased body fat, moon facies, striae (CS), loss of body hair, hypotension, skin hyperpigmentation (AD), hypothermia	Electrolyte abnormalities, enlarged sella turcica, exogenous steroid drug administration	62–64
Cushing's syndrome (CS)	Apathy, psychosis, severe dementia, depression		
Addison's disease (AD)			

* CSF = cerebrospinal fluid; † BUN = blood urea nitrogen; ‡ EEG = electroencephalogram.

TABLE 4-5   Intoxications in the Elderly

Drugs	Other Agents
Antihypertensive	Ethyl alcohol
Anticonvulsants	Illicit drugs
Antiparkinson	Heavy metals—mercury,
Antipsychotic	lead
Digitalis	Organic solvents
Patent medicines—	Carbon monoxide
antihistamines	
Sedative hypnotics	
"Minor" tranquilizers	
Sedative/Hypnotics	
Lithium and bromide	

Nutritional Deficiencies

The classic nutritional deficiencies that produce nervous system diseases have become rare in the United States. These include a lack of folate and B vitamins, especially B-12, as well as Vitamin E. Most deficiency conditions exist in concert with chronic alcoholism or advanced systemic diseases, such as malignancy or profound malabsorption syndrome. As a general rule, peripheral polyneuropathies are a prominent feature of nervous system disease resulting from nutritional deficiency. Despite its rare occurrance, serum Vitamin B-12 and folate levels are a routine part of evaluation in dementia since these deficiencies are treatable (see Volume I, Chapter 22 and Volume II, Chapter 12).

Alzheimer's Disease

Broadly defined, Alzheimer's disease accounts for 50–60% of all dementia in persons over 65 years of age.[63] Current nomenclature confines 1) The Alzheimer designation to persons with an onset of symptoms at younger than age 65; and 2) Senile dementia of the Alzheimer's type (SDAT) to persons whose symptoms begin after 65 years of age. This distinction based upon age is arbitrary and of doubtful clinical or scientific merit. Among persons older than age 65, only about 5% suffer from severe memory or intellectual impairment. Two points bear emphasis: 1) Senile dementia is not inevitable in elderly persons; and 2) The pathologic changes seen in Alzheimer's disease and SDAT are the same. Confusion as to what constitutes normal aging is justified since many of the pathologic features

of Alzheimer's disease appear in a "normal" aging brain; the distinction between disease and "normality," in part, is one of degree.[64] This long-established observation has raised questions as to whether Alzheimer's disease reflects an accelerated or premature form of the natural aging process, or if aging allows increased susceptibility to some as yet unknown but pathologic process. Recent advances in research into the pathogenesis of Alzheimer's disease lend support to the latter viewpoint.

Clinical Course

The patient with Alzheimer's disease experiences three phases of illness.[65] In the initial phase, the patient becomes aware of intellectual or memory impairment, but the mild symptoms are not noticed by family and friends. With progression into the second phase, close family and friends begin to notice the patient's difficulties with memory, intellect, and judgment. Finally, in the third stage the patient loses awareness of the illness, but the symptoms are so advanced as not to be missed by those around the patient. Detection of dementia during the early phases often is difficult and requires recognition of the subtleties of presentation and a thorough approach to evaluation and diagnosis.

During the initial stage, difficulties with failing intellect and memory are sometimes ignored and, instead, complaints center on trivial somatic symptoms such as tension headache, abdominal discomfort, and various musculoskeletal aches and pains. A prior long-standing affliction may become the focus of medical attention, leading to extensive investigations and consultation with a number of physicians. Frequently, no pathologic explanation for the complaint is discovered and, likewise, symptomatic therapy affords little relief. All too often this diversion of attention causes physicians to ignore clear-cut signs of intellectual or memory impairment.

With loss of cognitive function, alarmed family members often bring the patient for medical attention. Sometimes, however, because of embarrassment or to avoid conflict they may "cover" over difficulties for the patient. In obtaining medical history, a physician should be alert to this possibility, especially if the patient provides vague or sketchy details and relies on a spouse or other informant to "fill in" specific details. Eliciting all information initially from the patient will avoid this pitfall. The history can be confirmed or amplified by conversation with additional informants.

Alzheimer's disease is characterized by a relentless progression over 2–10 or more years. Besides difficulties with memory, judgment, and intellect, language function—including aphasia—may be apparent early in the course of illness. Motor findings include apraxia, increased tone, tonic rigidity, myoclonic jerks, and hyperactive reflexes, often with accompanying Babinski signs. In occasional cases, focal motor signs may be found early in the course of illness and rarely seizures are encountered. So-called vegetative reflexes, which include snout, grasp, suck, and palmomental, are an invariant finding at one time or another, however, these are of dubious value early in the course of illness since all are also found in normal elderly persons.[66]

Pathology

At autopsy, an Alzheimer's diseased brain usually demonstrates a global atrophy. The cerebellum and brainstem are spared. On sectioning, the lateral and third ventricles appear dilated, but major cerebral arteries and white matter are normal. Microscopic examination shows a mild loss of small cortical neurons, although a massive loss of cortical neurons does not occur in Alzheimer's disease.

The two major features that comprise the microscopic hallmark of Alzheimer's disease are neuritic (senile) plaques and neurofibrillary tangles (*see* Figures 4-1, 4-2). The latter are made up of paired helical filaments that appear within the nerve cell bodies with a special predilection for pyramidal cells of the frontal and temporal cortex. Ammon's horn involvement is invariable. Neuritic plaques are clusters of degenerating nerve axons around an amyloid core. They

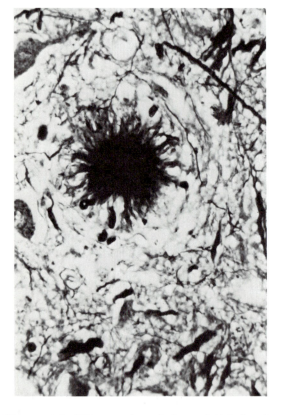

FIGURE 4-1 Microscopic pathology of Alzheimer's disease: silver stained section of frontal cortex showing a "senile plaque."

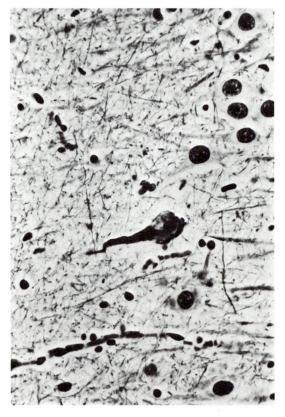

FIGURE 4-2 Microscopic pathology of Alzheimer's disease: silver stained section of hippocampus showing neurofibrillary tangles within neuronal cell bodies.

are usually located adjacent to a capillary and, typically, are surrounded by astrocytes. They distribute throughout the neuropil of the cerebral cortex, hippocampus, and amygdala. Additional microscopic findings of uncertain significance include granulovacuolar degeneration and Hirano bodies within hippocampal neurons (*see* Figure 4-3).[67]

Pathogenesis

Although the cause of Alzheimer's disease remains unknown, important neurochemical and neuroanatomic features have been identified that may lead to an eventual understanding and effective treatment. Several investigators have found that cerebral cortex and hippocampus tissue removed from persons with Alzheimer's disease has a 60–90% reduction in the enzyme choline acetyltransferase (CAT), which synthesizes acetylcholine (ACh).[68–70] The loss of cholinergic activity in these regions seems to be quite specific since other neurotransmitter systems in the brain are not so affected. Neuroanatomic studies suggest that the brain regions where CAT activity is reduced receive cholinergic input from a projection pathway whose neuronal cell bodies are located within the basal forebrain. Neuritic plaques are proportional in number to clinical dementia and to the degree of cholinergic loss.[71] The possible relation of the neuritic plaque to the basal forebrain cholinergic projection has been schematized as shown in Figure 4-4.[72] It would appear that a fundamental aspect of Alzheimer's disease is the selective degeneration of a population of cholinergic neurons whose cell bodies are located within the basal forebrain. The cause(s) of this selective neuronal degeneration and its relation to the other major neuropathologic finding—neurofibrillary tangles—has not been determined. Despite the compelling evidence that a selective dysfunction of cholinergic projections to the cerebral cortex may be the fundamental lesion in Alzheimer's disease, therapeutic efforts directed at increasing brain ACh are still unresolved.[76]

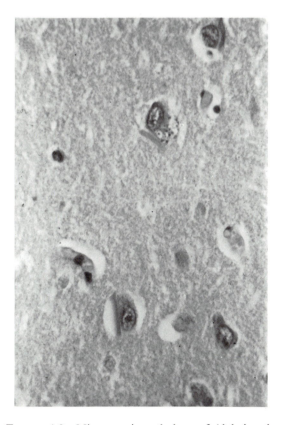

FIGURE 4-3 Microscopic pathology of Alzheimer's disease: section of hippocampus showing neuron with granulovacuolar changes and a linear Hirano body. A second neuron (low center) contains a pencil shaped Hirano body, but little granulovacuolar change.

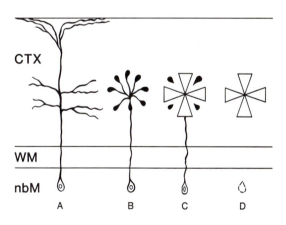

FIGURE 4-4 Development and evolution of a neuritic "senile" plaque in Alzheimer's disease. Cerebral cortex CTX receives acetylcholine input from neurons whose cell bodies are located within the basal forebrain (nucleus basalis of Meynert ηbM) (A). Axon and nerve terminals of these neurons become dystrophic (B) and eventually produce a plaque containing a central core of amyloid (C) surrounded by neurites. When advanced, the basal neurons degenerate leaving only the amyloid remnant (D). WM, white matter. (From Price, et al, used by permission).

Evaluation of the Demented Patient

The evaluation of the demented patient requires careful attention to the details of the presentation and progression of symptoms, the physical neurologic examination, and (often) the psychiatric examination. The presence of systemic illness, multiple medications, and focal neurologic findings should raise suspicion that the dementia may be secondary to a potentially treatable illness. However, the absence of these features does not exclude a treatable cause.

Routine radiologic and laboratory studies, including a chest x-ray film, hemogram, sedimentation rate, fluorescent treponemal antibody (FTA), electrocardiogram (ECG), serum electrolytes, and screening measures of the renal, hepatic, and pulmonary function help to exclude systemic causes. Additional specific determinations of thyroid function, drug levels, toxic screens, arterial blood gases, and determinations of Vitamin B-12 levels should be obtained whenever appropriate. Neurologic studies include brain CT scan, electroencephalogram (EEG), lumbar puncture, and psychometric testing. In special cases, cerebral angiography may prove useful.

Role of the Brain CT Scan

The value of a CT scan of the brain in diagnosing structural brain lesions is great. There is no better method of demonstrating primary or metastatic tumors of the brain, brain abscess, subdural hematoma, or hydrocephalus. The CT scan is frequently helpful in the diagnosis of multiinfarct dementia and other stroke syndromes, although does not in general provide insight into the cause of the vascular pathology. In toxic and metabolic encephalopathies the CT scan is usually performed to exclude one of the above structural lesions. Although it is of unsurpassed value in identifying focal brain lesions, the CT scan is not predictive of clinical neurologic function and is of less value in diffuse brain diseases. This is especially true for cerebral atrophy which can, by CT scan criteria, appear to be "advanced" in persons with normal neurologic function.[74] In Alzheimer's disease, "diffuse cortical atrophy," with an enlarged ventricular system or so-called hydrocephalus ex vacuo, is the usual CT scan finding; however, not infrequently, the CT scan is within the normal range for the patient's age. As a general rule, all patients with undiagnosed dementia, especially of a recent onset, should undergo CT scanning.

Yield

Despite thorough evaluation, a definitive antemortem diagnosis of cause in dementia is not always established. From a practical standpoint, the important "yield" in a differential diagnosis of dementia are those cases that have a treatable and potentially reversible cause. In this sense, the yield depends upon several important factors, which include the presentation and duration of symptoms of intellectual decline. An extensive review of several clinical series points to the importance of these symptoms and the population base from which the patient comes for medical attention.[75]

In a hospital-based outpatient population presenting with dementia, Malletta and Pirozzolo diagnosed Alzheimer's dementia in 43% of the patients;[76] a depressive disorder was caused in 24%, multiinfarct dementia in 10%, and alcoholism in 7%. Overall, potentially reversible causes were identified in almost one third of the population studied (30%). In a somewhat more select group of patients, Smith and Kiloh found a potentially reversible cause for dementia in 11.5% of 200 cases who were less than 64 years old (77). They found, as did others, a reversible cause more often in younger age groups, so that only 3.8% of cases over 64 years of age had a potentially reversible dementia. Reversible causes for dementia are found most often in those individuals with a recent onset of symptoms.[6] There is no doubt that most elderly individuals with symptoms of dementia will eventually prove to have Alzheimer's disease. Nonetheless, this fact should not dissuade the clinician from a thorough evaluation and consideration of differential diagnosis in all patients with impairment of cognitive function.

References

1. Royal College of Physicians, Committee on Geriatrics: Organic mental impairment in the elderly: implications for research, education and the provision of services. *J R Coll Physicians Lond* 15:141–167, 1981.

2. Kay DWK, Beamish P, Roth M: Old age mental disorders in Newcastle Upon Tyne. I. A study of prevalence. *Br J Psychiatry* 110:146–158, 1964.

3. Editorial: Dementia: the quiet epidemic. *Br Med J* 1:1–2, 1978.

4. Katzman R: The prevalence and malignancy of Alzheimer's disease: a major killer. *Arch Neurol* 33:217–218, 1976.

5. Katzman R: Introduction: comments on epidemiological and socioeconomic implications, in Katzman R (ed): *Congenital and Acquired Cognitive Disorders*. New York, Raven Press, 1979, pp 1–4.

6. Marsden CD: The diagnosis of dementia, in Isaacs AD, Post F (eds): *Studies in Geriatric Psychiatry*. New York, John Wiley & Sons, 1978, p 95.

7. Seltzer B, Sherwin I: "Organic brain syndromes": an empirical study and critical review. *Am J Psychiatry* 135:13–21, 1978.

8. Kiloh LG: Pseudo-dementia. *Acta Psychiatr Scand* 37:336–351, 1961.

9. Ron MA, Toone BK, Garralda ME, et al: Diagnostic accuracy in presenile dementia. *Br J Psychiatry* 134:161–168, 1979.

10. Straub RL, Black FW: Neurobehavioral syndromes associated with focal brain lesions, in *Organic Brain Syndromes*. Philadelphia, Davis Co, 1981, pp 213–266.

11. Victor M, Adams RD, Collins GH: in Plum F, McDowell FH (eds): *The Wernicke-Korsakoff Syndrome: a Clinical and Pathological Study of 245 Patients, 82 with Post-mortem Examinations*. Philadelphia, Davis Co, 1971, chap 2, pp 16–34.

12. Horel JA: The neuroanatomy of amnesia. *Brain* 101:443–445, 1978.

13. Fisher CM, Adams RD: Transient global amnesia. *Acta Neurol Scand* 40(suppl 9):9–83, 1964.

14. Fogelholm R, Kivalo E, Bergstrom L: The transient global amnesia syndrome. *Eur Neurol* 13:72–84, 1975.

15. Benson DF: *Aphasia, Alexia and Agraphia*. New York, Churchill Livingstone, 1979, pp 71–77.

16. Frackowiak RSJ, Pozzilli C, Legg NJ, et al: Regional cerebral oxygen supply and utilization in dementia: a clinical and physiological study with oxygen-15 and positron tomography. *Brain* 104:753–778, 1981.

17. Kaplan JG, Katzman R, Horoupian D, et al: The syndrome of progressive dementia, amyotrophy and visual deficits: micro-infarction of the nervous system. *Neurology* 30:390–397, 1980.

18. Tomlinson BE, Blessed G, Roth M: Observations on the brains of demented old people. *J Neurol Sci* 11:205–242, 1970.

19. Adams RD, Fisher CM, Hakim S, et al: Symptomatic occult hydrocephalus with normal cerebrospinal fluid pressure. *N Engl J Med* 273:117–126, 1965.

20. LeMay M, Hochberg FH: Ventricular differences between hydrostatic hydrocephalus and hydrocephalus ex vacuo by computed tomography. *Neuroradiology* 17:191–195, 1979.

21. Ostertog CB, Mundinger F: Diagnosis of normal pressure hydrocephalus using CT and CSF enhancement. *Neuroradiology* 16:216–219, 1978.

22. Sohn RS, Siegel BA, Gado M, et al: Alzheimer's disease with abnormal cerebrospinal fluid flow. *Neurology* 23:1058–1065, 1973.

23. McKissock W, Richardson A, Bloom WH: Subdural hematoma. A review of 389 cases. *Lancet* 1:1365–1369, 1960.

24. Richards T, Hoff J: Factors affecting survival from acute subdural hematoma. *Surgery* 75:253–258, 1974.

25. Little JR, MacCarty CS: Colloid cysts of the third ventricle. *J Neurosurg* 39:230–235, 1974.

26. Keschner M, Bender MB, Strauss T: Mental symptoms in cases of tumor of the temporal lobe. *Arch Neurol Psychiatry* 35:572–596, 1936.

27. Holmes G: Discussion on the mental symptoms associated with cerebral tumors. *Proc R Soc Med* 24:997–1008, 1931.

28. Brewer NS: Brain Abscess: A review of recent experience. *Ann Int Med* 12:197–205, 1975.

29. Merritt HH, Adams RD, Solomon HC: *Neurosyphilis*. Oxford University Press, New York, 1946.

30. Chajek T, Fainaru M: Behcet's disease. Report of 41 cases and review of the literature. *Medicine* 54:179–196, 1975.

31. Pattison EM: Uveo-meningoencephalitic syndrome (Vogt-Koyanagi-Harada). *Arch Neurol* 12:197–205, 1965.

32. Delaney P: Neurologic manifestations in sarcoidosis. *Ann Int Med* 87:336–345, 1977.

33. Udani PM, Dastur DK: Tuberculosis encephalopathy with or without meningitis: Clinical features and pathological correlations. *J Neurol Sci* 10:541–561, 1970.

34. Kocen RS, Parsons M: Neurological complications of tuberculosis. Some unusual manifestations. *Quart J Med* 39:17–30, 1970.

35. Lewis JL, Rabinovich S: The wide spectrum of cryptococcal infection. *Am J Med* 53:315–322, 1972.

36. Cupps TR, Fauci AS: Central nervous system vasculitis, in Smith, Lloyd H. Jr (ed): *The Vasculitides,* Vol 21 in Major Problems in Internal Medicine. Philadelphia, WB Saunders & Co, 1981.

37. Gibbs CJ Jr, Gadjusek DC: Infection as the etiology of spongiform encephalopathy (Creutzfeldt-Jakob disease). *Science* 165:1023–1025, 1969.

38. Brooks BR, Jubelt B, Swarz JR, et al: Slow viral infections. *Ann Rev Neurosci* 2:309–340, 1979.

39. Prusinger SB: Novel proteinaceous infectious particles cause scrapie. *Science* 216:136–144, 1982.

40. Duffy PE, Wolf J, Collins G, et al: Possible person-to-person transmission of Creutzfeldt-Jakob disease. *N Engl J Med* 290:692–693, 1974.

41. Gajdusek DC, Gibbs CJ Jr, Asher DM, et al: Precautions in medical care of, and in handling materials from, patients with transmissible virus dementia (Creutzfeldt-Jakob disease). *N Engl J Med* 297:1253–1258, 1977.

42. Baringer JR, Gajdusek DC, Gibbs CJ Jr, et al: Transmissible dementias: Current problems in tissue handling. *Neurology* 30:302–303, 1980.

43. Blass JP, Plum F: Metabolic encephalopathies in older adults, in Katzman R, Terry RD (eds): *The Neurology of Ageing*. FA Davis Co., Philadelphia, 1983, chap 9, pp 189–220.

44. Flenley DC: Clinical hypoxia: causes, consequences, and correction. *Lancet* 1:542–546, 1978.

45. Blass JP, Gibson GE: Consequences of mild, graded hypoxia. *Adv Neurol* 26:229–250, 1979.

46. Corday E, Irving DW: Effect of cardiac arrhythmias on the cerebral circulation. *Am J Cardiol* 6:803–808, 1960.

47. Zieve L, Nicoloff DM: Pathogenesis of hepatic coma. *Ann Rev Med* 26:143–157, 1975.

48. Schenker S, Breen KJ, Hoyumpa AM: Hepatic encephalopathy: current status. *Gastroenterology* 66:121–151, 1974.

49. Victor M, Adams RD, Cole M: The acquired (non-Wilsonian) type of chronic hepatocerebral degeneration. *Medicine* 44:345–396, 1965.

50. Wilson SAK: Progressive lenticular degeneration: a familial nervous disease associated with cirrhosis of the liver. *Brain* 34:295–509, 1912.

51. Marshall JR: Neuropsychiatric aspects of renal failure. *J Clin Psychiatry* 40:45–51, 1979.

52. Locke S, Merrill JP, Tyler HR: Neurological complications of uremia. *Arch Int Med* 108:519–530, 1961.

53. Alfrey AC, Le Gendre GR, Kaehny WD: The dialysis encephalopathy syndrome. *N Engl J Med* 294:184–188, 1976.

54. Noriega-Sanchez A, Martinez-Maldonado M, Haiffe RM: Clinical and electroencephalographic changes in progressive uremic encephalopathy. *Neurology* 28:667–669, 1978.

55. Newmark SR, Himathongkam T, Shane JM: Hyperglycemic and hypoglycemic crisis. *JAMA* 231:185–186, 1975.

56. Garcia MJ, McNamara PM, Gordon T, et al: Morbidity and mortality in diabetics in the Framingham population. *Diabetes* 23:105–111, 1974.

57. Arieff AI, Carrol HJ: Nonketotic hyperosmolar coma with hyperglycemia: clinical features, pathophysiology, renal function, acid-base balance, plasma cerebrospinal fluid equilibria and effect of therapy in 37 cases. *Medicine* 51:73–94, 1972.

58. Olivarius B, Roder E: Reversible psychosis and dementia in myxedema. *Acta Psychiatr Scand* 46:1–13, 1970.

59. Thomas RB, Mazzaterri EL, Skillman TG: Apathetic thyrotoxicosis: a distinctive clinical and laboratory entity. *Ann Int Med* 72:679–685, 1970.

60. Spillane JP: Nervous and mental disorders in Cushing's syndrome. *Brain* 74:72–94, 1951.

61. Glaser GH: Psychotic reactions induced by corticotropin (ACTH) and cortisone. *Psychosom Med* 15:280–291, 1953.

62. Raskin NH, Fishman RA: Neurologic disorders in renal failure. *N Engl J Med* 294:143–148, 204–210, 1976.

62. Thompson TL II, Moran MG, Nies AS: Psychotropic drug use in the elderly. *N Engl J Med* 308:134–138, 1983.

63. Terry RD, Davies P: Dementia of the Alzheimer's type. *Ann Rev Neurosci* 3:77–95, 1980.

64. Tomlinson BE, Blessed G, Roth M: Observations on the brains of non-demented old people. *J Neurol Sci* 7:331–356, 1968.

65. Appel SH: Alzheimer's disease and dementia. *Neurology Clinics* 4:3–11, 1982.

66. Jacobs L, Gossman MD: Three primitive reflexes in normal adults. *Neurology* 30:184–188, 1980.

67. Hirano A, Dembitzer HM, Kurland LT, Zimmerman HM: The fine structure of some intraganglionic alterations. *J Neuropath Exp Neurol* 26:167–182, 1968.

68. Bower DM, Smith CB, White P, Davison AN: Neurotransmitter-related enzymes and indices of hypoxia in senile dementia and other abiotrophies. *Brain* 99:459–495, 1976.

69. Davies P, Maloney AJR: Selective loss of central cholinergic neurons in Alzheimer's disease. *Lancet* 2:1403, 1976.

70. Perry EK, Perry RH, Blessed G, et al: Neurotransmitter enzyme abnormalities in senile dementia. *J Neurol Sci* 34:247–265, 1977.

71. Perry EK, Tomlinson BE, Blessed G, et al: Correlation of cholinergic abnormalities with senile plaques and mental test scores in senile dementia. *Br Med J* 2:1457–1459, 1978.

72. Price DL, Whitehouse PJ, Struble RG, et al: Ba-

sal forebrain cholinergic systems in Alzheimer's disease and related dementia. *Neurosci Commentaries* 1:84–92, 1982.

73. Etienne P, Daston D, Gauthier S, et al: Alzheimer disease: Lack of effect of lecithin treatment for 3 months. *Neurology* 31:1552–1554, 1981.

74. Earnest MP, Heaton RK, Wilkinson WE, et al: Cortical atrophy, ventricular enlargement and intellectual impairment in the aged. *Neurology* 29:1138–1143, 1979.

75. Hutton JT: Clinical nosology of the dementing illness, in Maletta GJ, Pirozzolo FJ (ed): *The Ageing Nervous System*. New York, Praeger, 1980, pp 149–174.

76. Pirozzolo F: Neuropsychological assessment of dementia. *Neurology Clinics* 4:12–18, 1982.

77. Smith JS, Kiloh LG: The investigation of dementia: Results in 200 consecutive admissions. *Lancet* 1:824–827, 1981.

CHAPTER 5

Abnormalities of Posture and Movement

John G. Nutt, M.D.

Posture and Gait

Alterations of posture and gait commonly accompany aging and are indicators of the health and biologic age of an individual. They may also be disabling, by decreasing confidence, restricting mobility, and causing injuries. Posture and gait may be compromised by cardiovascular, arthritic, and orthopedic disorders, but most commonly are impaired by neurologic disease. The neurologic disturbances producing posture and gait abnormalities can be categorized under three headings: 1) Afferent or sensory dysfunction; 2) Efferent or motor dysfunction; and 3) Central or integrative dysfunction.

Humans depend primarily on three sensory modalities for orienting themselves in space: proprioceptive, vestibular, and visual. The sensory input is redundant, and posture and gait are generally normal in the absence of one or even two of the sensory modalities. However, if all are compromised, or there is erroneous or conflicting input (such as in acute vestibular disease or the initial use of bifocals), postural and gait disturbances may result. The more common sensory causes of postural difficulties, the accompanying signs, and the characteristic gaits are summarized in Table 5-1.

Disturbances in the efferent or motor system are manifest by weakness and alterations in muscle tone. Primary muscle disease (dystrophy, myopathy, or myositis) affects proximal muscle symmetrically. Weakness of the muscles of the pelvic girdle produces exaggerated lumbar lordosis, waddling gait, and particular difficulties in rising from chairs and negotiating stairs. Motor neuropathies commonly affect distal musculature, but they may also involve proximal muscles (most dramatically seen in the diabetic amyotrophy or radiculoplexopathy). Both muscle and peripheral nerve disorders are associated with normal or decreased muscle tone. Weakness on the basis of corticospinal tract damage is associated with hyperactive reflexes, Babinski signs, and increased ("spastic") tone. The salient features of these motor abnormalities and the associated gait disturbances are summarized in Table 5-2.

The central integration of sensory input and motor output for postural responses and ambulation uses the cerebral hemispheres, basal ganglia, cerebellum, and vestibular nuclei. Diseases affecting these structures may produce characteristic postural and gait disturbances, as well as involuntary movements, alterations in muscle tone, and disruption of voluntary and automatic motor acts. In addition, there are gait abnormalities in elderly persons, often termed senile gaits, that cannot be explained by either "peripheral" abnormalities or any of the classic "central" gait disorders. "Central" gait disorders are summarized in Table 5-3. Spastic, ataxic, and senile gaits are considered below; parkinsonian, marche de petits pas, and apractic gaits are discussed in the section on parkinsonism.

Spastic Gaits

The hemiparetic gait with unilateral spasticity is easily recognized: the circumduction of the leg, reduced arm swing, flexed posture of the arm,

TABLE 5-1   Sensory Abnormalities Producing Postural and Gait Disturbances

Modality	Lesion	Signs	Gait
Proprioceptive	Peripheral nerves	Loss of position sensation, stocking glove sensory loss, decreased or absent DTRs,* positive Romberg sign	Ataxic
	Spinal posterior columns	Loss of position sensation other signs of spinal cord dysfunction	Ataxic
Vestibular	Peripheral: labyrinth and vestibular nerve	Nystagmus, hearing deficits, past pointing	Weaving "drunken"
	Central: vestibular nuclei and pathways	Nystagmus, past pointing, cerebellar and other cranial nerve signs	Weaving or ataxic
Visual	Lens, vitreous, retina, extraocular muscles	↓Visual acuity, diplopia, or deficient downgaze	Tentative, uncertain

* DTRs = deep tendon reflexes.

TABLE 5-2   Motor Abnormalities Producing Postural and Gait Disturbances

Lesion	Signs	Gait
Muscle	Proximal weakness, normal DTRs*	Waddling
Distal motor nerve	Distal weakness, decreased DTRs	Slapping, foot drop, steppage
Proximal motor nerve or roots	Patchy weakness, proximal and distal	Waddling and/or slapping
Corticospinal tracts	Distal > proximal weakness, increased DTRs, increased tone, Babinski sign	Circumduction, "spastic"

* DTRs = deep tendon reflexes.

TABLE 5-3   Central or Integrative Dysfunction Producing Postural and Gait Disturbances

Lesion	Signs	Gait
Corticospinal tracts	Weakness, increased DTRs,* and tone	"Spastic," stiff legged, circumduction
Frontal lobes	Dementia, perseveration, hand and foot grasp reflexes	"Apractic"
Deep white and grey matter	Corticospinal tract signs, pseudobulbar palsy, history of "strokes"	Marche de petits pas
Basal ganglia	Tremor, rigidity, bradykinesia	Parkinsonian
	Choreic movements of face, trunk, limbs	Dancing or choreic
Cerebellum	Limb dysmetria, intention tremor	Ataxic
Multiple central and peripheral sites	Absence of other significant central or peripheral disturbances to explain gait disorder	"Senile"

* DTRs = deep tendon reflexes.

and extended leg are very characteristic. On examination, the presence of the ipsilateral weakness, hyper-reflexia, and hypertonus confirms the diagnosis. Hemiparkinsonism can produce diagnostic confusion if not accompanied by tremor, because parkinsonism commonly starts with unilateral hypertonus, absent arm swing, and foot drag. Reflexes may even be brisker on the affected side. Hemiparkinsonism can be differentiated from hemiparesis by a careful evaluation of tone (plastic rigidity versus the velocity-sensitive spastic "catch") and the presence of other subtle parkinsonian signs (masked facies, soft voice, and mild contralateral rigidity).[1]

Paraparesis with spasticity produces a gait characterized by: 1) Bilateral circumduction; 2) Short steps; 3) Narrow base; and if severe, 4) Scissoring. The bilaterally brisk reflexes, Babinski signs, and hypertonus are diagnostic. A coexisting, mild peripheral neuropathy may dampen ankle jerks and mislead the clinician.

Spasticity is caused by chronic metabolic, degenerative, and structural lesions disrupting the corticospinal tracts anywhere from the cortex to the spinal cord. If the etiology is not historically obvious, this problem is best evaluated in conjunction with a neurologic consultant.

Therapeutic efforts should be directed to bracing, ambulation aids, and gait training. Antispasticity agents such as baclofen, diazepam, and dantrolone sodium generally produce weakness and disequilibrium at doses that reduce spasticity and, consequently, are of little assistance in the potentially ambulatory patient; however, they may be worthwhile in patients confined to wheelchairs and bed.

Ataxic Gait

Cerebellar ataxia is characterized by a wide-based stance and irregularity of the amplitude and timing of steps, particularly on turns. An unsteady, weaving gait without a wide base may be seen with acute vestibular lesions (peripheral or central), midline cerebellar lesions, and sedative-hypnotic intoxication. It is important to recognize that gait ataxia need not be accompanied by abnormalities of other coordination tests, such as the finger-to-nose or heel-to-shin tests.

Treatable etiologies of ataxia among the geri-

atric population include thiamine or Vitamin B-12 deficiency, hypothyroidism, sedative-hypnotic intoxication, and the Arnold Chiari malformation.[2] Other than the recognition of these remediable entities, treatment consists of insuring safe living quarters and providing for mobility with a walker or wheelchair.

Senile Gaits

"Senile" gait is not a diagnosis but a label for the unsteady gait of older persons that cannot be attributed to orthopedic causes or the other neurologic causes detailed in Tables 5-1, 5-2, and 5-3. Most commonly, this takes the form of a shortened stride and "en bloc" turning. These changes may be non-specific, for they can be observed in younger individuals who are uncertain of their footing (e.g., when walking in the dark). A second form of "senile gait" is the insecure gait; which is an unwillingness to walk without the assistance of another person, the gait appearing relatively normal when the patient is assisted. Finally, difficulty initiating gait, short shuffling steps, and unsteady turns, features that might suggest parkinsonism, marche de petits pas, or gait apraxia, are observed in patients who have none of the other stigmata of the disorders associated with these gait disturbances.

There are several hypotheses to explain "senile" gaits. One is that the commonly observed loss of ankle tendon reflexes and the diminished vibratory sensation represent a mild peripheral neuropathy producing the gait disturbance.[3] As this degree of peripheral neuropathy does not cause a significant gait disruption in younger individuals, it is unlikely that this is the sole cause of senile gait.

A second hypothesis attributes senile gait to normal pressure hydrocephalus.[4] The evidence supporting this is an increased ventricular span on computed tomography (CT scan) compared to a geriatric population with no gait disturbance and an improvement in gait following removal of cerebrospinal fluid (CSF) by lumbar puncture. However, the criteria for making a diagnosis of normal pressure hydrocephalus remains problematic and, in most clinicians' experience, normal pressure hydrocephalus is an uncommon cause of gait disturbance. Furthermore, ventricular shunting for normal pressure hydrocephalus is associated with significant morbidity and mortality.[5,6]

A third hypothesis is that multiple, minor neurologic deficits result in the gait and postural instability. There is a progressive loss of Betz cells, purkinje cells, dopaminergic neurons, and spinal motor neurons with aging.[1] Furthermore, there are age-related alterations in sensation,[7] motor power,[7] monosynaptic reflexes,[7] vestibular reflexes,[8] and control of body sway.[9] No single abnormality is sufficient to destabilize posture and gait, but the combination of all these minor deficits may do so.

Pharmacologic intervention is of no benefit and is often detrimental in these patients. Antiparkinsonian agents do not help, and sedatives, antivertiginous drugs, and, occasionally, antihypertensives exacerbate their imbalance. Treatment of contributing musculoskeletal disorders is worthwhile.[10] Gait training is of limited benefit; however, teaching the patient to make wide turns and to use caution in confined spaces such as closets and bathrooms may avoid falls. The living quarters should be evaluated for loose rugs, obstructions, handrails, and lighting to minimize accidents.

Parkinsonism

Epidemiology

Parkinson's disease is exceedingly common in the geriatric population; estimates are that 1 in 100 individuals over the age of 50 are parkinsonian.[11] The peak incidence occurs in the 7th decade, and the majority of reported cases have their onset between 45–75 years of age. The sexes are affected equally.

Pathology

Parkinsonism is caused by a disruption of dopaminergic neurotransmission. Processes that destroy the pigmented dopaminergic neurons of the substantia nigra, disrupt the synthesis, storage, and release of dopamine, alter the postsynaptic dopamine receptors, or damage the postsynaptic striatal neurons can produce clinical parkinsonism. The most common form of parkinsonism in the geriatric population is idiopathic Parkinson's disease, which is character-ized by the loss of pigmented neurons in the substantia nigra and locus coeruleus. Eosinophilic inclusion bodies, termed Lewey bodies, are present in the remaining pigmented neurons of these structures, as well as in neurons of the nucleus basalis, the dorsal nucleus of the vagus, and the autonomic ganglia.[12] The loss of cortical and nucleus basalis neurons, and the presence of neurofibrillary tangles in cortical neurons in demented parkinsonian patients, raises a question of the relationship between Alzheimer's disease and Parkinson's disease.[13,14]

Clinical Features

Four groups of signs characterize parkinsonism. The first is tremor. Classically a 4–6 Hz tremor is present when the limb is supported or suspended (i.e., arm resting in lap or hanging by the side), and is abolished by complete relaxation (such as during sleep) or by voluntary movement of the limb. The tremor generally begins insidiously in one hand, then spreads to the ipsilateral foot, subsequently to the contralateral limbs, and perhaps to the tongue and jaw. In addition to the resting tremor, many patients have a faster 6–9 Hz action tremor. The presence of tremor is neither sufficient nor required for a diagnosis of parkinsonism. The diagnosis of parkinsonism in patients with tremor alone, and no bradykinesia or rigidity, is hazardous and generally reflects a confusion with essential tremor. Conversely, although it is a common presenting sign, tremor may never develop in the course of Parkinson's disease.

The second cardinal feature of parkinsonism is rigidity. The rigidity is "plastic" or "lead pipe" and is perceived as a constant or ratchety (cogwheeling) resistance to passive movement of a joint. Rigidity is often detected first in the nuchal musculature. All muscles may eventually be affected, but the distribution of rigidity need not be symmetrical. Rigidity must be differentiated from spasticity and gegenhalten (paratonia). In spasticity, the resistance to passive joint movement tends to be greater the faster the limb is moved and to increase initially, and then melt away. In "gegenhalten" or "paratonia," there is a variable resistance because the patient cannot relax the limb and moves it either against or with the examiner. The later tone abnormality is common in dementing illnesses. Although it is teleologically attractive to attribute many of the bradykinetic and postural parkinsonian features to the rigidity, there is a poor correlation between the severity of rigidity and other parkinsonian signs.

The third feature is bradykinesia, which encompasses the slowness of voluntary movements and the loss of automatic or associated movements. Voluntary movements may be visibly slowed. Repetitive dextrous movements become irregular in tempo and amplitude, leading to scratchy, small handwriting (micrographia), difficulty with hand tools (especially screwdrivers) and eating utensils, and problems with dressing and grooming. The blink rate is decreased, facial expression is fixed, and the voice is soft and monotonous. Speech, however, is sometimes hurried—a festination of sound production that is reminiscent of the festinating gait. A reduced frequency of unconscious swallowing is responsible for drooling. The normal fidgety movements, readjustments of sitting or standing posture, crossing and uncrossing of the legs while sitting, and the arm swing while walking are reduced or absent.

The final feature is static and kinetic postural abnormalities. Characteristically, the parkinsonian patient assumes a flexed posture (simian posture) with flexion of the knees, trunk, elbows, wrists, and metacarpal-phalangeal joints. Fixed spinal deformities (scoliosis) may develop. When standing or sitting, the trunk may unconsciously drift to the side or back. Inadequate defensive postural responses to perturbations of equilibrium lead to propulsion, retropulsion, and falls.

The mental status of parkinsonian patients is classically thought to be normal. James Parkinson, in the original description of "paralysis agitans" stated that "the senses are left intact." However, it has become increasingly clear that dementia is more common in patients with parkinsonism than in an age-matched control group.[15] An anatomic basis for this is suggested by the recent observations of cortical and nucleus basalis cell loss, senile plaques, tangles, and granulovacuolar degeneration suggesting a relationship to Alzheimer's disease.[13,14]

The dementia associated with parkinsonism does not have unique features that allow a clear separation from other dementias, although focal deficits (aphasia, agonosia, and apraxias) occur less frequently than in Alzheimer's disease. It is important not to confuse the slow responses and dysarthria that are common in parkinsonism with true dementia. In addition to the functional difficulties produced by dementia, drug therapy is often complicated by the condition; many of the antiparkinsonian medications increase confusion and precipitate hallucinations or frank psychosis in these patients.

Differential Diagnosis

The clinician is faced with two diagnostic branch points in evaluating a hypokinetic motor disorder. First, does the patient have parkinsonism at all? Disorders that may superficially resemble parkinsonism include hypothyroidism and depression with psychomotor retardation. Disorders that are more difficult to separate from parkinsonism are the "marche de petits pas" of the hypertensive lacunar state[16] and the gait apraxia of frontal lobe disease[17] and normal pressure hydrocephalus.[18] The marche de petits pas is a narrow-based shuffling gait accompanied by postural imbalance. Other features of parkinsonism (tremor, bradykinesia) are generally absent, and other evidence of vascular disease (history of "small strokes," pseudobulbar palsy, and corticospinal tract signs) is present. Gait apraxia is characterized by a difficulty with gait initiation, a narrow or wide-based gait with short sliding steps, and a prominent foot grasp (tonic foot response). This form of gait disturbance is accompanied by perseveration in motor acts, grasp reflexes, and dementia. It has been associated with frontal lobe disease and normal pressure hydrocephalus. The gait disturbance of parkinsonism, marche de petits pas, and gait apraxia are often indistinguishable clinically and are only differentiated by associated signs. Essential tremor, discussed later in this chapter, must also be differentiated from parkinsonism.

Secondly, if the patient does have parkinsonism, is it the common, idiopathic form of the syndrome, is it secondary to an identifiable cause, or is it part of another neurologic entity? Table 5-4 summarizes some of the secondary causes of parkinsonism and Table 5-5 the system degenerations that may have parkinsonism as a major component of the clinical picture.

TABLE 5-4 Secondary Parkinsonism

Etiology	Features Differentiating from IPD*
Neuroleptics	History of neuroleptic usage
Reserpine	History of reserpine usage
Encephalitis[19]	History, pupillary and extraocular abnormalities, oculogyric crises, other neurologic signs
Head trauma	History, other neurologic signs
Carbon monoxide poisoning	History, dementia

* IPD = idiopathic Parkinson's disease.

The differentiation between the various parkinsonian syndromes is important; only idiopathic Parkinson's disease responds reliably to L-Dopa. In other forms of parkinsonism, L-Dopa is less beneficial and commonly produces confusion, hallucinations, or psychosis without benefiting the parkinsonism. Parkinsonism secondary to neuroleptic drugs is reversible (over days to months) following withdrawal of the offending drug.

Despite the many etiologies of parkinsonism, the idiopathic form is by far the most common. The practiced geriatrician can confidently make this diagnosis based on the individual's history and examination. If the history or examination suggest another etiology or a more widespread neurologic dysfunction, then a neurologic consultation should be obtained.

Treatment of Parkinsonism

The therapy for Parkinson's disease may be considered under three headings: Who? When? What?

Who

Approximately 85% of idiopathic Parkinson's disease patients will respond, to some extent, to L-Dopa or to L-Dopa + carbidopa (Sinemet). The response is generally minimal in other parkinsonian syndromes; these patients often experience adverse psychiatric effects with this drug. It may still be elected to try L-Dopa in these patients, but it should be done cautiously with the drug being withdrawn if no obvious benefit accrues.

When

The efficacy of L-Dopa wanes with continued therapy. Psychiatric side effects and a fluctuating response to the drug ("on-off phenomenon") commonly develop with prolonged use and may limit the usefulness of the drug.[23] There is a concern that the drug itself may be responsible for these problems. Therefore, many neurologists choose to wait until the parkinsonian symptoms become a significant hindrance to the patient's life style before initiating L-Dopa therapy.[24]

What

The secondary or subsidiary antiparkinsonian agents (anticholinergics, amantadine, and di-

TABLE 5-5 Neurologic Syndromes in Which Parkinsonism May be a Prominent Feature

Disorder	Features Differentiating
Multiple System Atrophy[20] (Shy-Drager, olivopontocerebellar degeneration, striato-nigral degeneration)	Autonomic dysfunction (particularly orthostatic hypotension) corticospinal and cerebellar signs
Progressive supranuclear palsy[21]	Paresis of voluntary vertical gaze (particularly downgaze), marked postural instability with relatively preserved locomotion
Alzheimer's disease[22]	Early and prominent dementia preceding motor abnormalities, other focal cortical signs
Creutzfeldt-Jacob disease	Rapidly progressing illness with dementia, cerebellar signs, upper and lower motor neuron signs, and myoclonus
Rigid Huntington's disease	Family history of Huntington's disease

phenhydramine) offer mild to moderate relief of parkinsonian symptomatology and are often employed as the initial or adjunct therapy. All these drugs have anticholinergic actions, and they are particularly useful in patients with sialorrhea or tremor. However, the anticholinergic side effects must be carefully considered in a geriatric population, because the drugs may exacerbate angle closure glaucoma, cause urinary retention in patients with prostatic hypertrophy, aggravate constipation, and produce psychiatric and cognitive difficulties. If some preparation of L-Dopa is added later, it is worthwhile to try to discontinue anticholinergics, as their combination with L-Dopa is generally no more effective than L-Dopa alone; also, the side effects of the anticholinergics may be avoided. Abrupt cessation of anticholinergics will, sometimes, markedly exacerbate parkinsonism and, therefore, these drugs should be gradually withdrawn.

L-Dopa is generally prescribed in combination with the peripheral decarboxylase inhibitor carbidopa (the combination is marketed as Sinemet—with carbidopa to L-Dopa ratios of 10 : 100 mg, 25 : 100 mg, and 25 : 250 mg) to lessen the peripheral side effects of L-Dopa, nausea and cardiac arrhythmias. The drug is best started at low doses (one-half or one 25 : 100 mg tablets three times per day), and then slowly increased over the ensuing weeks to a dose giving a satisfactory response without side effects (usually in the range of 600–1,500 mg of L-Dopa administered daily in 3–6 doses). The most common causes for apparent therapeutic failure are: 1) Rapid increase in drug dosage leading to unacceptable nausea or other side effects; 2) Failure to increase the dose until a benefit accrues or side effects prohibit further increases; 3) Therapeutic response judged from effects on tremor, the symptom most resistant to L-Dopa; and 4) The patient does not have idiopathic parkinsonism.

The clinical experience with dopamine agonists such as bromocriptine and pergolide is encouraging. At this time, however, they are not first-line antiparkinsonian drugs, and they are reserved for patients whose response to L-Dopa is limited by rapid swings between being underdosed and overdosed ("on-off" and "wearing off phenomena") and/or by dyskinesia. Orthostatic hypotension and psychiatric side effects can be prominent with dopamine agonists. They should be used with caution in patients with postural hypotension, dementia, or psychiatric illness.

Abnormal Involuntary Movements

Tremor

Tremor is categorized by the activity that maximizes the tremor. A rest tremor is that tremor most evident when the limb is inactive, lying in the lap, or hanging at the side. A postural or action tremor is most evident when an antigravity posture is being maintained, often most dramatically as the patient holds a tea cup. Kinetic or intention tremor is a rhythmic movement present in a limb as it approaches a goal, and it is characteristic of cerebellar dysfunction.

The majority of tremor occurring in the geriatric population is due to three entities: parkinsonism, benign essential tremor, and metabolic tremor.

Parkinsonian rest tremor is considered above. Mention has been made of the fact that these patients may have a postural tremor alone or in combination with a rest tremor.

Benign essential tremor is primarily a postural tremor, but it may also be present at rest and with intention. Onset occurs from early adulthood to senescence. It commonly affects the upper extremities, head, voice, and only rarely the legs. The amplitude may vary from barely noticeable to very wide. The tremor is aggravated by emotional tension and fatigue. A family history of tremor is generally obtained. A most characteristic feature is the amelioration of the tremor by alcohol; a fact that most patients discover for themselves and sometimes employ therapeutically. The neurologic examination is unremarkable except for the tremor and, specifically, there is no rigidity or other evidence of parkinsonism and no evidence of cerebellar disease. The handwriting is large and irregular (tremorous), rather than small as in parkinsonism.[25]

Propranolol in doses of 20–320 mg/day is the drug of choice for this disorder. It reduces the amplitude, but does not abolish the tremor.[26] The drug must be given with caution in patients with congestive heart failure, asthma, and insu-

TABLE 5-6 Common Metabolic and Toxic Causes of Tremor

Hyperthyroidism
Uremia
Liver failure
Alcohol withdrawal
Lithium
Tricyclic antidepressants
Caffeine, theophyline
Isoproterenol
Sodium valproate

lin-dependent diabetes. The selective β_1 antagonists have been used successfully to treat tremor in patients with bronchospasm. Other mild sedatives, such as phenobarbital and diazepam, also may be used to advantage.

A variety of toxic and metabolic insults accentuate the normal physiologic tremor to produce an irregular postural tremor, which may be associated with asterixis (*see* Table 5-6).

Choreoathetosis

Choreiform movements are "spontaneous" or "involuntary" brief muscle contractions (jerks) that produce simple movements, such as flexion or extension of a finger, and/or complex semi-purposeful movements, such as raising the hand to the face. These choreatic movements may occur when the limb is at rest or may be superimposed on voluntary movements. Facial, respiratory, truncal, and limb muscles may be involved. The temporal and spatial pattern is generally irregular; this differentiates the movements from tics, which are stereotyped. Athetosis is similar to chorea except that the movements are slower and often blend one into another, which leads to a sinuous or writhing quality rather than the jerky movements of chorea. The distinction between the two is often difficult and has no pathologic significance.

The more common etiologies of choreoathetosis are listed in Table 5-7. The disorder most frequently encountered by the geriatrician is tardive dyskinesia. Meige syndrome, described below, is often confused with tardive dyskinesia.

Myoclonus

Myoclonic movements are exceedingly brief, shock-like contractions of muscle that may lead to almost undetectable movement or produce large excursions of the limb or trunk. They are

TABLE 5-7 Choreoathetosis in the Geriatric Population

Etiology	Features
Drug induced	
Neuroleptics	History of drug use, predomi-
Reserpine	nantly affects face, lips, and
L-Dopa	tongue
Other psychoactive drugs	
Metabolic	
Hyperthyroidism	Abnormal thyroid function tests
Hypocalcemia	Low serum calcium
Miscellaneous	Abnormal liver function tests
Vascular	
Subthalamic or perisubthalamic stroke	Sudden onset of hemichorea or hemiballismus
Vasculitis	ANA,* elevated ESR,† angio-
Polycythemia	graphic evidence of vasculitis RBC‡ mass
Infectious	
Encephalitis (acute and as a sequelae)	CSF§ pleocytosis (acute phase)
Creutzfeldt-Jacob disease	Dementia, other neurologic signs

* ANA = positive antinuclear antibody; † ESR = erythrocyte sedimentation rate; ‡ RBC = red blood cell; § CSF = cerebrospinal fluid.

TABLE 5-8   Etiology of Myoclonus

Metabolic
    Hypoxic encephalopathy
    Uremic encephalopathy
    Hepatic encephalopathy
    Other, including drug intoxication
Infectious
    Acute viral encephalitis
    Creutzfeldt-Jacob disease
Idiopathic seizure disorders
Benign
    Sleep jerks (nocturnal myoclonus)
    Hiccups

irregular in timing and distribution. Some forms are induced by touch, noise, or intentional movements. Myoclonic movements must be differentiated from tics (which are repetitive stereotyped movements), from chorea (which is less shock-like), from asterixis (which is caused by brief electromyogram [EMG] silence and loss of muscle tone), and from irregular tremor. Myoclonus may arise from disorders of the spinal cord, brainstem, and hemispheres; it is, thus, variably associated with cortical electroencephalogram (EEG) abnormalities. Myoclonus may be benign, as exemplified by the "sleep jerks" that most people experience as they fall asleep or by hiccups. However, myoclonus is often an accompaniment of idiopathic epilepsy, central nervous system infections, Creutzfeldt-Jacob disease, and metabolic disorders, particularly hypoxic encephalopathy[27] (*see* Table 5-8).

Dystonia

Dystonic movements are characterized by slow, protracted muscle contractions that produce abnormal postures of limbs and axial structures. The dystonic contractures are often bizarre, are commonly exacerbated by emotion and stress, and may only appear during certain motor acts. These features commonly lead to the erroneous diagnosis of a functional or hysterical disorder. Another feature that confuses the diagnosis of dystonia is that many patients with dystonia will have a postural tremor or other "jerky" movements.

A classification of dystonia is presented in Table 5-9. Generalized dystonia is uncommon in the geriatric population; however, the focal dystonias occur in this age group, and Meige syndrome is almost exclusively an illness of elderly persons.

Meige syndrome is named after a French neurologist who described "midline spasms" manifest by a forceful, involuntary closure of the lids (blepharospasm), involuntary opening of the jaw, and tongue protrusion. A variety of other manifestations are now recognized including retraction of the corners of the mouth, contraction of the platysma, jaw clenching, lip pursing and torticollis. Any of these movements may be the only manifestation of the syndrome and, particularly, blepharospasm is often a solitary sign. Meige syndrome is only of cosmetic importance to many patients, but in some the blepharospasm sufficiently interferes with vision to prevent driving, reading, or watching TV. The oromandibular involvement may

TABLE 5-9   Dystonia

Etiology	Features
Generalized Torsion dystonia (dystonia musculorum deformans)	Widespread axial and limb musculature involvement
Focal —Meige blepharospasm oromandibular dystonia	See text
—spasmodic dysphonia[31]	Strained, forced voice
—torticollis[32]	Involuntary rotation, flexion, or extension of neck
—writer's cramp[33] and writer's tremor	Appearance of a dystonic posture or tremor with attempted writing

produce dysarthria and dysphagia.[28] The entity most commonly confused with Meige syndrome is tardive dyskinesia. The blepharospasm and prolonged jaw opening or tongue protrusion is not classic for tardive dyskinesia, but it certainly may occur in that disorder. The history of neuroleptic use, and the appearance of the movements while on neuroleptics or shortly after their withdrawal, is the sine qua non for tardive dyskinesia. Spontaneous oral and facial dyskinesias occur in elderly persons that do not appear to be part of Meige syndrome or related to neuroleptic use; but the frequency is controversial.[29]

The onset of Meige syndrome occurs commonly in the 6th and 7th decades, and females are more commonly affected than males. The course is, in general, slowly progressive with long periods of stability. Although other facial and cervical muscles may eventually become involved, it is distinctly rare for the dystonia to spread to the limbs or trunk.

Treatment is of limited efficacy. Some patients respond to anticholinergics, benzodiazepines, or neuroleptics.[28] Blepharospasm may be treated surgically by destruction of the fibers of the facial nerve that innervate the orbicularis oculi, but with resultant facial weakness.[30]

Tics

Tics are repetitive, stereotyped movements that generally involve the face, respiratory musculature (leading to snorts, grunts, and calls), neck, and shoulder. The movements can be voluntarily reproduced and, likewise, suppressed. The patient consciously experiences a need to make a movement. The nervous twitch of the periorbital musculature is the most common tic; this, as well as other tics, are often accepted as "mannerisms" and not brought to the physician's attention. Generally, tics are benign and not indicative of central nervous system disease, although they may be a sequelae of encephalitis. Geriatricians should be aware that Tourette's syndrome, characterized by multiple tics and involuntary vocalizations with onset in childhood,[34] continues through life and, thus, may be encountered in older age groups. A disorder that may be confused with tics and occurs almost exclusively in older age groups is

hemifacial spasm.[35] It is characterized by rapid clonic contractions of facial musculature, usually unilateral, that cannot be willfully suppressed, although they may be exacerbated by anxiety and fatigue. This disorder appears to result from a lesion about the facial nerve exit zone from the pons, and it may be produced by tumor, demyelination, or blood vessels impinging on the nerve. This may respond to tegretol or to surgical placement of a sponge between the nerve and any adjacent vessels.[36]

References

1. Gilbert GJ: A pseudohemiparetic form of Parkinson's disease. *Lancet* 2:442–443, 1976.
2. Friede RL, Roessmann V: Chronic tonsilar herniation. *Acta Neuropath* 34:219–235, 1976.
3. Sabin TD: Biologic aspects of falls and mobility limitations in the elderly. *J Am Ger Soc* 30:51–58, 1982.
4. Fisher CM: Hydrocephalus as a cause of disturbances of gait in the elderly. *Neurology* 32:1358–1363, 1982.
5. Hughes CP, Siegel BA, Coxe WS, et al: Adult idiopathic communicating hydrocephalus with and without shunting. *J Neurol Neurosurg Psychiat* 41:961–971, 1978.
6. Black PM: Idiopathic normal-pressure hydrocephalus: Results of shunting in 62 patients. *J Neurosurg* 52: 371–377, 1980.
7. Jenkyn LR, Reeves AG: Neurologic signs in uncomplicated aging (senescence). *Sem Neurol* 1:21–30, 1981.
8. Woollacott MH, Shumway-Cook A, Nashner L: Postural reflexes and aging, in Mortimer LA, Pirozzolo G, Maletta F: (eds): *The Aging Motor System*. New York, Praeger, 1982, pp 98–119.
9. Sheldon JH: The effect of age on the control of sway. *Geront Clin* 5:129–138, 1963.
10. Steinberg FU: Gait disorders in old age. *Geriatrics* 134–143, March 1966.
11. Kurland LT: Epidemiology: Incidence, geographic distribution and genetic considerations, in Fields WS (ed): *Pathogenesis and Treatment of Parkinsonism*. Springfield, Ill, Charles C Thomas, Publisher, 1958, pp 5–49.
12. Alvord EC: The pathology of parkinsonism, in Minekler J (ed): *Pathology of the Nervous System*. New York, McGraw-Hill Book Co, 1968, pp 1152–1161.
13. Boller F, Mizutani T, Roessman U, et al: Parkinson disease dementia and Alzheimer disease: Clinicopathological correlations. *Ann Neurol* 7:329–335, 1980.

14. Hakim AM, Mathieson G: Dementia in Parkinson disease: A neuropathologic study. *Neurology* 29:1209–1214, 1979.

15. Loranger AW, Goodel H, McDowell FH: Intellectual impairment in Parkinson's syndrome. *Brain* 95:405–412, 1972.

16. Critchley M: Arteriosclerotic parkinsonism. *Brain* 52:23–83, 1929.

17. Meyer JS, Barron DW: Apraxia of gait: A clinico-physiological study. *Brain* 83:261–284, 1960.

18. Estanol BV: Gait apraxia in communicating hydrocephalus. *J Neurol Neurosurg Psychiat* 44:305–308, 1981.

19. Rail D, Scholtz C, Swash M: Post-encephalatic parkinsonism: Current experience. *J Neurol Neurosurg Psychiat* 44:670–676, 1981.

20. Bannister R, Oppenheimer DR: Degenerative diseases of the nervous system associated with autonomic failure. *Brain* 95:457–474, 1972.

21. Steele JC: Progressive supranuclear palsy. *Brain* 95:693–704, 1972.

22. Pearce J: The extrapyramidal disorder of Alzheimer's disease. *Europ Neurol* 12:94–103, 1974.

23. Marsden CD, Parkes JD: Success and problems of long-term levodopa therapy in Parkinson's disease. *Lancet* 1:345–349, 1977.

24. Fahn S, Calne DB: Considerations in the management of parkinsonism. *Neurology* 28:5–7, 1978.

25. Critchley E: Clinical manifestations of essential tremor. *J Neurol Neurosurg Psychiat* 35:365–372, 1972.

26. Winkler GF, Young RR: Efficacy of chronic propranolol therapy in action tremors of the familial, senile or essential varieties. *N Engl J Med* 290:984–988, 1974.

27. Swanson PD, Luttrell CN, Magladery JW: Myoclonus—A report of 67 cases and a review of the literature. *Medicine* 41:339–356, 1962.

28. Marsden CD: Blepharospasm-oromandibular dystonia syndrome (Brueghel's syndrome). *J Neurol Neurosurg Psychiat* 39:1204–1209, 1976.

29. Kane JM, Weinhold P, Kinon B, et al: Prevalence of abnormal involuntary movements ("spontaneous dyskinesias") in the normal elderly. *Psychopharmacology* 77:105–108, 1982.

30. Frueh BR, Callahan A, Dortzbach RK, et al: The effects of differential section of the seventh nerve on patients with intractable blepharospasm. *Trans Am Acad Ophth Otolaryngol* 81:595–602, 1976.

31. Aminoff MJ, Dedo HH, Izdebski K: Clinical aspects of spasmodic dysphonia. *J Neurol Neurosurg Psychiat* 41:361–365, 1978.

32. Patterson RM, Little SC: Spasmodic torticollis. *J Nerv Ment Dis* 98:571–599, 1943.

33. Sheehy MP, Marsden CD: Writers' cramp—A focal dystonia. *Brain* 105:461–480, 1982.

34. Shapiro AK, Shapiro E, Wayne HL: The symptomatology and diagnosis of Gilles de la Tourette's syndrome. *J Am Acad Child Psychiat* 12:702–723, 1973.

35. Ehni G, Wollman HW: Hemifacial spasm. *Arch Neurol Psychiat* 53:205–211, 1945.

36. Jannetta PJ, Abbasy M, Maroon JC, et al: Etiology and definitive microsurgical treatment of hemifacial spasm. *J Neurosurg* 47:321–328, 1977.

CHAPTER 6

Headache and Facial Pain

JOHN P. HAMMERSTAD, M.D.

Headache is one of the most common symptoms for which patients consult physicians. It is estimated that at least 80% of the population will suffer from headaches at some time in their lives, with severe headaches reported by 50% of females and 40% of males.[1] The prevalence of headache declines with age. In a survey in Wales, 66% of females and 53% of males at age 55 reported headaches, while 55% of females and 21% of males at age 75 reported headaches in the previous year.[2] Although the incidence of headache decreases beyond middle age, headaches due to cerebrovascular disease, cervical osteoarthritis, tumors, and giant cell arteritis are more frequent; headache remains a common problem for the geriatrician. Rupture of a saccular aneurysm declines with age, but other sources of intracranial hemorrhage, especially hypertensive hemorrhage, remain important. The geriatrician should keep these disorders in mind when faced with a complaint of headache in elderly persons.

General Approach to the History and Examination

The history and examination can be misleading in distinguishing a benign headache as a primary disorder from a headache as a symptom of a more serious disease requiring early recognition and treatment. A serious symptomatic headache may seem seductively benign early in its course; vigilance is paramount, although always difficult because of the overwhelming majority of benign headaches. A few headache patterns should always arouse suspicion and more careful scrutiny. Generally, in the geriatric population, benign headaches have been present many years. If it can be established that the headache is genuinely different from any experienced before, it deserves special attention. The same is true for a headache that may start out as a banal pain easily relieved by aspirin, but is steadily progressive in severity and frequency. The presence of other neurologic symptoms (e.g., unilateral hearing loss and tinnitus secondary to an acoustic schwannoma) or constitutional symptoms and signs (fever, malaise, weight loss, and so on) should launch a systematic evaluation. Although the majority are benign (90%), the "cough headache" induced by a valsalva maneuver (such as coughing, sneezing, or straining) or the positional headache (headache consistently produced by a particular position) may be associated with an intracranial neoplasm, subdural hematoma, Chiari malformation, or basilar impression.[3]

In addition to neurologic examination and vital signs (especially temperature and blood pressure), particular attention should be given to the cervical spine, carotid and superficial temporal arteries, temporomandibular joints, teeth, and ocular pressure. Laboratory evaluation is guided by the history and examination. However, in elderly persons it is a good practice to always include a complete blood count (CBC) and erythrocyte sedimentation rate (ESR) to screen for giant cell arteritis. The computed tomography (CT scan) has supplanted the routine skull x-ray film, but because of its expense and low yield when used as a routine screening device, it need not be obtained in a patient with a benign history and negative examination. A lumbar puncture is indicated when there is fever or other evidence of infection after a CT scan has excluded an intracranial abscess.

Benign Headache

In general, benign primary headaches are divided into muscle contraction (tension) and vascular categories. Clinically, there is a considerable overlap in the syndromes, which is reflected in the frequently used diagnosis of mixed tension-vascular headache. Contraction of the neck and occipital scalp muscles may occur with a migraine, and nausea may accompany a non-throbbing band-like tension headache. Also, recent evidence suggests that vascular factors may play a role in tension headache. Inhalation of amyl nitrite or intravenous (IV) infusion of histamine to produce vasodilatation not only invariably induces or exacerbates a headache in migrainous patients, but it also produces a headache in a significant proportion of tension headache patients when compared to control groups.[4,5] As yet, undefined neurovascular changes that occur with aging may account for the onset of typical tension headaches in an elderly patient who had no previous disposition.

Muscle Contraction Headache

Most of the population has experienced a headache in response to emotional stress, fatigue, and exposure to a variety of other noxious environmental factors. When it becomes a frequent, almost daily constant aching, tight pressure or band-like sensation, it is termed a chronic tension headache. A new onset of tension headache was uncommon in elderly persons who accounted for 3% of 466 patients given that diagnosis in an outpatient clinic.[6]

Special attention should be given to psychological factors. Headache is a common somatic complaint of depression. For less serious psychological disorders, counseling in conjunction with relaxation training is often beneficial. Electromyogram (EMG) recording with auditory feedback has become a popular form of relaxation therapy, but there is no evidence that it produces any specific benefit.[7] While psychotherapy is underway to remove the factors producing the tension, symptomatic relief usually can be obtained with heat, massage, and non-opiate analgesics. Benzodiazipines are generally not indicated because they may contribute to depression, and intoxication with these drugs is a greater risk for elderly persons due to their slower hepatic drug catabolism. Amitriptyline can be effective, independent of its antidepressant action.[8]

There is no foolproof way of distinguishing a muscle contraction headache secondary to stress and tension from that produced by cervical osteoarthritis and spondylosis, although the latter are more commonly occipital and associated with neck pain and stiffness and sometimes radiate into the fronto-temporal region. The presence of crepitus and radiographic changes of arthritis-spondylosis is no guarantee of a causal relationship. When suspected, however, it should be treated with a cervical collar, nonsteroidal antiflammatory agents, heat, and massage. Vigorous manipulation should be avoided, because it usually is ineffective and exposes the patient to a risk of a stroke by damaging the vertebral artery as it passes through the bony foramina of the cervical vertebrae. Response to traction is variable and should be abandoned if relief is not prompt or pain is exacerbated. Unless there is an associated occipital neuralgia with paresthesias, sectioning of the greater occipital nerve is of no value, because the pain arises in diseased upper cervical joints and is not due to a compression of upper cervical roots.[9]

Just as cervical disorders may cause pain referred to fronto-temporal regions, disorders of the cranial and facial structures may, on occasion, produce neck stiffness and occipital headache. Some examples are temporomandibular joint disease and glaucoma, though the local pain is generally more prominent and should draw attention to the affected structure.

Migraine

There is a widely held notion that migraine lessens in severity or ceases altogether with the passage of time, especially in postmenopausal females. As a general rule it is probably true;

but when this issue was specifically studied, the data gathered did not provide much comfort for the older migraineur. In this study, 9 of 18 patients (50%) over 64 years of age continued to have attacks; of 40 patients in whom menopause had occurred, only 4 had noted a definite improvement or cessation of the attacks.[10] There may be a change in character, however, which should not be construed as an ominous sign. The onset of migraine is unusual after age 50 and other vascular causes should be excluded.[11]

Migraine is classified according to the presence or absence of prodromal symptoms or aura and the presence of neurologic signs during the course of the headache (*see* Table 6-1). When there is a previous history of migraine or migraine equivalents (*see below*) starting earlier in life, even if there is a hiatus of several years one may accept them as a migraine. Also, attacks that may have ceased earlier in life may reappear in a modified form. This is the one instance in which a change in character of the headache is not necessarily a cause for concern. For example, aura or migraine accompaniments may change in character or appear for the first time in association with an otherwise typical vascular headache.

A transient, focal neurologic disturbance with inconspicuous or no headache at all is a well-recognized and accepted migrainous phenomenon and is termed migraine equivalent. The disturbances that occur are the same as those associated with classic and complicated migraine (i.e., scintillating scotomata and fortification spectra, homonymous hemianopia,

TABLE 6-1 Descriptive Classification of Migraine

Classic
Visual disturbance or focal neurologic symptoms precede headache 10–60 minutes and subsides as hemicranial headache builds.

Common
No aura, may be bilateral. Includes most premenstrual and facial migraine.

Migraine equivalent
Gradual onset and resolution of focal neurologic symptoms similar to a migrainous aura or prodrome, without any headache.

Complicated
Visual or neurologic deficit persists during the headache and sometimes well after the headache has subsided. This includes hemiplegic, ophthalmoplegic, and vertebrobasilar migraine.

aphasia, paresthesias, dysarthria, hemiplegia, and brainstem symptoms). These transient episodes are, in general, easily recognized as migraine equivalents in younger patients, but in older patients they may be differentiated from transient ischemic attacks (TIAs) with difficulty.

A case study of 120 persons over 40 years of age, with no prior history of migraine, who had transient episodes of neurologic symptoms compatible with migrainous accompaniments provide useful guidelines.[12] By appropriate studies and cerebral angiography, cerebral thrombosis, embolism and dissection, epilepsy, thrombocythemia, polycythemia, and thrombocytopenia were excluded. The most reliable symptom in excluding TIA is the scintillating scotoma or fortification spectra, which refers to the slowly enlarging scotoma surrounded by luminous angles or shimmering that slowly changes shape and moves across the visual field to the periphery. The build up of the scotoma over 5–30 minutes clearly distinguishes it from the transient scintillations of posterior, cerebral artery ischemia due to embolism or thrombosis. If the patient is observant, one usually can determine by alternately closing each eye that it is homonymous; thus retinal ischemia is excluded.

Another useful observation is the persistence of positive visual symptoms when the eyes are closed, which is consistent with a cerebral and not a retinal source of the symptoms. In other cases, there was a progression from one accompaniment to another. For example, visual symptoms may progress to paresthesias, then to dysphagia or brainstem symptoms, sometimes with an intervening delay of 5–30 minutes. This is not like TIAs, in which the several manifestations occur simultaneously. In some cases, the paresthesias occurred without visual phenomena. A reliable sign of migrainous paresthesias is the march of numbness that takes from 15–25 minutes, which is rare in stroke and much longer than the more rapid march of the focal sensory seizure.

Treatment
The choice of intermittent therapy for the acute attack, versus continuous therapy for prophylaxis against attacks, depends on the frequency, duration, and severity of the attacks and consequent disability. They are not mutually exclu-

sive, however. For example, ergotamine may be necessary for an occasional acute attack during continuous therapy with propranolol or amitriptyline. In general, a frequency of attacks greater than 2–3 times per month is an indication for prophylactic therapy. A less frequent attack rate may also necessitate prophylactic therapy if the attacks are especially severe or prolonged, or if the attacks lack an aura, are accompanied by early vomiting, or are full-blown upon awakening and, thus, prevent effective use of ergotamine.

Therapy for Acute Migraine
Ergotamine in its various formulations is still the most effective drug for aborting an acute attack. Because of delayed gastric emptying and intestinal absorption in migraine, parenteral or rectal administration is more effective than oral preparations. However, this is inconvenient for many persons whose activities prevent the use of suppositories. The sublingual form has a more rapid onset of action than the coated oral preparations and may be preferred by these individuals. There is a wide range of sensitivity to the centrally mediated emetic effect of ergotamine, and the dose should be individualized to find the effective subnauseating dose. Generally, 2–3 mg is required, and every effort should be made to give the maximum-tolerated dose immediately, since repeat doses are generally ineffective if the first has failed to abort the attack.

The use of ergotamine in the geriatric population has limitations because of its vasoconstrictive properties. It is best not to use it in patients with coronary artery, peripheral vascular, renal, or hepatic diseases. Hypertension is a relative but not absolute contraindication for its use.[13]

Interval Therapy
Several drugs may be effective in the prophylaxis of migraine. Amitriptyline (or other tricyclics with serotonergic activity) or propranolol are generally used initially, followed by trials of ergonovine, cyproheptadine, and finally methysergide, which is the most toxic of these drugs and should be used with great care in the geriatric patient. Ergonovine is a useful alternative to ergotamine, especially for interval therapy, because it produces less nausea and vaso-

constriction. The only definite contraindictions to its use are peripheral vascular disease and Prinzmetal's angina.[13]

Cluster Headache

The onset of cluster headache for the first time is unusual in the geriatric population (only about 10% of reported cases have onset above age 50).[14] However, it is important to distinguish this treatable headache from "sinus" headaches or more serious intracranial and vascular disorders. As the name implies, the headaches typically occur in clusters up to several times per day for weeks or months, with remissions of months to many years. A chronic variant without prolonged remissions occurs in about 15% of patients with cluster headache.[15] An even less common variant is distinguished by its frequency (5–20 headaches per day) and response to indomethacin; it is known as chronic paroxysmal hemicrania.[16]

Unlike a migraine, a cluster headache is invariably unilateral, centered about the eye, rapid in onset and offset, and generally lasts from 15 minutes to 2 hours. The pain is intense, boring or tearing in quality, non-throbbing, and unaccompanied by nausea and vomiting except in occasional cases. It is often, but not invariably, accompanied by local autonomic instability, such as conjunctival injection, lacrimation, and nasal stuffiness. In about 40–50% of subjects studied, the attacks occur with clock-like regularity, usually at night. Infrequently, the headaches switch sides from cluster to cluster, but rarely during a cluster.

Methysergide and ergotamine are the most effective drugs for treating periodic cluster headaches. Despite the drawbacks of their use in the geriatric patient, they can be most useful in the cluster headache that lasts a few weeks when prophylaxis for 3–4 weeks is followed by gradual withdrawal. If the headaches recur, the cycle is repeated. Ergotamine works best in the patient with the time-locked attack when the drug can be taken 30–60 minutes ahead of the anticipated headache. This seems to work particularly well with nocturnal attacks when a suppository can be taken at bedtime. In some patients, this strategy is unsuccessful because the attack is only delayed until the effect of the drug wears off. When ergotamine and methysergide fail, steroids may be effective in doses of 20–40 mg/day of prednisone. Inhalation of oxygen may be used to abort an acute attack. These agents should not be used in the chronic cluster headache patient. Lithium has been proven to be effective in more than 60% of subjects studied with chronic cluster headache, but it has not been as successful in episodic cluster headaches.[17] A trial of indomethacin is worthwhile in case it proves to be the chronic paroxysmal hemicrania variant. Amitriptyline, propranolol, and cyproheptadine are of no benefit.

Symptomatic Headache

Intracranial Neoplasm

The brain itself and much of the meninges are not pain sensitive. Headache from intracranial disorders arises from traction or displacement of proximal portions of the cerebral and dural arteries, the large veins, the dural sinuses. These pain-sensitive structures are innervated by the trigeminal nerve in the supratentorial compartment, and by the 9th and 10th cranial nerves and the upper three cervical nerves in the infratentorial compartment. Therefore, supratentorial tumors often produce frontal headaches, while posterior fossa tumors produce occipital headaches. When the headache is lateralized, it is often homolateral to the tumor. A headache is more likely to be the first symptom of a tumor located below the tentorium than of one above it. Unfortunately, most tumor headaches do not differ in intensity, location, or character from benign headaches. Features that should arouse suspicion include a headache that is definitely new or is different in character from previous headaches. Although the majority of headaches that awaken one from sleep are benign, these also should be viewed with greater concern, especially the morning headache associated with nausea and vomiting that improves as the day progresses. A cough or exertional headache is a severe transient pain that is often maximal at the vertex produced by coughing, sneezing, straining, bending, lifting, and so on. Usually, it is a benign headache although it may be associated with a neoplasm, especially in the posterior fossa. It has also been reported in association with Chiari malfor-

mation, basilar impression, and subdural hematoma.[3] One distinctive headache syndrome is commonly associated with a ventricular tumor, especially a colloid cyst of the third ventricle. This is a paroxysmal headache of sudden onset and severe intensity, often associated with a loss of consciousness, vomiting, or weakness of the legs ("drop attacks").

Subdural Hematoma

There is nothing distinctive about the headache associated with subdural hematoma. In fact, in some cases, the patient may not complain of a pain, but rather a heaviness or fullness in the head. Subdural hematoma should be suspected when there is an associated drowsiness or an acute to subacute decline in mentation. The offending traumatic event may be trivial and not even a direct blow to the head. Therefore, failure to elicit a history of trauma should not prevent consideration of a chronic subdural hematoma. Other neurologic symptoms and signs produced by the hematoma may be subtle, but when present they should lead to further investigation with a CT scan. There are occasional instances in the development of chronic, bilateral subdural hematomas when the hematoma is isodense with brain tissue and produces a "hypernormal" appearance or a CT scan (i.e., small ventricles and lack of a sulcal pattern expected for the age of the patient).

Giant Cell Arteritis

Giant cell arteritis (temporal or cranial arteritis) is a relatively common disorder of elderly persons. Over the age of 50, it has an estimated annual incidence of 17 per 100,000 persons and a prevalence of 130 per 100,000. The 20–30% incidence of permanent bilateral blindness in untreated patients underscores the importance of recognition and timely treatment with corticosteroids. Blindness is caused by an ischemic optic neuropathy as a result of inflammation of the ophthalmic and posterior ciliary arteries. Visual failure generally occurs early in the course (i.e., 4–7 weeks after the onset of the headache), is usually monocular initially, and abrupt in onset in over 50% of the patients studied. In other patients, the visual loss may be gradual over several days or be preceded by transient obscurations. When one eye is affected, the second is affected in 75% of the patients 1 day to 3 weeks later.[18]

Headache is considered the most common initial and characteristic symptom. However, it is not uncommon for the headache to be preceded by polymyalgia rheumatica and other constitutional symptoms of malaise, anorexia, and weight loss. When present, jaw or lingual claudication is virtually pathognomonic. Pharyngeal and limb claudication may also occur.

The headache may be unilateral or bilateral and is most commonly temporal in location, although other areas of the cranium, including the occiput, may be involved. The headache is generally steady, non-throbbing, and often sharp and boring. The patient is often aware of a tenderness of the scalp and reports tender nodules or thickened scalp vessels. The latter complaint can be verified by observing the nodular thickening and erythema over the distribution of the superficial temporal artery. The pulsations of the involved temporal artery are usually diminished or absent. When present, a characteristic feature of the headache is its aggravation by exposure to cold.

The syndrome of polymyalgia rheumatica has clearly been demonstrated to be a part of giant cell arteritis (see Volume I, Chapter 19). This may precede the headache by several weeks. The diagnosis is supported by an elevated ESR that is greater than 50 mm/hour in 95% of reported cases. The definitive diagnosis is made by an examination of the temporal artery biopsy. Because the involvement may be segmental ("skip lesions"), an adequate length of artery (greater than 4 cm) should be serially sectioned at several intervals.[20] In some cases, a biopsy of the other temporal artery will be positive when the first biopsy is negative.

When visual symptoms have occurred, a medical emergency is present and requires immediate treatment with high-dose corticosteroids. Daily high-dose therapy is continued until the patient is asymptomatic and the sedimentation rate is normal. If alternate-day therapy is used, the patient must be monitored carefully because of a relatively high frequency of control failure on alternate-day therapy.[21] Although giant cell arteritis is a self-limited disease, one should not discontinue the steroids

before 1 year at the earliest. Sometimes, treatment for 3 years or longer is required.[22] For this reason, it is best to confirm the diagnosis via biopsy when committing an elderly patient to long-term steroid therapy.

Cerebrovascular Disease

Headache, often severe, is a regular feature of intracerebral hemorrhage and embolic infarction. Headache may also accompany atherosclerotic, occlusive cerebrovascular disease as part of a stroke, TIA, or internal carotid artery occlusion, with or without infarction or TIA. It is generally a dull, non-throbbing headache localized to the retro-orbital and frontal region in anterior circulation disease, and to the occiput in posterior circulation ischemia. Headache occurs in approximately 30% of patients with internal carotid artery occlusion and may be accompanied by an ipsilateral Horner's syndrome.[23] A unilateral headache and facial pain, with ipsilateral Horner's syndrome and tenderness over the affected carotid artery, also may be associated with a dissection of the carotid arterial wall[24] or follow carotid endarterectomy.[25]

Carotidynia has been described as an idiopathic syndrome with a peak incidence in the 4th through 6th decades, which usually affects females.[26] Tenderness and swelling over the underlying carotid artery is accompanied by a deep, dull aching pain in the neck or jaw with an episodic, throbbing ipsilateral headache. It is doubtful that it is a distinct entity since carotid pain and tenderness may accompany migraine, giant cell arteritis, or the disorders mentioned in the previous paragraph. It is treated with the same drugs used for migraine.

Headache also occurs in approximately 25% of patients with TIAs.[27] This gives rise to a dilemma in geriatric patients with a previous history of migraine, especially vertebrobasilar TIAs, when the visual accompaniments may mimic migraine equivalents. Features that may distinguish the two were discussed in the section on migraine. Although monocular blindness may be seen in younger patients with migraine (retinal migraine), in an elderly patient it should be considered due to atherosclerotic disease until proven otherwise. Lacunar infarcts due to a small vessel disease are not accompanied by headache, probably because these vessels are not innervated.

The relationship between headache and hypertension is controversial. Hypertension alone is not believed to cause a headache unless the diastolic pressure is above 140 mm Hg.[28] However, there is a subgroup of patients with the classically described nocturnal or morning headache whose headaches disappear during the course of treatment. This group had a slightly higher blood pressure (highest blood pressure recorded averaged 196/125 mm Hg versus 191/119 mm Hg) before treatment. Treatment produced a greater drop in blood pressure than the study group as a whole.[29] Also, in patients with a previous history of vascular headaches, hypertension often causes headaches, which are relieved by lowering blood pressure.

Headache Due to Extracranial Disease

A headache may arise as a referred pain from a disease of the paranasal sinuses, teeth, and the temporomandibular joint. Headaches due to acute sinusitis is seldom difficult to diagnose because of the localized pain over the affected sinuses, the localized percussion tenderness, and exacerbation with stooping or bending over. Although headache is often blamed on chronic sinusitis, it is seldom a cause of chronic headache when there are no nasal symptoms. One exception is when the sphenoid sinus is affected, which may produce a frontal headache and is overlooked on an x-ray film when a clouding of the sinus is attributed to a congenital anomaly.[30]

Orbital Pain

Pain centered in the orbital and frontal regions may be due to intracranial aneurysms, an orbital tumor, or orbital granuloma (Tolosa-Hunt syndrome); however, a more common cause is glaucoma, which should always be considered in elderly persons.[31] The pain is generally most intense upon arising in the morning and may be associated by typical blurred vision and halos around lights. On occasion, the headache is described as an occipital or fronto-temporal dull, aching pain that is indistinguishable from a muscle contraction headache. A cluster headache is often centered in the orbit; its features are discussed in the previous section.

Ear Pain

Cranial nerves 5, 7, 9, and 10 innervate the ear, and any irritation or destruction of these nerves may present as a pain felt in the ear or mastoid area. For example, Bell's palsy may be accompanied by a pain in the ear, especially in the mastoid region. Aneurysms and metastatic or primary tumors affecting nerves 9 and 10 also may produce a pain felt deep in the ear. Glossopharyngeal neuralgia is one of the idiopathic cranial neuralgias that can cause pain in the ear radiating into the throat.

The temporomandibular joint syndrome caused by arthritis, bruxism, or malocclusion may be described by the patient as ear pain.[32] Upon careful questioning, the pain is usually located anterior to the tragus, and it generally radiates into the temporal region, jaw, and throat. It may be accompanied by a spasm and tenderness of the muscles of mastication. It is generally increased by chewing and talking. Crepitus and subluxation of the joint on jaw opening is often present. Treatment is individualized according to probable cause. Bite blocks are often helpful for the patient with bruxism or minor malocclusion (*see* Volume I, Chapter 34). Edentulous patients should have their prosthesis revised or replaced. Mild arthritis can be treated with the usual anti-inflammatory agents, and so on. Severe arthritis may necessitate replacement with an artificial joint.

Facial Pain

Severe, unilateral facial pain is most commonly seen in the middle-aged and elderly population, largely due to the age-specific incidence of idiopathic trigeminal neuralgia. However, it is not uncommon for the patient to see a neurologist only after extensive evaluation for sinus and dental disease. Sinus disease is seldom, if ever, a cause of severe lancinating pain, and an abscessed tooth can be readily revealed by percussion of the affected tooth. Once it is appreciated that the pain is truly neuralgic, the task is to differentiate between idiopathic and symptomatic trigeminal neuralgia.

Trigeminal Neuralgia

Idiopathic trigeminal neuralgia is characteristically seen in the middle-aged and elderly population. When it occurs before 40 years of age, it is usually a symptom of multiple sclerosis or some other structural lesion. The pain of idiopathic trigeminal neuralgia is characteristically a brief, severe, and lancinating pain lasting a few seconds to 1 minute. The paroxysms of pain are in the distribution of one or more divisions of the trigeminal nerve, most commonly in the second or third divisions or a combination of the two, and uncommonly in the first division. The paroxysms are characteristically triggered by stimuli in the territory of the affected division ("trigger zones"). Common triggers are a light touch, a cold breeze on the face, chewing, and hot or cold liquids in the mouth. This results in the reluctance of the patient to wash, shave, or eat. In between paroxysms, the patient is symptom free. Once asleep, the patient is not awakened by the pain, but it may commence immediately upon awakening. There are usually remissions of a few weeks to several months.

Trigeminal neuralgia secondary to serious intracranial disease may be described as a typical tic-like pain, but it is often more continuous, deep, and boring in character.[33] It may awaken the patient from a sound sleep and trigger zones are often not present. Sensory or motor abnormalities do not occur in idiopathic tic douloureux and, if present, a careful investigation is required. A variety of lesions may produce an irritation of the trigeminal nerve and an associated sensory loss, including an aneurysm of the basilar artery, metastatic tumors in the region of the gasserian ganglion, primary tumors of the posterior fossa such as acoustic or trigeminal neuroma, meningioma, or epidermoid lesions. An aneurysm or tumor in the cavernous sinus may also cause facial pain as well as headache. Invasion of the sinus by nasopharyngeal carcinoma often produces trigeminal pain and sensory loss as an early symptom. With the advent of antibiotics, osteomyelitis of the apex of the petrous temporal bone (petrositis) is uncommon, but it should be considered when there is an associated 6th nerve palsy (Gradenigro's syndrome). Pain and sensory loss of the forehead due to lesions of the first division may be produced by orbital granuloma (Tolosa-Hunt syndrome) or pericarotid lesions, which are associated with a unilateral Horner's syndrome (Raeder's paratrigeminal neuralgia).

In a sense, all idiopathic trigeminal neuralgia may be "symptomatic." When the posterior fossa is explored for surgical relief of the pain, a large proportion of trigeminal nerves are distorted by vascular structures. Placement of a small piece of sponge between the nerve and the offending vessel has produced a high rate of success and it is rapidly becoming the most popular surgical procedure for the relief of trigeminal neuralgia.[34]

Although some patients become refractory and require surgical intervention, medical therapy with phenytoin (Dilantin) and carbamazepine (Tegretol) may be successful in some patients. Often, only intermittent therapy is required since spontaneous remissions are common. After 1 or 2 months of therapy, the drug may be tapered and resumed only when the pain returns. Recently baclofen (Lioresal) has been reported as an effective treatment.[35]

Other Neuralgias

The pain of glossopharyngeal neuralgia has the same characteristics as trigeminal neuralgia, but it is located in the throat and triggered by talking and swallowing. It also may respond to Dilantin, Tegretol, or Baclofen. If these are unsuccessful, a division of the glossopharyngeal nerve and upper rootlets of the vagus near the medulla is the treatment of choice.

Postherpetic neuralgia due to herpes zoster ophthalmicus or geniculate herpes (herpes of the external auditory meatus and pinna with tinnitus, vertigo, deafness, and facial palsy) may subside several weeks or a few months after the herpetic eruption subsides. Unfortunately, the pain may become chronic and intractable, especially in elderly patients. It is one of the most difficult pains to alleviate. Phenytoin and carbamazepine are seldom helpful. The most successful medical therapy to date has been a combination of a tricyclic antidepressant and a neuroleptic major tranquilizer (fluphenazine is most commonly used). The neuroleptics must be used with great caution in elderly persons because of the considerable incidence of sedation, pseudodementia, extrapyramidal syndromes, and the increased risk of tardive dyskinesia.

When all the classic pain syndromes and local sources of pain have been excluded, there are a residual number of cases that are collected under the term "atypical facial pain." Some of these cases are attributed to sphenopalatine neuralgia (Vidian or Sluder's neuralgia), especially if the pain is centered at the root of the nose and accompanied by excessive lacrimation or nasal discharge. Some of these are migraine syndromes; however, if appropriate therapy is unsuccessful, cocainization followed by neurectomy of the sphenopalatine ganglion may be tried, although this has seldom provided a lasting relief of symptoms.

References

1. Ziegler DK, Hassanein RS, Couch JR: Characteristics of life headache histories in a nonclinic population. *Neurology (NY)* 27:265–269, 1977.
2. Waters WE: The Pontypridd headache survey. *Headache* 14:81–90, 1974.
3. Rooke ED: Benign exertional headache. *Med Clin North Am* 52:801–808, 1968.
4. Martin PR, Mathews AM: Tension headaches: psychophysiological investigation and treatment. *J Psychosom Res* 22:389–399, 1978.
5. Krabbe AA, Olesen J: Headache provocation by continuous intravenous infusion of histamine. Clinical results and receptor mechanisms. *Pain* 8:253–259, 1980.
6. Lance JW, Curran DA, Anthony M: Investigations into the mechanism and treatment of chronic headache. *Med J Aust* 2:909–914, 1965.
7. Bruhn P, Olesen J, Melgaard B: Controlled trial of EMG feedback in muscle contraction headache. *Ann Neurol* 6:34–36, 1979.
8. Couch JR, Ziegler DK, Hassanein R: Amitriptyline in the prophylaxis of migraine. *Neurology (Minneap)* 26:121–127, 1976.
9. Edmeads J: Headaches and head pains associated with diseases of the cervical spine. *Med Clin North Am* 62:533–544, 1978.
10. Whitty CWM, Hockaday JM: Migraine: a follow up study of 92 patients. *Brit Med J* 1:735–736, 1968.
11. Selby G, Lance JW: Observations on 500 cases of migraine and allied vascular headache. *J Neurol Neurosurg Psychiatry* 23:23–32, 1960.
12. Fisher CM: Late-life migraine accompaniments as a cause of unexplained transient ischemic attacks. *Canad J Neurol Sci* 7:9–17, 1980.
13. Raskin NH, Appenzeller O: Headache, in Smith LH (ed): *Major Problems in Internal Medicine*. Philadelphia, WB Saunders & Co, 1980, vol 19, pp 122–127.
14. Kudrow L: *Cluster Headache, Mechanisms and Management*. Oxford, Oxford University Press, 1980.
15. Ekbom K: Chronic migrainous neuralgia, diagnostic and therapeutic aspects. *Headache* 11:97–101, 1971.
16. Mathew NT: Indomethacin responsive headache syndrome. *Headache* 21:147–150, 1981.
17. Ekbom K: Lithium for cluster headache: review of literature and preliminary results of long-term treatment. *Headache* 21:132–139, 1981.
18. Hollenhorst RW, Brown JR, Wagener HP, et al: Neurologic aspects of temporal arteritis. *Neurology (Minneap)* 10:490–498, 1960.
19. Sorensen PS, Lorenzen I: Giant-cell arteritis, temporal arteritis and polymyalgia rheumatica. *Acta Med Scand* 201:207–213, 1977.
20. Klein RG, Campbell RJ, Hunder GG, et al: Skip lesions in temporal arteritis. *Mayo Clinic Proc* 51:504–510, 1976.
21. Hunder GG, Sheps SG, Allen GL, et al: Daily and alternate-day corticosteroid regimens in treatment of giant-cell arteritis. *Ann Int Med* 82:613–618, 1975.
22. Beevers DG, Harpur JE, Turk KAD: Giant-cell arteritis—the need for prolonged treatment. *J Chron Dis* 26:571–584, 1973.
23. Fisher CM: Headache in cerebrovascular disease, in Vinken PJ, Bruyn GW (ed): *Handbook of Clinical Neurology*. Amsterdam, North Holland, 1968, vol 5, pp 124–156.
24. West TET, Davies RJ, Kelly RE: Horner's syndrome and headache due to carotid artery disease. *Brit Med J* 1:818–820, 1976.
25. Pearce J: Headache after carotid endarterectomy. *Brit Med J* 2:85–86, 1976.
26. Raskin NH, Prusiner S: Carotidynia. *Neurology* 27:43–46, 1977.
27. Grindal AB, Toole JF: Headache and transient ischemic attacks. *Stroke* 5:603–606, 1974.
28. Badran RHA, Weis RJ, McGuiness JB: Hypertension and headache. *Scott Med J* 15:48–51, 1970.
29. Traub YM, Korczyn AD: Headache in patients with hypertension. *Headache* 17:245–247, 1978.
30. Birt D: Headaches and head pains associated with diseases of the ear, nose, and throat. *Med Clin North Am* 62:523–531, 1978.
31. Behrens MM: Headaches associated with disorders of the eye. *Med Clin North Am* 62:507–521, 1978.
32. Reik L, Hale M: The temporomandibular joint

pain—dysfunction syndrome: a frequent cause of headache. *Headache* 21:151–156, 1980.

33. Needham CW: Major cranial neuralgias and the surgical treatment of headache. *Med Clin North Am* 545–557, 1978.

34. Janetta PJ: Microsurgical approach to the tri-geminal nerve for tic Douloureux. *Prog Neurol Surg* 7:180–200, 1976.

35. Fromm GH, Terrence CF, Chatta AS, et al: Ba-clofen in trigeminal neuralgia. Its effect on the spinal trigeminal nucleus: a pilot study. *Arch Neurol* 37:768–771, 1980.

CHAPTER 7

Neuromuscular Diseases

DAVID P. GARDNER, M.D., PH.D.

Disorders of the Spinal Cord

Disease of the spinal cord is often referred to by the generic term myelopathy or, when inflammation is suspected, myelitis. The narrow confines of the bony vertebral canal may increase the risk of neurologic damage whenever the cord is directly injured or becomes swollen as a result of inflammation. Although the cord ends at the L1-L2 interspace, the same principles apply to the cauda equina, which lies within the bony canal at the lumbar and sacral levels.

There are numerous causes of myelopathy, the most common being trauma, mechanical compression, nutritional or metabolic factors, and various degenerative conditions. The frequency of disease varies depending on age; for example, multiple sclerosis occurs more frequently in young persons and amyotrophic lateral sclerosis primarily affects older persons.

All these diseases will produce symptoms reflecting a pathology of two structures: the long tracts (e.g., corticospinal and posterior column) or the gray matter, especially the anterior horn cells. Although the ventral and dorsal roots and the dorsal root ganglia are classified as part of the peripheral nervous system, diseases of the spinal cord will frequently affect them, thus producing characteristic symptoms. A disease may affect the cord throughout its length (as in Vitamin B-12 deficiency) or the pathology may be limited to a particular level, in which case the term transverse myelopathy is applied, or transverse myelitis if inflammation is suspected.

The rapidity of onset (acute, subacute, or progressive) is an extremely important diagnostic clue to the etiology of the symptoms.

Clinical Manifestations

Diseases of the spinal cord produce identical clinical manifestations whether occurring in old or young persons. In elderly persons, however, subtle symptoms may be dismissed or blamed on "arthritis" or other malady that age brings. This is especially true when the complaint is weakness, one of the cardinal signs of myelopathy. One of the most difficult judgments for the clinician to make is in trying to decide whether true neurogenic weakness exists in an already arthritic hand, or whether the leg weakness in a patient convalescing from a hip fracture represents merely pain and disuse or has its origin in a cord pathology incurred in the same accident that caused the fracture. Muscle wasting is another sign of pathology within the vertebral canal, particularly when the roots are involved. However, this judgment also may be difficult to determine in patients of advanced age, especially in the presence of weight loss or cachexia, which causes a generalized loss of muscle mass. Although weakness is common in myelopathy (especially leg weakness), the patient may direct his complaints toward the functional aspects of the symptoms. For example, he may complain of tiredness in the legs or difficulty walking. A complaint of "poor balance" may, on closer questioning, reveal that the patient is having increasing difficulty walking without stumbling, especially on rough ground.

Indeed, a history of frequent, unexplained falls may be the first clue to a myelopathy. It may, in retrospect, be difficult to determine whether the falling was the cause or the result of the spinal cord pathology. When the motor deficit involves an upper limb, there may be symptoms of clumsiness or impaired manual dexterity related to work or hobbies. Tasks involving buttons, shoelaces, watchbands, and so on may become difficult and inordinately time consuming.

Compromise of the posterior column white matter or spinothalamic tracts usually results in impaired sensation with a great variety of adjectives being employed by patients to describe the symptoms. For example, it may be said that the involved extremity is "numb," "dead," or "like lead." Sensations of "tightness," "stiffness," or "tingling" may be described. Frequently, the complaint of "numbness" may be out of proportion to the demonstrable deficit and may even be the term chosen by the patient to describe weakness. At times, colorful similies will be used; the involved extremity skin area will be said to feel like "a crust" or "a rind." There may be a feeling of "thickness," or that there is "too much skin," or that an unseen glove is covering the affected part. Odd paresthesias (altered sensations) may be described, such as the feeling that a "spider web" is touching the skin.

In the case of complete cord transection or destruction, there will be complete anesthesia caudal to the lesion. For a variable period of time after the lesion, however, sensations of pain may be experienced in the extremities. These sensations, in cord transection, have been found to originate in the proximal stump of the severed cord. Another sensation that is common with cord lesions is the feeling that a "band" of numbness or tightness is present around the chest or abdomen. Lhermitte's sign (actually a symptom) is a feeling of electric shock down the back and, occasionally, in the extremities on flexion of the neck. Although most frequently seen in multiple sclerosis, it is not uncommon in cervical spondylosis and has been described as occurring in combined degeneration (Vitamin B-12 deficiency). Deficits resulting from myelopathy may be ill-defined and patchy. Examination of the patient with a suspected myelopathy should include a diligent search for a "sensory level" (i.e., a level on the trunk below which sensation is impaired and above which it is normal). Frequently, this level will be represented in an extremity, usually in an upper limb. When only a small area is involved, occurrence of the deficit in an area that overlaps the distribution of several peripheral nerves helps to betray the true myelopathic nature of the lesion.

Besides motor and sensory disturbances, the third cardinal feature of myelopathy is altered bowel, bladder, and sexual function. Impaired micturition usually is the first symptom, although subtle anorectal dysfunction (such as the inability to distinguish flatus from feces) may be an early complaint if specifically asked about. A history of impaired sexual function also must be specifically questioned and frequently is neglected when interviewing elderly patients.

Lesions of the descending autonomic and ascending sensory pathways in the spinal cord cause impaired bladder emptying, which ranges from anuresis to urinary urgency to incontinence. These symptoms result from a combination of impaired motor control of bladder emptying and sphincter muscles and a failure of sensory information from bladder receptors in reaching higher control centers. As a rule, progressive spinal cord lesions are associated with a small, hyperactive bladder producing symptoms of poor control, urgency, and incontinence. Lesions at the lower thoracic or lumbar levels that affect the roots of the cauda equina rather than the spinal cord are associated with a large, flaccid hypofunctioning bladder, which produces symptoms of hesitancy, diminished stream, or anuresis requiring catheterization. Following acute, severe spinal cord injury, a classic pattern of symptoms evolves. Initially, in the stage of "spinal shock," there is urinary retention. This is followed, after a variable period of time, by overflow incontinence and, finally, by reflex or automatic emptying. In addition to the clinical history, cystometrographic techniques are available to aid in defining the type of abnormality, especially when there is uncertainty regarding the location of the lesion (e.g., spinal cord versus cauda equina).

Finally, examination of myotatic (deep tendon) reflexes and muscle tone, both increased in lesions of the spinal cord, is essential. Superficial reflexes should be evaluated; some are absent in myelopathy (abdominal and cremasteric), whereas the normal plantar response is converted into an abnormal reflex, the Babinski response.

Important Causes of Myelopathy in Elderly Persons

Spondylosis

The term spondylosis refers to degenerative changes in the architecture of the osseous and fibrocartilaginous structures of the vertebral column wrought by advancing age and/or osteoarthritis.[1] Obviously, this process may be accelerated by the presence of specific diseases, such as rheumatoid arthritis, Marie-Strumpell ankylosing spondylitis, Paget's disease, and so on. Spondylosis is a common cause of spinal cord compression occurring after middle age; compression of roots may occur as well. Although the course of the disease is usually insidious, it may be punctuated by acute disc protrusions or a sudden compromise of spinal vascular supply. The symptoms vary with the level of the lesion, with the cervical and lumbar regions being most commonly involved and the thoracic region being less involved.

Cervical spondylosis may produce a mixture of motor symptoms that reflect an involvement of both roots and spinal cord tracts (lower and upper motor neurons). Damage to the corticospinal tract results in spasticity (heightened reflexes, increased resistance to passive stretch, weakness, and poor motor control). Involvement of cervical ventral roots causes weakness, atrophy, and a loss of reflexes. Injury to dorsal roots causes pain, which may radiate into the affected extemity, and other sensory symptoms (paresthesias are more common than anesthesia). Sensory disturbances in the legs reflect a dysfunction of the ascending cord pathways (posterior columns and spinothalamic tracts). Pain in the nuchal region and chronic occipital "tension headache" are common features.

When a cervical disc has herniated, there may be a history of a sudden "snap" or "pop" that is often associated with physical activity. Discs usually involve cervical levels C5-C7. A direct or lateral compression of the head usually produces pain (Spurling's sign). Cervical traction produces relief and is the initial treatment of choice in cervical disc protrusions. When the pain is unremitting, or when significant atrophy or signs of damage to the spinal cord occurs, surgical removal of the herniated disc material is indicated. A myelogram is employed as a prelude to surgery.

Lumbar spondylosis produces only pain in the majority of patients. When an injury to the roots of the cauda equina occurs, it usually is the result of lumbar disc degeneration and herniation. An injury of nerve roots in the cauda equina produces pain, sensory symptoms, and a lower motor neuron type of weakness in the involved extremity. On occasion, the osteophytes of lumbar spondylosis, superimposed on a congenitally narrow lumbar canal, will result in symptomatic stenosis.[2] In these cases, symptoms of pain in the buttocks, thighs, and legs may simulate vascular claudication, especially if they occur when walking. The symptoms are relieved by flexion of the lumbar spine, which diminishes the degree of stenosis.

Trauma

Trauma is the most frequent cause of spinal cord pathology, especially in the cervical region. The presence of spondylosis, which is prevalent in elderly persons, adds considerably to the hazard of damage to the spinal cord or roots. Falls or even a relatively minor trauma may be the cause of such an injury. Although associated vertebral fracture/dislocations may be apparent from x-ray films, the phenomenon of spinal cord contusion or even bleeding (hematomyelia) without fracture is well known. Odontoid dislocation, a common occurrence in the presence of vertebral disease (especially Paget's), may be overlooked unless specifically sought with appropriate x-ray procedures, myelography, or computed tomography (CT scans). Although a whiplash injury may cause a myelopathy, it more commonly causes pain, which is often chronic, due to an injury of nuchal muscles and ligaments.

Vascular Disease

Ischemia due to atherosclerosis or other vascular diseases affects the spinal cord less frequently than the brain. Occasionally, during a hypotensive episode, infarction of the spinal cord will occur in "watershed" areas such as the high thoracic region. Specific spinal stroke syndromes may occur in conjunction with a dissecting aortic aneurysm or vasculitis; both of these may affect critical spinal branches of the intercostal arteries, thus causing a picture of weakness and dissociated sensory loss (loss of pain and temperature, but preservation of vibratory and discriminative sensation) below the level of the lesion. This is known as the anterior spinal artery syndrome.

The most important vascular complication is a hemorrhage in the area of the spinal canal, which occurs in patients with bleeding diatheses or those taking anticoagulants. The most common vascular complication is an epidural hematoma, which may cause a rapid cord compression and represents a surgical emergency. Although an epidural hematoma may occur spontaneously, a lumbar puncture is frequently a precipitating cause and should be performed with caution, if at all, in high-risk patients. In anticoagulated patients, a lumbar puncture should be performed only after discontinuation of anticoagulants; these may be resumed 2 hours after the procedure, or longer if the tap is traumatic.[3]

Amyotrophic Lateral Sclerosis (ALS)
Progressive degenerative disorders affecting the motor neurons of the motor cortex, brainstem, and spinal cord are referred to collectively as motor system disease. In adults from middle age to later life, amyotrophic lateral sclerosis (ALS) is the principal representative of this group of diseases.[4] The onset is insidious, but it may be described as sudden if it has only recently come to the patient's attention. Weakness may present as wrist drop, foot drop, poor grip, impaired manual dexterity, or a frequent choking on liquids. In retrospect, cramps (especially in the feet, calves, and hands) are early presenting symptoms. Because sensory impairment (apart from the mild loss of vibratory sensation seen in elderly persons) is lacking, myopathy and myasthenia gravis may enter into the differential diagnosis. However, it usually is cervical spondylosis, which in elderly persons presents the most difficult differential diagnostic problem. Cervical spondylosis frequently causes simultaneous signs of lower motor neuron disease in upper extremities (wasting) and upper motor neuron disease (spasticity, Babinski signs) in lower extremi-

ties, thus masquerading as ALS. The occurrence of the two diseases together complicates matters even more. A scrupulous search for signs of brainstem involvement (e.g., fasciculations of the tongue) will often, but not always, betray the presence of ALS. Many patients will undergo a decompressive laminectomy for a diagnosis of cervical spondylosis only to deteriorate from the ravages of ALS. Nevertheless, it must be remembered that the former disease is treatable, whereas no convincing treatment for ALS has ever been demonstrated.

Hereditary Degeneration
Degeneration of the corticospinal tracts occurs in families, although rarely, as a dominantly or sporadically inherited condition. It involves the slow progression of weakness and spasticity without sensory symptoms. This type of myelopathy is thought to represent a variant of motor neuron disease and is often designated primary lateral sclerosis.

Vitamin B-12 Deficiency
and Other Nutritional Disorders
The best known nutritional myelopathy is that caused by Vitamin B-12 deficiency, which is most often seen in connection with pernicious anemia (*see* Volume I, Chapter 22). Failure to absorb Vitamin B-12 due to a lack of intrinsic factor, postgastrectomy states, or diseases of the terminal ileum causes both hematologic and neurologic pathologies, the latter being referred to as subacute combined degeneration. The lesions of Vitamin B-12 deficiency are of the demyelinating type and primarily affect the spinal cord and optic nerves. Occasionally, small lesions of the cerebral white matter have been described, but the relationship of these to the dementia seen in pernicious anemia is uncertain. The posterior column white matter of the spinal cord is the earliest area to be affected followed by the corticospinal tracts and spinothalamic tracts. A peripheral neuropathy is also present, but its manifestations are often overshadowed by symptoms of posterior column dysfunction. Loss of vibratory and position sensation, particularly in the lower extremities, is the earliest sign. Reflexes may be increased or diminished, depending on the degree of corticospinal tract disease and peripheral neuropathy. As the disease progresses, the gait be-

comes ataxic and all aspects of sensation become impaired, both in the arms and legs. Occasionally, megaloblastic anemia may be absent, especially when folate has been administered.[5]

Thiamine deficiency has been associated with sensory myelopathy, but symptoms referable to a neuropathy usually overshadow those which may be caused by spinal cord involvement.

Most nervous system pathology attributed to vitamin deficiency is thought to result from a combination of vitamin deficiencies and, possibly, from protein-calorie malnutrition.[6]

Neoplasms and Paraneoplastic Syndromes

Intramedullary, intradural, and extradural tumors account for 5%, 40%, and 55%, respectively, of all tumors affecting the spinal cord.[7] Tumors of neural origin (spinal cord or peripheral nerve) probably occur less frequently than lymphomas, carcinomas, and other non-neural tumors, unless one includes meningiomas. Metastatic lesions account for 16–66% of spinal cord tumors.[8] The relative frequencies of primary versus metastatic tumors that affect the spinal cord are outlined in Tables 7-1 and 7-2.

It is worth noting that an even larger percentage of space-occupying lesions of the spinal canal is accounted for by epidural hematomas, abscesses, extruded discs, and similar nonneoplastic lesions, which occasionally may simulate tumors.

The most common primary tumors are neurofibromas and the meningiomas. Since tumors arising within the spinal cord (intraspinal, mainly gliomas) are rare, most neoplasms will damage the spinal cord by means of extrinsic compression. The potential benefit from surgical intervention is therefore quite favorable, particularly when the lesion is discovered early and is benign. Unfortunately, the effects of spinal cord compression progress rapidly, and delay in diagnosis, together with the limited regenerative capacity of the spinal cord, frequently results in a poor prognosis. Since a myelogram is occasionally followed by a rapid deterioration due to an increased compression by the tumor, it is important to have facilities and personnel for surgery readily available.[9] A myelogram should be done whenever there are signs of a compressive cord lesion or even when a high index of suspicion exists, such as in a cancer patient who develops back pain. CT scans have not yet replaced myelography, but they may be a useful ancillary procedure, particularly in distinguishing an epidural tumor from a hematoma and especially in the lumbar region. Occasionally, plain x-ray films of the spine will disclose a bony erosion of pedicles or neuroforamina.

The treatment of choice for benign tumors within the spinal canal is surgery. In malignant tissue, the prognosis with radiation therapy alone is as good or better than with surgical therapy alone, irrespective of the histologic type.[10] Steroids also are beneficial when administered with radiation therapy.[11]

On occasion, degeneration of the spinal cord occurs as a remote or paraneoplastic effect of carcinoma.[12,13] The most common syndrome is a symmetric degeneration of the posterior columns causing a loss of vibration and position sense. The pathogenesis of this syndrome is unclear, and it is frequently difficult to separate from the effects of nutritional deficiency associ-

TABLE 7-1 Relative Incidence of Primary Tumors Causing Spinal Cord Compression[9]

Tumor	Percent of Total
Schwannomas	30
Meningiomas	26
Gliomas (including ependymomas)	23
Sarcomas	11
Hemangiomas	6
Others	4

TABLE 7-2 Relative Incidence of Metastatic Tumors Causing Spinal Cord Compression[10]

Tumor	Percent of Total
Breast	22
Lung	16
Prostate	11
Kidney	9
Lymphoma	6
Myeloma	6
Melanoma	5
Gastrointestinal	4
Other	22

ated with cancer or the effects of radiation on the spinal cord.[14]

In rare instances, a rapid, severe, and ascending degeneration of the spinal cord occurs as a paraneoplastic effect of carcinoma. This syndrome usually progresses to a flaccid, areflexic paraplegia and terminates fatally in a matter of days or weeks. The pathologic correlate of this syndrome is a patchy necrosis primarily affecting the lumbosacral and posterior regions of the spinal cord. Myelography usually is negative. Cerebrospinal fluid (CSF) examination usually reveals an elevated protein level, occasionally with pleocytosis and red blood cells.[15,16]

Disorders of the Peripheral Nervous System

Neuropathies

Diseases of peripheral nerves may affect the neuron (perikaryon or axon), the Schwann cell myelin sheath, or the surrounding connective tissue and blood vessels. Neuropathies may be divided into axonal or demyelinating types, depending on which tissue is predominantly involved. Although this classification is pathologically useful, from the standpoint of nerve conduction velocity testing most neuropathies involve damage to both the axons and myelin.

Clinical Features of the Neuropathies

As in diseases of the central nervous system, afflictions involving peripheral nerves cause weakness and sensory disturbances. When there is a generalized involvement of the peripheral nervous system, as in diabetic polyneuropathy, the symptoms of weakness are diffuse. When one or more single nerves are involved (mononeuropathy or mononeuritis multiplex), manual muscle testing will reveal a pattern of weakness that is helpful in identifying the affected nerve or root. With peripheral nerve diseases, as with anterior horn cell diseases, there is muscle atrophy, which is predominantly distal. Some neuropathies, such as that produced by leprosy, mainly cause sensory symptoms that also are more distal than proximal.

Neuropathic disease also causes fasciculations, which can be seen as visible muscle twitches. These are rarely as prominent as in motor neuron disease.

Finally, neuropathy causes loss of reflex. Since these effects also are prominent distally, ankle jerks are the earliest affected myotatic (tendon jerk) reflexes. Loss of the autonomic reflexes causes the appearance of dry, "dystrophic" skin on the hands and feet; more serious autonomic dysfunction may produce orthostatic hypotension, cardiac arrhythmias, and even cardiac arrest.

Common Neuropathies in Elderly Persons

Diabetic Neuropathy   Diabetes mellitus is the most common cause of neuropathy in most age groups, including elderly persons. Four main types occur:[17]

1. Distal, symmetric, and primarily sensory neuropathy
2. Autonomic neuropathy
3. Proximal, asymmetric, painful, and primarily motor neuropathy
4. Cranial mononeuropathy

The severity of the neuropathy is related only roughly to the severity of the diabetes, but the prevailing view is that some improvement may occur with optimal control of serum glucose.

The pathogenesis of distal, symmetric, and diabetic neuropathy (the most common type in diabetes) is disputed, with various theories proposed ranging from small vessel (vasa nervorum) disease to osmotic damage from sugar alcohols.[18] There is a general agreement that the painful, acute, and proximal neuropathies of diabetes and the cranial neuropathies are the result of neural infarcts.[19,20] The above list omits the more exotic manifestations of diabetic neuropathy, such as thoracic polyradiculopathy (which may present as acute abdominal pain[21]) and the various individual mononeuropathies[22] or diabetic neuropathic cachexia.[23] Apart from improved diabetic control, the chronic, painful, and diabetic neuropathies are best managed symptomatically; an approach that has included transcutaneous stimulation[24] and administration of various combinations of tricyclic antidepressants and phenothiazines.[25] With regard to the latter, it should be noted that there is an overlap between the symptomatology of painful diabetic neuropathy and depressive illness.[26]

Neuropathies of Alcoholism and Nutritional Deficiency The symptoms of alcoholic peripheral neuropathy, as with those of diabetes, include painful burning sensations. They are invariably distal, symmetrical, and involve mainly the lower extremities, particularly the feet. Indeed, the painful sensations (dysesthesias) of the soles of the feet are frequently so severe that they prevent a reliable assessment of plantar responses. The pathogenesis is thought to be related to the nutritional deficiency of alcoholism, particularly to B-vitamin deficiency (B-1, B-6, B-12), but also possibly to a deficiency of pantothenic acid and niacin. There is also debate as to whether there is a direct toxic effect of ethanol on nerves.[27] Neuropathy occurs in B12 deficiency but is frequently overshadowed by the concomitant cerebral and spinal manifestations.

Inflammatory Polyneuropathy or Guillain-Barré (GB) Syndrome Guillain-Barré (GB) syndrome is probably the most common cause of acute paralytic illness in civilized countries. Persons at any age may be affected and, although no consistent predisposing factors have been identified, there is frequently a history of recent viral illness. The overall mortality rate, mainly due to respiratory insufficiency, is about 5%;[28] however, this is probably higher in elderly persons, particularly in the presence of a concurrent, chronic pulmonary disease.

The diagnosis of GB syndrome can be difficult,[29,30] and many patients in early stages of the disease have been diagnosed in emergency rooms as having hyperventilation syndrome or other functional illness only to return in 24 hours with absent reflexes and respiratory distress. Other causes of subacute, severe, and generalized weakness (such as myasthenia gravis, myasthenic syndrome, potassium deficiency, botulism, diphtheria, tick paralysis, or toxin ingestion) also must be considered.

The earliest symptoms are weakness, paresthesias, and pain that begins distally. Although progression of the weakness has been described as "ascending," in reality it is centripetal, which affects arms as well as legs. With progression, cranial nerves (particularly the facial nerves) may be affected and deep tendon reflexes are progressively lost. Rarely, extraocular muscles are affected, which cause a complete or partial ophthalmoplegia.[31] For reasons that are not entirely clear, fluctuating autonomic symptoms occur, mainly in the form of wide swings in blood pressure and heart rate.[32,33] Fatal arrhythmias have occurred.[34]

The disease may progress for 1–3 weeks, after which improvement occurs. Significant discomfort in the back and extremities may be present during the course of the disease and may persist as a neuralgic pain, especially in the feet, for many months thereafter. During the height of the disease, a typical cell-protein dissociation in the spinal fluid (high protein with a low normal cell count) may be demonstrated. Treatment of the acute phase of illness is supportive; steroids and plasmapheresis have been used without demonstrable success.[35–37] In a small percentage of patients, a chronic, relapsing polyneuropathy persists after the acute illness; it is frequently steroid and plasmapheresis responsive.[38]

Paraneoplastic Neuropathy Neuropathy may occur in association with carcinoma or other malignant diseases. An occult malignancy should be suspected when an unexplained polyneuropathy occurs in an elderly patient (*see* Table 7-3). Paraneoplastic neuropathies are mainly of two varieties: 1) A symmetric axonal degeneration similar to diabetic neuropathy; and 2) A severe, predominantly sensory neuropathy reflecting degeneration of the dorsal root ganglion.[39] Both of these types are most commonly associated with small cell anaplastic carcinoma of the lung. An acute GB-like syndrome and a chronic inflammatory polyradiculopathy also have been described in association with neoplastic disease.[40]

In rare instances, amyloid polyneuropathy is seen in association with multiple myeloma,[41] although carpal tunnel syndrome is a relatively frequent occurrence.[42] In Waldenstrom's macroglobulinemia, mononeuritis multiplex is seen, which is presumably due to microinfarction of the neural vessels.[43]

Since the various paraneoplastic syndromes rarely occur in isolation, encephalitis, cerebral ataxia, or myasthenic syndrome all may be seen

TABLE 7-3 Paraneoplastic Neuropathies

Sensory neuropathy
Occurs in 20% of paraneoplastic neuropathies.
Usually seen with small cell carcinoma, but also
with carcinoma of the esophagus and cecum.

Mild, distal, sensorimotor polyneuropathy
Most common type of paraneoplastic neuropathy. Identical to other common neuropathies,
such as in diabetes. Usually of little clinical
significance to the patient.

Acute and subacute sensory and motor neuropathy
Usually occurs with carcinoma of the lung, but
also of the colon, bladder, pancreas, stomach,
and cervix. Difficult to distinguish from Guillain-
Barré Syndrome.

Remitting and relapsing motor and sensory
neuropathy
The association with carcinoma of the lung is
relatively low (15%). There is an association with
seminoma of the testis. Similar to chronic, relapsing polyneuropathy with demyelinating features.

Paraneoplastic pandysautonomia
Severe, usually acute or subacute development
of autonomic dysfunction. The association is
with various malignancies. Recovery following
irradiation of tumor has been reported.

1. Polyarteritis nodosa
2. Giant cell arteritis
3. Granulomatous vasculitis:
   Churg-Strauss allergic granulomatosis, sarcoidosis, Wegener's granulomatosis
4. "Connective tissue disease":
   Systemic lupus erythematosis, rheumatoid
   arthritis, progressive systemic sclerosis, Sjogren's syndrome, and mixed connective tissue disease.
5. Other:
   Hypersensitivity angiitis, Kohlmeier-Degos
   arteritis

The vasculitides usually are generalized, although they may be limited to the nerve, muscle, or central nervous system.[48,49] Thus, when
a vascular disease is suspected in a patient with
polyneuropathy, a sural nerve biopsy will (in
most cases) substantiate the diagnosis.[50]

The treatment of choice for the vasculitis
neuropathies is high-dose steroids.[47] It is frequently necessary to add cyclophosphamide or
other immunosuppressive agents to the regimen
to achieve a maximum therapeutic effect.[51]

Toxic and Metabolic Neuropathies Various
drugs, heavy metals, and industrial agents that
cause neuropathies are listed in Table 7-4.

These agents can cause a polyneuropathy.
Demyelination may be marked (as with lead intoxication) or relatively minor (as with acrylamide). Some toxins primarily affect small pain,
temperature, and autonomic fibers (Kepone);

in combination with polyneuropathy. A frequently encountered diagnostic difficulty is distinguishing neuropathy as a remote effect of
cancer from a direct invasion of a nerve, especially nerve roots, by tumor cells. The latter
complication is virtually limited to metastatic
carcinoma and lymphoma, particularly histio-
cytic lymphoma.[44]

Many chemotherapeutic agents used in the
treatment of cancer also are potent neurotoxins
that may produce a polyneuropathy or, minimally, a loss of myotatic reflexes.

Vascular Disease and Neuropathy Scattered
peripheral nerve infarcts produce a clinical picture of mononeuropathy multiplex, which in diabetes mainly affects the femoral, sciatic, or
cranial nerves. Severe, peripheral vascular disease will cause numbness in the extremities, but
only after the disease has progressed to the pre-
gangrenous stage and all tissues are suffering
the consequences of ischemia.[45,46]

Generalized vasculitis can produce either a
mononeuropathy multiplex or a symmetric, distal polyneuropathy; the latter is often a sequela
of the former.[17,47]

TABLE 7-4 Chemical Agents Causing
Neuropathies

Medications
Isoniazid, nitrofurantoin, cytotoxic agents (especially vincristine), phenytoin, chloramphenicol,
disulfiram, amitriptyline, hydralazine, dapsone,
thalidomide, glutethimide.

Heavy metals
Lead, thallium, mercury, arsenic, gold.

Industrial agents
Acrylamide, organophosphorus compounds,
carbon disulfide, trichloroethylene, n-hexane,
carbon monoxide, methyl bromide, DDT, Lin-
dane, PCBs, carbon tetrachloride, dichloro-
phenoxyacetic acid (2,4-D), pentachloro-
phenolate, methyl n-butyl ketone, 2,5
hexanedione, kepone, hexachloraphene,
triethyltin.

some, predominantly motor fibers (Dapsone, lead). Some toxins have a predilection for certain nerves, such as that of lead for radial nerves, or trichloroethylene, which mainly affects the trigeminal nerve. The majority of toxic agents cause a mixed sensorimotor polyneuropathy with varied involvement of other organ systems.[52–54]

Chronic neuropathies due to metabolic derangements (uremia, porphyria, hypothyroidism) are pathologically indistinct from those caused by toxins, including alcohol. The precise biochemical events leading to the degeneration of nerves is similarly unclear.[55–57] In all cases of chronic neuropathy due to toxic or metabolic causes, there is a predominantly distal, random dropout of nerve fibers with varying degrees of demyelination.

Clinically, the toxic metabolic neuropathies initially cause sensory symptoms, usually beginning in the feet and spreading to the hands and more proximal areas as the pathology progresses. An early manifestation may be the onset of isolated compression palsies (particularly carpal tunnel syndrome and ulnar groove compression) to which patients with chronic polyneuropathies are notoriously susceptible. A complaint of severe discomfort in the feet, usually described as a burning sensation, is a frequently early complaint and may be intensified by the application of only light stimuli or the placement of the foot upon the floor. Other sensations include a "heavy" or "wooden" feeling in the feet and legs. These same sensations frequently accompany the neuropathies of diabetes, alcoholism, and vitamin deficiency. With further progression, the motor system becomes involved with atrophy of the distal muscles and complaints of weakness. The loss of reflexes, again predominantly distal, may reflect a degeneration of muscle spindle-afferent fibers rather than a loss of motor fibers per se.

Electrodiagnosis

The electrodiagnosis of a chronic peripheral neuropathy will invariably reveal evidence of denervation when needle electrodes are inserted into the small muscles of the hands and feet. With advancing diseases, more proximal muscles may be affected, although involvement of the hip or shoulder girdle musculature is more typical of a nerve infarction, root disease, or plexus pathology. With nerve conduction techniques, absent or small amplitude potentials can be demonstrated in distal muscles, which reflects the dropout of motor nerve fibers. Nerve conduction velocity measured in the calf, forearm, and so on is either normal, borderline, or mildly reduced. In neuropathies that are primarily demyelinating, such as GB syndrome or chronic relapsing polyneuropathy, the conduction velocities may be markedly reduced. This is a finding that is helpful in narrowing the range of diagnostic possibilities. The interpretation of such tests must allow for the relatively slower conduction velocities and lower-evoked potential amplitudes found in elderly persons.[58]

Nerve Root Compression
(Spondylotic Radiculopathy)

Although nerve roots can be affected by numerous processes causing pain and neurologic dysfunction (e.g., tumors, trauma, viruses, diabetes), by far the most common cause of nerve root problems in elderly persons is spondylosis. The generally accepted cause of symptoms in both cervical and lumbar radiculopathy is encroachment on the intervertebral foramen by degenerated disc material, osteophytic spurs, or other hyperplastic or hypertrophic connective tissue. Other mechanisms, such as traction, angulation, or inflammation of the nerves, may also play a role.[59] Nerve root compression syndromes usually involve cervical roots C5-T1 and lumbar roots L4-S1. Each syndrome is associated with specific neurologic symptoms and signs, which are subject to interpatient variation because of slight differences in the segmental level of innervation.[1,60–62] Thus, the diagnosis and localization of spondylotic nerve root compression is mainly clinical, with the predominant presenting symptom being neck or back pain.

With cervical root compression, the pain usually is more severe on one side and may be aggravated by tilting the head to that side (Spurling's sign), an action causing a further narrowing of the involved intervertebral foramen. When multiple nerve roots are involved, the neck pain may be diffuse, bilateral, and associated with chronic, occipital, muscle-contraction type headaches. With acute nerve root compression, as with herniated disc material, there usually is a radiation of pain into the shoulder, scapular region, and (occasionally) the anterior chest (the latter simulates referred cardiac pain). Paresthesia in the appropriate dermatomal distribution is the most common sensory complaint, with actual anesthesia being rare. Absence or diminution of the myotatic reflexes helps to localize the lesion (C7-C8 for the triceps and C5-C6 for the biceps and brachioradialis). Manual testing may reveal a weakness in muscles innervated by the involved nerve root(s).

The picture of pain, paresthesia, weakness, and reflex change also is characteristic of lumbar nerve root compression. The pain is frequently worse on one side of the lumbosacral area. It may radiate to the hip, buttock, thigh, leg, or even the foot. The pain is made worse by movement, by coughing or sneezing, or by various maneuvers that stretch the involved roots (straight-leg raise, neck flexion, pressure over the sciatic notch, and so on). The knee jerk reflex (L3-L4) or the ankle jerk reflex (S1-S2) may be diminished or absent. Rarely, when multiple roots are involved or there is cauda equina compression from stenosis of the bony canal (Verbiest's syndrome), urinary and anal sphincter function may be compromised.[2] When this finding is present, however, another diagnosis (such as a tumor of the lumbar spinal canal) should be considered. As mentioned earlier, cervical spondylosis includes signs of nerve root and spinal cord dysfunction, either separately or together, and for this reason a diagnosis of motor neuron disease may be suggested.

Radiologic investigation is helpful in localizing the vertebral level of involvement. Narrowing of the intervertebral foramina on oblique projections in cervical x-ray films correlates with the level of root involvement. Lumbar spine x-ray films may reveal a narrowing of the intervertebral distance at the level of disc herniation. A myelogram with oil or water-soluble contrast media is generally performed in patients whose course is sufficiently severe to warrant surgical intervention, or in those whom the diagnosis is in doubt. Recently, CT scans have been used as an alternative to myelography with encouraging results, particularly in the lumbar region.[63]

Electromyography is useful, not only in identifying the diseased nerve root but in separating at an early stage root lesions that cause denervation from those in which weakness is due only to mild compression (neurapraxia). Such information is important in determining the need for surgical intervention.

Spondylosis commonly affects older persons, the incidence of disease being relatively small prior to 50 years of age. Males are more commonly affected than females. Mainstays of conservative therapy include bed rest, heat, muscle relaxants, anti-inflammatory compounds, and (most important in the case of cervical radiculopathy) traction.

Plexopathy

Diseases of the brachial or lumbosacral plexuses are uncommon and may have various causes.[64,65] The clinical presentation may be one of pain in the shoulder or buttock, with signs of patchy neurologic dysfunction in the extremities reminiscent of multiple radiculopathy. Alternatively, the clinical picture may be one of a painless wasting of an extremity, which suggests a "focal" motor neuron disease or a spinal cord tumor. Symptoms may be acute, subacute, or chronic and insidious. In elderly persons, the most common causes of plexopathy are diabetes mellitus, direct invasion by cancer, radiation "plexitis" resulting from cancer therapy, or traction injury due to either trauma or prolonged stretching (e.g., shoulder hyperabduction) during surgical procedures. Various other causes of plexopathies in elderly persons are listed as follows:

Diabetic "amyotrophy"—most commonly affects distribution of the femoral nerve
Tumor infiltration, particularly carcinoma at the apex of the lung
Radiation injury
Trauma
Autoimmune (postvaccinal) plexitis
Idiopathic plexopathy
Viral plexitis (varicella-zoster? coxsackie?)
Outlet syndrome (e.g., compression of the lower brachial plexus by a cervical rib or band; compression of the sciatic portion of the lumbosacral plexus by the fibrotic pyriformis muscle)

Mononeuropathies

Isolated nerve palsies (mononeuropathies) that affect individual nerves are common in patients with a pre-existing polyneuropathy, particularly elderly persons who are often suffering from a chronic disease, diabetes, vitamin deficiency, multiple neurotoxic medications, or cachexia due to various causes. In such patients, a slight, additional nerve trauma at points of pressure or angulation causes a local demyelination and loss of axons, which leads to varying degrees of weakness, sensory loss, and pain. A number of well-recognized syndromes have been described; two of the most common are carpal tunnel syndrome and ulnar elbow-compression palsy. Both of these syndromes, if severe, can cause a marked impairment of hand function as a result of muscle wasting and can be corrected by relatively minor surgical procedures. In addition, the symptoms of the mononeuropathies are particularly protean and may masquerade as other disease processes (e.g., carpal tunnel syndrome may present as a shoulder pain, and thoracic intercostal neuropathy may simulate an abdominal visceral pathology).[21,66] Foot drop due to compression of the common peroneal nerve at the head of the fibula is another common neuropathy in elderly persons. It is likely to occur after a severe weight loss, which causes a loss of protective subcutaneous fat, and renders the nerve liable to compression (particularly in patients who habitually cross their legs).

Most mononeuropathies cause a mixed sensory and motor dysfunction; but some, such as meralgia paresthetica (compression of the lateral-femoral cutaneous nerve in the region of the anterior-superior iliac spine), cause a pure sensory syndrome that may produce such severe pain as to cause patients to seek emergency attention.[66,67] Individual cranial nerves also may be affected. Nerve conduction tests can be helpful in identifying the involved nerves and sites of compression. These conditions often can be ameliorated by treatment of the underlying disease process, by physical therapy, or by administration of medications aimed at attenuating neurogenic pain (e.g., tricyclic antidepressants, carbamazepine, or phenytoin).

In some patients, multiple mononeuropathies—both chronic and recurrent—may occur.[66,68] This picture, so-called mononeuritis or mononeuropathy multiplex, is associated with certain diseases (see Table 7-5) and its presence may be helpful diagnostically.[69]

TABLE 7-5   Causes of Mononeuropathy Multiplex

Diabetes mellitus

Systemic lupus erythematosis

Sarcoidosis

Vasculitides
  Progressive systemic sclerosis, polyarteritis nodosa, rheumatoid arthritis, giant cell arteritis, Sjogren's syndrome, mixed connective tissue disease

Granulomatous angiitis
  Wegener's granulomatosis, allergic granulomatosis, tuberculoid leprosy

Amyloidosis

Waldenstrom's macroglobulinemia

Viral neuritis
  Epstein-Barr virus, Varicella-Zoster virus

Of interest is the specificity by which certain cranial nerves are affected by certain diseases; for example, the facial nerve in sarcoidosis, the trigeminal nerve in several "connective tissue" diseases, and the oculomotor nerve in diabetes.

Diagnosis of Neuropathies
The serum chemistry profile, peripheral smear and red blood cell indices, sedimentation rate, serum protein electrophoresis, glucose tolerance test, thyroid functions, Vitamin B-12 and folate levels, and CSF examination are all important in the evaluation of neuropathies. In addition, testing of cellular immunity and a search for occult cancer may be indicated in specific cases. A practical knowledge of the neurotoxicity of commonly used medications and the careful taking of a toxic exposure history may occasionally lead to a diagnosis.

Nerve biopsy (usually the sural nerve) may be useful when the suspected diagnosis is vasculitis, sarcoidosis, amyloidosis, hypothyroidism, leprosy, chronic demyelinating neuropathy, or other severe and progressive neuropathies of unknown etiology.

In addition to localizing the lesion in isolated mononeuropathies, nerve conduction testing may identify the type of polyneuropathy (axonal versus demyelinating). Similarly, an electromyographic examination may be useful in separating neuropathies from radiculopathies and in identifying the particular nerve roots, trunks, or cords involved.

Muscle Disease

Diseases of the skeletal muscles are generically subsumed under the designation of myopathies. The hallmark of myopathic disease is weakness without a loss of sensation. Thus, the differential diagnosis of myopathies includes only two other categories of neurologic disease: disorders of the neuromuscular junction and motor system diseases (broadly including motor neuron diseases and "pure" motor neuropathies). Another common symptom (or sign) of muscle disease is symmetric muscle wasting. Attaching diagnostic significance to muscle wasting in elderly persons, of course, means taking into account the degree of weight loss and cachexia relating to a patient's general health. In polymyositis, muscle pain also may be a significant complaint. Two major categories of muscle diseases are of importance in elderly persons: inflammatory and metabolic.

Inflammatory Myopathies (*see also* Volume I, Chapter 19)

In older patients, the most common inflammatory myopathies are polymyositis and dermatomyositis, which usually appear in the 5th and 6th decades. These diseases begin with a variety of symptoms, which include fever, malaise, or non-specific gastrointestinal complaints. In dermatomyositis, the characteristic rash, if present, allows a diagnosis to be made with confidence. Diffuse aches and pains are present to a greater or lesser degree, particularly in the larger muscles. There is usually pain on palpation of the muscles. Weakness usually begins over the course of several weeks, but it may be more acute, thus rendering the patient unable to walk within a matter of days. A frequent complaint is the inability to hold an extremity in a prolonged antigravity position, such as the arm over the head when brushing the hair. The natural history of dermatomyositis and polymyositis is variable, with extremes ranging from a complete remission to a prolonged disease and death in a matter of months due to inanition and respiratory failure.[70] Esophageal and cardiac involvement, the latter causing arrhythmias, are not uncommon.[70,71]

A diagnosis of inflammatory myopathy rests, in addition to the clinical picture, on the demonstration of elevated serum "muscle" enzymes (especially creatine kinase). These enzymes may, however, be within the normal range during inactive or mild phases of the disease. The erythrocyte sedimentation rate (ESR) may be elevated, which also parallels the activity of the disease. Electromyogram (EMG) examination gives the most helpful information during active phases of the diseases, showing abundant fibrillations, high-frequency discharges, and sharp waves. While not specific for polymyositis, the additional finding of short-duration, polyphasic motor units and abnormal recruitment is highly suggestive of the disease.[72] On taking a muscle biopsy specimen, similar inflammatory changes are seen in polymyositis and dermatomyositis, with an infiltration of leukocytes into endomysial connective tissue.[73] Apart from a rash, perifascicular muscle fiber atrophy, which appears to be more prominent in dermatomyositis than in polymyositis, represents a pathologic distinction between two otherwise clinically similar muscle diseases.

There is a frequent association between polymyositis/dermatomyositis and "collagen-vascular" diseases such as systemic lupus erythematosis, Sjogren's syndrome, and scleroderma. In an older patient, the association between cancer and myositis, especially dermatomyositis, is well recognized. The association is most often with bronchogenic carcinoma, is rarely seen in patients under 40 years of age, and is greatest (10–50%) in older patients.[56] When dermatomyositis is associated with a malignancy, improvement following treatment of the tumor has been described.[74]

Polymyositis or dermatomyositis should be initially treated with prednisone in doses of 1–2 mg/kg per day. Some clinicians prefer to add various immunosuppressive drugs to this regimen, including azathioprine, cyclophosphamide, and even methotrexate (irrespective of an association with malignancy).[70] Treatment is based on a monitoring of symptoms and signs; creatine kinase levels; and the erythrocyte sedimentation rate.

Polymyalgia rheumatica, another muscular disease of elderly persons, also affects females more frequently than males. This disease, unlike polymyositis, is poorly defined, pathologically, and presents with pain, aching, and stiffness out of proportion to the actual weakness.

Arthralgia, weight loss, fever, and depression may be present. The single most useful laboratory abnormality is an elevated sedimentation rate (ESR), although this finding may not always be present. A striking association exists between polymyalgia rheumatica and temporal (giant cell) arteritis. Identification of the latter disease is important, not only because of the severe headaches encountered but also because of the potential for blindness caused by an occlusion of ophthalmic vessels. Treatment with prednisone causes a dramatic response with a rapid abolition of symptoms, and it also protects against visual impairment.[70,75]

Although less common in civilized countries, parasitic infections (trichinosis, cysticercosis from Taenia solium, and toxoplasmosis) may cause severe inflammatory myopathy.

Transient myositis due to viral infection, especially influenza, is well recognized; however, the role of other viruses, such as coxsackie B, in myopathic disease may be underestimated.[70] Although a myopathy is associated with sarcoidosis, most patients having this complication are probably asymptomatic.

Metabolic Myopathies

This category includes a vast number of disorders with heterogeneous clinical pictures. A list of metabolic causes of myopathies in older patients is given in Table 7-6.

Metabolic myopathies are characterized by a proximal weakness without sensory loss. The weakness may be fixed or slowly progressive. Fatigue, aching, and cramps during or following exercise are common complaints. Occasionally, myoglobinuria may be present, for example, following a bout of alcoholic binge drinking.

Most metabolic myopathies, in contradistinction to polymyositis, are mild and may be overlooked in the presence of more severe medical complications. Myasthenia-like weakness or actual myasthenia gravis may coexist with several of the metabolic myopathies, especially dysthroid and drug-induced syndromes, and should be suspected when severe weakness or respiratory distress is present.

Muscle weakness may result from a serum potassium imbalance caused, for example, by diuretics, vomiting, or hyperaldosteronism. The episodic weakness caused by heredi-

TABLE 7-6   Metabolic Myopathies in Elderly Persons

Endocrine disturbances
  Hyperthyroidism
  Hypothyroidism
  Hyperparathyroidism
  Cushing's syndrome
  Addison's disease
Toxic myopathies
  Alcoholism
  Drug-induced (corticosteroids, mineralocorticoids, aminoglycosides, β-blockers, chloroquine, diuretics, clofibrate, epsilon-aminocaproic acid, vinca alkaloids, cimetidine, lithium, tricyclics, chlorpromazine, anticonvulsants, penicillamine, monoamine oxidase inhibitors, inhalational anesthetics, succinylcholine)
  Industrial toxins
Disturbances of potassium balance or transport
  Hereditary periodic paralysis
  Acquired potassium imbalance
Abnormalities of mitochondrial function
  Luft's disease
  Oculocraniosomatic muscular dystrophy
  (Kearns-Sayre syndrome)

tary periodic paralysis is thought to be due to an abnormal transport of electrolytes across the sarcolemmal membrane and may be associated with decreased, increased, or normal serum potassium levels. All forms of periodic paralysis can be treated with acetozolamide, which diminishes the frequency and severity of the attacks.[76] Episodic weakness identical to periodic paralysis, except for the lack of an identifiable hereditary pattern, also has been described as occurring with thyrotoxicosis. As a rule, hereditary forms of periodic paralysis begin in adolescence or in the 3rd decade. The symptoms tend to diminish in severity with advancing age, except in those cases where episodic paralysis is replaced by a permanent proximal weakness typical of any metabolic myopathy.

A rare cause of skeletal muscle weakness associated with a hypermetabolic state and normal thyroid functions is Luft's disease, which is thought to be due to an intramitochondrial uncoupling of oxidative phosphorylation.[70] Oculocraniosomatic neuromuscular disease of Kearns and Sayre (also thought to represent mitochondrial metabolic dysfunction) is somewhat more common, may be present in the elderly patient, and is distinctive for the easily recognizable syndrome of retinitis pigmentosa, heart block, and ophthalmoplegia.[70]

Most metabolic myopathies respond, or at least stabilize on treatment of the underlying medical condition or withdrawal of the offending drug.

A diagnosis of chronic metabolic myopathy may be aided by an EMG, particularly when polyphasic potentials and typical short-duration, low-amplitude abundant motor units are recorded. However, the EMG usually reveals non-specific abnormalities or supportive, rather than diagnostic, evidence of a myopathy.

A muscle biopsy specimen gives variable findings in metabolic myopathy. The most common findings are architectural changes in muscle histology with a slight variation in fiber size, basophilic staining, nuclear rearrangement, and "moth-eaten" or frankly necrotic fibers. The periodic paralyses, thyrotoxicosis, hypokalemia, and acute alcoholic myopathy show vacuolar degeneration of the muscle. Cushing's syndrome, steroid myopathy, and disuse atrophy from any cause will result in a selective loss of type II fibers. A muscle biopsy specimen in disorders of mitochondrial metabolism may show an abundance of so-called "ragged red fibers," which are characteristic of that group of disorders.

An uncommon but serious myopathic disorder may accompany a malignant hyperpyrexia. This condition usually accompanies surgery and is associated with halothane and succinylcholine administration. Generally, temperature elevation and increased muscle tone (especially masseter muscles) is noticed during or shortly after induction of anesthesia. Unless rapidly treated, there is an explosive rise in temperature accompanied by muscular rigidity, acidosis, rhabdomyolysis, and usually death. Treatment consists of cooling measures, steroid administration, and a reversal of acidosis. Administration of dantrolene sodium, 7–10 mg/kg given intravenously, also has been suggested.[70]

Disorders of Neuromuscular Transmission

It is difficult to estimate the true incidence/prevalence of disorders affecting the neuromuscular junction. The prevalence of myasthenia gravis (MG) has been estimated to be 0.5–5 per 100,000, but a large number of undiagnosed individuals are suspected to be affected.[77] In patients over 40 years of age, the incidence of MG is the same for both sexes, whereas in younger age groups there is a marked preponderance of female sufferers outnumbering male patients 3:1 or 4:1. Although the highest incidence is in the third decade, a second incidence peak occurs in the seventh decade, often associated with thymoma. The myasthenic syndrome of Eaton and Lambert (ELS) occurs principally in elderly persons because of the association with cancer and, in particular, with small cell carcinoma of the lung.[78] A third category is drug-induced disorders of neuromuscular transmission, which are particularly likely to occur in elderly persons, perhaps because of the greater probability of the use of an offending drug and the higher frequency of factors that lower the safety margin for neuromuscular transmission (e.g., electrolyte imbalances).

Myasthenia Gravis (MG)

Normal neuromuscular transmission depends on the occurrence of an orderly sequence of steps. First, the release of an adequate number of molecules of acetylcholine (ACh) from the prejunctional nerve terminal must occur in response to an action potential. Second, the ACh molecules must cross the neuromuscular junction and interact with receptors on the postsynaptic membrane of the motor end-plate. Third, interactions between ACh molecules and receptors on the postsynaptic membrane must generate small potentials (miniature end-plate potentials [MEPPS]) that summate electrically to produce a sufficient shift in the resting membrane potential (threshold voltage), which causes a depolarization (action potential) of the muscle membrane and a subsequent contraction of the muscle.

In MG, there is a reduction in the number of active ACh receptors on the postsynaptic membrane. In addition, there is a loss of the normal number of folds or convolutions within the postsynaptic membrane. These pathologic changes are probably mediated immunologically. Although alterations of both cellular and humoral immunity can be demonstrated, the salient laboratory abnormality of practical importance is the presence of circulating ACh receptor antibodies in 80% of MG patients.[79]

The clinical hallmark of MG is episodic weakness. In 50% of MG patients, the initial symptoms involve the eyes, causing ptosis or diplopia. In another one third of MG patients, the first symptoms may involve other bulbar muscles, which causes difficulty in swallowing, speaking, chewing, or holding up the chin. A smaller group of patients will have a generalized weakness as the first symptom. Fatigability, the second most characteristic feature of MG, may become apparent when muscle strength returns following a short rest, only to be replaced by weakness after a few minutes of exercise.

The diagnosis of MG rests upon the presence of the typical clinical features, but several diagnostic tests are helpful. These are the resolution of objective weakness (such as ptosis on sustained upgaze) following the intravenous (IV) injection of edrophonium chloride (Tensilon), a rapidly acting inhibitor of acetylcholinesterase, or the demonstration of an abnormal electrical decrement recorded from an affected skeletal muscle (especially several minutes after exercise) on repetitive stimulation of the motor nerve supplying that muscle.

Treatment of MG, based on our knowledge of its pathogenesis, is designed to increase the probability of neuromuscular transmission by facilitating the effect of available ACh. Accordingly, any one of several acetylcholinesterase inhibitors is used; the most common one is pyridostigmine (Mestinon) given in divided doses ranging from 120–600 mg/day. In patients with a more severe disease, treatment must be directed at the immune system by using steroids, occasionally with immunosuppressives such as azathioprine. Obviously, malignant thymoma, which is present in approximately 10% of all patients with MG, is a mandatory indication for thymectomy. Myasthenic crisis (profound generalized weakness with potential respiratory compromise) usually occurs in a setting of diminishing anticholinesterase benefit and is best managed by solicitous attention to respiratory function with frequent bedside spirometry, transfer to the intensive care unit when vital capacity drops below 15 ml/kg of body weight, and (if necessary) intubation and ventilation until the crisis is resolved. Assiduous prevention of electrolyte imbalances, administration of steroids/immunosuppressives, and particularly plasmapheresis, all can be of value in the management of myasthenic crisis. It should be noted that there is much individual variation and controversy surrounding the treatment of MG, particularly regarding the need for timing of the thymectomy and management of the crisis. The above outline should be taken as an introduction to aspects of treatment with more detailed information being sought elsewhere.[77]

Eaton Lambert Syndrome (ELS)

The myasthenic syndrome of Eaton and Lambert also is characterized by weakness. Clinically, however, there are several notable features of ELS that are not seen in MG. First, the weakness is more characteristically progressive than episodic. Second, although bulbar muscles may be affected (most commonly ptosis), it is most characteristic for generalized weakness to occur that affects, primarily, proximal limb muscles, especially in the lower extremity. Third, the response of patients with ELS to anticholinesterases, unlike MG, is frequently only fair to nil. Finally, there are other symptoms that occur with variable frequency, such as a dry mouth and paresthesias; the latter represents a polyneuropathy with which the disease is associated.

The most striking clinical feature of ELS is its association with malignant neoplasms. The most common tumor is small cell carcinoma of the lung, although other carcinomas have been described. In many patients (perhaps as many as 50%), a tumor cannot be found even after a diligent search. However, it must be realized that the onset of weakness may precede discovery of a tumor by months or even years.

In ELS, as in MG, there is a failure of neuromuscular transmission. This failure occurs, however, because of an ineffective release of ACh from the presynaptic nerve terminal, rather than a loss of receptors in the postsynaptic membrane. The pathogenesis of ELS is not understood, although the production by the tumor of a blocking substance or antibody that interferes with a calcium-mediated release of ACh has been postulated. Although no humoral factor has been consistently identified in ELS, a diagnosis can be established by repetitive nerve stimulation, which reveals a diminished muscle action potential following a single shock and markedly incrementing potentials during repetitive rapid shocks.

Both MG and ELS patients are exquisitely sensitive to the administration of drugs that interfere with normal neuromuscular transmission. Indeed, the first manifestation of weakness may be a prolonged respiratory paralysis following the administration of a neuromuscular blocking agent during surgery. As mentioned previously, patients with ELS have only a modest improvement with anticholinesterase. Some symptomatic relief can be obtained by administration of quanidine hydrochloride, which augments the release of ACh from the peripheral nerve terminals. In general, the prognosis of ELS is poor, although a brief recovery from weakness has been reported following removal of the tumor. Plasmapheresis also has been reported to decrease the weakness, but only transiently; numerous exchanges were required before improvement occurred.[80]

Drugs Causing Myasthenic Weakness

Many drugs will unmask MG or make a patient with diagnosed MG weaker by interfering with neuromuscular transmission. Occasionally, these medications will induce a myasthenic weakness in an otherwise normal individual.

TABLE 7-7   Drugs that Induce a Myasthenic Syndrome

Antibiotics
   colistin, clindamycin, kanamycin, lincomycin, neomycin, streptomycin, tobramycin, tetracyclines, polymyxin B
Cardiovascular drugs
   lidocaine, quinidine, trimethaphan, procainamide, propranolol, oxprenolol, practolol
Antiheumatic drugs
   chloroquine, D-penicillamine
Psychotropic drugs
   lithium, phenelzine, promazine, chlorpromazine
Anticonvulsants
   phenytoin, trimethadione
Hormones
   ACTH, corticosteroids, thyroid hormones, oral contraceptives
Others
   aprotinin, acetylcholinesterase inhibitors, oxytocin, methoxyflurane, tetanus antitoxin

This occurrence of myasthenic weakness following the administration of one of these medications should, however, alert the clinician to the possibility of pre-existing MG. The medications most frequently responsible are antibiotics, particularly aminoglycosides. A partial list of offending drugs is given in Table 7-7.[81]

References

1. Brain WR, Northfield DWC, Wilkinson M: Neurological manifestations of cervical spondylosis. *Brain* 75:187–192, 1952.
2. Wilson CB: Neurogenic claudication, in Weinstein PR, Eni G, Wilson CB (eds): *Lumbar Spondylosis*. Chicago, Year Book Medical Publishers, 1977, pp 134–145.
3. Ruff RL, Dougherty JH: Evaluation of acute cerebral ischemia for anticoagulation therapy: computed tomography or lumbar puncture. *Neurology (NY)* 31:736–740, 1981.
4. Juergens SM, Kurland LT: Epidemiology, in Mulder DW (ed): *The Diagnosis and Treatment of Amyotrophic Lateral Sclerosis*. Boston, Houghton Mifflin Co, 1980, pp 35–51.
5. Adams RA, Victor M: Diseases of the nervous system due to nutritional deficiency, in *Principles of Neurology*. New York, McGraw-Hill Book Co, 1981, pp 718–719.
6. Farmer TW: Neurologic complications of vitamin and mineral disorders, in Baker AB, Baker LH (eds): *Clinical Neurology*. Philadelphia, Harper & Row Publishers Inc, 1979, chap 42, p 2.
7. Adams RA, Victor M: Diseases of the spinal cord, in *Principles of Neurology*. New York, McGraw-Hill Book Co, 1981, chap 35, p 638.
8. Vieth RG, Odon GL: Extradural spinal metastases and their neurosurgical treatment. *J Neurosurg* 3:501–508, 1965.
9. Weiss HD: Neoplasms in, Samuels MD (ed): *Manual of Neurologic Therapeutics,* ed 1. Boston, Little Brown & Co, 1978, pp 215–245.
10. Gilbert RW, Kim J, Posner JB: Epidural spinal cord compression from metastatic tumor: diagnosis and treatment. *Ann Neurol* 3:40–51, 1981.
11. Posner JB, Howieson J, Cvitkovic E: "Disappearing" spinal cord compression: oncolytic effect of glucocorticoids (and other chemotherapeutic agents) on epidural metastases. *Ann Neurol* 2:409–413, 1977.
12. Norris FH: Remote effects of cancer on the spinal cord, in, Vinken PJ, Bruyn GW (eds): *Handbook of Clinical Neurology*. Elsevier Press, North-Holland. 1979, vol 38, chap 27, pp 669–677.

13. Victor M: The effects of nutritional deficiency on the nervous system: a comparison with the effects of carcinoma, in Brain WR, Norris FH (eds): *The Remote Effects of Cancer on the Nervous System*. New York, Grune & Stratton, 1965, pp 134–161.

14. Godwin-Austen RB, Howell DA, Worthington B: Observations on radiation myelopathy. *Brain* 98:557–568, 1975.

15. Mancall EL, Rosales RK: Necrotizing myelopathy associated with visceral carcinoma. *Brain* 87:639–656, 1964.

16. Richardson EP: Case records of the Massachusetts General Hospital. *N Eng J Med* 294:26, 1447–1454, 1976.

17. Asbury AK, Johnson PC: Diabetic neuropathies, in, *Pathology of Peripheral Nerve*. Philadelphia, WB Saunders & Co, 1978, pp 96–109.

18. Thomas PK, Eliasson SG: Diabetic neuropathy, in Dyck PJ, Thomas PK, Lambert EH (eds): *Peripheral Neuropathy*. Philadelphia, WB Saunders & Co, 1975, pp 956–981.

19. Raff MC, Sangalang V, Asbury AK: Ischemic mononeuropathy multiplex associated with diabetes mellitus. *Arch Neurol* 18:487–489, 1968.

20. Asbury AK, Aldredge H, Hershberg R, et al: Oculomotor palsy in diabetes mellitus: a clinico-pathologic study. *Brain* 93:555–560, 1970.

21. Sun SF, Streib EW: Diabetic thoracoabdominal neuropathy: clinical and electrodiagnostic features. *Ann Neurol* 9:75–79, 1981.

22. Aguayo AJ: Neuropathy due to compression and entrapment, in Dyck PJ, Thomas PK, Lambert EH (eds): *Peripheral Neuropathy*. Philadelphia, WB Saunders, 1975, pp 688–713.

23. Ellenberg M: Diabetic neuropathic cachexia. *Diabetes* 23:418–423, 1974.

24. Thorsteinsson G, et al: Transcutaneous electrical stimulation: a double-blind trial of its efficacy for pain. *Arch Phys Med Rehab* 58:8–13, 1977.

25. Davis JL, Lewis SB, Gerich JE, et al: Peripheral diabetic neuropathy treated with amitriptyline and fluphenazine. *JAMA* 238:2291–2292, 1971.

26. Turkington RW: Depression masquerading as diabetic neuropathy. *JAMA* 243:1147–1150, 1980.

27. Asbury AK, Johnson PC: Metabolic and toxic polyneuropathies, in *Pathology of Peripheral Nerve*. Philadelphia, WB Saunders & Co, 1978, p 86.

28. Asbury AK, Johnson PC: Acute idiopathic polyneuritis and related disorders, in *Pathology of Peripheral Nerve*. Philadelphia, WB Saunders & Co, 1978, p 20.

29. Asbury AK: Diagnostic considerations in Guillain-Barre syndrome. *Ann Neurol* 9(suppl):1–5, 1981.

30. (Announcement) Criteria for diagnosis of Guillain-Barre syndrome. *Ann Neurol* 3(suppl 6):565–566, 1978.

31. Fisher CM: An unusual variant of acute idiopathic polyneuritis (syndrome of ophthalmoplegia, ataxia and areflexia). *N Engl J Med* 255:57–65, 1956.

32. Lichtenfeld P: Autonomic dysfunction in the Guillain-Barre syndrome. *Am J Med* 50:772–780, 1971.

33. Walshe TM: Disease of nerve and muscle, in Samuels MA (ed): *Manual of Neurologic Therapeutics*. Boston, Little Brown & Co, 1978, pp 368–370.

34. Emmons PR, Blume WT, DuShane JW: Cardiac monitoring and demand pacemaker in the Guillain-Barre syndrome. *Arch Neurol* 32:59–61, 1975.

35. Hughes RAC, Newson-Davis JM, Perkin GD, et al: Controlled trial of prednisone in acute polyneuropathy. *Lancet* 2:750–753, 1978.

36. Hughes RAC: Treatment of acute inflammatory polyneuropathy. *Ann Neurol* 9(suppl):125–132, 1981.

37. Osterman PO, Fagius J, Safwenberg J, et al: Treatment of the Guillain-Barre syndrome by plasmapharesis. *Arch Neurol* 39:148–151, 1982.

38. Dalakas MC, Engel WK: Chronic relapsing (dysimmune) polyneuropathy: pathogenesis and treatment. *Ann Neurol* 9(suppl):134–142, 1981.

39. Asbury AK, Johnson PC: Metabolic and toxic neuropathies, in *Pathology of Peripheral Nerve*. Philadelphia, WB Saunders & Co, 1978, chap 4, pp 80–82.

40. Lisak RP, Zweiman B, Mitchell M, et al: Guillain-Barre syndrome and Hodgkin's disease: three cases with immunologic studies. *Ann Neurol* 1:72–78, 1977.

41. Benson MD, Cohen AS, Brandt KD, et al: Neuropathy, M components and amyloid. *Lancet* 1:10–12, 1975.

42. Adams RA, Victor M: Diseases of peripheral nerves, in *Principles of Neurology*. New York, McGraw-Hill Book Co, 1981, chap 45, p 915.

43. Julien J, Vital C, Vallat J, et al: Polyneuropathy in Waldenstrom's macroglobulinemia. *Arch Neurol* 35:423–425, 1978.

44. Griffin JW, Thompson RW, Mitchinson MJ, et al: Lymphomatous leptomeningitis. *Am J Med* 51:200–208, 1971.

45. Hutchinson EC, Liversedge LA: Neuropathy in peripheral vascular disease: its bearing on diabetic neuropathy. *Quart J Med* 25:267–270, 1956.

46. Daube JR, Dyck PJ: Neuropathy due to peripheral vascular disease, in Dyck PJ, Thomas PK, Lambert EH (eds): *Peripheral Neuropathy*. Phil-

adelphia, WB Saunders & Co, 1975, chap 35, pp 714–733.

47. Moore PA, Fauci AS: Neurologic manifestations of systemic vasculitis: a retrospective and prospective study of the clinicopathologic features and responses to therapy in 25 patients. *Am J Med* 71:517–524, 1981.

48. Tarvik A, Berntzen J. Necrotizing vasculitis without visceral involvement. *Acta Med Scand* 184:69–73, 1968.

49. Cupps TR: Central nervous system vasculitis, in *The Vasculitides. Major Problems in Internal Medicine.* Cupps TR & Fauci AS (eds) Philadelphia, WB Saunders & Co, 1981, vol 21, chap 10, p 123.

50. Wres SJ, Sunwoo IN, Oh SJ: Sural nerve biopsy in systemic necrotizing vasculitis. *Am J Med* 71:525–526, 1981.

51. Fauci AS, Katz P, Haynes BF, et al: Cyclophosphamide therapy of severe, systemic necrotizing vasculitis. *N Engl J Med* 301:235–238, 1979.

52. Le Quesne P: Neuropathy due to drugs, in Dyck PJ, Thomas PK, Lambert EH (eds): *Peripheral Neuropathy.* Philadelphia, WB Saunders & Co, 1975, chap 62, pp 1263–1280.

53. Goldstein NP, McCall JT, Dyck PJ: Metal neuropathy, in Dyck PJ, Thomas PK, Lambert EH (eds): *Peripheral Neuropathy.* Philadelphia, WB Saunders & Co, 1975, chap 61, pp 1227–1262.

54. Hopkins A: Toxic neuropathy due to industrial agents, in Dyck PJ, Thomas PK, Lambert EH (eds): *Peripheral Neuropathy.* Philadelphia, WB Saunders & Co, 1975, chap 60, pp 1207–1226.

55. Asbury AK: Uremic neuropathy, in Dyck PJ, Thomas PK, Lambert EH (eds). *Peripheral Neuropathy.* Philadelphia, WB Saunders & Co, 1975, vol 2, chap 48, pp 982–992.

56. Ridley A: Porphyric neuropathy, in Dyck PJ, Thomas PK, Lambert EH (eds): *Peripheral Neuropathy.* Philadelphia, WB Saunders & Co, 1975, vol 2, chap 46, pp 942–955.

57. Bastron JA: Neuropathy in disease of the thyroid, in Dyck PJ, Thomas PK, Lambert EH (eds): *Peripheral Neuropathy.* Philadelphia, WB Saunders & Co, 1975, vol 2, pp 999–1006.

58. Desmedt JE, Cheron G: Somatosensory evoked potentials to finger stimulation in healthy octogenarians and in young adults: wave forms, scalp topography, and transit times of parietal and frontal components. *Electroenceph Clin Neurophysiol* 50:404–425, 1980.

59. Cailliet R: *Neck and Arm Pain.* Philadelphia, FA Davis, 1981.

60. Keegan TJ: Variations of symptoms with herniation of intervertebral discs. *Nebraska MJ* 43:191, May 1958.

61. Wilkinson M: *Cervical spondylosis,* ed 2. Philadelphia, WB Saunders & Co, 1971.

62. Murphey F, Simmons JCH, Brunson B: Surgical treatment of laterally ruptured cervical disc. *J Neuro Surg* 38:679–683, 1973.

63. Genant AK, Chafetz N, Helms CA: *Computed Tomography of the Lumbar Spine: Diagnostic and Therapeutic Implications for the Radiologist, Orthopedist and Neurosurgeon.* University of California, 1982.

64. Tsairis P, Dyck PJ, Mulder DW: Natural history of brachial plexus neuropathy. *Arch Neurol* 27:109–117, 1972.

65. Sanders BA, Sharp FR: Lumbosacral plexus neuritis. *Neurology (NY)* 31(suppl 4):470. 1981.

66. Kopell HP, Thompson WAL: *Peripheral Entrapment Neuropathies.* Baltimore, Williams & Wilkins Co, 1963.

67. Kitchen C, Simpson J: Meralgia paresthetica: a review of 67 patients. *Acta Neurol Scand* 48:547–555, 1972.

68. Aguayo AJ: Neuropathy due to compression and entrapment, in Dyck PJ, Thomas PK, Lambert EH (eds): *Peripheral Neuropathy.* Philadelphia, WB Saunders & Co, 1975, vol 1, chap 34, pp 688–713.

69. Dyck PJ, Low PA, Stevens JC: Diseases of peripheral nerves, in Baker AB, Baker LH (eds): *Clinical Neurology.* Hagerstown, Harper & Row Publishers Inc, 1971, vol 3, chap 38, pp 1743–1810.

70. Brooke MH: *Clinician's Guide to Neuromuscular Disease.* Baltimore, Williams & Wilkins Co, 1977, pp 138–194.

71. Schaumberg HH, Nielson SL, Yurchak PM: Heartblock in polymyositis with proven involvement of the heart. *N Engl J Med* 284:480–481, 1971.

72. Johnson EW (ed): *Practical electromyography.* Baltimore, Williams & Wilkins Co, 1980, pp 110–134.

73. Dubowitz V, Brook MH: *Muscle Biopsy: A Modern Approach.* Philadelphia, WB Saunders & Co, 1973.

74. Barus BE: Dermatomyositis and malignancy. *Ann Int Med* 84:68–70, 1976.

75. Rowland LP, Layzer RB: Muscular dystrophies, atrophies and related diseases, in Baker AB, Baker LH (eds): *Clinical Neurology.* Hagerstown, Harper & Row Publishers Inc, 1977, chap 37.

76. Griggs RC: The myotonic disorders and periodic paralysis *Adv Neurol* 17:151–161, 1977.

77. Lisak RP, Barchi RL: Myasthenia gravis, in *Problems in Neurology,* Philadelphia, WB Saunders & Co, 1982, vol 11.

78. Eaton LM, Lambert EH: Electromyography and electric stimulation of nerves in diseases of the motor unit: Observations on myasthenic syndrome associated with malignant tumors. *JAMA* 161:1117–1121, 1957.

79. Lindstrom JM, Lambert EH: Content of acetylcholine receptor and antibodies bound to receptor in myasthenia gravis, experimental autoimmune myasthenia gravis, and Eaton-Lambert syndrome. *Neurology (NY)* 28:130–138, 1978.

80. Denys EH, Dau PC, Lindstrom JM: Neuromuscular transmission before and after plasmapheresis in myasthenia gravis and the myasthenic syndrome, in Dau PC (ed): *Plasmapheresis and the Immunobiology of Myasthenia Gravis*. Boston, Houghton Mifflin Co, 1979, pp 248–257.

81. Argov Z, Mastaglia FL: Disorder of neuromuscular transmission caused by drugs. *N Engl J Med* 301:409–414, 1979.

CHAPTER 8

Ophthalmology

LARRY F. RICH, M.S., M.D.

Normal Changes in the Aging Eye

To an elderly person, vision is no less important than it is to a younger individual. Vision may be more crucial to an elderly person, for as aging proceeds and the acuity of other senses becomes blunted, the need for adequate visual orientation increases. Yet, advancing years take their toll on the visual system as well; ocular disease, visual loss, and blindness itself are far more common in elderly persons. The incidence of potentially blinding eye diseases increases dramatically after age 40 and astronomically after age 65. The need for frequent eye examinations increases proportionately.

The physician who treats elderly patients must anticipate visual problems and be aware of the effect that diminished vision has on a patient's capabilities and life style. Nurses, social workers, and paramedical assistants may have an advanced awareness of subtle visual changes in a given patient, because they are in daily contact with that individual. Therefore, communication between all health care personnel is essential.

The ocular system evolves throughout life and certain aging changes are expected and are normal. The distinction between normal aging changes and disease states often is difficult. Nevertheless, the physician must recognize that significant visual loss is not necessarily a part of aging and satisfactory vision may remain throughout an individual's life. An awareness of "normal" changes and their sometimes subtle transformation into frank disease may aid in recognizing, treating, and preventing visual dis-orders in a particular patient and in maintaining an elderly individual's contact with his or her environment so that social withdrawal is prevented.

In elderly persons, as with emaciated individuals, the fat cushion behind the globe of the eye atrophies and produces a recession of the eye into its orbit. This may be exacerbated when the patient assumes a supine position. The skin of the eyelids becomes wrinkled, which in combination with atrophy of orbital fat produces a deepening of the upper lid sulcus. The eyelids become lax, thinner, and may droop. Upper eyelid skin folds may become so flaccid as to obstruct the superior or temporal visual fields.[1]

Normally, the skin and musculature of the eyebrow become lax, compounding the problem of upper eyelid redundancy. With ptosis, the contribution of a sagging eyebrow must be assessed.

The lower eyelid loosens similarly and may actually fall away from the globe, in which case it is definitely abnormal. A more subtle change occurs when the inner puncta no longer lie against the globe and adequate tear drainage is prevented. In these cases, the tears spill over the eyelid margin onto the cheeks (epiphora), compelling the patient to wipe the lower eyelids frequently. If the patient wipes away tears with a laterally directed motion, a greater stretching of the eyelid occurs and the puncta are pulled further away from the globe. Whenever lid laxity is encountered, the physician should encourage the patient to blot the tears medially toward the inner canthus to push the lower eyelid inward, thus preventing a worsening of the problem.

The eyelids may be so loose that they fall away from the globe only when the patient is in a prone position or the head is positioned downward, as in reading. In examining the eyelids of a patient with epiphoria, the physician should attempt to accentuate eyelid abnormalities with prone or downward positioning.

Assessment of eyelid movement during blinking often is overlooked. In some elderly individuals, the blink rate is diminished, particularly in conditions such as Parkinson's disease. Blinking serves two major purposes: 1) It distributes the tear film across the globe, providing nourishment to the ocular surfaces; and 2) It is a vital part of the pumping mechanism in tear drainage. Looseness of the eyelids, malposition of the puncta, alterations of blink frequency, or habits of excessive squeezing of the eyelids interfere with these functions and can lead to true disease states.

The tear film comprises three layers: 1) An inner mucin layer; 2) The middle aqueous layer, which forms the bulk of the tear film; and 3) An outer lipid layer.[2] Any three of these layers may become abnormal, but the most common abnormality of the tear film is a deficiency of the aqueous layer. Physiologically, a diminution of the aqueous component of tears occurs with advancing years. Postmenopausal females are particularly prone to this disorder, which implicates a role of estrogen withdrawal in dryness of the eyes. In milder states, decreased tear production may merely dull the luster of the cornea, causing the commonly observed "loss of gleam" in the eye of an elderly person. In moderate dryness states, the patient may experience a burning sensation, a gritty feeling of the eyes, or a vague ocular discomfort. If dryness is the cause, the symptoms worsen the longer the eyes remain open and are typically most pronounced during the evening hours. In more severe cases, a true keratitis sicca results. Ocular dryness is generally managed with artificial tear preparations.

The conjunctiva, the thin membrane covering the anterior portion of the globe (*see* Figure 8-1), loses its elasticity with age as does the skin, primarily from changes in the collagenous structure of its stroma and the keratinization of the surface. Normally, with age, it becomes yel-

lowed due to fat deposition. Large collections of fatty tissue and hyalinization of the conjunctiva in the interpalbebral fissure vicinity are more common in individuals who have lived or worked outdoors most of their lives. These are actinic changes and, when localized to the conjunctiva, are termed pingueculae; a pterygium is an overgrowth of conjunctiva-like scar tissue beyond the corneoscleral junction (limbus) onto the cornea.

The cornea is the main refracting element of the eye, and changes in its structure may readily influence visual function. Gerontoxin, or arcus senilis, is a peripheral corneal lipid deposition. In its earlier stages, this condition may be noted on examination only when magnification is used. Typically, it is more pronounced superiorly and inferiorly and progresses to a complete ring years later. Also typically, there is a zone of clear cornea, known as the lucid interval, between the lipid deposition and the limbus.[3] The condition is bilateral and symmetrical except when there is a severe, unilateral carotid vascular disease, in which case there is a less prominent arcus senilis on the side of the more compromised blood flow. An obvious arcus should be considered abnormal in an individual younger than 35 years of age and should lead the physician to evaluate the patient's serum triglyceride and cholesterol levels.[3] Arcus senilis can be confused with more severe disorders, such as peripheral corneal thinning and certain ulcerative states; however, these often are accompanied by pain or changes in vision.

The corneal endothelium, which is the innermost monolayer of corneal cells, is most responsible for the maintenance of corneal clarity. Normally, the population density of this cell layer diminishes with age;[4] but if trauma occurs, additional endothelial cells die, and the cornea may eventually decompensate and loose transparency. Loss of corneal endothelial cells due to age alone does not normally lead to corneal decompensation unless these other factors are superimposed.

The sclera, as with the conjunctiva, often becomes the repository for various fats and pigments. This may produce a yellowish or grayish discoloration of the globe. If the deposition is not uniform, a mottled appearance may result.[1] This must be differentiated from scleral thinning, which is an abnormal condition not associated with aging that gives the globe a characteristically blue tinge. Typically, the rigidity of the sclera increases with age, producing a profound impact on the measurement of intraocular pressure.[2,4]

Pressure inside the eye must exceed that of the atmosphere to prevent a collapse of the globe. Normal values of intraocular pressure are between 10–22 mm Hg, but variations (1–2 mm Hg) occur with heartbeats and respirations. Wider swings (2–5 mm Hg) occur as diurnal variations.[2]

Intraocular pressure is determined by the rate of aqueous humor formation in the ciliary body and by aqueous humor outflow, which occurs primarily through the trabecular meshwork into the canal of Schlemm (see Figure 8-1). Hence, maintenance of intraocular pressure is a dynamic process.

With increasing age, the rate of aqueous humor formation decreases slightly, but the resistance to outflow of fluid from the eye increases. Thus, intraocular pressure rises slightly with advancing age but, as a general rule, is remarkably stable.[6]

The depth of the anterior chamber diminishes with age as the lens increases in thickness.[5] Increasing lens thickness does not cause an elevation in intraocular pressure unless the lens has changed rapidly and dramatically, displacing the iris against the trabecular meshwork.[4] Similarly, a tumor inside the eye does not grow fast enough to increase intraocular pressure unless it directly invades the aqueous outflow pathways. A sudden hemorrhage into the eye or into a tumor may alter the pressure.[4]

The lens of the eye is a unique structure with regard to aging. In embryologic life, the lens placode invaginates from the surface ectoderm to form the lens vesicle so that the apices of the cells point inward and their bases are externalized.[4] Unlike other cells of ectodermal origin, such as hair and nail cells, lens fibers derived from these epithelial cells cannot be sloughed off.[4] Rather, they are compacted centrally as the lens continues to grow throughout life with successive annulation of new lens fibers. A dense nucleus of older fibers surrounded by a cortical layer of newer fibers results.

Although it is living, the lens is avascular; its nourishment is derived from the surrounding aqueous humor. Transient changes in a person's health may alter the clarity of growing lens fibers. In this way, isolated opacities result and, if the cataractogenic effect subsides, transparent lens fibers will subsequently be laid

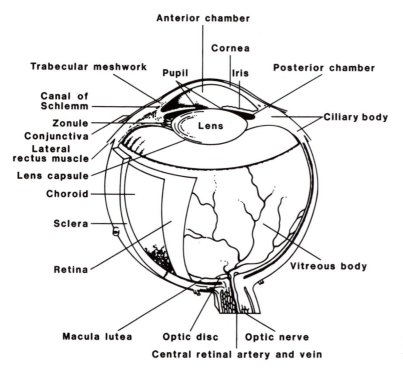

FIGURE 8-1 Internal structures of a normal human eye.

down. The opaque "island" becomes a permanent record of the disturbance; the more superficial the opacity, the more recent its occurrence.

The density of the lens nucleus increases with age due to a loss of water, a compression of older fibers, and a conversion of lower-weight crystalline proteins into higher-weight, insoluble albuminoid proteins. This results in a higher lens weight with increased age; a lens in a 65-year-old may weigh 2 1/2 times more than it did at birth.[4] Transparency decreases with age.

A transparent, homogeneous capsule surrounds the entire lens. Beneath the anterior lens capsule and between the capsule and cortex are the lens epithelial cells, which throughout life migrate peripherally toward the equatorial region where they convert to lens fibers.[4] The lens and its capsule, although not composed of elastin, are in fact elastic; this allows the lens to change shape when accommodating for near vision. During the process of accommodation, the circular fibers of the ciliary body muscle contract, causing a decreased circumference of the muscular ring and less tension on the zonules connecting the ciliary body and lens capsule. Loosening tension on the zonules allows the lens to assume a more spherical-producing, increased anterior-posterior diameter. The greater convexity of the lens in the accommodated state increases its dioptric power, which allows closer objects to come into focus on the retina.[2] With advancing age, the lens becomes less elastic due to an increased density of its nucleus and cortex and a diminished elasticity of the capsule. When the ciliary body muscle contracts in an older individual, the lens is less able to increase convexity, and powers of accommodation are subsequently diminished. Thus, the amplitude of accommodation, which is the amount that the eye can alter its refraction, slowly decreases until it is essentially lost in late middle age (*see* Figure 8-2).[8] As a person ages, the nearest point to which that person can focus gradually recedes. If clear vision is to be maintained, plus-power lenses in the form of reading eyeglasses or bifocals are necessary. This is the result of normal aging changes that slowly, but invariably, occur in every human; the condition is called presbyopia.

The uvea comprises three structures: the iris, ciliary body, and choroid (*see* Figure 8-1). The iris controls the size of the pupillary aper-

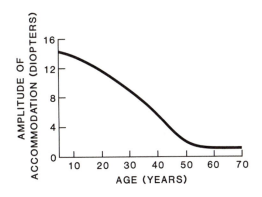

FIGURE 8-2   The amplitude of accommodation versus age.

ture, the average diameter of which gradually increases up to the 15th year of age, but decreases thereafter until the minimal average diameter is reached in the 6th decade.[1] The aged iris thins and rigidifies[5] due to fibrosis and hyalinization. The stroma of the iris atrophies and the posterior pigment layer of the iris degenerates with advancing age.[4]

The ciliary body, which has both secretory and muscular functions, thickens gradually with age. Beginning in middle age, connective tissue accumulation becomes more obvious in histologic sections of otherwise normal eyes.[9] The epithelia of the ciliary processes, which are responsible for secreting aqueous humor, become attenuated with age;[4] the production of aqueous humor concomitantly diminishes.[6]

The choroid is the most posterior portion of the uveal system. Its principal functions are to nourish the outer retina while providing a pathway for vessels that supply the anterior portion of the eye. Bruch's membrane, which is the innermost elastic layer of the choroid lying directly beneath the retina, exhibits the most dramatic changes of all choroidal tissues. Beginning in young adult life, accumulations of granular and filamentous material are found on Bruch's membrane. These changes are more prominent in the macula and the vicinity of the optic nerve and may lead to drusen, which are protruding collections of amorphous granular material between Bruch's membrane and the retina (*see* Figure 8-3).[4] In addition, the vascular elements of the choroid become more sclerotic and rigid with age, the stroma of the

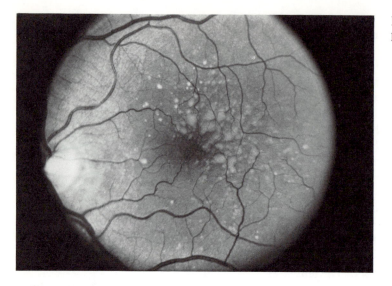

FIGURE 8-3 Ocular fundus in a patient with drusen.

choroid becomes less cellular, and connective tissue increases.

The vitreous humor is a semisolid gel that supports the retina and fills the posterior cavity of the eye. Although it is over 98% water, collagen and hyaluronic acid are responsible for maintaining its structure. The collagen content is highest where the vitreous is a gel near its attachments behind the ciliary body (the vitreous base) and, posteriorly, where it attaches to the macula and optic disc. The solid components of the vitreous undergo gradual shrinkage with age, leaving the posterior portion of the vitreous cavity filled with liquid vitreous. This frequently results in a separation of the solid vitreous from the macula and/or optic disc, which is called a posterior vitreous detachment. Visual symptoms such as flashes of light may follow, particularly during movements, and must be distinguished from early retinal detachments.[10] The distinction, therefore, between a "normal" vitreous detachment (a more physiologic process) and a retinal detachment (a clearly pathologic process) is not always clear from symptoms alone.

Aging changes in the retina are more likely to be seen as functional aberrations than as gross anatomic alterations. Anatomic changes do occur nevertheless. Loss of the normal pigment xanothophil in the macular area accompanies a reduction of central acuity to the 20/25 level in the 8th decade.[10] Earlier, there is a loss of the foveal light reflex on examination by ophthal-moscopy. A significant percentage of the adult population will exhibit senile, peripheral retinal degenerations, which seldom impair visual function or progress to actual retinal detachment.

As a rule, retinal arterioles develop sclerotic changes with aging, which are manifest on ophthalmoscopy both as a narrowing of the visible blood column and an increased visibility of the arteriolar wall light reflex (see Figures 8-4, 8-5). Unless the underlying venous column is compressed, these changes are not necessarily pathologic and are more indicative of advanced age.[10]

Functional changes commonly occur in the retina with advancing age. Visual threshold, which is defined as the least amount of light energy necessary to elicit a visual sensation in a dark-adapted eye, increases with age. Measurement of the electrical response of the retina to brief flashes of light (an electroretinogram) has demonstrated that the inner retinal neuron response ages with decreasing amplitude with each decade.[2] These changes are not entirely due to retinal aging alone, for a decreased transparency of the cornea, lens, and vitreous may play a role.[1] The ocular media reduce the amount of light reaching the retina unequally for various wavelengths within the visual spectrum; therefore, this threshold is not exclusively a function of retinal capacity.

"Dark adaptation" is the increase in light sensitivity of the eye that occurs in the dark.

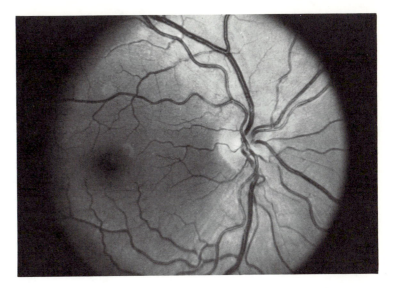

FIGURE 8-4 Photograph of a normal ocular fundus in a young adult.

After exposure to a bright light, the visual pigments are bleached. If then exposed to the dark, the eye requires 5–9 minutes for the cones to regenerate their maximal sensitivity to light, whereas 30 minutes or more are required for full dark adaptation of the rods. Higher age groups tend to dark-adapt more slowly. Even when the effect of lenticular nuclear sclerosis is eliminated by testing only patients with clear lenses, components of the human electroretinogram are altered with advancing age.[11] Furthermore, the visually evoked potential, which involves cortical activity, changes significantly with older age groups. This suggests a significant increase in the time needed by these subjects for cognitive processing.[12]

Optical considerations aside, older individuals exhibit a reduced contrast sensitivity to low spatial frequencies (i.e., they require more contrast to distinguish fine gratings of a given size than younger individuals[13,14]). Temporal resolution also is blunted by age. Flicker fusion frequency rates, where a light is intermittently flashed on and off at progressively faster rates until the flicker is too rapid to be seen and the light seems to be steady, drops significantly with aging. Changes of the ocular media and macular pigment, as well as retinal and central

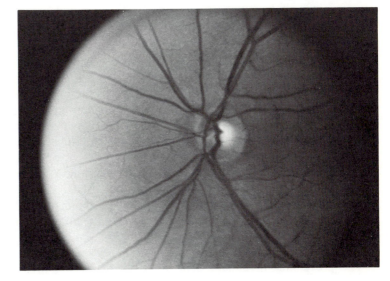

FIGURE 8-5 Photograph of a normal fundus in an elderly person.

nervous mechanisms, may be responsible for this decline.[2]

Color perception may be altered with advancing age by a variety of mechanisms. As the lens becomes more yellow with age, short wavelength light is filtered, producing a greater difficulty in detecting violet and blue light. This effect is compounded by alterations in macular pigmentation with age.[1]

Pathologic Conditions in the Aged Eye

Visual Loss in Elderly Persons —The Magnitude of the Problem

Visual impairment and blindness produce a tremendous impact on our society, both socially and economically. In the general population, nearly 11.5 million persons in the United States—1 of every 19—have some degree of visual impairment. Nearly 500,000 Americans, an incidence rate of 225 of every 100,000 persons, are legally blind.[15] Legal blindness is merely one category of the vision impairment spectrum. It includes persons whose corrected vision in their better eye is 20/200 or poorer, or whose visual field is restricted to no greater than 20 degrees in its widest diameter in their better eye.

Estimates of the economic impact of visual disorders are startling. The cost of professional care (including hospitalization, surgery, office visits and professional treatments, rehabilitation, benefits, and support for visually handicapped persons) exceeds $5 billion a year in this nation alone.[15]

Statistics on the prevalence of blindness have a particular significance for the geriatrician. Over 50% of all blind persons in the United States are 65 years of age or older. The prevalence of blindness rises sharply from 42 of every 100,000 persons for those under 5 years of age to 3,000 of every 100,000 persons for those 85 years of age or older. Furthermore, new cases of blindness are predominantly found in persons 65 years of age or older. Of the blind persons in the older age group (65 years of age or older), blind females outnumber blind males.[15]

The prevalence of blindness in the United States is lowest in the west and highest in the District of Columbia and the southern states. In general, states with a high proportion of nonwhites and elderly persons have higher prevalence rates.

For those persons 65 years of age or older, the leading causes of legal blindness are glaucoma, macular degeneration, senile cataracts, and diabetic retinopathy. New cases of legal blindness in the elderly age group are primarily due to macular degeneration.[15]

The visually impaired are persons who have some trouble seeing with one or both eyes even when wearing eyeglasses or corrective lenses. Of the more than 11 million Americans in this category 43% were 65 years of age or older. Cataracts are the leading cause of new cases of visual impairment. Glaucoma and general diseases of the eye follow as other causes of new cases of visual impairment.[15]

Diseases Causing Visual Loss in Elderly Persons

Glaucoma

Glaucoma is a progressive eye disease resulting from excessive pressure within the eye. It is the leading cause of blindness in the United States for persons of all ages. Over 2 million Americans (approximately 2% of the population) have glaucoma, and 1 of every 8 cases of blindness is due to this disease. The older a person becomes, the greater the risk for developing glaucoma; 3 of every 100 persons over age 65 have this disease.[15]

Glaucoma causes a visual loss by damaging the anterior portion of the optic nerve and the retinal nerve cells due to excessive pressure within the globe of the eye. Frequently, there are no symptoms, so glaucoma escapes detection unless regular eye examinations and pressure measurements are performed. Chronically elevated intraocular pressure first destroys the peripheral retinal nerve fibers; therefore, initial signs or symptoms may be decreased side vision or an inability to see in the dark. Central vision is typically spared until the end-stages of the disease. This type of visual loss cannot be restored. However, treatment can generally prevent a progression of the disease and, in some cases, can permanently eliminate the excessive pressure.

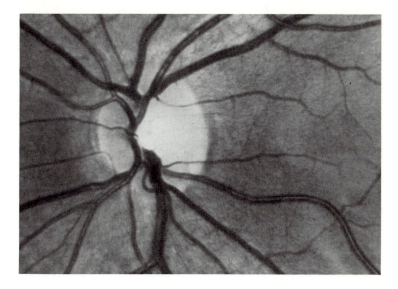

FIGURE 8-6 Photograph of a normal optic nerve head.

The diagnosis of glaucoma is based upon three characteristic clinical findings: increased intraocular pressure, atrophy and cupping of the optic nerve head, and visual field defects (*see* Figures 8-6 and 8-7). Elevations of intraocular pressure alone, without the accompanying changes in the nerve head or visual field, may not necessarily require treatment although they mandate close observation. Furthermore, there is a condition termed low tension glaucoma in which the intraocular pressure is not elevated, although the optic disc undergoes gliosis that is characteristic of glaucoma. In these rare cases, even intraocular pressures in the seem-

ingly "normal" range apparently lead to optic disc and nerve damage. Thus, the ophthalmologist does not treat intraocular pressure as an isolated phenomenon but aims to prevent optic nerve injury.

Clinically, glaucoma behaves as a pressure-induced, chronic optic neuropathy. Glaucoma is classified as open-angle and closed-angle types. Of all glaucomas, 95% are the open-angle variety, with angle-closure glaucoma accounting for the majority of the remainder (congenital glaucoma accounts for less than 1% of all cases). If the cause of the glaucoma is not clinically known, it is termed primary; if the cause is

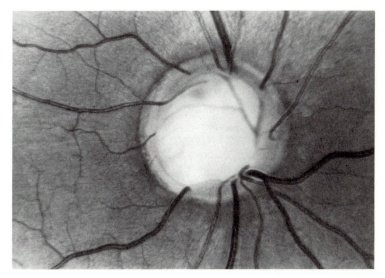

FIGURE 8-7 Photograph of an optic nerve head in a patient with a long-standing, uncontrolled glaucoma.

discernible, it is termed secondary glaucoma.[7] The cause(s) of primary open-angle glaucoma have not been identified, although the trabecular meshwork is known to be the site of the blockage in open-angle glaucoma. In open-angle glaucoma, the aqueous humor has free access from the ciliary body (where it is formed) through the posterior chamber, the pupil, into the anterior chamber, and to the trabecular meshwork without obstruction (see Figure 8-1). Angle-closure glaucoma, on the other hand, involves anatomic, intermittent obstruction of the trabecular meshwork region by the root of the iris. This occurs in individuals who have an anatomically shallow anterior chamber. When the pupil becomes partially dilated in people with this condition, the aqueous humor flow through the pupil becomes relatively blocked (relative pupillary block). This causes the pressure to rise in the posterior chamber, driving the iris against the cornea, closing the angle, and blocking aqueous outflow. These individuals typically have sudden elevations of intraocular pressure when the pupil is dilated, such as with emotional stress, or when mydriatic eyedrops are given. Rapid, marked elevations of intraocular pressure result; the patient will experience acute pain, a clouding of vision, and (not uncommonly) headache and nausea. The pain and stress of the attack may lead to a myocardial infarction.

It is important to realize that the vast majority of glaucomas, the open-angle variety, do not produce acute elevations of intraocular pressure with pain; therefore, patients are not aware of their condition. The disease can be detected only if frequent ocular examinations are performed.

Once a diagnosis of glaucoma has been made, therapy is aimed at the underlying pathophysiology. In the vast majority of cases, this involves the use of topical pharmaceutical agents.

There are several classes of drugs used in the treatment of glaucoma.[17] Miotics, such as pilocarpine and carbachol, constrict the pupil and stimulate the longitudinal muscle fibers of the ciliary body, thus opening the trabecular meshwork pores. Miotics, therefore, decrease resistance to the outflow of aqueous humor and, in the case of narrow-angle glaucoma, prevent the iris root from mechanically blocking the trabecular meshwork. There are a variety of parasympathomimetic drugs that are useful for this purpose, and they usually must be taken for the remainder of a person's life. They have undesirable side effects, such as altered visual acuity due to induced myopia, headaches on initiating treatment, and dimming of vision from the smaller pupil. Longer-acting parasympathomimetic drugs, such as the anticholinesterases, minimize fluctuations in vision after drops are used. However, they have the disadvantage of being more highly toxic if accidentally taken internally and are therefore dangerous. They have also been implicated in the formation of cataracts.

Another approach to controlling intraocular pressure with drugs is to diminish inflow (i.e., to lower the rate of production to the aqueous humor[17]). Levo-epinephrine, in 1% or 2% concentrations, diminishes intraocular pressure when applied as topical drops. This decreases aqueous humor production through its vasoactive effects, but the drug also increases the outflow of aqueous humor through the trabecular meshwork. Its side effects include eye pain, headache, and conjunctival redness. Adrenochrome deposits may occur in the cornea and conjunctiva with prolonged use. A beta-adrenergic-blocking agent, timolol maleate, recently has been proven safe and effective in lowering intraocular pressure when applied topically. As with levo-epinephrine, this drug does not cause miosis and must be instilled only twice daily in the effected eye. Timolol maleate does not increase the outflow of aqueous humor, but does reduce its secretion. As with systemically administered beta-blockers, this drug is not to be used in individuals with a history of asthma or bradycardia.

Systemic medications are often used when topical medications alone are ineffective or contraindicated. Carbonic anhydrase inhibitors lower the production of aqueous humor by interfering with the equilibrium between carbonic acid and carbon dioxide. The flow of water across membranes is influenced by this equilibrium in tissues that contain the enzyme carbonic anhydrase. This enzyme is widely distributed throughout the body, and inhibitors of carbonic anhydrase, therefore, have widespread effects. Nevertheless, they are effective agents for reducing intraocular pressure. Side effects such as paresthesias in the extremities, anorexia, drowsiness, renal lithiasis, and blood dyscrasias are not uncommon. Confusion may occur in elderly patients taking these drugs.[17]

Agents that increase serum osmolality withdraw fluid from the eye and lower intraocular pressure. This mechanism is recognized in patients with diabetic ketoacidosis. The ophthalmologist may use osmotically active agents to decrease intraocular pressure and volume for a short period of time (e.g., to break an attack of angle-closure glaucoma or prior to some forms of intraocular surgery when lower pressure is desired). The osmotic agents most commonly used are glycerol and isosorbide, which may be given orally. These hyperosmotic agents are rapidly, but transiently, effective in lowering intraocular pressure. They cause polyuria. Isosorbide, unlike glycerol, is not metabolized and provides no calories, thus making it safer for use in diabetics. Mannitol is the alcohol of the sugar mannose and also is pharmacologically inert. However, it must be given intravenously as a 20% solution, and it has a transient effect on lowering intraocular pressure.

Surgical therapy for glaucoma is indicated when pharmacologic agents alone are insufficient in maintaining intraocular pressure at normal levels, or if there is a progression of glaucomatous field loss or optic nerve damage on maximal medical therapy. For patients who exhibit a poor compliance in the use of their medications (as often occurs in confused, elderly individuals), surgery may also become necessary.

Conventional glaucoma surgical procedures are designed to produce a fistula between the anterior chamber and the subconjunctival space through which the aqueous humor can egress from the eye.[7] Successful maintenance of this opening is the limiting factor. A significant number of patients will scar the opening closed, rendering them glaucomatous once again.

Cyclocryotherapy is a procedure in which the ciliary body is ablated by freezing. This is accomplished without making incisions on the eye, but it causes a moderately severe discomfort for days to weeks afterwards.

Before proceeding with conventional surgery, the ophthalmologist may be able to control intraocular pressure in many glaucoma patients by using laser treatment on the trabecular meshwork. Laser photocoagulation of the tra-becular meshwork, termed "laser trabeculoplasty," is gaining in popularity for treating certain glaucoma cases. This procedure is much less complicated for the patient, because it does not require hospitalization. Rather, the patient must remain quietly seated in front of a biomicroscope (slit lamp) for only 20–30 minutes, and minimal medication is necessary for control of pain.

Macular Degeneration

The macula is the central portion of the retina that surrounds the fovea centralis and is the area necessary for acute vision. It is located between the upper and lower temporal arcade of the vessels and extends temporally from the optic disc approximately 2 disc diameters. The photoreceptor population is markedly skewed in this region with a high concentration of cones and very few rods, thus making this the area responsible for high-resolution visual acuity.[4] A small lesion that would not affect vision if located peripherally may lead to a severe loss of visual acuity when present in the macula. Cones contain the pigments responsible for color perception; therefore, a functioning macula is necessary for color vision.

Anatomically, retinal vessels diminish in caliber as the fovea centralis is approached. Nourishment for the macula is derived principally from the underlying choroidal vasculature.[4] This is at least partially responsible for the unique involvement of the central retina in a variety of degenerative conditions termed macular degeneration.

In general, degenerations of the macula are easily seen with an ophthalmoscope (see Figure 8-8). However, the ophthalmoscopic appearance cannot be correlated with the level of visual acuity, for many conditions in this area that destroy vision are microscopic or subclinical. In recent years, a great deal has been learned about the causes of senile macular degeneration by using fluorescein angiography. This technique permits an evaluation of the retinal and choroidal vasculature, including areas of vessel leakage, regions of hypovascularization, or abnormalities of the pigment epithelium or Bruch's membrane (see Figures 8-9, 8-10). Consequently, inroads of therapy are now being developed and many forms of macular degeneration can be improved with laser

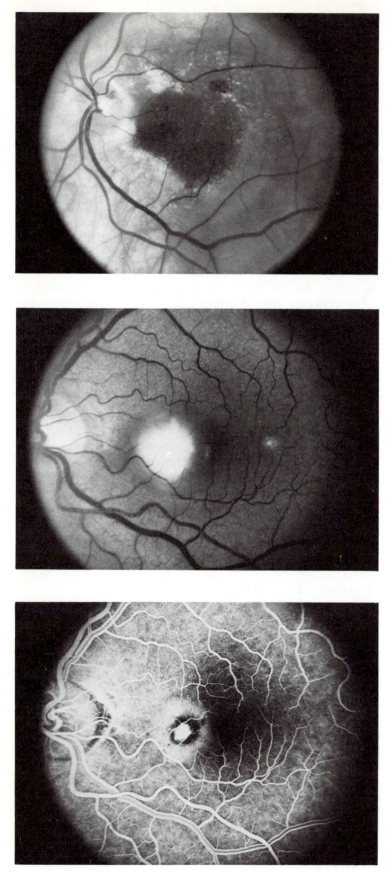

FIGURE 8-8 Photograph of an ocular fundus in a patient with macular degeneration.

FIGURE 8-9 Photograph of an ocular fundus with leakage of a retinal vessel and an accompanying edema.

FIGURE 8-10 Fluorescein angiogram of the ocular fundus shown in Figure 8-9. The bright area denotes the locus of leakage between the optic nerve and the macula.

FIGURE 8-11 Photograph of a senile cataract as seen with diffuse light and the patient's pupil dilated.

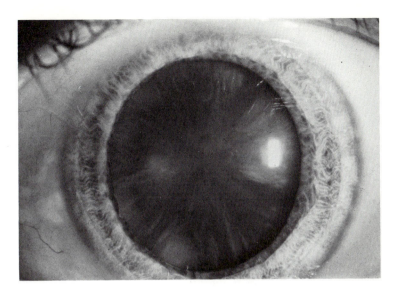

photocoagulation. Certain inflammatory conditions of the macula and central retina can be treated pharmacologically. Patients in whom laser and medical therapy is of no value may derive useful vision when provided with low-vision aids.

Macular degeneration is the second leading cause of blindness and affects 1 of every 9 blind persons. The vast majority of these patients are 65 years of age or older.[15] Unlike glaucoma, the symptoms of macular degeneration are readily noticeable to the patient as a loss of central acuity. With the continuing trend towards an older population, the proportion of blindness due to this disorder will increase in the future.

Cataracts

The term cataract is vastly misunderstood by many people, including physicians. Any opacity of the lens, whether it interferes with vision or not, is a cataract by definition. In the United States, 50% of the population over 40 years of age have some form of cataract, but cataracts are responsible for only 1 of every 12 cases of legal blindness.[15] The most common type of cataract is a senile cataract, which typically progresses slowly in a given individual (*see* Figures 8-11, 8-12). It is sometimes stated that if an individual lives long enough, a cataract will develop.

Although cataracts are most commonly asso-

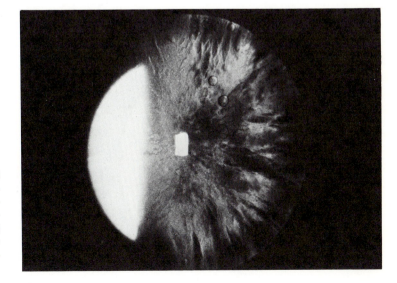

FIGURE 8-12 The same patient as shown in Figure 8-11. The cataract is photographed with a retroillumination similar to that encountered when viewing with an ophthalmoscope. The bright areas are light reflexes off the cornea and iris.

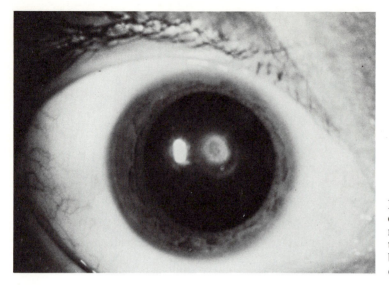

FIGURE 8-13 Corticosteroid-induced, posterior subcapsular cataract as seen with diffuse light and the patient's pupil dilated. The bright area is a light reflex off the cornea and should be ignored.

ciated with aging, younger persons may experience the same problem. Cataracts can occur in conjunction with other medical disorders or can result from physical, chemical or radiation injury. Many diseases, such as diabetes mellitus, hasten the development of cataracts. Some forms of cataract are iatrogenic; corticosteroid-induced lens changes are the most notorious (*see* Figures 8-13, 8-14).

There is no effective medical treatment for cataracts at this time. Certain types of cataracts can be prevented or their progression arrested; however, existing cataracts do not regress. Cataracts due to galactosemia, diabetes mellitus, hypoparathyroidism, or toxic ingestion of drugs can be prevented or their progression halted by controlling the underlying disease.

While there are no drugs to reverse cataract growth, some patients with cataracts will see better when the pupil is dilated. Vision will not be brought back to normal with eyedrops, but their use may permit the postponement of cataract extraction or allow the patient to function at a more normal level until surgery is indicated.

With modern microsurgical techniques, removal of cataracts is highly successful.[16] Indeed, cataract extraction is one of the most

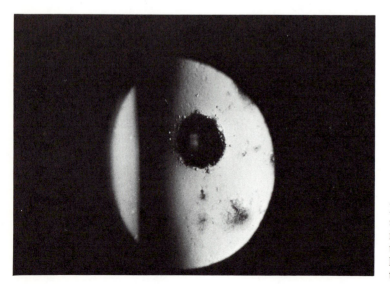

FIGURE 8-14 The same patient as shown in Figure 8-13. The cataract is photographed in retroillumination with the patient's pupil dilated. The corneal light reflex is the bright area at the left.

commonly performed surgical procedures in the United States; over 330,000 cases are performed each year, with the vast majority being done for elderly individuals.[15] Although 75% of all persons over 60 years of age probably have cataracts, only 15% will experience a significant visual loss and fewer than 5% will need surgery.[15]

Cataract surgery offers a successful restoration of vision in 95% of all cases. A common misconception, perhaps arising from surgical techniques of the past, is that a cataract must be "ripe" before it can be removed. At present, the decision to operate depends more on the amount of influence the cataract has on the patient's life style; some patients may require a lens extraction with visual acuity of 20/60, whereas others may not need surgery until visual acuity is 20/200 or less.

Visual loss due to cataracts is caused by the opacification of the lens, which interferes with the transmission of light through the eye on its way to the retina. But the lens contributes refractive power to the eye, and when the opacified lens is removed, the refractive error must be corrected with artificial means. In addition, spherical and chromatic aberrations are induced and astigmatism may result from the surgery. At present, there are four ways of correcting aphakia, which is the postoperative condition of an eye with its lens removed: spectacles (eyeglasses), contact lenses, intraocular lenses, and refractive corneal surgery. Each has its own indications and complications. For example, if a cataract has been present and is removed from only one eye (producing monocular aphakia), eyeglasses cannot be used, because the severe magnification that is induced results in a marked disparity in the image size presented to the refractively corrected aphakic eye and the uninvolved phakic eye. A spectacle lens used to correct aphakia magnifies images by approximately 25% and the brain cannot fuse to such disparate images.[16] Only by placing the refractive correction onto or into the eye is this induced magnification minimized, thus permitting cerebral fusion of the images.

Even when cataracts have been removed from both eyes, a refractive correction with aphakic spectacles is abnormal. Not only is the magnification induced, making objects appear closer than they really are, but distortion also results. Straight lines, such as doorways and walls, appear bowed. This produces the so-called "pin cushion effect". A midperipheral, annular-shaped visual field defect is produced by these spectacles, and objects moving from the peripheral visual field into the magnified central field appear to jump or dart into view; this is appropriately termed the "jack-in-the-box" phenomenon. Because of the characteristics of aphakic spectacles, patients corrected in this manner have a difficult time adjusting to their eyeglasses, particularly when walking or moving about. In elderly individuals who may be less adaptable than younger individuals, this adjustment period is trying.

Many of the problems in the correction of aphakia are minimized or eliminated by contact lenses. By placing the optical correction closer to the eye, the magnification is far less than it would be with the same correction via eyeglasses. Whereas an aphakic spectacle lens magnifies as much as 20–30%, a contact lens magnifies only 7% or 8%. In cases of monocular aphakia, this degree of magnification is not so severe as to prevent a fusion of images between the contact lens-corrected aphakic eye and the unoperated eye. Furthermore, there is little or no distortion or visual field limitation induced by aphakic contact lenses. Contact lenses do have their drawbacks, however. They often are irritating to the eyes and many patients are only able to wear them for a portion of the day. Spectacles, then, must be used as a supplement if functional vision is to be enjoyed throughout the day. Many elderly persons experience difficulty in handling contact lenses, particularly when they are aphakic and cannot see the tiny devices with uncorrected vision. Tremulousness, decreased dexterity, partial paralysis, or severe weakness may make the use of this modality inadvisable if it were not for recent advances in soft contact lens manufacturing. Many soft contact lenses now have been approved by the federal Food and Drug Administration for continuous (extended) wear in which the patient may leave the lens on the eye for weeks or months. Daily handling, therefore, is eliminated. These patients must return to the ophthalmologist's office at regular intervals for skilled removal of the lens, cleaning, and replacement on the eye. The use of extended-wear soft contact lenses is more risky than daily wear. Blood vessels may invade the normally avascular cornea and abrasions or infected ulcers may develop in the cornea. Furthermore, extended-wear contact lenses are not indicated in patients with extremely dry eyes, severe glaucoma, or greater than moderate levels of corneal astigmatism.

A rapidly changing and increasingly accepted mode of aphakic correction is the use of intraocular lenses (pseudophakos). The theoretical advantages of intraocular lenses are enormous. The refractive correction is placed at or near the physiologic lens plane inside the eye and magnification from refractive correction following cataract extraction is negligible. Patients also experience a recovery of vision almost immediately after surgery, although most patients require some form of minor adjustment in the form of eyeglasses. This type of aphakic correction produces a more natural type of vision than contact lenses or aphakic spectacles.

Many cataract patients cannot have an intraocular lens implanted for correction of their aphakia. Pseudophakos is inadvisable in patients with high myopia, glaucoma, corneal endothelial dystrophies, diabetic retinopathy, or retinal detachment. Because of possible late sequelae, intraocular lens use today is restricted primarily for elderly persons.

An experimental method of correcting aphakia, termed refractive keratoplasty, is being studied in many medical centers throughout the world. With these techniques, the corneal contour is surgically altered to correct the refractive error in aphakia. To date, the use of these procedures is limited and is most widely used for those patients in whom the other three modalities are contraindicated or unsuccessful.

Diabetic Retinopathy

A threat to every person with diabetes mellitus is the possibility of developing diabetic retinopathy. This disease affects the blood vessels of the eye and accounts for 1 of every 15 cases of blindness in the United States. Diabetic retinopathy ranks third, behind macular degeneration and glaucoma, as a leading cause of new cases of blindness.[15] Those persons most at risk for developing diabetic retinopathy are patients who have had diabetes for over 10 years. Nevertheless, diabetes mellitus often goes undetected for years, and retinopathy may be the presenting problem.

Visual loss due to diabetic retinopathy is often related initially to vascular changes in and around the macula (see Figure 8-15). Microaneurysms lead to hemorrhages and exudates, and related vascular abnormalities may produce a leakage of serous fluid or blood.[9] When one or more of these phenomena occur in the macular area, visual acuity deteriorates. With fluorescein angiography and laser photocoagulation, these areas often can be detected and treated, which restores the vision. In advanced cases of diabetic retinopathy, neovascularization occurs in, over, or beneath the retina

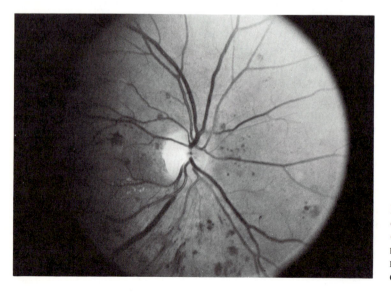

FIGURE 8-15 Photograph of an ocular fundus in a patient with early (background) diabetic retinopathy. Note the microaneurysms, blot hemorrhages, and exudates.

and is called proliferative retinopathy. This also is treatable with photocoagulation therapy. For reasons that are incompletely understood, panretinal photocoagulation (in which the chorioretinal layers anterior to the equator of the eye are ablated by photocoagulation) often preserves the central vision as proliferative neovascularization involutes postsurgically.

Corneal Disease

The cornea, like the lens and vitreous humor, must remain transparent if light is to reach the retina. Corneal disorders cause a visual loss less frequently than the previously mentioned ocular disease, but are often correctable with therapy.

Herpetic keratitis is the most common cause of corneal-induced blindness in this nation.[15] Repeated bouts of infection with herpes virus may lead to opacification of the cornea with a subsequent visual loss. Several pharmacologic and surgical means of treating herpes simplex keratitis are now available. Antiviral drugs shorten the course of superficial herpes keratitis but do not prevent recurrences.

Disorders of the corneal endothelium are not uncommon causes of corneal-induced blindness in elderly persons. Progressive, primary endothelial cell loss (Fuchs' corneal dystrophy) and endothelial damage following cataract surgery may lead to a corneal edema and blisters of the corneal epithelium. These blisters, or vesicles, may coalesce and form bullae that rupture and expose bare nerve endings, which produces severe pain. This pain may be intermittent in its early stages, but it eventually becomes chronic. The patient may become withdrawn due to the pain and photophobia.

Corneal scars and edematous or damaged corneas can, in many cases, be treated successfully with corneal transplantation. Visual acuity is often restored to near normal levels when a clear graft is obtained and an optical correction is prescribed.

Healing of corneal grafts is a very slow process, since the cornea is avascular and cells must migrate relatively long distances into the area of the wound. It is not uncommon, following corneal transplantation that 6–12 months of healing must transpire before functional vision can be obtained with eyeglasses or contact lenses. Yet, corneal transplants are performed in individuals in their 8th, 9th, or even 10th decade of life, with a subsequent improvement in their quality of life. Corneal transplant surgery is presently no more stressful for an individual than the removal of cataracts. Long periods of bed rest and hospitalization are not necessary, and excellent general health is not a prerequisite to corneal surgery.

Ocular Infections

The use of antimicrobial drugs in ophthalmology is guided by general knowledge. An awareness of ocular microbiology is helpful and sometimes essential, because certain microorganisms invade ocular tissues preferentially; selected eye structures may be more prone to infection with a specific microorganism. For example, by virtue of its avascularity, the cornea is an immunologically unique structure.

Obviously, the first requirement of treating ocular infection is to diagnose the cause. Although an external ocular infection produces a redness of the eye, there may be other causes for this symptom (such as acute glaucoma, iritis, and so on). Second, the selection of an appropriate antimicrobial agent depends upon a correct identification of the offending organism and a knowledge of those drugs to which it is sensitive. Finally, the toxic effect of drugs is particularly important in ophthalmology, because many highly effective antimicrobial agents cannot be used topically due to their ocular side effects. Certain topical agents may be used in lieu of more potent drugs due to their lack of toxicity.

Topical antibiotics are used prophylactically before surgery more frequently in ophthalmology than in other surgical specialities. The rationale is that sterilization of the eye preoperatively is highly desirable; a minute innoculum of bacteria that might not cause an infection in a skin incision may produce devastating consequences when present in the eye. Environmental contamination may occur due to either the normal flora of the ocular adnexa or airborne particulate matter while the eye is open during surgery. The intraocular contents are warm, moist, rife with nutrients, and relatively isolated from the circulation, thus producing a privileged site for microorganisms.

The use of drugs in treating human viral infections began in ophthalmology.[21] A selective inhibition of herpes simplex virus in the cornea was obtained by the topical administration of idoxuridine. Prior to this time, no medication had been shown to improve a viral infection without harming host cells significantly. Subsequently, other antiviral drugs have been developed, some of which are usable systemically (vidarabine).

Antiviral drugs are effective in decreasing the duration of herpes simplex keratitis, and they offer prophylaxis against reactivation of viral disease when topical corticosteroids are used for ocular inflammation. They are not without their complications, however, and a thorough knowledge of their side effects and contraindications is essential before use.

Antifungal drugs often are extremely toxic to ocular tissues. Treatment of intraocular fungal infections is disappointing, for the drugs are so toxic that the concentrations necessary to inhibit the microorganism frequently destroy ocular tissues. Newer antifungal agents, such as pimaracin, flucytosine, and ketoconazole show promise by virtue of their safer therapeutic index.

Ocular Inflammation

A variety of anti-inflammatory agents are useful in treating ocular disease or trauma. The site of inflammation, as well as the underlying cause, must be kept in mind when using such drugs. For example, inflammations of the eyelids or ocular surface are best treated with agents that penetrate the globe poorly. This minimizes the intraocular side effects and concentrates the drug where it is most needed. With infectious processes, it is always best first to attack the microorganism and use anti-inflammatory agents only when the infection is controlled and/or the inflammatory process itself is a threat to sight. The use of corticosteroids in ocular reactions should be limited to those situations in which the inflammation is severe enough to threaten a permanent structural change. Mild intraocular inflammation may require corticosteroid therapy, whereas moderately severe external inflammations may not require such treatment.

Corticosteroids are the primary ocular anti-inflammatory agents. There are multiple corticosteroid preparations available for ophthalmic use, and the physician must select an agent or mode of therapy appropriate to the condition. The patient's general health status influences this selection process.

Corticosteroids may be given topically in the form of eyedrops or ointments, as a periocular injection, or systemically.[18] In general, the intraocular penetration of topically applied corticosteroids depends on their relative lipid and water solubilities. A given compound may have great anti-inflammatory activity but poor penetration. This renders it unavailable for intraocular action and useful only in treating extraocular processes. Some compounds have biphasic solubilities; the lipid soluble phase allows the drug first to penetrate the corneal epithelium, whereas the aqueous phase permits passage through the corneal stroma, which maximizes intraocular concentration. Some liquid preparations are produced as solutions, whereas others are suspensions requiring vigorous shaking before use. Ointment forms have prolonged action by virtue of their greater contact time with the eye.

The systemic side effects commonly associated with oral corticosteroid administration generally do not follow topical use, even when given for long periods of time. Periocular injections of steroids are reserved for severe inflammatory processes in which systemic administration is contraindicated, or when maximal intraocular concentration is required and topical or systemic administrations are insufficient. These injections are useful for concentrating the drug in a given area of the ocular system.[18] They may be given in soluble forms, in which case they are present for a short time, or in the depot variety, which prolongs their action.

Systemic administration can be parenteral or oral. Their use should be guided by general medical principles. The major contraindication to the use of corticosteroids is a lack of a specific indication for their need; these drugs should never be given as a placebo or as "shotgun" therapy. Although typical complications such as psychosis, peptic ulcer disease, osteoporosis, and Cushingoid changes do not occur with topical use, local side effects are observed when the drug is applied to the eye. As systemic corticosteroids reduce the resistance of the body to infection, the same effect is noted in the eye with topical administration. In addition, activation of herpes simplex may occur with frequent, topical corticosteroid use.

Glaucoma may be induced by topical, periocular, or systemic use of corticosteroids, particularly after prolonged use.[17] A glaucomatous response to corticosteroid use is hereditarily determined and found in one third of the population.[19] The majority of patients with a known, primary open-angle glaucoma will experience additional elevations of intraocular pressure when topical corticosteroids are used. Angle-closure glaucoma patients do not respond in this manner unless they also carry the gene for chronic open-angle glaucoma. The gene is a dominant trait. When an individual is heterozygous, the response to corticosteroid use will be an elevation of intraocular pressure; when homozygous a person will develop chronic open-angle glaucoma.[17]

The degree of intraocular pressure elevation following corticosteroid use depends upon the potency of the steroid and the frequency and duration of its use. Researchers have sought to separate the anti-inflammatory activity from the pressure-elevating properties of corticosteroids. Hydromethylprogesterone, a progestational steroid, does not elevate intraocular pressure; however, it is a very weak anti-inflammatory agent. Perhaps it does not increase intraocular pressure when applied topically because it does not penetrate the eye to a significant degree. Fluorometholone, on the other hand, allegedly retains both anti-inflammatory potency and significant intraocular penetration, but it does not elevate intraocular pressure as the more potent agents.[20]

Anticholinergic preparations are of value in the treatment of anterior uveitis (iritis). Atropine is an effective drug that acts to reduce the pain of iritis, helps to prevent adhesions of the iris to adjacent structures, and reduces the permeability of inflamed vessels, which causes less exudation of protein and inflammatory cells.[17] The duration of action of atropine may be as long as 14 days. Other anticholinergic preparations with shorter durations of action have been developed for topical use. All anticholinergic drugs produce a paresis of accommodation, dilate the pupil, and can have systemic side effects such as dryness of the skin and mouth, fever, delirium, tachycardia, and cutaneous vasodilation.

Drugs that interfere with prostaglandins have great theoretic implications in ophthalmic use. Their inflammatory activity in the treatment of ocular disease is being investigated but has not, as yet, been shown to be of significant value. Their effect on glaucoma has been established in experimental animals but not in humans.

Adnexal Problems

Because aging changes of the eyelids often transform imperceptibly into disease states they are sometimes overlooked and may lead to blindness, or they become responsible for significant visual loss or discomfort. When alterations of eyelid function occur, the preservation of the eye and vision is endangered. The integrity of the ocular surface is maintained only if the globe is kept moist by a distribution of tears via repeated blinking. Repeated or prolonged exposure leads to dryness, provides an avenue for infection, and may cause thinning and perforation of the cornea.

Although normal aging involves a looseness of the skin and decreased muscle tone of the eyelid, if the eyelid falls away from the globe so that the eye is incompletely covered, tear distribution is compromised and localized dryness may occur. In some cases, excessive tearing from chronic irritation develops. In other cases, dryness leads to keratinization of the ocular surface or the complications listed above. Laxity of the lower eyelid that produces malposition is termed ectropion and usually is correctable by surgery (*see* Figure 8-16).[16]

Senile entropion is a condition in which the eyelid margin is turned inward onto the globe and the lashes irritate the eye (*see* Figure 8-17). The spastic variety of senile entropion is caused by an overaction of the orbicularis oculi muscle that is associated with weakness of its antagonists. This allows the eyelid to turn inwards. The atonic type of entropion is associated with a loss of tone of several eyelid muscles and may occur alone or in combination with the spastic variety. Entropion is frequently intermittent in its early stages. Asking a patient to forcibly squeeze the eyelids may reveal the tendency toward infolding. Temporary relief of the condition may be accomplished by taping the lower

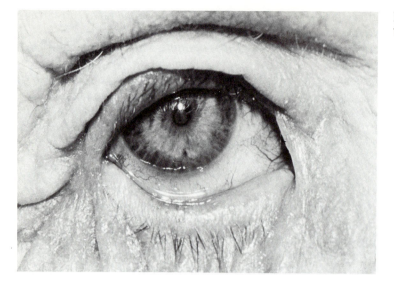

FIGURE 8-16   Senile ectropion of the lower eyelid.

eyelid, but a permanent cure requires surgical intervention.[16]

Incomplete eyelid closure may also result from a senile laxity of the eyelids. Thyroid disorders or 7th cranial nerve malfunction may cause or complicate the situation. If the underlying cause is temporary, the eye may be maintained on artificial tear drops and ointment lubricants, combined with taping the eyelids, until the underlying cause is corrected. In more permanent disorders, such as endocrine exophthalmos, a partial or total surgical closure of the eyelids (tarsorrhaphy) may be necessary.

An annoying problem to many elderly individuals is epiphora, which is an excessive tearing of the eye that spills over the eyelid margin onto the cheeks. This may be caused, paradoxically, by ocular dryness. In this situation, the baseline secretion of tears is inadequate, dry spots develop on the cornea producing an irritation, and reflex tearing occurs in copious amounts. Treatment in this situation is aimed at tear supplementation to prevent the development of dry spots.

Adequate tear drainage is prevented and epiphora results if the tear drainage system is blocked either through 1) A closure or malposition of the lacrimal puncta of the inner canthus;

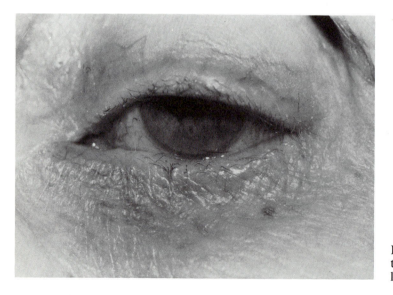

FIGURE 8-17   Senile entropion of the lower eyelid. Note the eyelashes touching the cornea.

or 2) An obstruction of the lacrimal canaliculi or lacrimal duct system.[7] These conditions are usually treated by surgical means, but they may be effectively managed with minor manipulations of the lacrimal drainage system, such as probing or dilation of the lacrimal passages.

Neurosensory Blindness

Ischemia or atrophy of the optic nerve accounts for over 5% of blindness in people over 65 years of age.[15] Ischemia of the optic nerve may produce a slight edema of the disc that is associated with an altitudinal (superior) field defect.

Temporal arteritis may lead to a sudden visual loss through optic nerve ischemia. It is characterized by a low-grade fever, headache, anorexia, and a pain or tenderness around the temporal vessels.[16] The erythrocyte sedimentation rate (ESR) is elevated, and there may be an associated leukocytosis and increased plasma fibrinogen. The arteritis of the internal elastic layer of the cranial vessels can lead to an abrupt obliteration of the vessel lumen. An immediate diagnosis is urgent and must not await the results of laboratory tests. Treatment should begin as soon as possible with high doses of systemic corticosteroids if vision is to be preserved.

Other forms of optic nerve disease, such as optic neuritis, may be idiopathic and associated with multiple sclerosis and lead poisoning. Intracranial mass lesions or vasculitides other than temporal arteritis may cause neurologic deficits that include optic atropy.

Low Vision Aids

Patients with subnormal vision and many legally blind individuals may be helped with telescopic lenses, special magnifiers, or specially devised optical and electronic devices that are now available.[22] Although the number of patients who can learn to use these devices may be small, a low-vision aid evaluation is often worthwhile. Particularly older patients, who may be less adaptable than younger individuals, frequently find that they are able to use nothing more than simple magnifying lenses. A patient should have reasonable expectations, an understanding of the underlying condition, and a high degree of motivation for success with low-vision aids. Low-vision aids merely allow a patient to maximize the use of his or her remaining vision.

Physicians should reassure macular degeneration patients that although central vision is lost, their condition will not lead to total blindness, and that they may be able to experience a better life if they can learn to use one of these aids. Hence, it is important for the physician to understand the distinctions between visual impairment, legal blindness, and total blindness.

References

1. Weale RA: *The Aging Eye*. London, Bartholomew Press for Harper & Row Publishers Inc, 1963.
2. Moses RA: *Adler's Physiology of the Eye: Clinical Application,* ed 5. St. Louis, The CV Mosby Co, 1980.
3. Grayson M: *Diseases of the Cornea*. St. Louis, The CV Mosby Co, 1979.
4. Hogan MJ, Alvarado JA, Weddell JE: *Histology of the Human Eye; An Atlas and Textbook*. Philadelphia, WB Saunders & Co, 1971.
5. Berens C: Aging changes in eye and adnexa. *Arch Ophthal* 29:171–209, 1943.
6. Brubaker RF, Nagataki S, Townsend DJ, et al: The effect of age on aqueous humor formation in man. *Ophthalmology* (*Rochester*) 88(suppl 3):283–288, 1981.
7. Newell FW: *Ophthalmology: Principles and Concepts,* ed 4. St. Louis, The CV Mosby Co, 1978.
8. Duane A: Subnormal accommodation. *Arch Ophtal* 54:568, 1925.
9. Hogan M, Zimmerman L: *Ophthalmic Pathology; An Atlas and Textbook,* ed 2. Philadelphia, WB Saunders & Co, 1962.
10. Keeney AH, Keeney VT: A guide to examining the aging eye. *Geriatrics* Feb 1980, pp 81–91.
11. Weleber R: The effect of age on human cone and rod ganzfeld electroretinograms. *Invest Ophthalmol Vis Sci* 20(suppl 3):392–399, 1981.
12. Beck EC, Swanson C, Dustman RE: Long latency components of the visually evoked potential in man: effects of aging. *Exper Aging Res* 6(suppl 6):523–545, 1980.
13. Sekuler R, Hutman LP: Spatial vision and aging. I: Contrast sensitivity. *J Gerontol* 35(suppl 5):692–699, 1980.
14. Hutman LP, Sekuler R: Spatial vision and aging. II: Criterion effects. *J. Gerontol* 35(suppl 5):700–706, 1980.

15. National Society to Prevent Blindness: *Vision Problems in the United States: A Statistical Analysis*. New York, National Society to Prevent Blindness, 1980.

16. Libow LS, Sherman FT: *The Core of Geriatric Medicine: A Guide for Students and Practitioners*. St. Louis, The CV Mosby Co, 1981.

17. Havener WH: *Ocular Pharmacology,* ed 2. St. Louis, The CV Mosby Co, 1970.

18. Aronson SB, Elliott JH: *Ocular Inflammation*. St. Louis, The CV Mosby Co, 1972.

19. Becker B, Hahn KA: Topical corticosteroids and heredity in primary open-angle glaucoma. *Amer J Ophthal* 57:543–547, 1964.

20. Leopold IH: Considerations of the topical use of corticosteroids in ophthalmology. Allergan Pharmaceuticals, Report Series No 81.

21. Kaufman H, Nesburn AB, Maloney ED: I.D.U. therapy of herpes simplex. *Arch Ophthal* 67:582–585, 1962.

22. American Foundation for the Blind: *Aids for the 80's: What They Are and What They Do*. New York, American Foundation for the Blind, 1981 (Publication No [ISBN]0-103-89128-7).

CHAPTER 9

Audiology

B. Z. RAPPAPORT, PH.D.

Many geriatric patients have difficulty in reporting an adequate history and in following specific instructions because of a problem in communication. This chapter will deal with the most pervasive of these problems, impaired hearing.

Scope of the Problem

Harris[1] states that hearing impairment ranks second only to arthritis as the most prevalent condition affecting the health of senior adults. In 1971, a Health Resources Administration survey found that 25% of the population of the United States had a significant hearing loss as a result of aging.[2] A 48% and 90% incidence rate of hearing loss was found in residents of two nursing homes.[3,4] Thus, particular attention to amplification and aural rehabilitation is indicated in our elderly population.

Effects of Age on Hearing

The common term used to describe hearing loss resulting from the effects of aging is presbycusis. In practice, this term encompasses a variety of processes and factors that contribute to a decreased auditory function in elderly persons. A classic cross-cultural study[5] evaluated and compared the hearing sensitivity in populations ranging from 10–70 years of age in New York, Dusseldorf, Cairo, and from a tribal population in an isolated area of the Sudan. The older people of the tribal population had significantly better hearing sensitivity than any of the other groups studied. It was concluded that factors such as environment, diet, and degree of stress contributed to the variability in hearing sensitivity seen among these sample groups.

Presbycusis will be considered in its physical (anatomic and physiologic) and psychosocial aspects. Both are necessary to build an adequate framework for understanding the factors that constitute presbycusis.

Anatomic and Physiologic Effects

In describing the physical effects of presbycusis, it is useful to divide the ear into its mechanical and sensory processes. For this purpose, mechanical relates to the anatomy and physiology of the outer and middle ear. Sensory processes will cover the cochlea, auditory nerve, brainstem, and cortex.

Mechanical
Perhaps the only change of clinical significance that occurs, with age, in the outer ear is the loss of elasticity in the cartilaginous portion of the pinna and external auditory canal. If the ear canal becomes occluded as the result of this loss of resiliance, it can effect sound transmission and produce a high-frequency hearing loss.[6]

The most prominent changes in the middle ear are progressive translucency and rigidity of the tympanic membrane and a loss of compliance of the ossicular chain.[7] These changes have no significant effect on auditory sensitivity.[8]

Sensory

Most changes affecting audition occur in the sensory processes of the ear and the neural pathways. Corso[9] described six general classes of morphologic changes in the auditory pathways that are identified as a function of age:

1. Sensory presbycusis: atrophy and degeneration of hair cells in the cochlea.
2. Metabolic presbycusis: atrophy of the stria vascularis, which affects the biochemical and bioelectric properties of the cochlea.
3. Mechanical presbycusis: reduction in the vibratory abilities of the cochlea.
4. Neural presbycusis: loss of neurons of the 8th nerve.
5. Vascular presbycusis: loss of blood supply to the cochlea.
6. Central presbycusis: loss of neurons in the auditory pathway of the brainstem and cortex.

The age of onset of presbycusis is extremely difficult to determine and is a subject of considerable debate. Degeneration of the hair cells of the basal cochlea has been reported in newborn infants,[10] which implies that the effects of aging may begin at birth or even in utero. Behavioral studies[11] have shown changes in the auditory sensitivity of high-frequency stimuli in adolescents and young adults that are not attributable to any identifiable external influence. This loss of ability to hear high-frequency auditory stimuli appears to be the characteristic finding of the degeneration of the cochlear processes. The functional result of this type of decreased cochlear ability is a reduction in the ability to understand or discriminate sounds of speech. This is most apparent when the individual with a high-frequency hearing loss is communicating in an environment with a competing auditory stimulus. For example, many patients complain of difficulties understanding conversations at social gatherings or against the background of home appliances.

Gaeth[12] coined the term "phonemic regression" to describe the inordinate decrease in the ability to discriminate speech relative to the loss of hearing sensitivity in elderly hearing-impaired patients. This disproportionately poor understanding of speech has been attributed to a degeneration of the 8th nerve, auditory brainstem, and auditory cortex. With the advent of more sophisticated audiologic evaluation techniques, it is possible to identify more subtle aspects of the neural processing of auditory information that contribute to presbycusis. Significant aspects are a decreased ability to handle degradation of the temporal parameters of hearing (compressed speech, sound localization) and the inability to extract meaningful information from its auditory background. Physiologic findings of presbycusis rarely occur independent of one another, and it is the audiologist's task to identify these components in determining a course of rehabilitation.

Psychosocial Effects

Sensory deficits of aging influence human behavior. The psychological effects of hearing loss have been discussed at different levels of behavior.[13]

Auditory Background

Auditory stimuli such as wind in the trees, coins in one's pocket, or the sounds of water in the plumbing serve as auditory background. Individuals do not overtly respond to these sounds, but use them at a subconscious level to keep in contact with the environment. When a hearing-impaired person loses touch with the auditory environment it promotes a dissociation from the active world. The desire to venture beyond a secure environment lessens and may be a factor leading to depression.

Warning

These are auditory cues that signal events requiring an overt response. The sound of an ambulance or fire engine are examples of warning signals. A reduction in the ability to hear this type of sound and, thus, respond appropriately can be a factor in an elderly individual's withdrawal from life-long activities such as driving a car or working at a particular job. Loss of the ability to detect warning signals may produce fearful behavior. The individual becomes concerned about the personal harm that may result or harm to others.

Symbolic

At the highest level of function, sound is used as a means of communication. Loss of hearing may produce a diminished ability to interact socially, force one to alter or stop recreational activities, and may significantly affect family relationships.

A reduced function of hearing in elderly persons often occurs concurrently with other sensory and motor deficits. Each has its independent effect as well as interrelating with other losses to influence behavior patterns of some elderly individuals.

Assessment of Auditory Function

Interviewing the Hearing-Impaired Elderly Patient

Prior to gathering audiologic data, it is beneficial to obtain a detailed history. The history should include medical, psychological, and social information pertinent to evaluating a patient's auditory function. A few observations about technique and basic information are warranted.

Many elderly patients visit an audiology clinic because of the insistence of family and friends. They deny the existence of a hearing problem by projecting the problem to others. "People just don't speak clearly to me," is a common phrase, as well as, "I can't understand these youngsters nowadays." The Denver Scale of Communication Function[14] is a useful tool for assessing an individual's impression of his auditory function. This 25 question survey covers areas relating to family, self, social/vocational, and communication. In addition to providing pertinent information, it is used as a measure of graded improvement throughout a program of aural rehabilitation.

Often, an elderly hearing-impaired patient is accompanied to the interview by a spouse, child, or significant other. It is frequently necessary to rely on these individuals to provide some or all of the history. However, the patient should be encouraged to supply as much of the information as possible, for the following reasons. First, it promotes self-esteem for the patient in terms of being responsible for his own treatment. Second, with a skilled interviewer, it demonstrates both to the patient and the significant others that there are techniques for improving the patient's communication skills. Suggestions that will substantially increase the ability of the hearing-impaired listener to understand the speaker include the following: choose a well-lit room that eliminates as much background noise as possible, maintain good eye contact with the patient, don't speak while looking down at a chart, and encourage the patient to maintain eye contact as well. Although a common fault, the interviewer need not speak loudly (especially with a patient who already is wearing a hearing aid), but should speak slowly and clearly without exaggerated lip movements or facial expressions. It often is helpful to rephrase a statement that is misunderstood rather than repeating it verbatim. This may eliminate words that are particularly difficult to hear because of their acoustical composition in relationship to the patient's hearing configuration.

The Auditory Evaluation

When pertinent information has been obtained from the interview, the audiologic evaluation can be initiated. An elderly patient may fatigue rapidly and, therefore, several abbreviated sessions are less tiresome than a single long one. Geriatric patients sometimes adopt their own response mechanisms for behavioral type tests that are different from those the audiologist recommends. For example, the patient may nod his head rather than raise a hand when a tone is heard. The examiner should be flexible enough to allow the patient his own response tool as long as the criteria for responding is appropriate. The patient may require repeated instruction throughout a test sequence and often will perform better when given positive verbal reinforcement for a correct response.

The following tests determine overall hearing sensitivity and assess the various levels and sites of auditory processing throughout the auditory system. The list is not complete, but encompasses those tests most commonly used.

Basic Tests

Audiologic evaluation can generally be divided into two major categories characterized by the types of auditory stimuli employed.

Pure-Tone Tests The use of a highly specified, well-controlled sinusoidal auditory stimulus or pure-tone permits an accurate measurement of the auditory system. The results of this type of test provide discrete bits of information that are frequency specific. The most basic of these evaluations is a pure-tone, air conduction threshold test. The auditory stimulus is presented to the patient through an earphone, and the overall sensitivity of the peripheral auditory system is determined. The same pure-tone stimuli can be presented to the patient with a bone conduction oscillator (usually placed on the mastoid). This evaluates cochlear function and, therefore, is a basic means for differentiating cochlear from middle or outer ear dysfunction.

Pure-tone threshold sensitivity typically decreases as age increases. This reduction in hearing acuity is frequency dependent; it first appears for higher-frequency stimuli and gradually progresses toward the lower end of the frequency spectrum. For similar ages, puretone thresholds for females are, on the average, better than for males (*see* Figure 9-1). It is not certain, however, how much this latter finding is influenced by occupational noise exposure.

Speech Tests While pure-tone tests generate frequency-specific information concerning auditory function, they do not provide much

knowledge regarding the ability to process the most important type of auditory stimulus: speech. Speech stimuli are generally presented via earphones and may be used, as are pure-tones, to measure acuity or assess the ability to understand or discriminate a verbal auditory message.

The Speech Reception or Spondee Threshold test measures a patient's threshold for hearing by identifying two-syllable words. It is similar to the pure-tone air-conduction threshold test in the frequency range that comprises the acoustic spectrum of speech.

The Speech or Word Discrimination test measures the ability of a patient to identify monosyllabic words that are presented at a comfortable listening level, in quiet. The Speech Reception Threshold and Word Discrimination tests of subjects ranging from 11–84 years of age show a decrement in both measures as a function of age.[15] A poor ability to discriminate speech that is secondary to degeneration of neurons within the brainstem and cortical auditory pathways is a serious handicap in elderly persons.

Many auditory tests are designed to differentiate between peripheral (conductive, cochlear) versus neural (8th nerve, brainstem, cortex) sites.

Site of Lesion Tests

Pure-Tone Tests A variety of tests that employ tonal stimuli are used in the differential diagnosis of hearing impairment. These tests, which are both behavioral (requiring an overt response from the patient) and objective (data collected without the patient's overt response), are used to evaluate cochlear 8th nerve and brainstem functions. They measure a patient's ability to detect small increments in intensity, make loudness judgments, quantify the rate of neural adaptation, and they assess the ability of a patient to localize an auditory stimulus in space or lateralize an auditory stimulus presented in earphones.

Speech Tests These tests are generally more popular as a method for evaluating brainstem and cortical auditory function. Typically, they analyze a patient's ability to handle a degraded speech message or to synthesize a message that has been acoustically divided in frequency,

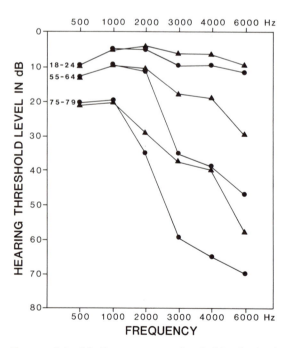

FIGURE 9-1 Median pure tone thresholds obtained from three different age decades for males (•) and females (▲).

with each portion presented to one ear simultaneously with the other portion. It is well known that an elderly patient's ability to process simple speech messages is generally not affected. The stress on the auditory system produced by altering the speech stimulus, however, often uncovers auditory processing deficits, which characterize elderly hearing-impaired persons.

Aural Rehabilitation and the Elderly Patient

Only 1% of the elderly patient population with hearing impairments have the type of ear pathology that is amenable to medical or surgical intervention.[7] The audiologist, therefore, is an essential person in the health care team for elderly persons.

As with any therapeutic approach, the total individual must be considered. This is especially true with an elderly patient. For example, the communication requirements of a 40-year-old professional with a mild hearing loss are not the same as a retired 80-year-old person with minimal social interactions and a similar hearing loss. The 40-year-old professional might benefit from a more aggressive approach with binaural hearing aids. The 80-year-old person, however, might benefit most from a monaural hearing aid or individual and family counseling. A major consideration is to simplify the use of prosthetic devices by an elderly patient. In working with a hearing-impaired elderly person, one needs to consider the extent to which the individual has projected his hearing loss onto others and the motivation for improvement of communicative skills. Considerable judgment and experience is necessary to determine how aggressive rehabilitation should be with a patient whose cognitive function is such that his communication skills are compromised more by processing deficits than by sensory ones.

Hearing Aids and Elderly Persons

The primary means of improving hearing in elderly patients is through the use of amplification with an appropriate hearing aid or aids. Most presbycusic-type hearing losses have a gradual onset and are long standing. Therefore, the patient often is not aware of the extent to which hearing has changed. The placement of amplification can be a traumatic event, which may result in a negative attitude toward hearing aid use. It is essential that an elderly patient and his or her significant others have a clear understanding of the benefits and limitations of hearing aid use. It is important for the patient to comprehend that a hearing aid is not a corrective device that will restore hearing to normal, and that listening to sounds through a hearing aid is much different than listening without one, especially in terms of the quality of sound. Through the careful selection of appropriate amplification, coupled with a program of aural rehabilitation, an elderly patient can expect to increase the ability to communicate with others. Patients who adamantly deny the existence of hearing loss, project the problem onto others, and who are incapable or unwilling to make changes, cannot be forced to use amplification. One has to be motivated to improve to derive maximum benefit from a hearing aid. The audiologist can instill some of this motivation in the patient, but the patient must assume responsibility for his care by assisting in this rehabilitation process.

Types of Hearing Aids

Hearing aids can be categorized by their packaging or electroacoustic characteristics. All hearing aids have some common components. Each hearing aid has a microphone that converts sound or vibration into electrical energy. It has an amplifier to boost or intensify this energy. It has a gain or volume control for personal adjustment of the intensity of the output of the hearing aid. It has a speaker that transduces the amplified electrical energy back into sound energy, and an ear mold that directs the sound from the hearing aid into the ear canal. The construction of each of these components influence the way in which sound is amplified. There are other features, such as tone controls, compression circuits, and induction coils, which further modify the hearing aid.

Hearing aids can be built in a variety of packages (*see* Figure 9-2). At present, the most popular package for a hearing aid is the postauricular or "behind-the-ear" type instrument. The hearing aid is hooked over the top and behind

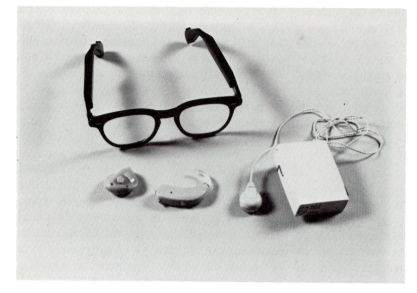

FIGURE 9-2   Hearing aids.

the pinna and is connected to a flexible piece of tubing that channels sound to the ear mold. A relatively recent development that is gaining in popularity is the "in-the-ear" type hearing aid. This instrument is a hearing aid within an ear mold that is worn within the concha and ear canal. These two instruments can be used for a wide range of mild to moderate hearing losses. They are, however, relatively small and present problems to some elderly patients in terms of manipulating the controls, inserting and removing the battery, and in placement of the hearing aid. Modifications can be made to these instruments, such as raising the volume control for easier adjustment and attaching handles to the ear mold to facilitate insertion and extraction.

Another common package for a hearing aid is one that is built into the temple of a pair of eyeglasses. Electroacoustically, it is similar to the postauricular and in-the-ear instruments. Its advantages are the ease of wearing both hearing aids and eyeglasses simultaneously. This feature may simplify its use by geriatric patients and can be a plus factor in the acceptance of amplification. A disadvantage is related to the visual problems that geriatric patients may experience and the frequency of required lens changes. When the patient is without his eyeglasses, he is also without his hearing aid. An added attraction of the eyeglass hearing aid relates to a special hearing aid modification known as a CROS (Contralateral Routing of Signal) hearing aid. This type of hearing aid is beneficial for patients with one extremely poor ear (for which amplification is of little value) and one relatively good ear. A CROS hearing aid places the microphone of the hearing aid on the poor ear side. The microphone is electrically connected to the amplifier and speaker located on the better ear side, and the sound is fed into the better ear. In this way, sound that occurs on the poor ear side is transmitted to the better ear. The electrical connection can be made through the frames of eyeglasses and can be worn without any additional equipment that would be required if this hearing aid were to be used in a non-eyeglass configuration.

Finally, for the most serious hearing losses, the use of a body-worn hearing aid may be required. This instrument has a relatively large package containing the microphone, amplifier, and gain controls. Typically, this is worn in a shirt pocket or a chest carrier. The output of the hearing aid is fed via electrical wire to a receiver attached to an ear mold. The severity of the hearing loss is what usually mandates the need for a larger hearing aid. However, the size of the instrument and its controls can facilitate hearing aid use for some elderly persons. Several manufacturers produce body-worn hearing aids that are less powerful specifically for this purpose.

Hearing Aid Evaluation
The basic criteria for selection of amplification were first delineated in 1946.[16] Basically, the evaluation requires an initial audiologic evaluation to determine the patient's threshold levels for pure-tones, Speech Reception Threshold, Speech Discrimination, the intensity level at which sound is most comfortable, and the intensity level at which sound is uncomfortable. These tests are accomplished by presenting stimuli through earphones. Several tests are accomplished with stimuli presented through various speakers located in a sound-treated examination room. The patient's auditory function is thereby evaluated under binaural listening conditions. These additional tests include the Speech Reception Threshold, Speech Discrimination under good listening conditions, and Speech Discrimination under poor listening conditions. The Speech Discrimination tests are accomplished with the stimulus presented at an intensity level approximating typical conversational speech. The Speech Discrimination test under a good listening condition is accomplished with the material presented without any competing conversational speech under optimal listening conditions. The Speech Discrimination test under poor listening conditions is the same type of test except that speech is presented against a background of variable intensity noise. The competing stimulus can take the form of masking noise, recordings of environmental noise or other people's voices. This test is intended to simulate a typical listening situation where there is some level of background noise from which the individual must extract the message.

All of the tests presented through the speakers or in a "sound field" are performed when the patient is not wearing a hearing aid. Results are then compared using the same tests, but with the patient wearing a number of hearing aids that the audiologist has selected for trial. Hearing aids are preselected, based on various criteria that the audiologist presumes will result in maximum performance. Some of these criteria are briefly described below.

Monaural versus Binaural Amplification
Based on the extent of the hearing loss, the symmetry of loss, and communication needs, the decision to wear one or two hearing aids can be reached by both the audiologist and patient. Another factor for the geriatric patient in this decision relates to the ability to manipulate two hearing aids to achieve an appropriate binaural gain setting.

Electroacoustic Parameters The frequency response, gain, and maximum power output are three of several variables that are selected to meet the needs of the individual. Most hearing aids have controls that allow the audiologist to vary these parameters. This is helpful for the geriatric patient whose tolerance for amplification may be initially poor but improving with use.

The Hearing Aid Package This needs to be considered from a practical standpoint as well as from a cosmetic one. A hearing aid that is not worn because of the vanity of the user is as good as no hearing aid at all. Within the limits of the other previously mentioned considerations, the patient's appearance with the hearing aid should be regarded.

Obviously, with elderly people living on a fixed income, the ability to purchase the necessary amplification must be considered. Ultimately, it is up to the patient to determine the affordability of one versus two hearing aids or a hearing aid versus no aid. The audiologist and physician should be familiar with agencies offering a graduated fee schedule or organizations that provide hearing aids to those who cannot afford them.

Once an appropriate hearing aid has been selected, and an ear mold has been fabricated, the patient should be instructed thoroughly in the proper use, care, and maintenance of the instrument. No matter how carefully this is accomplished, the majority of return visits by an older patient are due to a lack of understanding of the function of the hearing aid they have received. During this counseling, it is helpful to have another family member or friend present who is capable of assimilating the information. Occasionally, this significant other will have sole responsibility for making sure that the hearing aid is worn and maintained. This occurs when a cognitive deficit or physical disability prohibits the patient from performing these tasks. In these instances, it is essential to enlist the help of someone who can provide consistent care.

One of the most commonly asked questions is, "Do I need to use the hearing aid all of the time?" Philosophies differ with regard to the answer. The opinion of the author is that the goal of hearing aid use should be to wear the instrument all of the time during waking hours. The more accustomed one becomes to amplified sound, the more one is able to use amplified auditory information for communication. Those individuals who use hearing aids on a limited basis are typically those who are the least motivated and least successful users. Some patients require a "breaking in" period where they gradually increase the time periods per day during which the hearing aid is used. A standard approach is to advise patients to initially use their hearing aids two to three times per day for 1 hour each time in very controlled listening situations. For example, the hearing aid can be worn while conversing with one other individual in a quiet room. Another situation would be to use the hearing aid while listening to radio or watching television when the volume control has been set by someone with normal hearing. The time periods and difficulty of the listening experience can be gradually increased from this point.

Related to the question of how much to use the hearing aid is the question of how high to set the gain. The gain of the hearing aid should be at a level that permits maximum speech intelligibility without approximating the limit of tolerance for amplified sound. Tolerance may actually increase with the use of a hearing aid, and the geriatric patient can (if necessary) begin wearing the hearing aid with less than optimum gain. After confidence with the aid increases, the gain can then be increased to the patient's optimal level. The individual should be encouraged to find the best gain setting and leave the control alone once that point has been determined. Patients should be allowed to experience sounds that are both louder and softer than normal, which makes for a more natural listening experience. Adjusting the gain of a hearing aid to suit the situation detracts from this goal and, ultimately, from a hearing aid acceptance. Of course, there are certain conditions of intense sound environments (airports, power

tools, home appliances, and so on) that require the user to reduce the gain of the hearing aid.

The initial period of hearing aid use with an older patient should be monitored closely. A follow-up appointment no later than 2 weeks after the date of hearing aid receipt is advisable. Assessment should be made of the patient's progress with adjustment to the hearing aid. The ear mold may be causing some minor irritation and may require modification. The patient's abilities to operate the hearing aid should be re-evaluated and any questions should be answered. Depending on the findings, one or more follow-up appointments may be scheduled. It is critical to maximize the patient's chances for successful hearing aid use at the outset by minimizing the negative experiences they encounter. It is always valuable to include family members or friends in at least a portion of these subsequent visits. Their perception of the patient's adjustment to amplification are sometimes quite different from that of the patient. This additional information may assist the audiologist in making modifications.

Rehabilitation

The provision of amplification to a hearing-impaired elderly person is one aspect of what should be considered a total program of rehabilitation. It is important to stress, prior to hearing aid use, that amplification is not a panacea. A hearing aid does not restore hearing to normal. There are other supplemental forms of rehabilitation that also can improve communication. These include maximizing the use of visual information and manipulating one's environment to minimize auditory distractions. These aspects of aural rehabilitation can be employed with patients who, for one reason or another, are not candidates for amplification.

As with hearing aid acceptance, probably the most important factor in achieving some measure of success in aural rehabilitation is motivation. The patient that resists change, denies or represses his or her problem, or projects it onto others will not be amenable to changing long-standing patterns of behavior even though they may be detrimental. Two approaches may increase the patient's desire to change.

The first one requires that the audiologist be able to isolate and identify one or more specific situations in the patient's own daily routine that appear to cause difficulty. The patient may not be able to provide this information if he denies the existence of any loss of hearing. Therefore, the audiologist may need to make some observation or enlist the help of significant others and/or staff personnel at health care facilities. Once areas of specific difficulty are identified, the audiologist can devise a plan that will result in improved communication. If a patient experiences success, he or she may be more willing to acknowledge his or her own sensory deficit. Additionally, they may become motivated to generalize this improvement for other situations and to learn other ways of coping with their hearing loss.

A second approach that may increase one's desire to improve communication is through the use of group interaction. An elderly patient who is reticent to discuss problems individually with an audiologist may feel more comfortable in a group of people with similar problems. The composition of such a group should be fairly homogeneous in terms of age and degree of hearing loss. It is helpful at the outset to have at least one member of the group who is more experienced than the others to facilitate interaction.

Environmental Considerations
Once a patient is willing to work on improved communication, several areas can be identified where communication can be enhanced by environmental manipulation. The poorer the signal-to-noise ratio in any message, the less likely the message will be understood; that is, the higher the intensity of unwanted auditory stimuli, relative to the intensity of any auditory message, the more difficulty experienced in interpreting the message. This fact holds true for those of us with normal hearing. It is compounded for those with hearing loss. It is worsened even more for an elderly patient with a hearing loss because of existent auditory processing disorders, as well as pure peripheral sensory deficits.

Noise, in its generic sense, means any unwanted stimulus. Auditorily, noise can refer to the sound of a vacuum cleaner that interferes

with a husband and wife's conversation. It can be the sound of other voices at the dinner table while trying to communicate with just one individual. Another type of noise that is non-auditory in nature is distance. Beyond a distance of 6–10 feet, the space between speaker and listener becomes a deterrent to effective communication. This is especially true for the hearing-impaired individual who also has a visual deficit.

A patient can be trained to attenuate background noise, thereby improving the signal-to-noise ratio. At home, a patient should be encouraged to turn off the television or radio when trying to communicate with other family members. At social gatherings, such as church or civic club meetings, the individual should be instructed to position him or herself as close to the primary speaker as possible. Therapy, individually or in groups, can be centered around discussions of ways to manipulate one's own environment for optimum communication. Additionally, real life situations can be simulated with the use of tape recordings and, with the hearing aid in use, the patient can practice under controlled and increasingly more difficult listening situations.

It is generally helpful to discuss, both with the hearing-impaired patient and their significant others, the ways in which speaking will improve or detract from understanding the content of conversation. The natural tendency when talking to someone with a hearing loss is to raise your voice or, sometimes, to shout when you are not understood. It should be stressed that the best way to communicate is face-to-face, speaking slowly and clearly without exaggerated lip movements or facial expressions, and to reword a sentence that the listener has particular difficulty understanding.

Auditory Training and Speech Reading
The term "lip reading" has been used to describe the process whereby an individual gains linguistic information through the use of visual stimuli from the speaker. Traditionally, this meant attempting to train hearing-impaired persons to identify individual speech sounds, or phonemes, by their visual appearance on the speaker's lips. The current terminology, "speech reading," is intended to convey that

any visual information provided by the speaker, in addition to lip movement, can be used to supplement auditory information in determining the content of a spoken message. Controversy still exists as to whether one can actually be taught, through formal training, to extract specific information from visual cues. Two variables, visual acuity and short term memory, strongly correlate with speech reading ability and have significance for elderly persons. Several researchers have demonstrated that visual short term memory is decreased in elderly persons[17] and that they require longer stimulus durations to identify visual forms than do younger persons.[18] If any information about the use of visual stimuli can be taught, these two factors certainly contribute to making the task more difficult in an elderly population.

One fact remains clear and should be impressed upon an elderly patient. All of us, normal hearing and otherwise, use visual information in some manner to assist us auditorily. Frequently, elderly hearing-impaired patients with a long-standing hearing loss and other sensory and motor deficits have withdrawn from much of their social contacts. They become depressed and develop a posture with head bowed. It is remarkable, both to the patient and family alike, how much communication can be enhanced simply by urging the listener to maintain eye contact with the speaker.

Other techniques recommended for use with an elderly population generally involve a synthetic approach to speech reading and auditory training; that is, rather than breaking speech down into its basic components (speech sounds), training is concentrated on larger speech units (i.e., words, phrases, and sentences). The patient is taught to synthesize all information relative to the message. The knowledge of the topic of conversation, where the conversation is taking place, the gestures and facial expression of the speaker, all provide cues for understanding. Training a patient to be aware of these sources and to not become stymied by the inability to understand one or two words in a message is the goal of this approach.

Another tool suggested for use with elderly persons is that of subvocal rehearsal. This involves training a patient to mimic the articulatory movements visible from the speaker. The rationale for this approach is to provide additional proprioceptive information that may assist in improving intelligibility.

Communication Problems and Needs in an Institutional Setting

For an elderly patient who lives with family or nearby long-time established friends, a significant support system is available throughout the rehabilitation process. They are present to insure that the patient continues to use and maintain their hearing aids in an appropriate manner. They help to create listening situations in which the chances for maximum communication are optimized. They have developed some skill in speaking to a hearing-impaired person.

For an elderly individual who resides in a retirement community, these support systems may not be firmly established. It is for these patients that the audiologist may need to act as an advocate. Many programs exist where aural rehabilitation is brought to the community, such as in a "senior center." In retirement homes, or nursing homes, those staff providing care and having direct contact with patients should develop an understanding of the principles underlying communication needs of elderly persons. While this seems obvious, it is appalling to see the lack of use of amplification in these settings. Even when it is available, many nursing home residents do not use their hearing aids because nobody in the environment understands its operation or how to make minor repairs. The audiologist should provide in-service training for those who provide daily care to elderly persons.

The ultimate goal of all geriatric health care providers is to improve or maintain the quality of life of their patients. The extent to which adequate communication relates to the quality of life makes the audiologist an essential member of the geriatric health care team.

References

1. Harris CS: *Fact Book on Aging: A Profile of America's Older Population*. Washington, D.C., National Council on the Aging, 1978.
2. National Center for Health Statistics: *Prevalence of Selected Impairments, United States 1971*: U.S. Dept of Health, Education, and Welfare publication no. (HRA) 75-1527. Health Resources Administration, 1975.

3. Schow RL, Nerbonne MA: Hearing levels among elderly nursing home residents. *J Speech Hearing Dis* 45:24–32, 1980.

4. Chafee CE: Rehabilitation needs of nursing home patients: a report of a survey. *Rehab Lit* 28:377–382, 1967.

5. Rosen S, Plester D, El-Mofty A, et al: High frequency audiometry in presbycusis. *Arch Otolaryngol* 79:18–31, 1964.

6. Chandler JR: Partial occlusion of the external auditory meatus: its effect upon air and bone conduction hearing acuity. *Laryngoscope* 74:22–54, 1964.

7. Maurer JF, Rupp RR: *Hearing and Aging: Tactics for Intervention*. New York, Grune & Stratton, 1979.

8. Jerger J, Jerger S, Muldin L: Studies in impedance audiometry: I. Normal and sensorineural ears. *Arch Otolaryngol* 96:512–523, 1972.

9. Corso JF: Presbycusis hearing aids and aging. *Audiology* 16:146–163, 1977.

10. Johnsson LG, Hawkins JE: Sensory and neural degeneration with aging as seen in microdissections of the human inner ear. *Ann Otolaryngol* 81:179–183, 1972.

11. Fausti SA, Frey RH, Erickson DA, et al: A system for evaluating auditory function from 8–20 kHz. *J Acout Soc Amer* 66:1713–1718, 1979.

12. Gaeth J: A study of phonemic regression associated with hearing loss. Unpublished Doctoral Dissertation, Northwestern University, Evanston, Ill., 1948.

13. Ramsdell DA: The psychology of the hard-of-hearing and the deafened adult, in Davis H, Silverman R (eds): *Hearing and Deafness*. New York, Holt Rinehart & Winston Inc, 1966, pp 459–473.

14. Alpiner JG: Evaluation of communication function, in Alpiner JG (ed): *Handbook of Adult Rehabilitative Audiology*. Baltimore, Williams & Wilkins Co, 1978, pp 30–66.

15. Goetzinger C, Rousey C: Hearing problems in later life. *Medical Times* 87:771–780, 1959.

16. Carhart R: Selection of hearing aids. *Arch Otolaryngol* 44:1–18, 1946.

17. McGhie A, Chapman J, Lawson JS: Changes in immediate memory with age. *British J Psychol* 56:69–75, 1965.

18. Eriksen CM, Hamlin RM, Breitmeyer RG: Temporal factors in visual perception as related to aging. *Percep Psychophys* 7:354–356, 1970.

CHAPTER 10

Pulmonary Diseases

JAMES F. MORRIS, M.D.

Second only to the skin, the bronchopulmonary system is subject to environmental ravages. Every few seconds, the ambient air and all it contains is inhaled and in contact with a surface area equivalent in the adult to the size of a tennis court. Perhaps, in anticipation of environmental slings and arrows, natural in earlier days and man-made at present, we are endowed with one extra lung. With a normal aging process, the bronchopulmonary system should be adequate for about 90 years of continuous functioning. The lungs were initially thought to be designed only for acting as a fluctuating bellows, which results in the transfer of oxygen and carbon dioxide (CO_2). Additional biochemical and immunologic roles have been discovered, thus assigning the lungs a more active metabolic status.

Anatomy

The three main structural elements of the bronchopulmonary system include (obviously) both the airways and the lung parenchyma and (less obviously) the chest wall. The airways primarily provide a conducting function for the movement of inspired and expired gases. Gas transfer first appears only at the level of the respiratory bronchiole. The simultaneous progressive narrowing and branching of the airways produce a marked increase in the total cross-sectional diameter and a resulting decrease in the resistance to airflow. The ability of the airways to both dilate and lengthen during inspiration adjusts to the increasing tidal volume. The airways can be divided into those with cartilaginous support and those lacking it. These latter airways are the bronchioles, which are usually 2 mm or less in diameter. The supporting mechanism of the bronchioles is the tethering effect of the parenchymal elastic tissue. They are, thus, more susceptible to changes in lung inflation and intrathoracic pressure. In addition, airway lumens can be narrowed by a constriction of bronchial muscle, loss of supporting parenchymal tissue, thickening of bronchial epithelium by hypertrophy, edema or inflammation, and by obstructing bronchopulmonary secretions.

It is difficult to separate changes that are due to the aging process itself from those due to an accumulative exposure to toxic gases and particulates, antigenic substances, and microorganisms. The most easily demonstrable change is the loss of elastic lung parenchyma surrounding small non-cartilaginous airways. This causes a premature small airways closure that results in an increase in trapped or residual gas volume and a decrease in forced expired airflows. Specific age changes in the airways are more difficult to define. In the absence of specific lung diseases, a loss or changes in connective tissues appear to increase the compliance of the airways, which results in progressive enlargement of the bronchi, bronchioles, and alveolar ducts. In bronchial walls, aging increases the size of mucous glands and a calcification of cartilage.

The enlargement of the airway caliber is negated by the decrease in parenchymal support of the smaller airways, resulting in a net decrease in the diameter of the airways with progressive aging.

Decreased elastic recoil with a decreased distensibility results in a descent of the diaphragm and an expansion of the thorax. A common misconception is that these changes are produced by hyperinflation of the lungs when, in truth, they are due to the natural tendency of the chest cavity to enlarge unless opposed by the elastic recoil of the lung. The changes in the distribution of parenchymal elastic tissue result in panlobular emphysema, which is characterized by a progressive dilation of alveoli and an eventual disruption of their walls. In contrast to the centrilobular emphysema associated with cigarette smoking, the respiratory bronchioles are minimally involved, there is no inflammatory component, the distribution is predominantly in the lower lobes, the lungs are less compliant, and the changes are not severe. There is a similarity to the panlobular emphysema found in patients with homozygous alpha$_1$-antitrypsin deficiency who appear to have accelerated lung senescence. The balance of forces between elastase and antielastase is proposed as the determinant of alveolar disruption. Aging, tobacco smoke and other air pollutants, many pulmonary infections, and deficiency of antiproteases, tip the balance in favor of elastase and the development of various forms of emphysema.

The chest wall has been relatively neglected regarding its contribution to ventilation. Macklem has referred to it as the last unexplored organ in the body.[1] The muscles of respiration consist of the intercostal and accessory muscles, the diaphragm, and the abdominal muscles. During quiet breathing, the diaphragm is responsible for ventilatory work, with the other respiratory muscles helping to stabilize the chest wall and abdomen.[2] During exertion, all the respiratory muscles are needed; the degree of involvement related to the level of work being done. With aging and a decline in physical activity, muscle atrophy can lead to a diminished exertional capacity. Changes in skeletal portions of the chest wall include calcification of costochondral joints and a decreased chest wall compliance.

Lung Defense Mechanisms

An individual inhales an average tidal volume of 500 ml about 18,000 times daily, or about 9,000 liters of ambient air. The lungs have a complex defense system to protect them against inhaled particles, gases, microorganisms, and products of combustion.[3] When defense mechanisms are overwhelmed or are lacking, respiratory diseases result. In addition to inhaled noxious agents, the lung must defend itself against biochemical substances in the pulmonary capillary blood that can result in damage to the alveolar capillary membrane.

Aerosols settle out in the airway via the mechanisms of impaction, sedimentation, or diffusion, and are influenced by particle size, airway caliber and configuration and the velocity of airflow. Gases penetrate into the airway according to their water solubility (less soluble penetrate further distally).

Non-specific defense mechanisms include the regulation of temperature and humidity, clearance mechanisms, mucus, and cellular defenses. Responses to specific antigens include local antibody production and cell-mediated immunity.

Both mechanisms are progressively impaired by the aging process. Thus, elderly persons are more vulnerable to viral and bacterial respiratory infections from reduced humoral antibody response and to fungal pneumonia, tuberculosis, and lung cancer due to impaired cell-mediated immunity.

Respiratory viral infections predispose to acute bacterial bronchitis and pneumonia. The principal mechanism occurs by temporarily suppressing pulmonary bactericidal activity. Indirectly, defense mechanisms are adversely affected by the impairment of mechanical transport out of the lung. Aging appears to increase the susceptibility to respiratory infections by poor antibody response and a reduced clearance of particles.

Inhaled tobacco smoke blunts the effectiveness of both non-specific (phagocytic) and specific (immunologic) defense mechanism systems of the lung. This impairment may be responsible for a smoker's increased susceptibility to bronchopulmonary infections; it hampers the handling of other inhaled particulates by the lung. The functions of alveolar macrophages and lymphocytes are adversely affected by cigarette smoke.

Inhaled particulates and gaseous agents other than that found in tobacco smoke also suppress pulmonary defense mechanisms. Noxious agents act singly or in combination. For example, irritant gases may be absorbed onto particulates, deposited in the lung, and phagocytized by alveolar macrophages. Adverse effects of environmental agents include the inhibition of phagocytosis and antibody production. Susceptibility to both viral and bacterial infectious may be increased. Both the effects of cigarette smoke and of environmental pollutants are increased by prolonged exposure and are, thus, worse in older adults.

Chronic diseases of the lungs, heart, kidney, bone marrow, and other organ systems, which are more common in elderly persons, are associated with an increased susceptibility to lower respiratory infections. Conditions such as hypoxia, acidosis, malnutrition, uremia, and cold exposure impair alveolar macrophage functions.

Pulmonary Function

A reserve capacity is built into most body organs. For breathing, it appears that one lung is perfectly adequate in early adult life, with the other representing a spare. Considerable lung disease is required to produce a significant impairment of pulmonary function. As in other organs, diffuse damage results in a greater functional loss than focal damage. The principal symptom of pulmonary function impairment is dyspnea or shortness of breath. It represents an awareness of breathing that usually is an unconscious act. Dyspnea does not always mean pulmonary dysfunction.[4] First, it may be appropriate for the level of exertion and the work of breathing required. Second, dyspnea may result from any deficiency in the entire oxygen transport system.

Ventilation

The principal components of ventilation are lung volumes and air flows. Figure 10-1 shows static lung volumes and capacities in normal individuals. Note that the capacities consist of two or more lung volumes. The determinants of lung volumes are represented by the respiratory muscles, elastic properties of the lung and chest wall, and caliber of the airways. The degrees of inspiratory and expiratory pressures generated by respiratory muscles influence lung volumes. Other influences include age, body position, height, and sex. Even in younger persons, assuming a supine position reduces vital capacity and functional residual capacity primarily by a cephalad shift of the diaphragm. When one is in an upright position, aging decreases the vital capacity and increases the residual volume.[5,6] Only minor changes occur in functional residual capacity and total lung capacity. Increased residual volume represents trapped gas that is

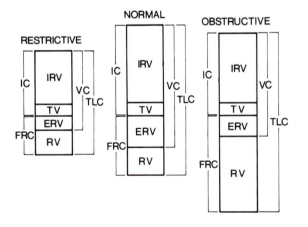

IC: Inspiratory Capacity
FRC: Functional Residual Capacity
VC: Vital Capacity
TLC: Total Lung Capacity

IRV: Inspiratory Reserve Volume
TV: Tidal Volume
ERV: Expiratory Reserve Volume
RV: Residual Volume

FIGURE 10-1   Lung volumes and capacities in health and disease.

probably caused by early airway closure, increased thoracic cage rigidity, and decreased lung elastic recoil.[7]

Expired gas flows are determined by forces that are exerted by respiratory muscular effort and lung elastic recoil, and are influenced by the airway diameter. As lung volume diminishes, gas flow becomes nearly independent of muscular effort. Conditions that reduce elastic recoil or patency of the airways impair forced expiratory flows. With advancing age, total lung capacity is maintained and contributes to the preservation of large airway diameter.[8] Changes in elastic tissues of the lung result in a decrease of elastic recoil and an increase in its compliance or distensibility. At high lung volumes, the smaller airways have a decreased airway resistance. As expiration achieves lower lung volumes, resistance to airflow increases and smaller airways prematurely close. The volume of gas remaining in the lung as airways close is termed the closing volume. It normally is not within resting tidal volumes, as it is less than the functional residual capacity. As aging results in a reduced elastic recoil, the closing

volume increases and, in the supine position, encroaches on the tidal volume.[9] The third force influencing flows is respiratory muscular effort, which decreases with aging. Thus, all flows are reduced; those at high lung volume are due to a diminished elastic recoil and airway diameter.[10]

Figures 10-2 and 10-3 indicate the five spirometric tests that are useful in measuring ventilatory function: the FVC, FEV 1, FEF 200–1,200, FEF 25–75%, and FEF 75–85%.[11] FVC = forced vital capacity; FEV 1 = forced expiratory volume in one second; FEF 200–1,200 = forced expiratory flow rate between 200 and 1200 cc's; FEF 25%–75% = forced expiratory flow rate between 25% and 75% of vital capacity; FEF 75%–85% = forced expiratory flow rate between 75% and 85% of vital capacity. Figure 10-4 and 10-5 show the age-related decline in four of these measurements based on a cross-sectional study of healthy non-smoking adults.[12] There are two flaws in such studies; first, a longitudinal study is preferable, but obviously difficult to achieve. Second, normal predicted values usually are expressed as a linear

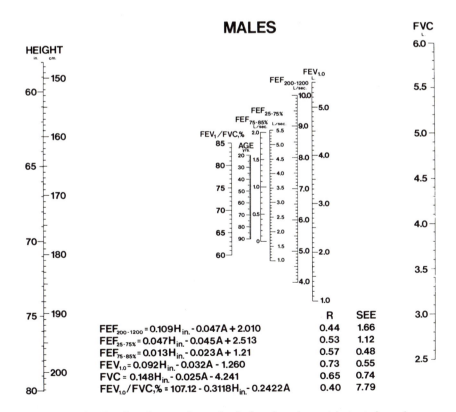

$$FEF_{200\text{-}1200} = 0.109H_{in.} - 0.047A + 2.010 \qquad R\ 0.44 \quad SEE\ 1.66$$
$$FEF_{25\text{-}75\%} = 0.047H_{in.} - 0.045A + 2.513 \qquad 0.53 \quad 1.12$$
$$FEF_{75\text{-}85\%} = 0.013H_{in.} - 0.023A + 1.21 \qquad 0.57 \quad 0.48$$
$$FEV_{1.0} = 0.092H_{in.} - 0.032A - 1.260 \qquad 0.73 \quad 0.55$$
$$FVC = 0.148H_{in.} - 0.025A - 4.241 \qquad 0.65 \quad 0.74$$
$$FEV_{1.0}/FVC,\% = 107.12 - 0.3118H_{in.} - 0.2422A \qquad 0.40 \quad 7.79$$

FIGURE 10-2 Predicted normal standards for six spirometric tests in males.

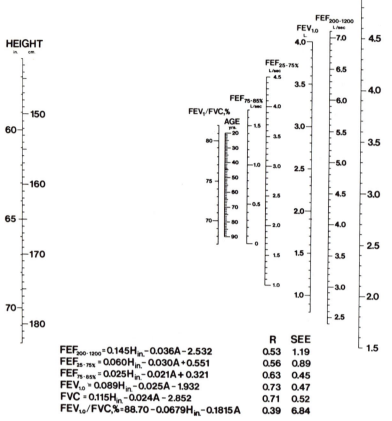

FEMALES

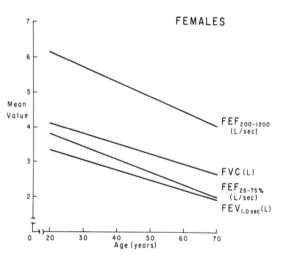

FIGURE 10-3 Predicted normal standards for six spirometric tests in females.

	R	SEE
$FEF_{200-1200} = 0.145H_{in.} - 0.036A - 2.532$	0.53	1.19
$FEF_{25-75\%} = 0.060H_{in.} - 0.030A + 0.551$	0.56	0.89
$FEF_{75-85\%} = 0.025H_{in.} - 0.021A + 0.321$	0.63	0.45
$FEV_{1.0} = 0.089H_{in.} - 0.025A - 1.932$	0.73	0.47
$FVC = 0.115H_{in.} - 0.024A - 2.852$	0.71	0.52
$FEV_{1.0}/FVC,\% = 88.70 - 0.0679H_{in.} - 0.1815A$	0.39	6.84

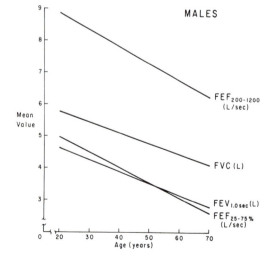

FIGURE 10-4   Decline of four spirometric tests with increasing age in males.

FIGURE 10-5   Decline of four spirometric tests with increasing age in females.

regression equation, although a curvilinear function is more appropriate. The decrement of flows and volumes are not the same for each year of the life span. The difficulty of obtaining an adequate study of representative elderly subjects has yet to be resolved. A normal variation from predicted sample means is substantial despite an accounting for sex, height, and respiratory health. Selection of a fixed value such as 1.65 times the mean value may result in negative-predicted values for expiratory flows in elderly persons. Serial studies in an individual subject would be preferable for observing the course of pulmonary function, which is influenced not only by age, but by diseases due to smoking, air pollution, and infections. Table 10-1 lists regression equations that are useful for calculating the equivalent lung age. This represents the age in which the observed test results would be normal for a person of the same age, sex, and height. For example, the FEV 1 of a 52-year-old cigarette smoker would be normal for a 75-year-old male of similar height, but without ventilatory impairment. These calculations may provide a motivation for cessation of smoking. A variety of spirometers are available, ranging from simple volume displacement devices to computerized electronic systems. The American Thoracic Society has established standards of accuracy to which all devices should conform.[13]

Alveolar Gas Exchange

The essential function of the lungs is to exchange oxygen (O_2) and carbon dioxide (CO_2) across the alveolar capillary membrane. This process requires not only both ventilation and blood perfusion suitable to the metabolic activity of the body, but also the matching of ventilation and perfusion as perfectly as possible.

"Dead space" ventilation represents wasted ventilation. The ratio of dead space to tidal volume best expresses the degree of abnormality. In adult life, this increases approximately 0.17% per year from a normal of 25%. In aging lungs, both ventilation and perfusion are distributed unevenly, resulting in a decreased arterial PO_2 of about 0.42 mm Hg per year for patients in the supine position.[14] Because of earlier airway closure during expiration, arterial PO_2 is always lower in the supine position than when seated.[15] In an upright patient, perfusion of lung bases diminishes with age, which results in an increased ventilation-perfusion ($\dot{V}/\dot{Q}$) ratio. There usually is no significant change in arterial pH or PCO_2. Exchange of CO_2 is linearly influenced by alveolar ventilation. Other than hypoventilation, elimination of CO_2 is relatively uninfluenced by disease processes that produce a $\dot{V}/\dot{Q}$ mismatch, diffusion impairment, or vascular shunting. Aging does not result in CO_2 retention.

Pulmonary Circulation

The entire output of the right ventricle of the heart passes through the pulmonary arterial circulation. The pulmonary arteries, containing the venous blood, supply the gas exchange portion of the lung, beginning at the level of the respiratory bronchiole. Pulmonary arteries lack precapillary sphincters common to systemic arterioles. The mean pulmonary arterial pressure

TABLE 10-1   Equivalent Lung Age

Males	
FVC	Lung age = 5.920H − 40.000(Obs. FVC) − 169.640
FEV 1	Lung age = 2.870H − 31.250(Obs. FEV 1) − 39.375
FEV 200–1,200	Lung age = 2.319H − 21.277(Obs. FEF 200–1,200) + 42.766
FEF 25–75%	Lung age = 1.044H − 22.222(Obs. FEF 25–75%) + 55.844
Females	
FVC	Lung age = 4.792H − 41.667(Obs. FVC) − 118.833
FEV 1	Lung age = 3.560H − 40.000(Obs. FEV 1) − 77.280
FEF 200–1,200	Lung age = 4.028H − 27.778(Obs. FEF 200–1,200) − 70.333
FEF 25–75%	Lung age = 2.000H − 33.333(Obs. FEF 25–75%) + 18.367

H = height, in inches.

at rest is about 19 mm Hg. Because of the ability to recruit collapsed pulmonary capillaries as cardiac output increases, exercise normally produces little rise in mean arterial pressure. Pulmonary capillary blood volume is about 75 ml at rest and 200 ml during exercise, which reflects the cardiac stroke volume. With age, the pulmonary capillary blood volume remains unchanged, as does total lung perfusion. The loss of pulmonary capillaries either from emphysema or normal aging does not cause pulmonary hypertension. This contrasts with hypoxemia, which induces pulmonary arterial constriction and an elevation of pressure. Perfusion of the lung in the upright position is influenced by gravity, with a pressure and perfusion greater in the lower part of the lung; this represents about 70% of the total lung area. Because of this relative increase in pressure, flow in these pulmonary capillaries is independent of alveolar pressure. The decrease in the diffusing capacity for oxygen with advancing age in both males and females is presumably due more to decreasing perfusion at lung bases with a consequent increase in the $\dot{V}/\dot{Q}$ ratio than to a loss of surface area of the alveolar capillary membrane.

Control of Ventilation

Breathing is regulated by peripheral and central chemoreceptors acting as sensors and central nervous system areas acting as controllers.[16] The primary oxygen sensors are the carotid bodies, which respond to hypoxemia. The control of CO_2 is less clear. Investigators have reported the peripheral chemoreceptor contribution to regulating ventilatory response to hypercapnia ranges from 20–50%. The central chemoreceptors in the brainstem account for the remainder of the response to abnormal PCO_2. The mechanism of sensing the CO_2 level is by the formation of carbonic acid and the acidification of brain extracellular fluid. Other acids can similarly affect the brainstem controller. For example, if hypoxemia-induced hyperventilation is severe, lactic acid production may influence a further increase in ventilation by acting both on the carotid body chemoreceptor and the brainstem controller. In addition to hypoxemia, hypercapnia, and acidemia, receptors in the upper airway and lung also influence

respiration, thus responding to chemical and mechanical stimuli. Studies of aging have indicated an overall diminution in response to low O_2, high CO_2, and mechanical loads, which is presumably due to a functional decline of both peripheral and central chemoreceptors.

Sleep Apnea Syndrome

Since 1965, there has been a burgeoning interest in breathing disorders in adults during sleep. As techniques of polysomnography are more widely used, the occurrence of the sleep apnea syndrome is now known to range from normal individuals to those whose existence is threatened. Apnea is defined as the cessation of all airflow at the nose and mouth for at least 10 seconds. The syndrome requires at least 30 such apneic episodes per night. Obstructive apnea results from occlusion of the upper airway in the face of persistent efforts to breathe. Central apnea occurs in the absence of any breathing effort. In mixed apnea, airflow ceases with an early absence of breathing effort, followed by a resumption of unsuccessful ventilatory effort in the latter part of the episode. Physiologic and clinical consequences may be disastrous and include daytime somnolence, changes in mental status and personality, erythrocytosis, pulmonary hypertension, and cardiac arrhythmias. Incidence is higher in males and postmenopausal females. Risk factors include obesity, older age, and use of central nervous system depressants. Snoring has been identified as a risk factor and an important signal in those with obstructive apnea.[17] Because of its risk for nocturnal mortality and hypoxemia-induced morbidity, symptoms suggesting sleep apnea should be investigated by experts with the experience and facilities to perform polysomnography. For details of these evaluation methods and therapeutic interventions, refer to the section in Chapter 14 on sleep disorders. Recognition of this common and serious syndrome, which becomes worse with advancing age and weight, may avert considerable nocturnal deaths and morbidity.

Exercise Training

Exercise capacity usually is indicated by the body's maximal oxygen capacity or uptake ($\dot{V}O_2$ max). To provide oxygen to the working muscles, the oxygen transport system moves oxygen from ambient air to muscle mitochondria. The system involves the interrelationship of the lungs, chest wall, heart, vessels, and hemoglobin.[18] The effects of aging adversely affect all the involved mechanisms to varying degrees. Although it is difficult to separate from illnesses whose incidence rate increases with age, exercise or aerobic capacity deteriorates with age after attaining physical maturity.[19] In younger persons, cardiac output appears to be the limiting factor in endurance performance. Of the two components of cardiac output, stroke volume is both the limiting and trainable factor in comparison with heart rate. With increasing age, the cardiac output decreases about 8% each decade. The large reserve in ventilatory capacity has been shown not to be a limitation in exercise performance in young persons. But with age, a stiffening of the chest wall with a loss of compliance combines with decreased muscle strength, vital capacity, and maximum-forced expiratory flows to provide a limitation of exercise capacity.[18] Hemoglobin does not routinely decrease sufficiently with age to impair oxygen transport.[19]

In addition to the effects of aging and disease, the increasingly sedentary life style common to older people contributes to the loss of aerobic capacity and, thus, endurance function. In a study of healthy older subjects prior to and after endurance conditioning,[20] DeVries showed their trainability in the 7th and 8th decades. Both cardiac and respiratory function improved in terms of improved cardiac output and exercise ventilation. The latter has not been sufficiently appreciated when the studies have involved younger subjects. The respiratory pump also can undergo disease and be reversed by training inspiratory muscles.[21] Other beneficial effects include a reduction in systolic and diastolic blood pressures and a reduction in the resting muscle potential level, which is referred to as a "tranquilizer" effect.[22] Decreased physical dependency and improved self-image are less quantitative, but nonetheless are important results of exercise programs. Other components of physical fitness that also should be considered are flexibility, strength, agility, and balance. These may require special programs, such as calisthenics. Despite the justifiable enthusiasm for exercise programs for elderly persons, particular precautions are advisable because of their inherently greater risks of cardiovascular and musculoskeletal diseases. Activities that use large muscle groups in rhythmic activity (such as walking, jogging, or swimming) are preferable to those involving bursts of activity, small muscle groups, and static muscle contraction. Prior to each activity, muscle stretching techniques are essential as is a slow and careful warm-up. An elderly individual should monitor his or her pulse rate in the prescribed target zone, which usually is 70% of the predicted heart rate (220 − age in years times 70%); however, under no condition is it to exceed 170 beats per minute. Cooling down after exercise should be done as slowly as warming up. A study of highly trained, older endurance athletes, in comparison with younger athletes revealed a lower maximum heart rate and $\dot{V}O_2$ max of 15% less in the older athletes.[23] The identical O_2 pulse ($\dot{V}O_2$/heart rate) suggested that the reduction in $\dot{V}O_2$ max was due to the lower maximum heart rate than to either the reduced maximum stroke volume or maximum arteriovenous difference. Heath, et al estimated 9% of $\dot{V}O_2$ max was lost each decade after age 25.[23] The average decline in the trained older athletes was 5% per decade; thus, the amount of decline in aerobic capacity and endurance can be reduced by weight control and appropriate exercise.

Obstructive Pulmonary Diseases

Chronic obstructive pulmonary disease (COPD) encompasses a group of diseases having in common an obstruction to expired airflow.[24] Although not a direct major cause of death, COPD does lead to respiratory impairment and cor pulmonale. It results in considerable work disability and hospitalization. As such, it is an important economic burden to individuals and society.

The term COPD applies to a range of diseases, but it generally includes asthma, chronic bronchitis, and emphysema. Other diseases, such as bronchiectasis and cystic fibrosis, are far less common. Asthma, chronic bronchitis, and emphysema may overlap and interact; elements of all three may be present. For clarity, the diseases will be discussed separately.

Asthma

Hyper-reactivity of the airways can cause sudden transient attacks of bronchospasm. Other elements of airway obstruction, such as mucus hypersecretion and mucosal edema, may be present. If neglected or subject to frequently recurring attacks, or complicated by bronchial infections or cigarette smoking, chronic airway obstruction may develop. This end-result may appropriately be termed chronic asthmatic bronchitis. Typical paroxysmal asthma, due to an allergy to specific antigens, characteristically occurs at an early age and may wane with maturity. Asthma developing in middle age or later always should be investigated as a possible manifestation of an underlying collagen-vascular disease. With advancing age, bronchial hyper-reactivity may be provoked by a wider range of stimulants that include cold air, exercise, dust, viral respiratory infections, and others.

Chronic Bronchitis

The essential characteristics are excessive bronchial mucus production and a chronic cough that persists for at least 2 successive years in the absence of any specific disease. This may lead to airflow obstruction via the mechanisms of viscid secretions, mucosal edema, and cellular proliferation, to some element of smooth muscle spasm, and to a loss of support of the bronchial walls by inflammatory changes in cartilage and connective tissues. Infection and allergy play minor roles, but the overwhelmingly associated factor is inhaled tobacco smoke. The early pathologic changes occur in the small bronchioles and proceed centripetally to the larger bronchi. Thus, it begins as bronchiolitis and develops with time into bronchitis. The combination of mucus hypersecretion and inflammation of the bronchial mucosa produces airway obstruction. Because the distribution of bronchial obstruction is non-uniform, ventilation-perfusion mismatching may occur, which leads first to hypoxemia and later to CO_2 retention. Chronic bronchitis usually precedes parenchymal emphysema and the diseases coexist. Aging by itself does not cause chronic bronchitis. If exposed to noxious, inhaled materials such as cigarette smoke, the greater the number of "pack/years," the greater the likelihood of having chronic bronchitis.

Emphysema

This process is best defined as an enlargement of air spaces that are distal to the terminal non-respiratory bronchiole with a destruction of alveolar walls. The two principal types are centrilobular and panlobular. As the term suggests, centrilobular emphysema begins as an inflammatory process in the respiratory bronchiole surrounded by alveoli. As the inflammation increases and the bronchiole dilates, the adjacent alveoli also dilate and undergo a disintegration of the walls. A confluence of the destroyed alveoli reduces the elastic forces and the surface area available for gas exchange. Because the bronchioles are held open mechanically by the tethering of the lung parenchyma, the changes of emphysema result in an early closure of small peripheral airways during exhalation, especially when forced. Thus, obstruction of airflow can result from an intrinsic blockage due to chronic bronchitis, or a premature airway collapse due to emphysematous destruction.

A second type of emphysema is panlobular. Here, alveolar dilatation and destruction occurs uniformly throughout the acinus in the presence of normal bronchioles. It tends to be prevalent in lower lung areas in contrast to centrilobular emphysema, which favors upper lobes. Panlobular emphysema is associated with aging, but in the absence of specific pulmonary diseases it usually does not severely impair pulmonary function; perhaps, this is due to the reserve capacity of the lungs. Because emphysema does not produce as non-uniform a ventilation as chronic bronchitis, it ordinarily does not cause alveolar hypoventilation or $\dot{V}/\dot{Q}$ mismatch with abnormalities of the arterial blood gases. As previously mentioned, chronic bronchitis and emphysema, when associated with cigarette smoking, usually coexist; both contribute to abnormalities of ventilation and gas exchange.

Management

Therapy for elderly patients with COPD is limited and directed toward a control of symptoms, an increase of physical activity and independence, and independent self-care with a reduction of hospitalization. Despite the inability to achieve a cure, these important objectives can benefit the lives of older COPD patients.

The asthmatic component is uncommonly of the atopic or extrinsic type, and little effort should be expended in identifying specific allergens and subsequent desensitization. Excellent drugs are available to achieve and maintain satisfactory bronchodilation (*see* Table 10-2).

Bronchodilators
Theophylline drugs are valuable both for chronic oral dosage and for acute intravenous use. Patient compliance and a consistent control of airway caliber have been achieved by sustained-release preparations. An oral dosage given twice daily has become standard practice. The dosage, however, varies considerably with age, body size, and drug metabolism. Blood levels of 10–20 μg/ml are considered desirable and should be used as guides for therapy. Once an apparently stable dose is achieved, changes in smoking habits and concomitant drugs such as erythromycin and cimetidine may change blood levels of theophylline.

Beta-adrenergic Drugs
If maximum ventilatory function is not attained by orally administered theophylline drugs, or if they are poorly tolerated, the use of an inhaled or oral beta-adrenergic drug is indicated. Some clinicians prefer to initiate therapy with these drugs. A combination of theophylline and beta-adrenergic drugs may produce an optimal ventilation with fewer side effects.

Principal beta-adrenergic drugs are metaproterenol, terbutaline, and albuterol. The oral doses may have to be reduced in older patients to minimize side effects, beginning with 2.5 mg of terbutaline, 2 mg of albuterol, and 10 mg of metaproterenol, each given three times daily.

The use of a metered dose inhaler can provide effective bronchodilation with few, if any, side effects. The reason for a lack of maximal effectiveness has been the failure to use them properly. The two requirements are patient education and proper instructions. New studies provide the basis for the instructions in Figure 10-6 for metaproterenol and albuterol. Further modifications in these techniques may be made as newer information is available. Some physicians recommend placing the inhaler in the mouth with the lips closed around it. The two most important instructions are to inhale the aerosol slowly and to hold the breath at full lung inflation for 10 seconds. Shim and Williams suggest that an inhaled beta-adrenergic drug can produce a greater benefit than the same drug

TABLE 10-2 Useful Drugs for Airway Obstruction

Drug	Route	Dosage
Adrenergic		
Metaproterenol	oral	20 mg q 8 h
(Alupent, Metaprel)	inhalation	2 inhalations q.i.d.
Albuterol	oral	2–4 mg t.i.d. or q.i.d.
(Proventil, Ventolin)	inhalation	2 inhalations q 4–6 h
Terbutaline	oral	2.5–5 mg q 8 h
(Brethine, Bricanyl)	subcutaneous	0.25 mg q 4–8 h
Theophylline	oral	300–600 mg q 12 h to maintain
(Slow release)		plasma level 10–20 mcg/ml
	intravenous	4–6 mg/kg/day initially
Glucocorticoids		
Prednisone	oral	begin with 60–80 mg/day
		and reduce to 10–15 mg/day
		each a.m.
Methyl prednisolone	intravenous	20–40 mg q 8 h
Beclomethasone	inhalation	2 inhalations q.i.d.
(Beclovent, Vanceril)		

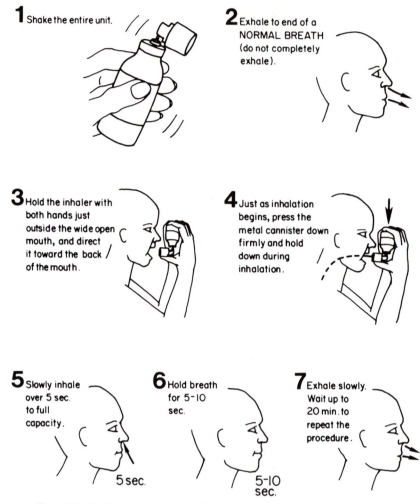

1 Shake the entire unit.

2 Exhale to end of a NORMAL BREATH (do not completely exhale).

3 Hold the inhaler with both hands just outside the wide open mouth, and direct it toward the back of the mouth.

4 Just as inhalation begins, press the metal cannister down firmly and hold down during inhalation.

5 Slowly inhale over 5 sec. to full capacity.

5 sec.

6 Hold breath for 5-10 sec.

5-10 sec.

7 Exhale slowly. Wait up to 20 min. to repeat the procedure.

James Morris, M.D., V.A. Medical Center, Portland, Oregon
April, 1982

FIGURE 10-6   Instructions for patients to properly use metered dose inhalers containing metaproterenol or albuterol.

taken orally, providing that the inhaled drug is used properly.[25]

Anticholinergic Drugs

Inhaled atropine, in doses of 0.025–0.05 mg/kg have been used when beta-adrenergic drugs have failed.[26] There is an ill-defined subset of patients with reactive airway disease who are responsive to atropine. As yet, no atropine-like drug has been released for use in the United States. Such an agent should have few anticholinergic side effects, such as dry mouth or tachycardia. Elderly patients are at greatest risk for atropine side effects.

Corticosteroids

Although not technically considered bronchodilators, corticosteroids can benefit those persons with reactive airway disease. Asthmatic patients will benefit most, and those with emphysema have no benefit. Corticosteroids have not been shown to improve chronic bronchitis, perhaps because of the progression from chronic asthmatic bronchitis to mucous gland hyperplasia and hypersecretion.[27] Corticosteroids do have a proven value in acute exacerbation of chronic bronchitis. A major therapeutic advance was the introduction of relatively insoluble, inhaled corticosteroids, chiefly beclomethasone. Its effective use helps to reduce or omit systemic corticosteroids as maintenance therapy. It is essentially free from side effects, other than oral candidiasis. Beclomethasone is particularly beneficial to elderly patients who are most vulnerable to the side effects of systemic corticosteroids. The use of disodium cromoglycate has been of negligible benefit in adult patients.

Non-pharmacologic Therapy

A variety of therapeutic modalities have been recommended for COPD patients. Two that have shown demonstrable success have been oxygen therapy and exercise, occasionally used together. Oxygen therapy at home is required by relatively few patients when strict criteria are used (*see* Table 10-3). During sleep, most individuals hypoventilate relative to their waking state. Sleeping COPD patients commonly develop a serious hypoxia, which may go unrecognized unless monitored by an ear oximeter. Complications, such as sustained pulmonary hypertension with cor pulmonale and congestive heart failure, may develop.[28] The decision to use home oxygen for an elderly patient should be based on firm clinical and laboratory criteria. The major disadvantages are cost, limitation of physical activity, the potential for CO_2 retention, and possible oxygen toxicity. A recent multicenter study showed an improved survival if oxygen was used continuously rather than for 12 hours daily.[29] Less desirable alternatives limit oxygen use to times of sleeping or exercising. Refillable, lightweight, and portable oxygen cylinders are available for increasing

TABLE 10-3   Indications for Outpatient Oxygen Therapy

Resting arterial oxygen tension (PaO2) below 50 mm Hg (at sea level breathing room air).

Resting PaO2 below 55 mm Hg with evidence of hypoxic organ dysfunction, including erythrocytosis, cor pulmonale, sleep, or mentation disturbances.

Resting PaO2 greater than 55 mm Hg, but less than 55 mm Hg during an exercise training program.

Patients not meeting the above criteria, but with hypoxic organ dysfunction or hypoxemia (PaO2 less than 55 mm Hg), which is benefited by oxygen therapy

---

Patients residing at high altitudes have lower arterial PO_2 and O_2 saturation values.

the range of activities. Liquid gas containers also provide both home and portable oxygen therapy, but at an increased cost. An alternative to gas cylinder or liquid container oxygen is the oxygen extractor. This device provides a safe, dependable, and relatively economic source of oxygen. Drawbacks include a vulnerability to electric power failure and the inability to fill portable cylinders.

Various forms of physical therapy are used for COPD patients, many of which are of dubious value. These include breathing training, postural drainage, and chest percussion or vibration. There is no real controversy regarding the many benefits of exercise training. Because of associated medical problems in elderly persons that may impose limitations, exercise therapy may have to be carefully tailored to the individual patient. Walking, swimming, and bicycling are particularly well suited for an older COPD patient. The goals are an increased exercise tolerance with less physical dependence and a reduction of exertional dyspnea. For an elderly patient, a return to gainful employment is uncommon. However, reductions in the need for hospitalization and an improvement in the quality of life are attainable. An increase in survival and an improvement in pulmonary function are more difficult to prove.

The most important element of patient education is to promote the cessation of smoking; otherwise, the progression of COPD is inevitable. An important component of the antismoking cessation program is pulmonary function testing. Confronting an older patient with the amount of loss of ventilatory function compared with non-smokers of similar age can provide a strong motivation to quit. As in many chronic illnesses affecting the older patient, realistic goals should be set and measures directed toward halting a further deterioration and promoting a functional performance within limits imposed by structural changes.

Restrictive Pulmonary Diseases

Causes

Restricted lung expansion can result from voluntary hypoventilation, such as that due to the pain of breathing. Other causes include age-re-

TABLE 10-4 Causes of Interstitial Lung Disease

Inorganic dusts
Organic dusts
Toxic gases and fumes
Drugs
Poisons
Infections
Chronic heart or kidney failure
Collagen-vascular diseases
Granulomatous diseases
Vasculitides
Idiopathic

lated changes in muscles or joints of the chest or in the pleura and the lung parenchymal interstitium. The latter cause the greatest physiologic impairment, primarily in gas exchange. Table 10-4 lists the known and unknown causes of interstitial lung disease, the most common of which is idiopathic pulmonary fibrosis.

Idiopathic Pulmonary Fibrosis

This usually is clinically evident in the 6th decade and is manifested by an increasing dyspnea on exertion. A dry cough is a common feature. Changes on physical examination and chest x-ray films may be minimal in the early stages. As the disease progresses, inspiratory crackles, increased transmission of breath sounds, prolongation of expiration, and reduced chest expansion develop. The chest x-ray film shows a variety of changes, usually diffuse reticular and reticulonodular patterns. In advanced stages, multiple translucencies may suggest a honeycomb appearance.

Measurement of arterial PO_2 and calculation of the alveolar-arterial PO_2 gradient after exercise are the most sensitive measures of interstitial disease impairment.[30] Less consistently, abnormalities are found in lung volumes, expired flows, diffusion capacity, lung compliance, and resting arterial blood gases.

Diagnosis

The assessment for activity of the inflammatory process is critical. The approach to the evaluation and treatment of interstitial lung disease has been systematized.[31] The value of obtaining a lung biopsy specimen depends on obtaining a representative tissue sample of the general pulmonary disease process. Some areas of the lung may show an active inflammation, while others are in an advanced fibrotic stage. The value of an initial open-lung biopsy procedure is to determine a specific cause of the interstitial lung disease, such as pneumonoconiosis or rheumatic lung disease.

Newer procedures have been advocated to assess inflammatory activity. Gallium-67 scintigraphy is both sensitive and specific for alveolitis. It is valuable in determining the degree of active inflammation, in measuring by serial studies the effectiveness of therapy directed against the alveolitis, and in detecting a relapse. Bronchoalveolar lavage, when properly done, will consist of 97% alveolar fluid and only 2% bronchial fluid. Determination of the percentage of the cell types may help determine both the presence and nature of alveolitis. The procedure requires fiberoptic bronchoscopy and is relatively easy and safe to perform. Serial use of both techniques is valuable in monitoring the success of therapy.

Management

Using the methods described above, with special emphasis on postexercise arterial blood gas studies and gallium-67 scintigraphy, an assessment of alveolitis and the degree of its physiologic impairment may be made. A major decision is whether there is a specific cause of the interstitial disease or if it is idiopathic. An inciting exposure to drugs, dusts, or chemicals should be eliminated. In the majority of cases, the cause will be unknown and the choice will be to begin a prolonged aggressive therapy directed toward the prevention of pulmonary fibrosis and a loss of functioning acini. In addition to the degree of active inflammation and impairment of pulmonary function, the goals of the patient must be considered. Corticosteroids are the primary drugs currently used to affect the inflammatory and immunologic derangements. Because of the need for high dosages over prolonged periods, the hazards for elderly patients include osteoporosis with vertebral compression fractures, an increased susceptibility to infections, an exacerbation of diabetes, hypertension, tuberculosis, peptic ulcer disease, and hypoadrenalism. Therefore, some frail elderly patients with significant disabilities due to other disorders are not treated. There is no accepted regimen for drug therapy, but some clinicians would advocate an aggressive approach.[31] Alternative drugs, such as cyclophosphamide and azothioprine, have been used in cases of corticosteroid failures. Beside refractoriness to prednisone therapy, relapse is a significant problem and may require repeated doses of an antiinflammatory therapy. The prospect for a progressive worsening of interstitial fibrosis is an increasing hypoxemia that requires inhaled oxygen. An inability to maintain a PaO_2 of at least 60 mm Hg may result in the classic sequence of pulmonary hypertension, erythrocytosis, and cor pulmonale.

Bronchopulmonary Infections

Acute Bronchitis

In contrast to chronic bronchitis, acute bronchitis usually is an infectious process, barring an acute exposure to irritant chemicals. The cause usually is non-bacterial. In an older patient, viruses are more common than mycoplasma. Acute bronchitis may be part of a more extensive involvement of respiratory epithelium, such as laryngotracheobronchitis. For patients with a seriously impaired pulmonary function, such as those with COPD, the widespread narrowing of airways due to mucosal inflammation and bronchial secretions may cause severe alveolar hypoventilation or $\dot{V}/Q$ mismatch. Therapy is non-specific in the absence of a bacterial or mycoplasmal cause and includes bronchodilators, systemic hydration, and ventilatory support as needed. The routine use of antimicrobial drugs in acute exacerbations of chronic bronchitis is controversial, but their use appears to offer no convincing benefit.[32]

Pneumonia

Pneumonia has traditionally been more prevalent in elderly persons and is the leading infectious cause of death. In 82% of adult cases of bacterial pneumonia, there are underlying conditions that predispose to bronchopulmonary infection.

In elderly persons, it is largely assumed that bronchopulmonary clearance mechanisms suffer from the aging process.[33] These include macrophage and mucociliary functions. Decreased production of serum immunoglobulins against certain pathogens such as pneumococcal serotypes could partially account for an increased susceptibility to bacterial pneumonias. Most of these pneumonias result from minor aspirations of microorganisms colonizing the nasopharynx. Diminution of the gag reflex with aging could predispose to an aspiration even without the addition of sedative drugs.

Diagnosis

The microorganisms to be considered as causes of bacterial pneumonia are listed in Table 10-5. Because an elderly patient may be in a health care facility, hospital, or nursing home, a distinction should be made between community-acquired or nosocomial infection. In the community, Streptococcus pneumoniae during the year and influenza A virus during epidemic seasons are most likely to occur. In a health care facility, gram-negative bacilli should be suspected as well as pneumococci. Hemophilus influenza commonly colonizes the airway in older patients with chronic bronchitis.[34] These are virtually always non-typable strains that are considered incapable of causing pneumonia. Because of their presence in bronchopulmonary secretions, they often are mistakenly implicated as causing pneumonia in older patients. Their presence in body fluids (blood, pleural effusion) does establish causation in occasional cases of H. influenza pneumonia.

TABLE 10-5 Causes of Bacterial Pneumonia

Aerobic gram-positive cocci
  Streptococcus pneumoniae
  Staphylococcus aureus
  Streptococcus pyogenes
Aerobic gram-negative bacilli
  Klebsiella enterobacter
  Escherichia coli
  Proteus
  Pseudomonas aeruginosa
  Acinetobacter
  Serratia marcescens
  Legionella pneumophila
Anaerobic bacteria
  Peptostreptococcus
  Fusobacteria
  Bacteroides

The clinical presentation of pneumonia in elderly patients may not be typical. Fever, productive cough, malaise, and physical findings may be muted. Chest x-ray films, however, should reveal airspace consolidation in bacterial pneumonia. Similarly, gram stains of a sputum smear should reveal a predominance of a single aerobic bacterial species. The adequacy of the sputum specimen should be verified as having less than 10 epithelial cells and, ideally, more than 25 granulocytes per low-power microscopic field. Alternatives to expectorated sputum are, of necessity, invasive. They include nasotracheal suctioning, transtracheal suctioning, fiberoptic-bronchoscopic aspiration and brushing, and percutaneous "skinny" needle aspiration. Sputum culture is essential to definitively identify the microorganisms and to perform antimicrobial susceptibility tests, especially against Staphylococcus aureus and gram-negative bacilli. Blood and pleural fluid cultures are invaluable in indicating the causative bacteria of pneumonia.

Chest x-ray films establish the diagnosis of pneumonia. They also can reveal unusual parenchymal destruction; either necrotizing pneumonia or abscess. Because these are rarely seen in pneumococcal pneumonia, a consideration of infection from staphylococci, gram-negative bacilli, and anaerobic microorganisms is vital. Associated pleural effusion should be aspirated to determine if empyema that requires drainage is present.

Treatment

Because of the potential mortality and severe morbidity of bacterial pneumonia in elderly patients, prompt effective treatment must be stressed. Initial antimicrobial therapy should be influenced by the gram-stained sputum smear and modified as cultural and drug susceptibility data become available (*see* Table 10-6). The dosage may have to be adjusted in the presence of renal impairment, especially when an aminoglycoside drug is used. For hospitalized patients, the intravenous route is desirable, at least initially. This is particularly true in older patients who may have uncertain drug levels in using oral medications because of either undependable absorption from the gastrointestinal tract or erratic ingestion. Duration of antimicrobial therapy varies with the type of infection and the microorganism. For example, most pneumococcal pneumonias require only 5–7 days, gram-negative bacilli 2 weeks, staphylococcal infections 4 weeks, and anaerobic lung abscesses 6 weeks. Patients may be switched to intramuscular or oral routes as the infection is controlled.

In an older patient, especially one with a

TABLE 10-6   Antibiotic Treatment of Bacterial Pneumonia

Organism	First Choice	Alternatives
Streptococcus pneumoniae	Penicillin G	Erythromycin (also treats Mycoplasma and Legionella) Cephalosporins
Staphylococcus aureus	Nafcillin	Cephalosporins Mezlocillin
Klebsiella	Cephalosporin and Aminoglycoside	Mezlocillin or Chloramphenicol and Aminoglycoside
Escherichia coli	Ampicillin and Aminoglycoside	Cephalosporin
Pseudomonas	Carbenicillin and Aminoglycoside	Cephalosporin
Serratia	Carbenicillin or Ticarcillin and Aminoglycoside	Cefoxitin and Aminoglycoside
Anaerobic bacteria	Penicillin G	Clindamycin

chronic pulmonary impairment, prophylaxis for pneumococcal pneumonia is most feasible at this time. Two principal measures are immunization with antipneumococcal vaccine (providing 90% protection) and 250 mg of oral penicillin V twice daily (offering 100% protection). For patients at high risk for acute respiratory failure due to pneumococcal pneumonia, both preventive measures should be considered.

Aspiration Pneumonia

Pulmonary aspiration is a disturbingly common event. In hospitalized patients, it can reproduce different clinical syndromes and frequently is fatal. It occurs commonly in situations that include stupor, coma, alcohol or drug intoxication, nasogastric tube feeding, general anesthesia, seizure disorders, cardiopulmonary resuscitation, and esophageal motility disorders. Frequently, the aspiration is not observed or is overlooked. The damage done by pulmonary aspiration may involve airway obstruction, chemical pneumonitis, or infection. The upper airway is normally protected by gag and cough reflexes. A number of conditions interfere with these defenses, which range from coma to normal sound sleep. In elderly persons, a diminution in the sensitivity of the cough and gag reflexes weaken these vital defenses, particularly during sleep, and are further weakened by alcohol, sedatives, and hypnotic drugs.

Clinical Features

Clinical syndromes depend upon the type of material aspirated. They can be separated into non-toxic substances, toxic or acidic substances, and infected oropharyngeal secretions. Non-toxic substances vary in the degree of damage produced. Clear liquids usually produce minimal or transient damage, unless found in large amounts. Large particles (usually poorly chewed food) obviously can obstruct major airways and usually are quickly recognized. Gastric contents are a mixture of partially digested food and gastric secretions and cause chronic injury. The long-term effects of foodstuff aspiration seem limited, except for bronchiolitis obliterans.[35] Damage can be done to the lung even when the aspirate is close to a neutral pH. The subsequent administration of corticosteroids can interfere with localization of the lung damage and prolong acute inflammatory changes.

Toxic substances in the lung usually result from aspirating fasting-gastric secretions with a pH below 2.5. The normal gastric pH range is 1.5–2.4, which can cause severe damage to the alveoli and airways. In an elderly patient, degrees of achlorhydria may result in a gastric secretion of pH above 2.5, which then falls into the non-toxic substance category. The effects of aspirating toxic substances are similar to a burn injury. Interstitial and alveolar edema result in hypoxemia. Vasodilation and edema of the bronchial epithelium narrows the lumen, causes ventilation-perfusion mismatch, and contributes to hypoxemia. The end-result may be severe fibrosis of the smaller airways and the lung parenchyma.[36] The sequelae of aspirating infected oropharyngeal secretions depend on the predominating bacteria and their numbers. Community-acquired aspiration pneumonia usually is caused by anaerobic bacteria, which are either alone or mixed with aerobes. This is particularly true in patients with gingival infection (peridontitis), which harbors large numbers of anaerobes. Hospital-acquired aspiration pneumonia may be caused by aerobic bacteria (especially gram-negative enteric bacilli) alone or mixed with anaerobes in a dentulous patient.

Chest x-ray films commonly show a non-specific bronchopneumonia that is segmental rather than lobar, and with its location corresponding to the dependent area when aspirating. The subsequent course is influenced by the infecting microorganisms; however, in the case of anaerobic bacteria or gram-negative enteric bacilli, necrotizing pneumonia and lung abscesses are common.

Therapy

Some clinicians recommend antimicrobial therapy in all cases of aspiration pneumonia, while others prefer to wait until clear evidence of bacterial infection is obtained. Selection of drugs may be guided by the following:

Dentulous patients with definite community-acquired pneumonia, especially if necrotizing or with a lung abscess, should be treated for anaerobic infection (4–6 weeks of at least 6 million units of penicillin daily, or clindamycin, 600 mg every 8 hours). If cultures reveal an aerobic bacillary infection, more appropriate antimicrobials are used.

Hospital-acquired aspiration pneumonia should be regarded as either an aerobic or mixed aerobic-anaerobic infection. Initially, combination drugs such as clindamycin plus an aminoglycoside or a broad-spectrum cephalosporin are useful until sputum cultures are definitive.

Prevention

Aspiration can occur in any patient and even in normal individuals during sound sleep, but especially in patients with predisposing conditions. Possible preventive measures include a head-down position if unconscious, oral antacids to raise gastric pH above 2.5, intubation to protect the airway, and dental extraction to reduce the chance of anaerobic lung infection.

Influenza

Despite the availability of effective vaccines, influenza remains as a serious cause of morbidity and mortality. Influenza A virus and influenza B virus cause only a fraction of respiratory infections each year, but are unique in that they are responsible for periodic widespread outbreaks of febrile respiratory infections in both children and adults. The illness usually produces a fever, chills, headaches, cough, and myalgia. It may last several days or 1 week or longer and usually has a complete recovery. Complications include pneumonia, myocarditis, pericarditis, encephalitis, and aseptic meningitis.

Efforts to prevent or control influenza typically have been directed toward protecting those who are at the greatest risk of death or serious illness. These individuals include those over 65 years of age and chronically ill adults. The mortality rate is 1 in 100 of those 65 years of age or older in the presence of chronic illness. The chief problem, other than a compliance with vaccination, is a variation in the influenza antigens, usually antigen A. This can take the form of an antigenic drift, which is a minor change where the vaccine has a real but diminished usefulness. It also can have an antigenic shift about every 10 years, when a new vaccine must be prepared. In years without antigenic variation, vaccination can provide up to 85% protection against the viruses contained in the vaccine.[37] Older individuals have a lower antibody response than younger persons. Local re-

actions, including erythema and induration, are infrequent and mild. Fewer than 1% of persons vaccinated develop systemic reactions such as fever and myalgia. Considering the hazards to elderly patients, physicians should encourage its annual use.

The use of antiviral agents is limited to influenza A, and both prophylactic and therapeutic effects have been achieved. Amantadine has been available since 1967 and a derivative, rimantadine, is awaiting Food and Drug Administration (FDA) approval. Amantadine has been shown to be 91% effective in preventing influenza A virus infection.[38] It is beneficial for elderly patients or for those with serious chronic illness who are exposed to influenza A virus. It can be used in place of a vaccination or as a supplement. As a therapeutic agent, it has about 50% effectiveness on the course of influenza A virus.[39] Considering the 5% prevalence rate of central nervous system side effects (usually mild and reversible), only severe cases of influenza should be treated with amantadine. For the usual self-limited, uncomplicated case of influenza in an older patient, symptomatic therapy with an adequate hydration and one to two aspirin tablets every 4 to 6 hours usually suffices. With evidence of pneumonia, it is important to distinguish between influenza viral pneumonia and a bacterial suprainfection. Pneumococci and staphylococci account for most of all the community-acquired, post-influenzal bacterial pneumonias.

Tuberculosis

Despite the marked reduction in tuberculosis, it still remains the number one fatal communicable disease in the United States. Among all infectious diseases, only pneumonia exceeds its annual fatality rate. Modern chemotherapy is extraordinarily effective and should be successful in all cases that are caused by drug-susceptible Mycobacterium tuberculosis. Why then does tuberculosis continue to cause about 28,000 new cases annually and result in 3,000 deaths? Some of the reasons include a noncompliance with therapy regimens, drug-resistant disease, and misdiagnosis.

A unique quality of tuberculosis is the ability of the infection to remain inactive over decades and then reactivate. The balance between the virulence of the microorganisms and the cell-mediated immunity of a patient determines the course of this life-long infection. The diminution of cell-mediated immunity is characteristic of the aging process and may be reflected in a decreased reaction to tuberculin testing. The booster effect of a repeat tuberculin test performed 1–4 weeks after a non-diagnostic reaction has been more marked in older populations.[40] Thus, it is not surprising that reactivation tuberculosis is increasingly seen among older individuals.[41] Additional reasons, other than naturally waning immunity, are the development of certain diseases such as diabetes, malignancies, the taking of immunosuppressive drugs such as corticosteroids, malnutrition, and alcoholism.

Diagnosis

As tuberculosis has decreased in prevalence, it has become concentrated in urban areas that are characterized by low social and economic levels. For many physicians, it presents infrequently enough to be easily misdiagnosed. To add to this problem, unusual clinical and x-ray presentations have become more common. Typically, tuberculosis in adults presents on chest x-ray films as a destructive process located in the upper lobar apical and posterior segments and, less commonly, in the lower lobar superior segments. With a progression of the disease, other areas may be affected. With infiltrates of upper-lobar anterior segmental, middle lobar, and lower lobar, a diagnosis may not be made. Finally, the relative infrequency of tuberculosis may result in primary infections in older adults; perhaps this explains the mid- and lower lung fields involvement and pleural effusion.[42] Miliary disease as a manifestation of reactivation tuberculosis has been increasingly observed in elderly patients.[43]

Despite atypical presentations on a chest x-ray film, it still is the best screening examination for tuberculosis.

The definitive diagnosis remains a positive sputum smear for typical acid-fast bacilli, with a confirmation by culture technique. Tuberculin testing via standard 5 Tuberculin Unit (TU) Mantoux technique in older persons may result in false-negative reactions, despite positive reactions to control antigens such as mumps, candida or trichophytin. Two recommended procedures are to repeat the 5 TU test to achieve a booster effect or to repeat it with the second-strength 250 TU test. A negative reaction to a 250 TU test in the presence of a positive control test virtually rules out tuberculous disease.

Therapy

A better understanding of the basic mechanisms of drug action provides a rational basis for currently used therapeutic programs. Principles of therapy include the use of a combination of bactericidal drugs, which affect metabolically different microbial populations by means of specific actions. The experience in Arkansas and prior field trials have crystallized in an initial treatment regimen. The current recommendation of the Center for Disease Control and the American Thoracic Society is isoniazid in doses of 300 mg and rifampin in doses of 600 mg taken once daily for 9 months.[44]

After 1 month of daily therapy, twice weekly dosages of isoniazid (15 mg/kg) and rifampin (600 mg) can be substituted. This regimen requires negative sputum cultures after the first 3 months of therapy followed by 6 more months of combination drugs. The short course program is used only with combinations of bactericidal drugs. Attempts to reduce the duration of treatment any further will require the addition of two other bactericidal drugs, such as streptomycin and pyrazinamide. Because both isoniazid and rifampin are potentially hepatotoxic, a patient should routinely have a careful check for hepatitis each month. As a minimum, this should include questions regarding symptoms of hepatitis and examination for scleral icterus and hepatic tenderness. The question of when to release a patient from isolation to a hospital ward or nursing home is unsettled, but 2–4 weeks of therapy or negative sputum smears are usually cited as adequate. Otherwise, physical activity should be unrestricted. Adequate nutrition is important despite the great efficacy of current drug therapy.

Preventive Therapy

The use of isoniazid, 300 mg/day for 1 year, recommended for those infected by tubercle bacilli (as shown by a positive tuberculin test without radiologic or microbiologic evidence of

TABLE 10-7   Indications for Preventive Therapy of Tuberculosis

---

Household members and other close associates of newly diagnosed patients.

Tuberculin skin test converters within the past 2 years.

Positive tuberculin skin test reactors with abnormal chest x-ray films consistent with tuberculosis.

Positive tuberculin skin test reactors with associated diseases or situations, such as corticosteroid or other immunosuppressive therapy, diabetes, silicosis, gastric resection with weight loss.

Positive tuberculin skin test reactors below age 35.

---

disease), is ideally suited to prevent reactivation.[45] Since the recognition that isoniazid can cause serious hepatitis, such a prophylaxis has become more selective. Toxic hepatitis is distinctly age related. After 35 years of age the case rate increases to about 64 years of age, where it has a 2.3% rate of occurrence. Therefore, in elderly tuberculin reactors, considering the number of potential years for reactivation and the high risk of isoniazid hepatitis, a significant risk factor (see Table 10-7) should be required before preventive therapy. The otherwise healthy, well-nourished elderly tuberculin reactor has a greater morbidity and mortality risk due to isoniazid than tuberculosis.

Neoplastic Disease

Bronchogenic Carcinoma

Lung cancer has become infamous as the leading cause of cancer deaths in males and is rapidly overtaking breast cancer as the leading cause in females. The annual death rate from lung cancer now exceeds 100,000 in the United States and continues to rise. It also is characterized by a short duration from diagnosis to death. The 5-year survival rate of 5–10% has changed little in the past 30 years despite advances in the diagnosis and treatment. This renders more urgent the necessity of preventing this epidemic disease. Despite minor contributions of occupational and atmospheric exposure, tobacco smoking remains the major cause.

Age is a critical factor in the clinical recognition of lung cancer. Because it probably requires the inhalation of tobacco smoke for at least 20 years, lung cancer rarely occurs in persons younger than 35 years of age and less than 5% of reported cases are younger than 40 years of age.[46] The majority of cases are manifest in the 6th and 7th decades. Unfortunately, when diagnosed, the tumor has achieved about 80% of its ultimate growth and has a high probability of having produced lymphatic or hematogenous metastases. The major cell types in order of frequency are squamous cell, adenocarcinoma, small cell, and large cell carcinoma. All but adenocarcinoma are closely correlated with cigarette smoking. Adenocarcinoma includes bronchioloalveolar carcinoma, and it has shown the most rapid increase in frequency. The basis for this increase in unknown, but it may be related to environmental pollution such as urban asbestosis.

Diagnosis

A major problem in recognizing lung cancer is that in the early stages, symptoms may be nonexistent or resemble those of chronic bronchitis. In later stages, symptoms may reflect a distant spread of the tumor. Frequent screening chest x-ray films have not been shown to improve survival. Despite this, chest x-ray films remain the best initial means of detecting bronchogenic carcinoma. A variety of presentations exist; probably the two most common varieties are the solitary pulmonary nodule and a hilar mass. Body-section x-ray films or laminograms are useful to detect calcification, to localize the lesion, to determine the presence of additional tumor masses, and to evaluate the relationship of the tumor of the chest wall. Special views such as 55° hilar laminograms and computerized tomography (CT scans) of the mediastinum are useful to detect lymph node metastases. Gallium-67 scans have been recommended to detect mediastinal metastases, but they have had a limited acceptance because of the lack of specificity.

Sputum cytology is useful for exfoliative endobronchial masses, especially central squamous cell carcinomas, but the false-negative rate is substantial. The fiberoptic bronchoscope introduced in 1970 has become the most valuable means of obtaining tissue confirmation.

Technologic improvements, such as narrower outside diameters, improved optics, and greater tip flexion have continued to improve its usefulness. Combining endobronchial or transbronchial biopsy and brushing techniques achieves a tissue diagnosis in up to 85% of subsequently proven tumors.[47] In addition, the assessment of the proximity to the main carina, deformity by mediastinal lymph node metastases, and vocal cord paralysis can assist in staging the anatomic extent and potential for surgical resection. Percutaneous needle biopsy procedures have become safer with the development of thin and ultrathin needles.[48] "Liquid biopsy" specimens can be obtained by aspiration with only a small risk of serious complications. Pneumothorax occurred in 8% of those using ultrathin needles, of which only 2 of the 4 patients required a chest tube.[48] This is an important consideration in a high-risk older patient.

Surgical diagnostic procedures include cervical mediastinoscopy, mediastinotomy, and thoracotomy. The role of mediastinoscopy and, to a lesser extent, mediastinotomy is controversial. A more aggressive removal of hilar and mediastinal nodes in association with a lung resection has brought these two staging procedures into question. As a means of obtaining a tissue diagnosis, it has become less frequently performed as the use of fiberoptic bronchoscopy and percutaneous needle biopsy has increased. If small cell carcinoma is suspected in a centrally located lesion with negative bronchoscopic results, a bone marrow biopsy procedure is indicated before a surgical procedure.[49] If the biopsy specimen is negative, mediastinoscopy or mediastinotomy should precede a thoracotomy. The most frequent indication for the two staging procedures is to determine non-resectability in elderly or impaired patients who are at a high risk for surgical complications. In these patients, the presence of mediastinal metastases provide justification to forego a thoracotomy.

Pulmonary function testing is important before a lung resection in an elderly patient who may have a considerable impairment of ventilation or gas exchange. The combination of measuring the forced expiratory volume in 1 second (FEV 1) and a radionuclide-perfusion lung scan has been advocated to help determine operability.[50]

Treatment

Three modalities are available, but obviously with a survival rate of 5 years being between 5–10% of reported cases, success is limited. One study indicates that elderly patients may be more concerned about immediate survival than at 5 years postoperatively. This contrasts with the attitude of a young medical house staff.[51] Failure of the staff to appreciate the values of an elderly patient with lung cancer may seriously impair the quality of his or her remaining life.

Surgery Particularly in cases of squamous cell carcinoma, pulmonary resection represents the best chance for a cure or long-term survival. With adenocarcinoma or large cell carcinoma, surgical cures are fewer because of the greater tendency towards lymphatic and hematogenous spread. This spread is almost uniform with small cell carcinoma, rendering surgery useless except for the possibility of a small peripheral nodule. The principal limitation of a successful surgical resection is an unrecognized extra-pulmonary spread of the carcinoma. Of additional concern is the operative mortality of patients over 65 years of age, which is reported to be approximately twice that of younger patients undergoing lobectomy or pneumonectomy.[52]

Radiation Therapy Megavoltage radiation by either cobalt or linear accelerator sources is valuable for palliation of complications. These include pain due to bone metastases, superior vena caval obstruction, central nervous system metastases, and obstructive pneumonia. Postoperative radiation therapy, especially in the presence of hilar or mediastinal nodal metastases, often is done, but without firm evidence of any benefit. Curative irradiation of inoperable tumors also is attempted as a poor alternative to surgery, especially in elderly patients.[53]

Chemotherapy Single or combination chemotherapy for treatment of non-small cell carcinoma has been a disappointment in improving the quality and length of survival.[54] It cannot be recommended at this point, except in investigative protocols with new drug regimens. For an elderly patient with a limited life expectancy a truly informed consent is essential to justify the possible impairment of nutrition and well-being. Small cell carcinoma, however, has emerged as the only cell type with a potential for non-surgical cure.[55] Aggressive use of combination chemotherapy plus prophylactic brain irradiation and the selective use of chest irradiation, is justified for those patients with an adequate functional status. Most, if not all, chemotherapy can be accomplished on an outpatient basis.

Between 90–95% of all lung cancer patients will eventually die of it. For these approximately 95,000 Americans, the challenge is to provide relief of pain, personal support, encouragement, and realistic discussion of their prospects. For those untold numbers of persons not yet manifesting lung cancer, the prevention via cessation of cigarette smoking and the early detection via use of careful history taking, sputum cytology, chest x-ray films, and fiberoptic bronchoscopy are available.

Pulmonary Vascular Disease

Pulmonary Thromboembolism

The prevalence of pulmonary embolism is estimated to be 650,000 cases annually in the United States; 38% of these are fatal.[56] In an autopsy series, only 40–60% are recognized antemortem.[57] The source of the emboli is primarily in the upper leg, specifically the popliteal, femoral, and iliac veins. Other potential although less likely sources are the pelvic veins, calf veins, upper extremity veins, and cardiac chambers. Conditions that predispose to venous thromboembolism are more common in elderly persons. These include immobilization, prolonged bed rest, hip fractures, obesity, congestive heart failure, COPD, and malignancy.

Diagnosis
Clinical manifestations are non-specific. Some apply to the embolic event, such as dyspnea, tachypnea, and tachycardia. Other manifestations, such as pleuritic chest pain and hemoptysis, pertain to a pulmonary infarction. Electrocardiography may show only a sinus tachycardia. The chest x-ray film usually is normal, less often shows "congestive atelectasis" with elevation of a hemidiaphragm, and pulmonary infarction only about 10% of the population studied.[56] Hypoxemia may be the only abnormal laboratory value and is present in

about 90%. It must be recognized that advancing age reduces arterial PO_2 and increases the alveolar-arterial PO_2 gradient. A perfusion lung scan, if normal, virtually rules out a significant pulmonary embolism. In an older patient, a normal lung scan is much less likely to be obtained because of scarring, panlobular emphysema, or COPD. Classically, a ventilation-perfusion lung scan will show a segmental or greater area of non-perfused lung that is ventilated. This produces the physiologic consequences of wasted ventilation. Pulmonary angiography is the most reliable diagnostic method, but is invasive and carries a small but significant hazard. The finding of a filling defect that is larger than a subsegment or the cutoff of a pulmonary arterial branch is characteristic. The confirmation of a pulmonary embolus is essential if anticoagulant therapy is particularly hazardous to an individual patient due to a potential for bleeding complications.

Because most pulmonary emboli originate in the proximal leg veins, attempts are warranted to demonstrate deep venous thrombosis (DVT). Three effective techniques include 1) Contrast venography; 2) Radionuclide venography and thromboscintography; and 3) Impedance phlebography or plethysmography. The radionuclide venogram can be performed as part of the perfusion lung scan. It provides a good visualization of the deep veins of the lower extremity without the risk of thrombophlebitis, which accompanies contrast venography. A comparison of impedance phlebography with conventional radiographic venography shows an excellent agreement.[58] Impedance phlebography has two advantages: being non-invasive and a mobile procedure suitable for the bedside, outpatient clinic, or emergency room. Figures 10-7 and 10-8 provide diagnostic guidelines for patients with a suspected DVT and/or pulmonary embolism. Individual patients may not be suitable for these algorithms. For example, a critically ill patient at a high risk for bleeding may undergo pulmonary angiography directly.

Treatment
The usual treatment of pulmonary embolism is intravenous heparin initially, followed by orally given warfarin. Preventive treatment consists of low-dose subcutaneous heparin, 5,000 units every 12 hours. This is given to high-risk pa-

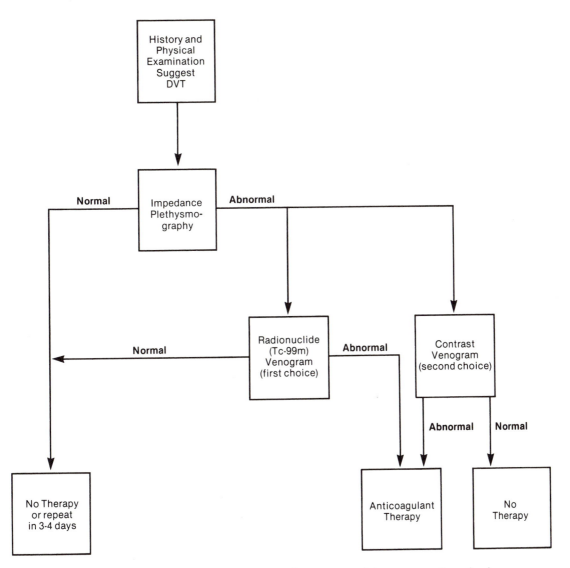

FIGURE 10-7 Suggested diagnostic approach to suspected deep venous thrombosis.

tients, especially those who remain immobile for at least 48 hours. When a venous thromboembolism is demonstrated, intravenous heparin is given (preferably continuously) in a dosage that maintains the partial thromboplastin time (PTT) 1.5 to 2.5 times the normal control. The advantages of continuous over intermittent administration include less bleeding and the ability to monitor PTT without regard to the time of perfusion. Oral warfarin is begun after a few days, but the heparin infusion should be maintained for about 5 days until warfarin is fully effective. The duration of anticoagulant therapy after an initial DVT or pulmonary embolism is controversial. Recommendations range from 10 days to 1 year, but 3–6 months are most commonly advised. In a recent study evaluating subcutaneous heparin versus oral warfarin in the long-term treatment of DVT, two thirds of the recurrent venous thromboembolism occurred after 3 months of effective anticoagulant therapy.[59] Thrombolytic therapy has not been widely used for pulmonary emboli, perhaps because of its expense and the potential hazards of bleeding. Neither justify withholding this effective therapy when indications for it exist. The two major indications are an acute, massive pulmonary embolism or when it seriously

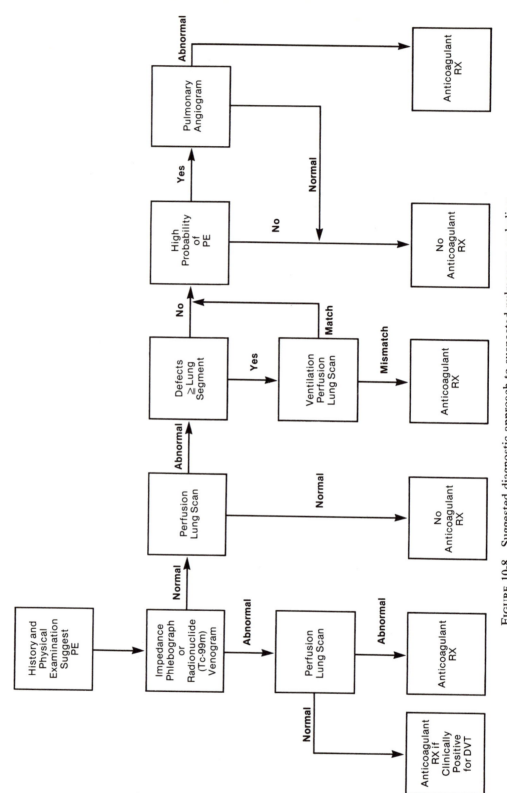

FIGURE 10-8   Suggested diagnostic approach to suspected pulmonary embolism.

compromises circulatory dynamics.[60] Contraindications are conditions predisposing to hemorrhage.

References

1. Macklem PT: Respiratory muscles: the vital pump. *Chest* 78:753–758, 1980.
2. Luce JM, Culver BH: Respiratory muscle function in health and disease. *Chest* 81:82–90, 1982.
3. Green GM, Jakab GJ, Low RB, et al: Defense mechanisms of the respiratory membrane. *Am Rev Resp Dis* 115:479–514, 1977.
4. Pierson DJ, Hudson LD: Evaluation of dyspnea. *Geriatrics* 36:48–62, 1981.
5. Kent S: The aging lung Part 1. Loss of elasticity. *Geriatrics* 124–130, Feb 1978.
6. Manderly JL: Effect of age on pulmonary structure and function of immature and adult animals and man. *Fed Proc* 38:173–177, 1979.
7. Jones RL, Overton TR, Hammerlindl DM, et al: Effects of age on regional residual volume. *J Appl Physiol: Respirat Environ Exercise Physiol* 44:195–199, 1978.
8. Knudson RJ, Clark DF, Dennedy TC, et al: Effect of aging alone on mechanical properties of the normal adult lung. *J Appl Physiol: Respirat Environ Exercise Physiol* 43:1054–1062, 1977.
9. Dhar S, Shastri SR, Lenora RA: Aging and the respiratory system. *Med Clin North Am* 60:1121–1139, 1976.
10. Kent S: Decline of pulmonary function. *Geriatrics* 33:100–111, Mar 1978.
11. Morris JF: Spirometry in the evaluation of pulmonary function. *West J Med* 125:110–118, 1976.
12. Morris JF, Koski A, Johnson LC: Spirometric standards for healthy nonsmoking adults. *Am Rev Resp Dis* 103:57–67, 1971.
13. Gardner RM, et al: Snowbird workshop on standardization of spirometry: a statement by the American Thoracic Society. *Am Rev Resp Dis* 119:831–838, 1979.
14. Sorbini C, Grassi V, Salmas F, et al: Arterial oxygen tension in relation to age in healthy subjects. *Respiration* 25:3–10, 1968.
15. Ward RJ, Tolas AG, Benveniste RJ, et al: Effect of posture on normal arterial blood gas tensions in the aged. *Geriatrics* 21:139–143, Feb 1966.
16. Berger AJ, Mitchell RA, Severinghaus JW: Regulation of respiration. *N Engl J Med* 297:92–97, 134–143, 194–206, 1977.
17. Block AJ: Is snoring a risk factor? Editorial. *Chest* 80:525, 1981.
18. Wasserman K, Whipp BJ: Exercise physiology in health and disease. *Am Rev Res Dis* 112:219–249, 1975.
19. Astrand PO: Human physical fitness with special reference to sex and age. *Physiol Rev* 36:307–335, 1956.
20. deVries HA: Physiological effects of an exercise training regimen upon men aged 52 to 88. *J Gerontol* 25:325–336, 1970.
21. Belman MJ, Mittman C: Ventilatory muscle training improves exercise capacity in chronic obstructive pulmonary disease patients. *Am Rev Resp Dis* 121:273–280, 1980.
22. deVries HA: Tips on prescribing exercise regimens for your older patients. *Geriatrics* 34:75–81, April 1979.
23. Heath GW, Hagberg JM, Ehsani AA, et al: A physiological comparison of young and older endurance athletes. *J Appl Physiol: Respirat Environ Exercise Physiol* 51:634–640, 1981.
24. Oregon Thoracic Society (an) *Chronic Obstructive Pulmonary Disease,* ed 5., New York, American Lung Association, 1981.
25. Shim C, Williams MH Jr: The adequacy of inhalation from canister nebulizers. *Am J Med* 69:891–894, 1980.
26. Marini J, Lakshminaryan S: The effect of atropine inhalation in "irreversible" chronic bronchitis. *Chest* 77:591–596, 1980.
27. Sahn SA: Corticosteroids in chronic bronchitis and pulmonary emphysema. *Chest* 73:389–396, 1978.
28. Wynne JW, Block AJ, Hemenway J, et al: Disordered breathing and oxygen desaturation during sleep in patients with chronic obstructive lung disease (COLD). *Am J Med* 66:573–579, 1979.
29. Nocturnal Oxygen Therapy Trial Group: Continuous or nocturnal oxygen therapy in hyperemic chronic obstructive lung disease. *Ann Int Med* 93:391–398, 1980.
30. Keogh BA, Crystal RG: Pulmonary function testing in interstitial pulmonary disease. *Chest* 78:856–865, 1980.
31. Crystal RG, Gadek JE, Ferrans VJ, et al: Interstitial lung disease: current concepts of pathogenesis, staging and therapy. *Am J Med* 70:542–568, 1981.
32. Nicotra MB, Rivera M, Awe R: Antibiotic therapy of acute exacerbations of chronic bronchitis. *Ann Int Med* 97:18–21, 1982.
33. Phair JP, Kauffman CA, Bjornson A, et al: Host defenses in the aged. Evaluation of components of the inflammatory and immune responses. *J Infect Dis* 138:67–73, 1978.
34. Haas H, Morris JF, Samson S, et al: Bacterial flora of the respiratory tract in chronic bronchitis: comparison of transtracheal, fiberbronchos-

copic, and oropharyngeal sampling methods. *Am Rev Resp Dis* 116:41–47, 1977.

35. Wynne JW, Reynolds JC, Hood IC, et al: Steroid therapy for pneumonitis induced in rabbits by aspiration of foodstuff. *Anesthesiology* 87:466–474, 1977.

36. Wynne JW, Modell JH: Respiratory aspiration of stomach contents. *Ann Int Med* 87:466–474, 1977.

37. Williams GO: Vaccines in older patients. Combating the risk of mortality. *Geriatrics* 35:55–64, Nov 1980.

38. Dolin R, Reichman RC, Madore HP, et al: A controlled trial of amantadine and rimantadine in the prophylaxis of influenza A infection. *N Engl J Med* 307:580–584, 1982.

39. VanVoris LP, Betts RF, et al: Successful treatment of naturally occurring influenza A/USSR/77 H1N1. *JAMA* 245:1128–1131, 1981.

40. Thompson NJ, Glassroth JL, Snider DE, et al: The booster phenomenon in serial tuberculin testing. *Am Rev Resp Dis* 119:587–597, 1979.

41. Stead WW: The pathogenesis of pulmonary tuberculosis among older persons. *Am Rev Resp Dis* 91:811–822, 1965.

42. Miller WT, McGregor RR: Tuberculosis: frequency of unusual radiographic findings. *Am J Roentgenol* 130:867–875, 1978.

43. Khan MA, Kovnat DM, Bachus F, et al: Clinical and roentgenographic spectrum of pulmonary tuberculosis in the adult. *Am J Med* 62:31–38, 1977.

44. Stead WW, Dutt AK: Chemotherapy for tuberculosis today. *Am Rev Resp Dis* 125 (part 2):94–101, 1982.

45. Farer LS: Chemoprophylaxis. *Am Rev Resp Dis* 125(part 2):102–07, 1982.

46. Matthay RA, Balmes JR: Lung cancer: a persistent challenge. *Geriatrics* 37:109–131, 1982.

47. Zavala DC: Diagnostic fiberoptic bronchoscopy: techniques and results of biopsy in 600 patients. *Chest* 68:12–19, 1975.

48. Zavala DC, Schoell JE: Ultrathin needle aspiration of the lung in infectious and malignant disease. *Am Rev Resp Dis* 123:125–131, 1981.

49. Bruya T, Morris JF, Barker AF: Bronchoscopy and bone marrow examinations. An efficient strategy to establish the diagnosis of small cell carcinoma of the lung. *Chest* 79:423–426, 1981.

50. Ali MK, Mountain CF, Ewer MS, et al: Predicting loss of pulmonary function after resection for bronchogenic carcinoma. *Chest* 77:337–342, 1980.

51. McNeil BJ, Weichselbaum R, Parker SG: Fallacy of the five-year survival in lung cancer. *N Engl J Med* 1397–1401, 1978.

52. Peterson BA, Kennedy BJ: Aging and cancer management Part 1: clinical observations. *CA* 29:322–332, 1979.

53. Coy P, Dennelly GM: The role of curative radiotherapy in the treatment of lung cancer. *Cancer* 45:698–702, 1980.

54. Spiro SG: The management of lung cancer. *Lung* 160:141–155, 1982.

55. Greco FA, Richardson RL, Snell JD, et al: Small cell lung cancer: complete remission and improved survival. *Am J Med* 66:625–630, 1979.

56. Bell WR, Simon TL: Current status of pulmonary thromboembolic disease: pathophysiology, diagnosis, prevention, and treatment. *Am Heart J* 103:239–262, 1982.

57. Freiman DG, Suyemoto J, Wessler S: Frequency of pulmonary embolism in man. *N Engl J Med* 272:1278–1280, 1965.

58. Hull R, Hirsh J, Sackett DL, et al: Cost effectiveness of clinical diagnosis, venography, and noninvasive testing in patients with symptomatic deep vein thrombosis. *N Engl J Med* 304:1561–1567, 1981.

59. Hull R, Delmore T, Carter C, et al: Adjusted subcutaneous heparin versus warfarin sodium in the long-term treatment of venous thrombosis. *N Engl J Med* 306:189–194, 1982.

60. Sharma GV, Cella G, Parisi AF, et al: Thrombolytic therapy. *N Engl J Med* 306:1268–1276, 1982.

Chapter 11

Cardiology

Edward S. Murphy, M.D.

Henry DeMots, M.D.

Cardiovascular disease is the principal cause of mortality and morbidity in the elderly population. Heart disease is the largest single cause of death in persons over the 65 years of age, with over one third of all deaths directly related to heart disease.[1] In the United States, 72% of cardiovascular deaths occur in patients 65 years of age or older.[2] The vast majority of these deaths are due to coronary artery disease. Nearly 50% of the population over 65 years of age shows some evidence on examination of cardiac disease, whether by a history of chest pain, prior myocardial infarction, heart murmurs, or electrocardiographic abnormalities.[3]

The Aging Cardiovascular System

The Physiologic Changes of Aging

Precise description of normal physiologic changes in cardiac functions that occur with aging is difficult because of the high prevalence of heart disease in elderly people. In one study, there was clear evidence of heart disease in 50% of persons studied who were 65–74 years of age and 60% in those older than 75 years of age.[3] With the decline in total body mass and metabolizing cells that begins at 30 years of age, there is a decrease in lean body mass that is reflected in a reduced, total oxygen consumption at rest and during exercise.[4] Cardiac function must be considered in relation to these changes.

The physiologic alterations related to the normal aging process involve changes in each of the major determinants of cardiac performance.

Although the resting heart rate changes little with age, the maximal heart rate during exercise generally declines with age.[5] With progressive aging, there is a steady, gradual decrease in resting cardiac output. The blood volume declines and the circulation time increases. This produces a decrease in cardiac output of approximately 1% per year.[6] Non-invasive studies of the ejection fraction, velocity of fiber shortening by echocardiography, and nuclear isotope studies have indicated no changes in myocardial performance at rest; however, as an individual gets older, the increase in the ejection fraction with exercise that is seen in younger people is diminished or even absent.[7,8]

During exercise, there is a smaller increase in cardiac output in elderly persons due to a decrease in the maximum heart rate.[9] Also during exercise, systolic and mean arterial pressures rise more in elderly than in young persons. The filling pressures of the left side of the heart, as judged by pulmonary capillary wedge pressure, are similar in both old and young persons at rest; but with exercise, wedge pressures rise to higher levels in older patients, which indicates an impairment to left ventricular filling during stress. Echocardiographic studies confirm a gradual impairment of left ventricular filling with a decrease in the E-F slope of the anterior mitral leaflet.[10] Impaired diastolic filling may explain why older individuals are more likely than younger ones to develop breathlessness and other symptoms of left ventricular failure during tachycardia.

The best measurement of overall cardiovascular performance during exercise is maximal oxygen consumption. Both cross-sectional and longitudinal studies have demonstrated in both physically active and sedentary men that there is a 1% per year decline of maximal oxygen consumption (VO_2 max).[7] Although total muscle mass decreases with age, a decline of VO_2 max persists even when corrected for this factor. Although an increase in the inspired oxygen concentration does not increase VO_2 max in normal young males, it may do so in elderly persons. Thus, respiratory function may limit oxygen consumption in older persons.

The effect of age on the ability to direct flow from the periphery towards areas that need increased perfusion during stress is not clear, because only the distribution of cardiac output during rest has been studied.[7] Renal blood flow declines by 55% between the 4th and 9th decades. This decline is considerably more than the fall in cardiac output and is associated with the loss of nephrons. Cerebral blood flow also declines by an average of approximately 16% between 20 and 70 years of age. Details of changes in splanchnic blood flow are not available, but it is likely that the blood flow to the liver decreases in proportion to the basal metabolic rate; that is, about 15% between 25 and 65 years of age. Changes in the pulmonary circulation and muscle blood flow due to aging are also relatively slight.

In summary, with progressive aging there is a mild slowing of heart rate, a reduction of cardiac output, and a slowed rate of left ventricular filling at rest. During exercise, there is a decrease in peak heart rate, stroke volume, and (in some patients) even the ejection fraction, with an increase in pulmonary capillary wedge pressures.

Pathologic Changes in Elderly Patients

An elderly patient may have any of the cardiac abnormalities found in a younger individual. Even patients with major congenital abnormalities occasionally live to an advanced age. In any pathologic series, the distribution of the findings represents the overall prevalence of the disease in the community. Thus, coronary artery disease with infarction, ventricular hypertrophy most commonly associated with hypertension, valvular disease, and cor pulmonale make up the vast bulk of pathologic findings.[11–13]

Normal Aging Changes

Although heart weight remains proportional to body weight with advancing age, in the absence of underlying cardiac disease, other changes are known to occur. Lipofuscin is a yellow-brown pigment of unknown significance that is not found in the heart during early age, but is widely distributed in elderly persons.[11] There is increasing density and sclerosis of the collagen of fibrous skeleton of the heart with the development of small areas of calcification. The atrial endocardial surface and the atrial side of the tricuspid and mitral valves progressively thicken with age.

In the cardiac valves, nodular thickening on the lines of closure of the atrioventricular (AV) valves are noted, as well as palpable ridges along the attachments of the aortic cusp.[14] The thickening and nodularity produce an increased stiffness at the base of the aortic cusp, which is the most likely cause of the common systolic ejection murmur found in elderly persons. Similar changes of a lesser degree occur in tricuspid and pulmonary valves.

Calcification of the mitral valve ring, which occurs particularly in females 75 years of age and over, is an additional frequent change probably related to age. In addition, minor degrees of mucoid degeneration of the posterior mitral leaflets can occur.[14]

There is a decreasing elasticity of the aorta with age. This is accompanied by an increase in the caliber of the aorta, which is observed at autopsy and clinically.[7] This reduction in elasticity is associated with an increase in both the velocity of propagation of pulse waves and the rapidity of upstroke of the pressure pulse in the central arterial pressure chamber. These alterations are due to changes in the aortic media and do not reflect atherosclerosis.

Coronary Artery Disease

Coronary artherosclerosis is the most important cause of heart disease in middle-aged and older persons. Nonetheless, it is worth emphasizing that not all elderly patients have ischemic heart disease. If those patients with cardiac failure are analyzed, only 50% have ischemic disease that is usually associated with localized transmural infarctions or, occasionally, diffuse concentric subendocardial fibrosis with three-vessel disease.[13] In a selected subset of non-hospital sudden deaths, the frequency of ischemic heart disease is as high as 62% in patients 65 years of age or older.[11] The pathology of ischemic heart disease is generally the same in persons under or over 65 years of age. Clinically unsuspected, ischemic pathology may emerge at autopsy in as many as 20% of the elderly population.

Myocardial Hypertrophy

The second most common pathologic finding is that of myocardial hypertropy. Although it often is associated with hypertension, other factors such as aortic valvular or ischemic heart disease may contribute to this. The age-related increase in relative heart weight is associated with an age-related increase in systolic blood pressure.

Amyloidosis

Senile cardiac amyloidosis is a subgroup of primary amyloid disease that appears to have distinctive age and pathologic characteristics; it also is immunologically distinct from other forms.[15] It is generally encountered in individuals older than 70 years of age and may be demonstrated in almost 50% of people in this age group.[11] By using light and electron microscopy, the earliest deposits are observed in atrial capillaries and in interstitial areas of the subendomyocardium. In severe instances, the size and number of foci of the amyloid deposition increases, and eventually they cause myofibrillar atrophy via compression. Small deposits may occur in the valves, but rarely is the conducting system affected. Extracardiac deposits generally occur only in patients with severe cardiac involvement.

Valvular Disease

Degenerative valvular disease can take the form of either calcification or mucoid degeneration,[14,16] which is generally limited to left-sided heart valves. Degenerative calcification is one of the most common findings of cardiac pathology in elderly persons and is identified microscopically in the hearts of about one third of patients over 75 years of age. The calcification first appears at the base of the aortic cusps and is probably related to the repeated mechanical stress in normal valve action. With increasing severity, the deposits extend towards the free margins of the cusp, but they rarely involve the free edges. Large masses in calcification can distort a three-cusp aortic valve without evidence of previous inflammation. The precise, underlying pathologic disturbance that triggers the progressive calcification is not clear. There is some evidence that even minor irregularities of the aortic valve may contribute to the progressive calcification and stenosis found in elderly patients.[17,18]

Mitral annular calcification has been reported at autopsy in as many as 10% of all patients over 50 years of age.[11,14,19] Its frequency increases with age. Females are affected approximately four times as frequently as males, which is the exact reverse of an aortic valve abnormality. Although mitral annular calcification usually is an incidental finding, it may be associated with mitral insufficiency, conduction abnormalities, bacterial endocarditis, or even (rarely) mitral stenosis.[20,21] It may be a contributing factor to congestive heart failure in elderly persons.

Mucoid degeneration primarily affects the mitral valve and is characterized by the normally dense valve fibrose that becomes a loose, anachromatically staining connective tissue.[11] This softening permits a stretching of the mitral leaflet under normal intracardiac pressure. This progresses until there is a large floppy leaflet prolapsing into the left atrium during systole. Severe mucoid degeneration in the mitral valve has been found in about 1% of autopsies performed on patients over 50 years of age, and it probably is equally distributed between males and females. These changes can produce a floppy valve with prolapse, and even an aneurysmal protrusion of the posterior mitral leaflet. A mitral systolic murmur is heard in almost all affected patients; but, it is not associated with a clinically significant mitral insufficiency in almost 50% of all patients in whom the lesion is found at autopsy. The primary cause of serious difficulty is the development of a chordal rupture, which can occur spontaneously or be associated with infective endocarditis.

Non-bacterial thrombotic endocarditis is associated with a disseminated malignancy and other wasting diseases, particularly carcinoma of the pancreas, colon, or lung.[22] It is characterized by vegetations on the closure lines at the cusp, which almost always are mitral or aortic. Macroscopically, the vegetations are indistinguishable from those of bacterial endocarditis. Microscopically, they differ in the absence of microorganisms and inflammation, and by the lack of a destruction of the underlying valve cusps. The vegetations often are endothelialized. Occasionally, organization or calcification may be seen. In general, non-bacterial thrombotic endocarditis is a minor aspect of a terminal disease, although systemic emboli have been reported in 14–60% of all cases.[11]

Bacterial endocarditis is an important valvular disease of elderly persons but the pathology is similar in both elderly and young persons. Occasionally, other inflammatory valvular diseases may be seen, such as rheumatoid, ankylosing spondylitis, syphilis, or (rarely) carcinoid disease.

Conduction System

Pathologic changes in the conduction system in older persons are so common as to be regarded as virtually normal, and they are the likely cause of some age-related electrocardiographic changes.

With age, the number of pacemaking cells in the sinus node diminishes so that by 75 years of age an individual may only have 10% of the pacemaker cells that he had when younger.[23] In addition, the amount of fibrous tissue within the atrial myocardium, increases with age with a diminution in the number of muscle fibers and a development of some adipose tissue infiltration.

There has, as yet, been no age-related changes described in the AV node. In the bundle of His and its branches, there appear to be distinct age-related changes that may produce a loss of over 50% of the fibers in the His bundle. Mechanical strain in the area of the upper ventricular septum, which produces an increasing fibrosis followed by sclerosis and microcalcification, is believed to be the mechanism of this process and has been described by Lev as "sclerosis of the left side of the cardiac skele-

ton."[23] Any cause of left ventricular hypertrophy, especially hypertension, accelerates this process. The more distal branches show some decrease in fine fibrous tissue and elasticity with age, but are less dramatic.

Chronic AV block of an unknown etiology is usually shown to be caused by a slowly progressive loss of conduction fibers in the bundle branches without demonstrable myocardial or vascular disease. The loss of conduction fibers leads to replacement fibrosis.[23] Two distinct forms have been highlighted in the literature; 1) Lev's disease, which is a loss of conduction fibers in the proximal left bundle and occasionally the bifurcating bundle; and 2) LeNegre's disease, which is a diffuse disease involving middle and distal portions of the conduction system. There often is a considerable overlap in sex, incidence, age, and pathology. The etiology and pathogenesis of the damage is unknown.

The Cardiac Evaluation of Elderly Persons

Although cardiovascular disease is the major cause of the morbidity and mortality among the elderly population, the etiology of a particular cardiac problem in an individual patient frequently is not determined. Such terms as senile cardiomyopathy and arteriosclerotic cardiovascular disease are used to explain congestive heart failure or other cardiac problems of elderly persons without adequate documentation. Although some degree of myocardial function may be lost due to aging, a specific cardiac disease or diseases almost always can be identified by a careful history and clinical evaluation in any patient. Most cardiac diseases in elderly persons are due to the same pathologic processes that occur in younger patients; however, the manifestations may be more severe due to a longer duration of the disease or because more than one cardiovascular disease usually is present in a geriatric patient.

History

A precise and detailed history from an elderly patient remains a keystone in the clinical evaluation. It requires patience and care to extract this history. Poor memory, altered pain perceptions, perhaps a less active life style, and the diminished expectations of elderly persons may deter a physician from optimal evaluation of disease-imposed limitations.

Breathlessness, or dyspnea, on exertion remains the predominant complaint, and it often overshadows other cardiovascular symptoms such as chest pain. As discussed earlier in this chapter, there are pulmonary and cardiovascular changes in aging that make breathlessness occur earlier as part of the natural history of cardiovascular disorders in elderly patients. In addition, an underlying pulmonary disease, such as emphysema, chronic bronchitis or asthma, musculoskeletal disorders or central nervous system diseases, malnutrition, or chronic illness, may complicate the assessment of any particular symptom.

A differential diagnosis of chest pain in an elderly patient includes many conditions, such as poorly fitting dentures, temporo-mandibular arthritis, temporal arteritis, hiatal hernia, esophageal difficulties, peptic disease, and shoulder or neck arthritis.

One of the most difficult complaints to evaluate and explain are episodes of weakness, giddiness, light-headedness, or even prolonged syncopal episodes. This will be discussed in more detail subsequently.

Edema may occur frequently in an elderly patient as a result of chronic venous insufficiency or even hypoproteinemia. If edema is a predominant presenting complaint, right-sided heart failure due to pericardial constriction, idiopathic cardiomyopathy, or tricuspid valve disease should be considered as seriously as the usual left-sided diseases.

A cerebrovascular accident may be a presenting symptom of a systemic embolus due to a cardiac source such as bacterial or non-bacterial endocarditis, a left ventricular aneurysm, atrial fibrillation, or even systemic emboli from a chronic atrial fibrillation or sick sinus syndrome.

Physical Exam

An examination of the cardiovascular system requires an analysis of the arterial pressure and pulse, venous pressure and pulse, precordial palpation, and auscultation of the heart. Critical evaluation of each of these components, as well as a review of an electrocardiogram (ECG) and chest x-ray film, allows a physician to establish the significance of a physical finding. Other tests, including echocardiography, fluoroscopy, or nuclear cardiovascular studies, may be necessary on occasion.

Blood Pressure and Arteries

It is particularly important in an elderly patient to evaluate arterial pressure in both the lying and standing position, to examine the pulse and the blood pressure in both arms to evaluate the presence of an obstructive disease of the great vessels, and to diagnose orthostatic hypotension. Of all normal, asymptomatic elderly patients, 11–24% demonstrate a decline of 20 mm Hg or more in their systolic pressure when they stand.[24,25] Generally, symptomatic postural hypertension is not observed until the standing systolic pressure is below 110 mm Hg.

A description of the carotid upstroke is an important part of the examination of an elderly patient with a systolic murmur. It may be particularly difficult to evaluate this in an elderly person, because many have non-compliant stiff arteries and produce an especially brisk upstroke. The perception of any delay in the carotid pulse in an elderly patient should make the physician suspicious of an important hemodynamic obstruction either of the aortic valve or the great vessels. The rapid rise and fall of the carotid impulse may mimic aortic regurgitation as found in younger patients, but it is often found in an elderly patient without aortic regurgitation. The presence of a thrill in the carotid artery invariably identifies the presence of severe aortic stenosis. Often, the thrill only can be felt in the carotid artery, as the other sites of transmission may be so separated from the chest wall by tissue or emphysematous lung changes as to blunt the detection of the thrill. Other pathologic findings that are associated with an abnormal arterial pulsation (such as pulsus alternans, pulsus paradoxicus, or a bifid pulse) have similar meaning in elderly and young persons.

An uncommon but occasionally confusing observation is the kinked right carotid syndrome, in which the right carotid pulsation is unusually prominant. This often is mistaken for a right carotid aneurysm, but it is in fact just a manifestation of a long, tortuous right carotid artery. It is a benign disorder.

Venous Pressure

The venous pressure and pulse can be reliably evaluated in an elderly patient, although the left jugular pressure occasionally may be somewhat higher because the left innominate vein may be compressed in systole between the enlarged aorta typical of old age and the back of the sternum. This pseudo-obstruction is relieved by a deep inspiration. If the venous pulsations can be identified as exceeding 10 cm above the level of the right atrium, venous hypertension is clearly present and due to either heart failure or a superior vena caval obstruction. The significance of the abnormalities of venous pulsation are the same in elderly and young persons.

Precordial Examination

Palpation of the heart remains a critical part of the examination of an elderly patient. Because of the difficulty of localizing a heart murmur in an elderly patient, palpation of the precordium and in the neck and suprasternal area is important in locating a thrill. Palpation may identify a palpable first heart sound that is characteristic of mitral stenosis or a pulmonic component secondary to severe pulmonary hypertension. The palpation of the left-ventricular presystolic outward movement is characteristic of an accentuated atrial filling, is an important sign of left ventricular disease, and is the most reliable way of distinguishing "the normal" fourth heart sound from a pathologic sound.[26]

Cardiac Auscultation

The principles of cardiac auscultation that apply in the examination of younger patients have the same significance in elderly patients. A delay of the aortic component of the second heart sound is associated with a delay of the left ventricular ejection after right ventricular ejection, for example with left-bundle branch block or a failing left ventricle. A widely split, fixed second heart sound also indicates the high likelihood of an atrial septal defect, which is the most common, clinically significant congenital heart defect in elderly persons. A fourth heart sound, when loud and associated with a palpable presystolic lift, is a sign of a poorly compliant left ventricle, which is commonly due to a left ventricular hypertrophy or a left ventricular ischemia. A third heart sound is always abnormal.

The Systolic Murmur

Although some investigators report the incidence of systolic murmurs in elderly persons to be as high as 80%, the true prevalence rate is probably closer to 30%.[27] Most systolic murmurs originate from the aortic area and are attributed to a dilation of the ascending aorta or a thickening and deformity of the aortic cusp, usually without a hemodynamically significant stenosis. The murmurs may be best heard at the apex, rather than at the base, because of the chest deformities of elderly patients. The murmur is usually grade 1 or 2 out of 6 in intensity, peaks early, and is of short duration. It usually radiates poorly towards the carotid artery. The second heart sound usually is physiologically split and there is a brisk carotid upstroke. The most important differential diagnostic consideration is a hemodynamically significant valvular aortic stenosis. Other causes of systolic murmurs include hypertrophic cardiomyopathy and mitral diseases, particularly mitral prolapse.

In evaluating any systolic murmur, the associated clinical findings as well as the ECG, chest x-ray film, and (occasionally) echocardiogram are important in assessing the significance of a murmur.

Diastolic Murmurs

A diastolic murmur always is abnormal. The diastolic decrescendo-blowing murmur along the left sternal border nearly always indicates an aortic regurgitation. A diastolic rumble at the apex usually indicates a mitral stenosis secondary to a rheumatic etiology, although patients with calcific mitral annulae may also have occasional diastolic rumbles.[21]

Radiologic Exam

A radiologic examination of the heart continues to have an important part to play in cardiac diagnoses in elderly persons. A cardiothoracic ratio that exceeds 50% correlates with cardiac enlargement. The most striking change in the chest x-ray film is the elongation and increased tortuousity of the aorta, which occurs with advancing age and increasing atherosclerosis. The descending thoracic aorta often appears tortuous and unfolded, and it may be mistaken for an aneurysm of the descending thoracic aorta. Descending thoracic aneurysms are relatively uncommon and can be diagnosed by a computerized tomography (CT scan) or angiography. The superior mediastinum may appear to be wide on the postero-anterior (PA) chest x-ray film due to a tortuousity and elongation of the brachiocephalic arteries. Calcification of the aortic knob that occurs in 25–60% of elderly patients is not significant. Calcification of the ascending aorta, however, may be associated with syphilitic aortitis or, more commonly, an atherosclerotic disease of the ascending aorta. The pulmonary vasculature is essentially the same in elderly patients as in younger patients.

If calcification in the aortic valve is noted on a plain x-ray film, it is almost certainly associated with a hemodynamically severe aortic stenosis. However, a calcification in the mitral annulus is common and does not necessarily identify a hemodynamically important lesion. Tricuspid and pulmonic valvular calcifications are rare. Occasionally, calcification is noted in the pericardium and may be associated with a constrictive pericardial disease. Calcification also may be observed in the coronary arteries. In younger patients, calcification in the coronary arteries is associated with a high specificity with a severe atherosclerotic disease.[28] In patients 70 years of age or older, the presence of calcifications is less specific for severe atherosclerosis.[29] Occasionally, myocardial infarctions or aneurysms may become calcified.

Electrocardiogram (ECG)

In large samples, 57% of the electrocardiograms (ECG) showed abnormalities in elderly patients.[30] The prevalence of electrocardiographic abnormalities is described in Table 11-1.[31,32] Longitudinal studies have identified only minor changes in aging healthy people.[33] Therefore, virtually all the electrocardiographic abnormalities occur in association with cardiac disease, some of which will be clinically important. The

TABLE 11-1 Prevalence of ECG Abnormalities in Elderly Persons

	Percent (%)
Left axis deviation	11
Right axis deviation	1
First degree AV block	9
Right bundle branch block	5
Left bundle branch block	3
ST-T changes	16
Premature atrial beats	10
Premature ventricular beats	6
Atrial fibrillation	8

prognostic significance of a specific electrocardiographic abnormality essentially remains that of the underlying heart disease. ST-segment and T-wave changes (ST-T), left-bundle branch block, interventricular conduction defects, and atrial fibrillation show a highly significant correlation with clinical heart disease. Left anterior hemiblock, right-bundle branch block, and myocardial infarction also represent anatomic and, often, clinical heart disease.

Ambulatory Electrocardiography

Twenty-four hour ambulatory monitoring is a very useful test to evaluate symptoms such as syncope, dizziness, or light-headedness in elderly patients. Recent studies of ambulatory electrocardiography in elderly people are summarized in Table 11-2.[34–37]

TABLE 11-2 Prevalence of Abnormal Rhythms in Elderly Persons

	Percent (%)
Sinus tachycardia	77
Sinus bradycardia	26–89
Marked sinus bradycardia (less than 40 beats/min)	2
Sinus pause	2
AV block	0–2
Supraventricular ectopic beats	
Frequent	22–54
Supraventricular tachycardia	13
Atrial fibrillation or flutter	1–3
Ventricular ectopic beats	
Isolated	78
Frequent	12–15
Multiform	8–35
Couplets	11–23
Ventricular tachycardia	0–4

Stress Testing

Electrocardiographic stress testing can be valuable in eliciting the symptoms of coronary ischemia, in assessing cardiovascular impairment, and in obtaining useful prognostic information.[35,36] Unfortunately, many elderly patients are limited in their exercise capacity by other associated diseases of the musculoskeletal or neurologic system. In addition, the baseline ECG often is abnormal, thus limiting an interpretation of ST-segment changes with exercise. An exercise test should be performed in a flexible manner to accommodate physical limitations and anxiety in an elderly patient. Nonetheless, stress testing still can be useful in determining an ischemic threshold and in assisting the physician and patient in deciding on an appropriate therapy. Its relatively poor specificity limits its usefulness as a diagnostic test, and its predictive accuracy is dependent upon the pretest likelihood of disease.[37]

Echocardiography

Echocardiography non-invasively provides important diagnostic information about cardiac structural abnormalities. Both M-mode and two-dimensional studies can evaluate left ventricular function, the presence of any structural abnormalities of the aortic and mitral valve, and lesions on the right side of the heart. Recently, the range-gated doppler technique has become generally available.[38] This technique is useful in localizing the site of heart murmurs. It is extremely sensitive in detecting aortic, mitral, and tricuspid regurgitation. It may have some value in assessing the hemodynamic severity of lesions, but further investigations must be done before this is convincingly established.

The echocardiographic assessment of the normal, adult aging population demonstrated that, with increasing age, there was a decreased mitral valve E-F slope indicating an impaired left ventricular filling, an increased aortic root diameter, and an increased left ventricular wall thickness.[10] The left ventricular cavity size did not change.

One problem of echocardiographic studies is that complete echocardiograms may be obtained in only two thirds of elderly persons because associated lung diseases or chest deformities limit the optimal sound wave transmission. Nevertheless, it is a useful tool for evaluating left ventricular size and wall motion, pericardial effusion, and valvular disease, or in evaluating cardiac sources of emboli.[39]

One of the most difficult clinical problems in elderly persons is evaluating aortic outflow obstruction. An echocardiogram can identify the aortic valve thickening, calcification, and reduced leaflet motion. The reduced leaflet motion may, however, merely reflect a reduced cardiac stroke volume or cardiac output that is secondary to an impaired left ventricular performance, diminished intravascular volume, severe hypertension, or another etiology. In addition, in elderly persons, the leaflets are commonly thickened, the aortic orifice is small and asymmetric in severe aortic stenosis, and small changes in the valve area can have major hemodynamic consequences. Thus, the echocardiographic description of the aortic valve, either M-mode or two dimensional, usually does not quantify the severity of an aortic valve stenosis. The finding of a wide aortic leaflet separation of 15 mm or more in elderly persons makes severe aortic stenosis unlikely.

An echocardiogram can reliably identify rheumatic disease of the mitral valve, ruptured chordae, and mitral valve prolapse.

An echocardiogram remains the most valuable tool in determining the presence or absence of pericardial effusion. Unfortunately, an echocardiogram is not able to reliably evaluate the hemodynamic significance of the pericardial fluid, because echocardiographic parameters are all indirect and cannot absolutely confirm pericardial tamponade. This is particularly true of a constrictive pericarditis in which there may be only the non-specific finding of a thickened pericardium without a pericardial effusion.

An echocardiogram can be valuable in identifying the presence of valvular vegetations in endocarditis. Vegetations must be 2 mm or larger to be identified.[40] The sensitivity of the echocardiogram in identifying vegetations is between 50–80%.

An echocardiogram can identify idiopathic-hypertrophic cardiomyopathy. The characteristic abnormalities are an asymmetric septal thickening and a systolic anterior septal motion of the mitral leaflet that is often associated with contact with the septum as well as a notching of the aortic valve in midsystole, which indicates a partial closure of the aortic valve.[41]

In other clinical situations in elderly persons, an echocardiogram may demonstrate thrombi that are usually associated with an old myocardial infarction or cardiomyopathies, the presence of atrial myxoma, or previously unsuspected findings such as congenital heart disease (most commonly an atrial septal defect).

Nuclear Cardiology

Nuclear cardiovascular studies can provide valuable diagnostic and management guidance in elderly persons. The most commonly used test is the exercise thallium study, which can identify the presence of coronary artery disease by demonstrating a perfusion defect either during rest or exercise.[42] Unfortunately, in the presence of other associated cardiovascular diseases such as aortic stenosis or cardiomyopathy, the specificity of the thallium defect declines.[43] Nonetheless, it can be a valuable technique for evaluating a chest pain syndrome, particularly in an individual with an abnormality of the ECG (such as a left-bundle branch block, Wolff-Parkinson-White Syndrome (WPW) or the presence of digoxin), which obscures the evaluation of routine exercise testing. The thallium test tends to become abnormal at a lower level of exercise than an ECG. Thus, in someone with an impaired exercise performance due to non-cardiovascular conditions, a thallium test may be more likely to give diagnostically valuable information.

Radionuclide angiography has been validated as an accurate non-invasive method for measuring the left ventricular ejection fraction and ventricular volumes.[44] The evaluation of left ventricular volume and ejection fractions via this technique provides a useful tool in evaluating cardiovascular symptoms and assists in management decisions. A normal individual who exercises has an increase in his left ventricular ejection fraction. Port, et al have demonstrated a decline of the left ventricular ejection fraction during exercise in 50% of an elderly population studied.[8] Unfortunately, the specificity of this abnormality for any particular cardiovascular disease is less than 60%.[45]

Cardiac Catheterization

Although there have been great strides in non-invasive studies, which can characterize the cardiovascular impairment of elderly patients, invasive studies are currently required to identify abnormalities of coronary anatomy, to quantitate the severity of an aortic stenosis, and to evaluate hemodynamic responses to valvular heart disease. Although there is some debate, as a general rule, patients being considered candidates for cardiac surgery require invasive cardiovascular studies. These studies can be performed accurately and safely in an elderly patient.

Major complications of invasive studies in elderly persons are damage to vessels, volume shifts, and a usually reversible nephrotoxicity of contrast agents.[46] With careful monitoring and appropriate precautions, detailed cardiac studies can be performed. In fact, they may be essential in an elderly patient, because multiple anatomic abnormalities and physiologic disturbances are often present in this population.[13] Before making definitive plans for medical or surgical management, it is imperative that all the pathologic and physiologic details are identified.

Congestive Heart Failure

The prevalence of heart failure in persons older than 75 years of age is 10 times its prevalence in persons 45–64 years of age.[47] The prevalence of heart failure in those 65–74 years of age is four times that of individuals 45–64 years of age. Of all ambulatory patients with congestive heart failure, 75% are over the 60 years of age. The physiologic changes associated with aging that were described earlier in this chapter do not result in a symptomatic heart failure at rest. They may, however, produce symptoms when the heart is stressed, or in association with other cardiovascular disease.

Autopsy studies on the hearts of patients dying of cardiac failure emphasize the important observation that a specific pathologic process can be identified in 90% of all cases with two or more pathologic processes present in 65% of patients who died of cardiac failure.[13] Table 11-3 lists the pathologic findings of patients who die of cardiac failure.

TABLE 11-3 Prevalence of Cardiac-Pathologic
Abnormalities in Elderly Patients with and without
Cardiac Failure*

	With Cardiac Failure (%)	Without Cardiac Failure (%)
Ischemic heart disease	48	18
Recent infarction	22	0.5
Calcific valve disease	45	28
Aortic stenosis	9	2
Aortic calcification	23	18
Mitral calcification	35	22
Hypertension	35	11
Cor pulmonale	9	2
Rheumatic disease	8	2
Others:		
Senile amyoid	18	6
Thrombotic endocarditis	11	2
Mucoid degeneration of mitral	6	3

* Of all patients with cardiac failure, 65% have two or more
pathologic processes.

A diagnosis of cardiac failure in elderly patients may be more difficult than in younger patients, because symptoms may be misleading. Breathlessness may be due to many factors that include pulmonary diseases, chest wall abnormalities, or other conditions. Breathlessness also may be a consequence of a transient, exertionally related angina rather than as a consequence of irreversible abnormalities of ventricular performance, and it might be better treated with anti-ischemic agents. Pedal edema can be due to etiologies other than cardiac failure. These include renal and hepatic diseases and abnormalities of the leg veins. Examination of the neck veins may be impaired by an anatomic venous compression. The liver may be palpable because of abnormalities of the thoracic cage or diaphragm. Rales may be present in an individual because of a chronic pulmonary disease. Auscultatory evidence of an S3 gallop indicates left ventricular failure; however, an S4 gallop is commonly heard regardless of the presence or absence of a cardiac pathology, perhaps due to decreased ventricular compliance.

The principles of management of cardiac failure in elderly persons are similar in a patient of any age: 1) Identify the etiology of the cardiac failure either by clinical examination, non-invasive tests, or invasive studies if required; 2) Meticulously search for a precipitating factor (such as an infection, diet change, anemia, or new drug) that may have aggravated the cardiac failure; 3) Initiate a specific therapy if possible, such as aortic valve replacement for aortic stenosis, or a non-specific therapy such as diuretics, digitalis, and vasodilators if no specific therapy is available.

Angina and Coronary Artery Disease

In patients 65 years of age or older, the prevalence of coronary heart disease, on the basis of a clinical examination, is about 20% in males and females.[48] On the basis of pathologic and angiographic observations, the prevalence of a coronary disease in elderly persons is 30–50%.[49]

Risk Factors

Age itself is a risk factor for the development of atherosclerotic disease. The Framingham study shows that patients who otherwise would be categorized as having low risk atherosclerotic disease develop atherosclerotic disease with advancing age.[50] The atherosclerotic risk increases from approximately 1% at 40 years of age to 10% at 70 years of age in patients at "low risk." In contrast, high-risk males have a 60% probability of having atherosclerotic disease at 40 years of age and an 80% probability by 70 years of age. The Framingham study emphasizes that although age is an independent risk factor, the other risk factors (such as systolic hypertension, elevated serum cholesterol, glucose intolerance, and active cigarette smoking or ECG abnormalities) remain additional risk factors for cardiovascular disease.[50]

In elderly persons, an elevated blood pressure stands out as the major risk factor. Unfortunately it is not safe to await the appearance of target organ involvement in elderly hypertensive persons before treating them, because 50% of cardiovascular sequelae in males and 40% of the cardiovascular sequellae in females appear before such evidence can be detected by routine examination.[50] Thus, hypertension is the most potent, most common, and most treatable contributing risk factor for cardiovascular diseases in elderly persons.

Data on the role of physical activity in the development of a cardiovascular disease are inconsistent. Certainly, regular physical activity seems desirable, but there is no clear evidence that it is associated with reduced morbidity and mortality.

Obesity has little effect on cardiovascular morbidity and mortality as an isolated factor. Certainly, weight reduction would reduce the cardiac workload and improve exercise tolerance in patients with an already compromised circulation, and it is advisable.

Although cigarette smokers have a slightly higher coronary mortality at 75–84 years of age, the relative risk attached to smoking diminishes with advancing age.[50] The benefit of quitting smoking is provided by prospective studies that document a reduced incidence of coronary attacks in persons who gave up smoking; but, this effect has not been demonstrated in patients over 65 years of age. Interestingly, the overall death rate is considerably lower in persons who give up smoking despite the lack of change in the rate of new coronary attacks. Thus, there is adequate reason to advise elderly persons to give up cigarettes, even if it does not reduce the risk of coronary attacks.

Cholesterol elevation is a weak predictor of cardiovascular risks in elderly persons, and there is no convincing evidence that even lowering the cholesterol level decreases the risk.[50] Patients with diabetes mellitus have an increased risk of cardiac failure that is secondary to abnormal myocardial function.[51] There is little evidence that the control of hyperglycemia, either by oral agents or insulin, improves cardiovascular mortality.

Neither coffee nor moderate alcohol use seem to be associated with an increased cardiovascular risk. The reduction of emotional stress would seem reasonable, but there is little definitive evidence to support this recommendation. Available evidence demonstrates no benefit from the prophylactic use of aspirin or beta-adrenergic blocking agents in asymptomatic patients.

Prognosis

Once coronary disease is identified as being present, the prognosis is related to the extent of the atherosclerotic disease and the performance of the left ventricle.[52] The more extensive the atherosclerotic disease and the more severely damaged the left ventricle, the worse the prognosis. On the basis of a clinical history alone, the presence of angina identifies the patient who is at risk for a 4% annual mortality, with an additional 4–5% non-fatal infarction rate each year. If there is an extensive atherosclerotic disease and a damaged left ventricle, identified either by the presence of cardiac failure on examination or by laboratory tests, the mortality rate may increase to as high as 30–40% per year.

Clinical Presentation

Coronary artery disease is primarily presented in four ways. It may present as sudden cardiac death, angina, acute myocardial infarction, or cardiac failure.

Almost 50% of the sudden cardiac deaths in a community will occur in individuals who have had no prior history of cardiac disease.[53] The overwhelming majority of sudden cardiac deaths are due to atherosclerotic coronary diseases, which usually is extensive. Pathologic studies often identify evidence of old myocardial infarctions. With improved community emergency services, some people who would otherwise be victims of sudden cardiac death are surviving. In patients who survive a sudden cardiac arrest, only 20% will have evidence of a transmural infarction.[54] The precipitating event is most likely a ventricular tachycardia or ventricular fibrillation, and there is a very high rate of a recurrent collapse. The most powerful predictors of survival of the initial event are the time to initiation of cardiopulmonary resuscitation (CPR) as well as the age of the patient; the more prompt initiation of CPR has a favorable prognosis and advancing age is an adverse prognostic factor.[55] The optimal management of the survivors of sudden death syndrome is not clear at present, but some combination of anti-arrhythmic therapy and, perhaps, a coronary artery bypass grafting in suitable candidates is appropriate.[56]

A typical history of exertional angina may be difficult to obtain in an elderly individual, because activity may be limited by other factors. Breathlessness on exertion is a manifestation of coronary ischemia that is common in elderly persons and may be erroneously attributed to cardiac failure, chronic lung diseases, or deconditioning. In addition, the chest pain may mimic other common problems of elderly persons. Table 11-4 lists the differential diagnostic considerations in individuals complaining of chest discomfort. To complicate matters, there is often radiological corroboration of cervical arthritis or a hiatal hernia with reflux in elderly persons. It remains for the clinician to sift through the history and physical examination of a patient to establish the appropriate diagnosis.

Angina or symptoms of myocardial ischemia, either at rest or with minimal exertion such as postprandial or nocturnal angina, have the same significance in elderly and young patients; that is, the symptoms usually are associated with extensive atherosclerotic disease and tend to be associated with an increased risk of infarction or death.[57] Rapidly progressive or sustained angina attacks have a similar ominous prognosis.

The physical examination of a patient with a suspected coronary disease should focus on ruling out other components of the differential diagnosis. These include aortic stenosis, hypertrophic cardiomyopathy, or severe hypertension. Also, associated conditions that might compromise medical management should be sought, such as peripheral arterial and venous diseases and orthopedic and central nervous system problems with a resultant orthostatic hypotension.

The pathophysiology of ischemic cardiac symptoms, whether angina or breathlessness, is a consequence of the development of myocardial ischemia due to an imbalance between myocardial oxygen supply and demand.[58] The most common etiologic factor is fixed atherosclerotic lesions; however, vasospasm of the coronary vessels, and thromboembolic accidents or emboli, may precipitate anginal episodes or even myocardial infarction. One also must consider factors that contribute to myocardial oxygen demand. The most common are hypertension, fluid overload contributing to cardiac dilatation, and other conditions such as fever, anemia, or thyrotoxicosis that accentuate the myocardial oxygen demand. The optimal management of a patient with ischemic heart disease requires the control of each of those factors that contribute to the ischemic disease and its symptoms. Both the supply components and the demand components of myocardial oxygenation should be approached with an appropriate medical or even surgical therapy.

Laboratory evaluation consists of an ECG and chest x-ray film. Electrocardiographic stress testing has a limited diagnostic value, but it may have prognostic information on the duration of exercise and the heart rate, blood pressure, and ST-segment response to exercise.[35,36] An echocardiogram and nuclear cardiologic studies may be useful in selected circum-

TABLE 11-4   Differential Diagnosis of Chest Pain

Psychogenic
  Depression
  Anxiety
  Hyperventilation
Cervical
  Arthritis
  Herniated disc
  Cervical rib
Neurologic
  Herpes zoster
  Radiculitis
  Thoracic outlet syndrome
Musculoskeletal
  Rib fracture
  Arthritis and bursitis
Thoracic
  Pulmonary hypertension
  Pulmonary embolism/infarction
  Pneumothorax
  Pleuritis
Cardiovascular
  Myocardial infarction
  Angina
  Dissecting aneurysm
  Pericarditis
  Cardiomyopathy
  Valvular disease
Gastrointestinal
  Hiatal hernia
  Peptic diseases
  Pancreatitis
  Biliary tract disease

stances, such as evaluating left ventricular performance or excluding other cardiovascular diseases.

Sublingual nitroglycerin is mainstay therapy for an acute attack of symptomatic ischemic disease. Long-acting nitrates, beta-blockers, and calcium channel-blocking agents can be valuable in protecting against recurrent attacks, and they may prolong life.[59] Unfortunately, an older patient is more likely to have orthostatic hypotension and may not tolerate conventional dosages of nitrates; thus, the individualization of therapy is critical. Beta blockade can be valuable; but, again, caution is required. An elderly patient's resting heart rate usually is lower and the incidence of the sinus and AV node dysfunction is greater than in younger patients. The risk of provoking a symptomatic bradyarrhythmia remains extremely low. Most patients can tolerate beta blockade, even if they have had cardiac failure, after they have been appropriately treated with digitalis and diuretics and with cautious reinstitution of beta blockade. Occasional, troublesome side effects of beta blockade can include depression, excessive fatigue, and even hyperglycemia (especially if aggravated by hypokalemia) that leads to a non-ketotic hyperosmolar coma.[60,61] Underlying contributing conditions that can precipitate or aggravate angina (such as hypertension, congestive heart failure, anemia, and thyrotoxicosis) should, of course, be adequately treated.

Calcium antagonists recently have been introduced in this country with good results in treating patients with angina.[62] Both verapamil, nifedipine, and diltiazam can diminish the frequency of anginal attacks during rest or exertion.

Elderly patients can derive the same symptomatic benefits from coronary bypass grafting as younger patients. Coronary bypass surgery is justified for otherwise fit and reasonably active older patients whose angina, despite optimal medical therapy, continues to compromise their life style. Operative mortality does tend to be slightly higher in older patients (4–12% compared to 4% or less in younger patients).[63–65] Associated conditions such as cerebral vascular disease or renal failure can contribute to the perioperative mortality and morbidity rates.

Acute Myocardial Infarction

In an elderly patient, the most common presentation of an acute myocardial infarction is a sudden onset of breathlessness or an exacerbation of heart failure, rather than the classic symptom of a sustained episode of chest pain.[49,66] Table 11-5 lists the modes of presentation of an acute myocardial infarction in an elderly person. The age of a patient remains a major prognostic variable in surviving an acute myocardial infarction. Patients 70 years of age or older have a hospital mortality rate of 25–35%, which is twice that of younger patients.[67]

The physical findings of patients with an acute myocardial infarction may be non-specific and range from no new findings to evidence of severe cardiac failure, peripheral emboli, or evidence of hypoperfusion. A pulmonary embolism and a dissecting aortic aneurysm should be considered, as well as a ruptured intra-abdominal viscus.

An ECG and serial cardiac enzyme determinations remain the mainstay of diagnostic testing. In occasional circumstances, nuclear medicine or other studies may assist in establishing a diagnosis when the history, ECG, or enzyme data is compromised by a cardiac arrest with resuscitation, a chronic left-bundle branch block, or an absence of a reliable history or enzyme determinations.[68]

Ventricular rhythm disturbances remain the most common cause of mortality in non-hospitalized acute infarction, and aggressive antiarrhythmic therapy is warranted in any age group. As with most medications, greater caution must be exercised in elderly persons because of an

TABLE 11-5 Clinical Features of Acute Myocardial Infarction in Elderly Persons

Predominant Clinical Feature	Percent (%)
Sudden dyspnea or exacerbation of cardiac failure	20–27
Chest pain alone	25
Chest pain with dyspnea	20–45
Other	
Syncope	8
Stroke	7
Weakness, vertigo, vomiting, confusion.	35

increased susceptibility to drug toxicity. The central nervous system threshold for lidocaine toxicity may be lower and the metabolism may be slower in older patients, which causes an increased risk of central nervous system depression and seizures.[69] We recommend the prophylactic use of lidocaine even in elderly patients, but at a reduced dosage and with a greater alertness for signs of confusion or disorientation. (See Volume I, Chapter 39.) The management of the complications of myocardial infarction are similar in elderly and young patients.[70]

A cardiac rupture, an uncommon but catastrophic complication, is found most frequently in elderly persons.[11] It usually occurs 3–12 days following an infarction, is often heralded by the reappearance of chest pain, and is associated with sinus rhythm at the onset of hypotension (i.e., electrical mechanical dissociation).

An elderly patient recovering from a myocardial infarction presents several problems. A prolonged coronary care unit (CCU) stay with an associated isolation and disruption of normal eating and sleeping habits may cause an acute psychosis or confusion. Intravenous (IV) lines and other life support devices may be disconnected. A patient may get out of bed and fall. The acute psychosis or confusion can be induced by cerebral hypoxia or a reaction to sedatives or other medications, particularly lidocaine. Excessive analgesia for sedation or chest pain can cause a respiratory depression or hypotension. Prolonged bed rest may result in atelectasis, pneumonia, a venous thrombosis, a pulmonary embolism, and a profound deconditioning that markedly impairs elderly patients, thereby preventing a return to full functional status. Finally, anticoagulation carries an increased risk of cerebral, gastrointestinal, and pericardial bleeding in elderly persons.[71] Nonetheless, because of the risk of venous thrombosis,[72] low-dose heparinization (5,000 units subcutaneously Q12 hours) is recommended in all patients admitted to a CCU with an acute myocardial infarction; it is continued until the patient is fully ambulatory.

Despite these problems, an elderly patient may gain the same benefits from a CCU as a younger patient. Elderly patients can recover from an infarction and return to an active life.

Valvular Heart Disease

Aortic Stenosis

Aortic stenosis is the most important and most common valve abnormality of elderly persons. The etiology of this valve abnormality is most likely a congenital malformation of the valve in which the cusps are traumatized by altered flow patterns. Over a period of many years, this results in an increasing fibrosis, thickening, and (ultimately) calcification of the valve leaflets.[18] The degree of congenital abnormality can range from the typical bicuspid valve, which usually presents at an earlier age, to more mild abnormalities in which there may be only a partial fusion of two of the aortic cusps.[17] Although tricuspid valves predominate in patients with aortic stenosis over 70 years of age, the precise anatomic disturbance may be difficult to delineate in a severely diseased, calcified stenotic valve. Occasionally, rheumatic valve disease may be present in an elderly patient.

The primary disturbance of aortic valve stenosis is a restriction of left ventricular emptying. As a consequence, the ventricle progressively hypertrophies, prolongs systolic ejection, but ultimately fails and progressively dilates. During the period of adequate compensation by ventricular hypertrophy and prolongation of systolic ejection, the patient usually is asymptomatic. The most typical symptom that develops is either a chest pain similar to angina pectoris of ischemic heart disease, exertional syncope, or breathlessness on exertion. Each of these symptoms is associated with a failure of the compensatory mechanisms for aortic stenosis; they indicate the onset of an ominous phase of the disease, with death usually ensuing within a few months to years. Only in rare instances (approximately 5%) is sudden death the initial symptomatic presentation of aortic stenosis.[73] The absence of angina does not exclude severe, associated coronary disease.[74] Some patients may have only a mild aortic stenosis and severe coronary disease. Late stages produce left ventricular failure and, subsequently, right ventricular failure.

The classic physical findings consist of a slowly rising, systemic arterial pulse, often with a palpable anacrotic notch, and a systolic thrill that is localized to the left upper sternal border and radiates well into the carotid arteries. Palpation of the precordium may show a sustained, left ventricular impulse, often with a palpable atrial filling component. A late-peaking systolic ejection murmur, a single or paradoxically split second heart sound, and an audible fourth heart sound often are present and tend to correlate with the severity of the stenosis.[75] In the presence of left ventricular failure, a third heart sound may be evident.

In the elderly patient the peripheral signs may be misleading and the examination of the heart may be difficult. The peripheral signs of the delayed carotid upstroke may be masked by the increased stiffness of the great vessels. In addition, one third of all patients with a severe valvular aortic stenosis will be hypertensive[69]; 10% of all patients will, in fact, be severely hypertensive, and so the expected low pulse pressure or low pressures are not present. In addition, due to the chest deformities of elderly patients, the heart murmur may be maximal at the apex of the heart, but still radiate well to the neck. The intensity of the heart murmur usually is not a reliable sign in that soft heart murmurs may be associated with severe valvular stenosis. However, very loud heart murmurs (grade 4 or more with a thrill) usually indicate a severe stenosis. The intensity of the heart murmur is a function of stroke volume. An individual with cardiac failure and a rapid heart rate may have a very small stroke volume and a very faint grade 1 or 2 heart murmur in the presence of a severe valvular aortic stenosis.

A physician should be particularly suspicious of an aortic stenosis in any elderly patient who has cardiac failure with a systolic heart murmur, if there is evidence of a ventricular overload (i.e., an ECG of left ventricular hypertrophy (LVH) with secondary T-wave changes).

Evidence of a left ventricular hypertropy via an ECG is present in 88–95% of all patients with severe valvular aortic stenosis and ECG is rarely normal.[74] The echocardiogram, as discussed previously, is of limited value in assessing the severity of aortic stenosis in elderly persons. A chest x-ray film that shows evidence of an aortic valve calcification would strongly support the diagnosis of a severe aortic valvular stenosis. The absence of calcium on fluoroscopy in the region of the aortic valve virtually rules out severe valvular aortic stenosis in an elderly patient.

The major differential diagnostic considerations of aortic stenosis in elderly persons include aortic sclerosis due to a thickening of the valve without an actual outflow obstruction, hypertrophic cardiomyopathy, and mitral valve disease. Patients with an aortic sclerosis should not have LVH on ECG, unless it is secondary to hypertension. Patients with an aortic sclerosis often have a preserved physiologic split of the second heart sound and an early peaking systolic ejection murmur.

Gastrointestinal bleeding due to malformation of blood vessels in the colon have been described in association with aortic stenosis.[76]

The importance of establishing the correct diagnosis of aortic stenosis lies in the fact that its surgical treatment is effective.[74] It prolongs and improves life, even in patients severely disabled with cardiac failure. Hemodynamic studies are important to determine the precise degree of stenosis. The risk of underestimating the severity of the disease and missing a correctable lesion is otherwise great. The operative mortality in elderly patients can be less than 10% with a 10-year survival of 50%, as opposed to the 10-year survival of a non-operated patient of virtually 0%.[74,77] Even patients with cardiac failure and a severely reduced ejection fraction can exhibit a significant improvement after the operation with a normalization of the ejection fraction.[74]

Aortic Regurgitation

Aortic regurgitation can occur either in an acute or chronic form. Acute aortic regurgitation in elderly persons usually is caused by either infective endocarditis or aortic root dissection. In the absence of a left ventricular hypertrophy and dilatation, the abrupt development of aortic regurgitation with resultant left ventricular volume overload produces an acute onset of cardiac failure and, often, cardiovascular collapse.[78] These individuals with acute aortic regurgitation do not have evidence of ventricular hypertrophy, a large pulse pressure, or pandiastolic murmurs. The onset of cardiac failure due to acute aortic regurgitation is a medical emergency that requires an aggressive attitude towards catheterization and valve replacement, even in elderly patients. Without surgery, these patients will typically expire acutely, or if they survive the acute episode, they remain at high risk of sudden death. Operative mortality in most series is 20–30%, but it is justified by the non-operative mortality of 70–100%.[78]

Chronic aortic regurgitation develops as a consequence of a deformity of the aortic leaflets (which may be congenital, rheumatic, postendocarditic, secondary to myxomatous disease) or an inflammatory disease such as ankylosing spondylitis; it also may be caused by a dilation of the aortic root and annulus that is secondary to syphilitic aortitis, Marfans Syndrome, or annuloaortic ectasia. Even severe aortic regurgitation can be associated with a long asymptomatic period. The most initial common symptoms are fatigue or breathlessness on exertion, followed by a more severe cardiac failure. The time interval from the appearance of the first symptom to the fully developed cardiac failure varies widely.[79]

Anginal chest pain is relatively uncommon in early aortic valve regurgitation disease unless it is associated with an additional cardiac pathology such as coronary disease or an associated aortic stenosis.

In contrast to acute aortic regurgitation, the physical findings of chronic aortic regurgitation are generally reliable in assessing its severity. Still, in 20% of all cases, the physical findings will erroneously underestimate the severity of aortic regurgitation or the extent of a left ventricular dysfunction.[80] On physical examination, there often are findings of a hyperdynamic and volume-overloaded circulation with a bobbing head, visible precordial heaves, and widened pulse pressure with a typical diastolic murmur. The ECG shows evidence of a left ventricular hypertrophy; a chest x-ray film shows an enlargement of the heart. The echocardiogram generally confirms this and may also give some evidence as to the etiology of the aortic valve disease. Early closure of the mitral valve is more common in the acute form[78]; but in any case, it is associated with an impending cardiovascular collapse and should be interpreted as an ominous sign indicating the patient requires a prompt evaluation and operation.[78]

The optimal management of an individual with chronic aortic regurgitation is a subject of controversy.[81] The major goals of management are the improvement of symptoms and the preservation of left ventricular performance. Symptomatic improvement often can be obtained with the use of digitalis and diuretics. Vasodilators, particularly hydralazine, have been demonstrated, in a few selected patients, as producing a dramatic improvement in cardiac dilatation.[82] Aortic valve replacement can improve symptoms and may cause a reduction in heart size and an improvement of the ejection fraction. Chronic, severe volume overload, however, may produce severe, irreversible ventricular damage.[83] Occasionally, left ventricular damage may even be irreversible before clinical symptoms are severe enough to draw attention to the lesion. In following an asymptomatic patient with aortic regurgitation, it is important to follow the signs of ventricular enlargement and function using an echocardiogram and nuclear-gated blood pool studies.[84] If the individual has findings of a large pulse pressure, an enlarging or markedly enlarged heart, evidence of left ventricular hypertrophy on an ECG, and evidence of a progressive cardiac dilatation and reduced systolic function demonstrated by echocardiogram or gated blood pool study, an operation usually is warranted. This depends on the individual clinical circumstances and the rehabilitative potential of the patient.[81,83,84] In chronic aortic regurgitation, when there is an enlarging heart, a pulse pressure of 100 mm Hg or more, and an ECG evidence of LVH, the patient has a 30% chance of developing cardiac failure or dying within 1 year.[85]

Rheumatic Heart Disease

Although rheumatic heart disease usually is acquired before 20 years of age, the clinical problems may not arise for many decades and severe cardiac symptoms may not be present until the individual is elderly. The role of recurrent rheumatic inflammation in chronic rheumatic heart disease is being debated. The American Heart Association advises life-long penicillin prophylaxis for streptococcal infections in patients with rheumatic heart disease to protect against reinfection and reinflammation.[86] Rheumatic heart disease may primarily involve the aortic valve with a mixed stenosis and regurgitation or an isolated regurgitation; most commonly, it is recognized as a mitral valve disease predominantly mitral stenosis. This mitral stenosis may be associated with other valvular diseases, including mitral regurgitation, aortic stenosis, regurgitation, or even tricuspid valve disease.

Mitral Stenosis

Attempts must be made to identify patients with an undiagnosed mitral disease by a careful clinical evaluation of patients with atrial fibrillation, systemic emboli, or pulmonary hypertension and right-sided heart failure. A careful auscultatory examination, as well as echocardiography, can virtually always identify a patient with mitral stenosis. The typical auscultatory findings are those of the pandiastolic rumble and an accentuated first heart sound. The accentuated first heart sound may be found less commonly in older patients because of an impaired mobility of the mitral leaflet. The rhythm is often atrial fibrillation and an ECG may show evidence of right ventricular overload in the form of a prominant R or R prime in V1 with a right axis deviation. A chest x-ray film may show evidence of pulmonary hypertension, increased interstitial markings with left atrial enlargement, and evidence of right ventricular enlargement. Calcium may be evident in the mitral valve. An echocardiogram is the most important non-invasive diagnostic tool, and it will reliably identify a rheumatic mitral stenosis by thickened mitral leaflets and a reduced filling rate with fusion of the anterior and posterior leaflets. Two-dimensional echocardiography permits a reasonably good assessment of the severity of a mitral stenosis.[87] The most precise diagnostic tool, however, remains a cardiac catheterization with a determination of pressure gradient and flow across the mitral valve.

The natural history of mitral stenosis is related to the severity of the stenosis, the presence of associated pulmonary hypertension, and other cardiac diseases compromising left ventricular performance. The natural history is complicated by the occurrence of systemic embolism at a rate of 4–8% per year.[88,89] Other complications include atrial fibrillation, pulmonary hypertension, pulmonary hemorrhage, and endocarditis. The dominant symptoms are breathlessness on exertion, fatigue, and (ultimately) pulmonary edema and right heart failure. An occasional patient with severe mitral stenosis will present only with severe right heart failure and fatigue; the pulmonary edema component may not be present because of a severe increase in pulmonary vascular resistance.

It is important to control the ventricular response to atrial fibrillation either with digoxin, propranolol, or verapamil. Effective rate control, particularly with exercise, allows a maximum diastolic time for flow and minimizes the diastolic gradient.

A systemic embolism can be a catastrophic presentation of a mitral stenosis. The emboli are not necessarily related to the severity of mitral stenosis, but over 70% of these emboli occur in patients with atrial fibrillation.[89] Treatment of a systemic embolism is basically medical and requires life-long anticoagulant therapy, generally with coumadin. Recent evidence suggests that antiplatelet agents may be of some benefit.[88] The role of prophylactic anticoagulation in patients who develop atrial fibrillation with a mitral stenosis remains controversial, but is probably warranted.

Mitral valve surgery is indicated in the presence of cardiac failure, severe pulmonary hypertension, or severe mitral stenosis. Mitral commissurotomy is desirable, but usually cannot be accomplished because of the calcification of the valve in elderly persons. Mitral valve replacement can be performed with an acceptable mortality of about 10% with reasonably good, long-term results, even in elderly persons.[90,91] Unfortunately, these patients remain at risk for systemic emboli and often require chronic anticoagulation if they have had systemic emboli or remain in atrial fibrillation.

Mitral Regurgitation

Mitral regurgitation may be a consequence of rheumatic heart disease or other lesions, such as a myxomatous degeneration of the mitral valve, mitral prolapse, a spontaneous rupture of the chordae tendinae, postinfarction mitral regurgitation, postendocarditic mitral regurgitation, a calcification of the mitral annulus, or dilatation of the left ventricle with resultant secondary regurgitation.

Myxomatous degeneration of the mitral valve occurs in elderly persons and may present as either an isolated prolapse or as spontaneous rupture of the chordae. Of all age groups, including elderly persons, 6% have physical findings of mitral prolapse either with a systolic click or a late systolic murmur.[92,93] Mitral regurgitation in these patients, when present, is usually mild and without the associated signs of cardiac overload. An x-ray film generally is normal and an ECG usually is normal, although there occasionally are inferior non-specific ST-T abnormalities. An echocardiogram can confirm this diagnosis. Mitral prolapse may occur as a primary valvular disturbance or may occur secondary to rheumatic disease or following a myocardial infarction. In a mitral valve prolapse that is secondary to myxomatous disease of the leaflets, symptomatic rhythm disturbances may occasionally develop. Progressive, hemodynamically important mitral regurgitation may develop either secondary to progressive prolapse or to ruptured chordae. These patients are at risk for developing infective endocarditis, even if the regurgitation is only mild.[94] Cerebral emboli have been described with prolapse.[95] Ordinarily, an elderly patient with a mitral valve prolapse should be subjected to minimal intervention. Protection from endocarditis via standard prophylaxis is indicated however.

Mitral regurgitation due to a rupture of the chordae may develop as a consequence of a pre-existing abnormality of the valve or secondary to infective endocarditis. A spontaneous chordal rupture typically presents as the sudden appearance of a heart murmur of a mitral regurgitation that is often associated with signs of cardiac failure. The heart murmur is holosystolic, but may radiate toward the spine or to the base of the heart, thus mimiking an aortic stenosis. The ECG may be initially normal, but it subsequently will show evidence of ventricular overload and eventually will develop atrial fibrillation. Cardiomegaly is not initially present, but it will subsequently develop. An echocardiogram, especially the two-dimensional type, can establish a diagnosis of a ruptured chordae. It is important to investigate for endocarditis by obtaining blood cultures. The prognosis of a ruptured chordae is related to the severity of the volume overload. A mitral valve replacement or repair generally is necessary in patients with severe regurgitation. In patients who are

not suitable candidates for mitral valve surgery, vasodilator therapy with hydralazine or another afterload-reducing agent may provide some symptomatic relief.

Severe left ventricular dysfunction can cause secondary mitral regurgitation. It is important to distinguish a severely damaged left ventricle from a postinfarction mitral regurgitation, which occasionally is due to a reversible ischemia or a very localized area of infarction. The treatment of mitral regurgitation that is a consequence of a severe left ventricular dysfunction usually is medical. However, there are occasional patients in whom left ventricular damage is localized to a papillary muscle, so that the residual left ventricular function is adequate to justify surgical correction.

Mitral annular calcification is a common process in elderly persons and is more common in females.[19] Its precise etiology is unknown, but it is believed to be a degenerative process. The calcification may limit leaflet mobility and normal annular changes during systole, and it may produce hemodynamic consequences (more commonly mitral regurgitation, but occasionally stenosis).[21] The calcium usually is easily seen radiographically, with lesser degrees recognized fluoroscopically or echocardiographically. Ordinarily, medical therapy usually is satisfactory, but, there is an occasional patient for whom a mitral valve replacement might be required. These patients are also at risk for bacterial endocarditis and systemic embolus.[96,97]

Bacterial Endocarditis

Bacterial endocarditis is now a common disease of elderly persons.[98] The major problems in bacterial endocarditis are a delayed recognition of the disease and management of complications, especially cardiac failure.[99] A delay in diagnosis in elderly persons usually occurs because the fever is low grade or even absent, or because presenting symptoms (such as arthritis, confusion, fatigue, weakness, systemic emboli, or dementia) are non-specific. Heart murmurs may be present only in two thirds of the patients, and fever in 80–90%.[100–102] Even in patients with a fever, the clinical diagnosis may be made or suspected in only about one-third; an underlying valvular disease may be identifiable in only two-thirds. Endocarditis may be a consequence of hospitalization in an elderly patient, with the development of bacteremia from an infected IV or urologic catheter system. Blood cultures may be negative.[103]

Therapy for bacterial endocarditis is based upon an accurate microbiologic diagnosis, parenteral administration of antibiotics, careful daily examinations, and an adjustment of the specific antimicrobial therapy with blood culture confirmation of efficacy.[104] Careful attention should be given to identification and treatment of the portal of entry.

Mortality remains high (30–60%) in elderly persons and severe complications, such as congestive heart failure (50% mortality) or systemic emboli, indicate an ominous prognosis.[105] Cardiac failure is present in 90% of all deaths and usually is due to a new regurgitant lesion.[105] Although the surgical mortality is 25%, the nonsurgical mortality of patients with moderate to severe cardiac failure ranges from 60–100%; therefore, an aggressive treatment of cardiac failure, usually with a valve replacement, is justified even in elderly persons. Because the development of severe cardiac failure can be acute and catastrophic, patients should be evaluated for cardiac surgery at the earliest sign of cardiac failure. Other indications for cardiac surgery are more complex and might include recurrent emboli and a failure to achieve a microbiologic cure.[106]

Long-term Management

All patients with valvular heart disease, whether elderly or young, should have their functional capacity optimized, complications minimized, left ventricular function preserved, and their life span prolonged. In an attempt to achieve these goals, it is important to review several issues in each individual with a valvular heart disease: 1) Is the hemodynamic state optimal? 2) Is an antibiotic prophylaxis required for prevention of endocarditis? (This is required for

TABLE 11-6 Prophylaxis of Infective Endocarditis

	Initial Therapy	Subsequent Therapy
Dental and upper respiratory tract procedures		
Regimen A	Aqueous penicillin G (1 million units) plus procaine penicillin G (600,000 units) IM*	Penicillin V, 500 mg p.o.† Q6H for 8 doses
or	Penicillin V (2 g p.o.)	Penicillin V, 500 mg p.o. Q6H for 8 doses
or	Erythromycin 1 g p.o.	Erythromycin, 500 mg p.o. Q6H for 8 doses
or	Vancomycin (1 gm IV over 30 min)	
Regimen B Prosthetic Values	Aqueous penicillin G (1 million units) plus procaine penicillin G (600,000 units) IM *plus* streptomycin (1 g IM)	Penicillin V, 500 mg p.o. Q6H for 8 doses
Gastrointestinal and genitourinary surgery and instrumentation	Aqueous penicillin G (2 million units) or ampicillin (1 g) IM or IV†† *plus* gentamicin (1.5 mg/kg up to 80 mg IM or IV) or streptomycin (1 g IM)	Repeat Q8H for 2 additional doses (Q12 if streptomycin used)
or	Vancomycin (1 gm IV over 30 min) *plus* streptomycin (1.0 g IM)	May repeat for 1 dose

* IM = Intramuscular route.
† p.o. = *per os* (by mouth)
†† IV = Intravenous route.

dental and urologic work in most patients with a valvular heart disease.) (*See* Table 11-6.)[107,108] 3) Is antibiotic prophylaxis against rheumatic fever required?[81] 4) Is anticoagulation required? (Generally, in the presence of systemic emboli, prosthetic valves, or mitral stenosis and atrial fibrillation, it is justified. It is usually not warranted in other circumstances.) 5) Are the presenting complaints or symptoms and findings of the patient due to the valvular disease, or as a consequence of some other associated condition?

Miscellaneous Conditions

Hypertrophic Cardiomyopathy

Hypertrophic cardiomyopathy is a disorder characterized by a marked septal hypertrophy, often with myofibril disarray.[109] It can have both obstructive and non-obstructive components. The precise role of the obstruction in the disorder is debated, but the predominant symptomatic problem in these patients is some combination of angina, breathlessness, and often syncope. One third of all patients with a hypertrophic cardiomyopathy are over the 60 years of age at the time of their diagnosis.[110] The diagnosis typically was not recognized previously, due to either the patient not being seriously symptomatic or the clinical features suggesting either coronary or valvular disease.

The clinical presentation will most commonly be angina, syncope, or breathlessness. The angina usually is indistinguishable from a typical, ischemic heart disease pain, although it occasionally may have a postexertional feature. Syncope is most commonly due to marked positional shifts that limit venous return and either aggravate the outflow gradient or precipitate a low cardiac output and syncope. Serious rhythm disturbances (either ventricular, atrial, or bradyarrhythmias with AV block) may contribute to the syncope in some individuals.[110–112] The breathlessness and congestive heart failure that occur usually are due to the markedly elevated, left ventricular, end-diastolic pressure and usually is not associated with a reduced ejection fraction. Clinical signs include a bifid carotid pulse, a fourth heart sound with a sustained papable atrial impulse at the apex, and a systolic ejection murmur that typically radiates to the neck, but also may mimic mitral regurgitation. The murmur usually is accentuated with a Valsalva maneuver or with the use of amyl nitrate. Occasionally, these changes in the heart murmur may be subtle and masked by other conditions, such as cardiac failure. Of all affected patients, 24% may have diastolic murmurs of aortic regurgitation.[113] Mitral regurgitation may be present. The heart murmur commonly fluctuates to a great degree and may be barely audible when the patient is well hydrated; however, if a person should become dehydrated due to illness, the heart murmur and symptoms may be markedly accentuated.

Pertinent laboratory abnormalities include an abnormal ECG with a left ventricular hypertrophy or abnormal Q-waves.[114] A chest x-ray film may be unremarkable or mitral annular calcification, which has an increased association with hypertrophic cardiomyopathy, may be noted.[115] The echocardiogram is the most useful diagnostic test and shows evidence of a marked septal hypertrophy and the outflow obstruction in the form of a systolic anterior motion of the mitral valve.[41] Cardiac catheterization findings are variable, ranging from a supernormal ejection fraction with a variable outflow gradient accentuated by valsalva, amyl nitrate, or isoproterenol, to a dilated heart with poor left ventricular performance, or an elevated left-ventricular diastolic pressure without an outflow gradient.[109]

The annual mortality rate ranges from 2.5–5% per year.[116] The presence of breathlessness, exertional chest pain, and syncope indicate a worse prognosis. Management should address the symptoms, primarily with beta blockade (often in large doses), controlling symptomatic rhythm disturbances, and educating the patient to avoid sudden shifts in position that would accentuate the tendency to syncope. Calcium blockers, specifically verapamil and nifedipine, may have some value.[117,118] Prophylaxis for endocarditis is indicated. Gratifying symptomatic and hemodynamic improvement has been reported after a septal myotomy and myomectomy, even in elderly patients with a hypertrophic cardiomyopathy, and may have a role in selected patients.[119]

Amyloidosis

Amyloidosis is a family of disorders of the immune system that can be an important cause of progressive heart failure.[120] Clinically, amyloid heart disease can mimic constrictive pericarditis, ischemic heart disease, valvular disease, or refractory cardiac arrhythmias of unexplained origin. A diagnosis is established by obtaining a biopsy specimen of appropriately selected, involved tissue. There are no pathognomonic electrocardiographic, radiologic, angiographic, or echocardiographic signs. The usual clinical presentation is that of a rapidly progressive heart failure. The typical findings are an ECG with low voltage, atrial arrhythmias, and an echocardiographically normal-size left ventricle with thickened, speckled, and often poorly contracting walls.[121] The average survival time after the onset of symptoms is approximately 14 months. There is no specific therapy for cardiac amyloidosis, and its management does not differ in principle from that of congestive heart failure and arrhythmias due to other causes. Digitalis seems to be poorly tolerated.

Congenital Heart Disease

Occasionally, previously unrecognized congenital heart diseases may first present in elderly persons. The most likely lesion permitting survival to an old age, and then present as cardiac failure, is an atrial septal defect.[92] Symptoms occur as a consequence of volume overloading of the right side of the heart due to long-standing left-to-right shunting at the atrial level. The volume passing through the pulmonary circulation may be two to four times larger than the systemic circulation, which results in a right ventricular dilatation and (ultimately) right-sided heart failure. Pulmonary hypertension may ensue in some patients and contribute to the failure. An atrial septal defect often is misdiagnosed, because it is not thought of and the patient is thought to have chronic rheumatic heart disease or idiopathic cardiomyopathy. Cardiac failure and atrial rhythm disturbances are common complaints in these elderly persons. A physical examination demonstrates a widely split second heart sound with a prominent right ventricular heave, often with a sys-

tolic ejection murmur in the pulmonary area. An ECG usually reveals an incomplete or complete right-bundle branch block, often with right axis deviation and first degree block. A chest x-ray film shows an enlargement of the main pulmonary artery and right heart chamber, with pronounced (often giant), dilated pulmonary artery branches. An echocardiogram demonstrates an enlargement of right ventricle and paradoxic septal motion due to right-ventricular volume overload. The definitive diagnosis must be confirmed by catheterization. A natural history of patients with atrial septal defect varies widely, but symptomatic deterioration ultimately is to be expected in virtually any individual with an atrial septal defect. Since the risk of surgical correction is very small, an operation is justified, even in asymptomatic patients. After surgery, symptomatic improvement can be marked, even if severe cardiac failure was present beforehand.[122] Unfortunately, the atrial rhythm disturbances persist despite successful surgery. Other congenital heart diseases are rare in elderly persons.

Vascular Diseases

Peripheral vascular diseases often are associated with an ischemic cardiac disease, and heart disease is a major cause of morbidity and mortality in patients with a peripheral vascular disease.[123] Careful attention should be directed at the optimal management of an elderly patient's cardiovascular status when being evaluated for therapy for peripheral vascular disease (*see* Volume I, Chapter 33).

Aortic Dissection

Aortic root dissection can have a dramatic catastrophic presentation in an elderly patient.[124] It may present as syncope, myocardial infarction, pericardial tamponade, stroke, cardiovascular collapse, or as a severe unrelenting chest pain. A diagnosis is based most commonly upon angiographic studies, but recent improvements in CT scanning indicate an increasing role for that technique in the diagnosis of dissection. The management of dissection, involving the ascending aortic root, primarily is surgical as these tend to extend and be unstable. The management of dissection that involves the descending thoracic aorta primarily is medical, as these tend to stabilize with an effective control of blood pressure.

Pericardial Disease

Pericardial diseases may present in an elderly person as an acute inflammatory illness, asymptomatic pericardial effusions, pericardial tamponade, or constriction. A diagnosis of pericarditis ordinarily is based on the clinical symptoms of pericarditis and associated pericardial rub with electrocardiographic changes. The most common etiologies are viral infection, myocardial infarction, medications, uremia, or tumor infiltration.

Pericardial tamponade often presents in elderly persons as an acute catastrophic consequence of some other illness, although idiopathic pericarditis occasionally may be an underlying etiology.[125] The diagnosis is established by the typical findings of a pulsus paradoxicus and an elevated venous pressure. Echocardiography and hemodynamic evaluation may be helpful in confirming these findings, but are not essential in initiating effective therapy. The presence of pericardial tamponade as manifested by these findings justifies a pericardiocentesis and/or surgical pericardiectomy. An important consideration is the underlying etiology of the pericardial disease. The most important etiologies in an elderly patient include malignant diseases (most commonly lung tumor), idiopathic pericarditis, and uremia.[125]

Pericardial constriction can be a more subtle disorder to detect as it typically presents with a history of months or years of fatigue and edema, and is often associated with breathlessness.[126] It is commonly misdiagnosed, because the symptom complex is erroneously attributed to other cardiovascular disorders or to cirrhosis. It typically has an elevated jugular venous pressure, but no pulsus paradoxicus. Once pericardial constriction is considered, a hemodynamic evaluation should be performed. Echocardiography can establish the presence of pericardial effusion, but it is not reliable in the evaluation of pericardial constriction or the hemodynamic significance of pericardial fluid. The major differential diagnostic consideration

is a restrictive cardiomyopathy such as amyloid. Myocardial biopsy specimens may be necessary to make the distinction. If there remains a high likelihood of pericardial constriction, surgical intervention is justified. Currently, the etiology is unknown in most cases.

The rare disorder of atrial myxoma can present in elderly persons.[127] The three major symptoms are either signs of mitral obstruction (either persistent or intermittent), evidence of an embolism, or constitutional symptoms. Diagnosis is now relatively easy with M-mode and two-dimensional echocardiography. Approximately 5% of all reported cases are found in patients 65 years of age or older. If there are no contraindications, surgical therapy is recommended.

Rhythm Disturbances

Cardiac rhythm disturbances are not unique to elderly persons, but they present special problems, because the older individual often has an underlying cardiovascular disease or a greater impairment of physiologic reserve and an altered pharmacologic response to drugs.

Recent studies suggest that aging may be associated with changes in cellular electrophysiology that are characterized by alterations in the action potential amplitude and the rate of the depolarization and altered repolarization.[128] These electrophysiologic changes are distinct from disease states and may be a factor in the increased frequency of rhythm disturbances in elderly persons.

The etiology of a rhythm disturbance and an underlying heart disease are important. For example, in aortic stenosis, the loss of the atrial contribution to ventricular filling during atrial fibrillation may be a catastrophe that must be corrected by prompt cardioversion. Ischemia, digitalis or antiarrhythmic agent excess, electrolyte disturbance, psychotropic drugs, hypoxia, thyrotoxicosis, infections, or a pulmonary embolism should be considered and reversible components corrected.

Before reviewing each of the major rhythm disturbances that might be management problems in elderly persons, it is important to note that studies in a healthy population of elderly subjects show a substantial prevalence of supraventricular ectopic beats and ventricular ectopic beats, both isolated and complex.[34-37] Even a marked sinus bradycardia and sinus pauses up to 1.9 seconds or an isolated transient AV block occasionally are noted.[34] Of the "normal" study group, 30% were shown to have multiform ventricular ectopic beats; 17% had greater than 100 ectopic beats with 7% of them greater than 60 in any given hour. Even 4 episodes of ventricular tachycardia were observed in an apparently normal population of elderly patients.

Supraventricular Rhythm Disturbances

A supraventricular rhythm disturbance can be identified in 50–90% of apparently normal, healthy elderly subjects.[34-37] Most are asymptomatic and without adverse hemodynamic or electrical consequences. For supraventricular arrhythmias, the hemodynamic consequences usually dictate the need and urgency for therapy.

Sinus tachycardia virtually is always due to another etiology, such as fever, infection, hypoxia, thyrotoxicosis, medication, cardiac failure, or ischemia. If no etiology is discovered, the physician should reconsider the possibility that it really is an ectopic atrial tachycardia or another automatic focus rather than sinus. There have, however, been isolated cases of sustained sinus tachycardia.[129]

Minor arrhythmias that do not require treatment include atrial or junctional premature contractions. These occur frequently in elderly patients and although the palpitations occasionally can be distressing to a patient, therapy is generally ineffective and not justified. Sinus arrhythmias and a wandering atrial pacemaker also can be observed in elderly patients. These are generally stable rhythm disturbances and do not justify therapy. There may be an occasional patient with a wandering atrial pacemaker who has troublesome symptoms, such as syncope. The wandering atrial pacemaker may be a manifestation of the failure of adequate sinus mechanisms and provide an indirect support of the sick sinus syndrome. Further evaluation and therapy is then justified.

Paroxysmal Supraventricular Tachycardia

Paroxysmal atrial tachycardia or paroxysmal supraventricular tachycardia (PSVT) usually are due to re-entry within the AV node, occasionally using a concealed extranodal pathway or, less likely, an automatic ectopic atrial focus.[130] The treatment of the PSVT depends on the clinical circumstances. Treatment is directed toward both a termination of the arrhythmia and a prevention of recurrences. Vagal stimulation using carotid sinus pressure, often with the addition of a Valsalva maneuver, is the initial method of choice for the termination of PSVT. Pressor agents should not be used in elderly patients. Verapamil is the agent of choice for the acute termination of PSVT. Care must be taken to observe blood pressure and hemodynamic status during its use. Digitalis, quinidine, propranolol, and procainamide all can be subsequently used, singly or in combination, for acute termination and subsequent control. Direct current (DC) cardioversion is uniformly effective, and is the procedure of choice in the event of hemodynamic deterioration. Rapid atrial pacing also can be used for termination and may have a role in chronic suppression in selected patients. If chronic therapy is necessary, digitalis, propranolol, quinidine, or verapamil (singly or in combination) usually provide effective control. Occasionally, more detailed investigations that use programmed stimulation are necessary to provide optimal management.

Atrial tachycardia with an atrial rate of 150–200 beats per minute and an associated AV block is a digitoxic rhythm until proven otherwise. However, in 50% of the patients it may be due to an underlying heart disease or pulmonary disease and its complications, and it can be managed similarly to PSVT.

Multifocal atrial tachycardia with varying P-waves, PR-intervals, and R-R intervals with an atrial rate greater than 100 can be a troublesome rhythm in an elderly person.[131] It almost always is seen in patients with evidence of a severe cardiovascular or pulmonary disease. The major principle in its management is to distinguish it from atrial fibrillation and to correct the underlying, contributing pulmonary or cardiovascular condition with a particular focus on eliminating a toxic agent (i.e., aminophylline, terbutaline, and so on). Digitalis is not effective in controlling the rate.

Atrial Fibrillation

The incidence rate of atrial fibrillation in a large series of non-hospitalized elderly patients range from 2–10%.[128] Approximately 70% of these patients had clinical evidence of heart disease. Atrial fibrillation occurs in 15–30% of hospitalized or chronic-care facility elderly populations; most have clinical evidence of heart disease. In addition to a consideration of the usual cardiac diseases, an elderly patient with atrial fibrillation must be evaluated for thyrotoxicosis. Rigorous evaluation in at least one study of an elderly population with atrial fibrillation found an incidence rate of thyrotoxicosis as high as 13%.[132]

Atrial fibrillation also may be a manifestation of the sick sinus syndrome. This should be considered when elderly patients have intermittent atrial fibrillation that is associated with long periods of asystole following termination, or when an individual with atrial fibrillation is seen with a history of frequent episodes of syncope or dizziness, perhaps associated with the spontaneous change in his or her rhythm. If atrial fibrillation is persistent, the symptoms of sick sinus syndrome may remit.

The therapy for atrial fibrillation should be directed toward the identification and correction of the underlying disease(s). If the underlying precipitant of atrial fibrillation is treated successfully, a spontaneous resolution of the arrhythmia may occur in 50% of all cases. After underlying etiologies are corrected, the treatment of persistent atrial fibrillation should be directed first at controlling the ventricular response, usually with digitalis, to maintain a resting and exercising ventricular response between 60 and 120 beats per minute. If termination of atrial fibrillation is indicated for hemodynamic reasons or to minimize the risk of thromboembolic complications, electrocardioversion is the method of choice. Patients should be selected for electrical cardioversion on the basis of their clinical status, chronicity of the arrhythmia, underlying disease, likelihood of recurrence of the atrial fibrillation, and the consequences of atrial fibrillation. Quinidine

may provide some protection from a recurrence, but chronic quinidine therapy should only be used in patients in whom there is a high likelihood of a recurrence of the atrial fibrillation or the consequences of atrial fibrillation are serious.[133]

The role of anticoagulation-using warfarin (Coumadin) during the electrical cardioversion of atrial fibrillation and chronic anticoagulation use in patients with an isolated atrial fibrillation has remained controversial. The goal of the coumadin anticoagulation is to minimize the risk of a systemic embolus either during cardioversion or in patients with chronic atrial fibrillation. In a large trial that evaluated coumadin in electrical cardioversion, the anticoagulated group had a significantly reduced incidence of systemic embolism during the cardioversion.[134] However, 50% of the embolic events occurred in patients with prior embolic episodes or an underlying rheumatic disease. The risk of a systemic embolism during the electrical cardioversion of a patient without a prior embolus or rheumatic disease would be approximately 2–3% versus 1% in anticoagulated patients. Thus, there is probably a protective effect of routine Coumadin anticoagulation for 3 weeks before the elective electrical cardioversion of atrial fibrillation; however, the gain is small and the risks of anticoagulation with Coumadin use, even for a short time, can be significant in elderly persons. Therefore, clinical judgment must be used to assess the estimated risk of a systemic embolus based on a history of prior embolic episodes, underlying etiology of heart disease, and an assessment of cardiac performance, versus the risk of anticoagulation. Those patients with prior embolic episodes, rheumatic mitral stenosis, dilated cardiomyopathies, and a markedly impaired cardiac performance have the greatest likelihood of developing a systemic embolus; anticoagulation is recommended in the absence of contraindications.

Similar problems arise in discussions of chronic anticoagulation in patients with chronic atrial fibrillation. Convincing data exists that there is an increased association of cerebrovascular events in patients with atrial fibrillation.[135] It is not yet established whether or not they are causally related. Until more information is available, chronic anticoagulation is advised for patients with an atrial fibrillation who have evidence of a rheumatic mitral stenosis, a prior systemic embolus, or who have a dilated cardiomyopathy. Some evidence suggests that antiplatelet agents provide a protective effect from a systemic embolism in patients with rheumatic heart disease.[88]

Atrial Flutter

Atrial flutter almost always is associated with an underlying heart disease. Direct electrical cardioversion of an atrial flutter usually is preferred, as it is the most effective means of re-establishing sinus rhythm. Although drugs such as digitalis or verapamil may work in controlling the heart rate, they usually require large doses that are often near toxic levels and are difficult to sustain for long. Atrial electronic pacing offers an alternative if an atrial electrode can be easily implanted.

Sinus Bradycardia

The heart rate tends to gradually slow with age, probably due to an increase in parasympathetic tone rather than an intrinsic disease. Although the prevalence of sinus bradycardia in a resting ECG is low, on 24-hour ambulatory monitoring in healthy elderly persons, almost 90% of the patients studied had at least one episode of a sinus bradycardia.[34] Heart rates below 40 beats per minute for 4 beats are rare. As an isolated finding, sinus bradycardia usually is benign. Studies of asymptomatic-isolated sinus bradycardia have demonstrated normal-resting cardiac hemodynamics, and an appropriate exercise duration.[136] A marked sinus bradycardia with a heart rate that is less than 40 beats per minute for more than six seconds (four beats) or pauses 2 seconds or more on an ECG is worrisome. An asymptomatic patient deserves careful observation and follow-up, but a symptomatic patient is a candidate for pacemaker insertion. In an asymptomatic patient, exercise stress testing, a 24-hour ECG, and an electrophysiologic evaluation of sinus node function may have a helpful role; but, the 24-hour ECG remains the optimal test.[137,138] Treatment of symptomatic sinus bradycardia requires an evaluation of the patient for contributing conditions, such as hypothyroidism, beta- or calcium

blockers. Acute therapy often can be in the form of atropine, (rarely) isuprel, and temporary pacing. Long-term pharmacologic therapy is ineffective, and permanent pacing is indicated when chronic therapy is required.

Sick Sinus Syndrome

The term "sick sinus syndrome" was introduced in 1967. It describes a rhythm disturbance that follows an electrical reversion of chronic atrial fibrillation. It was described as a "defective elaboration or conduction of sinus impulses characterized by chaotic atrial activity, changing P-wave contour, bradycardia interspersed with multiple and recurrent ectopic beats with runs of atrial and nodal tachycardia."[139] This disorder may manifest itself primarily as a persistent marked sinus bradycardia that is often less than 40–50 beats per minute or an intermittent or sustained sinus arrest with greater than 2-second sinus pauses with or without AV-junctional escape rhythms. A brady-tachycardia syndrome due to a combination of bradycardia with at least one bout of a paroxysmal supraventricular tachycardia (either atrial fibrillation, flutter, or another PSVT) usually is present. A routine ECG may confirm the sinus bradycardia and the ectopic and shifting P-waves with pauses; but, a routine ECG also may appear perfectly normal. The symptoms may be due to either the bradyarrhythmia or to the tachyarrhythmia. The sick sinus syndrome may be present in association with an acute process, such as an acute myocardial infarction, drug intoxication, electrolyte imbalance, or endocrine abnormalities. Syncope is the most frightening symptom and may be associated with either a bradycardia or tachycardia. In the absence of syncope, symptoms may be cardiac failure, angina pectoris, dizziness, or lightheadedness.

A diagnostic evaluation must be individualized. Electrocardiogram records with rhythm strips and 24-hour ECG recordings or exercise testing may provide a diagnosis. The electrophysiologic studies to measure sinus node recovery time and sinoatrial conduction time have a relatively low sensitivity in establishing a diagnosis; however, in equivocal cases, they may provide evidence of severe or multiple electrophysiologic abnormalities that might justify using a pacemaker. Also, other causes of syncope should be considered. Electrocardiographic- or ambulatory-monitoring documentation of an arrhythmia with associated symptoms remains the only definitive proof.

Asymptomatic patients generally require no treatment. This may also be true of patients with only sporadic fleeting dizziness or palpitations. Occasionally, antiarrhythmic therapy to relieve the palpitations may actually aggravate the sinus arrhythmia and precipitate a more serious symptom, such as syncope. Antiarrhythmic agents must be used with caution in the absence of an underlying ventricular pacer. If there is evidence of symptomatic bradyarrhythmias, a definitive therapy requires a permanent pacemaker. Ventricular pacing is the most commonly used mode; but, occasionally, ventricular pacing may lead to further problems with a loss of synchronized atrial systole that leads to adverse hemodynamic effects. Atrioventricular sequential pacing may help these patients.

Unfortunately, even after the most thorough evaluations, more than one third of all patients with pacemakers implanted due to sick sinus syndrome will fail to have a relief of their syncope symptom.[140] The prognosis of the sick sinus syndrome, with or without a pacemaker, is primarily dependent on the underlying heart disease.

In patients with the sick sinus syndrome, a physician should be alert for the development of a systemic embolism, in which case long-term anticoagulation therapy is justified.[141] At present, chronic anticoagulation of all patients with the sick sinus syndrome to protect against a systemic embolus is not justified.

An episodic sinus bradycardia or arrest may be due to a hypersensitive carotid sinus reflex. Carotid sinus hypersensitivity can be present in 20% of an older age group.[142] A precise definition of a carotid sinus hypersensitivity is difficult, since conflicting definitions of normal and abnormal responses to carotid sinus stimulation have been presented. For clinical purposes, an abnormal response may be considered when an asystole lasting 3 seconds or more results from 5 seconds of lightly applied carotid massage. The majority of patients with a hypersensitive carotid sinus reflex are asymptomatic. In symptomatic patients with a hypersensitive carotid

reflex, a closer investigation can reveal other causes of syncope, which include paroxysmal tachyarrhythmias, orthostatic hypotension, episodic heart block, or a central nervous system disorder. The bradycardia or asystole of a carotid sinus hypersensitivity usually is attributed to the effects of excessive vagal tone alone, as electrophysiologic testing of the sinus node demonstrates that these patients have normal sinus node function. Electronic pacemaker therapy is justified in patients with a symptomatic carotid sinus syncope. Rarely, patients have a vasodepressor response without a bradycardia to carotid sinus massage. There is no effective therapy for this type of response.

Electronic pacemakers have improved recently in reliability and durability, but several principles of electronic pacemaker implantation and follow-up should be emphasized. First, every attempt should be made to establish a clear indication for the implantation of a permanent pacemaker before its insertion. The clearest indication is a documented symptomatic bradyarrhythmia. The use of pacemakers in other circumstances should be acknowledged to be a therapeutic trial. Second, it should be recognized that the most common symptoms for which pacemakers are placed (i.e., syncope, light-headedness, or dizziness) have a high rate of spontaneous resolution and, as symptoms by themselves, provide little prognostic information in most clinical settings.[143] The adverse prognostic implications of syncope, dizziness, and light-headedness are related to the seriousness of the underlying heart disease and the etiology of the syncope. Third, pacemakers are expensive and have complications, some of which may be serious. Finally, the implantation of a pacemaker commits the patient and the physician to a program of regular evaluation of the clinical results, as well as the integrity of the pacemaker and lead system. Despite a high degree of reliability and durability of current pacemakers and leads, complications (such as lead failure, electrical/mechanical interference, infection, and adverse hemodynamic consequences) can impair effective pacemaker performance (occasionally) suddenly and catastrophically.

The newest AV sequential pacemakers, although having some theoretic advantages, probably are only essential in the management of a minority of patients with symptomatic bradyarrhythmias. Pacemakers can help control tachyarrhythmias in specially selected circumstances.

Premature Ventricular Complexes

The prevalence of premature ventricular complexes (PVCs) is increased in an older population (6–11% in routine ECG recordings)[34–37]; 70–80% will have evidence of PVCs with ambulatory monitoring. Complex ventricular rhythm disturbances with frequent PVCs of 100 or more per hour, multifocal PVCs, or couplets, can be found in approximately 30% of all elderly patients. Even ventricular tachycardia has been observed in 4% of an ambulatory healthy population of elderly patients. Thus, in a clinically normal elderly population, PVCs are ubiquitous; even complex forms are common. In an acute setting of a myocardial infarction or digitalis intoxication, treatment of PVCs is indicated because of the increased risk of electrical instability, the relatively short duration of this electrical instability, and the established effectiveness and safety of antiarrhythmic agents. In elderly patients with chronic cardiovascular diseases, or even without any apparent cardiovascular disease, the treatment of ventricular arrhythmias is a complex and difficult problem. The decision to treat ventricular arrhythmias in a chronic setting requires a knowledge of the natural history and prognosis of the underlying disease, a careful assessment of the patient's symptoms, coupled with an analysis of the potential risk for therapy. In patients who are asymptomatic and without any known heart disease, PVCs should not be treated. Treatment is indicated in patients who have symptomatic ventricular rhythm disturbances, particularly ventricular tachycardia or fibrillation. At present, antiarrhythmic therapy in patients with clinical heart disease and asymptomatic ventricular rhythm disturbances, usually is not warranted, even though these patients are recognized as being at an increased risk for sudden death. The sensitivity and specificity of PVCs as a predictor is poor, and the exact risk and benefits of antiarrhythmic therapy have not been established.

Antiarrhythmic agents can be hazardous and may, in fact, even aggravate a rhythm disturbance.[144] Once a decision has been made to initiate antiarrhythmic therapy, the best way to evaluate the effectiveness of the drug is unclear. Modes of evaluation have included the evaluation of drug levels, 24-hour ECG monitoring, exercise testing, and even detailed electrophysiologic studies. Each of these methods has potential problems and uniform recommendations cannot be made. The consequences of therapy failure, the clinical status of the patient, and the resources available to the physician are the major considerations in this decision.

Heart Block

Atrioventricular-nodal conduction disease as well as an intraventricular conduction disease increases in prevalence in older populations, with approximately 10% of a healthy elderly population having evidence of a first-degree AV block or intraventricular conduction disease that is either a right- or left-bundle branch block.[30] Although the presence of first-degree AV block has little association with an underlying heart disease, 80% of all patients with a bundle branch block will have evidence of a cardiovascular disease, with coronary disease being most common. The development of intraventricular conduction disease is associated with an increased incidence rate of cardiovascular complications. Intraventricular conduction disease, AV block, or bundle branch block progresses to complete a heart block at a rate of 1–2% per year.[143,145,146] In most circumstances, the development of the heart block is not catastrophic; usually, there are clear clinical signs of difficulty, and the patient can be managed easily and effectively. Even patients with syncope and evidence of a bundle branch block are not at an increased risk for cardiac death or the development of a complete heart block.[143]

The presence of a second- or third-degree AV block on a resting ECG is a definite abnormality in an elderly patient that requires further investigation and possible treatment. Second-degree AV block of the Wenckbach type requires consideration of extrinsic causes, particularly digitalis excess. If a patient is asymptomatic, specific therapy usually is not necessary, and these patients do well without pacemakers.[147] Symptomatic patients with Mobitz type II-AV block or with a complete heart block require permanent pacemaker therapy. The prognosis, once permanent pacing is established, is linked to that of the underlying heart disease. Patients with cardiac failure, a myocardial infarction, or angina pectoris have the worst prognosis.[148]

Syncope (See also Volume II, Chapter 7)

Syncope is a common clinical disorder that can be defined as the sudden temporary loss of consciousness.[149] This loss of consciousness results from an impairment in cerebral metabolism, which is the consequence of a brief deprivation of essential energy substrates, specifically oxygen and glucose. Syncope should really be considered a symptom complex rather than a primary disease state; it has many potential causes (*see* Table 11-7). Syncope can develop as a consequence of problems that are intrinsic to the cerebral circulation, an inadequacy of cardiac performance, a diminution of systemic pressure to a level less than that required to perfuse the brain, or as a result of a shortage of required energy substrates as constituents of blood delivered to the brain.

Obstruction of the cerebral blood flow generally is due to an anatomic etiology, such as an atherosclerotic plaque or clot. An obstruction may produce transient ischemic attacks (TIAs) or a stroke. Syncope alone is uncommon in most obstructive processes unless it is particularly extensive. More commonly, fainting that is associated with a cerebral occlusive disease is a result of some combination of other mechanisms, such as a decreased perfusion associated with a moderate postural hypotension plus a pre-existing occlusive disease. A cough or hyperventilation also can cause syncope by altering the cerebral perfusion.

The heart may be the cause of syncope by either a rhythm disturbance or an anatomic disturbance. Virtually any rhythm disturbance can precipitate syncope. Heart block, sinus bradycardia, ventricular tachycardia, and a carotid sinus syncope are the most common disturbances. The principal, anatomic cardiac lesions that are associated with syncope are obstructions to left ventricular outflow due to the aortic

TABLE 11-7   Differential Diagnosis of Syncope

Obstruction to cerebral blood flow	Cerebrovascular accident
	Transient ischemic attack (TIA)
	Tussive syncope
	Hyperventilation
Cardiogenic: heart rate, rhythm	Heart block
	Tachy-brady syndrome
	Vasodepressor syncope
	Carotid sinus sensitivity
	Supraventricular or ventricular tachycardia
Obstruction	Aortic stenosis
	Hypertrophic cardiomyopathy
	Pulmonary hypertension/embolus
Fall in blood pressure Cardiogenic Decreased stroke volume	Blood loss
	Adrenal insufficiency
	Postural hypotension
Decreased peripheral resistance	Vasodilator drugs
	Postural hypotension
	Vasovagal
Blood constituents	Hypoxia
	Anemia
	Hypoglycemia

the aortic valve disease or hypertrophic cardiomyopathy. In general, exertional syncope denotes a severe obstruction; however, syncope in aortic stenosis also can be due to a rhythm disturbance, tachycardia, bradycardia, or a failure to provide an adequate cardiac output during exercise, which results in a decreased cerebral perfusion.

The most common form of syncope is the common faint or vasodepressor syncope. Usually, there is a clinically recognized presyncopal syndrome of autonomic overactivity with pallor, sweating, an uncomfortable epigastric feeling, a blurring of vision, and a loss of hearing. Hemodynamically, the principal mechanism is not bradycardia, but peripheral arteriolar vasodilatation.

A reduction in blood pressure may result in syncope. The reduction in blood pressure ordinarily is due to either a reduction in cardiac output or a marked reduction in peripheral resistance. The decreased cardiac output can be due to either a reduction of the heart rate, or a decreased stroke volume. The decreased stroke volume may be caused by either decreased myocardial performance, obstruction to outflow, or decreased cardiac filling. Decreased ventricular filling may result from hypovolemia or a diminished venous tone. A decrease in peripheral vascular resistance may be produced by vasodilator drugs or a decreased sympathetic stimulation, as in orthostatic hypotension and vasodepressor syncope.

Finally, the cerebral blood flow may be adequate, but there may be a failure of critical constituents in the blood, primarily oxygen and glucose, for effective cerebral metabolism. Hypoxia or hypoglycemia usually produces a much more sustained and prolonged syncope rather than momentary losses of consciousness.

A history and physical examination can be sufficient for an accurate diagnosis in approximately 85% of all patients.[150] Selected tests, such as blood chemistries, ECGs, electroencephalograms (EEGs), and 24-hour ECG monitoring and CT scans, may be adequate to establish a diagnosis. There may be selected circumstances where a more detailed electrophysiologic evaluation may be helpful, but the history, physical, and specific tests will identify the etiology in the majority of patients. Interestingly, syncope does not recur in 50–70% of all

patients.[143,151] The highest risk subset of patients are those with cardiac causes, so a particular effort is generally directed at excluding serious cardiac diseases. Patients who have had a loss of consciousness on a vasovagal, psychogenic, or unknown basis generally are at a very low risk. Important, often-neglected aspects of the examination include carotid sinus syncope and a careful evaluation of orthostatic blood pressures.

One of the most devastating causes of syncope is idiopathic-orthostatic hypotension.[152] If there is an adequate intervascular volume and cardiac performance, this usually is due to a disorder of the autonomic nervous system with a failure of appropriate vasoconstriction and cardiac acceleration. Autonomic dysfunction may be neurogenic as with diabetes and idiopathic-orthostatic hypertension, or may be secondary to drugs (most commonly antihypertensives and antidepressants). After eliminating precipitating causes, therapy is directed towards elevating blood pressure in the upright posture. This may be accomplished by increasing the blood volume with supplemental salt, fluids, or with corticosteroids such as Florinef. Vasopressor agents and a mechanical augmentation of venous return with constricting garments to prevent peripheral pooling may help. Unfortunately, the condition generally remains refractory to therapy.

Therapeutic Problems

Even when the correct cardiovascular diagnosis has been made and a rational management plan has been developed, the effective and safe use of cardiac drugs or surgery in elderly persons presents a special challenge. Age-related biologic and physiologic changes in an elderly person often lead to altered pharmacokinetics. These changes, coupled with the unique features of illness in elderly persons as well as physical, psychological, and socioeconomic considerations, interfere with effective, safe drug therapy. The important principles of cardiovascular drug therapy in elderly persons and guidelines for the use of medications have been reviewed in Volume I, Chapters 38 and 39 as well as in recent review articles.[153,154]

Cardiac Surgery

After cardiac surgery was established as a generally safe and effective procedure in younger patients, it was gradually extended to elderly patients. The major, cardiac surgical interventions have been coronary artery bypass grafting and aortic valve and mitral valve replacement. Generally, each procedure is done separately in individual patients; occasionally, multiple procedures are performed in the same patient. The primary indication for coronary bypass surgery has been chronic stable angina with unsatisfactory medical control or unstable angina. Surgical mortality in elderly persons has ranged from 4.5–12%, compared to 1–4% in younger patients.[63–65] The major cause of death and morbidity have been myocardial failure (usually associated with a perioperative myocardial infarction), postsurgical bleeding, neurologic complications of either transient or prolonged periods of a depressed mental status, and strokes. There has been concern about the role of underlying, cerebral vascular diseases in patients who are undergoing coronary artery bypass surgery.[155] Despite the increased surgical mortality, the late results of coronary artery bypass surgery generally have been gratifying in elderly patients, with 70–90% of all patients having excellent symptomatic results.[63–65] Selected subjects have improved survival.

The selection of patients for coronary artery bypass surgery should be based on the physiologic age of the patient, the amount of jeopardized myocardium, the activity of the patient before limitations of a severe angina have occurred, the mental status and motivation of the patient to get back to an active life, and the absence of severe, associated disease processes, such as renal failure or a cerebral vascular disease. The major risk of cardiovascular surgery in an elderly person remains the same as in a young person (i.e., the adequacy of left ventricular function rather than age). With an appropriate selection of patients with adequate left ventricular function and distal coronary arteries suitable for bypass grafting, the excellent symptomatic relief and resulting improvement in the independence and quality of life justifies bypass surgery for elderly patients.

The primary indications for aortic valve replacement are the presence of a severe valvular

aortic stenosis that is usually associated with symptomatic limitation or a severe aortic regurgitation with either an impaired left ventricular performance or cardiac failure. It is important to note that the preoperative left ventricular function, aortic valve area, cardiac index, and hemodynamics are similar to a younger population.[74] Thus, an elderly patient does not have a unique hemodynamic response to aortic stenosis, but has a hemodynamic response identical to younger patients. Surgical mortality ranges from 2.7% to almost 20% in the earliest series studied.[63,74,91] The most common cause of surgical death in an elderly patient is acute myocardial failure that is usually associated with a perioperative infarction. Symptomatic improvement and survival in patients undergoing surgery for an aortic stenosis are excellent. The 10-year survival rate approaches 50%, which is comparable to the survival rate in younger patients populations.[74] Of all patients undergoing surgery, 90% are at the New York Heart Association functional class I or II, with patients with a coronary disease generally doing worse.

The most common cause of late problems are sudden cardiac death, cardiac failure, a myocardial infarction, endocarditis, a cerebral hemorrhage, a stroke, or problems with anticoagulation. Because of the increased risk of anticoagulation complications in elderly patients, biologic prostheses are preferred to avoid the requirement for chronic anticoagulation.

As with aortic valve replacement, mitral valve replacement has become safer for elderly patients in recent years, with surgical mortality falling from more than 30% initially to around 10–12%.[63,90,91] The cause of surgical mortality remains the same: a perioperative myocardial infarction. Right ventricular dysfunction is a consequence of severe pulmonary hypertension. Right ventricular failure can be an important complicating feature in some patients, which re-emphasizes that an excessive delay in valvular surgery is to be avoided. Myocardial function remains the same or deteriorates in patients receiving a mitral valve replacement for severe mitral regurgitation. Thus, a ventricular ejection fraction of less than 0.4 substantially increases the risk and impairs long-term results.[156] The functional improvement in patients can be good after a mitral valve replacement, but an intrinsic myocardial disease, problems with prosthetic perivalvular leaks, and calcified annulae may limit the improvement.

Late complications are similar to an aortic valve replacement. Cardiac failure is the most common cause of late death, and thromboembolic complications are a more common cause of morbidity and mortality in patients with a prosthetic mitral valve than in patients with an aortic prosthesis. Biologic valves are preferred in an elderly patient in the mitral position to allow anticoagulation to be individualized.

Cardiac surgery can offer a dramatic improvement in symptoms and even a survival of selected patients; however, care should be taken to select suitable candidates based upon physiologic age coupled with rehabilitative expectations.

Non-Cardiac Surgery

An additional important and common problem is the evaluation of a cardiac patient for non-cardiac surgery. There have been several, excellent recent reviews of this topic.[157,158] Risk factors can be divided into two classes. The first is the type of surgery to be performed, with intraperitoneal, intrathoracic, or aortic surgery and emergency surgery having the highest risk. The second class is the patient variable. The most powerful, adverse risk factors are the presence of cardiac failure, a recent (less than 6 months) myocardial infarction or unstable angina, evidence of severe underlying cardiovascular disease that is generally demonstrated by frequent premature beats, or evidence of severe valvular aortic stenosis. The risk of a perioperative myocardial infarction in patients with peripheral vascular disease is approximately 4% and is the major cause of death.

As a general rule the cardiac operative risk, for a patient due to his cardiac disease, in a non-cardiac surgical procedure is approximated by his or her estimated 1-year survival on the basis of his cardiac disease. Thus, a patient with severe cardiac failure, with an impaired left ventricular performance on the basis of extensive coronary disease, may have a surgical risk for a general non-cardiac surgical procedure as high as 30%, while an individual with chronic, stable, and well-controlled angina without evidence of cardiac failure will have a surgical risk of 4–5%.

Most patients will do well with good preoperative medical management and attention to the control of cardiac failure, relief of ischemia, protection against rhythm disturbance, and prophylactic antibiotics in patients with valvular lesions coupled with an aggressive postsurgical evaluation of hemodynamic and rhythm status. Cardiac surgery is justified before an elective, general surgical procedure in patients with severe aortic stenosis, unstable angina, or left main or severe coronary disease.[159]

References

1. Caird FI, Dall JLC, Kennedy RD (eds): *Cardiology in Old Age*. New York, Plenum Press, 1976, 1–10.
2. *National Program to Conquer Heart Disease, Cancer and Stroke*. Washington, DC, The President's Commission, 1964.
3. Kennedy RD, Andrews GR, Caird FI: Ischemic heart disease in the elderly. *Br Heart J* 39:1121–1125, 1977.
4. Shock NW: The physiology of aging, in Powers JH (ed): *Surgery of the Aged and Debilitated Patient*. Philadelphia, WB Saunders & Co, 1968.
5. Kostis JB, Moreyra AE, Amendo MI, et al: The effect of age on heart rate in subjects free of heart disease. *Circulation* 65:141–145, 1982.
6. Brandfonbrener M, Landowne M, Shock NW: Changes in cardiac output with age. *Circulation* 12:557–566, 1955.
7. Gerstenblith G: Congestive heart failure, in Noble RJ, Rothbaum DA (eds): *Geriatric Cardiology*. Philadelphia, FA Davis, 1981, pp 131–144.
8. Port S, Cobb FR, Coleman E, et al: Effect of age on the response of the left ventricular ejection fraction to exercise. *N Engl J Med* 303:1133–1137, 1980.
9. Gerstenblith G, Lakatta EG, Weisfeldt ML: Age changes in myocardial function and exercise response. *Prog Cardiovasc Dis* 19:1–21, 1976.
10. Gerstenblith G, Frederiksen J, Yin FCP, et al: Echocardiographic assessment of a normal adult aging population. *Circulation* 56:273–278, 1977.
11. Pomerance A: Cardiac pathology in the elderly, in Noble RJ, Rothbaum DA (eds): *Geriatric Cardiology*. Philadelphia, FA Davis, 1981, pp 9–54.

12. Cosby RS, Mayo M, Peterson JA: The aging heart. *Western J Med* 134:186–189, 1981.

13. Pomerance A: Pathology of the heart with and without cardiac failure in the aged. *Br Heart J* 27:697–710, 1965.

14. Bloor CM: Valvular heart disease in the elderly. *J Am Geriatr Soc* 30:466–472, 1982.

15. Cornwell GG, Westermark R: Senile amyloidosis: A protean manifestation of the aging process. *J Clin Path* 33:1146–1152, 1980.

16. Pomerance A: Aging changes in human heart valve. *Br Heart J* 29:222–230, 1967.

17. Waller BF, Carter JB, Williams HJ, et al: Bicuspid aortic valve. *Circulation* 48:1140–1150, 1973.

18. Vollebergh FEMG, Becker AE: Minor congenital variations of cusp size in aortic valves. Possible link with isolated aortic stenosis. *Br Heart J* 39:1006–1011, 1977.

19. Fulkerson PK, Beaver BM, Auseden JC, et al: Calcification of the mitral annulus. *Am J Med* 66:967–977, 1979.

20. Hammer WJ, Roberts WC, deLeon AC: "Mitral stenosis: secondary to combined massive mitral annular calcific deposits and small hypertrophied left ventricle. *Am J Med* 64:371–376, 1978.

21. Osterberger LE, Goldstein S, Khaja F, et al: Functional mitral stenosis in patients with massive mitral annular calcification. *Circulation* 64:472–476, 1981.

22. Deppisch LM, Fayemi AO: Non-bacterial thrombotic endocarditis. *Am Heart J* 92:723–729, 1976.

23. Davies MJ: Pathology of the conduction system, in Caird FI, Dall JLC, Kennedy RD (eds): *Cardiology in Old Age.* New York, Plenum Press, 1976, pp 57–80.

24. Johnson RH: Blood pressure and its regulation, in Caird FI, Dall JLC, Kennedy RD (eds): *Cardiology in Old Age.* New York, Plenum Press, 1976, pp 101–126.

25. Caird FI, Andres GR, Kennedy RD: Effect of posture on blood pressure in the elderly. *Br Heart J* 35:527–530, 1973.

26. Tavel ME: The fourth heart sound—a premature requiem. *Circulation* 49:4–6, 1974.

27. Duthie EH, Gambert SR, Tresch D: Evaluation of the systolic murmur in the elderly. *J Am Geriatr Soc* 29:498–502, 1981.

28. Bartel AG, Ghen JT, Peter RH, et al: The significance of coronary calcification. *Circulation* 49:1247–1253, 1974.

29. Hamby RI, Tabeah F, Wisoff BG, et al: Coronary artery calcification: clinical implications and angiographic correlates. *Am Heart J* 87:565–570, 1974.

30. Fisch C: Electrocardiogram in the aged: an independent marker of heart disease. *Am J Med* 70:4–6, 1981.

31. Campbell A, Caird FI, Jackson TFM: Prevalence of abnormalities of electrocardiogram in old people. *Br Heart J* 36:1005–1011, 1974.

32. Fisch C: The electrocardiogram in the aged, in Noble RJ, Rothbaum DA (eds): *Geriatric Cardiology.* Philadelphia, FA Davis, 1981, pp 65–74.

33. Bachman S, Sparrow D, Smith LK: Effect of aging on the electrocardiogram. *Am J Cardiol* 48:513–516, 1981.

34. Fleg JL, Kennedy HL: Cardiac arrhythmias in a healthy elderly population. *Chest* 81:302–307, 1982.

35. Fortuin NJ, Weiss JL: Exercise stress testing. *Circulation* 56:699–712, 1977.

36. Schneider RM, Seaworth JF, Dohrmann ML, et al: Anatomic and prognostic implications of an early positive treadmill exercise test. *Am J Cardiol* 50:682–688, 1982.

37. Goldman L, Cook EF, Mitchell N, et al: Incremental value of the exercise test for diagnosing the presence or absence of coronary artery disease. *Circulation* 66:945–953, 1982.

38. Pearlman AS, Stevenson JG, Baker DW: Doppler echocardiography: applications, limitations, and future directions. *Am J Cardiol* 46:1256–1262, 1980.

39. Larson EB, Stratton JR, Pearlman AS: Selective use of two-dimensional echocardiography in stroke syndromes. *Ann Int Med* 95:112–114, 1981.

40. Wann LS, Hallam CC, Dillon JC, et al: Comparison of M-mode and cross-sectional echocardiography in infective endocarditis. *Circulation* 60:728–733, 1979.

41. Gilbert BW, Pollick C, Adelman A, et al: Hypertrophic cardiomyopathy: subclassification by M-mode echocardiography. *Am J Cardiol* 45:861–872, 1980.

42. Bodenheimer MM, Banka VS, Helfant RH: Nuclear cardiology II. The role of myocardial perfusion imaging using Thallium-201 in diagnosis of coronary heart disease. *Am J Cardiol* 45:674–684, 1980.

43. Bailey IK, Come PC, Kelly DT, et al: Thallium-201 myocardial perfusion imaging in aortic valve stenosis. *Am J Cardiol* 40:889–899, 1977.

44. Bodenheimer MM, Banka VS, Helfant RH: Nuclear cardiology I—Radio-nuclide angiographic assessment of left ventricular contraction: uses, limitations, and future directions. *Am J Cardiol* 45:661–673, 1980.

45. Gibbons RJ, Lee KL, Cobb F, et al: Ejection fraction response to exercise in patients with

chest pain and normal coronary arteriograms. *Circulation* 64:952–957, 1981.

46. D' Elia JA, Gleason RE, Aldary M, et al: Nephrotoxicity from angiographic contrast material. *Am J Med* 72:719–725, 1982.

47. Klainer LM, Gibson TC, White KL: The epidemiology of cardiac failure. *J Chronic Dis* 18:797–814, 1965.

48. Kitchin AH, Lowther CP, Milne JS: Prevalence of clinical and electrocardiographic evidence of ischemic heart disease in the older population. *Br Heart J* 35:946–953, 1973.

49. Rothbaum DA: Coronary artery disease, in Noble FJ, Rothbaum DA (eds): *Geriatric Cardiology*. Philadelphia, FA Davis, 1981, pp 105–118.

50. Kannell WB, Gordon T: Evaluation of cardiovascular risk in the elderly: the Framingham study. *Bull NY Acad Med* 54:573–591, 1978.

51. Regan TJ, Ahmed SS, Haider B, et al: The myocardium and its vasculature in diabetes mellitus. *Mod Concepts Cardiovasc Dis* 47:71–78, 1978.

52. Rahimtoola SH: Coronary bypass surgery for chronic angina. *Circulation* 65:225–241, 1982.

53. Kuller L, Perper J, Cooper M: Demographic characteristics and trends in arteriosclerotic heart disease mortality: sudden death and myocardial infarction. *Circulation* 52(suppl III):III–1—III–11, 1975.

54. Lown B: Sudden cardiac death: the major challenge confronting contemporary cardiology. *Am J Cardiol* 43:313–327, 1979.

55. Eisenberg MS, Hallstrom A, Bergner L: Long-term survival after out-of-hospital cardiac arrest. *N Engl J Med* 306:1340–1343, 1982.

56. Rapaport E: Prevention of recurrent sudden death. *N Engl J Med* 306:1359–1360, 1982.

57. Gerstenblith G, Ouyang P, Achuff SC, et al: Nifedipine in unstable angina. *N Engl J Med* 306:885–889, 1982.

58. Hillis LD, Braunwald E: Myocardial ischemia. *N Engl J Med* 296:971–978, 1034–1041, 1977.

59. Braunwald E, Muller JE, Klaner RA, et al: Role of beta-adrenergic blockade in the therapy of patients with myocardial infarction. *Am J Med* 74:113–123, 1983.

60. Conally ME, Kersting F, Dallery CT: The clinical pharmacology of beta-adrenoceptor-blocking drugs. *Prog Cardiovasc Dis* 19:203–234, 1976.

61. Nardone DA, Bouma DJ: Hyperglycemia and diabetic coma: possible relationship of diuretic-propranolol therapy. *South Med J* 72:1607–1608, 1979.

62. Antman E, Stone PH, Muller JE, et al: Calcium channel blocking agents in the treatment of cardiovascular disorders. *Ann Int Med* 93:875–903, 1980.

63. Jolly WW, Isch JH, Shumacker HB: Cardiac surgery in the elderly, in Noble RJ, Rothbaum DA (eds): *Geriatric Cardiology*. Philadelphia, FA Davis, 1981, pp 195–210.

64. Knapp WS, Douglas JS, Craver JM, et al: Efficacy of coronary artery bypass grafting in elderly patients with coronary artery disease. *Am J Cardiol* 47:923–930, 1981.

65. Hochberg MS, Levine FH, Daggett WM, et al: Isolated coronary artery bypass grafting in patients seventy years of age and older. *J Thorac Cardiovasc Surg* 84:219–223, 1982.

66. Pathy MS: Clinical presentation of myocardial infarction in the elderly. *Br Heart J* 29:190–199, 1967.

67. Norris RM, Brandt PW, Gaughey DE, et al: A new coronary prognostic index. *Lancet* 1:274–281, 1969.

68. Berger HJ, Zaret BL: Nuclear Cardiology. *N Engl J Med* 305:799–808, 855–865, 1981.

69. Pfeifer HJ, Greenblatt DJ, Koch-Weser J: Clinical use and toxicity of intravenous lidocaine: a report from the Boston collaborative drug surveillance program. *Am Heart J* 92:168–173, 1976.

70. Karliner JS, Gregoratos G: *Coronary Care*. New York, Churchill Livingstone, 1981.

71. Coon WW, Willis PW: Hemorrhagic complications of anticoagulant therapy. *Arch Int Med* 133:386–392, 1974.

72. Pitt A, Anderson ST, Habersberger PG, et al: Low dose Heparin in the prevention of deep-vein thromboses in patients with acute myocardial infarction. *Am Heart J* 99:574–578, 1980.

73. Ross J, Braunwald E: Aortic stenosis. *Circulation* 37(suppl V):V–61—V–67, 1968.

74. Murphy ES, Lawson RM, Starr A, et al: Severe aortic stenosis in patients 60 years of age and older: left ventricular function and 10-year survival after valve replacement. *Circulation* 64(II):II–184—II–188, 1981.

75. Voelkel AG, Kendrick M, Pietro DA, et al: Noninvasive tests to evaluate the severity of aortic stenosis. *Chest* 77:155–160, 1980.

76. Gelfand ML, Cohn T, Ackert JJ, et al: Gastrointestinal bleeding in aortic stenosis. *Am J Gastroenterol* 71:30–38, 1979.

77. Schway F, Bauman P, Mantley J, et al: The effect of aortic valve replacement on survival. *Circulation* 66:1105–1110, 1982.

78. Morganroth J, Perloff JK, Zeldis SM, et al: Acute severe aortic regurgitation. *Ann Int Med* 87:223–232, 1977.

79. Goldschlager N, Pfeifer J, Cohn K, et al: The

natural history of aortic regurgitation. *Am J Med* 54:577–583, 1973.

80. Karian CH, Greenberg BH, Rahimtoola SH: *Accuracy of Non-invasive Methods in the Assessment of Left Ventricular Size and Systolic Pump Function in Chronic Aortic Regurgitation.* Submitted for publication.

81. O'Rourke RA, Crawford MH: Timing of valve replacement in patients with chronic aortic regurgitation. *Circulation* 61:493–495, 1980.

82. Greenberg BH, Rahimtoola SH: Long-term vasodilator therapy in aortic insufficiency. *Ann Int Med* 93:440–442, 1980.

83. Greves J, Rahimtoola SH, McAnulty JH, et al: Pre-operative criteria predictive of late survival following valve replacement for severe aortic regurgitation. *Am Heart J* 101:300–308, 1981.

84. Ross J: Left ventricular function and the timing of surgical treatment in valvular heart disease. *Ann Int Med* 94:498–504, 1981.

85. Spagnuolo M, Kloth H, Taranta A, et al: Natural history of rheumatic aortic regurgitation. *Circulation* 44:368–371, 1971.

86. Kaplan EL, Bisno A, Derrick W, et al: Prevention of rheumatic fever. *Circulation* 55:223–225, 1977.

87. Martin RP, Rakowski H, Kleiman JH, et al: Reliability and reproducibility of two dimensional echocardiographic measurement of the stenotic mitral valve orifice area. *Am J Cardiol* 43:560–568, 1979.

88. Steele P, Rainwater J: Favorable effect of sulfinpyrazone on thrombo-embolism in patients with rheumatic heart disease. *Circulation* 62:462–465, 1980.

89. Pumphrey CW, Fuster V, Chesebro JH: Systemic thromboembolism in valvular heart disease and prosthetic heart valves. *Mod Concepts Cardiovasc Dis* 51:131–136, 1982.

90. Hochberg MS, Derkac WM, Conkle DM, et al: Mitral valve replacement in elderly patients: encouraging post-operative clinical and hemodynamic results. *J Thorac Cardiovasc Surg* 77:422–426, 1979.

91. Jamieson WRE, Dooner J, Munro AI, et al: Cardiac valve replacement in the elderly: a review of 320 consecutive cases. *Circulation* 64(suppl II):II–177—II–183, 1981.

92. Selzer A, Pasternak RC: Congenital and valvular heart disease, in Noble RJ, Rothbaum DA (eds): *Geriatric Cardiology.* Philadelphia, FA Davis, 1981, pp 169–183.

93. Higgins CB, Reinke RT, Gosink RT, et al: The significance of mitral valve prolapse in middle-aged and elderly men. *Am Heart J* 91:292–296, 1976.

94. Clemens JD, Horwitz RI, Jaffe CC, et al: A controlled evaluation of the risk of bacterial endocarditis in persons with mitral valve prolapse. *N Engl J Med* 307:776–781, 1982.

95. Barnett HJM, Boughner DR, Taylor DW, et al: Further evidence relating mitral valve prolapse to cerebral emboli. *N Engl J Med* 302:139–144, 1980.

96. Burnside JW, DeSanctis RW: Bacterial endocarditis on calcification of mitral annulus fibrosus. *Ann Int Med* 76:615–618, 1972.

97. Pantely GA, Housman LB, DeMots H, Rahimtoola SH: Monocular blindness secondary to calcific embolization. *Chest* 69:555–556, 1976.

98. Finland M: Current problems in infective endocarditis. *Mod Concepts Cardiovasc Dis* 41:53–58, 1972.

99. Wilson WR, Guiliani ER, Danielson GK, et al: General considerations in the diagnosis and treatment of infective endocarditis. *Mayo Clin Proc* 57:81–85, 1982.

100. McAnulty JH, Rahimtoola SH, DeMots H, et al: Clinical features of infective endocarditis, in Rahimtoola SH (ed): *Infective Endocarditis.* New York, Grune & Stratton, 125–148, 1977.

101. Thell R, Martin FH, Edwards JE: Bacterial endocarditis in subjects 60 years of age and older. *Circulation* 51:174–182, 1975.

102. Appelfeld MM, Nornick RB: Infective endocarditis in patients over 60. *Am Heart J* 88:90–94, 1974.

103. Van Scoy RE: Culture negative endocarditis. *Mayo Clin Proc* 57:149–154, 1982.

104. Wilson WR, Guiliani ER, Danielson GK, et al: Management of complications of infective endocarditis. *Mayo Clin Proc* 57:162–170, 1982.

105. Pelletier LL, Petersdorf RG: Infective endocarditis: a review of 125 cases from the University of Washington Hospitals, 1963–1972. *Medicine* 56:287–313, 1977.

106. Dinubile MJ: Surgery in active endocarditis. *Ann Int Med* 96:650–659, 1982.

107. Kaplan EL, Anthony BF, Bisno A, et al: Prevention of bacterial endocarditis. *Circulation* 56:139A–143A, 1977.

108. Everett ED, Hirschmann JV: Transient bacteremia and endocarditis. A review. *Medicine* 56:61–77, 1977.

109. Ross J, Shabetai R, Curtis G, et al: Non-obstructive and obstructive hypertrophic cardiomyopathies. *West J Med* 130:325–349, 1979.

110. Krasnow N, Stein RAL: Hypertrophic cardiomyopathy in the aged. *Am Heart J* 96:326–336, 1978.

111. Canedo MI, Frank MJ, Abdulla AM: Rhythm disturbances in hypertrophic cardiomyopathy: prevalence, relation to symptoms and management. *Am J Cardiol* 45:848–854, 1980.

112. Bharti S, McAnulty JH, Lev M, et al: Idiopathic hypertrophic subaortic stenosis and split His potentials. *Circulation* 62:1373–1380, 1980.

113. Whiting RB, Powell WJ, Dinsmore RE, et al: Idiopathic hypertrophic subaortic stenosis in the elderly. *N Engl J Med* 285:196–200, 1971.

114. Savage DD, Seides SF, Clark CE, et al: Electrocardiographic findings in patients with obstructive and non-obstructive hypertrophic cardiomyopathy. *Circulation* 58:402–408, 1978.

115. Kronzon I, Glassman E: Mitral ring calcification in idiopathic hypertrophic subaortic stenosis. *Am J Cardiol* 42:60–66, 1978.

116. McKenna W, Deanfield J, Faurqui A, et al: Prognosis in hypertrophic cardiomyopathy: role of age and clinical, electrocardiographic and hemodynamic features. *Am J Cardiol* 47:532–536, 1981.

117. Rosing DR, Epstein SE: Verapamil in the treatment of hypertrophic cardiomyopathy. *Ann Int Med* 96:670–672, 1982.

118. Lorell BH, Paulus WJ, Grossman W, et al: Modification of abnormal left ventricular diastolic properties by Nifedipine in patients with hypertrophic cardiomyopathy. *Circulation* 65:499–507, 1982.

119. Koch J, Maron BJ, Epstein SE, et al: Results of operation for obstructive hypertrophic cardiomyopathy in the elderly. *Am J Cardiol* 46:963–966, 1980.

120. Glenner GG: Amyloid deposits and amyloidosis. *N Engl J Med* 302:1283–1292, 1333–1343, 1980.

121. Buja LM, Khoi NB, Roberts WC: Clinically significant cardiac amyloidosis. *Am J Cardiol* 26:394–405, 1970.

122. Sutton MSJ, Tajik AJ, McGoon DC: Atrial septal defect in patients ages 60 years or older: operative results and long-term post-operative follow-up. *Circulation* 64:402–409, 1981.

123. Spittell JA: Recognition and management of chronic atherosclerotic occlusive peripheral arterial disease. *Mod Concepts Cardiovasc Dis* 50:19–23, 1981.

124. Dalen JE, Pape LA, Cohn LH, et al: Dissection of the aorta: pathogenesis, diagnosis, and treatment. *Prog Cardiovasc Dis* 23:237–245, 1980.

125. Guberman BA, Fowler NO, Engel PJ, et al: Cardiac tamponade in medical patients. *Circulation* 64:633–640, 1981.

126. Hirschmann JV: Pericardial constriction. *Am Heart J* 96:110–122, 1978.

127. Guillet P, Baconnet C, Labrousse A, et al: Left atrial myxoma in the elderly. *J Am Geriatr Soc* 29:453–459, 1981.

128. Heger JJ: Cardiac arrhythmias in the elderly, in Noble RJ, Rothbaum DA (eds): *Geriatric Cardiology*. Philadelphia, FA Davis, 1981, pp 145–159.

129. Bauernfeind RA, Amat-Y-Leon F, Dhingra RC, et al: Chronic nonparoxysmal sinus tachycardia in otherwise healthy persons. *Ann Int Med* 91:702–710, 1979.

130. Morady F, Scheinman MM: Paroxysmal supraventricular tachycardia. *Mod Concepts Cardiovasc Dis* 51:107–117, 1982.

131. Shine KI, Kaster JA, Yurchak PM: Multifocal atrial tachycardia. *N Engl J Med* 297:344–347, 1968.

132. Forfar JC, Miller HC, Toft AD: Occult thyrotoxicosis: a correct cause of "idiopathic" atrial fibrillation. *Am J Cardiol* 44:9–12, 1979.

133. Sodermark T, Sjogren OEA, Olsson A, et al: Effect of Quinidine on maintaining sinus rhythm after conversion of atrial fibrillation or flutter. *Br Heart J* 37:486–492, 1975.

134. Bjerkelund CJ, Orning OM: The efficacy of anticoagulant therapy in preventing embolism related to D.C. electrical conversion of atrial fibrillation. *Am J Cardiol* 23:208–216, 1969.

135. Wolf PA, Dawber TR, Thomas HE, et al: Epidemiologic assessment of chronic atrial fibrillation and risk of stroke: the Framingham study. *Neurology (NY)* 28:973–977, 1978.

136. Agrus NS, Rosin EY, Adolph RJ, et al: Significance of chronic sinus bradycardia in elderly people. *Circulation* 46:924–930, 1972.

137. Rliffel JA, Bigger JT, Cramer M, et al: Ability of Holter electrocardiographic recording and atrial stimulation to detect sinus nodal dysfunction in symptomatic and asymptomatic patients with sinus bradycardia. *Am J Cardiol* 40:189–194, 1977.

138. Gann D, Tolentino A, Samet P: Electrophysiologic evaluation of elderly patients with sinus bradycardia. *Ann Int Med* 90:24–29, 1979.

139. Lown B: Electrical reversion of cardiac arrhythmias. *Br Heart J* 29:469–473, 1967.

140. Wohl AJ, Laborde J, Atkins JM, et al: Prognosis of patients permanently paced for sick sinus syndrome. *Arch Intern Med* 136:406–408, 1976.

141. Fairfax AJ, Lambert CD, Leatham A: Systemic embolism in chronic sinoatrial disorder. *N Engl J Med* 295:190–192, 1976.

142. Walter PF, Crawley IS, Dorney ER: Carotid sinus hypersensitivity and syncope. *Am J Cardiol* 42:396–403, 1978.

143. McAnulty JH, Rahimtoola SH, Murphy ES, et al: Natural history of "high risk" bundle branch block. *N Engl J Med* 307:137–143, 1982.

144. Velebit V, Podrid P, Lown B, et al: Aggravation and provocation of ventricular arrhythmias by antiarrhythmic drugs. *Circulation* 65:886–894, 1982.

145. Dhingra RC, Wyndham C, Amat-Y-Leon F, et al: Incidence and site of atrioventricular block in patients with chronic bifascicular block. *Circulation* 59:238–246, 1979.

146. Dhingra RC, Wyndham C, Deedwania PC, et al: Effect of age on atrioventricular conduction in patients with chronic bifascicular block. *Am J Cardiol* 45:749–756, 1980.

147. Strasberg B, Amat-Y-Leon F, Dhingra R, et al: Natural history of chronic second degree atrioventricular nodal block. *Circulation* 63:1043–1049, 1981.

148. Fitzgerald WR, Graham IM, Cole T, et al: Age, sex, and ischemic heart disease as prognostic indicators in long-term cardiac pacing. *Br Heart J* 42:57–60, 1979.

149. Noble RJ: The patient with syncope. *JAMA* 237:1371–1376, 1977.

150. Day SC, Cook FF, Funkenstein H, Goldman L: Evaluation and outcome of emergency room patients with transient loss of consciousness. *Am J Med* 73:15–23, 1982.

151. Gulamhusein S, Naccarelli GU, Ko PT, et al: Valve and limitations of clinical electrophysiologic study in assessment of patients with unexplained syncope. *Am J Med* 73:700–705, 1982.

152. Thomas J, Schirger A, Fealy RD, et al: Orthostatic hypertension. *Mayo Clin Proc* 56:117–125, 1981.

153. Ouslander JG: Drug therapy in the elderly. *Ann Int Med* 95:711–722, 1981.

154. Greenblatt DJ, Sellers EM, Shader RI: Drug disposition in old age. *N Engl J Med* 306:1081–1088, 1982.

155. Ropper AH, Wechsler LR, Wilson LS: Carotid bruit and the risk of stroke in elective surgery. *N Engl J Med* 307:1388–1390, 1982.

156. Phillips HR, Levine FH, Carter JE, et al: Mitral valve replacement for isolated mitral regurgitation. *Am J Cardiol* 48:647–654, 1981.

157. Goldman L, Caldera DL, Nussbaum ST, et al: Multifactorial index of cardiac risk in noncardiac surgical procedures. *N Engl J Med* 297:845–850, 1977.

158. Rose SD, Corman LC, Mason DT: Cardiac risk factors in patients undergoing noncardiac surgery. *Med Clin North Am* 63:1271–1287, 1979.

159. McCollum CH, Carcia-Rinaldi R, Graham JH, et al: Myocardial revascularization prior to subsequent major surgery in patients with coronary artery disease. *Surgery* 81:302–305, 1977.

Chapter 12

Hypertension

Walter J. McDonald, M.D.

The past 3 decades have witnessed major achievements in the field of medicine. Perhaps two of the greatest achievements have been: 1) The documentation that elevated blood pressure is a major risk factor in the development of cerebrovascular, cardiovascular, and renal diseases; and 2) The demonstration that antihypertensive therapy can significantly diminish that risk. Clinical research in hypertension has dramatically increased, but as yet little effort has been directed toward elderly persons. As a result, the dogmas that hypertension is a benign disease in old age, that it is the natural result of aging, that old people need higher blood pressures to perfuse aging organ systems, and that antihypertensive therapy is of no value and too dangerous in persons over 65 years of age, are all too frequently heard. An analysis of 100 studies on the effect of antihypertensive therapy showed that 84% of these studies specifically excluded subjects over 69 years of age.[1] The mean age of elderly persons included in the remaining 16% of these studies was 64 years! Because hypertension is so common in elderly persons, because the number of elderly persons is increasing, and because of the devastating social, emotional, and financial impact of the consequences of hypertension, it is imperative that the issues involved in the management of hypertension in this age group be addressed.

Consequences and Definition of Hypertension

What constitutes an abnormal, as opposed to a normal, physiologic state can be defined by either two standard deviations from the mean or by the pathologic consequences that are associated with that state. Elevated blood pressure, by the nature of its high incidence in western civilizations, must be defined by the latter.

The question to be answered is whether elevated blood pressure constitutes a significant-enough risk factor to warrant a consideration of therapeutic intervention. On this point, there is no reason to equivocate; both systolic and diastolic hypertension increase the risk of cerebrovascular, cardiovascular, and renal diseases. A synopsis of data relevant to this point in elderly persons is contained in Table 12-1.

Classic hypertension, defined as the elevation of diastolic blood pressure, has been studied most frequently. Perhaps, the most careful and conclusive data are derived from the Framingham Study.[2] In an analysis of cardiovascular events, it was shown that in persons over 64 years of age, diastolic blood pressure elevations of 90–109 mm HG carried an almost 2-fold higher risk of untoward events. In diastolic pressures higher than 110 mm Hg, the risk was almost tripled. Several other findings are worth noting. First, although the ratio of risk in hypertensive versus normotensive study subjects decreased with age, in absolute terms hypertension in elderly persons was associated with a greater risk of cardiovascular events. Second, an inspection of Table 12-1 shows that the increased risk in elderly females was at least as great as in elderly males. This underscores the folly of the frequently stated belief that hypertension in geriatric females is a well-tolerated condition.

Limited data are available from the National Cooperative Pooling Project.[3] This study was the result of pooling data from five separate

TABLE 12-1 Risks Associated with Elevated Diastolic or Systolic Blood Pressure

Study	Age (years)	Sex	Blood Pressure Studied (mm Hg)	Risk Studied	Follow-up	Increased Risk of Higher Pressure (%)
Diastolic						
Framingham[2]	65–74	M*	<90 vs. >90–109	Cardiovascular events	18 years	77
			<90 vs. >110			130
		F	<90 vs. >90–109			88
			<90 vs. >110			217
National Cooperative Pooling Project[3]	60–64	M	<80 vs. >94	First major coronary event	10 years	270
Systolic						
Colandrea, et al[6]	69	M & F	<140 vs. >160	Cardiovascular mortality	4 years	590
Chicago People's Gas Company[7]	40–59 (Average age 65 at end of study)	M	<140 vs. >140	Total mortality: Cardiovascular-renal mortality	15 years	70
				Coronary mortality		88
Chicago Stroke Study[8]	65–74	M & F	<180 vs. >180	Total Mortality: Cardiovascular-renal mortality	3 years	103 59 69
				Coronary mortality		98

* M = male, F = female, and M & F = male and female.

studies of a similar design. All five found a consistent relationship between diastolic blood pressure and the risk of a first major coronary event. These data are briefly summarized in Table 12-1. For all increments in diastolic blood pressure, there was an increased risk of coronary events. For diastolic blood pressures greater than 94 mm Hg, there was almost a 3-fold increased risk compared to subjects with diastolic pressures less than 80 mm Hg. The risk was greater in subjects 60–64 years of age than in younger subjects.

The relationship of an elevated diastolic blood pressure to premature morbidity holds for other end-points as well, including fatal coronary heart disease, stroke, and mortality from all causes.[4] Additionally, hypertension may be an etiologic factor in multi-infarct dementia.[5]

Although not as well studied as diastolic hypertension, systolic hypertension also has an impact on survival in old age. A major effect is a related cardiovascular disease. Cardiac work is related to the product of three variables:

1. Systolic blood pressure
2. Heart rate
3. Stroke volume

Thus, an elevated systolic blood pressure should be expected to contribute to heart failure and to increase myocardial oxygen demand, which leads to angina and a myocardial infarction. It seems likely that systolic blood pressure also should contribute to vascular damage, as the tension developed during systole, is greater (though of a shorter duration than during diastole), and is thus potentially more damaging.

The National High Blood Pressure Education Program Coordinating Committee, in evaluating the data concerning the impact of systolic blood pressure on morbidity and mortality, concluded that systolic blood pressure greater than 180 mm Hg increased the risk of stroke or death due to a coronary heart disease by 2 1/3 times in persons 65–74 years of age.[5] Table 12-1 contains a partial listing of the data that support this conclusion.

In a prospective study of over 10,000 elderly people[6], only 72 subjects were found who fulfilled the criteria of a systolic blood pressure greater than 160 mm Hg and a diastolic blood pressure less than 90 mm Hg. The study subjects were matched with individuals with systolic blood pressures less than 140 mm Hg and diastolic blood pressures less than 90 mm Hg. Over a 4-year follow-up period, there was a significant 6-fold higher risk of cardiovascular mortality in the hypertensive group. Myocardial infarctions, angina, and stroke were increased 2–3-fold, although these increases were not statistically significant due to the small number of subjects studied.

Similar numerical problems were avoided in the Chicago People's Gas Company Study.[7] In this study 782 subjects with systolic blood pressures greater than 140 mm Hg were compared to 194 subjects with systolic blood pressures less than 140 mm Hg. The follow-up period was 15 years, at which time the average subject was 65 years of age. All subjects were free of clinical coronary artery diseases at the onset. Increases in mortality from all causes, cardiovascular-renal causes, and coronary heart disease of 70%, 90%, and 100% respectively were observed in the hypertensive group. Unfortunately, this study included no females and the end-point of the described data was 65 years of age.

The Chicago Stroke Study[8] included both males and females over 65 years of age with systolic hypertension. Systolic hypertension was defined as a systolic blood pressure over 180 mm Hg associated with a diastolic blood pressure less than 95 mm Hg. The 3-year risks for death from all causes, cardiovascular-renal causes, and coronary artery diseases are shown in Table 12-1. A significantly increased risk in all three categories was observed among hypertensive subjects. Supportive data are found in the Society of Actuaries Study[9] as well as the Framingham Study.[2]

Based on a review of currently available data, it seems both conservative and reasonable to conclude that diastolic blood pressures above 90 mm Hg and/or systolic blood pressures above 160 mm Hg (and possibly 140 mm Hg) are associated with an increased risk of cardiovascular-renal morbidity and mortality.

Prevalence

Both classic hypertension and isolated systolic hypertension are common geriatric problems. The National High Blood Pressure Education

TABLE 12-2   Frequency of Diastolic and Systolic Hypertension

Study	Age (years)	Blood Pressure Criteria	Incidence (%)			
			Males		Females	
			White	Black	White	Black
Diastolic Hypertension						
CHEC Survey[11]*	60–64	<95 mm Hg	18.2	31.8	14.9	31.0
	>65	<95 mm Hg	15.1	28.6	14.0	27.6
Systolic Hypertension						
National Health	65–74	>160 mm Hg systolic and	15.0	25.5	30.7	38.9
Examination Survey[12]	75–79	<95 mm Hg diastolic	26.9	38.6	32.9	43.1

* CHEC = Community Hypertension Evaluation Clinic Survey.

Program Coordinating Committee[5] concluded that about 40% of all elderly white persons and more than 50% of all elderly black persons in the United States have either isolated systolic hypertension (160/90 mm Hg) or classic hypertension (diastolic blood pressure greater than 90 mm Hg). These data derive largely from the United States National Health Survey.[10]

The prevalence of elevated diastolic blood pressures is perhaps best documented in the Community Hypertension Evaluation Clinic (CHEC) Survey.[11] This study, based upon a single blood pressure measurement, documented the blood pressure of a large segment of the United States population between 1973 and 1975. These data are briefly summarized in Table 12-2. Diastolic hypertension was found to be most common in the age range 50–59 years of age, with the incidence declining thereafter. Above 65 years of age nearly 15% of all white persons and 30% of all black persons were found to have diastolic blood pressures greater than 95 mm Hg. These findings are consistent with the findings of the Hypertension Detection and Treatment Study.[12]

For systolic hypertension, the data are less clear. Koch-Weser[13] defines a disproportionate elevation of systolic blood pressure as a systolic blood pressure greater than [(diastolic pressure − 15) × 2]. This definition would include all patients with isolated systolic hypertension, as well as those with a systolic elevation that is inordinately high in relation to the diastolic blood pressure. The same investigator[1] reported that in the hypertension clinic setting, 43% of all patients over 64 years of age had disproportionate elevations of systolic pressure; roughly 50% of these patients had isolated systolic hypertension. In contrast, in patients younger than 45 years of age, disproportionate elevations of systolic pressure were found in 15% of all patients, while only 1% had isolated systolic hypertension.

The 1960–1962 National Health Examination Survey[10] assessed the frequency of systolic hypertension in a broad spectrum of the non-institutionalized population in the United States. In this study, systolic hypertension was defined by a systolic blood pressure greater than 160 mm Hg with an accompanying diastolic blood pressure less than 95 mm Hg. The findings (*see* Table 12-2) confirm that isolated systolic hypertension is rare before 55 years of age but that by 75–79 years of age, approximately 30–40% of all males and females are affected. These figures may be high, because they represent only a single blood pressure determination. This is confirmed by the study of Colandrea[6], who found an initial incidence rate of 19% in elderly persons; the figure fell to 3% on repeat measurement.

Regardless of the exact incidence of systolic or diastolic hypertension, it may be stated with certainty that hypertension is an extremely common problem in the geriatric population.

Effect of Therapy

While it is important to appreciate that hypertension is both a risk factor and one with a relatively high frequency, it is at least as important

TABLE 12-3 Efficacy of Antihypertensive Therapy

Study	Age (years)	Entry Blood Pressure (mm Hg)*	End-point Evaluated	Decreased Incidence in Treated Patients (%)
Veterans Administration Cooperative Study[14]	60–75	90–114	Cardio-cerebrovascular renal and large-vessel morbidity	54
Hypertension Detection and Follow-up Program[12,15]	60–69	>90	Death	16.4
(16)	60–69	>90	First non-fatal stroke	45.5
Carter[17]	60–74	>110 or >160 (systolic)	Mortality	None
Hypertension-Stroke Cooperative Study Group[18]	All ages (40% above age 60)	>140 (systolic) or >90	Stroke recurrence Cardiovascular and Renal Morbidity and Mortality	None

* Diastolic unless otherwise noted

to establish that therapy can favorably alter the risk. Table 12-3 summarizes information about efficacy of therapy.

The Veterans Administration Cooperative Study[14] was one of the first studies to randomly and prospectively imply the therapeutic benefits from antihypertensive therapy in older persons. Of those subjects studied, 81 were between 60–75 years of age. The therapy for this group of patients was highly effective. In particular, therapy for those patients with diastolic blood pressures between 90–104 mm Hg was much more effective in the elderly versus the younger patients. Several other important points emerged. First, a history of prior cardiovascular-renal disease only enhanced the effectiveness of therapy. This is evidence against the argument that obstructive vascular disease renders therapy more dangerous. Second, subjective complaints relating to drug side effects were equally common in both treated and control group patients after the second clinic visit. Thus, it would appear that at least from a subjective standpoint, antihypertensive therapy is well tolerated in elderly persons. This landmark study, unfortunately, had several major flaws. First, no females were included; second, the number of elderly patients was extremely small.

The Hypertension Detection and Follow-Up Program Study[12,15] addressed the above-men-

tioned weaknesses (see Table 12-3). All age groups up to 69 years of age were evaluated, and 2,376 patients 60–69 years of age were randomized into either an intensive stepped-care antihypertensive regimen (stepped care) or referred to their usual source of medical care (referred care). Therapeutic goals were diastolic blood pressures less than 90 mm Hg for study subjects with an initial diastolic blood pressure greater than 100 mm Hg or a decrease of 10 mm Hg for study subjects with entry diastolic blood pressures between 90–100 mm Hg. As a group, older patients achieved these goals as readily as younger patients, with 75% of stepped-care and 55% of referred-care patients attaining the preset target blood pressures. There was a 16.4% reduction in mortality in the more aggressively and effectively treated stepped-care group. Further analysis of the data[16] demonstrated a significant decrease in fatal and non-fatal strokes in elderly persons. Therapy was most beneficial in older patients with regard to this end-point.

Other less extensive studies also have addressed the question of therapeutic efficacy with difficult conclusions. Carter[17] studied the effect of hypotensive therapy in patients who had suffered a preceding ischemic stroke. A small number of the study patients were between 60–79 years of age. Analysis of the data suggested no benefit of therapy in elderly versus young patients. This was particularly true for patients with isolated systolic hypertension. Carter concluded that systolic hypertension in persons over 60 years of age with a previous stroke should not be treated aggressively.

The Hypertension-Stroke Cooperative Study Group[18] examined a similar question in a group of 205 patients who had survived a previous stroke. This study failed to demonstrate a beneficial effect of antihypertensive therapy from the standpoint of either mortality or prevention of a recurrent stroke. A benefit was suggested, however, for those patients over 70 years of age. It also should be noted that there was no detrimental effect of therapy, and that there was a decreased incidence of congestive heart failure in treated subjects.

The question of therapeutic efficacy in elderly persons may be resolved by the European Working Party on High Blood Pressure in the Elderly[19], which was formed to assess the effect of antihypertensive therapy in hypertensive study subjects older than 60 years of age. Several years into the study, a significant reduction in blood pressure has been achieved in those undergoing therapy, but there has yet to be any significant impact on prognosis. The study is designed to run 7 years or until a significant difference between the treated and untreated groups is observed.

Systolic hypertension, although probably associated with an increased morbidity and mortality, remains to be better studied with regard to the effects of antihypertensive therapy. Until this occurs, firm recommendations for the treatment of systolic hypertension cannot be based on hard information and must be merely inferred.

In summary, the current statement by the National Institutes of Health High Blood Pressure Coordinating Committee[5] states that therapeutic intervention should be undertaken in those patients with a diastolic blood pressure greater than 90 mm Hg. The goal should be a diastolic blood pressure less than 90 mm Hg or a decrease of at least 10 mm Hg if pretreatment values are between 90–100 mm Hg. Isolated systolic hypertension should be treated if systolic blood pressures are above 160 mm Hg. The systolic blood pressure should be lowered to 140–160 mm Hg initially, with a further attempt at reduction if tolerated. As a rule, these levels will be well tolerated if reduction is attempted cautiously and gradually.

Pretreatment Evaluation

In approaching a hypertensive patient, six questions must be answered before therapy is undertaken:

1. Is the patient truly hypertensive?
2. Is there evidence of hypertensive sequelae? (heart, brain, kidney, large vessels?)
3. Are there other cardiovascular risk factors that must be addressed?
4. Are other risk factors or detrimental habits present?
5. Are there conditions that affect drug selection?
6. Is there a secondary cause of hypertension?

Is the Patient Truly Hypertensive?

This may be the most difficult and time-consuming part of the evaluation. It may take months to establish that a patient is hypertensive. As a minimum, in the absence of hypertensive sequelae, blood pressure should be taken three times on 3 separate days before establishing a diagnosis.[5] The blood pressure cuff must be an adequate size, and blood pressures must be obtained with the patient in the recumbent, seated, and upright positions. The seated blood pressure generally is used as the reference blood pressure, but orthostatic changes also must be noted and taken into consideration during therapy. A pronounced, pretreatment orthostatic change (>30/20 mm Hg) may suggest a diagnosis of autonomic dysfunction, dehydration, or very rarely pheochromocytoma or primary aldosteronism. Of greater importance, it should suggest caution when using drugs that exacerbate these changes (diuretics and some sympatholytic drugs). The pretreatment evaluation also should include a documentation of blood pressure in both arms and at least one leg. If blood pressure is found to be higher in one arm, that arm should be used for subsequent measurements. Lower blood pressures in other extremities generally result from obstructing atherosclerotic lesions; these result in artificially low estimates of central blood pressure.

Isolated, low-extremity pressures also must be considered when employing pharmacologic agents. A decreased cardiac output resulting from the use of agents, such as propranolol, may exacerbate atherosclerosis-related symptoms, such as claudication. The incorrect or inadequate assessment of pretreatment blood pressure is probably the greatest source of subsequent problems in treating a hypertensive elderly patient.

Is There Evidence of Hypertensive Sequelae?

This second most important aspect of a hypertensive evaluation helps to guide both the aggressiveness of therapy as well as the selection of pharmacologic agents. A history should explore evidence of cardiovascular, cerebrovascular, renal, or major arterial diseases. A physical examination should include funduscopic, heart, and lung examinations, as well as a search for bruits and diminished pulses. The abdominal examination should include a palpation for an abdominal aneurysm. A laboratory may be employed to seek evidence of renal disease (urinalysis and creatinine) and heart disease (electrocardiogram [ECG] and chest x-ray film).

Are Other Risk Factors or Detrimental Habits Present?

Pertinent historical findings include diabetes, estrogen use, cigarette smoking, heavy salt, or alcohol intake. Obesity should be documented on a physical examination. A laboratory is useful in documenting diabetes and hypercholesterolemia. Treatment of these risk factors and habits is an important aspect of antihypertensive therapy.

Are There Conditions That Will Affect Drug Selection?

Sequelae related to obstructive vascular diseases such as syncope or claudication suggest the use of pharmacologic agents that do not decrease the cardiac output, while a history of angina may favor the use of beta-blockers. A history of renal disease, diabetes, previous antihypertensive therapy, or findings of profound

orthostatic changes, diminished pulses, hyperuricemia, or ECG abnormalities will influence the choice of drugs, as described below. A history of cigarette smoking, obesity, or the excess use of alcohol may suggest non-pharmacologic modes of treatment.

Is There a Secondary Cause of Hypertension?

This is the last on the list of goals for hypertensive evaluation for three reasons[5]: 1) Most hypertensive elderly persons can and should be treated medically; 2) Few patients have a surgically correctable cause of hypertension; and 3) Elderly patients generally are less tolerable of surgical intervention than younger subjects. The onset of hypertension after 55 years of age or accelerated hypertension after 65 years of age suggest a secondary cause. As a rule, patients should be extensively evaluated only if their blood pressure cannot be controlled medically. In this case, if the patient is a surgical candidate, an appropriate initial evaluation probably should be limited to a hypertensive pyelogram and a 24-hour urine test for metanephrine.

Table 12-4 lists the most useful history, physical, and laboratory parameters in the evaluation of a hypertensive patient.

Pathophysiology

Blood pressure is related to cardiac output and total peripheral resistance by the equation:

$$\text{Mean Arterial Pressure} = \text{Cardiac Output} \times \text{Total Peripheral Resistance}$$

Cardiac output and total peripheral resistance are, in turn, dependent on a number of interdependent variables, which include intrinsic myocardial and vascular diseases, extracellular volume, sympathetic nervous system activity, the renin-angiotensin-aldosterone system, and the kidney and baroreceptor reflexes, among others. With aging, changes take place in many of these variables.

Certainly, cardiac performance may diminish with age.[20] Whether this decrease is of a histochemical origin or simply related to atherosclerosis, fibrosis, or other processes, is not

TABLE 12-4   Initial Evaluation of the Hypertensive Patient (relative value indicated by + signs)

Parameter	Is Hypertension Present?	Hypertensive Sequellae?	Risk Factors or Habits	Drug Selection	Secondary Causes
History					
Family history	+				+
Cardiovascular disease	+	+++		++	
Cerebrovascular disease	+	+++		++	
Renal disease	+	++		++	
Diabetes			++	+++	
Duration of hypertension	++				++
Previous therapy	++			+++	
Other medications			+		++
Impotence				++	
Smoking			++		
Sodium intake			+++		
Alcohol intake			++		
Weakness					+
Orthostatic symptoms				+++	++
Physical					
Height and weight			+++		+
Blood pressure:					
Orthostatic	++			+++	++
Arms and legs	+++			+++	+
Fundoscopic	+	+++			++
Pulses		+		++	
Bruits		+		++	+
Heart	+	+		++	
Lungs		+		+++	
Abdomen (aneurysm)		++		++	
Neurologic		+++		++	
Laboratory					
Urinalysis		++			++
Electrolytes				+++	++
Creatinine		++		+++	++
Cholesterol			+		
Glucose			+	+++	+
Uric acid			+	++	
ECG*		+++		+++	
CBC				++	
Chest x-ray film		+		+	

* ECG = electrocardiogram, CBC = complete blood count.

known. Regardless, cardiac output in normal 65-year-old persons is but 70% of that in 25-year-old persons. Peripheral resistance also rises with age. This is partly related to structural changes in the vascular tree,[21] such as the loss of elastic fibers and increased collagen, calcium, and atheroma deposition in the aorta. It also is postulated that the walls of the precapillary arterioles, believed to be primarily responsible for an elevation of peripheral resistance in essential hypertension, are diffusely thickened.

The aging kidney loses mass and blood flow, and has a declining glomerular filtration rate beyond 40 years of age.[22] As a result, an elderly patient has a diminished ability to excrete and to conserve sodium as well as to concentrate urine.[23]

Both blood and extracellular volume diminish with age.[21] Renin activity and serum aldosterone levels generally decline[24], while plasma norepinephrine increases.[25] The baroreceptor function becomes blunted, especially in an elderly hypertensive person.[21]

The purpose of this brief review of blood pressure-determining physiologic changes that occur with advancing age is to point out that it is unreasonable to expect that young and elderly hypertensive subjects have the same pathophysiologic changes or respond in a similar fashion to antihypertensive drugs. Comparing older (mean age 67) and younger (mean age 35) hypertensive patients, it has been found that older subjects have significantly greater reductions in cardiac output (17%), left ventricular ejection rate (18%), renal blood flow (29%), and total blood volume (12%).[26] Significant increases in elderly persons were found in the total peripheral resistance (18%) and plasma norepinephrine (24%). Thus, established hypertension in geriatric patients appears to have a similar, but exaggerated, hemodynamic pattern that is relative to the pattern found in younger hypertensive patients.

Isolated systolic hypertension, however, appears to be hemodynamically different in young versus elderly hypertensive subjects.[27,28] The elderly patient with systolic hypertension has a normal, age-adjusted cardiac output and peripheral resistance, but a decreased arterial compliance.[28] In contrast, younger patients have a normal cardiac output, peripheral resistance, and arterial compliance, but a decreased left ventricular ejection time. Systolic hypertension, thus, appears to relate to a decreased arterial compliance in older subjects and a decreased left ventricular ejection time in younger subjects. Confirmatory studies show that systolic hypertension in elderly persons is related to a disappearance of the dicrotic notch, which is a measure of aortic distensibility.[29] These differences should be considered when designing a therapy for a geriatric hypertensive patient with isolated systolic hypertension.

Therapy

In establishing a plan of therapy for individual patients, one must consider not only the pathophysiology of the hypertensive state, but also the information gleaned from the evaluation. Non-pharmacologic manipulation should be considered first.

Non-Pharmacologic Therapy

Whether or not diuretics are employed in the treatment of hypertension, salt restriction is of value.[30] While a reduction of sodium chloride intake to 4–5 grams/day often is cited as the target, there is evidence that a decrease to 10 grams/day will achieve a 5–10 mm Hg decrease in blood pressure.[31] The diminished sodium intake serves the added function of decreasing the amount of sodium delivered to the distal tubule and, thereby, the amount of potassium excreted during diuretic therapy. *See* Volume II, Chapter 12 for a discussion of the sodium content of foods. To determine the efficacy of this approach, 1–2 months should be allowed to elapse. In some instances, the collection of a 24-hour urine sample for sodium may help determine compliance.

Weight loss also reduces blood pressure.[32] Newer information suggests that altering one's dietary composition may be of additional value. For example, diets high in fat and carbohydrates may be associated with a higher sympathetic nervous activity and a diminished sodium excretion.[33]

Other modalities that are of value include a reduction of nicotine and caffeine.[30] Exercise may be of some value, but it must be advised with caution and common sense. Older patients should go slowly.

More research must be done with stress reduction techniques, such as relaxation therapy and biofeedback, before they can be confidently recommended. Nonetheless, individuals undergoing unusually high levels of stress might benefit from such approaches.

Pharmacologic Therapy

The same stepped-care regimen is recommended for both older and younger patients.[5,34] A diuretic is generally employed first, then adding an adrenergic-inhibiting agent, and (finally) a vasodilator. This approach is outlined in Table 12-5. In elderly persons, initial doses should be smaller, and increments and changes should be made over weeks to months rather than days to weeks. Information gleaned from the evaluation of and knowledge of individual drug pharmacology should be employed to modify the approach (*see* Table 12-6). Few studies have

TABLE 12-5   Stepped Care
Approach

Step 1	Diuretic
Step 2	Beta-blockers
	Atenolol
	Metoprolol
	Nadalol
	Propranolol
	Clonidine
	Methyldopa
	Prazosin
	Rauwolfia compounds
Step 3	Hydralazine
Step 4	Captopril
	Minoxidil

looked specifically at the use of antihypertensive agents in elderly persons, but certain aspects of these drugs are more relevant for elderly persons.

Diuretics

These agents should be employed initially in most elderly hypertensive persons. They are inexpensive and probably have the fewest intolerable side effects.[35] Furthermore, they do not interfere directly with mentation or with already blunted orthostatic reflexes.

The effectiveness has been well established, as diuretics were the first-choice antihypertensive agent in the Veterans Administration Cooperative Study,[14] the Hypertension Detection and Follow-Up Study,[12] and the European Working Party Study.[19,36] They are effective not only in lowering blood pressure, but also in decreasing mortality. In the European Working Party Study, only 15% of all patients required more than a diuretic to achieve good blood pressure control.[36]

A thiazide diuretic is preferred over either loop-acting diuretics or longer-acting agents.[37] Loop diuretics should be used only when the creatinine clearance is less than 25 cc/minute. Thiazides, under most circumstances, are at least as effective as longer-acting agents. Diuretics that act over a longer period of time carry the risk of causing nocturia, while loop diuretics carry the added risks of extracellular volume depletion and acute urinary incontinence.

No diuretic is, however, risk free. Because elderly persons are less capable of conserving sodium, they also are more prone to volume depletion. This probably is the most frequently encountered problem when employing these drugs in elderly persons, and it carries the risk of a decreased organ perfusion and orthostatic hypotension. Hypokalemia is a second significant problem, especially in the geriatric population.[37] Unfortunately, this age group also tends to become potassium intoxicated more readily as well. It is suggested that either a potassium-sparing diuretic or potassium supplementation be used in conjunction with thiazides in elderly patients with obstructive pulmonary disease, serum potassium levels less than 3.0 mEq/L, and in patients with hypokalemia-related symptoms or who take digitalis preparations. Hypokalemia must be looked for carefully especially in the first 3 months.

Other diuretic-associated side effects include the impairment of glucose tolerance[38] and the elevation of uric acid and creatinine.[19,36] The significance of these minor laboratory abnormalities remains unknown. If they do occur, it generally will be in the first 3 months of therapy.[36]

A final concern derives from one report in which elderly patients with modest hypertension treated with thiazides had a 2-fold increase in mortality, myocardial infarctions, and sudden death when compared to patients treated with diet or beta-blocking drugs.[39] This deleterious effect was not seen in similarly treated patients with severe hypertension. Because these data differ so markedly from other studies, a further evaluation is necessary before the results are generally accepted. If diuretics cannot be used, beta-blockers, clonidine, or prazosin may be effective when used alone.

Beta-Blocking Drugs

The role of beta-blockers in the treatment of geriatric hypertension is somewhat controversial. While there is some evidence of a reduced responsiveness to these agents with advancing age,[40] their use is advocated by most authorities.[37,41–44]

In general, plasma half-lives of beta-blockers are prolonged in old age.[45-47] Lipid-soluble agents, such as metoprolol and propranolol, depend heavily on hepatic metabolism for their elimination; hepatic blood flow is diminished 40–50% by age 60.[48] Water-soluble agents, excreted primarily by the kidneys, also have a prolonged half-life related to a decreased renal blood flow. The resultant effect (an increased plasma drug level) appears to be offset by a relative resistance to beta blockade in old age.[40]

Extra caution must be employed in elderly persons because of an increased tendency toward bradycardia, heart block, glucose intolerance, bronchospasm, and congestive heart failure. All of these conditions may be exacerbated by beta blockade. These untoward effects usually will appear early on, if at all.[42-43] An additional concern that is particularly applicable to the elderly population is a tendency for these drugs to influence cortical function, which causes somnolence and depression.[45] On balance, however beta-blockers appear to be relatively safe and effective drugs for elderly persons if used with proper precautions.

Other Adrenergic-Inhibiting Agents

Guanethidine should be avoided because of its tendency to cause orthostatic hypotension. This is less of a problem with methyldopa, prazosin, clonidine, and reserpine.[14,49] However, methyldopa, clonidine, and reserpine, act within the central nervous system; particular attention must be paid to the appearance of somnolence, depression, and nightmares. With prazosin, the clinician must be aware that a small percentage of patients treated will develop tachycardia and hypotension with the administration of the first dose. This effect rarely recurs and can be minimized by administering the first dose at bedtime.

Vasodilators

Hydralazine must be used with caution because of its tendency to exacerbate angina. It does not, however, cause the same degree of tachycardia as it does in younger patients.

Other Drugs

Insufficient experience has been accumulated with minoxidil and captopril use in elderly patients to comment on except to state that their use, at present, should be limited to refractory hypertension.

A suggested approach to pharmacologic management is presented in Table 12-6.

General Concerns

1. Keep the treatment schedule simple. It rarely is necessary to administer drugs more than twice daily.
2. Change doses and drugs infrequently and over weeks to months.
3. Watch carefully for side effects, especially changes in mentation.
4. Watch for drug interactions; most common and/or serious ones are listed below:

diuretics   + cardiac glycosides = hypokalemia + digitalis toxicity

  + anticoagulants = may decrease hypoprothrombinemic effect

  + steroids = hypokalemia
  + salicylates = salicylate toxicity
  + lithium = lithium toxicity
  + insulin = impaired glucose tolerance

beta-blockers   + insulin = impaired glucose tolerance, may mask hypoglycemia

Methyldopa, clonidine, reserpine + tricyclics = attenuated antihypertensive effect
Reserpine, methyldopa, + monoamine oxidase (MAO) inhibitors = attenuated hypotensive effect and/or paradoxical hypertensive crisis.

5. Be aware of special concerns of elderly persons, such as fixed incomes, isolation, dietary problems, impediments in eyesight, hearing, mentation, and dexterity.

TABLE 12-6 A Suggested Approach in Elderly Persons

Step	Drug	Initial Dose	Maximum Dose	Relative Contraindications	Most Common and/or Serious Side Effects
1. (Begin with)	Hydrochlorathiazide	25 mg QD†	100 mg QD	GFR <25 cc/min, orthostatic hypotension, hypokalemia, diabetes, erythrocytosis, gout	Volume depletion, hypokalemia, glucose intolerance, drug interactions (see text), nocturia, incontinence
2. Add one	Propranolol Metoprolol (or other beta-blocker)	40 mg BID 50 mg BID	160 mg BID 200 mg BID	Bradycardia, diabetes, obstructive[1] pulmonary disease, claudication, heart failure	Bradycardia, diabetes, asthma, heart failure, claudication, somnolence, depression, sleep disturbances, sexual disturbances
	Clonidine	0.1 mg HS	0.4 mg BID	Tricyclic drugs, depressed mentation, orthostatic hypotension	Dry mouth, altered mentation, orthostatic
	Methyldopa	250 mg QD	1 g BID	Depressed mentation, orthostatic hypotension, tricyclic and MAO drugs	Altered mentation, sexual disturbances, orthostatic hypotension
	Reserpine	0.1 mg QD	0.2 mg QD	Depressed mentation, depression, orthostatic hypotension, tricyclic and MAO drugs	Depression, depressed mentation, sexual disturbances
	Prazosin	1 mg HS	5 mg BID		Orthostatic hypotension and tachycardia with first-dose, sexual disturbances
3. Add	Hydralazine	25 mg BID	100 mg BID	Angina	Angina, lupus-like syndrome

* Metoprolol may have less of a negative effect on diabetes, claudication, or obstructive pulmonary disease.
† QD = once daily, BID = twice daily, HS = at bedtime, GFR = glomerular filtration rate, MAO = monoamine oxidase.

References

1. Koch-Weser J: Arterial hypertension in old age. *Herz* 3:235–244, 1978.
2. Kannel WB, Gordon T: Evaluation of the cardiovascular risk in the elderly: the Framingham Study. *Bull NY Acad Med* 54:573–591, 1978.
3. Pooling Project Research Group: Relationship of blood pressure, serum cholesterol, smoking habit, relative weight and ECG abnormalities to incidence of major coronary events. Final report of the Pooling Project. *J Chron Dis* 31:201–306, 1978.
4. Dyer AR, Stamler J, Shekelle RB, et al: Hypertension in the elderly. *Med Clin North Am* 61:513–529, 1977.
5. National High Blood Pressure Education Program Coordinating Committee: *Statement on Hypertension in the Elderly*. Bethesda, MD High Blood Pressure Information Center, National Institutes of Health, 1980.
6. Colandrea MA, Friedman GD, Nichaman ME, et al: Systolic hypertension in the elderly—an epidemiologic assessment. *Circulation* 41:239–247, 1970.
7. Stamler J, Berkson D, Lindberg H: Risk factors: their role in the etiology and pathogenesis of atherosclerotic disease, in Wissler R, Geer J (eds): *The Pathogenesis of Atherosclerosis*. Baltimore, Williams & Wilkins Co, 1972, pp 41–119.
8. Shekelle B, Ostfeld A, Klawans H: Hypertension and risk of stroke in an elderly population. *Stroke* 5:71–75, 1974.
9. *Build and Blood Pressure Study 1959*. Chicago, Society of Actuaries, 1959, vol 1.
10. *Blood Pressure of Adults by Race and Area: United States 1960–62*. Rockville, MD, National Center for Health Statistics, 1964, series 11, no 5.
11. Stamler J, Stamler R, Riedlinger W, et al: Hypertension screening of 1 million Americans: Community Hypertension Evaluation Clinics (CHEC) Program, 1973–75. *JAMA* 235:2299–2306, 1976.
12. Hypertension Detection and Follow-up Program Cooperative Group: Five year findings of the Hypertension Detection and Follow-up Program, I. Reduction in mortality of persons with high blood pressure, including mild hypertension. *JAMA* 242:2562–2571, 1979.
13. Koch-Weser J: Correlation of pathophysiology and pharmacotherapy in primary hypertension. *Am J Cardiol* 32:499–551, 1973.
14. Veterans Administration Cooperative Study Group on Antihypertensive Agents: Effects of treatment on morbidity in hypertension. III. Influence of age, diastolic pressure and prior cardiovascular disease; further analysis of side effects. *Circulation* 45:991–1004, 1972.
15. Hypertension Detection and Follow-up Program Cooperative Group: Five year findings of the Hypertension Detection and Follow-up Program, II. Mortality by race, sex, and age. *JAMA* 242:2572–2579, 1979.
16. Hypertension Detection and Follow-up Program Cooperative Group: Five year findings of the Hypertension Detection and Follow-up Program, III. Reduction in stroke incidence among persons with high blood pressure. *JAMA* 247:633–638, 1982.
17. Carter AB: Hypertensive therapy in stroke survivors. *Lancet* 1:485–489, 1970.
18. Hypertension-Stroke Cooperative Study Group: Effects of antihypertensive therapy treatment on stroke recurrence. *JAMA* 229:409–418, 1974.
19. Amery A, Berthaux P, Birkenhager W, et al: Antihypertensive therapy in patients above age 60 years (Fourth Interim Report of the European Working Party on High Blood Pressure in elderly: EWPHE). *Clin Sci Mol Med* 55:2635–2703, 1978.
20. Lakatta E: Alterations in the cardiovascular system that occur in advanced age. *Fed Proc* 38:163–167, 1979.
21. Niarchos AP, Laragh JH: Hypertension in the elderly. *Mod Concepts Cardiovasc Dis* 49:43–48, 1980.
22. Hollenberg NK, Adams DF, Solomon HA, et al: Senescence and the renal vasculature in normal man. *Circ Res* 34:309–316, 1974.
23. Epstein M, Hollenberg NK: Age as a determinant of renal sodium conservation in normal man. *J Lab Clin Med* 87:411–417, 1976.
24. Thomas GW, Ledingham JGG, Ecilin LJ, et al: Reduced plasma renin activity in essential hypertension: Effects of blood pressure, age, and sodium. *Clin Sci Mol Med* 51:185s–188s, 1976.
25. Sever PS, Osikava B, Birch M, et al: Plasma noradrenalin in essential hypertension. *Lancet* 1:1078–1081, 1977.
26. Messerli FH, Glade LB, Dreslinski GR, et al: Hypertension in the elderly: Haemodynamic, fluid volume and endocrine findings. *Clin Sci* 61:393s–394s, 1981.
27. Adamopoulos PN, Chrysanthakopoulis SG, Frohlich ED: Systolic hypertension; Nonhomogeneous disease. *Am J Cardiol* 36:697–701, 1975.
28. Simon AC, Safar MA, Levenson JA, et al: Systolic hypertension: hemodynamic mechanism and choice of antihypertensive treatment. *Am J Cardiol* 44:505–511, 1979.
29. Kannel WB, Wolf PA, McGee DI, et al: Systolic blood pressure, arterial rigidity and risk of

stroke: The Framingham Study. *JAMA* 245:1225–1229, 1981.

30. Bentley DW, Izzo JL: Hypertension in the elderly. *J Am Geriatr Soc* 30:352–359, 1982.

31. Morgan T, Adam W, Gillies A, et al: Hypertension treated by salt restriction. *Lancet* 1:227–230, 1978.

32. Reisen E, Abel R, Modan M, et al: Effect of weight loss without sodium restriction on the reduction of blood pressure. *N Engl J Med* 298:1–5, 1978.

33. DeHaven J, Sherwin R, Hendler R, et al: Nitrogen and sodium balance and sympathetic nervous system activity in obese subjects treated with low-caloric protein or mixed diet. *N Engl J Med* 302:477–482, 1980.

34. The 1980 Report of the Joint National Committee on Detection, Evaluation and Treatment of High Blood Pressure. *Arch Intern Med* 140:1280–1285, 1980.

35. O'Brien DK, Pattee J: Hypertension in older patients—what drugs to use and when. *Geriatrics* 36:111–120, 1981.

36. Amery A, Berthaux P, Birkenhager W, et al: Antihypertensive therapy in patients over age 60. *Acta Cardiologica* 33:113–134, 1978.

37. O'Malley K, O'Brien E: Management of hypertension in the elderly. *N Engl J Med* 302:1397–1401, 1980.

38. Amery A, Berthaux P, Bulpitt C, et al: Glucose intolerance during diuretic therapy. *Lancet* 1:681–683, 1978.

39. Morgan TD, Adams WR, Hodgson M, et al: Failure of therapy to improve prognosis in elderly males with hypertension. *Med J Aust* 2:27–31, 1980.

40. Vestal RE, Wood AJJ, Shand DG: Reduced adrenoreceptor sensitivity in the elderly. *Clin Pharmacol Ther* 26:181–186, 1977.

41. Gavras I, Gavras H: Special considerations in treating hypertension in the elderly. *Geriatrics* 35:34–40, 1980.

42. Cooper J: Blood pressure control in the elderly. *J Royal Coll Geriatr Pract* 26:745–749, 1976.

43. Persson I: Treatment of hypertension in the elderly with pindalol and clopamide. *J Am Geriatr Soc* 26:337–340, 1978.

44. Franciosa JA, Simon G, Eckhoff PA: Hypertensive complications—a common geriatric problem. *Geriatrics* 35:65–73, 1980.

45. Lowenthal DT, Affrine MB: Cardiovascular drugs in the geriatric patient. *Geriatrics* 36:65–74, 1981.

46. Kendall MJ, Brown D, Yates RA: Plasma metoprolol concentrations in young, old and hypertensive subjects. *Brit J Clin Pharmacol* 4:497–499, 1977.

47. Castleden CM, George CF: The effect of aging on the hepatic clearance of propranolol. *Br J Clin Pharmacol* 7:49–54, 1979.

48. Sherlock S, Bearn AG, Billring BH, et al: Splanchnic blood flow in man by the bromosulfalein method: The relation of peripheral plasma bromosulfalein level to the calculated flow. *J Lab Clin Med* 35:923–932, 1970.

49. Ouslander JG: Drug therapy in the elderly. *Ann Intern Med* 95:711–722, 1981.

CHAPTER 13

Peripheral Vascular Disease

MICHAEL SPILANE, M.D.

Arteriosclerosis Obliterans

Arteriosclerosis obliterans is a chronic degenerative disease that affects the large blood vessels of the legs; it has etiologic factors similar to those of arteriosclerotic disease in coronary and cerebral vessels. The disease becomes symptomatic when obstructions lead to tissue ischemia.

This disease is infrequently symptomatic in patients under 45 years of age, and the incidence rate increases with advancing age. Females develop the disease less frequently than males and generally at an older age.[1] Diabetes mellitus, hypertension, and cigarette smoking are significant risk factors.

Symptoms

The principal symptom of arteriosclerosis obliterans is pain. The discomfort is termed "intermittent claudication" and is highly characteristic in its pattern of precipitation by exertion and relief by rest. It is first noticed only with unusually strenuous exertion, but it may progress to a disabling situation wherein pain occurs even with minimal activity. Most patients characterize the discomfort as aching or cramping, but others complain that the limb becomes numb, dead, or lame. Total relief of pain is achieved within minutes after the onset of rest. The patient is then able to resume exertion equivalent to the exertion that initially provoked the symptom. The location of the discomfort depends on the site of the arterial obstruction and the resulting ischemia to major muscle groups. Most commonly, the discomfort is in the calf of the leg. The hip and buttock is next in order of frequency and reflects the disease in the aorto-iliac area. Pain in the foot or thigh is less common.

In younger patients, it is seldom difficult to determine by a history that a patient has intermittent claudication. With older patients, the assessment is complicated more often. Elderly persons may be less precise in describing their symptoms or they have symptoms from a coexisting disease, such as arthritis or neuritis, which masks the exertion-pain and rest-relief characteristics of claudication. Older patients may not even mention the symptom, but attribute it to arthritis or to "growing old." Some elderly persons are spared the symptom, despite the disease, because their activity level is limited by other factors.

In advanced peripheral vascular disease, patients may experience pain at rest. This probably involves an ischemia to the nerves as well as to the muscles. The pain is often severe and resistant to analgesia. With its most common occurrence in the foot or lower calf, the discomfort frequently has a dysesthetic effect. It is worse with recumbency and improves with the legs in a dependent position. Patients may sleep in a sitting position to avoid unbearable pain. Patients with rest pain always have evidence, on physical examination, of a marked peripheral vascular disease.

Arterial insufficiency resulting in tissue breakdown and ulceration causes severe pain. An important exception is in diabetic patients with an anesthesia caused by a coexisting peripheral neuropathy.

Physical Signs

Abnormalities may exist on examination of the peripheral vascular system in asymptomatic patients. This is particularly true in elderly patients where absent pedal pulses and audible femoral bruits are relatively common. The significance of these abnormalities in asymptomatic patients should not be exaggerated. In patients with symptoms of a peripheral vascular disease, abnormalities almost always will be demonstrable via a physical examination (*see* Table 13-1).

An examination of the peripheral vasculature not only enables a physician to confirm the presence of a disease, but also allows a reasonable assessment of both the sites of vascular obstruction and the overall severity of the ischemic process.

A palpation of pulses, in conjunction with auscultation for bruits, is the most important means of establishing the presence of a disease and of localizing the sites of obstruction. It is important to examine a patient before and after exercise. Abnormalities will be accentuated and, occasionally, will be apparent only after exercise. Femoral pulsations normally increase in strength after exertion; a failure of this response is an important observation. Existent pedal pulses may diminish or disappear after exertion; normally, they are more readily palpable.[2] The "dropped pulse" phenomenon is explained by a limited blood flow that supplies a postexertional vascular bed of low resistance. It

should be remembered that the resiliency of blood vessels in older patients is decreased, and pedal pulses may be difficult to palpate even though the blood flow is not significantly diminished.

Bruits exist when a narrowing of blood vessels causes a turbulence in blood flow. The sound of a bruit radiates in the direction of the blood flow to the extent that a bruit produced by an aorto-iliac obstruction will be heard over the femoral artery as well as in the hypogastric area. Although bruits are most commonly heard during systole, a diastolic component exists when a substantial pressure gradient continues to exist, even in diastole. A diastolic bruit indicates a marked obstruction or poor collateral filling of the obstructed vessel. The diastolic component may be detected only in the postexertional state.

An ischemic extremity often undergoes color changes. The distal extremity may be pale and bloodless, but more often it exhibits a red or blue tone that results from blood in the superficial capillaries, which have dilated in response to the ischemia. The extremity feels cool and is dry, which is unlike the observations associated with similar color changes in patients with a benign vasomotor instability. Hair loss is common, and nails may be dystrophic. In an advanced disease, muscle atrophy and tissue ulceration may exist.

Certain maneuvers are used to estimate the overall severity of the circulatory inadequacy. A triad of observations that consist of the de-

TABLE 13-1 Recording Physical Findings*

	Hypo-gastric	Femoral	Popliteal	Posterior Tibial	Anterior Tibial	Pallor	Venous Filling	Color Return
L	+ / +	2 / + / ++	0 / 1 /	0 / 0 /	0 / 0 /	Moderate	30 sec	25 sec
R	+ / +	3 / + / ++	2 / 2 /	2 / 0 /	2 / 0 /	Slight	15 sec	10 sec

* A suggested format to display results of the peripheral arterial vascular examination.
Rest/Exercise Pulse 1–4 (4 = normal)
   +   systolic bruit
   ++ systolic-diastolic bruit

gree of pallor with leg elevation, the venous filling time, and the time until return of color with dependency, can be simply made. The extent of these physical abnormalities correlates with the degree of ischemia to the distal extremity. The extremities of a supine patient are elevated by the examiner and the degree of pallor is noted after 60 seconds. The patient then quickly sits up and dangles his or her legs while the examiner documents both the time necessary for blood to fill the veins of the feet and the time taken until full color returns to the feet. Normally, venous filling and return of color are completed within a few seconds; times in excess of 60 seconds are seen in a severe ischemic disease.

Ulceration

When ulceration exists on the extremity of any patient, it is essential to determine the correct etiology. Arterial insufficiency is but one of several common causes of ulcerations: in addition, ischemia may promote ulceration, even if it is not the primary cause. The prognosis is considerably better if factors other than arterial insufficiency are causative. Table 13-2 lists both the common causes of lower extremity ulceration and the differential characteristics. In elderly persons, it is not uncommon that two or more causes are operative in the development of an ulceration. Foot deformities, decreased sensation, and arterial insufficiency are a common grouping. If ischemia plays a major role in the etiology of an ulcer, a physical examination will reveal marked abnormalities in the peripheral circulation. To the degree that such findings are absent, other causes likely exist. In a diabetic person with a peripheral neuropathy, pressure-induced ulceration is commonly seen, particularly in association with corns and callouses. The treatment and prognosis for such ulcerations are considerably different than for ischemic ulcerations.

Differential Diagnosis

If an adequate history is possible, and if a thorough examination is performed, it is relatively easy to determine whether the symptoms are related to a peripheral vascular disease. Arthritic symptoms may be induced by exertion, but the pain is not relieved after a brief rest. Benign, nocturnal leg cramps are not associated with abnormalities of the vascular system on examination, and their absence during the day is quite unlike the rest pain of an ischemia. Although they are common in elderly persons and sometimes coexist with arterial insufficiency, conditions such as a peripheral neuropathy, venous insufficiency, and sciatica seldom pose a diagnostic difficulty.

The cauda equina syndrome (spinal claudication or neurogenic claudication) is a relatively uncommon condition that occurs in elderly persons, and it is thought, with uncertainty, to be

TABLE 13-2 Differential Diagnosis of Ulceration of the Lower Extremity*

Disease	Location	Description	Pain	Prognosis
Venous insufficiency	Lower third of calf, ankle	Large, shallow, weeping, marginated, beefy red base. Odorous if secondary infection is present	Usually tolerable, often mild	Good
Arterial insufficiency	Acral points Toes, malleoli, heel	Deep, dry, necrotic escar	Severe unless peripheral neuropathy coexists	Poor
Peripheral neuropathy	Pressure points Often associated with corns, callouses, bunions, foot-toe deformities	Associated infection: Deep, draining, may exist under a callous	Minimal	Good if osteomyelitis is not present

* Differential characteristics of the most common etiologies of lower extremity ulceration in elderly patients.

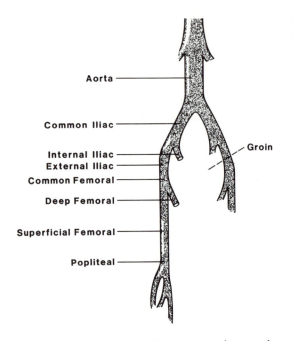

FIGURE 13-1 Anatomy of major arteries to the lower extremity.

caused by an ischemia of the spinal cord that is secondary to osteophytic deformities of the vertebral column. Symptoms are unlikely to be confused with a classic intermittent claudication. Patients with the cauda equina syndrome experience exertionally related symptoms that are described as a general lameness, instability, or weakness of the legs. There may be associated back pains with a radiation to the legs that is typically present at rest as well as with exertion. Unlike intermittent claudication, symptoms are not relieved by stopping and standing; the patient must sit down or lie down to achieve relief; usually, more than a few minutes are required before activity can be resumed without symptoms. Symptoms are often precipitated by standing without movement. An examination after exertion reveals generalized muscle weakness or, less often, specific neurologic abnormalities. The peripheral vascular examination may be normal.

Collateral Circulation

As an obstruction slowly develops in the large arteries of the lower extremities, the collateral circulation also develops to shunt blood to the postobstructed vessel. Were it not for the collateral vessels shunting blood around obstruc-

tions, many patients who experience only claudication would, instead, suffer a limb-threatening ischemia. Multiple vessels exist as potential collateral channels for obstructions in the aorto-iliac area. These collateral channels supply a sufficient blood flow to the distal extremity to prevent a severe ischemia, even in the presence of a marked aorto-iliac obstruction. Further down the vascular tree, the next significant, potential collateral channels are tributaries of the deep femoral artery. They shunt blood around obstructions in the superficial femoral and popliteal vessels. Although the deep femoral artery may be partially obstructed at its origin, it seldom is diseased beyond this point; thus, it is often able to assist its obstructed neighbor. Below the popliteal artery, opportunity for development of collateral circulation is poor. The more distal the obstruction the less likely that collateral channels will exist that can bring blood to a patent downstream vessel. Where major obstructions exist at several levels, collateral channels prove insufficient.

Combining the knowledge of collateral circulation with the results of physical examinations allows a reasonably accurate assessment of the location of obstructions. If an examination reveals disease of the aorto-iliac vessels, the nutritional status of the feet is good, and venous filling is prompt, it is likely that the significant disease is limited to the aorto-iliac vessels. If an additional major obstruction existed distally, two sites of collateral circulation would be needed to bring blood to the feet and more overt physical findings would exist. If serious findings do exist, such as ulceration or a markedly prolonged venous filling time, then it is likely that an obstruction exists in more distal vessels as well as in the aorto-iliac area. If evidence of severe ischemia to the feet exists, it is almost a certainty that the disease is widespread.

Patterns of Obstructive Disease

Although attempts have been made to classify arterial obstructions according to their location and number, variations among individual patients are so common that the classifications are more useful for research than for clinical purposes. Certain general patterns of obstructive disease are as follows:

Obstructions most often exist in multiple areas. Isolated major obstructions may exist.

Isolated aorto-iliac obstructions occur most often in non-diabetic males 50–65 years of age. Hypertension and cigarette smoking often coexist.

Serious disease below the popliteal artery is most common in diabetic patients.

The most common sites of obstruction in non-diabetic patients are: aorto-iliac vessels, origin of common femoral artery, common femoral artery, and distal popliteal artery.

In patients over 70 years of age, the disease is seldom segmental and isolated.

Diabetic patients are prone to develop disease at multiple sites and in more distal vessels.

Diabetic patients may develop a small-vessel angiopathy in association with arteriosclerosis obliterans.

Special Diagnostic Procedures

Non-invasive, vascular laboratory procedures are available to assist in an accurate diagnosis.[3,4] Ultrasound and plethysmographic techniques are most often used. These testing modalities can add precision in an assessment of the severity of disease and in its location; but, seldom are these modalities necessary to make the initial diagnosis. The results of the procedures infrequently lead to a significant alteration of basic decisions with regard to treatment.

Angiography is an effective means of defining the vascular anatomy and of localizing obstructive lesions. It is of great assistance to vascular surgeons in planning appropriate surgical procedures. An arteriogram has a significant morbidity risk in patients with diabetes mellitus and renal diseases. It is unreasonable to do an angiographic procedure unless it will influence therapeutic decision making; it is not needed to make a diagnosis of a peripheral vascular disease.

Prognosis

Patients with intermittent claudication have a significantly shortened life expectancy; for the most part, this is attributable to an associated atherosclerosis of the coronary and cerebral vessels.[1,5] If a patient with claudication is non-diabetic, the risk of extremity amputation is only 5% over 5 years of follow-up.[5,6] Diabetic patients have a markedly increased risk of subsequent amputation. When followed over time, a majority of all patients are found to have stable or even improved claudication symptoms.[1,7] Even with a stability of symptoms, the underlying disease, when assessed by objective means, does appear to progress.[8]

Medical Therapy

No medications have been shown to be effective in treating the symptoms of arteriosclerosis obliterans.[9] Given the potential side effects of medications such as vasodilators, it is wise to avoid their use. Certain medications, such as beta-adrenergic blocking agents and ergotamines, may precipitate or aggravate symptoms.

Medical treatment should be directed at improving cardiac output, controlling hypertension, and regulating blood sugar in patients with diabetes mellitus. Every effort should be made to convince a patient to discontinue smoking.

Patient education is vital and may need to be frequently reinforced. Elderly persons in particular are prone to precipitate a disaster by actions that should be avoided. Patients should not trim their own toenails; relatives should be taught how to do this. Corns and callouses should be treated only by professionals. The feet should be soaked daily for 15 minutes and dried thoroughly. Shoes should be loose and examined for obstructing objects before being worn. Patients should not walk barefoot, either indoors or outdoors. Cotton socks should be changed daily. Heating pads should not be placed on the lower legs, and water should always be pretested for heat with the hand. Salves and creams should be used only after the approval of a physician. Medical help should be sought for any rashes or dermatologic conditions that affect the extremities.

On the physician's part, care should be directed to searching for potential problems. Dermatophytosis should be treated. Nail care should be provided and corns and callouses carefully trimmed and treated. Shoes should be inspected.

It is a too frequent occurrence that a limb-threatening foot ulceration develops from an avoidable cause.[10] The importance of patient education and preventive measures justifies relatively frequent physician visits for a patient with an ischemic extremity.

Surgical Treatment

Surgical procedures can be effectively used to relieve the pain of an intermittent claudication and to prolong the viability of a severely ischemic extremity. Most often, a diseased vessel is bypassed via the use of either a synthetic tube or an autologous vein. Vessels also may be rechanneled by an endarterectomy. The procedure chosen depends on the anatomy and physiology of the diseased vessels and on the ability of the patient to tolerate this surgery. The basic surgical goal is to begin a reconstruction at a site where input pressure is high, and to end it at a site where outflow vessels are unobstructed. Procedures on the aorto-iliac vessels entail abdominal and retroperitoneal approaches with their attendant risks, but long-term results are excellent.[11–13] Bypass grafts from one femoral artery to the other femoral artery, or from a femoral artery to a more distant artery, are performed with a lower surgical mortality rate.[14–16] Using a subcutaneous track to the leg, distant vessels (such as the axillary artery) can be used as the input source.[17] Such approaches are chosen in patients in whom abdominal surgery entails a high risk and where more accessible vessels are diseased. The longer the graft and the smaller the vessel at the distal reconstruction site, the less likely the graft will subsequently remain patent.[18]

Percutaneous balloon-catheter dilatation and reconstruction of an obstructed artery can be used as an isolated procedure or in combination with bypass grafting.[19] The best results are obtained when the lesion is short, in a large vessel, not highly calcified, and only partially obstructing.

Decision Logic

The major decisions required in the treatment of arteriosclerosis obliterans relate to surgical intervention. The estimate of risk versus benefit for an individual patient often is difficult. For an elderly person with claudication as the only symptom, the surgical risk is best considered to be greater than the benefit. Most elderly patients with claudication adapt well to the symp-

tom and suffer an acceptable decrease in the quality of life. If these patients are non-diabetic, they also can be reassured that the danger of losing an extremity because of the progression of the disease is quite small.

Claudication that severely restricts activity may justify a surgical procedure if the patient otherwise would be much more active. Even in this circumstance, advancing age and the known existence of cerebral or coronary atherosclerosis should weigh against a decision for surgical intervention.

For patients with pain at rest or distal ulcerations, surgical intervention is more compelling. Unfortunately, these patients often have advanced and diffuse arterial disease in the lower extremities, and surgical restoration of adequate circulation is not easily achieved. If a patient's general health status allows, it is still reasonable to attempt to improve blood flow via a surgical procedure. Long-term limb salvage can be expected in a majority of all patients and the surgical mortality rate is generally less than 5%.

In certain instances, it is most wise to proceed directly with amputation. This includes the presence of an extensive ulceration and a previous failure of surgical approaches. If amputation is chosen, rehabilitation considerations become important from the time the amputation level is determined.[20]

The ideal surgical candidate is the rare patient without any known cerebrovascular or coronary artery disease who has a localized proximal obstruction with patent distal vessels. This patient may have weak or absent distal pulsations, but he or she will have good nutrition in the feet and a prompt venous filling time. The surgical risk is low, and the surgeon can realize the goals of placing a short graft that begins at the high input pressure and ends at non-diseased vessels. However, this patient should have claudication as the only symptom; if an adaptation to the symptom is possible without a serious impact on the quality of life, then even a low risk may not justify intervention.

In elderly patients, surgical procedures most often will be performed for limb salvage or for intractable rest pain. These patients will have absent pulses, trophic changes of the feet, and prolonged venous filling time. Coexisting cerebral and coronary vascular disease will be the rule. Surgical compromise will be necessary and the surgical risk will be significant.

Acute Obstruction

Vessels leading to the lower extremities may suddenly occlude as the result of an embolus or thrombosis. If the occluded vessel is of a substantial size, a serious limb ischemia will exist since collateral circulation has not had time to develop. Symptoms may be erroneously attributed to conditions such as phlebitis, muscle strain, or neuritis. In most instances, an acute occlusion occurs in the presence of previous arteriosclerosis obliterans; well-documented results of a previous vascular examination greatly facilitate an appreciation of new findings. In frail elderly persons, an acute vascular obstruction may be better managed conservatively with the use of anticoagulants in a hospital setting. If major tissue death is imminent, surgical intervention is necessary. In all cases of acute arterial obstruction, surgical consultation is indicated.

Venous Insufficiency and Edema

Edema of the lower extremities is a commonly encountered problem in elderly patients. The cause is often multifactorial.[21] Previous phlebitis and an occlusive venous disease may lead to chronic and severe venous stasis and leg swelling. Incompetent venous valves are more common in elderly persons and result in edema via the transmission of gravitational forces to peripheral venules. Inactivity and a lack of muscle tone interferes with the important role of muscle contraction in pumping venous blood toward the heart. Congestive heart failure and other fluid retention states can independently cause edema or can aggravate existent venous stasis.

In most cases, edema is mild and a result of venous insufficiency; patients note an increased swelling as the day progresses and a resolution following night-time recumbency. Salt restriction, leg elevation during the day, and elastic stockings usually are sufficient treatments. Diuretic drugs should be used only when these treatments fail or when sodium-retaining diseases exist. If diuretics are highly successful in clearing edema, congestive heart failure may also be present. Edema that is secondary to local venous disease responds less well to diuretic therapy.

When edema is severe, preventive care is necessary to avoid skin ulcerations. Edema fluid impairs the metabolic processes of the skin and causes it to become atrophic and susceptible to breakdown. A minor trauma can lead to ulceration. Patients should wear garments that cover the lower legs and ankles to avoid skin penetration from contact with sharp objects or from insect bites. Daily application of moistening cream is helpful. Medicated lotions should be used only with a doctor's advice. Heating pads should never be applied to edematous skin.

Skin ulceration is a common complication of severe edemas, particularly when it is caused by venous insufficiency. The ulcers are characteristic and should not be confused with ulcers that are secondary to arterial ischemia (see Table 13-2). They occur on the lower aspect of the tibial region or near the ankle. Though pain exists, it is most often non-severe; the absence of serious pain may cause a delay in a patient who is seeking medical attention. On presentation, venous ulcers may be large and often are secondarily infected. The presence of weeping serous fluid and beefy red granulation tissue at the base of the ulcer are characteristics that differentiate venous ulcers from those caused by arterial insufficiency.

With appropriate treatment, the prognosis of venous ulcerations is relatively good. Even patients with an extensive ulceration are unlikely to require leg amputation. Advanced ulcerations can be controlled and sometimes healed, but their recurrence is frequent. Attention is best directed at treating edematous extremities to avoid ulcerations. When tissue breakdown is imminent, the patient should be advised to remain recumbent to control swelling and to allow the skin an opportunity to strengthen. If an ulceration is already present, intense care is needed. The ulcers should be debrided of superficial material and antibiotics should be administered if an inflammation of the surrounding tissue exists. Wet to dry dressings should be administered three times daily. Salves and creams are best avoided. The patient should be instructed on the need for strict bed rest. Occlusive, medicated dressings such as an Unna paste boot frequently are helpful in elderly persons. They help to control the edema and eliminate the need for soaks and dressing changes by the patient. Although a weekly re-application of the paste dressing is best done by nursing personnel, the patient himself or a family member may be capable of the task. Even large ulcerations can be treated on an outpatient basis, if a patient is compliant with overall treatment recommendations. When compliance cannot be assured, home nursing visits and support from family members may prevent hospitalization or short-term admission to a nursing home. Surgical approaches may be helpful in the treatment of refractory, venous stasis edema and venous ulcerations.[22]

References

1. Peabody CN, Kannel WB, McNamara PM: Intermittent claudication. *Arch Surg* 109:693–697, 1974.
2. DeWeese JA: Pedal pulses disappearing with exercise. *N Engl J Med* 262:1214–1217, 1960.
3. Bernstein EF, Fronek A: Current status of noninvasive tests in the diagnosis of peripheral arterial disease. *Surg Clin North Am* 62:473–487, 1982.
4. Strandness DE: The use and abuse of the vascular laboratory. *Surg Clin North Am* 59:707–717, 1979.
5. Juergens JL, Barker NW, Hines EA: Arteriosclerosis obliterans: review of 520 cases with special reference to pathogenic and prognostic factors. *Circulation* 21:188–195, 1960.
6. Schadt DC, Hines EA, Juergens JL, et al: Chronic atherosclerotic occlusion of the femoral artery. *JAMA* 175:937–940, 1961.
7. Imparato AM, Kim G, Davidson T, et al: Intermittent claudication: its natural course. *Surgery* 78:795–799, 1975.
8. Warren R, Gomez RL, Marston JAP, et al: Femoropopliteal arteriosclerosis obliterans—arteriographic patterns and rates of progression. *Surgery* 55:135–143, 1964.
9. Coffman JD: Vasodilator drugs in peripheral vascular disease. *N Engl J Med* 300:713–717, 1979.
10. Weis AJ, Fairbairn JF: Trauma, ischemic limbs and amputation. *Postgrad Med* 43:111–115, 1968.
11. Gomes MR, Bernatz PE, Juergens JL: Aortoiliac surgery. *Arch Surg* 95:387–394, 1967.
12. Darling RC, Brewster DC, Hallett JW, et al: Aorto-iliac reconstruction. *Surg Clin North Am* 59:565–578, 1979.
13. Jones AF, Kempczinski RF: Aortofemoral bypass grafting. *Arch Surg* 116:301–305, 1981.
14. Dick L, Brief DK, Alpert J, et al: A 12-year experience with femorofemoral crossover grafts. *Arch Surg* 115:1359–1365, 1980.
15. Maini BS, Mannick JA: Effect of arterial reconstruction on limb salvage. *Arch Surg* 113:1297–1304, 1978.
16. Mannick JA: Femoro-popliteal and femoro-tibial reconstructions. *Surg Clin North Am* 59:581–596, 1979.
17. Holcroft JW, Conti S, Blaisdell FW: Extraanatomic bypass grafts. *Surg Clin North Am* 59:649–658, 1979.
18. Callow AD: Current status of vascular grafts. *Surg Clin North Am* 62:501–513, 1982.
19. Roberts B, Ring EJ: Current status of percutaneous transluminal angioplasty. *Surg Clinic North Am* 62:357–372, 1982.
20. Thompson RG, Keagy RD, Compere CL, et al: Amputation and rehabilitation for severe foot ischemia. *Surg Clin North Am* 54:137–154, 1974.
21. Dale WA: The swollen leg. *Curr Probl Surg* 1–66, 1973.
22. Linton RR: The postthrombotic ulceration of the lower extremity: its etiology and surgical treatment. *Ann Surg* 138:415–433, 1953.

CHAPTER 14

Gastroenterology

FREDERIC W. SMITH, M.D.

Although an older patient has a greater incidence of some gastrointestinal disorders, such as carcinoma of the esophagus, stomach, and colon, age itself does not shorten the list of disorders that produce dysphagia, abdominal pain, gastrointestinal bleeding, or weight loss. Age, however, frequently does make the process of diagnosis and treatment more difficult or hazardous. An older patient's symptoms may be superimposed on a background of chronic complaints from which the physician must select what is new and significant. Communication problems in an older patient due to hearing loss, stroke, dementia, a reluctance to complain, or an inability to bring attention to new complaints, may result in a delay of days to months in obtaining necessary medical attention. In addition, with increasing age, the decreased tolerance to infection, shock, polypharmacy, and the stress of surgery, magnifies errors and delays in diagnosis and treatment.

Diagnostic Investigations

The examination of an older patient should include specific questions about difficulty in swallowing, food sticking or causing pain, loss of appetite, epigastric pain, change in bowel habits, and the presence of blood in the stool. If answers cannot be obtained from patient, they frequently can be obtained from family members or nursing personnel. The patient's weight should be recorded, he or she should have a hematocrit or hemoglobin determination, and a stool specimen should be tested for occult blood. Iron deficiency anemia in an older person always should be considered secondary to gastrointestinal blood loss until proven otherwise.

Diagnostic tests should be selected to provide the best diagnostic information at the least cost, risk, and discomfort to the patient. Thus, a barium enema, sigmoidoscopy, and fiberoptic endoscopy are initial useful procedures for evaluating such complaints as dysphagia, epigastric pain, a change in bowel habits, or blood in the stool; they are well tolerated by most patients.[1] Abdominal ultrasound and computerized tomography (CT scan) allow the visualization of the gallbladder, the larger intra- and extrahepatic bile ducts, cysts and space-occupying lesions of the liver, and tumors and pseudocysts of the pancreas.[2,3] Although CT scans may, on occasion, show lesions that are not apparent on abdominal ultrasound examinations, their findings generally overlap. Ultrasound usually is the initial procedure of choice because of its availability, ease of accomplishment, and lower cost. It is preferable to the oral cholecystogram as an initial procedure for the demonstration of gallstones.

Other procedures may be needed when initial studies are unrevealing or non-diagnostic. Esophageal manometry and cineradiography of the act of swallowing may be helpful in evaluating dysphagia. The biliary ductal system can be outlined by the percutaneous, transhepatic injection of the ducts with a contrast agent using a thin, flexible needle (the "skinny needle" technique); both the biliary and pancreatic ducts may be visualized by injecting a contrast agent through the papilla of Vater using an endoscopically guided catheter (ERCP).[4,5] Angiography, particularly superselective angiography in which small peripheral arteries are injected, can define obscure bleeding points such as colonic telangiectasias and provide useful information about pancreatic carcinomas, islet cell tumors of the pancreas, or primary or metastatic cancers of the liver.[6] These latter three procedures are invasive, relatively uncomfortable or painful, and have hemorrhage, infection, or (in the case of angiography) arterial occlusion as significant risks.

Biopsy specimens are easily obtained with the standard endoscopes. Areas of the small bowel that are inaccessible to a fiberscope may be biopsied by using special capsules and tubes such as the Crosby capsule and the Rubin tube, which permit the tissue diagnosis of such conditions as sprue, Whipple's disease, or small bowel lymphoma.[7] In addition to a standard liver biopsy, which usually takes a random sampling of tissue from a right intercostal approach, biopsy specimens from small intrahepatic masses may be safely obtained with thin, cutting needles and ultrasonic guidance.[8] A similar technique can be used for percutaneous biopsies of pancreatic masses.[9]

Peritoneoscopy allows the visualization of portions of the anterior parietal peritoneum, omentum, and much of the surface of the liver and gallbladder. It occasionally obviates the need for surgical exploration in a poor-risk patient by demonstrating a metastatic tumor or by allowing the directed biopsy of small nodules on the peritoneum or the surface of the liver.[10]

Liver scans, using such radioisotopes as ^{99m}Technetium, are non-invasive and can demonstrate filling defects within the liver that are not diagnostic, but which may represent primary or metastatic carcinomas, cysts, abscesses, regenerating nodules, or areas of infarction.[11] The scan may aid in directing a needle biopsy. Technetium-99m iminodiacetic acid (^{99m}Tc-HIDA), a recently developed radiopharmaceutical, is rapidly cleared through the hepatobiliary system, allows the imaging of the gallbladder and biliary tree, and can be useful in the differential diagnosis of jaundice.[12]

The number of available tests and studies is impressive. Because of considerations of risk, discomfort, and cost, the potential information to be derived from a study must be relevant to clinical management.

Fiberscopes, in addition to their use in diagnosis, have an important role in treatment. Endoscopic polypectomy is now a common procedure for the safe removal of polyps throughout the colon and stomach.[13] They are frequently used in removing foreign bodies from the esophagus and stomach, and can assist in dilating tight esophageal strictures. In patients with an unresectable esophageal carcinoma, fiberscopes are used to pass a plastic tube through the tumor area to maintain a lumen and provide palliation of obstructive symptoms.[14] In selected patients, endoscopic papillotomy, with cutting of the sphincter of Oddi, allows the removal of obstructing common duct stones.[15] Electrocautery and lasar photocoagulation, under endoscopic guidance, are of occasional use in controlling hemorrhage from telangiectasias, ulcers or other discrete lesions of the gastrointestinal tract.

The Esophagus

Carcinoma

Progressively severe difficulty in swallowing solid foods over a period of weeks to months associated with marked weight loss are common symptoms of esophageal carcinoma. Although diagnosis is frequently made via a barium swallow, fiberoptic endoscopy with biopsy will usually confirm the diagnosis.

Because of poor survival rates with any modality of treatment and the morbidity and mortality that are associated with surgical resection, radiation therapy frequently is the treatment of choice for an older patient. It may give weeks to months of palliation, with relief of obstructive symptoms.[17,18] Other forms of palliation include the passing of metal dilators of the Sippy type through the area of obstruction, or the placing of a funnel-shaped plastic tube of the Celestine type, either surgically or endoscopically, through the tumor area.[19,14]

Hiatal Hernia with Reflux

Reflux symptoms frequently are described as "heartburn." This consists of an intermittent, burning retrosternal pain, which is characteristically present for months to years. The patient usually will obtain significant relief with antacids, and his symptoms are worse in the recumbent position. Reflux is commonly associated with a sliding hiatus hernia and the symptoms are made worse by ingesting fruit juices, alcohol, and aspirin-containing compounds. An upper gastrointestinal series will usually demonstrate the sliding hiatus hernia and the associated reflux. Endoscopy should be reserved for patients with atypical or unusually severe symptoms that are non-responsive to therapy.

In most instances, an antireflux regimen will provide symptomatic relief.[20] This consists of frequent antacids, a 6–8-inch elevation of the patient's bed, avoidance of known irritants, and taking only antacids during the 2 hours before bedtime. Some patients feel better by substituting suspenders for belts and avoiding girdles or abdominal binders. Tobacco, fats, and chocolate should be avoided because they weaken the lower esophageal sphincter. In addition to antacids, cimetidine (Tagamet), has been useful as has metoclopramide (Reglan) [21,22] (see the subsequent discussion in this chapter and in Volume I, Chapter 38 on the use of cimetidine in the elderly). Surgical procedures for decreasing gastroesophageal reflux should be reserved for patients with intractable symptoms and associated severe, distal esophagitis.

Benign Esophageal Stricture

A benign esophageal stricture is most often associated with reflux esophagitis and develops over a period of months to years.[23] Superimposed on symptoms of reflux esophagitis is a slowly progressive dysphagia for solid foods. X-ray film examination usually will demonstrate a smoothly tapered narrowing of the distal esophagus, which is adjacent to a sliding hiatus hernia. Although the x-ray film is characteristic, an endoscopic examination with biopsy should be done to rule out carcinoma. Particularly in older patients, strictures can be managed satisfactorily with esophageal dilatation using dilators that range from metal Sippy olives to mercury-filled rubber bougies.[24] Dilatation can be repeated at intervals of weeks to months, as necessary, to maintain a satisfactory diameter, and patients should follow an antireflux program. Surgical treatment rarely is necessary and should be reserved for strictures that cannot be successfully dilated.

Lower Esophageal Ring

A lower esophageal ring (Schatzki ring) is a thin, shelf-like fibromuscular ring that is circumferentially located around the lower esophagus in the region of the gastroesophageal junction. These rings are thought to be an acquired structural abnormality and may cause obstructive symptoms.[25] Typically, patients with a ring have episodic bouts of obstruction, which are usually associated with swallowing large pieces of food. The rings can be demonstrated by a barium swallow and usually are adjacent to a sliding hiatus hernia. Symptomatic rings can be managed by stretching or splitting them with bougies similar to those used in the management of esophageal strictures.

Foreign Bodies

Sudden esophageal obstruction due to swallowing food or small foreign bodies, such as tablets or capsules, always should suggest the presence of carcinoma or stricture. Some foreign bodies, however, because of their size or shape, may obstruct a normal esophagus. In any patient with a history that suggests obstruction due to a foreign body, no attempt should be made to dislodge the object by blindly passing a nasogastric or other tube. A barium swallow is the initial procedure of choice; if an obstructing object is identified, an attempt for more specific identification and removal can be made with a fiberoptic endoscopy.[26] Under direct vision, the foreign body frequently can be removed with a forceps or a wire loop or broken up into pieces that can be passed. In some patients, an examination with a large, rigid esophagoscope under general anesthesia may be required for removal.

In a patient with persistent retrosternal pain that is associated with the foreign body, or which appears following removal, the possibility of perforation should be considered. A chest x-ray film should be examined for mediastinal air and the patient should be followed closely for signs of sepsis. Esophageal perforation, regardless of age, is a surgical emergency that in most instances requires prompt exploration.

Zenker's Diverticulum

An occasional cause of esophageal obstruction, which increases in frequency with age, is a Zenker's diverticulum. This is a diverticular outpouching of the esophagus that opens immediately above the superior esophageal sphincter and extends down into the superior mediastinum. With enlargement of the sack and filling with ingested food and secretions, pressure on the esophagus may produce symptoms of intermittent obstruction. In addition, the patient will commonly complain of regurgitating food into his or her mouth or onto a pillow. The treatment of a symptomatic diverticulum is surgical removal or cricopharyngeal myotomy.[27]

Motor Disorders of the Esophagus

Motor disorders are suggested by difficulty in initiating swallowing, intermittent sensations of food arresting in the esophagus or passing slowly, and, occasionally by recurrent bouts of severe retrosternal pain that is associated with swallowing.[28] Obstructive symptoms, however, progress slowly or not at all, and food usually will pass by itself or with the assistance of a swallow of water. X-ray film and endoscopic examination show no evidence of an organic lesion.

Disorders of the cricopharyngeal muscle are a common cause of dysphagia in older patients, with the muscle failing to relax in a coordinated sequence with the act of swallowing.[29] Food, particularly liquids, appears to obstruct high in the throat at the level of the larynx; patients may have a continuing problem with aspiration and repeated episodes of pneumonia. They may need supervised or assisted feedings, should eat in the sitting position, and should have food prepared in the consistency that gives them the least difficulty. Some patients may require prolonged periods of feeding through a nasogastric tube. Etiologies are diverse and include cerebrovascular accidents and insufficiencies, muscle hypertrophy and spasm, myasthenia gravis, myotonic dystrophy, and scleroderma. Diagnosis depends on the clinical picture and cineradiography of the act of swallowing. Cricopharyngeal myotomy gives the most predictable relief.

Achalasia, or cardiospasm, refers to an esophageal motor disorder in which there is increased pressure in the lower esophageal sphincter, a failure of the sphincter to relax normally, and a loss of coordinated peristalsis in the esophageal smooth muscle.[30] These defects produce a dysphagia for both solid and liquid food. Over a period of time the esophagus will show a generalized dilatation and a characteristic, smoothly tapered narrowing at its distal extremity. Because of retained food in the esophagus, regurgitation is common at night, and aspiration may be associated with recurrent bouts of pneumonia. The dysphasia usually is slowly progressive and without symptoms that suggest esophageal reflux. Although the x-ray film may be characteristic, confirmation of the diagnosis should be made via esophageal manometry.

Some relief of symptoms can be obtained with periodic dilatations using a large bougie. More permanent, non-surgical relief may be obtained with a bag dilatation of the lower esophageal sphincter. This is accomplished by positioning a special balloon in the area of the sphincter, and inflating it either pneumatically or hydraulically in an effort to rupture muscle bundles. Although there is a small risk of esophageal perforation, the procedure provides symptomatic relief for a period of years. The alternative therapy is surgery, the Heller procedure, in which the sphincter is weakened by longitudinal surgical incisions.[31]

Diffuse esophageal spasm is a disorder of motility in which the patient experiences recurrent bouts of pressing, retrosternal pain, which at times may be severe.[3] In some patients, the swallowing of hot or cold liquids will initiate episodes of pain, but such episodes may appear in an unpredictable fashion that is not necessarily associated with swallowing. A barium swallow may demonstrate uncoordinated contraction waves (so-called corkscrew contractions) over the distal two thirds of the esophagus; manometric studies during an episode of pain show simultaneous contractions in the distal esophagus with a marked increase in intraluminal pressure. The treatment of diffuse esophageal spasm is frequently unsatisfactory; however, in some patients, nitroglycerin, calcium channel blockers such as nifedipine, or periodic dilatation with bougies has given relief.

Stomach

Gastric Carcinoma[33]

Gastric carcinoma has a diverse symptomatology. Patients may present with epigastric pain that initially resembles the pain of a typical peptic ulcer; that is, a periodic and recurrent pain relieved to some extent with food and antacids. Over a period of time, however, the pain becomes persistent, without significant relief from food or antacids, and with a gradually increasing loss of appetite. Guaiac-positive stools are common, as is hypoalbuminemia. Physical examination may demonstrate a palpable epigastric mass. An upper gastrointestinal series may show finding that range from a small benign-appearing ulcer to an obvious intragastric mass. Because there is no reliable x-ray film technique for differentiating benign from malignant ulcers, all such lesions should be examined endoscopically, with multiple biopsy specimens taken from the ulcer margin and brush cytology of the ulcer base. The treatment of gastric carcinoma is surgical, with either subtotal or total gastrectomy. Approximately 10% of all patients with gastric cancer can be expected to survive for 5 years.

Benign Gastric Ulcers

Typically, gastric ulcers present with recurrent epigastric pain that is variably relieved with food and antacids. Although x-ray film examination of the stomach usually will demonstrate ulcer, endoscopy with biopsy should be carried out to insure its benign nature. Although most patients with benign gastric ulcers will have normal or low gastric acidity, treatment with a standard antacid on an hourly basis usually is

effective, with healing taking place in most instances over a period of 6–12 weeks.[34] In addition to antacids, attention should be paid to the patient's general nutrition, and aspirin and aspirin-containing compounds should be avoided. Cimetidine (Tagamet), appears to be equally as effective as antacids.[35]

Because of the reliability of endoscopic biopsy and cytology, surgical treatment of the ordinary gastric ulcer can no longer be advocated on the basis of the risk of a malignancy. Although most ulcers will heal over a 6–12-week period, a small percentage (particularly in older patients) may require additional time for healing. Delayed healing by itself is not an indication for surgical intervention. Surgery, however, may be needed in the management of ulcer-associated hemorrhage, obstruction, or perforation.

Gastric Polyps

Gastric polyps usually are asymptomatic and are detected during an upper gastrointestinal evaluation for anemia or a complaint unconnected with the polyps. Because of the risk of carcinoma, they should be examined endoscopically and either biopsied or removed.[36]

Gastric Bezoars

Gastric bezoars usually represent matted intragastric masses of vegetable matter or hair. Bezoars composed of vegetable matter (phytobezoars) are more common in elderly persons, probably because of decreased gastric acidity, and in patients who have had partial gastric resections.[37] Symptoms range from a feeling of epigastric fullness in the epigastric area to recurrent attacks of pain, nausea, and vomiting. Bezoars can produce gastric outlet obstruction and may be associated with ulceration and perforation. An upper gastrointestinal series demonstrates a large intragastric mass, and its nature can be confirmed endoscopically. For bezoars composed of vegetable matter, intragastric cellulase may break up and dissolve even relatively large masses.[38] Bezoars may be broken up endoscopically, using wire loops or forceps, into sizes that will pass through the stomach or be grasped and removed through the mouth.[39] Surgery should be reserved for bezoars that because of size or composition cannot be dissolved or broken up.

Gastric Paresis

Gastric paresis refers to a decrease in gastric motility which produces various degrees of gastric retention.[40] Retention commonly is associated with vomiting, loss of appetite, and with a feeling of fullness. It is found in patients with diabetic neuropathy and in those taking anticholinergic drugs; it is sometimes associated with immobilization, severe pain, trauma, sepsis, uremia, hypokalemia, and hypocalcemia. Nasogastric suction, intravenous (IV) fluid replacement or hyperalimentation may be necessary until the underlying etiology can be identified and corrected. In patients with gastric retention that is related to diabetes, the oral administration of metoclopramide (Reglan) has proved useful.[41]

The Postgastrectomy Patient[42,43]

By maintaining an adequate dietary intake, patients who have undergone a subtotal gastric resection usually tolerate the malabsorption that is a consequence of the procedure. In older people, however, an adequate diet may not be maintained because of an inadequate socioeconomic situation, coexisting chronic diseases, poor dentition, or depression. Gastric atrophy, which increases with age, contributes to the malabsorption of iron and Vitamin B-12. Such patients may exhibit varying degrees of anemia, osteomalacia, and weight loss.

The dietary intake should be carefully monitored and, where appropriate, the patient should be encouraged to increase the size and/or frequency of his or her meals. Multiple small feedings may be better tolerated than three large meals daily. A diet high in protein and low in concentrated sweets is sometimes necessary to minimize the symptoms of the postgastrectomy syndrome (weakness, faintness, diarrhea, and tachycardia), which may persist even years after the procedure. Orally administered iron and vitamin supplementation, particularly fat-soluble vitamins, and Vitamin B-12 injections may be necessary to correct specific deficiencies.

An upper gastrointestinal series and endos-copy should be part of the evaluation of the symptomatic postgastrectomy patient. Afferent loop stasis should be considered in Billroth II-type operations, since bacterial overgrowth may contribute to problems with absorption. Likewise, stomal dysfunction (with or without a marginal ulcer) can produce partial outlet obstruction and contribute to poor dietary intake. Such conditions often require surgical revision of the initial procedure. Gastric carcinoma occasionally may be seen in the gastric remnant.[44]

The Small Intestine

Duodenal Ulcer Disease

Duodenal ulcer disease is not unusual in elderly persons. Patients characteristically present with a history of recurrent, well-localized epigastric or right-upper quadrant pain, which can be relieved with food or antacids. The pain may have a seasonal pattern over a period of many years. In some individuals, however, the epigastric pain may be atypical or vague, with a poor or inconsistent localization. Gastrointestinal bleeding may be the first manifestation of an active ulcer. An upper gastrointestinal series is the diagnostic procedure of choice, with endoscopy reserved for cases in which x-ray film is not diagnostic, the presentation is atypical, or there is a poor response to therapy.

Antacids are effective but require frequent dosage and strict compliance. Treatment is most conveniently carried out with cimetidine (Tagamet) and maintained for approximately 8 weeks, at which time the majority of all patients will have healed their ulcer. When the drug is stopped, the recurrence rate approaches 50%; therefore, maintenance therapy of a lower dose, if tolerated, is suggested for an additional 2–3 months.[45] In an older patient, particularly those with associated liver or renal disease, the use of cimetidine may produce disorientation or confused states.[46] This side effect, however, appears to be directly related to blood levels. In many patients, the drug can be continued by reducing the dosage. An additional important consideration is the increase in blood levels when other drugs are given concomitantly with cimetidine; most importantly, the coumadin-type anticoagulants, anticonvulsants, aminophylline, and the benzodiazepine tranquilizers.[47]

Ranitidine (Zantac), a new H_2-receptor antagonist, may also be used, and appears to have advantages over cimetidine in the elderly patient. It may be taken in a twice a day dosage, and experience to date suggests that it has a decreased tendency to produce central nervous system and endocrine effects and that it does not raise blood levels of other drugs that a patient may be taking. If used, antacids should be given in an hourly dosage of 30 cc while awake. In individuals where low sodium intake is desirable, a low sodium antacid, such as Alterna-GEL, should be used. Again, treatment should be continued for 8 weeks, with additional treatment based on the patient's symptoms. A new agent, sucralfate (Carafate), recently has been approved for the management of duodenal ulcer diseases and appears to act by binding to the ulcerated area. Tests have shown it to be as effective as cimetidine.[48] Although there is, as yet, no wide experience with sucralfate, it appears to have few significant side effects.

Surgical treatment is reserved for patients with complications of a duodenal ulcer disease, such as gastric outlet obstruction, perforation, and hemorrhage.

Malabsorption Syndromes[49,50]

Malabsorption should be considered in any patient with an unexplained weight loss or anemia, or with a low serum albumin or calcium; it may be further suggested by an abnormal small-bowel barium study or by the presence of pancreatic calcifications on a plain x-ray film of the abdomen. Malabsorption results from a failure to prepare food for absorption, as in pancreatic insufficiency, or from an inability of the small bowel to absorb nutrients. Nontropical and tropical sprue, Crohn's disease, Whipple's disease, gastrointestinal lymphoma, and amyloidosis are some of the diagnostic considerations in this latter group.

The presence of significant malabsorption can best be determined by measuring stool fat excretion over a period of 48–72 hours. If fat absorption is abnormal, an oral D-xylose absorption test will determine if the absorption defect is most likely to be in the small bowel or is the result of pancreatic insufficiency. The test usually is normal in cases of pancreatic insufficiency and abnormal in those conditions affecting the small bowel. The precise diagnosis of the small bowel abnormality usually will require a small bowel biopsy, using a special biopsy tube or capsule.[7] Pancreatic insufficiency can be managed by enzyme replacement; specific and effective treatment, such as the gluten-free diet for non-tropical sprue, is available for many of the conditions that are associated with defective absorption.

Intestinal Ischemia and Infarction[51,52]

In an older patient who complains of severe, postprandial abdominal pain that is steady or cramping in nature, the possibility of abdominal angina should be considered. This clinical picture is secondary to arterial insufficiency of the small bowel and appears to be related to a significant narrowing of at least two of the three major arterial trunks that supply it. Weight loss is common and related to the patient's reluctance to eat because of the associated pain. In patients with a typical clinical picture, angiography should be performed. Where there is significant narrowing or obstruction of major arteries, surgical correction may be possible.

An acute occlusion of a mesenteric artery, which is either secondary to localized atherosclerotic disease or an embolus, may produce an infarction of the small bowel and a clinical picture that is characterized by the sudden onset of severe, periumbilical abdominal pain. The severity of the pain is notable for the lack of associated physical findings; it may radiate into the back and, with time, become more diffuse and steady. Leukocytosis and fever are common, and with the passage of time hypotension and shock will supervene. Flat x-ray films of the abdomen typically show a generalized ileus. Angiography rarely is of additional help. With a typical clinical picture, emergency surgery should be performed. Non-occlusive intestinal infarction may present with a similar clinical picture, but the ischemia is based on poor perfusion secondary to hypotension shock or congestive heart failure. Angiography may help demonstrate both the absence of an occlusion to major arterial trunks and poorly perfused bowel loops. Surgical intervention has little to offer.

Colon, Rectum, and Anus

Irritable Bowel Syndrome

A variety of bowel complaints for which no organic cause can be discovered are common in older persons and collectively make up the irritable bowel syndrome.[53] These include abdominal pain of a cramping nature, alternating periods of constipation and diarrhea, large amounts of mucus in the stool, and the passage of excessive amounts of gas. Although physical examination may reveal some tenderness to palpation over the colon, there are no consistent physical findings. It is important to rule out other gastrointestinal disorders and to appreciate the association with depression, medications, and thyroid dysfunction.

Management of the irritable bowel syndrome includes reassurance, once an organic disease has been ruled out, and the avoidance of laxatives and other drugs that are associated with diarrhea or constipation. The introduction of more bulk into the diet (in the form of fruit or vegetables) may be helpful, as may be the use of bulk-forming agents such as psyllium seed (Metamucil). Anticholinergic agents should be used with caution in an older patient because of the risk of urinary retention and glaucoma.

Carcinoma[54]

In an older patient, any change in the bowel pattern, blood in the stool, or guaiac-positive stools, should raise the possibility of carcinoma involving either the colon, rectum, or anus. Anemia is a common presenting finding with right-sided lesions, whereas left-sided tumors may produce a recurrent, crampy abdominal pain suggestive of partial obstruction. Physical examination may demonstrate a palpable or visible mass that involves the anus; in those patients with rectal carcinoma, the tumor often may be found on digital examination. The diagnosis usually can be made with a combination of anoscopy, sigmoidoscopy, and a careful barium enema examination.[55] Colonoscopy may be used if the barium enema is negative or its findings are equivocal.

Surgical resection for a localized tumor is the treatment of choice in patients who can tolerate surgery. Although radiation and chemotherapy ocassionally have provided palliation for non-resectable tumors, the overall results for survival have been disappointing.

Colonic Polyps

Colonic polyps may be demonstrated during an investigation for blood in the stools or may be found during a routine sigmoidoscopy. Large villous adenomas, in addition to their potential for malignancy, may be associated with significant losses of fluids, electrolytes, and proteins. Polyps, in most instances, can be removed endoscopically from any place in the colon.[13]

Ischemic Colitis

Ischemic colitis results from obstruction of the inferior mesenteric artery or its branches, and it increases in frequency with age.[56] Patients typically have left-sided or lower abdominal cramping pain and rectal bleeding. If the ischemia involves the rectosigmoid, sigmoidoscopy may show mucosal edema and friability, suggestive at times of active ulcerative colitis. Some patients will have a fever, an elevated white blood cell count, and physical findings that are suggestive of peritonitis. When such symptoms are progressive, surgical exploration may be necessary to rule out the presence of perforation or necrotic bowel. Other patients will show a gradual resolution of symptoms, and a barium enema examination may demonstrate areas of narrowing (so-called thumbprinting) and perhaps ulceration. With a resolution of symptoms, such changes may be reversible or a stricture may develop and require resection.

Appendicitis

Appendicitis in an older patient should be considered whenever a clinician is evaluating any poorly defined abdominal pain of recent onset. Temperature and white blood cell count elevations may be minimal and the pain poorly localized.[57] In addition, the diagnostic problem is sometimes compounded by a patient's inability to communicate adequately. Physical examination, however, may reveal a persistent, right lower quadrant tenderness to palpation, especially on digital rectal examination. In most instances, because of the risk of perforation, such tenderness should lead to surgical exploration.

Diverticular Disease of the Colon[58]

Colonic diverticula are found in approximately one third of all individuals over 60 years of age. The great majority of such diverticula are located in the sigmoid colon. Diverticulosis may be associated in some individuals with recurrent bouts of constipation and diarrhea and episodes of poorly defined, left lower quadrant pain. Symptoms appear to be related to abnormalities in the motility of the sigmoid colon, in which high intraluminal pressures are developed. Except for the presence of diverticula and (occasionally) a spiking, sawtooth-like mucosal pattern, the barium enema, sigmoidoscopy, and laboratory work are unremarkable. Some symptomatic relief may be obtained with bulking agents and anticholinergic drugs.

Diverticulitis, on the other hand, represents an inflammatory response to the perforation of a diverticulum into the surrounding tissue or freely into the peritoneal cavity. Patients typically will complain of left lower quadrant pain and will display physical findings that are consistent with peritoneal inflammation or peritonitis. Diagnostic evaluations should include a plain x-ray film of the abdomen for the presence of free air and sigmoidoscopy to rule out other conditions, such as rectal carcinoma. In most instances, a barium enema should be deferred until the acute inflammatory process subsides. Complications include hemorrhage, peritonitis, abscess formation, obstruction, and the formation of sinus tracts between a diverticulum and its adjacent structures, such as the bladder or vagina.

The management of a patient with acute diverticulitis usually will include broad spectrum antibiotics, nasogastric suction, and careful management of fluid requirements by IV infusion. Emergent or semi-emergent surgery is necessary for peritonitis, especially if there is no improvement with medical therapy, and where there appears to be an enlarging abscess. Elective surgery may be necessary after the acute attack in the management of obstructive symptoms and fistulas.

In patients responding to medical therapy, follow-up management should be essentially the same as for patients with asymptomatic diverticulosis. Elective surgery for the removal of the involved sigmoid colon should be reserved for patients with a recurrent attack or attacks, since as many as two thirds to three quarters of all patients never experience a second attack.[59]

Severe hemorrhage may occur from an otherwise asymptomatic diverticulum. Although such bleeding usually will cease spontaneously, the site of bleeding should be ascertained by visceral angiography. The study may not only define the site of bleeding, but permit intra-arterial administration of pitressin to control it. If the bleeding site cannot be defined by arteriography, a barium enema should be done to look for other sources of bleeding. In addition, the barium enema examination itself may, on occasion, arrest the bleeding from a diverticulum. The treatment of persistent, uncontrollable bleeding is surgical, with resection of the involved segment (if possible) or a blind hemicolectomy if the bleeding site cannot be precisely determined.

Constipation

Constipation refers to the infrequent passage of hard, dry stool.[60] Bowel movements may be difficult or painful. Factors such as increasingly sedentary habits, confinement to bed, diet, and medication, may cause constipation. Laxative abuse itself may be a contributory factor by decreasing normal colonic motility.[61] It is important to consider organic lesions, such as carcinoma, and to review medications for tranquilizers, anticholinergics, or narcotics. Medical conditions to consider include hypothyroidism and depression.

In re-establishing normal bowel habits, the physician should suggest that the patient attempt to have a bowel movement on a regularly scheduled basis, such as after breakfast when there may be assistance from the gastrocolic reflex. Simple measures include mild exercise (such as walking), adequate fluid intake, the addition of bran, fruits, vegetables, and similar bulk and fiber-providing items to the diet. During the period of retraining, particularly in patients who require constipating medication, some form of laxative may be temporarily necessary. Bulk-forming agents such as psyllium seed (Metamucil), or a wetting agent such as sodium docusate (Colace), may be effective and are not habit forming. Milk of magnesia, lactulose syrup (Chronulac), or cascara-containing laxatives may be used when more stimulation is needed.

When an older patient is confined to bed, fecal impactions may form. A rectal examination is indicated whenever there is failure to pass stools over a period of several days, and if found, the fecal impaction may be broken up with the examining finger, be partially extracted, and then treated with soapsuds or oil retention enemas. Barium impactions are not uncommon following barium x-ray film examinations and may be managed in a similar fashion.

Hemorrhoids[62]

Symptomatic hemorrhoids are not uncommon in an older patient. Symptoms include bleeding, prolapse of internal hemorrhoids, and thrombosis. Although internal hemorrhoids are the most common cause of painless rectal bleeding, any such bleeding requires an evaluation for carcinoma of the anus, rectum, or colon.

Prolapsed hemorrhoids appear as soft, reddish masses protruding from the anus, commonly after defecation or straining at stool. These may reduce spontaneously or else require digital replacement. Thrombosis of external hemorrhoids usually produces severe perianal pain, with a patient having difficulty in sitting and with bowel movements. Analgesics and sitz baths provide symptomatic relief, although with large hemorrhoids, a surgical evacuation may be required. Thrombosis of prolapsed internal hemorrhoids frequently produces symptoms severe enough to require hospitalization and hemorroidectomy.

Sitz baths and stool softeners give symptomatic relief for most patients with internal hemorrhoids; persistent bleeding or discomfort may be best managed by a hemorrhoidectomy using rubber band ligation, injections of sclerosing agents, or cryosurgery. In some patients, the size and number of the hemorrhoids will require surgical ligation and removal.

Anal Fissures[63]

Anal fissures represent a tear in the anal mucosa that is caused by passing hard, inspissated stool. Such fissures typically cause pain on defecation, but usually respond to a regimen of stool softeners, sitz baths, and analgesics. Oc-

casionally, the application of a weak solution of silver nitrate to the base of the fissure may be useful. Chronic, non-healing fissures, however, require some form of surgical treatment, such as a lateral sphincterotomy.

Anorectal Abscesses and Fistulae[64]

Anorectal abscesses arise most often from an infection in the anal crypts which extends into an adjacent tissue space. Patients typically have a persistent pain in the perianal area that increases with defecation, on digital rectal examination, and with walking or sitting. Such abscesses may be associated with the development of a fistula opening onto the perianal area. The preferred treatment is surgical incision and drainage. Although in older patients Crohn's disease of the colon or small bowel is an uncommon association with such abscesses and fistulae, this possibility should be considered in those patients who also complain of rectal bleeding, epigastric pain, or diarrhea. In such patients, Crohn's disease should be ruled out by doing both a barium enema and small bowel follow-through before surgical treatment is undertaken.

Pruritis Ani[65]

Perianal itching may be a difficult diagnostic and management problem. Possible etiologies are diverse, including such dermatologic conditions as psoriasis and contact dermatitis. In some patients, perianal itching appears to be associated with the intake of food items such as milk, alcohol, coffee, and chocolate. Candidiasis, which involves the moist perianal skin, may appear following the use of antibiotics and can produce pruritus. Symptomatic treatment may be effective and includes maintaining a dry perianal area, using a 1% hydrocortisone cream, eliminating suspected food items, and where candidiasis is present, the use of local or oral nystatin (Mycostatin).

Liver and Gallbladder

Liver function abnormalities, including jaundice, are common diagnostic problems in the geriatric population; in most instances, these will be related to carcinomas, cholelithiasis, drugs, alcohol, type B, or non-A, non-B viral hepatitis. Alcoholic cirrhosis, biliary cirrhosis, and cirrhosis that is associated with hemochromatosis occasionally may be seen.

In a jaundiced patient, the immediate clinical concern is to differentiate extrahepatic obstruction, in which surgical intervention may be needed, from intrahepatic cholestasis. With obstructive jaundice, the alkaline phosphatase usually will be elevated two or more times above normal. In extrahepatic obstruction, an abdominal ultrasound examination may show dilated extra- and intrahepatic ducts.[2] Although intrahepatic cholestasis (due in most instances to drugs, alcohol, or viral hepatitis) also will have a similar alkaline phosphatase elevation, ductal dilatation will not be seen. Biliary cirrhosis also has high alkaline phosphatase levels with non-dilated ducts, but it will additionally show the presence of antimitochondrial antibody. If the clinical picture and ultrasound examination are equivocal, it may be necessary to evaluate the ductal system via a transhepatic cholecystography or an endoscopic injection of the common bile duct (ERCP).

Hepatocellular jaundice has as its major abnormality a moderate to marked elevation of the transaminase (SGOT, SGPT) that is associated with only a slight elevation of the alkaline phosphatase. An ultrasound examination shows no evidence of ductal abnormalities. Drug history may suggest that a new drug was initiated coincidentally with the onset of the jaundice; where possible, such drugs should be withdrawn or substituted with other agents. Because hepatocellular damage has been associated with many drugs that are in common clinical use (including tranquilizers, antibiotics, and antihypertensive agents), all drugs should be suspect.[66] In addition, alcohol can produce liver function abnormalities that are consistent with most forms of liver disease. A hepatitis B surface antigen test should be ordered routinely to rule out type B hepatitis; although rare in older age groups, IgM antibody to hepatitis A can indicate a recent, acute hepatitis A infection. Because most cases of viral hepatitis arising from blood transfusions are currently non-A, non-B hepatitis (for which there are no serologic markers), this should be considered where there is a history of a recent blood transfusion.

Isolated, asymptomatic elevations of the alkaline phosphatase level should not be ascribed to age alone.[67] An alkaline phosphatase elevation of liver origin is accompanied by an increase in the gamma glutamyl transpeptidase (GGT) level, and it can be the initial manifestation of liver involvement with primary or metastatic carcinoma.

Gallbladder Disease

Recurrent attacks of postprandial, right upper quadrant pain suggest the presence of gallstones. Approximately 25% of all individuals older than 60 years of age have gallstones; of these individuals perhaps 50% are symptomatic.[68] In most instances, these can be demonstrated abdominal ultrasound or by an oral cholecystogram.[2] Cholecystectomy is the treatment of choice for symptomatic gallstones. Although there is some difference of opinion, asymptomatic gallstones in an older patient do not, by themselves, justify surgery unless the patient is diabetic. Here, an elective cholecystectomy is preferable to the risk of the severe sepsis that may be associated with the initial attack of acute cholecystitis.[69] The use of orally given chenodeoxycholic acid for the medical dissolution of gallstones has been disappointing.[70]

Acute cholecystitis, with fever, right upper quadrant tenderness, and a white blood cell count elevation, usually will need an emergent or semiemergent cholecystectomy after hydration and treatment with broad spectrum antibiotics. Although gallstones usually are present, acalcareous cholecystitis (cholecystitis without gallstones) may be seen in some patients, particularly those recovering from surgery or immobilized due to orthopedic or other procedures.[71]

In high-risk patients who develop common bile duct obstruction due to a retained gallstone, endoscopic papillotomy should be considered. In this procedure, a fiberoptic endoscope is used to place a cutting wire loop into the papilla of Vater to open it widely. Through this opening, a balloon-tipped catheter or Dormia basket may be introduced to remove the impacted gallstone.[15]

Pancreatic Carcinoma[72]

A pancreatic carcinoma should be considered in any patient with persistent epigastric pain and weight loss. Typically, the pain will radiate into the back, is made worse with food, and may be relieved to some extent by bending forward or doubling up in bed. In the majority of patients, jaundice will occur at some time in the course of the illness. Early symptoms of pancreatic carcinoma may involve such non-specific syndromes as depression and anxiety. Migratory thrombophlebitis occasionally is seen, most frequently with tumors that involve the body or tail of the pancreas. The diagnosis often can be made by using either abdominal ultrasound, CT scans, visceral angiography, or ERCP. Therapy, for the most part, is palliative. Surgery may be of use in relieving biliary tract obstruction or gastric outlet obstruction.

Gastrointestinal Bleeding

The source of gastrointestinal bleeding usually can be identified by using a combination of endoscopy, angiography, and barium studies. Severe, upper gastrointestinal hemorrhaging usually will be due to duodenal or gastric ulcers, a Mallory-Weiss tear of the esophagus, or esophageal varices. Severe bleeding occasionally may be seen from both esophagitis and gastritis. Fiberoptic endoscopy by itself usually will identify these lesions.[73]

Lower gastrointestinal bleeding most often is due to hemorrhoids, diverticula, vascular malformations particularly of the cecum and ascending colon, and neoplasms.[74] Bleeding can be severe and, at times, exsanguinating. Severe bleeding also can be occasionally encountered with ischemic colitis and from areas of small bowel ischemia or infarction. Where bleeding is intermittent or not severe, a barium enema and colonoscopy may be used to identify the source. With severe bleeding, angiography usually is the procedure of choice.

Although there can be no dogmatic approach to the management of severe upper or lower gastrointestinal bleeding, it should be recognized that an older patient tolerates blood loss poorly, and prompt blood replacement to bring the hematocrit close to normal levels should be a major therapeutic goal. Where the bleeding is persistent or recurrent, early surgical intervention would appear to be a major factor in improving the overall survival.[75]

The use of IV pitressin and the Sengstaken-Blakemore balloon are the usual medical measures for controlling a hemorrhage due to esophageal varices. In addition, in patients who are poor surgical risks, bleeding due to esophageal varices occasionally may be controlled by the use of angiographic or endoscopic techniques for injecting the varices with sclerosing and thrombosing agents.[76,77] Angiography also may be used (usually in a patient who is a poor surgical risk), in controlling Mallory-Weiss bleeding, bleeding due to peptic ulcers, diverticula, and vascular malformations. As mentioned previously, endoscopically directed electrocautery and laser photocoagulation also have been used in controlling bleeding from vascular malformations.[78]

Intestinal Obstruction[79]

Intestinal obstruction should be considered in any patient who has an onset of nausea and vomiting that is associated with cramping abdominal pain. These symptoms may appear suddenly or with progressive severity over a period of days. Patients typically will cease passing stool or gas; with colonic or distal small bowel obstruction, they become increasingly distended. There may be diffuse abdominal tenderness. With mechanical obstruction the bowel sounds typically will have a high-pitched, tinkling character and show periodic increases in activity. In adynamic ileus, bowel sounds will be absent.

The common causes to be considered include adhesions due to previous surgery, carcinoma, particularly of the colon, incarcerated hernias, colonic volvuli, and fecal impactions. Adynamic ileus, where there is an absence of intestinal peristaltic activity, may be associated with generalized sepsis, intestinal ischemia or infarction, peritonitis, and hypokalemia; or it may appear as a late manifestation of mechanical obstruction.

Plain x-ray films of the abdomen may suggest

the site of obstruction by showing the gas primarily localized to either the small bowel or colon, with the small bowel showing such findings as dilated, gas-filled loops and fluid levels; the colonic gas pattern occasionally will suggest either a cecal or sigmoid volvulus. A sigmoidoscopy and barium enema will usually localize the site of colonic obstruction. If colonic obstruction can be ruled out, a barium meal may be used in studying the upper gastrointestinal track.[80]

Although obstruction from a sigmoid volvulus occasionally can be relieved with a sigmoidoscope or colonoscope, mechanical obstruction will usually require surgical intervention. Patients should be appropriately prepared with adequate fluid and electrolyte replacement; where there is a marked distention, an attempt can be made at decompression by using a nasogastric or Miller-Abbott tube. Such decompression should likewise be attempted in patients with an adynamic ileus who are being studied or who are under treatment for the underlying etiology.

References

1. Belsito AA, Dickinson P: Fiberoptic esophagogastroscopy: a crucial diagnostic test in the elderly. *Geriatrics* 27:90–98, 1972.
2. Ferrucci JT Jr: Body ultrasonography. *N Engl J Med* 300:590–602, 1979.
3. Baert AL, Wackenheim A, Jeanmart L: Abdominal computer tomography, in *Atlas of Pathological Computer Tomography*. Berlin, Springer-Verlag, 1980, vol 2.
4. Pereiras R, Chiprut RO, Greenwald RA, et al: Percutaneous transhepatic cholangiography with the "skinny" needle: a rapid, simple, and accurate method in the diagnosis of cholestasis. *Ann Intern Med* 86:562–568, 1977.
5. Cotton PB: Cannulation of the papilla of Vater by endoscopy and retrograde cholangiopancreatography (ERCP). *Gut* 13:1014–1025, 1972.
6. Athanasoulis CA, Waltman AC, Novelline RA, et al: Angiography: its contribution to the emergency management of gastrointestinal hemorrhage. *Radiol Clin North Am* 14:265–280, 1976.
7. Trier JS: Diagnostic value of peroral biopsy of the proximal small intestine (current concepts). *N Engl J Med* 285:1470–1473, 1971.
8. Schwerk WB, Schnitz-Moormann P: Ultrasonically guided fine-needle biopsies in neoplastic liver disease: cytohistologic diagnoses and echo pattern of lesions. *Cancer* 48:1469–1477, 1981.
9. Goldstein HM, Zornoza J, Wallace S, et al: Percutaneous fine needle aspiration biopsy of pancreatic and other abdominal masses. *Radiology* 123:319–322, 1977.
10. Trujillo NP: Peritoneoscopy and guided biopsy in the diagnosis of intra-abdominal disease (clinical trends and topics). *Gastroenterology* 71:1083–1085, 1976.
11. Holder LE, Saenger EL: The use of nuclear medicine in evaluating liver disease. *Seminars in Roentgenology* 10:215–222, 1975.
12. Weissmann HS, Badia J, Sugarman LA, et al: Spectrum of 99m-Tc-IDA cholecystic patterns in acute cholecystitis. *Radiology* 138:167–175, 1981.
13. Shinya H, Wolff WI: Morphology, anatomic distribution and cancer potential of colonic polyps: an analysis of 7000 polyps endoscopically removed. *Ann Surg* 190:679–683, 1979.
14. Peura DA, Heit HA, Johnson LF, et al: The esophageal prosthesis in cancer. *Am J Dig Dis* 23:796–800, 1978.
15. Safrany L: Duodenoscopic sphincterotomy and gallstone removal (clinical trends and topics). *Gastroenterology* 72:338–343, 1977.
16. Rogers BH, Adler F: Hemangiomas of the cecum. Colonoscopic diagnosis and therapy. *Gastroenterology* 71:1079–1082, 1976.
17. Lowe WC: Survival with carcinoma of the esophagus. *Ann Intern Med* 77:915–918, 1972.
18. Pearson JG: The present status and future potential of radiotherapy in the management of esophageal cancer. *Cancer* 39:882–890, 1977.
19. Heit HA, Johnson LF, Siegel SR, et al: Palliative dilatation for dysphagia in esophageal carcinoma. *Ann Int Med* 89:629–631, 1978.
20. Brunnen PL, Karmody AM, Needham CD: Severe peptic oesophagitis. *Gut* 10:831–837, 1967.
21. Wesdorp E, Barelsman J, Pape K, et al: Oral cimetidine in reflux esophagitis: a double blind controlled trial. *Gastroenterology* 74:821–824, 1978.
22. Schulze-DeLrieu K: Drug therapy: metoclopramide. *N Engl J Med* 305:28–33, 1981.
23. Castell DO (moderator), Knuff TE, Brown FC, et al (participants): Dysphagia (clinical conference). *Gastroenterology* 76:1015–1024, 1979.
24. Wesdorp ICE, Bartelsman JFWM, den Hartog Jager FCA, et al: Results of conservative treatment of benign esophageal strictures: a follow-up study in 100 patients. *Gastroenterology* 82:487–493, 1982.
25. Schatzki R: The lower esophageal ring. *Am J Roentgenol Radium Ther and Nucl Med* 90:805–810, 1963.
26. Waye D: The endoscopy corner: removal of foreign bodies from the upper intestinal tract with

fiberoptic instruments. *Am J Gastroenterol* 65:557–559, 1976.

27. Ellis FH Jr, Schlegel JF, Lynch VP, et al: Cricopharyngeal myotomy for pharyngo-esophageal diverticulum. *Ann Surg* 170:340–350, 1969.

28. Henderson RD: *Motor Disorders of the Esophagus.* Baltimore, Williams & Wilkins, 1979.

29. Palmer ED: Disorders of the cricopharyngeus muscle: a review (progress in gastroenterology). *Gastroenterology* 71:510–519, 1976.

30. Castell DO: Achalasia and diffuse esophageal spasm. *Arch Intern Med* 136:571–579, 1978.

31. VanTrappen G, Hellemans J: Treatment of achalasia and related motor disorders. *Gastroenterology* 79:144–154, 1980.

32. Fleshler B: Diffuse esophageal spasm. *N Engl J Med* 52:559–564, 1967.

33. McNeer G, Pack GT: *Neoplasms of the Stomach.* Philadelphia, JB Lippincott, 1967.

34. Bynum TE, Hartsuck J, Jacobson ED: Gastric ulcer (current clinical concepts). *Gastroenterology* 62:1052–1060, 1972.

35. Englert E Jr, Freston JW, Graham DY, et al: Cimetidine, antacid, and hospitalization in the treatment of benign gastric ulcer. *Gastroenterology* 74:416–425, 1978.

36. Bone GE, McClelland RN: Management of gastric polyps. *Surg Gynecol Obstet* 142:933–938, 1976.

37. Rigler RG, Grininger DR: Phytobezoars following partial gastrectomy. *Surg Clin North Am* 50:381–386, 1970.

38. Stanten A, Peters HE Jr: Enzymatic dissolution of phytobezoars. *Am J Surg* 130:259–261, 1975.

39. McKechnie J: Gastroscopic removal of a phytobezoar. *Gastroenterology* 62:1047–1051, 1972.

40. Rimer DG: Gastric retention without mechanical obstruction. A review. *Arch Intern Med* 117:287–299, 1966.

41. Snape WJ Jr, Battle WM, Schwartz SS, et al: Metoclopramide to treat gastroparesis due to diabetes mellitus. *Ann Intern Med* 96:444–446, 1982.

42. Wall AJ, Ungar B, Baird CW, et al: Malnutrition after partial gastrectomy. *Am J Dig Dis* 12:1077–1086, 1967.

43. Morgan DB, Pulvertaft CN, Fourman P: Effects of age in the loss of bone after gastric surgery. *Lancet* 2:772–773, 1966.

44. Kobayashi S, Prolla JC, Kirsner JB: Late gastric carcinoma developing after surgery for benign conditions. *Am J Dig Dis* 15:905–912, 1970.

45. Bodemar G, Walan A: Maintenance treatment of recurrent peptic ulcer by cimetidine. *Lancet* 2:403–407, 1978.

46. Kimelblatt BJ, Cerra FB, Calleri G, et al: Dose and serum concentration relationships in cimetidine-associated mental confusion. *Gastroenterology* 78:791–795, 1980.

47. Patwardhan RV, Johnson RF, Sinclair AP, et al: Lack of tolerance and rapid recovery of cimetidine-inhibited chlordiazepoxide (Librium) elimination. *Gastroenterology* 81:547–551, 1981.

48. Martin F, Farley A, Gagnon M, et al: Comparison of the healing capacities of sucralfate and cimetidine in the short-term treatment of duodenal ulcer: a double-blind randomized trial. *Gastroenterology* 82:401–405, 1982.

49. Symposium on malabsorption. Sleisenger MH and Glickman RM, eds. *Am J Med* 67:979–1104, 1979.

50. Steinberg WM, Toskes PP: A practical approach to evaluating maldigestion and malabsorption. *Geriatrics* 33:73–85, (July) 1978.

51. Sullivan JE: Vascular disease of the intestines. *Med Clin North Am* 58:1473–1485, 1974.

52. Ottinger LW: Nonocclusive mesenteric infarction. *Surg Clin North Am* 54:689–698, 1974.

53. Chaudhary NA, Truelove SC: The irritable colon syndrome. A study of the clinical features, predisposing causes, and prognosis in 130 cases. *Q J Med* 31:307–332, 1962.

54. Winawer SJ, Sherlock P, Schottenfeld D, et al: Screening for colon cancer (clinical trends and topics). *Gastroenterology* 70:783–789, 1976.

55. Miller RE: The clean colon (editorial). *Gastroenterology* 70:289–290, 1976.

56. Marcuson RW: Ischemic colitis. *Clin Gastroenterol* 1:745–763, 1972.

57. Williams JS, Hale HW Jr: Acute appendicitis in the elderly: review of 83 cases. *Ann Surg* 162:208–212, 1965.

58. Almy TP, Howell DA: Diverticular disease of the colon. *N Engl J Med* 302:324–331, 1980.

59. Parks TG: Natural history of diverticular disease of the colon. *Clin Gastroenterol* 4:53–69, 1975.

60. Benson JA Jr: Constipation: A saga of arrested motion. *GI Tract (Warren-Teed)* 4:4–7, 1974.

61. Urso FP, Urso MJ, Lee CH: The cathartic colon: pathological findings and radiological/pathological correlation. *Diagn Radiol* 8:557–559, 1975.

62. Kaufman HD: Hemorrhoids: presentation and management. *Practical Gastroenterol* 4:51–57, 1980.

63. Shub H, Salvati E, Rubin R: Conservative treatment of fissure. *Dis Colon Rectum* 21:582–583, 1978.

64. Lindell TD, Fletcher WS, Krippaehne WW: Anorectal suppurative disease. *Am J Surg* 125:189–194, 1973.

65. Sullivan ES, Garnjobst WM: Pruritus ani: a practical approach. *Surg Clin Nor Am* 58:505–512, 1978.

66. Zimmerman HD: *Hepatotoxicity—The Adverse Effects of Drugs and Other Chemicals on the Liver.* New York, Appleton-Century-Crofts, 1978.

67. Kampmann JP, Sinding, J, Moller-Jorgensen I: Effect of age on liver function. *Geriatrics* 30:91–95, 1975.

68. Redinger R: Advances in the diagnosis and treatment of gallbladder disease in the elderly. *Geriatrics* 35(suppl 4):105–109, Apr 1980.

69. Schein CJ: Acute cholecystitis in the diabetic. *Am J Gastroenterol* 51:511–515, 1969.

70. Schoenfield LJ, Lachin JM, et al: Chenodiol (chenodeoxycholic acid) for dissolution of gallstones: The National Cooperative Gallstone Study: a controlled trial of efficacy and safety. *Ann Intern Med* 95:257–282, 1981.

71. Ottinger LW: Acute cholecystitis as a postoperative complication. *Ann Surg* 184:162–165, 1976.

72. Hermann RE, Cooperman AM: Cancer of the pancreas (current concepts in cancer). *N Engl J Med* 301:482–485, 1979.

73. Katon RM, Smith FW: Panendoscopy in the early diagnosis of acute upper gastrointestinal bleeding. *Gastroenterology* 65:728–734, 1973.

74. Smith GW: Lower GI bleeding in the elderly. *Postgrad Med* 69:36–44, 1981.

75. Foster JH, Hickok DF, Dunphy JE: Factors influencing mortality following emergency operation for massive upper gastrointestinal hemorrhage. *Surg Gynecol Obstet* 117:257–262, 1963.

76. Bengmark S, Borjesson B, Hoerels J, et al: Obliteration of esophageal varices by PTP. *Ann Surg* 190:549–554, 1979.

77. Sivak MV Jr, Stout DJ, Skipper G: Endoscopic injection sclerosis (EIS) of esophageal varices. *Gastrointest Endosc* 27:52–57, 1981.

78. Wolff WI, Grossman MB, Shinya H: Angiodysplasia of the colon: diagnosis and treatment. *Gastroenterology* 72:329–333, 1977.

79. Sufian S, Matsumoto T: Intestinal obstruction. *Am J Surg* 130:9–14, 1975.

80. Miller RE, Brahms F: Large amounts of orally administered barium for obstruction of the small intestine. *Surg Gynecol Obstet* 29:1185–1188, 1969.

CHAPTER 15

Fluid and Electrolyte Disorders

ROBERT M. PALMER, M.D.

Disorders of fluid and electrolyte balance are common in elderly persons. The types and clinical presentations of electrolyte disorders that occur in elderly compared to younger patients may differ substantially. An understanding of the physiologic changes that influence fluid and electrolyte balance in elderly persons, and the clinical consequences thereof, enables the clinician to provide appropriate care for an elderly patient. Potential abnormalities can be anticipated and frequently prevented. For a general and more comprehensive review of fluid, electrolyte, and acid-base metabolism, the reader is referred to standard textbooks.[1,2]

Regulation of Body Fluids and Electrolytes: Changes with Aging

Total body water (TBW) is distributed between two major compartments: extracellular fluid (ECF) and intracellular fluid (ICF). The ECF includes plasma, interstitial fluid and lymph, and transcellular fluids. The ICF accounts for the greatest contribution to TBW. In lean, healthy males, TBW accounts for 50–60% of body weight; approximately two-thirds is ECF. About 5% of body weight represents plasma volume, while 15% is extravascular ECF. The TBW content, though, diminishes with age, which reflects a decrease in ICF due to a loss of muscle mass.[3] Extracellular fluid volume, however, does not change significantly with aging, thereby representing a larger proportion of TBW in an older individual.

Electrolyte composition differs markedly between ICF and ECF (*see* Table 15-1). The maintenance of normal concentrations of electrolytes depends on numerous homeostatic mechanisms. Hydrostatic and osmotic pressure gradients, in accordance with the Starling equilibrium, have the greatest effect on fluid balance. Although serum albumin levels appear to decrease with age,[4] serum globulins increase and osmotic pressure appears not to decrease. Little is known about changes in transport mechanisms with aging. For example, while changes in the sodium-potassium-ATPase pump may occur with aging, intraerythrocyte concentrations of sodium and potassium are similar in young and elderly people.[5] Homeostatic mechanisms thus appear to remain intact in a healthy older person.

Nonetheless, physiologic changes that accompany the aging process may have profound effects on fluid and electrolyte balance during episodes of physical stress and illness. Some major changes with aging are summarized in Table 15-2.

Whereas a younger patient may tolerate plasma volume losses up to 20% without demonstrating symptoms of hypoperfusion or othostatic hypotension, an elderly patient often does not. Diminished baroreceptor sensitivity[5] and loss of arterial elasticity blunt an elderly patient's cardiovascular reflexes in response to acute volume depletion. Decreased maximum heart rates, and possibly reduced cardiac beta-receptor activity, contribute to the relatively decreased cardiac output of a volume-depleted geriatric patient. Not surprisingly then, an

TABLE 15-1 Electrolyte Composition of Body Fluids

Electrolytes	Extracellular Fluid (serum [mEq/l])	Intracellular Fluid (muscle [mEq/kg H_2O])
Cations		
Sodium	140–145	±10
Potassium	4	156
Calcium	5	3.3
Magnesium	2	26
Anions		
Chloride	100–104	±2
Bicarbonate	26	±8
Phosphate	2	95
Sulfate	1	20
Organic acids	6	—
Protein	16	55

TABLE 15-2 Some Physiologic Changes of Aging Affecting Fluid and Electrolyte Balance

Organ System	Change with Aging
Cardiovascular	Diminished baroreceptor sensitivity Increased peripheral vascular resistance Reduced beta-receptor activity
Renal	Reduced urinary concentration and dilution Reduced activity of renin-angiotensin-aldosterone system Impaired sodium handling Decreased renal blood flow
Metabolic-Endocrine	Decline in lean body mass Increased ratio of fat to muscle Altered ADH secretion in response to various stimuli
Gastrointestinal	Decreased hepatic blood flow Decreased digestive capacity Reduced muscle tone and motor function
Neuromuscular	Diminished intellectual capacity Loss of muscle mass
Pulmonary	Reduced vital capacity and expiratory volumes Reduced ventilatory response to hypoxia and hypercapnia

acute intravascular volume depletion due to diuretic therapy or gastrointestinal illness frequently produces serious symptoms in older patients. Conversely, elderly persons poorly tolerate acute increases in intravascular volume (e.g., from the infusion of intravenous [IV] fluids). Reduced ventricular compliance, increased peripheral resistance, and decreased compliance of vascular beds, may lead to acute left ventricular dysfunction or frank pulmonary edema following the IV infusion of large amounts of isotonic fluids or small amounts of hypertonic fluids.

Other adaptive mechanisms that are responsible for homeostasis of extracellular volume and electrolyte composition in elderly persons often are impaired. In particular, renal handling of sodium and water often is abnormal during acute alterations in salt and fluid intake. Studies of the renal response to an acute reduction in salt intake show that while older patients can conserve sodium and attain sodium balance, their response is considerably slower than in younger patients.[6] A reduction of urinary sodium excretion after salt restriction may take more than 24 hours in patients over 60 years of age, and produces a negative sodium balance in the interim. During an acute illness, sodium intake may be decreased in a confused or disoriented patient who is without access to sodium-containing fluids or who receives hypotonic infusions, which further depletes extracellular volume and may impair organ system function.[6] A salt-losing tendency of an aged kidney occurs due to nephron loss, with a resultant increased osmotic load per nephron and mild osmotic diuresis.[6] Sodium depletion, in turn, can produce disturbances in urinary-diluting ability, especially in patients with chronic renal insufficiency. Sodium depletion apparently limits water excretion by decreasing the delivery of salt to the ascending limb of the nephron and reducing the flow of fluid entering the collecting tubule.[7] The urinary-concentrating ability also may be impaired in elderly persons as a result of deteriorating renal function, loop diuretics, transient obstruction of the urinary tract, and malnutrition.[7] Severe protein malnutrition, which is not uncommon in an institutionalized or chronically ill geriatric patient, decreases the medullary urea concentration. This results in reduced water extraction from the descending limb. Potassium depletion, usually a consequence of diuretic use, but occasionally of malnutrition or starvation, also interferes with urinary concentration. These abnormalities, while not unique to elderly persons, are more common in older patients, often go unrecognized, and occasionally produce serious consequences.[8]

Age-related changes in the renin-angiotensin-aldosterone system also affect the homeostasis of fluids and electrolytes.[5,6] Basal and provoked plasma renin activity diminishes with aging. The reduced secretion of aldosterone may allow inappropriate losses of urinary sodium. More important, the loss of aldosterone leaves an elderly person susceptible to hyperkalemia. This is a particular concern in patients with renal insufficiency and in those given potassium salts or potassium-sparing diuretics.[6,9] The decrease in aldosterone secretion, urinary-concentrating and urinary-diluting capacity, and renal function with aging, are responsible for many of the clinical syndromes that are associated with disturbances in sodium and water balance.

As the glomerular filtration rate declines with age, the electrolyte balance can be disturbed by a decreased renal clearance of drugs.[10] Both lithium and chlorpropamide, for example, depend on renal clearance and affect the water balance. The loss of muscle mass with aging leads to a decreased creatinine production and a deceptively "normal" serum creatinine that fails to reflect a declining glomerular filtration rate. Fortunately, creatinine clearance can be estimated accurately, and drug dosages can be appropriately adjusted from the serum creatinine based on equations that account for age and sex[11] (see Volume I, Chapter 16).

The decline in lean body mass with aging has other clinical implications. The loss of the major intracellular electrolytes, potassium, and phosphate (see Table 15-1), leaves an elderly person potentially susceptible to hypokalemia and phosphate depletion. An increased ratio of fat to muscle,[5] and of extracellular water to intracellular water[12] with aging, alters the volume of distribution of drugs[10], and leaves an elderly person at an increased risk of intracellular dehydration due to drugs or an illness that decrease TBW. The loss of muscle mass with aging has been observed in numerous cross-sectional studies and is corroborated by longitudinal studies.[3,5,12] Whether muscle atrophy is an inevitable consequence of aging is unclear. Recent studies suggest that older males may retain the potential for gross muscle hypertrophy during progressive strength training,[13] which implies that a loss of muscle mass may be preventable. In any event, an elderly person generally has a relative decrease in total body nitrogen, total body potassium, and intracellular water.

Endocrinologic changes with aging are now beginning to be appreciated. Adrenal cortical secretion in response to adrenocorticotropic hormone (ACTH), for example, may be blunted.[5] The clinical significance of these physiologic changes is yet to be determined. In contrast, the secretion of arginine vasopressin (anti diuretic hormone or ADH) by the neurohypophysis may be exaggerated in an elderly person in response to various stimuli. There is an age-related increase in osmoreceptor sensitivity in elderly persons. However, elderly compared to young patients may show a failure of ADH secretion in response to volume-pressure (non-osmotic) stimuli such as orthostasis.[14] The interpretation of water balance is confounded by the altered sense of thirst and the defective renal-diluting mechanisms that cause water retention in these patients, who otherwise appear clinically euvolemic.[6,15]

The physiologic changes of aging in other organ systems may be directly or indirectly responsible for disturbances in electrolyte balance or acid-base homeostasis. Decreased hepatic blood flow in elderly persons[5,10] alters the clearance of drugs that undergo hepatic biotransformation. Reduced muscle tone and motor function of the gastrointestinal tract and decreased digestive capacity affect absorption and bioavailability of drugs. Neuromuscular alterations with aging potentiate electrolyte disturbances. An elderly person with an impaired intellectual capacity may be unable to respond appropriately to thirst mechanisms or to request water when it is inaccessible. Reductions in the vital capacity, expiratory volume, and ventilatory responses to hypoxia and hypercapnia,[5] leave an elderly person predisposed to acid-base disorders during acute life-threatening illnesses, such as pneumonia or congestive heart failure; for example, acute respiratory acidosis due to hypercapnia may be superimposed on acute metabolic acidosis as lactate accumulates during tissue hypoxia.[16] In summary, the physiologic changes in organ system function with aging can have a profound influence on the homeostatic mechanisms that are responsible for normal electrolyte and fluid balance. These changes are especially important in the presence of illness and drug therapy.

Regulation and Disorders of Sodium Balance

The normal regulation of water and sodium balance depends on the integrity of homeostatic mechanisms. Water moves freely between ICF and ECF compartments in response to osmotic gradients. Solutes, though, are less permeable because of active membrane pumps, molecular size, or electrical charge.[1,17] Solute concentration (osmolality) across the cell membranes is equalized by the distribution of body water in each compartment. In ICF, the major osmotic solutes include potassium, magnesium, phosphate, and protein, whereas in ECF the major osmotic solutes are sodium and its accompanying anions, chloride and bicarbonate (see Table 15-1). In healthy adults, about two thirds of TBW is in the ICF compartments and one-third is in the ECF compartments; with aging, the proportion of TBW in ECF increases as ICF decreases, but the concentration of the solutes

is unchanged. Since sodium and its salts are the major solutes of ECF, changes in their amounts determine ECF volume and produce osmotic shifts of water across the cell membranes. An increase of ECF sodium, for example, creates an osmotic gradient that shifts water out of cells, thereby decreasing ICF volume but maintaining osmotic equilibrium.[1] Conversely, a reduction of ECF sodium or an increase in free water produces an osmotic gradient that favors a shift of water intracellularly. A normal concentration of ECF sodium is, thus, maintained, and ECF osmolality reflects intracellular osmolality. With free access to water and salt, an elderly person should be able to maintain a normal ECF volume and osmolality. Under conditions of sodium restriction, ECF sodium is conserved through renal tubular reabsorption and a reduced secretion of sodium in sweat and stool. A loss of ECF water is prevented primarily by renal mechanisms, particularly reabsorption of water in the collecting tubules under the influence of antidiuretic hormone (ADH). There probably exists a set point for sodium homeostasis that can be re-set under conditions of a sodium surfeit or deficit.[18] Derangements in these homeostatic mechanisms frequently are iatrogenic, caused by drug or fluid therapies.

In addition to dietary factors and renal function, sodium and water balance are influenced by extrarenal factors. Hydrostatic pressure and colloid osmotic pressure play hemodynamically important roles in maintaining ECF volumes. For example, increases in hydrostatic pressure or decreases in colloid osmotic pressure favor increases in extravascular (interstitial) fluid at the expense of intravascular (plasma) volume. Catecholamines (norepinephrine) increase hydrostatic pressure and reduce plasma volume. Prostaglandins also influence hydrostatic pressures and modulate the renal handling of sodium.[19] Mineralocorticoids secreted by the adrenal gland (e.g., aldosterone) influence the renal handling of sodium and water at the distal tubule. The role of brain peptides and the importance of the central nervous system in the regulation of body fluids is now being elucidated.[20] The mechanisms that control the balance of sodium and water are complex, but elderly persons retain the capacity to maintain fluid balance until illness or iatrogenic complications intervene.

Hyponatremia

Hyponatremia (serum sodium < 135 mEq/l) is the most common disorder of water balance seen in a geriatric patient. The state of water excess termed hypo-osmolality, usually is brought to the clinician's attention by a laboratory finding of a low serum sodium. Mild hyponatremia usually is asymptomatic and may result from a mild defect or delay in urinary dilution during ingestion or infusion of hypotonic fluids. However, when hyponatremia accompanies marked hypotonicity and hypo-osmolality, non-specific symptoms of water intoxication may be seen, such as a depressed sensorium, confusion, lethargy, anorexia, weakness, muscle cramps, or even fasciculations.[21] These symptoms can be confused with many common illnesses in an elderly person, such as depression, sepsis, malignancy, or dementia. Severe or acute hyponatremia (serum sodium < 110 mEq/l) may produce seizures or stupor.[23] Since hyponatremia may occur in the setting of any physical stress such as fever, acute viral illness, surgery, or heart failure, its symptoms may be difficult to interpret. Indeed, hyponatremia (serum sodium < 135 mEq/l) occurs commonly in hospitalized patients.[22] The clinician, therefore, should be suspicious of its possibility in an appropriate clinical setting when an elderly patient presents with or develops vague symptoms and non-specific physical signs.

Logical approaches to the classification of hyponatremia are based on serum osmolality, ECF volume (*see* Figure 15-1), and mechanisms that produce the hyponatremia.[22] The etiology of hyponatremia can be derived from measuring (or estimating) serum tonicity and estimating ECF volume; hyponatremia is either isotonic, hypertonic, or hypotonic, and hypotonic hyponatremia is either isovolemic, hypervolemic, or hypovolemic. Serum osmolality (Osm) can be measured directly or estimated, based on the formula:

$$\text{serum Osm} = 2 \times \text{plasma sodium (mEq/l)} + \frac{\text{blood glucose (mg/dl)}}{18} + \frac{\text{blood urea}^{24}}{2.8}$$

Isotonic Hyponatremia

The serum osmolality is normal (280–295 mosm) and the ECF volume is normal. This situation occurs when there is a decrease in the fractional content of plasma (pseudohyponatremia) due to hypertriglyceridemia or paraproteinemia (e.g., myeloma). The osmolality and sodium concentration ([Na]) of the clear serum actually is normal when the protein or lipid is removed.[15,22] Isotonic infusions of glucose, mannitol, and glycine (initially restricted to ECF) dilute serum [Na] and represent iatrogenic causes of isotonic hyponatremia.

Hypertonic Hyponatremia

The serum osmolality is increased (>295 mOsm) and so is the ECF volume. This situation results from hyperglycemia, and transiently, from an infusion of hypertonic solutions that contain effective osmols.[15] Serum [Na] falls by 1.5 mEq/l for each 100 mg/dl increase in serum glucose. The treatment of isotonic and hypertonic hyponatremias is directed at correcting the underlying cause.

Hypotonic Hyponatremia

The serum osmolality is low (<280 mOsm) and the ECF volume either is normal, increased, or decreased. These are common and important causes of hyponatremia. The specific etiologies of hypotonic hyponatremia with reduced total body sodium include renal losses (diuretics, sodium-losing disorders, renal tubular acidosis), gastrointestinal losses (vomiting, diarrhea), or other causes ("third-spacing," adrenal insufficiency). Therapy consists of isotonic sodium repletion. Hypotonic hyponatremia with an increased total body sodium (expanded ECF) is seen in edematous states (congestive heart failure, cirrhosis, nephrotic syndrome) and in severe malnutrition ("dilutional" hyponatremia). Therapy consists of sodium and, if necessary, water restriction plus the judicious use of diuretics. Hypotonic hyponatremia with normal total body sodium and ECF occurs in acute water intoxication, excessive secretion of ADH, chronic renal failure, acute glucocorticoid insufficiency, hypothyroidism, and potassium depletion. Therapy depends on the etiology of the hyponatremia.

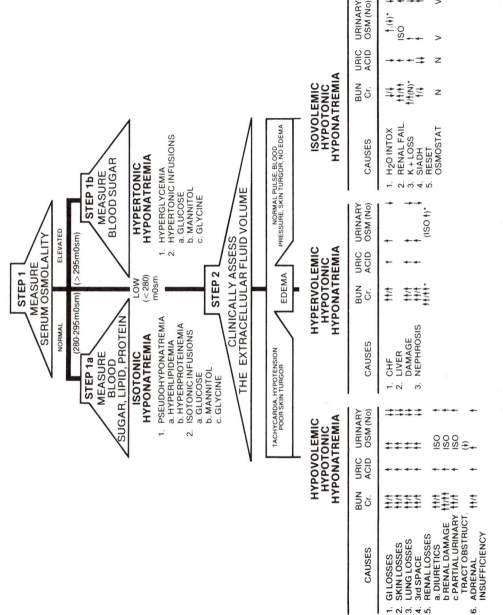

FIGURE 15-1 Diagnosis of fluid and electrolyte disorders. Abbreviations: mOsm = milliosmoles; ISO = isotonic; GI = gastrointestinal; CHF = congestive heart failure; K = potassium; N = normal, no change; V = variable; BUN = blood urea nitrogen; Cr = serum creatinine level. Adapted from Narins RG, Jones ER, Stom MC, et al: Diagnostic strategies in disorders of fluid, electrolyte and acid-base homeostasis. *Am J Med* 72:496–520, 498, 1982. Used by permission of author and publisher.

Diuretics

Of all drug therapies used in elderly patients, diuretics produce the greatest disturbances in fluid and electrolyte metabolism.[25] Hyponatremia due to diuretics probably results from several different mechanisms: 1) Avid reabsorption of sodium and water by the proximal tubule in response to the contraction of ECF volume; 2) Secretion of ADH in response to hypovolemia; 3) Severe potassium depletion (common in elderly persons) due to diuretics; and 4) Impairment of the urinary-diluting capacity.[8,24] Urinary losses of electrolytes may be replaced in error by hypotonic fluids (water via mouth or 5% dextrose in water via infusion) that contribute further to the hyponatremia. Most of the natriuresis and reduction in ECF volume from oral diuretics occurs in the first few days of therapy. If sodium intake is limited but free water is not, the risk of hyponatremia is markedly increased. Superimposition of other drugs that interfere with fluid balance or acute physical stresses (e.g., surgery) may lead to severe hyponatremia and water intoxication.[26] In contrast, the hyponatremia that is associated with chronic diuretic therapy usually is mild and asymptomatic.

Severe hyponatremia can be avoided in an elderly person if the clinician uses diuretics conservatively, in low doses, without severe sodium restriction or excessive free-water administration, and if serum electrolytes are monitored shortly after therapy is begun. Hyponatremia due to diuretics is best treated by stopping drug therapy, repleting ECF sodium, and replacing potassium losses. In extreme cases of hyponatremia with water intoxication, IV infusion of hypertonic (3%) saline may be life saving,[8] if infused in amounts that are sufficient to raise serum sodium by about 50% of the deficit within 8 hours. A more rapid correction may be dangerous in an elderly patient with cardiovascular disease and may require hemodynamic monitoring. The osmotic effects of hyponatremia are distributed throughout TBW; a calculation of the solute required for correction is based on an estimation of TBW.[24]

Other Drugs

Drugs other than diuretics may cause hyponatremia by affecting water excretion. These drugs act by stimulating ADH secretion or po-tentiating the renal effects of ADH. The list of suspected drugs is lengthy;[24,26] the most important ones used in elderly persons include the oral hypoglycemic agent chlorpropamide (Diabinese), carbamazepine (Tegretol) (used for tic doloreux, neuropathies, and seizure disorders), and the phenothiazines such as thioridazine (Mellaril). Treatment usually consists of simply stopping the offending drug.

Syndrome of Inappropriate Secretion of ADH (SIADH)

Excess secretion of ADH in response to osmotic and non-osmotic stimuli is common in elderly persons and is a result of normal aging.[6] However, when chronic hyponatremia occurs in the absence of appropriate physiologic stimuli that normally affect ADH secretion, SIADH should be suspected. The differentiation of primary SIADH from appropriate secondary elevations of ADH often is difficult or impossible under usual clinical circumstances. Furthermore, the specific etiologies of SIADH are diverse, ranging from ectopic secretion of ADH to abnormal secretion by the neurohypophysis.[27] The diagnosis of SIADH requires that hypo-osmolality and persistent ADH secretion occur in the absence of hypovolemia or hypotension. The basic abnormality in most cases is a failure to fully suppress ADH when the plasma osmolality falls below a normal threshold level. In the absence of direct laboratory measurements for ADH, the criteria for SIADH include: 1) Hypotonic hyponatremia; 2) Inappropriate antidiuresis (urine osmolality higher than anticipated for the degree of hyponatremia); 3) Normal renal function; 4) Normal adrenal and pituitary function; 5) Excretion of appreciable amounts of sodium when the patient is euvolemic; 6) Absence of clinical signs of hypovolemia and dehydration; 7) Absence of conditions causing edema or ascites; and 8) Correction of the hyponatremia and natriuresis by severe fluid restriction.[24] Urine osmolality usually exceeds plasma osmolality, and urine sodium is commonly >30–40 mEq/l. The diagnosis of SIADH may become easier to make in the future when the radioimmunoassay for arginine vasopressin (ADH) becomes widely available. However, in the appropriate clinical setting, the diagnosis can be readily suspected.

In elderly persons, abnormalities of the central nervous system are the most common causes of SIADH. Strokes, subarachnoid hemorrhages, seizures, head trauma, brain tumors, meningitis, encephalitis, and brain abscesses are causes of SIADH originating in the central nervous system. Pulmonary diseases (especially acute respiratory failure), severe pneumonias, active tuberculosis, and mycotic infections can produce this syndrome. Although less common, the ectopic production of ADH (or ADH-like substances) due to neoplasms receives considerable attention. An oat cell carcinoma of the lung is the most important of these neoplasms, while cancer of the prostate and pancreas are occasional causes of SIADH. Drug-induced isovolemic hyponatremia (discussed previously) produces a clinical picture that is similar to SIADH.

The therapy for SIADH depends on its cause and the severity of the hyponatremia. When hyponatremia is accompanied by clinical evidence of acute water intoxication, emergent therapy with hypertonic saline is warranted. Intravenous administration of hypertonic saline, given as a 3% (513 mEq/l) or 5% (855 mEq/l) solution at a rate of 3 ml/kg of body weight per hour for 2 hours, will raise serum sodium levels by 5–10 mEq/l.[27] Intravenous furosemide administration, concomitantly with hypertonic saline, has its proponents; but, it also may produce electrolyte disturbances and acute volume depletion, thereby minimizing its usefulness. Once the serum osmolality begins to rise, the hypertonic saline infusion can be slowed, and the serum sodium raised above 130 mEq/l over the ensuing 24–48 hours. Those patients with an abnormal diluting capacity due to drugs, intrinsic renal disease, or decreased osmotic gradients in the corticomedullary portions of the kidney are difficult to manage. Most patients with SIADH have a transient disorder and are, at most, mildly symptomatic. They can be managed satisfactorily with water restriction or IV infusion of normal saline solution. When the syndrome is chronic (e.g., oat cell carcinoma), other therapies may be employed. Salt supplements may suffice. Lithium carbonate has been used, but demeclocycline is considered the superior therapeutic agent and may obviate the need for severe water restriction.[28]

In general, while SIADH can produce profound hyponatremia, most cases of acute water intoxication are iatrogenic—a point that cannot be overstated. Also, before an elderly patient undergoes an exhaustive workup for possible SIADH, the clinician should first carefully review a patient's medication history and fluid intake. Diuretic therapy or an excessive infusion of hypotonic IV solutions is far more common than the ectopic production of ADH as a cause of hyponatremia. The rapid recognition of its likely etiology and the institution of appropriate therapy can reduce the morbidity of hyponatremia.[23]

Other Causes of Hyponatremia

Advanced organ diseases can produce hypervolemic hyponatremias in edematous patients. Congestive heart failure, hepatic cirrhosis, nephrotic syndrome, and severe hypoproteinemia due to nutritional or gastrointestinal disorders often present with asymptomatic hyponatremia. The total body sodium level is increased in these patients, but it is maldistributed so that the effective arterial plasma volume is reduced. Consequently, sodium reabsorption is increased and ADH levels often are elevated; urine output is reduced and urine sodium is less than 20 mEq/l. Therapy often is unsuccessful. Diuretics that work at two different sites in combination (e.g., metolazone and furosemide) often are helpful in reducing the edema of congestive heart failure, even in previously "refractory" cases. These patients usually require hospitalization with close attention to fluid balance and electrolytes.

Several endocrine disorders can produce hyponatremia. Adrenal insufficiency and myxedema are relatively uncommon causes of severe hyponatremia. Chronic hyponatremia and impaired water excretion may be seen in glucocorticoid insufficiency. Treatment consists of replacing the deficient hormone in each case.

Hypernatremia

Hypernatremia ([Na] > 150 mEq/l) occurs uncommonly in conscious people with free and ready access to water. Its presence is always accompanied by hypertonicity and hyperosmolality, although the patient's ECF volume may be normal, expanded, or depleted.[15] Hypervolemic hypernatremia results from an expansion of the ECF when the sodium gain is greater than the water gain. This situation is most commonly iatrogenic, secondary to IV infusions of hypertonic solutions such as sodium bicarbonate ([Na] = 1,000 mEq/l), which is given for treatment of acidosis. Less commonly, mild hypernatremia results from an exogenous or endogenous excess of mineralocorticoids (e.g., primary aldosteronism). In isovolemic hypernatremia, there is a loss of TBW with a relatively normal ECF volume. This form of hypernatremia most commonly results from the evaporative loss of water from the skin and respiratory tract. The febrile patient whose sensorium is depressed, and who is consequently unable to request water, is likely to present this way. Iatrogenic hypernatremia can result from replacement of hypotonic fluid losses with isotonic fluids. Because the ECF volume usually is near normal, these patients usually are not hypotensive when the hypernatremia is mild ([Na] < 160 mEq/l). Polyuric forms of isovolemic hypernatremia in elderly persons are uncommon; nephrogenic and central forms of diabetes insipidus usually are secondary to another disease process.

When the ECF volume depletion is characterized by water loss in excess of sodium loss, the result is hypovolemic hypernatremia. This form of hypernatremia occurs when hypotonic fluid is lost during the course of various renal and gastrointestinal disorders. In elderly persons, hypovolemic hypernatremia results most commonly from an acute gastroenteritis and from an osmotic diuresis. Increased urea formation, due to muscle catabolism during starvation or feeding protein-rich meals to catabolic patients, can produce an osmotic diuresis and hypernatremia. Glucosuria due to diabetes mellitus or an excessive infusion of hypertonic glucose is another cause of free water loss that leads to hypernatremia. Fever, tachypnea and reduced fluid intake in an elderly person can produce profound hypernatremia; the serum sodium concentration can exceed 200 mEq/l, yet the patient may survive if treated vigorously with fluids.[29] Of all the hypertonic states that can lead to hypovolemic hypernatremia, the most important is hyperglycemia.

Hyperglycemia will raise the osmolality of the ECF, and will produce an osmotic shift of water out of the cells and contract the ICF volume. The resultant expanded ECF volume should lower the serum sodium concentration by 1.5 mEq/l for every 100 mg/dl increase in serum glucose. In severe hyperglycemia, therefore, a "normal" or only slightly increased serum sodium is inappropriate, which indicates a considerable free-water deficit. The magnitude of this deficit can be estimated from standard formulas,[30] and the "true" or corrected serum sodium can be estimated as such:

$$\text{corrected serum [Na]} = \text{measured serum [Na]} + \left[\frac{\text{excess blood sugar (mg/dl)}}{100} \times 1.5 \right]$$

The combination of glucosuria with an osmotic diuresis and loss of ICF water produces a patient who is markedly dehydrated with depressed sensorium, hypotension, prerenal azotemia and (usually) tachycardia. Left untreated, the result is diabetic ketoacidosis or non-ketotic hyperosmolar coma.[31,32]

Polyuria and hypernatremia in the absence of hyperglycemia should arouse the clinician's suspicion of diabetes insipidus. Both nephrogenic and neurogenic (central) diabetes insipidus may present with polyuria, prerenal azotemia, normal urinary sodium excretion, and decreased urine osmolality. In elderly patients, most cases of central diabetes insipidus are acquired, being secondary to a disease of the central nervous system. Tumors or their treatment (e.g., surgery) may produce central diabetes insipidus; metastatic carcinoma due to lung or breast and primary tumors, such as a meningioma, are common causes. Vascular abnormalities, trauma, and granulomatous diseases such as sarcoidosis are less frequently implicated as causes of central diabetes insipidus.[27] Irrespective of the etiology, symptoms can be attributed to a deficiency of ADH secretion. Clinical manifestations can be variable, from mild polyuria and nocturia to extreme polyuria and thirst. The therapy is dictated by the severity of symptoms, etiology of the disease, and acceptability of the treatment to the patient. Primary therapy is hormonal replacement, with 1-deamino-8-D-arginine vasopressin (DDAVP) being the drug of choice for complete central diabetes insipidus.[33] Adjunctive therapies for patients with partial central defects include thiazide diuretics, chlorpropamide, and (less commonly) clofibrate. The differentiation between neurogenic diabetes insipidus and nephrogenic diabetes insipidus (where renal response to ADH is diminished) or primary polydipsia may become easier with the introduction of a radioimmunoassay for ADH.[34]

Nephrogenic diabetes insipidus results from the failure to either maintain the osmotic gradient in the renal medulla or use the gradient in the presence of adequate ADH.[33] Abnormalities of urinary concentration may be seen in disorders that decrease fractional solute reabsorption by the ascending portion of Henle's loop (e.g., urinary tract obstruction), increase urinary fractional solute excretion (e.g., post-obstructive diuresis), increase solute loss from the renal medulla (e.g., polydipsia), produce resistance to ADH (e.g., lithium, hypercalcemia, hypokalemia), or involve a combination of these mechanisms (e.g., amphotericin toxicity, analgesic nephropathy).[7] The therapy for nephrogenic diabetes insipidus consists of stopping the offending agent and treating the underlying disease. These elderly patients are prone to dehydration; therefore, access to free water must be available. Hormonal therapy is ineffective and drug therapies, with the occasional exception of thiazide diuretics, are not helpful.

Regulation and Disorders of Potassium Balance

Potassium is the major intracellular cation of the body. In healthy young adults, approximately 98% of total body potassium is intracellular. With aging and the loss of lean body mass (muscle), body potassium decreases. Even in apparently healthy patients over 65 years of age, total body potassium may decline by an average of 10%.[35] In hospitalized elderly patients, there are marked reductions in total body potassium and an increased ratio of body sodium to potassium.[36] The clinical significance of these changes is unclear; however, an elderly person may develop clinical evidence of potassium deficiency due to changes in dietary habits or the use of kaliuretic drugs, such as diuretics. Malnutrition (particularly in a chronically ill, alcoholic, edentulous, depressed, or institutionalized patient) and a dietary preference for foods low in potassium, contribute further

to potassium deficiency in elderly persons. Gastrointestinal and renal losses contribute to potassium deficiency; the excessive use of laxatives account for common intestinal losses and reduced tubular reabsorption that lead to obligatory urinary losses of potassium.[36,37]

Potassium homeostasis is conveniently divided into two inter-related systems, external and internal potassium balance.[38] Fluctuations in total body potassium levels are under external balance and determined by net differences in potassium intake and excretion. The distribution of potassium between ECF and ICF compartments depends on internal balance. The factors that influence external balance, such as renal and gastrointestinal changes with aging and dietary habits and medication use, have been alluded to already. Internal balance is determined by factors that influence the movement of potassium between fluid compartments.[37-39] Several factors alter internal potassium balance: 1) Acid-base disturbances that shift potassium into or out of cells; 2) Hypertonicity that shifts potassium out of cells; 3) The hormones insulin, aldosterone, catecholomines, glucagon, and growth hormones; and 4) Exercise that causes a release of potassium from muscles.[39] The secretion of insulin and aldosterone is influenced by plasma-potassium concentration; a deficiency of both hormones may precipitate hyperglycemia. Metabolic acidosis produces hyperkalemia, although the effects of mineral acids differ from those of organic acids. In lactic acidosis, for example, hyperkalemia parallels the severity of acidemia, but it probably correlates better with muscle catabolism (increasing potassium release into the ECF) and impaired renal function.[40] Epinephrine has a hypokalemic effect that is independent of insulin, aldosterone, or the renal excretion of potassium; the mechanism appears to be beta-adrenergic stimulation.[41] These mechanisms, which influence potassium balance, have important and sometimes confusing effects on plasma potassium levels in elderly persons. For example, while diuretics produce hypokalemia (a negative external balance), the addition of beta-adrenergic blockers (especially to insulin-deficient patients) may raise plasma potassium levels (internal balance favors a shift of potassium from the ICF to ECF) to misleadingly normal or near normal levels.

Hypokalemia

Hypokalemia may occur when the total body potassium level is normal, but it is most common when body potassium is depleted. There are numerous etiologies of hypokalemia,[15] but only a few are particularly common in elderly persons (see Table 15-3). The symptoms of hypokalemia are variable, ranging from none to severe muscle weakness or even paralysis. Most patients can tolerate a moderate reduction of potassium (5–10% of the total body potassium level) without symptoms. With larger losses, neuromuscular symptoms predominate, such as weakness, myalgias, cramps, restless legs, and (occasionally) fasciculations and paralysis.[21] In elderly persons, neuropsychiatric symptoms manifest as a depressive reaction with anorexia, apathy, and fatigue, or as a dementia with memory loss, disorientation, and confusion.[42] Severe potassium depletion produces dramatic abnormalities in organ function; cardiac and skeletal muscles and kidneys are especially susceptible to adverse consequences. The urinary-concentrating ability is impaired, which produces polyuria, nocturia, and a defect that is resistant to fluid restriction or the administration of ADH.[7] Cardiac manifestations of hypokalemia include ventricular arrhythmias and electrocardiographic abnormalities (depression of ST-segments, T-wave flattening or inversion, and prominent U-waves). Severe potassium depletion produces structural damage of the skeletal muscle, which leads to areflexia, respiratory paralysis, or even frank rhabdomyolysis. In addition, hypokalemia causes an exacerbation of glucose intolerance, especially in patients receiving thiazide diuretics.

Hypokalemia has numerous etiologies. Laboratory error is a rare cause of hypokalemia. Shifts in internal balance can produce a redistribution of potassium between cells (ICF) and plasma (ECF); the most common causes are metabolic alkalosis, insulin administration, and respiratory alkalosis. Potassium depletion is most commonly related to increased renal excretion and extrarenal losses of potassium (see Table 15-3). Decreased dietary intake is a rare cause of symptomatic hypokalemia in hospitalized patients who are maintained on a low-potassium diet for an extensive period and in a malnourished outpatient.

Diuretics are the most common cause of hypokalemia in elderly persons. Diuretics produce an immediate increase in potassium excretion. The mechanisms of the kaliuresis are complex, but involve an increased secretion of potassium in exchange for sodium. Elderly persons seem to be particularly prone to potassium deficiency due to diuretics. Although older studies have shown only mild losses of body potassium due to diuretic therapy, more recent studies suggest that potassium losses can be profound.[43] The prevention of potassium depletion can be attempted with the administration of a high-potassium diet (fruits and vegetables) or supplemental potassium chloride preparations (to replete concomitant chloride losses). Salt substitutes can be used in lieu of table salt. Modest potassium deficits can be corrected with a potassium chloride liquid or (when necessary) tablets. Intravenous potassium repletion is reserved for patients with severe hypokalemia, and impaired neuromuscular or myocardial function, or in those who are unable to eat. Potassium-sparing diuretics often are effective in preventing hypokalemia, but the risk of hyperkalemia is also greater in elderly persons.

Osmotic diuresis due to hyperglycemia,

TABLE 15-3 Causes of Potassium Deficit and Hypokalemia in Elderly Persons

Decreased dietary intake

Increased renal excretion
  Diuretics
  Osmotic diuresis
  Carbonic anhydrase inhibitors
  Metabolic alkalosis
  Ketosis/ketoacidosis
  Renal disorders—potassium wasting
    Renal tubular acidosis
    Drugs
  Endocrine disorders
    Primary aldosteronism
    Cushing's Syndrome
  Edematous states

Extrarenal losses
  Gastrointestinal
    Vomiting
    Laxative use (diarrhea)
    Colonic secretion
  Skin (sweating)

mannitol or urea infusions, or an increased urea excretion during protein catabolism, produces a marked kaliuresis. Potassium losses seen with starvation are, in part, due to the osmotic diuresis produced by urea. Ketoacids produced during starvation or diabetic ketoacidosis are anions that produce both an osmotic diuresis and an obligatory cation loss (especially sodium and potassium). The reduction of the ECF volume may lead to secondary aldosteronism and a further renal depletion of potassium. Therapy consists of fluid and electrolyte repletion as well as correction of the underlying disease process. Following muscle catabolism, potassium requirements are increased as muscle nitrogen is restored. This situation occurs, for example, when an elderly person is injured or has a stroke and is left immobilized and dehydrated for several days.

Renal tubular acidosis and renal toxicity of drugs can produce severe hypokalemia. Amphotericin B, for example, produces renal tubular dysfunction that leads to an increased exchange of potassium for hydrogen ions, and a clinical syndrome consistent with Type I renal tubular acidosis.[44] The coexistence of a metabolic acidosis and hypokalemia, in the absence of ketoacidosis, suggests the possibility of renal tubular acidosis.

Endocrine disorders are occasional causes of hypokalemia. Primary aldosteronism rarely has its initial presentation in an elderly patient; when it does, hypertension, metabolic alkalosis, and suppressed plasma renin activity accompany the hypokalemia. Hypokalemia in an untreated hypertensive patient, though, is more commonly associated with accelerated hypertension or renal artery stenosis. Cushing's Syndrome in an elderly person should make the clinician suspicious of an ectopic adrenocorticotropic (ACTH) hormone production (e.g., due to oat cell carcinoma of the lung). The excess production of mineralocorticoids due to ectopic ACTH secretion can produce marked hypokalemia.

Edematous states such as cirrhosis, congestive heart failure, and nephrotic syndrome are common causes of hypokalemia. The effective arterial plasma volume is reduced in these disorders. As a result, sodium is reabsorbed preferentially and kaliuresis occurs. Diuretic therapy may cause further potassium depletion.

Also, metabolic alkalosis probably contributes to the hypokalemia in these patients.[37]

Other renal causes of hypokalemia include antibiotics, carbonic anhydrase inhibitors, magnesium deficiency, and acute leukemia. High-dose sodium penicillin or carbenicillin therapy enhances potassium secretion; an increased delivery of fluid to the distal nephron results in the excretion of these relatively non-reabsorbable anions. Gentamicin also is known to produce kaliuresis through an uncertain renal mechanism. Lysozymuria that is associated with acute leukemia may produce renal potassium wasting.

Gastrointestinal illnesses are the principal causes of extrarenal potassium depletion. Vomiting produces hypokalemia through several mechanisms. The gastric losses of hydrogen and chloride produce a metabolic alkalosis that leads to renal potassium excretion. In addition, the loss of dietary and intestinal potassium (5–20 mEq/l), plus shifts of potassium intracellularly, contribute to the hypokalemia. Diarrhea, which is frequently due to acute gastroenteritis or laxative use, increases potassium excretion from the colon. A villous adenoma of the colon also can cause severe potassium depletion by increasing potassium secretion. Another extrarenal cause of potassium depletion is excessive sweating. However, because the concentration of potassium in sweat is so low (about 5–10 mEq/l), large amounts of sweat loss would be necessary before depletion becomes significant.

In most instances, the etiology of hypokalemia is easily determined. When the etiology is obscure, measurements of urinary electrolytes can be of diagnostic value. In general, given normal renal function, urinary potassium is <20 mEq/day and urinary sodium is >100 mEq/day when hypokalemia is due to extrarenal losses; urinary potassium is >20 mEq/day when hypokalemia is due to renal losses.[15]

Hyperkalemia

True hyperkalemia (serum potassium level >5.5 mEq/l) occurs most commonly when the internal balance favors the movement of potassium out of the cells and into the ECF compartment, or when renal excretion of potassium is decreased. Less commonly, it results from administration of an exogenous load of potassium, particularly when renal excretion is impaired. Hyperkalemia can result from derangements in the external balance due to an increased potassium intake (e.g., potassium salts, hemolysis during blood transfusions), renal failure, and hypoaldosteronism (e.g., Addison's disease). Alterations in the internal balance that produce hyperkalemia include metabolic acidosis, insulin deficiency and hypoaldosteronism, and tissue necrosis (e.g., rhabdomyolysis, hemolysis). In part, the acute hyperkalemia that is induced by hyperglycemia is related to concomitant hypertonicity. Some drugs may raise serum potassium concentrations by causing an efflux of potassium from the cells (e.g., beta-blockers). Digitalis toxicity can cause severe hyperkalemia. Renal prostaglandin inhibition by non-steroidal anti-inflammatory drugs is a potentially serious cause of hyperkalemia in elderly persons.[19]

There are several causes of a spurious elevation of serum potassium concentration. Hemolysis during venipuncture, before serum is separated from the clot, is the most common cause of "pseudohyperkalemia." During clotting, potassium is released from platelets and other cells, thus causing serum potassium to exceed plasma potassium concentrations by up to 0.5 mEq/l. With severe leukocytosis or thrombocytosis (e.g., myeloproliferative disease), the difference between plasma and serum measurements can be much greater. These differences can be demonstrated by comparing serum and plasma potassium levels from the same blood specimen.[15]

Acute hyperkalemia, in the absence of renal failure, occurs most commonly in elderly persons as a result of cellular catabolism and the administration of potassium-sparing diuretics or potassium-containing drugs (e.g., potassium supplements or potassium salts of antibiotics). Consequently, physicians should be alerted to the possibility of hyperkalemia when patients present with crush injuries or burns. Potassium supplements are especially likely to cause hyperkalemia in diabetic patients with hyporeninemic hypoaldosteronism.

The clinical manifestations of hyperkalemia usually are subtle until the serum potassium level is markedly elevated ($>6.5-7.0$ mEq/l). Symptoms and signs are non-specific and include apprehension, weakness, hyporeflexia, paresis, and fasciculations.[21] Electrocardiogram (ECG) abnormalities include peaked T-waves and, when hyperkalemia becomes life threatening, loss of P-waves and widening of the QRS complex.

For mild elevations of serum potassium levels, conservative therapy such as potassium restriction generally will suffice. When the potassium level exceeds 7.0 mEq/l or characteristic ECG changes of hyperkalemia appear, emergent therapy is warranted. For life-threatening hyperkalemia, infusions of calcium gluconate, glucose, and insulin, or sodium bicarbonate are indicated.[42,45] Treatment of hyperkalemia due to renal disease is discussed in Chapter 16.

In general, ambulatory geriatric patients rarely present to the clinician with severe hyperkalemia. Indeed, hyperkalemia in an elderly patient is most commonly iatrogenic, caused by potassium supplementations or infusions and the use of potassium-sparing diuretics. Thus, most cases are preventable.

Acid-Base Disorders

Disturbances of acid-base balance are common in elderly persons. These disturbances can be categorized conveniently as simple and mixed acid-base disorders.[16,46,47] Simple disorders include respiratory acidosis or alkalosis and metabolic acidosis or alkalosis. Mixed disorders include combinations of simple disorders. Homeostatic mechanisms normally maintain the blood within a narrow range of normal pH (7.36–7.44). Acidosis develops from the excessive retention of acids—either the retention of carbonic acid (H_2CO_3) that is produced from carbon dioxide (CO_2) or the accumulation of a fixed hydrogen (H^+) ion and its anion. A change in acid-base balance is compensated by the extracellular and intracellular buffer systems, respiratory compensation, and renal handling of excess acids and bases. For practical purposes, the serum bicarbonate concentration [HCO_3^-] reflects the metabolic response to changes in H^+ and its accompanying anions, while the pCO_2 of the blood reflects the respiratory response to changes in H_2CO_3. Buffers, such as phosphates and sulfates, can accept or donate H^+ ions, thereby modifying changes in pH. The interdependence of pH, HCO$_3^-$ and H$_2$CO$_3$ is reflected in the Henderson-Hasselbach equation:

$$pH = pK + \log \frac{(HCO_3^-)}{(H_2CO_3)}$$

An increase in [HCO$_3^-$] raises pH and causes a metabolic alkalosis, while a decrease in [HCO$_3^-$] lowers pH and causes a metabolic acidosis. Elevation of pCO$_2$ lowers pH and causes a respiratory acidosis, while a reduction of pCO$_2$ results in a respiratory alkalosis. The respiratory response (ventilation) to metabolic changes in pH is rapid but usually incomplete. In contrast, metabolic compensation (renal handling of HCO$_3^-$) is slower but nearly complete.[46] The addition of mineral acids (e.g., hydrogen chloride) produces a metabolic acidosis (hyperchloremic or normal anion gap acidosis). When a metabolic acidosis is due to the accumulation of anions and their respective protons (which consume bicarbonate), an anion gap acidosis results and serum [HCO$_3^-$] is decreased.

In healthy young adults, the compensatory response to simple acid-base disorders can be anticipated.[46] These generalizations, however, may be less reliable in an elderly population. As mentioned earlier, physiologic changes in aging influence the metabolic and respiratory response to changes in acid-base balance (see Table 15-2). Respiratory compensation for an acute metabolic acidosis (hyperventilation) may be blunted in an elderly person, thus leading to an inadequate compensation. The relative hypercapnia combined with the metabolic acidosis yields a pH lower than expected. The impact of such an incomplete compensation on the prognosis is unclear, but respiratory acidosis and metabolic acidosis frequently occur together in elderly patients with congestive heart failure, severe pneumonia, and acute respiratory failure. In a critically ill patient, acid-base disturbances are likely to be mixed. For example, diuretics produce a metabolic alkalosis (increased HCO$_3^-$) and may be used to treat a patient with congestive heart failure who has hypoxemia and a poor tissue perfusion that can produce a lactic acidosis (decreased HCO$_3^-$). The net result may be a normal or only slightly decreased HCO$_3^-$, while the pH is increased due to primary or compensatory respiratory alkalosis (hypocapnea). In general, though, the type of acid-base disturbance can be characterized through a measurement of blood pH, bicarbonate, and pCO$_2$. Of the various disorders, the differential diagnosis of metabolic acidosis seems most challenging, while metabolic alkalosis is most common.

Metabolic Acidosis

Metabolic acidosis is categorized according to the presence or absence of an anion gap.[48] The anion gap is estimated as Na − (Cl + HCO$_3^-$), and usually is 12 mEq/l ± 4. Normally, unmeasured cations and anions are present in the serum in small amounts (see Table 15-1). When an increase occurs in unmeasured anions such as sulfate, protein, organic acids, phosphate, or lactate, the result is an anion gap acidosis. On the other hand, an increase in unmeasured cations can produce a decrease in the anion gap (e.g., from myeloma protein or hypermagnesemia), but it is rarely associated with a clinically important disturbance of acid-base balance. Metabolic acidosis with a normal anion gap occurs in renal tubular acidosis, diarrhea (due to loss of bicarbonate or organic acid anions), and from the administration of chloride-containing acid (e.g., NH$_4$Cl). Metabolic acidosis is far more common, though, with an increased anion gap. In elderly persons, lactic acidosis is the most serious cause of this problem.

Lactic acidosis usually is associated with an apparent tissue hypoxia. Shock, hypoperfusion due to severe anemia and hemorrhage, congestive heart failure, and severe hypoxemia, can produce a severe metabolic acidosis due to marked increases in the serum lactate. Lactate accumulation after major motor seizures usually is transient, but it can cause severe acute acidosis. The acidosis of diabetic ketoacidosis is, in small part, due to lactate accumulation. Slight rises (usually inconsequential) in the serum lactate occur during exercise, carbohydrate infusions, and catecholamine administration.

The ingestion of drugs and toxins is an important cause of metabolic acidosis with an increased anion gap. Of these, aspirin intoxication is the most common and produces a mild elevation of the anion gap. Patients may use aspirin for a variety of reasons, some that are medically indicated and others that are not (e.g., as a sleeping aid). Aspirin intoxication may be a consequence of a deliberate or unintentional overuse and of delayed metabolism (excretion). With mild intoxication, for example, a confused patient may ingest toxic amounts of aspirin unaware of the adverse consequences. Aspirin intoxication usually is managed easily via diuresis, alkalinization of urine, and withholding of the drug; rarely are dialysis or hemodynamic monitoring necessary. Other intoxicants (and their anions) that are known to produce a metabolic acidosis with an anion gap include methanol (formate) and ethylene glycol (glycolate).

Ketoacidosis produces a mild or moderate metabolic acidosis through the retention of the anions, β-hydroxybutyrate and acetoacetate. Diabetic ketoacidosis is the most obvious cause of an increased anion gap, but starvation ketosis and alcoholic ketosis may be more common. Ketosis is detected by finding a positive nitroprusside test (strip or tablets) of the urine or by elevated blood levels of β-hydroxybutyrate. Since the urine may be negative by a dip-stick test, the addition of a few drops of hydrogen peroxide will oxidize urinary β-hydroxybutyrate to the nitroprusside-positive acetoacetate.[15] Finally, renal failure decreases the serum bicarbonate through the retention of organic acids, sulfates, and phosphates. In general, with a reasonable history and physical examination and use of a few simple tests, the cause of an elevated anion gap acidosis is easily ascertained, and appropriate therapy can be instituted.[46]

The hyperchloremic metabolic acidoses (normal anion gap) often are associated with either hyperkalemia or hypokalemia. A hypokalemic acidosis occurs most frequently with renal tubular acidosis and diarrhea; carbonic anhydrase inhibitors (e.g., acetazolamide) and ureteral diversions are less common causes. A hyperkalemic acidosis is seen in early renal failure and hypoaldosteronism.

Metabolic Alkalosis

Metabolic alkalosis in an elderly person usually is a consequence of excessive losses of acid (e.g., vomiting) or a contraction of ECF, thus increasing serum bicarbonate (e.g., diuretic therapy). Chloride losses due to secretory diarrhea or vomiting produce a saline-responsive form of alkalosis that is best corrected by reexpanding the ECF volume with normal saline solution. The renal alkalosis that is produced by diuretics and poorly reabsorbable anions (e.g., carbenicillin) also is saline responsive. Chloride is retained and a sodium and bicarbonate diuresis ensues. On occasion, a saline-unresponsive alkalosis results in severe potassium depletion or excess secretion of aldosterone. A severe metabolic alkalosis (e.g., pH > 7.55) causes neuromuscular irritability and occasional abnormalities on an ECG, particularly when associated with reduced levels of ionized calcium. A patient with a mixed respiratory and metabolic alkalosis is especially at risk for these complications. For example, patients with congestive heart failure often have a primary respiratory alkalosis and receive diuretic therapy that leads to a mixed alkalosis. In this setting, severe alkalosis also can sensitize a patient to digitalis toxicity. Careful attention to blood gases and ECG monitoring helps prevent serious complications of alkalosis.

Respiratory Acidosis and Alkalosis

Respiratory acidosis results from hypoventilation and the consequent retention of CO_2. Hypoventilation is most commonly due to cardiopulmonary diseases (asthma, obstructive lung disease, pneumonia, congestive heart failure), which increase H_2CO_3 production and $[H^+]$. The depressed ventilation due to drugs (e.g., opiates, barbiturates) is a more subtle and preventable cause of respiratory acidosis. Treatment is directed at increasing ventilation by correcting the underlying problem and using assisted ventilation when necessary.[46]

Respiratory alkalosis results from hyperventilation with an excessive loss of CO_2. Cardiopulmonary diseases can cause hyperventilation that leads to a respiratory alkalosis. Central causes include strokes, severe anxiety, metabolic encephalopathy, and gram-negative septicemia. Indeed, hyperventilation with respiratory alkalosis in confused or obtunded patients suggests a diagnosis of sepsis. Treatment, once again, is directed at the underlying cause. With severe alkalosis, rebreathing devices (e.g., masks) are useful.

Disorders of Calcium, Phosphorus, and Magnesium Balance

Calcium and phosphorus metabolism is discussed in Volume 1, Chapter 28. A few points warrant emphasis here. Hypercalcemia is commonly observed in elderly persons. Thiazide diuretics, hyperparathyroidism, and malignancies probably are the most common causes. Thiazides cause hypercalcemia through several mechanisms, which include hemoconcentration, enhanced renal calcium reabsorption, and (possibly) the augmented effects of parathyroid hormone (PTH) on bone. The hypercalcemia is reversed on discontinuing the thiazide diuretic. Changes in PTH levels and calcitonin secretion occur in elderly persons, and manifestations of hyperparathyroidism are variable.[49-51]

Hypocalcemia usually is a result of hypoalbuminemia; the serum calcium decreases by 0.8 mg/dl for every gram/dl decrease in serum albumin. Less commonly, hypocalcemia results from severe magnesium deficiency that impairs PTH secretion and its effects on bone. Hypoparathyroidism, which is usually secondary to surgical extirpation of the parathyroids, can cause hypocalcemia. Treatment consists of calcium and Vitamin D supplementation.

Hyperphosphatemia is less common than hypophosphatemia and usually is secondary to renal disease. Less commonly, hyperphosphatemia results from the use of enemas that contain phosphate, from rhabdomyolysis, or from IV phosphate infusion. Hypophosphatemia, in contrast, is relatively common in hospitalized patients and is due to gastrointestinal losses or an internal redistribution of phosphates (from ECF to ICF). The latter is most common when poorly nourished patients receive IV glucose. The infused glucose promotes acute cellular uptake of inorganic phosphates, which sometimes leads to severe hypophosphatemia.[52] Acute hypophosphatemia is frequently seen in starving patients and alcoholics and during IV hyperalimentation with phosphate-deficient solutions. The hypophosphatemia due to gastrointestinal losses usually is a result of secondary hyperparathyroidism that accompanies hypocalcemia and malabsorption of Vitamin D. Phosphate-binding antacids occasionally can cause reductions in serum phosphate. Other causes of mild hypophosphatemia in elderly persons include hyperparathyoidism, thiazide diuretic use, and respiratory alkalosis. Severe hypophosphatemia (phosphate < 1.0 mg/dl) produces severe biochemical disturbances that lead to neuromuscular dysfunction and hematologic abnormalities (paresis and hemolytic anemias), and it usually warrants phosphate therapy.

The interest in magnesium metabolism has increased in recent years. Elderly persons often have a dietary intake of magnesium below recommended levels and decreased serum levels. The clinical importance of these observations, however, is unclear.[53] Thiazide and loop diuretics perhaps are the most common causes of magnesium deficiency. Less commonly, hypomagnesemia results from dietary deficiencies, intestinal losses, and drug toxicities. A moderate to severe magnesium deficiency may result in hypocalcemia; PTH secretion is impaired and skeletal resistance to PTH occurs.[54] Therapy with magnesium sulfate is indicated when magnesium deficiency is symptomatic (e.g., when accompanying hypocalcemia). Symptomatic hypermagnesemia is uncommon and usually results from magnesium administration in patients with an impaired renal excretion.

References

1. Maxwell MH, Kleeman CR (eds): *Clinical Disorders of Fluid and Electrolyte Metabolism.* New York, McGraw-Hill Book Co, 1980.
2. Brenner BM, Rector FC (eds): *The Kidney.* Philadelphia, WB Saunders & Co, 1981.
3. Cohn SH, Vartsky D, Yasumura S, et al: Compartmental body composition based on total-body nitrogen, potassium, and calcium. *Am J Physiol* 239:E524–E530, 1980.
4. Shock NW: Physiologic aspects of aging in man. *Ann Rev Physiol* 23:97–122, 1961.
5. Masoro EJ (ed): *CRC Handbook of Physiology of Aging.* Boca Raton, FL, CRC Press, Inc, 1981.
6. Rowe JW: Aging and renal function, in *Annual Review of Gerontology and Geriatrics.* (Eisdorfer C ed.) New York, Springer-Publishing 1980, vol 1, pp 161–179.
7. Jamison RL, Oliver RE: Disorders of urinary concentration and dilution. *Am J Med* 72:308–322, 1982.
8. Ashraf N, Locksley R, Arieff AI: Thiazide-induced hyponatremia associated with death or

neurologic damage in outpatients. *Am J Med* 70:1163–1168, 1981.

9. Cox M, Sterns RH, Singer I: The defense against hyperkalemia: the roles of insulin and aldosterone. *N Engl J Med* 299:525–532, 1978.

10. Greenblatt DJ, Sellers EM, Shader RI: Drug disposition in old age. *N Engl J Med* 306:1081–1088, 1982.

11. Cockcroft DW, Gault MH: Prediction of creatinine clearance from serum creatinine. *Nephron* 16:31–41, 1976.

12. Bruce A, Andersson M, Arvidsson B, et al: Body composition. Prediction of normal body potassium, body water and body fat in adults on the basis of body height, body weight and age. *Scand J Clin Lab Invest* 40:461–473, 1980.

13. Moritani T, DeVries HA: Potential for gross muscle hypertrophy in older men. *J. Gerontol* 35:672–682, 1980.

14. Rowe JW, Minaker KL, Sparrow D, et al: Age-related failure of volume-pressure-mediated vaopressin release. *J Clin Endocrinol Metab* 54:661–664, 1982.

15. Narins RG, Jones ER, Stom MC, et al: Diagnostic strategies in disorders of fluid, electrolyte and acid-base homeostasis. *Am J Med* 72:496–520, 1982.

16. Bia M, Thier SO: Mixed acid base disturbances: a clinical approach. *Med Clin North Am* 65:347–361, 1981.

17. Humes HD, Narins RG, Brenner BM: Disorders of water balance. *Hosp Pract* 14:133–145, 1979.

18. Hollenberg NK: Set point for sodium homeostasis: surfeit, deficit, and their implications. *Kidney Int* 17:423–429, 1980.

19. Levenson DJ, Simmons CE, Brenner BM: Arachidonic acid metabolism, prostaglandins and the kidney. *Am J Med* 72:354–374, 1982.

20. Krieger DT, Martin JB: Brain peptides. *N Engl J Med* 304:876–885, 944–951, 1981.

21. Knochel JP: Neuromuscular manifestations of electrolyte disorders. *Am J Med* 72:521–535, 1982.

22. Flear CTG, Gill GV, Burn J: Hyponatremia: mechanisms and management. *Lancet* 2:26–31, 1981.

23. Arieff AI, Llach F, Massry SG: Neurological manifestations and morbidity of hyponatremia: correlation with brain water and electrolytes. *Medicine* 55:121–129, 1976.

24. Goldberg M: Hyponatremia. *Med Clin North Am* 65:251–269, 1981.

25. Madias NE, Zelman SJ: What are the metabolic complications of diuretic treatment? *Geriatrics* 37:93–104, 1982.

26. Moses AM, Miller M: Drug-induced dilutional hyponatremia. *N Engl J Med* 291:1234–1239, 1974.

27. Robertson GL, Aycinena P, Zerbe RL: Neurogenic disorders of osmoregulation. *Am J Med* 72:339–353, 1982.

28. Forrest JN, Cox M, Hong C, et al: Superiority of demeclocycline over lithium in the treatment of chronic syndrome of inappropriate secretion of antidiuretic hormone. *N Engl J Med* 298:173–177, 1978.

29. Goldszer RC, Coodley EL: Survival with severe hypernatremia. *Arch Int Med* 139:936–937, 1979.

30. Feig PU: Hypernatremia and hypertonic syndromes. *Med Clin North Am* 65:271–290, 1981.

31. Arieff AI, Carroll HJ: Nonketotic hyperosmolar coma with hyperglycemia: clinical features, pathophysiology, renal function, acid-base balance, plasma-cerebral fluid equilibria and the effects of therapy in 37 cases. *Medicine* 51:73–94, 1972.

32. Arieff AI, Carroll HJ: Cerebral edema and depression of sensorium in nonketotic hyperosmolar coma. *Diabetes* 23:525–531, 1974.

33. Singer I: Polyuria and diabetes insipidus. *Med Clin North Am* 65:303–320, 1981.

34. Zerbe RL, Robertson GL: A comparison of plasma vasopressin meausurements with a standard indirect test in the differential diagnosis of polyuria. *N Engl J Med* 305:1539–1546, 1981.

35. Lye M: Distribution of body potassium in healthy elderly subjects. *Gerontology* 27:286–292, 1981.

36. Cox JR: Potassium changes with age. *Gerontology* 27:340–344, 1981.

37. Cohen JJ: Disorders of potassium balance. *Hosp Pract* 14:119–128, 1979.

38. Cox M, Sterns RH, Singer I: The defense against hyperkalemia: the roles of insulin and aldosterone. *N Engl J Med* 299:525–532, 1978.

39. Sterns RH, Cox M, Feig PU, et al: Internal potassium balance and the control of the plasma potassium concentration. *Medicine* 60:339–354, 1981.

40. Fulop M: Serum potassium in lactic acidosis and ketoacidosis. *N Engl J Med* 300:1087–1089, 1979.

41. Rosa RM, Silva P, Young JB, et al: Adrenergic modulation of extrarenal potassium disposal. *N Engl J Med* 302:431–434, 1980.

42. Lindeman RD, Klingler EL: Combating sodium and potassium imbalance in older patients. *Geriatrics* 36:97–106, 1981.

43. Ram CV, Garrett BN, Kaplan NM: Moderate sodium restriction and various diuretics in the treatment of hypertension: effects of potassium

wastage and blood pressure control. *Arch Int Med* 141:1015–1019, 1981.

44. Sebastian A, Hulter HN, Kurtz I, et al: Disorders of distal nephron function. *Am J Med* 72:289–307, 1982.

45. Kunau RT, Stein JH: Disorders of hypo- and hyperkalemia. *Clin Neph* 7:173–190, 1977.

46. Narins RG, Gardner LB: Simple acid-base disturbances. *Med Clin North Am* 65:321–346, 1981.

47. Narins RG, Emmett M: Simple and mixed acid-base disorders: a practical approach. *Medicine* 59:161–187, 1980.

48. Emmett M, Narins RG: Clinical use of the anion gap. *Medicine* 56:38–54, 1977.

49. Insogna KL, Lewis AM, Lipinski BA, et al: Effect of age on serum immunoreactive parathyroid hormone and its biological effects. *J Clin Endocrinol Metab* 53:1072–1074, 1981.

50. Shamonki IM, Frumar AM, Tataryn IV, et al: Age-related changes of calcitonin secretion in females. *J Clin Endocrinol Metab* 50:437–439, 1980.

51. Fiatorone MA, Steel K, Egdahl RH: Hyperparathyroidism in the elderly. *J Am Geriatr Soc* 29:343–348, 1981.

52. Agus ZS, Goldfarb S: Clinical disorders of calcium and phosphate. *Med Clin North Am* 65:385–399, 1981.

53. McConway MG, Martin BJ, Nugent M, et al: Magnesium status in the elderly on hospital admission. *J Clin Exp Gerontol* 3:367–379, 1981.

54. Rude RK, Singer FR: Magnesium deficiency and excess. *Ann Rev Med* 32:245–259, 1981.

CHAPTER **16**

Nephrology

THOMAS A. GOLPER, M.D.

Physiologic Changes in the Senescent Kidney

Morphologic Changes

Between the 4th–8th decades of life, the kidneys lose about 20% of their weight, with a greater loss occurring in the cortex.[1] Particularly in the medulla, there is a generalized increase in interstitial fibrosis. In vessels larger than arterioles, progressive reduplication of elastic tissue and a thickening of the intima occurs. These changes are similar to those that are observed with chronic hypertension; but, they are present even in the absence of systemic arterial hypertension. They are followed by a subendothelial deposition of hyaline in the afferent (preglomerular) arterioles of the cortex. Hyalinization results in an obliteration of the vessel lumen, a loss of blood flow, and the ultimate collapse of the glomerular tuft. As glomeruli sclerose in the juxtamedullary region, anatomic continuity between afferent and efferent arterioles develops. As a result, the blood flow to the medulla is maintained, but the cortical flow is compromised.

About 50% of all glomeruli are lost through the vascular process described above. At the same time, other events transpire throughout the nephron with their own functional implications. Both glomerular and tubular basement membranes focally thicken and reduplicate. Tubular cells undergo a fatty degeneration. Proximal convoluted tubules collapse because of tubular wall atrophy that is associated with a cloudy swelling of tubular cells. Diverticula develop in the distal convoluted tubule. These may enlarge to become simple cysts and can become loci for bacterial growth.

A significant ultrastructural change in the senescent kidney is the mesangial deposition of macromolecular material, mainly IgM. It has been proposed that the glomerular capillary becomes more permeable with aging and that the mesangial clearing of globulins is impaired with a resulting accumulation. The physiologic significance of this finding is not known.

Renal Blood Flow

Total renal blood flow is maintained through the 4th decade, but it thereafter declines 10% per decade.[2] This decline in the blood flow represents a decrease in the perfusion per gram of renal tissue, and it is not merely a reflection of the diminished renal size.[3] Decreased renal perfusion in senescence occurs predominantly in the cortex, with a relative sparing of a deeper medullary blood flow. Although there is a mild fall in cardiac output in aging, the decrement in the renal blood flow is best explained by intrarenal morphologic changes.

Glomerular Filtration Rate (GFR)

From the 4th–6th decades, there is a linear decrease in creatinine clearance of 6.5 ml/minute/1.73m^2/decade. Beyond 60 years of age, the decrement in the GFR approaches 17 ml/minute/1.73m^2/decade.[4,5] The reduction of creatinine clearance with age is accompanied by a parallel reduction in the total daily urinary creatinine excretion, which reflects a decreased muscle mass. Muscle mass, creatinine production, release, and excretion are all reduced. Therefore, an unchanged serum creatinine is found despite a decrease in creatinine clearance.

In elderly study subjects with asymptomatic bacteriuria, the GFR was 18% lower than in non-infected age-matched subjects.[6] Furthermore, when followed for 22 months, the rate of fall of the GFR was three times faster in the elderly subjects with asymptomatic bacteriuria.

Sodium Handling

Senescence significantly impairs a kidney's capacity to conserve and excrete sodium (Na). Subjects over 60 years of age require 31 hours to lower urinary sodium excretion in response to sodium deprivation. Study subjects under 30 years of age accomplish the reduction in urinary sodium in 18 hours.[2] The renal blood flow and GFR decrements in senescence do not explain this inability to conserve sodium. It is presumed to be partially related to the increased solute load per nephron, as in other forms of renal insufficiency. Renin and aldosterone levels are lower in elderly subjects.[7] The entire renin-aldosterone system responds sluggishly in senescence and may contribute to the defect in sodium conservation. Renal prostaglandins also may have a contributory role.[8] Primarily because of the lower GFR, an aging kidney is less able to excrete an acutely administered sodium load compared to younger kidneys. Therefore, elderly persons are less able to rapidly adapt to changes in salt intake, which leads to either extracellular volume depletion or circulatory overload.

Potassium Handling

The impaired renin-aldosterone system and decreased GFR create a situation in which potassium excretion could be impaired. However, the sodium wasting seen in senescence may balance these factors, since distal sodium delivery also is a key determinant of potassium secretion. Thus, there may be a tendency toward either potassium retention or kaluresis in aging, depending on which factors are dominant in an individual patient.

Glucose Reabsorption

The maximum rate of the renal tubular reabsorption of glucose in the 9th decade is 40% of that observed in the 3rd decade.[9] This has only a minor clinical significance.

Renal Acidification

In the basal state, there are no major differences in acid excretion and urine pH between elderly and younger male subjects.[10] However, after an acute acid load (NH_4Cl), older males excrete less acid and the urine pH (4.9) is not decreased as much as that observed in the younger males (pH 4.5). Furthermore, ammonium excretion is reduced in elderly persons even after correction for the GFR. These data are consistent with the renal acidification defect commonly seen in cases of early to moderate renal insufficiency, regardless of age.[11] A decreased number of ammonium-producing renal cells, a decreased protein and phosphorus intake, decreased muscle mass (decreased titratable acid production), and an impaired aldosterone system all contribute to the impaired renal excretion of acid in senescence. Clinical repercussions are only seen during an acid stress, as in diabetic ketoacidosis or shock. In this setting, hyperkalemia may develop.

Concentration and Dilution

Older patients are less able to concentrate their urine after either water deprivation or the administration of an antidiuretic hormone (ADH).[12] At 80 years of age, the maximum urine concentration is 850 mosm/kg, which is about 70% of that achieved by 30-year-old study subjects. Since the urine concentration does not rise with ADH administration, the concentration defect is clearly renal in origin. The age-related decrement in the GFR is the most likely cause. Also, the shunting of blood towards the renal medulla may result in medullary solute "washout" and, thus, contribute to the concentration defect. Under conditions of free access to water, this concentration defect is insignificant. Under conditions of water deprivation or high-insensible or other water losses the risk of hypernatremia and a true water depletion are great. Furthermore, the presence of asymptomatic bacteriuria in an apparently normal elderly person is associated with a further significant reduction of the maximum urinary osmolarity, ranging from 625–826 mosm/kg.[13]

Antidiuretic hormone responses change in elderly persons.[14] Although a hypertonic saline solution (a secretory stimulus) induces a similar rise in serum osmolarity, older study subjects experience an ADH rise twice that of the younger subjects. Ethanol (an inhibitory stimulus) does not inhibit ADH secretion in elderly subjects as it did in the younger group. These data support the concept that the clinically observed excess of ADH secretion in elderly persons is a result of normal aging. The risk of water intoxication and hyponatremia is high in the presence of fever, psychological stress, acute viral illness, anesthesia, and surgery; all are situations where ADH secretion is stimulated.

Clinical Assessment of Renal Function in Elderly Persons

Creatinine Clearance (Ccr)

Creatinine is produced and released into the blood stream at a constant rate by skeletal muscle. When the serum creatinine level is stable, the amount of creatinine excreted daily is proportional to the lean muscle mass; 14–22 mg/kg/day in an adult female, 20–25 mg/kg/day in an adult male. There can be a daily variation of 25% in creatinine excretion. Therefore, clinical decisions should not be based on a single, isolated Ccr collection.

The following formula can be used to predict the Ccr from the serum creatinine level, body weight, and patient's age. It is reasonably reliable without a timed urine collection.[15]

$$Ccr = \frac{(140 - age) \times (body\ weight\ in\ kg)}{72 \times serum\ creatinine\ in\ mg/dl}$$

This result should be multiplied by 0.85 for females.

Serum Creatinine

The reduction in the Ccr with age is attended by a parallel reduction in daily urinary creatinine excretion, which reflects the decrease in lean muscle mass. The resulting net effect is no significant change in the serum creatinine level with aging.[4] The interpretation of a serum creatinine level must, therefore, include a bedside estimate of a patient's lean muscle mass.

Blood Urea Nitrogen (BUN)

The blood (serum) urea nitrogen (BUN) level varies considerably on a day-to-day basis, because it is dependent on the dietary protein intake and urine flow rate. When urine flow is reduced, urea has time to back-diffuse from urine to blood, which decreases urea clearance. The BUN normally rises only a few mg/dl with aging.

BUN/Serum Creatinine Ratio

This ratio normally is between 5 and 20. In the geriatric population, the BUN/Creatinine ratio is elevated when:

1. Dietary protein intake is increased.
2. Catabolic states exist where endogenous protein is broken down, which includes gastrointestinal bleeding, starvation, Glucocorticosteroid therapy, massive tissue ischemia, and severe trauma such as burns or crush injuries.
3. The urine flow rate is reduced as in prerenal azotemia (congestive heart failure, nephrotic syndrome, volume depletion, and [occasionally] hepatic cirrhosis), or in a urinary tract obstruction.
4. Tetracycline is ingested concomitant with a renal insufficiency.
5. Urinary diversion into the gastrointestinal tract is created.

The BUN/Creatinine ratio is decreased in the geriatric population when:

1. Protein intake is low.
2. Liver disease leads to reduced urea production.
3. Dialysis removes urea more efficiently than it does creatinine.
4. Rhabdomyolysis occurs, whereby muscle cells release excessive amounts of creatinine.

Urinalysis

It is not unusual to see more epithelial cells and hyaline casts in the urine of elderly patients. However, the senescent kidney normally does not "leak" red or white blood cells, glucose, or protein into the urine. There is a slight decrease in the tubular reabsorption of glucose, but the serum glucose level must be elevated for glycosuria to be observed. Asymptomatic bacteriuria is more common in elderly persons, but is is not a normal accompaniment of aging.

Plain X-Ray Film of the Abdomen or KUB

On an x-ray film study of the abdomen (KUB), the kidneys of older people are not smaller than the kidneys of younger people, when compared to vertebral body dimensions.[16] Large kidneys on a KUB usually imply a cystic disease, amyloidosis, early diabetes mellitus, or an acute hydronephrosis. Small kidneys usually imply a chronic renal disease. Asymmetric renal sizes can be seen in a renovascular disease, infection, and obstruction, as well as in many other disorders. A plain x-ray film sometimes reveals vascular and prostatic calcifications and radioopaque urinary tract stones.

Intravenous Pyelography (IVP)

This examination remains the best standard for defining the urologic and nephrologic gross anatomy. Nonetheless, the decision to employ this procedure requires that the information to be gained outweighs the risks involved. Radiographic contrast agents are hyperosmolar and induce an osmotic diuresis. In addition, the increased serum osmolarity draws extravascular water into the vascular space, which possibly precipitates a circulatory congestion. In elderly persons, there is a high incidence of renal injury associated with IVPs.[17] Since elderly persons often have diminished GFRs, but normal serum creatinine levels, pre-existing renal insufficiency frequently is unappreciated by the physician before requesting a radiocontrast examination. Most nephrologists feel that although age does not necessarily predispose a patient to a contrast agent nephropathy, renal insufficiency accompanying aging is a major risk factor. Other risk factors include situations that decrease renal perfusion (volume depletion, low cardiac output, hypotension, and vascular disease), multiple myeloma, diabetes mellitus, hyperuricemia, hyperuricosuria, proteinuria, the concomitant use of nephrotoxic drugs, and

a known hypersensitivity to radiocontrast agents. The indications, risks, and alternatives should be weighed in each case. Routine use of IVPs in elderly persons is not appropriate. When other studies will not suffice and precautions have been taken, an IVP can be performed. The avoidance of both multiple contrast studies (upper gastrointestinal series, cholecystogram, and so on) over several days and of volume depletion (e.g., from cleansing enemas) lowers the risk of a contrast agent nephropathy. The administration of hypertonic mannitol 1 hr after the contrast material may be effective in preventing acute renal failure.[18]

Arteriography

This procedure carries the same risk of developing a contrast agent nephropathy. There is an additional risk of a vascular injury, including atheroemboli, thrombotic emboli, and a direct catheter trauma to the vascular wall. These complications are more likely to occur in elderly persons because of atherosclerotic blood vessels.

Computed Tomography (CT scan)

A CT scan without contrast is a valuable alternative diagnostic tool for patients with a serious risk of a reaction to radiocontrast agents. It is even more effective when contrast agents can be employed.

Ultrasonography

This non-invasive procedure is essentially risk free and helpful in evaluating abnormalities that are frequently seen in the geriatric population. Obesity may obscure accurate imaging; otherwise, the B-mode scanning with gray scale imaging is accurate in the assessment of a urinary tract obstruction and renal masses.[19,20] Posterior views should be attempted if abdominal views are inadequate.

Radionuclide Imaging

Radioactively labelled technetium that is chelated by diethylenetriamine penta-acetic acid (^{99m}Tc DTPA) is filtered and excreted the same as inulin, which allows a delineation of renal outlines. It also marks the renal transit time, which is prolonged when there is a reduced GFR, renovascular constriction, volume depletion, and urinary obstruction. Radioiodinated hippuran is excreted by filtration and secretion, and it is helpful in evaluating the renal blood flow and tubular secretion. There is a relatively low radiation exposure. Imaging is not as precise as in an IVP, but in the geriatric population, the lower risks favor the renogram.

Radioisotope renograms are a helpful, adjunctive diagnostic tool in geriatric uronephrology to assess the relative blood flow to each kidney (renovascular disease), the size, shape, position, and function of each kidney, the evaluation of masses such as tumors or abscesses, the effect of lower urinary tract disease on renal function, and the status of renal transplants. Abnormal renograms in 25 of 35 elderly study subjects demonstrated focal areas of diminished uptake.[16] The focal scan defects were considered to be ischemic areas secondary to vascular insufficiency. The deterioration of renal function seen with aging was found to be asymmetric, unrelated to intrinsic glomerular disease, and did not alter kidney size.

Renal Biopsy

When less invasive tests fail to establish a diagnosis, a renal biopsy procedure may be performed. The indications, alternatives, and risks[21] are not different for the geriatric population. A closed (percutaneous) renal biopsy procedure requires a few days of bed rest following the procedure. Increased postbiopsy activity may explain the higher complication rate in younger patients.[22] An open surgical biopsy has less risk of a postbiopsy hemorrhage, but requires usually up to 7 days of postbiopsy hospitalization.

Diagnostic Approach to the Geriatric Patient with a Renal Disease

Proteinuria

The initial task in the evaluation of proteinuria in elderly persons is to obtain information about the involvement of other organ systems, such as the genitourinary tract, heart, lungs, intes-

tines, bones, joints, and skin. Hypertension, diabetes, weight loss, and drug ingestion may be related to proteinuria.

A laboratory evaluation should exclude an orthostatic component, with a 24-hour urine collection (split by posture) for protein and creatinine clearance. Over 150 mg/day of protein in the urine is abnormal, but it may not require extensive evaluation. If the serum albumin level is not less than 3.5 grams/dl, a systemic complication of the proteinuria is less likely. Proteins with molecular weights lower than albumin are present in the urine in excessive amounts in such disorders as ischemic nephrosclerosis with proximal tubular damage, chronic interstitial nephritis (including pyelonephritis), and increased protein production states (such as multiple myelomas or acute leukemia). If the nephrotic syndrome is present, a more extensive evaluation includes a urine culture test, a urine and serum protein electrophoresis (for light chains), an SMA-12 chemistry panel, hemogram, antinuclear antibody test (ANA), antistreptococcal antibody battery, serum complement test, and a 2-hour postprandial blood sugar test. A renal biopsy procedure may be necessary.

Pyuria

More than a 3 white blood cells (WBC)/high power field on a repeated urinalysis usually reflects renal pathology that includes various forms of acute and chronic renal and systemic infections, chronic interstitial nephritis, analgesic nephropathy, prostatitis and nephrolithiasis. In addition to a careful history of drug ingestion, specific cultures may be needed for unusual organisms. An imaging study and bladder/prostate evaluation may be necessary.

Hematuria

When hematuria is accompanied by cellular casts, the glomerulus almost always is the origin of the blood. In the absence of casts, isolated hematuria can be secondary to infections, calculi, prostatic diseases, trauma, neoplasms, and an interstitial nephritis, as well as from a glomerular source (concomitant proteinuria). The highest priority must be given to excluding neoplasms. An isolated hematuria is urologic until proven otherwise, and imaging studies and a cystoscopy are necessary. The magnitude of the hematuria generally is not helpful diagnostically.

Glomerular Diseases

Mechanisms of Glomerular Injury

Three major mechanisms lead to glomerular damage: 1) The deposition of circulating immune complexes (CIC); 2) The in situ immune complex formation of antibodies against glomerular or circulating antigens; and 3) A cell-mediated injury. Often, an acute antigenic stimulus will result in smaller-sized immune complexes; these tend to localize in the subepithelial space (i.e., they get through the basement membrane). A chronic antigenic stimulus frequently results in the accumulation of complexes within the basement membrane (intramembranous). Large complexes do not pass the basement membrane and, therefore, localize subendothelially.

Classification of Glomerular Disease

Glomerular disease is initially detected by an abnormal urinalysis that reveals cells, casts, or protein (*see* Table 16-1). Nephrotic diseases are characterized by proteinuria (usually greater than 3.5 grams/day), hypercholesterolemia, hypoalbuminemia, and edema. Because edema in an elderly person often signifies congestive heart failure, a diagnosis of a nephrotic syndrome may be delayed. A nephrosis is seen in disorders where there is an increased glomerular permeability to protein. There usually is only minimal cellular proliferation, leukocyte infiltration or necrosis. In addition to the clinical features above, one might observe a lipiduria, mild or microscopic hematuria, but rarely a marked hematuria or red cell casts. Renal vein and other deep venous thromboses are not uncommon in cases of nephrosis. Occasionally, a nephrotic syndrome may present with pulmonary emboli. The GFR may be normal or modestly impaired on initial presentation.

The clinical features of acute nephritic diseases (*see* Table 16-1) in elderly persons are not very different from those seen in younger patients.[23,24] The most common manifestations are edema, dyspnea, circulatory congestion, infection and non-specific symptoms such as anorexia, nausea, vomiting, diarrhea, and muscle pain. Azotemia, oliguria, hypertension, hematuria, and varying degrees of proteinuria usually follow shortly thereafter.[23,24] Initially, patients are thought to have cardiac failure or infection, and renal disease is not considered. Furthermore, since many elderly patients are afflicted with such degenerative diseases as diabetes, hypertension, cardiac failure, and peripheral vascular diseases, the presence of azotemia, proteinuria, edema, and even hematuria often are attributed to an extrarenal pre-existing disorder.

Hemoptysis often is observed in elderly patients with a severe heart disease, bronchitis, malignancies, infections, endocarditis, circulatory congestion, pulmonary emboli, and certain vasculitides. Rapidly progressive glomerulonephritis (RPGN) is the most frequently observed, serious glomerulopathy of senescence.[25] Therefore, the presence of hemoptysis

TABLE 16-1 Glomerular Disease Classification by Presentation

Nephrotic	Nephritic
Membranous	Membranoproliferative
Minimal change	Vasculitis
Focal glomerulosclerosis	SLE*
Diabetes	IgA
Amyloidosis	Acute (postinfectious)
Occasionally membranoproliferative	Rapidly progressive
Occasionally vasculitis	Cryoglobulinemia
Occasionally SLE	

* SLE = systemic lupus erythematosus.

in association with the nephritic picture guides the clinician to consider a primary renal disease.

The major differential diagnosis of glomerulopathies is between primary renal diseases and systemic diseases with renal manifestations. Other primary renal diseases (i.e., diseases with a major extraglomerular pathology) occasionally can present with features similar to the nephrotic and nephritic diseases described above. A review of the causes of renal diseases in 115 elderly patients who had renal biopsy procedures is presented in Table 16-2.[25] These patients are not a representative sample of nephrology consultations in the geriatric population, but only those who ultimately underwent a biopsy procedure. Table 16-3 shows the clinical presentation of these patients and illustrates the significant overlap.

An IVP or other imaging study may detect large kidneys, which suggests diabetes or an

TABLE 16-2 Biopsy Proven Renal Disease in 115 Elderly Patients[25]

Primary glomerular disease	
Idiopathic crescentic GN*	19
Glomerulosclerosis	16
Membranous gn	15
Minimal change GN	9
Focal proliferative/mesangiopathic GN	7
Diffuse proliferative GN	5
Chronic GN	5
Membranoproliferative	2
	78
Extra-glomerular renal disease	
Interstitial nephritis	4
Acute tubular necrosis	2
Obstructive nephropathy	2
Atheromatous embolic disease	1
Gentamicin nephrotoxicity	1
	10
Systemic disease with renal involvement	
Vasculitis	6
Amyloidosis	5
Wegener's granulomatosis	4
SLE† with Nephritis	2
Scleroderma	2
Essential cryoglobulinemia	2
Other (myeloma, hemolytic-uremic syndrome, thrombotic thrombocytopenic purpura, sarcoidosis, lymphoma, macroglobulinemia—one each)	6
	27

* GN = glomerulonephritis.
† SLE = systemic lupus erythematosus.

amyloidosis if a nephrosis is present. The serum complement has proven to be helpful, as it is depressed in only a few renal disorders. Table 16-4 lists several diseases in which various components of the serum complement are abnormal. Other laboratory investigations may help clarify a diagnosis without a kidney biopsy. When a diagnosis can be clinically made because of a known underlying disorder (e.g., poststreptococcal infection, diabetes, amyloidosis, and so on) or in the presence of bilaterally shrunken kidneys and renal insufficiency, a biopsy may not be necessary. However, when a diagnosis is needed for a prognosis or for therapeutic intervention, a renal biopsy must be performed.

Diseases Usually Causing Nephrosis (see Table 16-1)

Membranous Glomerulonephropathy

This disorder is histologically characterized by IgG and C3 disposition in the glomerular capillary wall. It has a variety of causes that include systemic lupus erythematosus (SLE), carcinomas, drugs, and infections. Many cases are idiopathic, which accounts for 38% of all cases of nephrotic syndrome in patients over 60 years of age.[26] A complete remission can be expected in about 25% of all patients, while another will have a partial remission, another 25% will remain nephrotic, and the final 25% will progress to end-stage renal disease (ESRD).[27] There is a high incidence of renal vein thromboses (possibly associated with a proximal renal tubular acidosis) in membranous nephropathies with a nephrotic syndrome.[28] There is an increased incidence of neoplasia in patients with a membranous glomerulopathy.[26,29] Serologic studies tend to be normal. Prednisone in large, alternate day doses (80–120 mg) may be helpful in inducing a remission of the nephrotic syndrome and may help preserve renal function.[30]

Minimal Change Disease

This entity usually is not associated with any recognized antecedent events. It accounts for 23% of all cases of nephrosis in elderly persons.[26] Epithelial foot process fusion is seen on

TABLE 16-3 Classification of Patients According to Their Final Diagnosis and the Clinical Problem at Initial Evaluation[25]

Number	Final Diagnosis	Total Number of Patients	Major Clinical Problem at Initial Evaluation			
			Acute Renal Failure (<2 mo)	Chronic Renal Failure (>2 mo)	Nephrotic Syndrome (urine protein >3.5 g/day)	Hematuria and Proteinuria (<3.5 g/day)
1	Crescentic GN*	19	17	2	—	—
2	Membranous GN	15	—	—	13	2
3	Minimal change nephrotic syndrome	9	—	—	9	—
4	Focal proliferative GN	7	1	—	1	5
5	Diffuse proliferative GN	5	1	1	1	2
6	Chronic GN	5	1	1	2	1
7	Membranoproliferative GN	2	—	—	2	—
8	Glomerulosclerosis	16	1	6	2	7
9	Vasculitis	6	3	—	—	3
10	Amyloidosis	5	2	—	3	—
11	Wegener's granulomatosis	4	4	—	—	—
12	Interstitial nephritis	4	2	2	—	—

* GN = glomerulonephritis.

TABLE 16-4 Serum Complement in Glomerulonephritis

GN*	C1q	C4	C3
Acute postinfectious	↓	↓	↓ ↓
Membranoproliferative	↓ or N	↓ or N	↓ ↓ ↓
SLE†	↓	↓	↓ ↓
Endocarditis	↓	↓	↓ ↓
Idiopathic crescentic	?	?	↓

↓ Occasionally slightly decreased
↓ ↓ Decreased
↓ ↓ ↓ Markedly depressed
N Normal.
* GN = glomerulonephritis.
† SLE = systemic lupus erythematosus.

electron microscopy, but whether this is the primary defect or is secondary to the proteinuria is not clear. There is a loss of negative charges in the capillary basement membrane. In elderly patients, one must always consider hematologic neoplasms when minimal-change nephrotic syndrome is detected via renal biopsy.[31] This disease usually is responsive to glucocorticosteroids; but even when not, it does not often progress to ESRD.[26,32]

Focal Glomerulosclerosis

Early in the course of this disease, juxtamedullary glomeruli sclerose. A biopsy procedure may miss the involved glomeruli, and an early diagnosis of minimal-change disease might be mistakenly made. The correct diagnosis becomes evident as the disease progresses. No therapy has been shown to ameliorate the nephrotic syndrome or renal failure of glomerulosclerosis. IgM and C3 are deposited in the involved glomeruli. Foot processes are fused in all glomeruli. Local tubulo-interstitial damage can be severe and extensive.

Diabetes Mellitus

The natural history in maturity-onset diabetes is variable and may be accompanied only by hyperglycemia and glycosuria. Conversely, an identical course to that of type I diabetes may be seen. Juvenile-onset diabetes (type I) usually results in a nephrotic syndrome 15–20 years later. In the years before a nephrosis, the GFR may actually rise for unclear reasons.[33] Once proteinuria begins, ESRD develops in 3–5 years.

In diabetics, there is an increased risk of a contrast agent nephropathy, especially when the GFR is less than 50 ml/minute.[17] It is important to evaluate every diabetic for a neurogenic bladder and infection, since both may further comprise renal function. Hyporeninemic, hypoaldosteronemic, and hyperkalemic renal tubular acidosis is commonly observed when moderate renal failure ensues.[11] A devastating complication that often accompanies infection is renal papillary necrosis. The mainstays of therapy for the renal disease of diabetes are careful control of blood sugar, prompt treatment of infections and hypertension, avoidance of toxic agents, and preventing urinary obstructions and stasis.

Amyloidosis

Amyloid fibrils deposit in glomerular capillary loops and the mesangium. In primary amyloidosis, these fibrils are light chains with a composition similar to that of Bence-Jones proteins. In secondary amyloidosis, the fibrils are a non-immunoglobulin protein, serum amyloid A, which appears to be an acute phase reactant. A primary amyloidosis often is related to plasma cell dyscrasias and occurs primarily in patients over 50 years of age.[34] A secondary amyloidosis is associated with chronic inflammatory diseases such as rheumatoid arthritis, diabetes, ulcers, chronic urinary tract infections (as occurring in a neurogenic bladder), bronchiectasis, osteomyelitis, tuberculosis, inflammatory bowel disease, or Familial Mediterranean fever. Other organs are involved and biopsy specimens of the liver (90%), rectum (60–80%), gingiva (60%), and skin (50%), may be diagnostic, thus obviating the need for a renal biopsy procedure, which is positive in over 90% of all cases. All nephrotic patients, over 50 years of age should have urine and serum protein electrophoreses. Amyloidosis of the kidneys rarely is reversible, but treatment of the primary disease is mandatory for any chance of improving the renal status.[35,36] In one series, amyloidosis was the most frequent cause of secondary nephrotic syndrome in patients over 60 years of age.[26]

Diseases Usually Causing Nephritis (*see* Table 16-1)

Membranoproliferative Glomerulonephritis

This disease is unusual in the geriatric population.

Vasculitis

This disease may present with a nephritic picture and will be discussed in the section on vascular disease.

Systemic Lupus Erythematosus (SLE)

Lupus nephritis usually takes one of four histologic patterns: mesangial, focal proliferative, diffuse proliferative, or membranous. Hematoxylin bodies in peripheral capillary loops are very suggestive of SLE. With nephritis, native or single-stranded DNA may be primary antigens. Classic pathway complement activation occurs with a low C3 and C4 disposition (*see* Table 16-4). A low C3 and DNA binding frequently parallel the severity of the renal lesion. Although IgG is the most frequently seen glomerular immunoglobulin, IgM, IgA, C3, and C4 frequently are detected.[37] Deposits that are subendothelial carry the worst prognosis. Renal histopathology is common, even in the absence of clinical signs. Lupus nephritis may present with a nephritic or nephrotic picture, which is usually consistent with the lesions seen in biopsy specimens. Of all patients with SLE, 50% have an impaired GFR at presentation; eventually, 75% of all patients develop some renal insufficiency. In elderly patients, the manifestations usually are non-renal.[38] The tubulointerstitium also can be affected, which leads to distinct tubular syndromes such as renal tubular acidosis (RTA) or hyperkalemia.[39] The prognosis is determined both by renal and extrarenal involvement. Impressive responses occur with combined prednisone and azothiaprine therapy.[40]

IgA Nephropathy

This nephritic disorder is a disease of young persons. Nonetheless, 4 of 7 patients with "focal proliferative GN" is one geriatic series suffered from an IgA nephropathy (*see* Table 16-2).[25] IgA, IgG, and C3 are deposited focally in the mesangium and are associated with focal mesangial hypercellularity. When IgA is deposited in glomeruli, the differential diagnosis is essentially Henoch-Schonlein purpura, SLE, IgA nephropathy, and (occasionally) a membranous glomerulopathy. Of these patients, 15–40% will have a progression to ESRD. The disease usually begins with a gross hematuria following upper respiratory infections. Less commonly, it may present as a nephrotic syndrome or similar to an acute glomerulonephritis.[41] No known therapy alters the course of IgA nephropathy.

Acute Postinfectious Diffuse Proliferative Glomerulonephritis

An exudative, diffuse proliferative lesion with subepithelial IgG and C3 "hump" deposits characterize the histology of this disorder. In some patients, an acute nephritic picture is seen 7–21 days after streptococcal skin or throat infections, shunt infections, varicella and other viral illnesses, hepatitis B, abscesses or pneumococcal infections. Antistreptolysin O and antiDNAase B titers are both helpful in establishing a streptococcal etiology. The acute nephritic picture in elderly persons can be easily confused with the degenerative diseases of other organ systems. Oliguria may be a key feature of acute glomerulonephritides with a depressed serum complement level in the acute phase (*see* Table 16-4).[23] It is important to treat the underlying infection, but prednisone does not modify the course of the renal disease. Because of severe renal insufficiency and oliguria, the most common cause of death is a pulmonary edema that is secondary to circulatory congestion. If older patients can survive the initial insult (with dialysis therapy if necessary), the prognosis usually is good.[23–25] Thus, the emphasis should be on supportive care and dialysis to sustain them through this self-limited illness.

Idiopathic Rapidly Progressive Crescentic Glomerulonephritis (RPGN)

Idiopathic-crescentic glomerulonephritis was the most common diagnosis in the report of renal biopsy results in geriatric patients (*see* Tables 16-2, 16-3).[25] The term RPGN is an operational definition for a nephritic syndrome that progresses to renal insufficiency over a period of weeks. Some disorders mentioned above and some forms of vasculitis can behave the same as the idiopathic form. In a renal biopsy series, only 1 patient had hemoptysis and antiGBM antibodies were detected in only 1 of 11 patients.[25] The serum complement level can be mildly depressed, but it is not a characteristic feature (see Table 16-4). The histology is dominated by epithelial and endothelial cell proliferation, granulocytic exudation, interstitial damage, and crescents.[42] Although the prognosis is generally poor,[24] there are no reports of pulse steroid or plasmapheresis therapy for RPGN in the elderly population. There are data to support a trial of such therapy in the general population.[43]

Essential Mixed Cryoglobulinemia

IgG-IgM antigen-antibody complexes that precipitate when cold and dissolve on rewarming contribute to the development of glomerulonephritis. Chronic infections (e.g., hepatitis B surface antigenemia) and neoplasms (myeloma) must be excluded if cryoglobulins are detected. In the glomerulus, there is mesangial and endothelial cell proliferation, and also a basement membrane deposition of IgG, IgM, and complement. The presentation may vary from vague constitutional symptoms with an abnormal urinalysis to an acute oliguric-nephritic syndrome with a renal insufficiency. The avoidance of exposure to the cold and treatment of the underlying disease are the main components of therapy. With an acute severe disease, steroids, immunosuppressive agents, and plasmapheresis may be effective.[44]

Tubulo-Interstitial Renal Disease in Elderly Persons

There are three reasons to study this group of disorders. Particular acid-base and electrolyte disturbances accompany interstitial diseases.[45] Possibly one third of all patients with end-stage renal disease (ESRD) have had a primary chronic interstitial process that contributed to

their renal failure.[46] Thirdly, many forms of interstitial nephritis are easily treated. The causes of tubulo-interstitial nephropathies are listed in Table 16-5. These include glomerulonephritis, and vascular and obstructive diseases.

Acute Tubulo-Interstitial Nephritis

As shown in Table 16-5, there are many causes of this acute deterioration of renal function. An important early distinction in an evaluation is the presence of recent drug ingestion or allergic signs or symptoms. Acute, allergic tubulo-interstitial nephritis is particularly prevalent in elderly patients. Penicillin and its derivatives, cephalosporins, rifampin, sulfa-containing antibiotics and diuretics, several anticonvulsants, allopurinol, phenacetin, azothiaprine, and nonsteroidal anti-inflammatory drugs, are the most common precipitating agents. The latent period from the initial exposure to the clinical manifestations varies from 3–21 days. The major signs and symptoms, with frequency of occurrence, are erythrocyturia (91%), leukocyturia (83%), eosinophiluria (82%), mild to moderate proteinuria (82%), eosinophilia (80%), fever (77%), fever and eosinophilia (68%), rash (43%), rash and eosinophilia (38%), rash and fever (34%), gross hematuria (34%), and the classic triad of rash, fever, and eosinophilia (31%).[47] Oliguria develops in 20–50% of all afflicted patients, and evidence of tubular injury with salt wasting, an RTA, or impaired potassium excretion are not uncommon.

A differential diagnosis includes glomerulonephritis and acute tubular necrosis. Early in the course of the disease, the urine sodium concentration may be low. As the disease progresses and oliguria ensues, the urine chemistries appear more like those found in acute tubular necrosis.[48,49] Histologically, there is edema and mononuclear cell infiltration of the interstitium. Eosinophils and giant cells are not unusual. Evidence of tubular necrosis and regeneration is universal. A gallium-67 scan reveals a significant renal uptake after 48 hours.[49] Red cell casts are unusual in an acute interstitial nephritis. However, a biopsy specimen may be necessary to make a definitive diagnosis. An acute interstitial nephritis usually resolves itself spontaneously, albeit slowly.[50] Prednisone therapy markedly shortens the duration of impaired

TABLE 16-5   Causes of Tubulo-interstitial Nephropathies[45]

Acute Tubulo-Interstitial Nephritides

Associated with drugs
  Methicillin
  Penicillin and derivatives
  Cephalosporins
  Sulfa derivatives
  Antitubercular drugs
  Antiepileptic drugs
  Allopurinol
  Phenacetin

Associated with immunologic diseases
  Transplant rejection
  Sjogren Syndrome
  Systemic lupus erythematosis
Idiopathic

Associated with infection
  Bacterial
  Granulomatous
    Tuberculosis and leprosy
    Sarcoid
    Leptospirosis
    Toxoplasmosis
    Syphilis
    Mycetoma
  Viral (especially mononucleosis)
Secondary to interstitial inflammation
  Pyelonephritis
  Acute tubular necrosis
  Toxic
Secondary to primary glomerular disease
  or vasculitis

Chronic Tubulo-Interstitial Nephropathies

Metabolic
  Hypercalcemia
  Hyperuricemia
  Sickle cell
  Paroxysmal nocturnal hemoglobinuria
  Hyperoxaluria
Neoplastic
  Multiple myeloma
  Leukemia
  Lymphoma

Immunologic
  Sjogren Syndrome
  Systemic lupus erythematosis
  Transplant rejection
Toxic
  Analgesic
  Balkan
Hereditary
  Polycystic
  Medullary cystic

renal function. In elderly patients with a decreased organ reserve, a shortened course of renal failure may make a distinct difference in the functional outcome.

Chronic Interstitial Nephritis (*see* Table 16-5)

Although the causes vary, the final common renal injuries are tubular atrophy and dilatation, interstitial fibrosis, mononuclear cell infiltration, and periglomerular fibrosis.[46] Changes that are compatible with an arteriolar nephrosclerosis are present in about 25% of all patients. A chronic interstitial nephritis was the cause of ESRD in one third of the cases in one reported series.[46] The clinical and laboratory characteristics include a urinary sediment with pyuria (casts only present during acute infections), urinary protein excretion less than 2 grams/day (1+ to 3+ by dip-stick), a minimal microscopic hematuria, non-cellular casts, occasional hyperchloremic acidosis, occasional massive salt

wasting and radiologic evidence of interstitial or calyceal abnormalities, asymmetrical scarring, or papillary necrosis. This presentation may not necessarily differ much from the one seen in chronic glomerulonephritis, except that normotension and acid-base electrolyte abnormalities are more common in a chronic interstitial nephritis. The previously accepted idea that chronic or recurrent urinary tract infections cause chronic interstitial nephritis or ESRD recently has been less emphasized. In the setting of an obstructive process or other structural abnormality, however, infections probably do cause chronic damage.

The exclusion of multiple myeloma should have a high priority in the presence of a proximal renal tubular acidosis. Lupus and acute myelogenous leukemia also can present this way. The distal nephron group of chronic interstitial nephritides are clinically characterized by salt wasting, hyperkalemia, and hyperchloremic acidosis. Amyloidosis, certain antibiotics, hypercalcemia, hypergammaglobulinemia, chronic urinary obstruction, and granulomatous infections cause this clinical picture. The medullary dysfunction group is characterized by polyuria due to an impaired urinary concentration. An analgesic nephropathy, hypercalcemia, hyperoxaluria, sarcoidosis, and/or hypokalemia can lead to medullary dysfunction.

Analgesic Nephropathy

The frequency of arthralgias in old age increases the risk of long-term analgesic use and abuse. There is a relative risk to developing a chronic interstitial nephritis and ESRD from the regular use of large amounts of combined analgesics. No single drug ingredient is responsible. One must assume that almost any analgesic ingredient can cause the disorder. The newer non-steroidal anti-inflammatory drugs are definitely included. In addition to a decreasing medullary blood flow, these drugs may inhibit the hexose monophosphate shunt, which leads to an oxidative injury of medullary cells. This probably occurs because these drugs are concentrated in the medulla, especially in water-deprived states. The renal damage is dose-dependent, which leads ultimately to a papillary necrosis, chronic interstitial nephritis, and ESRD. Patients with an analgesic nephropathy are predominantly female (4:1, female to male), anemic, and have a history of upper gastrointestinal ailments, headaches, and psychiatric disturbances.[51] Hypertension is not unusual and may even be severe, as it is attributed to the high incidence rate of renal vascular atheromatous diseases in an analgesic nephropathy.[52] An IVP may reveal a papillary necrosis in 25–40%, small kidneys in 50–65%, and normal kidneys in 5–15% of all examined patients. The differential diagnosis of a papillary necrosis includes sickle-cell anemia, diabetes mellitus, renal tuberculosis, an obstructive uropathy, and an acute pyelonephritis.

Daily ingestion of analgesic drugs over many years leads to this condition. Careful questioning of a patient and the family may be necessary to elucidate this history. Serum tests for salicylates and acetaminophen are available. Establishing a diagnosis is important, since a discontinuation of the offending agents usually stabilizes or leads to improved renal function.

In a large, reported series, 74% of the patients studied stopped analgesic abuse, 18% took occasional doses, and 8% continued to use the drugs.[53] A decline in renal function was associated with a malignant hypertension, greater than 2 grams/day of proteinuria, and a decreased renal size. Age, clinical gout, recurrent urinary tract infections, and renal medullary calcification did not appear to influence the clinical course of the patients. Transitional cell carcinomas of the renal pelvis and bladder occur at an alarming rate in these patients.[54] This creates a major diagnostic problem, since hematuria is frequent and an IVP may be useless when renal function is significantly impaired. This situation probably requires a retrograde pyelographic study. It seems prudent to aggressively treat any infections despite the lack of correlation with the progression. The mainstays of therapy are a discontinuation of the analgesics, blood pressure control, and a conservative management of renal insufficiency.

Acute Uric Acid Nephropathy

The hypercatabolic states of lymphoproliferative and myeloproliferative disorders, rhabdomyolysis, seizures, tissue necrosis, and the treatment of neoplasms with chemotherapy and/or radiation, are associated with a profound hyperuricemia. In the setting of a low urine pH and concentrated urine, uric acid may precipitate in the nephron lumina, thus causing an intrarenal obstruction. Oliguria or anuria may occur rapidly in this setting. Initially, symptoms may be non-specific, such as nausea, vomiting, and lethargy.[55] In one reported series, the mean serum-uric acid level was 20 mg/dl (a range of 12–36).[55] Occasionally, flank pain is present. The urinalysis can be normal, but urate crystals may be seen. The differential diagnosis includes an acute tubular necrosis (ATN) due to any cause, rhabdomyolysis, and severe prerenal azotemia. A spot urine sample for the urate-to-creatinine ratio may be helpful, as a ratio greater than 1 is associated with an acute urate nephropathy.[56] Renal tubular cells and granular and epithelial casts support a diagnosis of ATN. If the dip-stick hemoglobin level is positive, then urine should be specifically tested for myoglobin.

The prognosis is good if treated early. In chemotherapy for myeloproliferative disorders, allopurinol will decrease urate synthesis, but to be preventive, it must be given before chemotherapy begins. In any case, allopurinol therapy should be started to decrease any further urate production. The urine volume should be maintained and an attempt made to alkalinize the urine. Acetazolamide (250 mg given intravenously, Q6H) plus sodium bicarbonate ($NaHCO_3$) (100 mEq/1.73 m^2/day) is an effective regimen. Hemodialysis may hasten recovery, because it helps clear the uric acid.

Chronic Urate Nephropathy

Despite intensive investigation, it is still not clear what role chronic hyperuricemia plays in causing chronic interstitial nephritis. A chronic urate nephropathy that is associated with gout has been described. However, recent long-term studies have shown that hyperuricemia and/or gout rarely result in kidney damage unless there is coexistent hypertension, ischemic heart disease, or a primary pre-existing renal insufficiency.[57] In fact, hyperuricemia may be a marker of renal vascular involvement in patients with essential hypertension.[58] Among elderly males followed for 10 years, hyperuricemia was not a recognizable cause of renal failure.[59] Other investigators have found aging to be a factor in the progression of renal dysfunction in hyperuricemia.[60]

The early impairment of urine concentration is sometimes the only finding. A hyperuricemia that is out of proportion to the degree of renal failure may be the only clue to the diagnosis. Murray and Goldberg define this as a serum urate: 1) Greater than 9 mg/dl with a creatinine level of 1.5 mg/dl; 2) Greater than 10 with a creatinine level between 1.5–2; and 3) Greater than 12 with a creatinine between 2.1–3.0 mg/dl.[46] Tophi and a mild proteinuria occasionally are noted. It is a diagnosis of exclusion, with an obstructive uropathy and hypertensive nephrosclerosis as the major disorders to be ruled out. Because of the risk of a urate stone formation, uricosuric drugs probably should be avoided in those patients who produce too much uric acid (daily excretion greater than 700 mg). Allopurinol is helpful in decreasing the production of uric acid, but xanthine and oxypurinol stones

can result from its use; encouraging a high urine output is prudent.

Hypercalcemic Nephropathy

Chronic hypercalcemia, usually due to primary hyperparathyroidism or malignancies, can eventually cause distal tubular dysfunctions, which include RTA, salt wasting, hyperkalemia, and a concentrating defect.[45] Early in the onset of hypercalcemia, there is a tendency towards a metabolic alkalosis and hypokalemia that is secondary to the primary salt loss. As renal injury ensues, the later findings develop. In addition to the findings seen in chronic interstitial nephritis, calcium deposits may be found in tubules, glomeruli, or blood vessels. Hypercalcemia can cause a nephrolithiasis and all the subsequent problems that are associated with stones (e.g., infection, obstruction, and so on). The symptoms of hypercalcemia usually appear at lower calcium levels in elderly persons. Whereas a younger patient may not notice a serum total calcium level of 11.5 mg/dl, an elderly person might present with confusion, depression, and constipation. Other symptoms include anorexia, nausea, and symptoms of a concentrating defect (i.e., polyuria and polydipsia). Hypertension and a band keratopathy may be observed. The differential diagnosis is discussed in Volume I Chapter 28.

Renal function may improve by normalizing the serum calcium level. The hemodynamic effects of calcium, the concentrating defect, and the washing out of obstructing tubular casts all improve the renal function, but calcium complex deposition in renal parenchyma cannot be reversed.[61]

Cystic Disease in the Geriatric Population

Adult polycystic kidney disease usually has manifested itself before reaching senescence. Occasionally, it first presents in an elderly person with renal pain, a gross hematuria, or urinary tract infection. Renal sodium conservation may be impaired. A progressive renal insufficiency is the usual course of the disease; by 65 years of age, 60% of all afflicted patients have advanced renal failure. Hepatic cysts and intracranial aneurysms often accompany a polycystic kidney disease. The major goals of treatment are controlling hypertension, keeping the urine sterile, and therapy for ESRD.

Simple Cysts

The approach to simple cysts is discussed in the section on neoplasms. Cysts can cause pain, hypertension, and hematuria, but they usually are an incidental finding. Because of a dilatation in the senescent tubule, the incidence of simple cysts increases with age. Rarely, erythrocytosis and infections may be associated with these cysts. The differential diagnosis includes polycystic kidney disease and masses, such as abscess or neoplasm.

Hypokalemic Nephropathy

Chronic potassium depletion can cause a concentrating defect and impaired urine acidification. This lesion usually is reversible.

Sarcoidosis

Sarcoidosis causes glomerulonephritis, hypercalcemia, hypercalciuria, nephrocalcinosis, and granulomatous infiltration of the renal interstitium. A mild to moderate proteinuria, microscopic hematuria, and sterile pyuria dominate the urinalysis findings. The urinary concentration impairment, RTA, and inappropriate glycosuria occasionally may be seen.[62]

Vascular Disease in the Senescent Kidney

Hypertension and Arteriolosclerosis

Patients with mild to moderate hypertension for many years develop a gradual decline in renal function (GFR) that is secondary to arterial and arteriolar thickening with eventual ischemic changes in the glomeruli. Tubular cells that are responsible for the active transport processes of the nephron are very sensitive to an inadequate blood supply. As a result, tubular loss, atrophy, dilatation, eventual interstitial fibrosis, and mononuclear cell infiltration can all ensue. Kidneys tend to be equally affected, bilaterally although diseases of larger vessels may actually prevent the high blood pressure from reaching

the intrarenal vessels symmetrically. Clearly, arteriolonephrosclerosis is secondary to a chronic exposure to high blood pressure.[63] However, pathologic changes of arteriolonephrosclerosis in interlobular arteries and arterioles occur in normal aging, even in the absence of hypertension. Hypertension may accelerate the aging process within the kidney, so that the severity of the vascular lesions with aging increases with the blood pressure.

Usually, other complications of hypertension prompt elderly patients to seek medical attention (e.g., cerebral or myocardial ischemias). The fall in GFR with aging may be more severe in patients with hypertension. A urinalysis may reveal proteinuria, usually less than 2 grams/day, and occasional white blood cells or casts. Renal imaging often reveals small kidneys and, sometimes, cortical scars. Physical examination often reveals other sequelae of chronic hypertension. The differential diagnosis includes an obstructive uropathy, chronic analgesic kidney disease, and other tubulo-interstitial nephropathies. Controlling the blood pressure is the mainstay of therapy. Avoidance of nephrotoxic analgesics and maintenance of a sterile urine seem especially prudent in those patients who already have a major tubulo-interstitial insult.

Malignant Nephrosclerosis

Marked hypertension, accelerating renal insufficiency, and evidence of a necrotizing glomerular injury characterize this disorder. This is a medical emergency that requires prompt intervention to preserve the renal function and to avoid other catastrophic complications of malignant hypertension. Patients over 50 years of age with underlying, untreated hypertension are most likely to acquire this problem. The differential diagnosis includes an RPGN, acute (postinfectious) glomerulonephritis, vasculitis, and renal emboli.

Large-Vessel Atherosclerotic Renal Vascular Occlusion

Large vessel atherosclerosis can contribute to renal insufficiency in elderly persons, but other complications of hypertension generally bring these patients to medical attention. Therapy for compromised renal function that is secondary to atherosclerosis of the main renal arteries has not been prospectively evaluated. Surgical renal artery revascularization has been successful.[64] It seems reasonable to avoid surgery when the renal artery disease is unilateral, the opposite kidney is normal, and hypertension is medically controllable. When total renal function is threatened, greater risks in revascularizing are justified.[65] Percutaneous, transluminal angioplasty in patients with a severe, unilateral, and atherosclerotic renovascular disease is under investigation.[66]

Renal Artery Embolism

Although tumor and fat emboli and dissecting aortic aneurysms can occlude the renal arteries, the most frequently occurring, clinically apparent renal emboli are either atheroemboli from cholesterol plaques or blood clots from a diseased heart.[67,68] An atherosclerotic renal vascular disease and renal trauma create endothelial damage where an in situ thrombus may form that can embolize or cause an ischemia without embolization.

Necrosis occurs after several hours of total occlusion, but occasionally, a partial recovery of renal function has been observed after many weeks of occlusion. As renal function falls, so does oxygen consumption; thus, some renal tissue may survive. In one reported series, 16 of 17 patients suffered from an atrial fibrillation, mitral stenosis, a recent myocardial infarction, or cardiac surgery[67]; 13 patients suffered from pain in the flank, abdomen, chest, or lower back. Nearly 50% had nausea and vomiting; 10 of 12 had fever, and all had leukocytosis and proteinuria. The microscopic or chemical hematuria on urinalysis was uniform and 10 of 12 patients had pyuria. The serum lactic dehydrogenase (LDH) level also was uniformly elevated. Only hemolysis, myocardial infarction, renal transplant rejection, or serious liver injury can elevate the LDH to the magnitude that is seen in renal artery embolization. The IVP or renal scan reveals normal-sized kidneys, but a non-visualization of the infarcted area.

In patients with heart disease, a renal embolus must be highly suspected with the above signs and symptoms. In patients with an acute myocardial infarction and renal underperfusion from heart failure, a diagnosis is more difficult. Those patients are least likely to tolerate a renal arteriogram. Radioisotope renograms and IVPs may be non-diagnostic. A longer duration of the LDH elevation is seen after a renal artery embolization than in a usual myocardial infarction.

The treatment still is somewhat disputed. An embolectomy is probably best reserved for patients with severe renal failure who have shown little improvement after 4–6 weeks of anticoagulation therapy.[67] Dialysis should be employed during this period, when needed.

Renal Cholesterol (Athero) Embolization

Patients with advanced, diffuse atherosclerosis shed atheroemboli to many organs. Since each kidney receives more than 1/10 of the cardiac output, the kidneys are a likely target for cholesterol emboli. Because of their irregular shape, atheroemboli lodge in small vessels and may not cause a complete occlusion. Of patients over 80 years of age, 12% have evidence of spontaneous renal atheroemboli.[69] The incidence rate is higher following an aortic manipulation in surgery or aortography. Despite this high incidence of histological involvement, a clinically appreciable cholesterol embolization is less common.[70]

Weeks of slowly evolving renal decompensation is the usual course of the disease. Showers of emboli produce significant infarctions, with similar signs and symptoms to those described for renal artery emboli. In addition to a progressive deterioration in the GFR, one may see episodic or sustained hypertension, an increased erythrocyte sedimentation rate (ESR), transient eosinophilia, microscopic hematuria, leukocyturia, and mild proteinuria. A physical examination may reveal evidence of extrarenal cholesterol embolization, such as cholesterol emboli in retinal arterioles, subcutaneous nodules, livedo reticularis, focal digital ischemia, or frank gangrene.

A differential diagnosis includes a vasomotor nephropathy (ATN) in those cases where the renal function deteriorates quickly. The urine sodium concentration should be low in renal embolization, as compared to an ATN. Also, ATN is a self-limited disease in which renal function improves within 1 month of the insult. In an atheroembolic renal disease, spontaneous improvement is very rare.[70] Evidence of other organ involvement with emboli may manifest as an acute pancreatitis, myocardial infarction, organic brain disease, transient ischemic attacks (TIAs) or stroke, duodenal ulceration or gangrenous extremities.[71]

Therapy is supportive. Hypertension should be treated, but anticoagulants are not helpful. Dialysis may prevent death due to uremia; usually though, the severe, diffuse, and atherosclerotic vascular disease limits survival. Prevention is the most practical approach. Physician awareness and the strict limitation of procedures that contribute to the shedding of emboli may reduce the frequency of renal atheroembolic diseases.

Systemic Vasculitis, Wegener's Granulomatosis

Systemic vasculitides are common causes of renal diseases as reported in some series of elderly patients.[25] Wegener's granulomatosis is a necrotizing, granulomatous (giant cell granulomas) vasculitis of the nasopharynx, paranasal sinuses, lungs, and renal glomeruli. Medium and small vessels of virtually any organ can be affected.[72] In the glomeruli, a focal-segmental fibrinoid necrosis and sclerosis accompany mesangial and endothelial cell proliferation. Occasionally, crescents are present. The vessels in a renal biopsy specimen may reveal the giant cell granulomas that are characteristic of Wegener's granulomatosis.

Presenting symptoms generally are non-specific (e.g., fever, weight loss, weakness, and arthralgias), but upper and lower respiratory symptoms suggest Wegener's granulomatosis. A careful examination of the respiratory tract for biopsy specimen lesions is critical. A biopsy specimen of such tissue yields a high probability of establishing a diagnosis, while a renal biopsy specimen usually is only confirmative of a vasculitic process.[73] Anemia, elevated ESR, leukocytosis, and a nephritic urine sediment are usual findings.[72,73] Chest x-ray films are abnormal in the majority of patients when nodules and infiltrates dominate the findings. Renal involvement is indicated by urinalysis and a serum creatinine elevation at onset in 80% of the patients.[73] A differential diagnosis of renal and respiratory involvement includes Goodpas-

ture's Syndrome and other vasculitides. The course for untreated patients is one of a progressive respiratory and renal functional deterioration. The initial degree of renal involvement as manifested by serum creatinine levels, proteinuria, and a light microscopic morphology correlates well with the eventual outcome.[73] Long-lasting remissions have occurred with cyclophosphamide therapy.[72] Dialysis and transplantation have also been successful.[74]

Systemic Vasculitis, Polyarteritis Nodosa (PAN)

Classic polyarteritis nodosa (PAN) is a necrotizing vasculitis of small and medium-sized muscular arteries, with segmental lesions especially at bifurcations or branches.[75] Allergic histories are uncommon, as are granulomatas in the lesions. Renal involvement is vasculitic (70%) and glomerulonephritic (30%); the latter probably is secondary to ischemia, since the lesion is a segmental fibrinoid necrosis. Occasionally, there is mesangial and endothelial proliferation and crescent formation. Immunofluorescent and electron microscopy examinations do not demonstrate evidence of immune deposits.

Aneurysmal dilatations up to 1 cm are seen in arteriograms of the medium-size vessels of the kidney, liver, and intestines, which is a finding virtually pathognomonic of PAN.[75,76] Hypertension (50%), gastrointestinal symptoms (60%), mononeuritis multiplex, livedo reticularis, arthralgias, fever, weight loss, weakness, angina (coronary arteritis), hepatic dysfunctions, and myalgias may accompany the renal findings of a nephritic disorder, renal insufficiency, and (occasionally) renal pain. A biopsy specimen of involved tissues (kidney, peripheral nerve, or testicle) that reveals a mononuclear fibrinoid necrosis without granulomas is diagnostic. The complement and antinuclear antibody studies are normal.

The survival rate in untreated patients is a few months.[77] The mean survival rate in corticosteroid-treated patients is 63 months; for patients receiving combined corticosteroids and immunosuppressive agents, the mean survival rate is 149 months.[77] Immunosuppressive therapy alone also has proven to be beneficial.[78]

Scleroderma

Scleroderma affects the skin, gastrointestinal tract, muscles, lungs, heart, and kidneys through obliterative vascular lesions. Although rare, it does occur in elderly persons.[25] The interlobular arteries of the kidney are most severely affected, and these lesions result in cortical microinfarcts. The glomeruli are ischemic with a fibrinoid necrosis, and the tubulo-interstititum as atrophic and fibrotic. In contrast to vasculitides, there are no inflammatory infiltrates in the vessel walls. The histologic picture may be impossible to differentiate from the one seen in malignant hypertension or a hemolytic-uremic syndrome.

Cutaneous involvement usually antedates visceral involvement. Renal involvement is predominantly manifested as severe hypertension and progressive renal failure. Proteinuria may be mild. It does not necessarily imply an impending renal failure; but over time, it is associated with a worse prognosis.[79] Abrupt hypertension is associated with a rapid deterioration, whereas moderate hypertension presenting later in the course of the disease has a less grave prognosis. Renal failure can be slowly progressive, but the superimposition of a renal vasoconstrictor stimulus may precipitate a rapidly progressive renal failure. The urinary sediment generally is benign except for mild proteinuria. When malignant hypertension and a rapidly progressive renal failure ensue, hematuria may appear.

Captopril may help stabilize both the renal function and hypertension.[80] No other form of therapy has been shown to alter the progressive downhill course. A bilateral nephrectomy with dialysis has been helpful in patients with an ESRD who still have severe, renin-mediated hypertension. Transplantation also has been successfully used[81]; but for elderly persons, dialysis would probably be the preferred therapy.

Hemolytic-Uremic Syndrome (HUS) and Thrombotic Thrombocytopenic Purpura (TTP)

Both of these disorders can affect elderly patients.[25] They are characterized by platelet consumption, progressive renal failure, microangiopathic-hemolytic anemia, small-vessel thombi, neurologic abnormalities, and constitutional symptoms. Therapy with corticosteroids, platelet inhibitors, plasmapheresis and exchange, and splenectomy has been successful in TTP.[82] The therapy of HUS, other than the supportive management of ESRD, is not year clear.[83,84]

The Kidneys and Neoplasms in Elderly Persons

Renal Cell Carcinoma (Renal Adenocarcinoma)

The peak years for discovery of this cancer are between 55–60 years of age.[85] It represents 2% of newly diagnosed cancers, has an incidence rate of 7.5 cases per 100,000 persons, and a 2 : 1 male predominance ratio.[85] The neoplasm originates from proximal tubular epithelium and may produce a proximal tubular antigen.[86] Flank pain (50%), hematuria (40%), and a renal mass (30%), all form the classic triad of symptoms; but, less than 15% of all patients actually display all three. Malaise, weight loss, anemia, fever, hypertension, cardiac failure, hypercalcemia, thrombophlebitis, abnormal liver chemistries, amyloidosis, neuromyopathies, and an elevated ESR are additional clinical features seen in some cases. Unusual presentations include an immune complex glomerulonephritis, chest pain, and renal hemorrhage.[87]

An initial evaluation probably includes an IVP and/or ultrasound study. For asymptomatic space-occupying lesions, so common in elderly persons with benign solitary cysts, an ultrasound examination and possible adjunctive cyst puncture are appropriate. When the internal surface of the cyst is smooth, a tumor is less likely to develop.[88] The CT scan may help in cysts with low-level internal echoes. Angiography is reserved for small or echogenic lesions when a cyst puncture fails or shows abnormalities of the cyst wall. Where renal cell carcinoma is highly suspected, angiography is definitely indicated. Surgery is the treatment of choice. Hormonal agents, chemotherapy, and radiation occasionally are palliative, but generally disappointing.[87]

Urothelial Neoplasia

These malignancies usually are managed by urologists, but are mentioned here because they can present similarly to renal cell carcinomas. The concern here is for the increasing incidence of urinary tract malignancies in patients who have chronically ingested large doses of analgesic medications.[54] The evaluation of a hematuria includes an IVP, cystoscopy, and (possibly) a retrograde pyelogram.

Renal Involvement By A Nonrenal Neoplasm

Myeloma

The kidneys in a multiple myeloma may be involved directly via amyloidosis, plasmacytomas, pyelonephritis, the tubular toxicity of light chains (RTA), and intratubular obstructions that are secondary to myeloma proteins (myeloma kidney). Indirect renal involvement may occur due to a urinary tract obstruction in plasmacytomas, nephrocalcinosis or diabetes insipidus from hypercalcemia, and uric acid nephropathy from hyperuricemia. Myeloma patients are particularly sensitive to nephrotoxins (e.g., radiocontrast agents, aminoglycoside antibiotics, and so on).

Nephrotic Syndrome

Hodgkin's disease, various carcinomas (the most common carcinomas such as of the lung, colon, and so on), non-Hodgkin's lymphoma, and certain leukemias sometimes are associated with the nephrotic syndrome.[26,29,31,89] Membranous and membranoproliferative glomerulonephritis can be associated with carcinomas, while Hodgkin's disease is associated with minimal-change glomerulopathy.

Miscellaneous Involvement

The kidneys frequently are involved, secondarily, in non-renal neoplasms by a direct tumor invasion of: 1) Renal parenchyma; 2) Ureters causing an obstruction; 3) The renal arteries causing hypertension or ischemia; and 4) The renal veins causing a renal vein thrombosis or a nephrotic syndrome. Hyperuricemia, hypercalcemia, excretion of toxic paraproteins, and amyloidosis may be associated with malignancies.

Treatment with radiotherapy and chemotherapy may produce direct physical and toxic effects on the kidneys.

Malignancies occur with increased frequency in elderly persons. Because the senescent kidney has reduced the functional reserve, the clinician must be particularly aware of any change in renal function in elderly patients with malignancies of any kind.

Drug-Related Syndromes

Almost every drug-related renal syndrome occurs with a greater frequency and severity in the geriatric population.[90,91] Table 16-6 is a list of nephrotoxic drugs and syndromes.

Acute Tubular Necrosis (ATN)

The most common abrupt decline in renal function due to drugs is an acute tubular necrosis (ATN) from aminoglycoside antibiotics. Polyuria and an inability to concentrate urine usually precede azotemia. Factors that predispose a patient to aminoglycoside nephrotoxicity include advancing age, pre-existing renal dysfunction, volume depletion, and a recent exposure to aminoglycosides or other nephrotoxins.[92] Other renal manifestations include proteinuria, glycosuria, hypomagnesemia, hypocalcemia, and hypokalemia. Guidelines for aminoglycoside administration recommend maintaining an expanded extracellular fluid (ECF) volume status during therapy, adjusting the dose for a compromised and/or changing GFR, cautious use in the presence of other nephrotoxins, and early discontinuation if culture results signify that a less nephrotoxic drug would be effective. Drug levels have not been particularly helpful in avoiding a renal injury. A peak level less than 8 μg/ml and a trough level below 2 μg/ml may be reasonable guidelines.

Other antibiotics, which include tetracycline, polymyxin B, sulfonamides, and amphotericin B, can lead to a similar renal insult even when used with appropriate doses. Solvents, metals, and other environmental toxins can cause an ATN. Cisplatin apparently causes renal failure through a tubular injury.[93]

TABLE 16-6 Nephrotoxic Syndromes and Associated Agents[91]

Proteinuria-Nephrosis
  Penicillin
  Gold
  Trimethadione
  Paramethadione
  Dapsone
  Pencillamine
  Probenecid
  Mercurial diuretics
  Tolbutamide
  Perchlorate
  Phenindione
  Rifampin
  Doxorubicin hydrochloride
  Fenoprofen
Proximal Tubule-Fanconi Syndrome
  Salicylates
  Aminoglycosides
  Tetracycline
Distal Tubule-Renal Tubular Acidosis
  Amphotericin B
  Penicillin
  Lithium
Concentrating Defects-Nephrogenic Diabetes Insipidus
  Demethylchlortetracycline
  Methoxyflurane
  Lithium
  Phenytoin
Papillary Necrosis
  Analgesics (non-narcotic)
    Salicylates
    Phenacetin
    Phenylbutazone
  Intravesicle formalin
Interstitial Nephritis
  Salicylates
  Phenacetin
  Acetaminophen
  Combination non-narcotic analgesics
  Fenoprofen
  Methicillin
  Ampicillin
  Furosemide
  Cephalosporins

(Continued):
  Sulfonamides
  Rifampin
  Polymyxin B
  Allopurinol
  Phenindione
  Nitrosureas
  Lithium
Hematuria
  Cephalosporins
  Penicillin
  Cyclophosphamide
Acute Renal Failure— ↓ GFR*
  Analgesics
    Aspirin
    Indomethacin
    Phenylbutazone
  Aminoglycosides
  Cephalosporins
  Tetracyclines
  Amphotericin B
  Polymyxin
  Iodinated contrast media
  Platinum complexes
  Bismuth compounds
  Methotrexate
  Epsilon amino caproic acid
  Phenytoin
  Phenindione
  Propranolol
  Dextran
  Phenazopyridine
  Bismuth
Chronic Renal Failure
  Analgesics (non-narcotic)
  Tetracycline
  Iodinated contrast media
  Nitrosureas
  Methoxyflurane
Calculi
  Phenazophyridine
  Allopurinol (indirectly)
  Ticrynafen
  Triamterene
  Phenylbutazone (indirectly)

* ↓ GFR = decreased glomerular filtration rate.

Obstructive Uropathy

Uric acid, xanthine, and oxypurinol may crystallize and precipitate in renal tubules. Uric acid is released in a massive cell destruction as in a tumor lysis due to chemotherapeutic agents. Xanthine and oxypurinol crystals can result from allopurinol therapy. Methotrexate and radioiodinated contrast agents exert their nephrotoxocity, at least partially, through intratubular obstruction. Methysergide has been reported to cause a retroperitoneal fibrosis with a ureteral obstruction.

Acute Glomerulonephritis

Penicillin and its derivatives, illicit IV street narcotics, and organic solvents have been associated with an acute nephritic syndrome.

Acute Interstitial Nephritis

Penicillin and its derivatives, many other antibiotics, most diuretics, many non-steroidal antiinflammatory drugs (NSAID), and analgesic and other miscellaneous drugs may cause a renal insufficiency (with or without oliguria) 7–14 days after exposure (see the section in this chapter on "Tubulo-interstitial Renal Disease in Elderly Persons").

Chronic Tubulo-interstitial Nephritis

Phenacetin, acetaminophen, aspirin (alone or in combination), and other NSAIDs, when ingested regularly over a period of years, ultimately can impair renal function because of chronic interstitial nephritis and papillary necrosis.

Nephrotic Syndrome

Anticonvulsants, NSAIDs, tolbutamide, probenecid, mercurial diuretics, gold, penicillamine, penicillin, rifampin, and doxorubicin have been reported to cause a nephrosis in certain patients. In most cases, the nephrosis is resolved on discontinuation of the offending agent.

Antidiuretic Drugs

Nicotine, chlorpropamide, tolbutamide, clofibrate, cyclophosphamide, morphine, barbiturates, vincristine, carbamazepine, acetaminophen, indomethacin, isoproterenol, and (probably) drugs that are functionally similar to these, impair renal water excretion in certain patients, which leads to water intoxication. Elderly persons are particularly prone to this complication because of their typical excessive ADH response to certain stimuli.

Drug-Induced Polyuria

Alcohol, phenytoin, norepinephrine, and lithium restrict the availability of ADH. An ADH-dependent impairment of renal concentration is caused by lithium, demeclocycline, methoxyflurane, colchicine, vinca alkaloids, amphotericin B, aminoglycosides, and vasopressinoic acid. A renal concentration impairment that is independent of an ADH is caused (again) by lithium and sulfonylureas such as tolazamide, glyburide, and acetohexamide.

Renal Tubular Acidosis (RTA)

Amphotericin B, penicillins, and lithium can cause a syndrome that resembles a distal renal tubular acidosis (RTA). Salicylates, aminoglycosides, and tetracycline causes a syndrome that resembles a proximal RTA. Bicarbonate wasting without other evidence of a proximal tubular dysfunction is an accompaniment of therapy with acetozolamide.

Creatininemia

Cimetidine, trimethoprim, and some newer cephalosporins impair creatinine secretion and lead to an elevation in the serum creatinine level without actually lowering the GFR.

Non-Steroidal Antiinflammatory Drug (NSAID) Renal Syndromes

Because of the frequency of use of these drugs in the geriatric population, specific attention must be given to their untoward renal effects.

Locally synthesized renal prostaglandins act to oppose a renal vasoconstriction.[94] They probably are operative in situations where vasoconstriction is stimulated, such as in a hemorrhage, endotoxemia, anesthesia, extracellular volume depletion, decompensated hepatic cirrhosis, congestive heart failure, or a nephrotic syndrome (conditions of decreased, effective arterial blood volume). Prostaglandin inhibition by NSAIDs allow the renal vasoconstriction to go unopposed with a resulting impaired renal blood flow. Clinically, a decrement in the GFR is seen. If the intrarenal hemodynamic alteration is severe, an ATN can result.[95] If the offending prostaglandin inhibitor is discontinued before the development of an ATN, the fall in the GFR is rapidly reversible.[96] This is especially important when there is pre-existing renal dysfunction.

Sodium and water retention are normal responses to prostaglandin inhibition in elderly persons.[8] This can lead to a resistence to antihypertensive drugs and diuretics and an aggravation of existing hypertension or cardiac failure.[97] This same mechanism may predispose these patients to hyperkalemia.

Acute, allergic interstitial nephritis with proteinuria and even a nephrotic syndrome has been described with at least five different NSAIDs.[96] The proteinuria is thought to be secondary to the release from T-lymphocytes of a vascular permeability factor. This complication is reversible on stopping the offending drug, and prednisone may hasten the recovery.

Papillary necrosis and chronic interstitial nephritis have been reported with the long-term use of at least three NSAIDs.[96] This occurred even in the absence of acetaminophen- or phenacetin-containing compounds.

The NSAIDs are valuable therapeutic tools. Their use in elderly patients should not be withheld; rather, a careful follow-up examination is absolutely necessary. Patients should be warned about fluid retention and oliguria. A urinalysis and serum creatinine level should be obtained shortly after the drug is started and at regular intervals thereafter. Some complications occur within days, while other complications may not be evident for months.

Acute Renal Failure (ARF) in Elderly Persons

Acute renal failure (ARF) in elderly persons is not an infrequent complication of other serious illnesses. Often, it is induced by a smaller insult than that causing ARF in a younger patient. The mortality rate from ARF increases with age.[97] For older patients who survive ARF, the recovery of renal function is slower and less complete than that seen in younger patients.[98] The causes can be classified into three broad categories as shown in Table 16-7.

Pathophysiology

There are no data regarding a different pathophysiology of ARF in older patients. Both toxic and ischemic insults may produce renal cellular damage or alter glomerular hemody-

TABLE 16-7   Classification of Acute Renal Failure

Prerenal
Decreased effective arterial blood volume
Low cardiac output
Renal
ATN*
Toxins
Renal ischemia
Vascular obstruction
Vasculitis
GN†
Malignant hypertension
Acute interstitial nephritis
Postrenal
Urinary drainage obstruction

* ATN = acute-tubular necrosis.
† GN = glomerulonephritis.

namics, thus initiating an ARF. As pointed out earlier, the renal blood flow falls with aging, which may explain why older patients experience an ARF with a smaller hemodynamic insult than in younger patients.[98] Toxic insults also affect an older patient to an extent greater than that seen in younger patients (e.g., radiocontrast agents and/or aminoglycoside antibiotics).

Prerenal Azotemia

This may be caused by many specific clinical situations, but the final common pathophysiologic mechanism is renal hypoperfusion. Any situation where the effective arterial blood volume is reduced (such as nephrosis, cirrhosis, volume depletion, and so on), or where the cardiac output is low (congestive heart failure and/or cardiogenic shock), will cause a renal hypoperfusion. A prerenal azotemia accounts for over one third of all cases of ARF that are seen in a general medical center.[99] Renal ischemia, if severe or of a long duration, can cause an ATN.

Two forms of prerenal azotemia require further comment. Urine volumes of 1–2 l/day were described in nine patients with a prerenal azotemia who had diagnostic indices consistent with a prerenal azotemia.[100] Renal function improved with a correction of the hemodynamic status. The major defect that blunted their ability to become oliguric (less than 400 cc/day) was an impaired urinary concentration. Miller, et al labelled this entity "polyuric prerenal failure." With their pre-existing, impaired urinary-concentrating ability, elderly persons are particularly prone to this disorder.

Hepatorenal syndrome consists of oliguric renal failure in the setting of severe liver failure. The major pathophysiology is a profound redistribution of blood flow within the kidney. The renal failure is functional; that is, no structural abnormalities exist, and such kidneys perform normally when transplanted into recipients with a normal liver function.[101] Urinary diagnostic indices are similar to those in a prerenal azotemia, and urine output may improve with volume expansion.

Postrenal

Urinary obstruction almost always is reversible. It is imperative that an aggressive approach be taken because of the risk of a permanent renal injury in elderly patients with an obstruction and a pre-existing, compromised functional renal reserve. In one reported series of ARF cases, 5% were postrenal.[99]

Renal

The many general renal causes of ARF are classified in Table 16-7. ATN refers to ac-

tual cellular damage of the renal tubular epithelium, while the less specific term, "vasomotor nephropathy," implicates a primary alteration of renal hemodynamics in the initiation of ARF. Unfortunately, there is no clear-cut distinction, so the terms are often used interchangeably. ATN can be characterized by oliguria, but a non-oliguric form has become increasingly recognized.[102]

Differential Diagnosis

The clinical history should address the presence or absence of diabetes mellitus, hypertension, analgesic abuse, respiratory illness, arthritis, circulatory insufficiency, liver disease, any drug exposure, recent surgery, and others toxin exposures. The medical record should be scrutinized for drug and fluid administration, diet, and body weight. A physical examination must emphasize an ECF volume assessment, cardiac status, and evidence of embolic phenomena or liver disease.

Urinary Diagnostic Indices

Table 16-8 summarizes both the urine and serum diagnostic indices. A prerenal azotemia is accompanied by a bland sediment with hyaline and finely granular casts. ATN is character-

TABLE 16-8   Diagnostic Indices of Acute Renal Failure (ARF)

	Oliguric ARF	Non-oliguric ARF	Prerenal Azotemia	Acute Obstructive Uropathy	Acute Glomerulonephritis
Serum BUN/CR*	10	10	20	10	10
Urine Na† (mEq/l)	>30	>30	<20	>30	<20
Specific gravity	1.010–1.015	1.010–1.015	>1.015	1.010–1.015	1.010–1.015
Urine osmolarity (mosm/l)	350	350	>450	350	350
U/P†† creatinine	<20	<20	40	<20	40
U/P urea	<5	<10	>10	10	10
Fractional sodium excretion (%)	>3	3	<1	>3	<1
Urine volume (ml/day)	50–400	400–3,000	50–2,000	0–2,000	50–2,000

* BUN/CR = Blood urea nitrogen/Creatinine ratio.
† Na = sodium.
†† U/P = urine/plasma.

ized by coarse granular casts and tubular epithelial cells. An acute nephritic sediment is more consistent with glomerular diseases. Pigments and crystals should be noted. The fractional excretion of sodium is the ratio of the clearance of sodium to the clearance of creatinine, which is multiplied by 100 to make the number a percent ($FF_{Na} = 100 \times (U_{Na}/P_{Na})/(U_{cr}/P_{cr})$.[103] That test and others (Table 16-8), in addition to the clinical picture, help clarify the diagnosis.[104]

Other Diagnostic Procedures

To exclude a urinary tract obstruction, a bladder catheter must be placed, followed by a KUB x-ray film and ultrasound examination. If results are not definitive, a retrograde pyelogram will be necessary. If there is a compatible setting for atheroemboli or a vascular accident, an isotope renogram is indicated. If the index of suspicion is high and the renogram is non-decisive, an arteriogram is indicated.

Therapeutic Trials

Volume challenges with 200 ml increments of physiologic saline are reasonable in elderly patients who appear hypo- or euvolemic. If edema is present, the colloid or blood may be a more effective volume expander. If volume depletion is strongly suggested by a history and urinary diagnostic indices, yet edema is present, then central venous or pulmonary capillary wedge monitoring may be indicated. Small increments of volume replacement are more prudent in elderly persons than large boluses. If no respiratory problems evolve, continued increments can be administered. Once euvolemia has been achieved, but oliguria persists, a trial of diuretics can be attempted. Furosemide, 200 mg via drip infusion over 30 minutes and repeated once after 2 hours, is an adequate trial. It is important to realize that, to date, a diuretic treatment in ARF is a limited therapy at best. Some data suggest that an oliguric ARF can be converted to a non-oliguric ARF via high-dose diuretics administered early in the course of the disease.[105] If a patient is not euvolemic, such therapy has little chance of success. Continuous therapy with large doses

of diuretics in patients who fail to respond to initial doses is neither indicated nor prudent.

Clinical Course

Three non-distinct phases occur: oliguric, diuretic, and recovery. The oliguric phase ranges from 2 days to 8 weeks with a mean of 14 days. The average daily urine output is 150 ml/day. Acidosis, hyperkalemia, and volume overload frequently accompany oliguria. In older patients with less muscle mass, the BUN and creatinine levels may not rise as rapidly as they would in younger patients. Body catabolism occurs in underfed patients to an extent that 0.5 to 1 pound per day would be lost if they excreted water from this metabolism. In oliguric, underfed patients, a stable weight implies water accumulation.

During the diuretic phase, the urine volume may gradually rise to a fixed volume. This may reflect a previous volume overload, solute osmotic diuresis, or renal tubular dysfunction. The GFR may remain low during the diuretic phase. The urinary concentration usually is impaired, so volume depletion is a potential problem.

During the recovery phase, the GFR improves slowly; however, concentration, dilution, and acidification may be impaired for some time. In elderly persons, the degree of recovery of renal function after an ARF is less and the recovery period is longer than in their younger counterparts.[98]

Treatment

In elderly patients with reduced muscle mass, there is little reserve before nutritional bankruptcy. Early intervention with hyperalimentation, enteral or IV, is indicated. Drug management is complicated both by senescence and renal failure. Lastly, an acute dialysis in ARF in an elderly person may not be easy. Hemodialysis requires vascular access and a stable cardiovascular system. There is a risk of rapid solute and water shifts that lead to hypotension, dysequilibrium, seizures, and strokes. Peritoneal dialysis is more gentle, slower, less efficient, and causes transperitoneal protein losses. The therapy in each case must be individualized.

End-Stage Renal Disease (ESRD) in Elderly Persons

Chronic or Acute Renal Failure

When confronted with a patient with renal failure, three questions must be addressed: 1) What caused it? 2) Is it reversible? and 3) Is it acute or chronic? Elderly patients often have a considerable medical history, which must be evaluated in answering these questions. The physical examination may give some clues as to the rapidity of onset of the renal failure. The sallow pigmentation of uremia is secondary to chromagen pigment accumulation, which takes weeks. The pale complexion of uremia usually is due to the anemia of renal failure. In the absence of a blood loss or red cell destruction, this takes weeks to months to develop. As expected, therefore, a laboratory evaluation will reveal an anemia in chronic renal failure. Conversely, anemia in an ARF implies a concomitant acute loss of red blood cells. The serum electrolyte pattern in ARF usually is an anion gap acidosis (normal sodium and chloride, low total CO_2 combining power), while in chronic renal failure, one may instead see a hyperchloremic (non-anion gap) acidosis. The senescent kidney acquires an acidification defect that resembles the RTA acidosis known as type IV.[11] As progressive, chronic renal failure ensues, this defect may become clinically apparent. In chronic renal failure, osteodystrophy develops; in an ARF, there is insufficient time for it to appear. A renal osteodystrophy may present as bone pain, spontaneous fractures, radiographic skeletal dimineralization, resorption of distal clavicles, and subperiosteal resorption of phalanges.

A classification of the causes of an acute exacerbation of chronic renal failure in elderly persons are listed in Table 16-9.

Signs and Symptoms of Uremia in Elderly Persons

The earliest symptoms of uremia are insidious and non-specific, including fatigue, malaise, and weakness. Appetite decreases with a specific dislike of meats, and it progresses to nausea and vomiting.[106] Hiccups indicate a neuropathy and usually antedate central nervous

TABLE 16-9   Chronic Renal Failure with Exacerbation, Possible Reversible Causes

Volume-Related	Metabolic
Too much	↑ Ca^{++}
Too little	↑ PO_4
Hypertension	↑ glu
Mechanical	↓ K^+
Arteries	↑ Uric acid
Veins	
Urinary drainage	Spurious creatinine
Pericardium	Ketonemia
Infections	Cimetidine
Systemic	Trimethoprim
Urinary tract	Tetracycline
	Cephalosporins
Allergy	Primary disease
Drugs	Flare-up
Toxins	Natural history
Environmental	
Therapeutic agents	A second renal disease
Diagnostic agents	

system symptoms such as confusion or seizures. Weight loss occurs unless edema fluid accumulates. Pruritis, pallor, and sallowness affect the skin. Blood pressure may rise, particularly if the initial renal disease is a glomerulopathy. Angina may occur as the red blood cell volume falls. Bleeding tendencies develop, but pericarditis is a late finding. When the initial renal disease predominantly involves the tubulo-interstitium, a salt and water losing condition may evolve; at end-stage, these patients are often volume depleted.

Conservative Management of ESRD

Elderly patients are sensitive to therapeutic manipulations, so some degree of foresight and caution are necessary. Adequate nutrition includes a caloric intake between 35–55 calories/kg/day, 1 gram/kg/day of high (essential amino acid) biologic value protein, and a potassium, sodium, and fluid restriction only if necessary. Appetite stimulation, as with ethyl alcohol and discontinuation of nicotine, should be attempted. Oral supplements of glucose-protein-vitamin-mineral solutions (e.g. Isocal) should be used to maximize caloric intake. Serum inorganic phosphorus levels should be brought under 5mg/dl via aluminum-containing antacids (e.g., Alternagel). Since these are constipating, a stool softener (with or without a cathartic stimulant) should be given simultaneously. Occasionally, oral sorbitol solutions (20–70%) are necessary to keep the bowels moving.

If the cardiopulmonary status will tolerate it, patients may do better at a "trace edema" volume status. This maximizes the GFR and prevents a prerenal azotemia. Obviously, if extra fluid accumulates in the lungs, it must be removed. High doses of the loop diuretics furosemide and ethacrynic acid may be necessary; but at high doses, both drugs are ototoxic. The combination of metolazone or chlorthalidone with a loop diuretic may produce dramatic effects. It is difficult to predict what may happen to the serum potassium level in this setting. Mechanisms for both K^+ retention and excretion are effective. Therefore, this electrolyte must be carefully observed.

Several complications of ESRD have to be addressed differently in elderly persons. The treatment of anemia in ESRD in elderly persons is not different than in younger patients (administration of vitamins, iron, androgens, and so on), except for transfusion requirements. Uncompensated anemia leads to angina and cardiac failure. The tolerable level of hemoglobin varies from one patient to another. Transfusions should be administered liberally to elderly patients with ESRD. The rationale for such an approach is to maximize the quality of life. Administering one unit of blood at a time is a prudent way to prevent circulatory congestion. In younger patients, either quinine or diazepam is effective for muscle cramps. In elderly persons, the frequent central nervous system side effects of diazepam limit its application. Quinine sulfate, 200 mg given three times daily, is effective and probably safer.

Dialysis in Elderly Patients

Many forms of dialysis are available, ranging from home continuous ambulatory peritoneal dialysis (CAPD), home machine peritoneal dialysis, center (dialysis unit) peritoneal dialysis, home hemodialysis, and center hemodialysis. Peritoneal dialysis requires a permanent access through the abdominal wall and at least 40 hours per week of dialysate within the abdominal cavity (peritoneum). This technique allows for a slow equilibration and removal of solutes and fluid, which is an ideal situation for the un-

stable cardiovascular system that is so frequently seen in elderly persons. Major disadvantages are the time required and the complication of peritonitis. CAPD or one of its variants is the dialysis of choice for many elderly ESRD patients. Hemodialysis, conversely, accomplishes an adequate diffusion and ultrafiltration in about 12 hours per week divided into three equal sessions. However, this efficiency is costly in that acute solute and volume changes occur over a short time span, which provokes untoward responses in vulnerable patients. Nonetheless, hemodialysis has been used safely and effectively in the geriatric ESRD population.[107,108] For the first 18–36 months, elderly patients do as well on hemodialysis as do younger patients. Thereafter, the mortality rate in elderly persons significantly accelerates. Cardiovascular and cerebrovascular diseases are responsible for much of the mortality of this population.

There are no absolute laboratory values to signify the initiation of dialysis. Most patients have intolerable symptoms at a GFR between 6–8 ml/minutes. At that point, renal replacement therapy is initiated. Some patients may decide not to have dialysis. Dialysis is not necessarily an "all or none" arrangement. Some patients may opt to discontinue therapy. The clinician should be supportive in allowing flexibility and occasional reversals of decisions; however, the clinician should discourage too frequent changes, which can be very hard on patients and their families. Compassionate and ethically sound decisions must be used to consider each patient individually (see Volume II, Chapter 22).

Transplantation

Transplantation in elderly persons has risks that are inherent in elderly persons. For example, diverticulosis occurs more frequently in elderly persons; they are less active and possibly more prone to the infections of an immune-compromised host. Nonetheless, the data regarding a transplantation in elderly persons are encouraging, with graft and patient survival comparing favorably to that in the general population.[109–111] Transplantation is a reasonable alternative to dialysis in an older patient with ESRD. Individualization of therapy is appropriate and patients should not be excluded from a transplantation procedure simply because of age.[111]

References

1. McLachlan MSF: The aging kidney. *Lancet* 2:143–146, 1978.
2. Epstein M: Effects of aging on the kidney. *Fed Proc* 38:168–172, 1979.
3. Hollenberg NK, Adams DF, Solomon HS, et al: Senescence and the renal vasculature in normal man. *Circ Res* 34:309–316, 1974.
4. Rowe JW, Andres R, Tobin JD, et al: The effect of age on creatinine clearance in men: cross-sectional and longitudinal study. *J Gerontol* 31:155–163, 1976.
5. Wesson LG: Renal hemodynamics in physiological states in *Physiology of the Human Kidney*. New York, Grune & Stratton, 1969, pp 96–108.
6. Marketos SG, Papanayiotou PC, Dontas AS: Bacteriuria and non-obstructive renovascular disease in old age. *J Gerontol* 24:33–36, 1969.
7. Weidemann P, DeMytteneau-Bursztein S, Maxwell MH: Effect of aging on plasma renin and aldosterone in normal man. *Kidney Int* 8:325–333, 1975.
8. Macias-Nunez JF, Garcia Iglesias C, Tabernero Romo JM, et al: Renal management of sodium under indomethacin and aldosterone in the elderly. *Age and Aging* 9:165–172, 1980.
9. Miller JH, McDonald RK, Shock NW: Age changes in the maximal rate of renal tubular reabsorption of glucose. *J Gerontol* 7:196–200, 1952.
10. Agarwal BN, Cabebe FG: Renal acidification in elderly subjects. *Nephron* 26:291–295, 1980.
11. Batlle DC: Hyperkalemic, hyperchloremic metabolic acidosis associated with selective aldosterone deficiency and distal renal tubular acidosis. *Sem in Nephrol* 1:260–274, 1981.
12. Rowe JW, Shock NW, DeFronzo RA: The influence of age on the renal response to water deprivation in man. *Nephron* 17:270–278, 1976.
13. Dontas AS, Marketos SG, Papanayiotou P: Mechanisms of renal tubular defects in old age. *Postgrad Med J* 48:295–303, 1972.
14. Helderman JH, Vestal RE, Rowe JW, et al: The response of arginine vasopressin to intravenous alcohol and hypertonic saline in man and the impact of aging. *J Gerontol* 33:39–47, 1978.
15. Cockcroft DW, Gault MH: Prediction of creatinine clearance from serum creatinine. *Nephron* 16:31–41, 1976.
16. Friedman SA, Raizner AE, Rosen H, et al: Functional defects in the aging kidney. *Ann Int Med* 76:41–45, 1972.
17. VanZee BE, Hoy WE, Talley TE, et al: Renal injury associated with intravenous pyelography in nondiabetic and diabetic patients. *Ann Int Med* 89:51–54, 1978.
18. Anto HR, Chou S-Y, Porush JG, et al: Infusion intravenous pyelography and renal function: effects of hypertonic mannitol in patients with chronic renal insufficiency. *Arch Int Med* 141:1652–1656, 1981.
19. Scheible W, Talner LB: Gray scale ultrasound and the genitourinary tract; a review of clinical applications. *Radiol Clin North Am* 17:281–300, 1978.
20. Lingard DA, Lawson TL: Accuracy of ultrasound in predicting the nature of renal masses. *J Urol* 122:724–727, 1979.
21. Wickre CG, Colper TA: Complications of percutaneous needle biopsy of the kidney: a review. *Am J Nephrol,* in press.
22. Diaz-Buxo JA, Donadio JV: Complications of percutaneous renal biopsy: an analysis of 1000 consecutive biopsies. *Clin Nephrol* 4:223–227, 1975.
23. Arieff AI, Anderson RJ, Massry SG: Acute glomerulonephritis in the elderly. *Geriatrics* 26(suppl 9):74–84, 1971.
24. Montoliu J, Darnell A, Torras A, et al: Acute and rapidly progressive forms of glomerulonephritis in the elderly. *J Am Geriatr Soc* 29:108–116, 1981.
25. Moorthy AV, Zimmerman SW: Renal disease in the elderly: clinopathologic analysis of renal disease in 115 elderly patients. *Clin Nephrol* 14:223–229, 1980.
26. Zech P, Colon S, Pointet P, et al: The nephrotic syndrome in adults over age 60: etiology evolution and treatment of 76 cases. *Clin Nephrol* 18:232–236, 1982.
27. Pierides AM, Malasit P, Morley AR, et al: Idiopathic membranous nephropathy. *Quart J Med* 46:163–177, 1977.
28. Cade R, Spooner G, Juncos Fuller T, et al: Chronic renal vein thrombosis. *Am J Med* 63:387–397, 1977.
29. Row PG, Cameron JS, Turner DR, et al: Membranous nephropathy: long term follow-up and association with neoplasia. *Quart J Med* 44:207–239, 1975.
30. Coggins CH and Collaborative Study Members: A controlled study of short-term prednisone treatment in adults with membranous nephropathy. *N Engl J Med* 301:1301–1306, 1979.
31. Eagen JW, Lewis EJ: Glomerulopathies of neoplasia. *Kidney Int* 11:297–306, 1977.

32. Moorthy AV: Minimal change nephrotic syndrome—a benign cause of proteinuria in the elderly. *Am J Med Sci* 275:65–73, 1978.

33. Friedman EA, Shieh SD: Clinical management of diabetic nephropathy, in Friedman EA, L'Esperance FA (ed): *Diabetic Renal Retinal Syndrome.* New York: Grune & Stratton, 1980, pp 135–158.

34. Kyle RA, Bayrd ED: Amyloidosis—review of 236 cases. *Medicine* 54:271–299, 1975.

35. Jones NF: Renal amyloidosis: pathogenesis and therapy. *Clin Nephrol* 6:459–464, 1976.

36. Ogg CS, Cameron JS, Williams DG, et al: Presentation and course of primary amyloidosis of the kidney. *Clin Nephrol* 15:9–13, 1981.

37. Bardana EJ, Pirofsky B: Recent advances in the immunopathogenesis of systemic lupus erythematosus. *West J Med* 122:130–144, 1975.

38. Baker SB, Rovira JR, Campion EW, et al: Late onset systemic lupus erythematosus. *Am J Med* 66:727–732, 1979.

39. DeFronzo RA, Cooke CR, Goldberg M, et al: Impaired renal tubular potassium secretion in systemic lupus erythematosus. *Ann Int Med* 86:268–271, 1977.

40. Wagner L: Immunosuppressive agents in lupus nephritis: a critical analysis. *Medicine* 55:239–250, 1976.

41. Clarkson R, Seymour AE, Thompson AJ, et al: IgA nephropathy: a syndrome of uniform morphology, diverse clinical features and uncertain prognosis.*Clin Nephrol* 8:459–471, 1977.

42. Morrin PAF, Hinglais N, Nabarra B, et al: Rapidly progressive glomerulonephritis: a clinical and pathologic study. *Am J Med* 65:446–460, 1978.

43. O'Neill WM, Etheridge WB, Bloomer A: High dose corticosteroids: their use in treating idiopathic rapidly progressive glomerulonephritis. *Arch Int Med* 139:514–518, 1979.

44. Gorevic PD, Kassab HJ, Levo Y, et al: Mixed cryoglobulinemia: clinical aspects and long term follow-up of 40 patients. *Am J Med* 69:287–308, 1980.

45. Cogan MG: Tubulo-interstitial nephropathies: A pathophysiologic approach—Medical Staff Conference, University of California, San Francisco. *West J Med* 132:134–140, 1980.

46. Murray T, Goldberg M: Chronic interstitial nephritis: etiologic factors. *Ann Int Med* 82:453–459, 1975.

47. Cotran RS: Tubulointerstitial nephropathies. *Hosp Prac* 1:79–92, 1982.

48. Van Ypersele de Strihou C: Acute oliguric interstitial nephritis. *Kidney Int* 16:751–765, 1979.

49. Linton AL, Clark WF, Driedger AA, et al: Acute interstitial nephritis due to drugs: review of the literature with a report of nine cases. *Ann Int Med* 93:735–741, 1980.

50. Galpin JE, Shinaberger JH, Stanley TM, et al: Acute interstitial nephritis due to methicillin. *Am J Med* 65:756–765, 1978.

51. Gault MH, Rudwal TC, Engles WD, et al: Syndrome associated with the abuse of analgesic. *Ann Int Med* 68:906–925, 1968.

52. Kincaid-Smith P: Analgesic abuse and the kidney. *Kidney Int* 17:250–260, 1980.

53. Nanra RS: Factors which influence the clinical course of analgesic nephropathy. *Abstr Seventh Int Congr Nephrol,* 1978, p D–16.

54. Gonwa TA, Corbett WT, Schey HM, et al: Analgesic-associated nephropathy and transitional cell carcinoma of the urinary tract. *Ann Int Med* 93:249–252, 1980.

55 Kjellstrand CM, Campbell DC, VonHartitzsch Buselmeier TJ: Hyperuricemic acute renal failure. *Arch Int Med* 133:349–359, 1974.

56. Kelton J, Kelley WN, Holmes EW: A rapid method for the diagnosis of acute uric acid nephropathy. *Arch Int Med* 138:612–615, 1978.

57. Yu T-F, Berger L: Impaired renal function in gout: its association with hypertensive vascular disease and intrinsic renal disease. *Am J Med* 72:95–100, 1982.

58. Messerli FH, Frohlich ED, Dreslinski GR, et al: Serum uric acid in essential hypertension: an indicator of renal vascular involvement. *Ann Int Med* 93:817–821, 1980.

59. Fessel WJ: Renal outcomes of gout and hyperuricemia. *Am J Med* 67:74–82, 1979.

60. Yu T-F, Berger L, Dorph DJ, et al: Renal function in gout: V Factors influencing the renal hemodynamics. *Am J Med* 67:766–771, 1979.

61. Benabe JE, Martinez-Maldonado M: Hypercalcemic nephropathy. *Arch Int Med* 138:777–779, 1978.

62. Muther RS, McCarron DA, Bennett WM: Granulomatous sarcoid nephritis: a cause of multiple renal tubular abnormalities. *Clin Nephrol* 14:190–197, 1980.

63. Heptinstall RH: *Pathology of the Kidney,* ed 2. Boston, Little, Brown & Co, 1974.

64. Libertino JA, Zinman L, Breslin DJ, et al: Renal artery revascularization: restoration of renal function. *J Am Med Assoc* 244:1340–1342, 1980.

65. Gifford RW, Stewart BH, Alfidi RJ, et al: Controlling atherosclerotic renovascular hypertension. *Geriatrics* 28(suppl 9):124–131, 1973.

66. Madias NE, Ball JT, Millan VG: Percutaneous transluminal renal angioplasty in the treatment

of unilateral atherosclerotic renovascular hypertension. *Am J Med* 70:1078–1084, 1981.

67. Lessman RK, Johnson SF, Coburn JW, et al: Renal artery embolism: clinical features and long term follow-up of 17 cases. *Ann Int Med* 89:477–482, 1978.

68. Wasser WG, Krakoff LR, Haimov M, et al: Restoration of renal function after bilateral renal artery occlusion. *Arch Int Med* 141:1647–1651, 1981.

69. Sieniewicz DJ, Moore S, Moir FD, et al: Atheromatous emboli to the kidneys. *Radiology* 92:1231–1240, 1969.

70. Smith MC, Ghose MK, Henry AR: The clinical spectrum of renal cholesterol embolization. *Am J Med* 71:174–180, 1981.

71. Kassirer JP: Atheroembolic renal disease. *N Engl J Med* 280:812–818, 1969.

72. Wolf SM, Fauci AS, Horn RG, et al: Wegener's granulomatosis. *Ann Int Med* 81:513–525, 1974.

73. Appel GB, Gee B, Kashgarian M, et al: Wegener's granulomatosis: clinical-pathologic correlations and long-term course. *Am J Kid Dis* 1:27–37, 1981.

74. Duross S, Davin T, Kjellstrand CM: Wegener's granulomatosis with severe renal failure: clinical course and results of dialysis and transplantation. *Clin Nephrol* 16:172–180, 1981.

75. Fauci AS, Haynes BF, Katz P: The spectrum of vasculitis: clinical, pathologic, immunologic and therapeutic considerations. *Ann Int Med* 89:660–676, 1978.

76. The enigma of periarteritis nodosa—Medical Staff Conference, University of California, San Francisco. *West J Med* 122:310–315, 1975.

77. Leib ES, Restivo C, Paulus HE: Immunosuppressive and corticosteroid therapy of polyarteritis nodosa. *Am J Med* 67:941–947, 1979.

78. Fauci AS, Katz P, Haynes BF, et al: Cyclophosphamide therapy of severe systemic necrotizing vasculitis. *N Engl J Med* 301:235–238, 1979.

79. Oliver JA, Cannon PJ: The kidney in scleroderma. *Nephron* 18:141–150, 1977.

80. Zawada ET, Clements PJ, Furst DA, et al: Clinical course of patients with scleroderma renal crisis treated with captopril. *Nephron* 27:74–78, 1981.

81. LeRoy EC, Fleischmann RM: The management of renal scleroderma: experience with dialysis, nephrectomy and transplantation. *Am J Med* 64:174–978, 1978.

82. Myers TJ, Wakem CJ, Ball ED, et al: Thrombotic thrombocytopenic purpura: combined treatment with plasmapheresis and antiplatelet agents. *Ann Int Med* 92(part 1):149–155, 1980.

83. Goldstein MH, Churg J, Strauss L, et al: Hemolytic-uremic syndrome. *Nephron* 23:263–272, 1979.

84. Morel-Maroger L, Kanfer A, Solez K, et al: Prognostic importance of vascular lesions in acute renal failure with microangiopathic hemolytic anemia (hemolytic-uremic syndrome): clincopathologic study in 20 adults. *Kidney Int* 15:548–558, 1979.

85. Garnick MB: Advanced renal cell cancer. *Kidney Int* 20:127–136, 1981.

86. Tannenbaum M: Ultrastructural pathology of human renal cell tumors. *Pathol Ann* 6:249–261, 1971.

87. Cronin RE, Kaehny WD, Miller PD, et al: Renal cell carcinoma: unusual systemic manifestations. *Medicine* 55:291–311, 1976.

88. Johnson KE, Plain CL, Facron E, et al: Management of intrarenal peripelvic cysts. *Urology* 4:514–518, 1974.

89. Gagliano RG, Costanzi JJ, Beathard GA, et al: The nephrotic syndrome associated with neoplasia: an unusual paraneoplastic syndrome. *Am J Med* 60:1026–1031, 1976.

90. Bennett WM, Plamp C, Porter GA: Drug-related syndromes in clinical nephrology. *Ann Int Med* 87:582–590, 1977.

91. Roxe DM: Toxic nephropathy from diagnostic and therapeutic agents—review and commentary. *Am J Med* 69:759–766, 1980.

92. Cronin RE: Aminoglycoside nephrotoxicity: pathogenesis and prevention. *Clin Nephrol* 11:251–256, 1979.

93. Blachley JD, Hill JB: Renal and electrolyte disturbances associated with cisplatin. *Ann Int Med* 95:628–632, 1981.

94. Henrich WL, Blachley JD: Acute renal failure with prostaglandin inhibitors. *Sem Nephrol* 1:57–60, 1981.

95. Fong HJ, Cohen AH: Ibuprofen-induced acute renal failure with acute tubular necrosis. *Am J Nephrol* 2:28–31, 1982.

96. Torres VE: Present and future of the nonsteroidal anti-inflammatory drugs in nephrology (editorial). *Mayo Clin Proc* 57:389–393, 1982.

97. McMurray SD, Luft FC, Maxwell DR, et al: Prevailing patterns and predictor variables in patients with acute tubular necrosis. *Arch Int Med* 138:950–955, 1978.

98. Hall JW, Johnson WJ, Maher FT, et al: Immediate and long-term prognosis in acute renal failure. *Ann Int Med* 73:515–521, 1970.

99. Rose BD: *Pathophysiology of Renal Disease.* New York, McGraw-Hill Book Co, 1981, pp 55–95.

100. Miller PD, Krebs RA, Neal BJ, et al: Polyuric

prerenal failure. *Arch Int Med* 140:907–909, 1980.

101. Gordon JA, Anderson RJ: Hepatorenal syndrome. *Sem Nephrol* 1:37–42, 1981.

102. Anderson RJ, Linas SL, Berns AS, et al: Nonoliguric acute renal failure. *N Engl J Med* 296:1134–1138, 1977.

103. Espinel CH: The FE$_{Na}$ test: use in the differential diagnosis of acute renal failure. *J Am Med Assoc* 236:579–581, 1976.

104. Miller TR, Anderson RJ, Linas SL, et al: Urinary diagnostic indices in acute renal failure: a prospective study. *Ann Int Med* 89:47–50, 1978.

105. Levinsky NG, Bernard DB, Johnston PA: Enhancement of recovery of acute renal failure: effects of mannitol and diuretics, in Brenner BM, Stein JH (eds): *Comtemporary Issues in Nephrology No. 6: Acute Renal Failure*. New York, Churchill Livingstone, 1980, pp 163–179.

106. Mitchell JC: Chronic renal failure in the elderly: what to look for when it starts. *Geriatrics* 35(suppl 11):28–34, 1980.

107. Walker PJ, Ginn HE, Johnson HK, et al: Long-term hemodialysis for patients over 50. *Geriatrics* 31(suppl 9):55–61, 1976.

108. Rathaus M, Korzets Z, Bernheim J: Results of regular hemodialysis treatment in the elderly: a retrospective study. *Dialysis and Transplant* 9:1015–1018, 1091, 1980.

109. Delmonico FL, Cosimi AB, Russell PS: Renal transplantation in the older age group. *Arch Surg* 110:1107–1109, 1975.

110. Kjellstrand CM, Shideman JR, Lynch RE, et al: Kidney transplant in patients over 50. *Geriatrics* 31(suppl 9):65–73, 1976.

111. Golper TA, Barry JM, Bennett WM, et al: Primary cadaver kidney transplantation in older patients: survival equal to dialysis. *Trans Am Soc Artif Int Organs* 24:282–285, 1978.

CHAPTER 17

Urological Disorders

EUGENE F. FUCHS, M.D.

Benign Prostatic Hyperplasia

Among the genitourinary problems of the geriatric population, benign prostatic hyperplasia is certainly the most common; it may represent the most common neoplasm of mankind. It is a disease of advancing age with an uncertain etiology. It is linked to testosterone production, which is indicated by the finding that males who are castrated before puberty will not develop benign prostatic hyperplasia; also, castrated adult males will have a regression of the hyperplastic process.

Histologic evidence of prostatic hyperplasia is unusual before 40 years of age. Thereafter, however, the incidence increases rapidly, with greater than 90% of all males at 90 years of age showing histologic evidence.[2] By measuring objective parameters such as the urinary flow rate, a bladder outlet obstruction can be demonstrated in virtually all elderly males with an intact hormonal function. The vast majority of this group will have little or no significant complaints to warrant a definitive therapy to relieve the obstruction. Approximately 10% of all males surviving into the 8th decade will require some form of therapy to ameliorate symptoms of a bladder outlet obstruction.[3]

Clinical Presentation

Symptoms that are due to benign prostatic hyperplasia occur because of a urethral compression by the enlarging gland. The increased voiding pressure resulting from an increase in outflow resistance subsequently causes a bladder muscle hypertrophy. At this time, the patient is unlikely to offer any complaints. Slowly, over time, the bladder decompensates and voiding pressure decreases. At this point, males begin noticing a decreased force and caliber of the voided stream and, perhaps, some hesitancy and postvoid dribbling. When bladder emptying becomes inefficient, incomplete emptying becomes the rule. Complaints of nocturnal and diurnal urinary frequency and the feeling of incomplete emptying are common. As increasingly larger residual volumes develop, they predispose to urinary tract infections, which are marked by a severe dysuria and even more attempts at urination. In an inflamed and congested state, the prostatic veins become dilated and, if ruptured, they will cause hematuria, which is a common reason to finally seek medical attention even when other symptoms are long-standing.

If the condition is allowed to progress, acute urinary retention is frequent. This is especially true: 1) Following excessive alcohol intake, the ingestion of diazepam, phenothiazines, beta and/or alpha agonists or antagonists, and other drugs that may inhibit bladder emptying; or 2) If voiding is delayed beyond regular intervals. Acute retention of infected urine may cause an acute, severe sepsis.

Physical Findings

It is not possible to determine the extent of a bladder outlet obstruction by the findings of a rectal examination. However, as a general rule, larger glands are more likely to be associated with symptoms of a bladder outlet obstruction. The typical finding on rectal examination is a homogeneous, enlarged gland without the usual palpable median sulcus. A microscopic examination of prostatic secretions may demonstrate inflammatory cells that are characteristic of a prostatic infection, which itself may increase a bladder outlet obstruction and the resulting symptoms. During a rectal examination, an evaluation of rectal tone is helpful, as it may reflect the intactness of bladder enervation.

Catheterization for removing residual urine may be helpful to evaluate the efficiency of voiding. If a residual urine of more than 60 ml is discovered, the patient is inefficiently voiding, probably due to an outlet resistance and a decompensation of the bladder muscle. It also is possible, however, that the patient has a neurogenic bladder due to an occult neurologic process for which he may need further evaluation.

Excretory urograms are not necessary in all patients with symptoms of a bladder outlet obstruction; but, it should be obtained in the presence of an infection, hematuria, or flank pain. Suspicion of an upper tract obstruction also warrants this study.

Treatment

Surgery is usually recommended for symptomatic patients who have increased residual urine. However, in the absence of a significant residual urine or urinary tract infection in a patient whose symptoms are not severe enough to impair his quality of life, a definitive procedure to relieve a bladder outlet obstruction is not indicated. These patients should be followed to monitor their symptoms. If they begin to have more hesitancy and nocturia, a urologic evaluation should be pursued. In the presence of an active urinary tract infection, symptoms of a bladder outlet obstruction may be masked by the irritation of the infection. In such an instance, it is appropriate to treat the infection; if the symptoms are largely relieved, a definitive procedure for relieving the outlet obstruction may not be necessary. However, if the infection is not easily cleared and the symptoms are not resolved satisfactorily, or if the infection rapidly recurs, a definitive procedure to relieve the problem should be considered.

The standard treatment for a significant bladder outlet obstruction is a resolution by either a transurethral resection or an open prostatectomy. The choice of the procedures rests with the urologist and depends on several factors, which include his personal skill, the size of the prostate, and a patient's overall condition. Results of a transurethral resection or open prostatectomy are excellent, with the majority of patients getting a satisfactory relief of their symptoms. Many will continue to experience nocturia once or twice per night, but the flow rates should be improved and the patients should void to completion.

As an alternative to a definitive therapy for relief of the outlet obstruction, a program of intermittent self-catheterization may be elected in some cases. This is generally chosen for patients who are not candidates for a surgical procedure because of complicating medical conditions, or in patients who adamantly refuse surgical therapy. Intermittent self-catheterization can be successfully done by a well-motivated patient with a relatively low morbidity. There is some risk of a chronic urinary tract infection, particularly if a patient does not diligently follow the protocol; but, it is significantly less than with an in-dwelling catheter.

If neither a surgical procedure or intermittent self-catheterization is a possibility, an in-dwelling urethral catheter may be the only resort. Once a decision is made to commit an individual to a permanent in-dwelling urethral catheter, proper care of the catheter must be assured. Drinking copious amounts of fluid, enough to produce a urinary output of at least 2–3 liters per day, will help prevent encrustations on the catheter and allow a free flow. The catheter should be replaced periodically, with the frequency depending on the type used. All patients with a permanent in-dwelling catheter have chronic urinary tract infections. However, the continuous use of antibiotics should be avoided, as they will induce the development of highly resistant organisms; should a complication of epididymitis, prostatitis, or pyelonephritis arise, the armamentarium of antibiotics would be greatly lessened.

The placement of a suprapubic catheter is an alternative to chronic, in-dwelling intraurethral catheters. Its placement requires a short surgical procedure and general anesthetic. In a patient for whom prolonged catheter drainage is anticipated, a suprapubic tube may be the best alternative since it allows the use of a much larger tube, and, consequently, less frequent changes. Attaining a high urine output and avoidance of antibiotics apply to a suprapubic tube as well as to an intraurethral catheter.

Urinary Incontinence

Few, if any, conditions are as frustrating and humiliating as urinary incontinence. It often is the proximate cause of social isolation, depression, and dependency. It significantly increases the demand for nursing care or the attention of care-givers at home. It predisposes to skin breakdown and pressure sores. It can be intermittent or persistent, and it is often reversible or at least controllable. With a basic understanding of the physiology of normal micturi-

tion and the various types of incontinence, physicians can successfully help many patients with this disorder.

Physiology of Normal Micturition[4]

Normal voiding patterns involve a period of urinary storage followed by a voluntary and timely evacuation of the bladder. This process requires a coordinated and orderly function of the autonomic, somatic, and central nervous systems. Inhibitory centers in the brain, which communicate via the cortical spinal tracts, inhibit bladder emptying and facilitate bladder storage. The sympathetic nervous system contributes primarily to bladder storage via beta receptors that are located primarily in the main body of the bladder, and by alpha receptors that are concentrated in the bladder neck (*see* Figure 17-1). When stimulated, the beta receptors

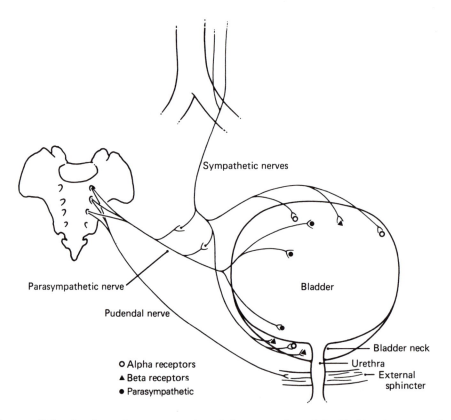

Sympathetic nerves

Parasympathetic nerve

Pudendal nerve

Bladder

○ Alpha receptors
▲ Beta receptors
● Parasympathetic

Bladder neck
Urethra
External sphincter

FIGURE 17-1 A schematic representation of the enervation of the bladder demonstrating the predominance of alpha receptors in the bladder base and beta receptors in the bladder detrusor muscle. The parasympathetic receptors are placed diffusely throughout the bladder. There also are extravesical communications between the parasympathetic and sympathetic system. The pudendal nerve to the external sphincter is of a somatic origin.

enhance the relaxation of the bladder. Alpha receptors, when stimulated, facilitate a closure of the bladder neck during periods of bladder storage. A somatic enervation to the external urinary sphincter via the pudendal nerve causes a contraction of the sphincter, thus adding to the total outlet resistance and contributing significantly to urinary continence. Voluntary and involuntary contractions of the external sphincter, via the pudendal nerve, also contribute significantly to the outlet resistance and the continence mechanism.

Bladder emptying is principally a function of the parasympathetic system, which by activating acetylcholine (ACh) receptors causes a contraction of the detrusor muscle. During evacuation, the bladder neck relaxes and opens because of a damping of sympathetic input. Somatic impulses are decreased, which allows the external sphincter to open, thus contributing to an efficient bladder emptying by further decreasing the outlet resistance.

A normal voiding frequency has an individual variation. In general, most individuals void four to five times during the course of their waking hours, and sleep through the night without awakening to empty their bladders. As a person ages, it is not unusual to arise once or twice per night to void, but with no other symptoms to suggest a pathology. The use of a diuretic will cause a decrease in the voiding interval. Patients with chronic congestive heart failure tend to mobilize fluid as they lie recumbent, which may be a cause of an increase in nocturia.

Bladder function can be objectively documented by using a cystometrography. A cystometrogram instrument records a bladder's response to slow filling, with either carbon dioxide (CO_2) or water, and documents resting voiding pressures (*see* Figure 17-2).

Normal continence is, thus, a matter of the pressure of an outlet resistance that exceeds the combined resting pressure of the bladder and the pressure of the abdominal contents exerted on the bladder. If, during any phase of urinary storage, the pressure of outlet resistance is less than the combined abdominal and bladder pressure, incontinence will result. Urinary incontinence can be divided into four subclassifications based on these concepts.

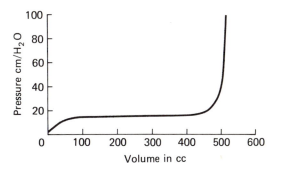

FIGURE 17-2 A normal cystometrogram curve. It should be remembered that the volume may vary up to several hundred cc to the right or left and still represent a normal bladder. The pressure generated by the detrusor muscle during contraction also may vary considerably, but still represent a bladder that functions normally.

Stress Incontinence[5]

Urinary stress incontinence results when a sudden and transient rise in abdominal pressure and (consequently) bladder pressure is not matched by a concomitant rise in the bladder outlet resistance. During these transient elevations in pressure, as with coughing, sneezing, or lifting, the patient experiences a loss of urine in an amount depending on the severity of the problem. These patients usually are multiparous females who experience incontinence during various exertional daily activities, but who remain dry during normal sleeping hours.

A typical patient will have a normal neurologic exam, normal cystometrogram, and minimal residual urine. On physical examination, it is common to discover the presence of a cystourethrocele, which may be a contributing factor although it probably does not cause incontinence.

The treatment of urinary stress incontinence is not indicated in females who only have an occasional loss of a small amount of urine. However, in females whose incontinence progresses to the point that they must wear protective devices to avoid soiling their clothes, some form of treatment is clearly needed. Females with mild stress incontinence may benefit by a pharmacologic manipulation with drugs that possess alpha-adrenergic activity (*see* Table 17-1).[6] These drugs enhance the closure of the bladder neck, thus increasing the outlet resistance and frequently correcting or improving

TABLE 17-1 Drugs Used to Treat Urinary Incontinence

Drugs	Dosages	Mechanisms of Action	Types of Incontinence	Potential Side Effects
Anticholinergic Propantheline	15–30 mg three times a day	Diminish uninhibited bladder contractions	Urge incontinence with uninhibited bladder contractions	Dry mouth Blurry vision Elevated intraocular pressure Constipation
Imipramine	25–50 mg three times a day			Postural hypotension, cardiac conduction disturbances (imipramine only)
Oxybutinin	5 mg three times a day	Increase bladder capacity	Stress incontinence with uninhibited bladder contractions	
Dicyclomine	10–20 mg three times a day			
Flavoxate Emepronium*				
Alpha-adrenergic agonists Pseudoephedrine	15–30 mg three times a day	Urethral sphincter contraction	Stress incontinence with sphincter weakness	Headache Tachycardia Elevation of blood pressure
Phenylpropanolamine	50 mg twice a day			Imipramine—see above
Imipramine	25–50 mg three times a day			
Cholinergic agonists Bethanechol	10–30 mg three to four times a day	Bladder contraction	Overflow incontinence with atonic bladder	Bradycardia, hypotension, bronchoconstriction, gastric acid secretion

Drug/Dosage	Mechanism of action	Type of incontinence	Side effects
Alpha-adrenergic antagonists Phenoxybenzyline — 20–200 mg four times a day	Urethral sphincter relaxation	Overflow incontinence with hyperactive urethral sphincter	Postural hypotension, nasal stuffiness, pupillary constriction
Estrogens Systemic Estrone — 0.3–0.625 mg every day Estradiol — 1–2 mg four times a day Topical Estrone — 1 g twice per week	Increase periurethral blood flow, muscle strength, and sphincter tone	Stress incontinence (female)	Endometrial cancer, elevated blood pressure, gallstones, cardiovascular (stroke, embolus, myocardial infarction)
Investigational Prostaglandin inhibitors Indomethacin — 25–100 mg twice a day Flubiprofen — 50 mg three times a day	Inhibit bladder contractions	Incontinence with uninhibited bladder contractions	Gastric irritation
Calcium antagonists Nifepidine — 10–20 mg twice a day Baclofen — 5–10 mg twice a day			Hypotension, reflex tachycardia, drowsiness (nifepidine) Weakness, insomnia, pruritis (baclofen)

* Not available in the United States; used in Europe.

SOURCE: Ouslander JG: "Urinary incontinence in the elderly." *West J Med* 135:482–491, 1981.

incontinence. Phenylpropanolamine hydrochloride (75 mg), and chlorpheneramine (12 mg [Ornade]) taken twice daily are most commonly used. In females with a severe urinary stress incontinence, drug therapy will not be effective; in these cases, surgical repair is indicated. A variety of surgical procedures have been devised to correct incontinence.[5,7]

It is unusual for males to develop pure urinary stress incontinence. When it does occur, it usually is after prostate surgery for a benign or malignant disease. Once again, pharmacologic manipulation can be tried. If this fails, a variety of anti-incontinence procedures using various prosthetic devices are available.

Urge Incontinence[8]

An uncontrolled loss of urine immediately preceded by an intense urge to void is classified as urgency incontinence. Patients with urge incontinence usually will complain of an extreme diurnal and, to a lesser extent, nocturnal urinary frequency. The loss of urine always is preceded by a strong urge to urinate, and is followed shortly by a sudden and forceful gush of a small volume of urine or, sometimes a complete emptying of the bladder. Symptoms may become so severe that the patient is completely homebound for fear of soiling himself in public.

The cause of this symptom complex is uninhibited bladder contractions due to a loss of central nervous system inhibition or to a local irritation of the bladder. Any condition that interrupts the inhibitory center of the brain or the cortical spinal tract can cause uninhibited bladder contractions (as an uninhibited neurogenic bladder), provided that the level of involvement is above the sacral reflex center (S2-S4). A local irritation of the bladder, particularly its base, also may produce symptoms that are indistinguishable from an uninhibited neurogenic bladder. An acute urinary tract infection with a subsequent inflammation of the bladder epithelium is the most common cause of uninhibited contractions due to bladder irritation. However, other inflammatory conditions of the bladder, such as tuberculosis and interstitial cystitis, can cause similar symptoms. The involvement of the bladder by a neoplastic process that is either primary to the bladder, secondary from a metastatic disease, or spread from adjacent structures, can cause a marked urinary urgency and urge incontinence.

On physical examination, findings may vary greatly, which depends on the extent of the primary cause. Patients with an uninhibited neurogenic bladder that is secondary to a loss of the central nervous system inhibitory centers may exhibit no other findings than an uninhibited neurogenic bladder. However, this would be quite unusual, as most patients will have enough adjacent areas involved to produce neurologic signs. Those patients with a spinal cord involvement also may have very selected spinal tracts involved, which produces very minimal physical signs. Once again, this is quite unusual; as a general rule, enough adjacent spinal tracts will be involved to produce positive neurologic signs.

In those patients with an inflammation or neoplastic involvement of the bladder, there will inevitably be correlative findings in the urine. Pyuria will be found in nearly all patients with an inflammation, which produces positive cultures if it is bacterial. Tuberculous inflammation or inflammation due to interstitial cystitis usually will have an associated hematuria, but the bacterial cultures will be negative. Hematuria will inevitably be present with a neoplastic process. Residual urine will be negligible, as these patients usually exhibit a complete emptying of the bladder. The key to a diagnosis of an uninhibited neurogenic bladder is in taking a careful history and doing a good physical examination to collaborate those findings with a cystometrogram. The cystometrogram curve inevitably will show a shift to the left and demonstrate uninhibited bladder contractions with relatively small volumes of urine. As the bladder becomes decompensated, the cystometrogram curve may shift to the right, which demonstrates a greater volume before the uninhibited contractions occur. Also, as the bladder decompensates, there may be a tendency to begin retaining urine due to the reduced pressure of the uninhibited contractions.

The proper treatment of patients with urge incontinence that is secondary to an uninhibited neurogenic bladder depends on marking an appropriate diagnosis. When the insult has involved the inhibition centers of the brain, it is unlikely that any therapeutic efforts will be successful in alleviating the insult. Nevertheless, these patients should have the benefit of an appropriate neurologic evaluation, if that has not already been accomplished by the time the symptoms have been recognized. When the pathologic process involves the spinal tracts in the spinal cord, it is more likely that a reversible process is involved.

The finding of a pyuria and hematuria in a patient with urge incontinence strongly suggests an inflammatory or neoplastic process and demands a thorough evaluation. Appropriate urine cultures along with an excretory urogram and cystoscopy often will assist in arriving at a correct diagnosis, correction of the problem, and alleviation of the symptoms.

Good symptomatic control of urge incontinence can be attained in most patients with urinary tract infections by using appropriate antibiotics. If a neoplasm is found, appropriate treatment usually will alleviate the symptoms. The use of anticholinergics[9,10] can suppress the contractions of an uninhibited neurogenic bladder. Propantheline is the most commonly used of this family of drugs. Oxybutynin chloride is another popular drug that has, in addition to its anticholinergic activity, a direct action on the smooth muscle to relieve uninhibited contractions. These drugs should be used with caution in elderly patients and in patients with cardiac conditions that may preclude the use of an anticholinergic agent. Patients may become constipated during therapy, and appropriate preventive measures should be taken. The additional side effects of dryness of the mouth and some blurring of vision also is common.

In elderly males with large obstructing prostates, the use of anticholinergic agents is particularly worrisome because an acute obstruction may result from a rapid decrease of detrusor tone. In such cases, a complete urologic evaluation is advisable before instituting drug therapy. Males who have obstructing prostates with a typical bladder trabeculation that is seen in patients who have been voiding against a high bladder outlet resistance for some time should undergo a transurethral resection of the prostate.

Total Urinary Incontinence

Total urinary incontinence is defined as a complete lack of control over the voiding function and the constant dripping of urine. Etiologies of this condition include a total loss of bladder outlet resistance or a urinary fistula formation that circumvents normal sphincteric mechanisms. A

typical patient will be either a male who has undergone some form of prostatectomy with complete destruction of the sphincteric mechanisms or a female who has undergone pelvic surgery and/or pelvic irradiation with the resultant vesicovaginal or ureterovaginal fistula. A loss of enervation of the pelvic diaphragm with a deactivation of the sphincteric mechanisms also can result in total urinary incontinence.

These are among the most miserable incontinent patients, as there is little they can do to ameliorate the situation. An evaluation of these patients usually reveals a person who is wearing some form of protective appliance; upon its removal, urine will be seen to drip steadily from the urethra. Residual urine can vary from nil in patients with normal bladders to a substantial amount in patients who have a concomitant flaccid neurogenic bladder. A urologic evaluation is mandatory in all patients with total urinary incontinence.

The treatment of this condition involves a surgical correction of urinary fistulas or somehow restoring or enhancing the sphincteric mechanism in those patients whose spincter muscles have been impaired. A variety of surgical techniques have evolved for increasing the bladder outlet resistance. Recent advancements in artificial urinary sphincters hold much promise in the treatment of these patients.

Overflow Urinary Incontinence

Paradoxical incontinence is defined as a frequent, uncontrolled loss of urine from an already full bladder. This can occur from an acute and/or chronic bladder outlet obstruction, a flaccid neurogenic bladder, and as a result of drug-induced acute retention; it can also occur in unconscious or demented patients.

Catheterization for residual urine will quickly establish the cause of the problem, as these patients usually will harbor residual urine in a large volume (occasionally up to more than 2 liters). It is common for the urine to be infected.

These patients should have their bladders acutely drained with an in-dwelling Foley catheter or a suprapubic tube, and have the urinary tract infection treated. After stabilization of their condition, patients should undergo a complete urologic evaluation to discover the cause of the acute and/or chronic retention.

Urinary Calculus Disease[11,12]

In the general population, the incidence rate of renal calculi is greater in males than in females, and it decreases in incidence as the population ages. In elderly persons, the incidence rate of calculus in males and females becomes approximately equal and assumes an even greater importance. The treatment for a small symptomatic renal or ureteral calculus is the same in all age groups. Most small calculi less than 0.5 cm at their greatest diameter will pass spontaneously, which requires only symptomatic treatment with analgesics. In an elderly individual with less reserve, however, close observation is mandatory; a complication of an obstructing calculus would be much more devastating than in a younger individual. An elderly patient with a symptomatic calculus disease should be initially hospitalized. If there is any indication of an infection proximal to the stone, some form of drainage procedure must be implemented to prevent life-threatening sepsis. On a successful passage of the calculus or surgical removal, consideration should be given to a metabolic screening to determine the cause of the calculus.

Staghorn calculi are more common in elderly persons, in whom the incidence rate is greater in females than males. The majority of calculi will be magnesium-ammonium phosphate (struvite) calculi that arise as a result of urinary tract infections. These stones must be removed surgically because of their high morbidity and mortality, which is a direct result of the calculus.[13] Sterilization of the urine should be attempted after the stone has been removed, followed by close monitoring for a recurrent infection.

Hematuria

Blood in the urine, whether microscopic or gross, always is an ominous finding. In an elderly person, hematuria is an especially worrisome symptom because of its high association with primary genitourinary malignancies or malignancies in adjacent organs that have invaded the genitourinary tract. The finding of a microscopic hematuria or a history of gross hematuria demands a complete urologic evaluation, which includes an excretory urogram and cystoscopy.

Hematuria can be associated with urinary tract infections, but once the infection is treated and the symptoms are relieved, the hematuria should disappear. A tuberculous infection of the bladder commonly presents as a hematuria and only can be diagnosed by appropriate cultures.

Anticoagulation therapy with coumadin commonly causes microscopic hematuria. It is important that these patients receive a thorough urologic evaluation for an occult genitourinary malignancy or other hidden causes of hematuria.

It should be stressed that a complete urologic evaluation includes an excretory urogram and cystoscopy. Only with a cystoscopy can the bladder be adequately evaluated for a malignancy or other causes of hematuria. Also, at the time of the cystoscopy, further studies may be completed to further evaluate the genitourinary tract.

Carcinoma of the Prostate

Carcinoma of the prostate is the third most common cancer found in American males; it currently accounts for greater than 60,000 new cases and more than 20,000 deaths annually. Despite several advances in treatment and a greater public awareness of prostatic carcinoma, only about 10% of all males with this condition have their disease detected early enough to effect a cure.

The etiology of prostatic carcinomas is unknown. There exists no known association between prostatic carcinoma and benign hyperplasia of the prostate or prostatitis, and there are no recognized carcinogenic agents for prostatic carcinoma. It occurs rarely before 45 years of age but by the 8th decade more than 50% of males examined in autopsy series will have a histologic evidence of a prostatic adenocarcinoma.[14] In the United States and Canada, adenocarcinoma of the prostate is more common in the black population than in the white population.[15] The black population in the United States has a greater incidence of this disease than an age-matched black population in Africa. Oriental males living in the United States have a lower incidence than American white persons, but a much higher incidence than in Oriental males living in the Orient.

Adenocarcinoma of the prostate accounts for greater than 95% of all prostate cancers, with the remaining small fraction being composed of squamous cell carcinomas, transitional cell carcinomas, and prostatic sarcomas.[16] Histologically, adenocarcinomas of the prostate usually are well differentiated, but the histology can range from well differentiated to undifferentiated anaplastic-appearing carcinomas. As a general rule, the more differentiated carcinomas grow more slowly and less aggressively than the anaplastic variety. An adenocarcinoma of the prostate, as with the prostate itself, usually is dependent on testosterone for growth. Androgen dependency tends to decrease as the tumor becomes more anaplastic. Well-differentiated adenocarcinomas usually retain the ability to produce acid phosphatase. As the carcinoma escapes the confines of the prostatic capsule and the acid phosphatase production continues, there is a rise in the serum acid phosphatase to above normal levels. As an adenocarcinoma of the prostate becomes more undifferentiated, and even in some well-differentiated carcinomas, the ability to produce acid phosphatase may be lost. This accounts for the observation that approximately 25% of all patients with a metastatic adenocarcinoma of the prostate will not demonstrate an elevated acid phosphatase level.[17]

The natural history of a prostatic carcinoma is one of local growth that eventually leads to an escape from the confines of the prostatic capsule to invade locally. Surgery before this occurs can be curative. Distant metastasis occurs first in the regional lymph nodes and bony pelvis or lower lumbar spine and, finally, to all distant sites.[18]

There are no early symptoms of a low-stage carcinoma of the prostate. An early detection depends entirely on a good physical examination with a digital rectal examination performed on a periodic basis beginning in the 4th decade.[19] Only then will a small nodule be discovered that is typical of a low-stage, and therefore curable, prostatic carcinoma. The rapid development and progression of symptoms of a bladder outlet obstruction is strongly suggestive of prostatic carcinoma, especially in males younger than 60 years of age.

The propensity to an early metastasis to the bones is the reason that many males present with bone pain as the first symptom. A local growth of the tumor into the prostatic urethra and the bladder or trigone may cause a hematuria and frequent urination, which is another common presenting symptom. A distal ureteral obstruction from a local growth of the prostate commonly causes an obstructive uropathy as the disease progresses. Death due to a carcinoma of the prostate commonly results from bone marrow replacement by the neoplasm, which causes severe anemia, liver involvement and liver failure, ureteral obstruction and renal failure, and pulmonary failure due to a metastasis to the lung.

The treatment of a prostatic carcinoma depends on the clinical stage of the disease at the time of presentation. At the time a diagnosis is suspected, a needle biopsy procedure of the prostate is done, either transrectally or transperineally, to document histologically the tumor characteristics. Once confirmed histologically, further staging is done by the traditional methods of a complete blood count (CBC), liver function tests, renal function tests, electrolyte screening, and a chest x-ray film. Because of the propensity for an early bony metastasis, a ^{99m}Technetium polyphosphate bone scan is mandatory. A serum acid phosphatase level should be determined in all patients suspected of having a prostatic carcinoma. If elevated, the patient has either a stage C or D disease. A normal acid phosphatase level does not rule out a metastasis. There are rare but well-recognized causes for acid phosphatase elevations that are unrelated to a prostatic carcinoma; among them are prostatic infarction, Gaucher's disease, Paget's disease, hyperthyroidism, and others.[20] Lymphangiography, computed tomography (CT scan), and a transrectal ultrasonography are becoming more popular in the staging of a prostate carcinoma; but, they are not yet in general use.

Once a clinical staging is complete, a rational approach can be made for treatment options. Table 17-2 outlines the standard treatment for various stages of the disease. Treatment options also must take into consideration the overall condition of the patient. An elderly individual who has an expected survival of less than 5 years, or who is severely disabled and likely to die soon of an unrelated disease, would not be a candidate for a radical prostatectomy. Because interstitial irradiation requires open surgery, that also would be contraindicated. External

TABLE 17-2 Staging of Prostatic Carcinoma

Stage	Clinical Characteristics	Treatment
A_1	Microfocal disease found in prostatectomy specimen, normal gland to palpation, acid phosphatase normal, no metastasis	No further treatment required
A_2	Diffuse disease found on prostatectomy specimen, normal gland to palpation, acid phosphatase normal, no metastasis	Total prostatectomy, interstitial or external beam irradiation
B_1	Solitary 1–1.5 cm nodule surrounded by normal prostatic tissue, acid phosphatase normal, no metastasis	Total prostatectomy, interstitial or external beam irradiation
B_2	On palpation, one or both lobes of prostate diffusely involved with tumor, acid phosphatase normal, no metastasis	Total prostatectomy, interstitial or external beam irradiation
C	On palpation, obvious tumor extension beyond prostatic capsule, no distant metastasis, acid phosphatase may be elevated slightly	Total prostatectomy, interstitial or external beam irradiation
D	On palpation, large diffusely nodular gland with obvious extension, distant metastasis present, acid phosphatase elevated in 75% of all cases	Irradiation to control local disease may be indicated, hormonal manipulation to relieve symptoms

beam irradiation is, however, an excellent option in these patients for local control of the disease.

Because 75% of all patients with prostate cancer have a carcinoma that is testosterone-dependent, depriving the prostate tissue of testosterone by suppressing its production or removing the testes will provide a good temporary control in those patients.[21] The goal of hormonal manipulation is to reduce the serum testosterone to anorchic levels. This can be achieved by administering 1 mg/day of diethylstilbesterol to suppress the luteinizing hormone. At a dose of 1 mg/day, the serum testosterone will be reduced to anorchic levels in 75% of males. The remaining group will require an increase of the dose to 1 mg three times daily before anorchic levels will be achieved. Alternatively, a bilateral orchiectomy can be done in those males willing to have the procedure, or in males who are not compliant in taking medication or whose cardiovascular status precludes the use of estrogens. Eventually, all men with a stage D disease will escape the hormonal control of their tumor and succumb to this progressive disease.

Conventional chemotherapy, either alone or in various combinations, has not proven to be an effective long-term treatment for an advanced carcinoma, and much work remains to be done in this area.[22] The use of these drugs adjuvantly with conventional irradiation or extirpative surgery has yet to be adequately studied; perhaps, they hold some hope for a yet to be determined subpopulation of patients with carcinoma of the prostate.

References

1. Walsh PC: "Benign prostatic hyperplasia, in Harrison H, Gittes R, Permutter A, Stamey T (eds): *Campbell's Urology,* ed 4. Philadelphia, WB Saunders & Co, 1979, vol 2, chapter 26, pp 949–961.

2. Harbitz TB, Haugen OA: Histology of the prostate in elderly males. *Acta Pathol Microbiol Scand* 80:756–768, 1972.

3. Lytton B, Emery JM, Heward BM: The incidence of benign prostatic hyperplasia. *J Urol* 99:639–645, 1968.

4. Bissada NK, Finkbeiner AE: Pharmacology of continence and micturition. *Am Fam Physician* 20(5):128–136, Nov 1979.

5. Stamey TA, Marshall JF: Urinary incontinence in the female, in Harrison H, Gittes R, Permutter A, Stamey T (eds): *Campbell's Urology,* ed 4. Philadelphia, WB Saunders & Co, 1979, vol 3, chap 75, pp 2272–2294.

6. Montague DK, Stewart BH: Urethral pressure profiles before and after ornade administration in

patients with stress urinary incontinence. *J Urol* 122(2):198–199, Aug 1979.

7. Kaufman JK, Raz S: The treatment of male urinary incontinence, in Harrison H, Gittes R, Permutter A, Stamey T (eds): *Campbell's Urology,* ed 4. Philadelphia, WB Saunders & Co, 1979, vol 3, chap 74, pp 2259–2271.

8. Kendall RA, Karafin L: Classification of neurogenic bladder disease. *Urol Clin North Am* 1(1):37–44, Feb 1974.

9. Knanna, OP: Disorders of micturition, neuropharmacologic basis and results of drug therapy. *Urol* 8:316–328, 1976.

10. Marks R, Bohr GA: How to manage neurogenic bladder after stroke. *Geriatrics* Dec 1977, pp 50–54.

11. Coe FL: *Nephrolithiasis: Pathogenesis and Treatment.* Chicago, Year Book Medical Publishers, 1978.

12. Drach, GW: Urinary lithiasis, in Harrison H, Gittes R, Permutter A, Stamey T (eds): *Campbell's Urology,* ed 4. Philadelphia, WB Saunders & Co, 1978, vol 1, chap 22, pp 779–878.

13. Sing M, Chapman R, Tressider GC, et al: The fate of the unoperated staghorn calculus. *Br J Urol* 45:581–585, 1973.

14. Rullis I, Shaeffer JA, Lilien OM: Incidence of prostatic carcinoma in the elderly. *Urol* 6:295–297, 1975.

15. Smith RL: Mortality attributed to cancer among Hawaiians and Filipinos of Hawaii and the racial groups of the United States and Hawaii. *J Nat Cancer Inst* 18:397–405, 1951.

16. Mostofi FK, Prince, EB: Tumors of the Prostate. In *Tumors of the Male Genital System.* Washington, Armed Forces Institute of Pathology, 1973, pp 177–194.

17. Mostofi FK, Prince EB: Malignant Tumors of the Prostate. In *Tumors of the Male Genital System.* Washington, Armed Forces Institute of Pathology, 1973, pp 196–252.

18. Elken M, Mueller HP: Metastases from cancer of the prostate. *Cancer* 7:1246–1248, 1954.

19. Klein LA: Prostatic carcinoma. *N Engl J Med* April 12, 1979, pp 824–833.

20. Catalona WJ, Scott WW: Carcinoma of the prostate, in Harrison H, Gittes R, Permutter A, Stamey T (eds): *Campbell's Urology,* ed 4. Philadelphia, WB Saunders & Co, 1979, vol 2, chap 31, pp 1098.

21. Walsh PC: Physiologic consequences of hormonal therapy in prostatic cancer. *Urol Clin North Am* 2(1):130–136, Feb 1975.

22. Johnson DE: Cancer of the prostate: Overview, in Johnson DE, Boileau MA (eds): *Genitourinary Tumors: Fundamental Principles and Surgical Techniques.* New York, Grune & Stratton, 1982, pp 1–31.

CHAPTER 18

Gynecology

E. PAUL KIRK, M.D.

Many women use an obstetrician-gynecologist as their primary health care providers. During the childbearing years, the relationship is normal if there are no serious medical problems. Whether or not the gynecologist remains a person's primary physician after menopause or assumes a consultant role, the special problems of an aging female are important and often reversible disorders.

Menopause

The identification of menopause as a landmark in an individual's life span is inevitable, if not always helpful. The climacteric period is one of diminishing ovarian function that is associated with physical changes, of which the cessation of menses is the most obvious. It introduces an era of altered reproductive capability in a female that is not matched in a male. For many females, fertility may have been lost some years before via a surgical intervention such as a hysterectomy or tubal ligation. In other females, infertility, whether deliberate or not, may have been the accepted life style. How any one individual copes with the different physical and emotional stresses of menopause depends on many different physical, psychological, and environmental variables. The spectrum of the experience will vary from a severe disruption of one's life style to an easy acceptance associated with a more comfortable sexuality that is free from the anxiety of unwanted pregnancy.

Estrogen therapy was, for many years, the mainstay of therapeutic intervention for a symptomatic climacteric person. The standard therapy was challenged in the 1970s by the awareness that continuous, unopposed estrogen therapy was associated, in some cases, with the development of an atypical endometrium or adenocarcinoma of the endometrium. As the evidence of the risks of estrogen therapy was being evaluated, so was the evidence demonstrating an important therapeutic benefit that was not merely symptomatic. A regimen of estrogen and progesterone therapy is effective in protecting against osteoporosis in susceptible individuals without unduly increasing the risk of uterine or breast cancer (*see* Volume I, Chapter 28).

Many females, therefore, pass beyond the years of the climacteric period with their natural aging process modified by hormone replacement. The gynecologic problems encountered may be divided into four main categories: 1) Structural support; 2) Epithelial dystrophies; 3) Epithelial inflammation; and 4) Malignant disease. In discussing the identification and management of a gynecologic problem in an elderly patient, it has to be appreciated that the simple identification of a problem is a gross oversimplification. This limitation applies particularly to a patient with a loss of structural support. This patient often describes symptoms in relation to their effect on function; with the cessation of menses, the focus of function may be directed towards the bladder or bowel function rather than the strict "sexual function" of the vagina. A careful review and understanding of the meaning of urologic or bowel symptoms of an elderly patient (together with appropriate investigations) is essential to a proper understanding of elderly patients.

Clinical Evaluation

An elderly gynecologic patient deserves special consideration in the clinical assessment. The gynecologic history will no longer focus on the menstrual pattern. However, it will pay particular attention to features that in a younger female may be considered unremarkable, but may carry considerable importance in an older female (e.g., the presence of a vaginal discharge). For a younger female, a pelvic examination may become almost routine; for an older female, there may be a temptation to avoid the examination for fear of causing physical discomfort when movement is limited, perhaps, by arthritis, a cerebrovascular accident, or a gross obesity; also, the examination may be avoided because of a misplaced fear of causing embarrassment. The important point, of course, is an insistence on high standards of careful history taking, followed by a disciplined approach to examination and (where necessary) investigation. A requirement with an elderly patient is a readiness on the physician's part to be flexible and considerate in providing the time and opportunity to take a full history and conduct the required examination. In particular, it may be necessary to allow a patient to assume an unusual position (perhaps the left lateral position rather than the standard lithotomy position), so that a thorough examination be completed without causing the patient discomfort. A speculum of an appropriate size should be carefully chosen, as there may be significant atrophy of the introitus or vagina. Discomfort in an examination may not be forgiven by a patient, so that it may be difficult to obtain consent for a second examination if needed.

The history should concentrate on four areas. Firstly, symptoms of vaginal bleeding or discharge. It is rare for any female several years past menopause to experience a vaginal discharge. A new discharge has to be investigated. Bleeding mandates, at the very least, an endometrial biopsy in addition to a careful visual examination of the vulva, vagina, and cervix. An inability to perform an office biopsy procedure (3–5% of all patients), which usually is due to a cervical stenosis, an enlarged uterus, an abnormal Papnicolaou smear, or persistent bleeding postbiopsy where no tissue was obtained, all are indications for in-patient dilata-

TABLE 18-1 Indications for Inpatient Dilatation and Curettage (D & C)

Cytology suggestive of a malignancy
Failed office biopsy procedure
Enlarged uterus
Persistent bleeding after negative office biopsy

tion and curettage (D & C) (*see* Table 18-1). It is not unusual for the curettage to be non-productive. In one review, a curettage for an investigation of postmenopausal bleeding in females over 60 years of age demonstrated carcinoma in 15 cases; in the remainder, bleeding was due to local proliferative changes or to atrophic changes.[1]

Secondly, the urinary tract symptomatology of an elderly patient may be complex, but a careful history of bladder function is an essential component of a gynecologic assessment. The purpose of the history is to separate, where possible, an intrinsic bladder dysfunction from an extrinsic one. Frequency of micturition may be due to a chronic infection, atrophic trigonitis, reduced bladder capacity, or habit. Incontinence may be due to a failure of the sphincteric muscle (stress), bladder dyssynergia (urge), or a neurogenic bladder (dribbling). Dysuria is invariably associated with an intrinsic lesion, whereas hesitancy or incomplete emptying may be associated with an anatomic displacement of the bladder or a urethral diverticulum. Hematuria usually signifies an intrinsic lesion, which may be superficial (e.g., a urethral carbuncle). Occasionally, an elderly person may have difficulty in separating bleeding from the urinary tract from bleeding from the genital tract. An examination of the urinary tract always should be considered when the investigations of a definite history of postmenopausal bleeding prove negative. In practice, it is not always possible to separate the urinary problem from the gynecologic problem. The impact of the aging process may alter the neuroregulation of bladder function at the same time, as there is a deterioration in the tone and function of the pelvic musculature. Cytometric evaluation often is necessary to provide an accurate diagnosis and the best chance of improvement.

The third symptom of significance is irritation. For some females, the irritation or soreness that is associated with atrophic vaginitis or with lichen sclerosus may be so intense as to be a constant distraction. Symptoms may be more severe than would be anticipated by the appearance of the area, which leads a patient to use some of a great variety of unhelpful topical applications. These cases often are refractory to treatment; if obsessional, they may benefit from either a non-directive or behavior modification type of psychotherapy.

Dyspareunia also may be a significant symptom in an elderly patient, when due either to an atrophic vaginitis or the changes of lichen sclerosus.

The last group of symptoms are those caused by structural laxity. Many sizeable prolapses virtually are symptom free, but others cause a dragging sensation in the low abdomen, some lower backache, difficulty with intercourse, or problems with evacuation of the bowel or bladder. In severe cases, a patient will be aware of a swelling in the vagina.

Structural Defects

The uterus is maintained in its pelvic position, being supported at the level of the cervix by the uterosacral and pubocervical ligaments. If these are weakened by the effects of childbirth or by tissue changes beyond the menopause, then the uterus will descend down the vagina. Eventually, it may occupy a position outside the vaginal introitus. A prolapse may be reduceable when occurring intermittently during activities such as defecation.

Many elderly females are unaware or unbothered by moderate degrees of uterine prolapse; but when symptoms occur, they may include a low abdominal dragging sensation, backache, the presence of a mass at the introitus, coital difficulties, and problems with emptying of the bladder or bowel, which sometimes requires intravaginal manipulation for successful evacuation. If the uterine prolapse is complete (procidentia) and has not been reduced, lichenification and ulceration of the cervical or vaginal mucosa is likely to develop and may lead to bleeding and discharge. A uterine prolapse may occur on its own or in association with a prolapse of the anterior vaginal wall (cys-

tocele and urethrocele) and posterior vaginal wall (enterocele and rectocele). The support of the anterior wall mainly is fascial while the posterior wall, particularly in its lower portion, is supported by the deep and (to a lesser extent) the superficial perineal muscles.

The goal of treatment for an elderly patient with a symptomatic prolapse should be to restore natural function. This involves correcting the prolapse, restoring voluntary and spontaneous bladder and bowel evacuation, and coital function. After many years of debate as to the management of choice, a consensus has been reached that surgery is indicated; a vaginal hysterectomy is the preferable operation. Emge,[2] reviewing the management of genital prolapse in 1966, reported that 50 years previously, Neugebauer had listed 400 different vaginal pessaries designed for the correction of a genital prolapse. Only a handful of different types are now available and should be reserved for temporary use in a patient awaiting surgery or where surgery is absolutely contraindicated. The vinyl ring, the Smith, Smith-Hodge, or Bellhorn pessaries are the models most commonly used these days. The choice should be made according to the length and width of the vagina and to the patient's comfort.

Serious complications may develop following the use of pessaries,[3] particularly if the pessary is not changed on a regular basis every 1–3 months. The comfort of a pessary should not be withheld, however, from a patient for whom surgery is an impossibility.[4]

A vaginal hysterectomy removes the prolapsing organ and provides access to its supporting ligaments. These are then shortened and used to support the vaginal vault. Care has to be taken to identify and correct any enterocele, which is the most common prolapse following hysterectomy; it can reach a considerable size in an elderly patient.

If the patient has previously had a hysterectomy and the prolapse is restricted mainly to the anterior or posterior walls of the vagina, then an anterior and posterior colpoperinorrhaphy is sufficient. When the surgery involves an extensive dissection of the bladder, then care must be taken to restore the correct urethro-vesical anatomic relationships or incontinence may result in a previously continent patient. The abdominal approach is best reserved for patients with a serious vault prolapse, with or without an enterocele, and an absent uterus.

The surgical management of a uterine or vaginal prolapse produces good results with a low morbidity.[5-7] Good results require careful preoperative assessment, improvements in anesthesia, and the appropriate use of prophylactic antibiotics and heparin. Preoperative care involves 1) Cytologic and histologic screening of the cervix and vaginal mucosa; and 2) Local hygiene with lactic acid, and Betadine douches, with a reduction of the procidentia by vaginal packing and the use of estrogens applied locally or systemically for 2–3 weeks before surgery. The recognition of the high incidence of an intraoperative thrombus formation in the pelvic and leg veins of females undergoing pelvic surgery often in the lithotomy position, has lead to the widespread use of microdose heparin to prevent postoperative thromboembolic phenomena. The reduction of vaginal bacterial colonizations presurgically by the use of antibiotics such as cephalosporins or metronidazole in addition to the local measures outlined above, together with a good surgical technique in ensuring hemostasis and limiting tissue damage, has led to a significant reduction in postoperative infectious complications.

The preoperative assessment should include the routine evaluation of a patient's nutritional, hematologic, and cardiopulmonary status. However, particular attention should be paid to the renal function and to the urinary tract, where chronic infection often is associated with stasis due to an anatomic distortion and poor bladder function. Radiologic studies are used preoperatively to chart the course of the ureters and to check the possibility of a ureteric obstruction, which may be associated with a gross displacement; the ureters sometimes are found outside the level of the introitus in severe procidentia.

The success of surgery in an elderly patient includes the short-term relief of symptoms and improvements in the life style together with a long-term prevention of recurrence. Numerous reports link short-term effectiveness with a minimal morbidity. While long-term results are more difficult to prove, the opinion is that surgery should not be withheld from an elderly pa-

tient unless the surgical or anesthetic risk is deemed to be extremely grave.

Epithelial Dystrophy and Inflammation

Lesions are categorized as red lesions, white lesions, and dark lesions.[8] Vulval problems of an elderly female are likely to be either associated with aging itself or with an inflammation that is sometimes secondary to a contact stimulus. Whenever an elderly patient presents with vulval symptoms of pain, irritation, dyspareunia, soreness, discharge, bleeding, or the appearance of a mass, an inspection is absolutely mandatory. Vaginal or vulvar carcinomas may be present with any of the symptoms listed above, and a high level of suspicion must be maintained with an early resort to a biopsy procedure and histologic diagnosis.

Atrophic vaginal changes occur in every female passing beyond the climacteric period without estrogen replacement. The epithelium is thin, with few layers, a preponderance of basal layers, and an absence of glycogen leading to a high pH of 6.5–7.5. Pathogenic bacteria, which commonly originate in the gut, often are found; but, not every female becomes symptomatic. For those that do, and in the absence of any other pathogen, such as trichomonas or candida (which are relatively rare in elderly persons), treatment with estrogens usually is successful. Vaginal application of an estrogen cream (Premarin, 1 gram at night) usually produces rapid relief. It must be understood, however, that local application leads to a significant absorption, and the same results can be obtained by the systemic administration of Premarin, 0.625 mg/day. The risk of prolonged estrogen administration has to be assessed whether it is given by the oral or vaginal route.

The vulva is not subject to the superficial changes of aging to the same extent as the vagina, although there is a reduction in the size of the labia. Together with some shortening and narrowing of the vagina, this may alter the appearance of the introitus, thus exposing the urethral meatus and sometimes leading to the direction of the urinary stream over the perineum. This may cause a contact dermatitis that is aggravated by contact with a variety of irritants found in clothing, detergents, medications, or associated with poor local hygiene. Such a dermatitis is best managed by avoiding excessive local therapy, obtaining a careful history to identify a particular irritant, and helping with local hygiene to guarantee cleanliness. Sometimes, the use of local hydrocortisone cream is necessary.

The vulva also may be involved in a number of infective processes, such as seborrheic dermatitis, folliculitis, or candidal vaginitis. The latter can be severe on the rare occasion when it presents in an elderly patient and where the possibility of associated diabetes mellitus needs to be investigated.

The important red lesion of the vulva is termed Paget's disease, which presents (as with many other dystrophies) with itching and soreness as the principal complaints, but with a distinctive appearance. The lesion is localized to the vulva and appears erythematous, with bands of islands of hyperkeratosis giving a patchy white appearance to the surface. A confirmatory diagnosis is obtained by a biopsy procedure. The condition is important because although it is not strictly malignant itself, it is associated with an underlying adenocarcinoma of the apocrine glands in one third of all cases. Treatment consists of an extensive vulvectomy after exclusion of any associated carcinoma with a careful follow-up to check for recurrence.

White lesions are reputedly the most typical lesion found in an elderly vulva. Over the years, different classifications of the leukoplakias have appeared and been modified. Once classification adopted by the International Society for the Study of Vulvar Disease is given in Table 8-2.[9] A diagnosis only can be made from a biopsy

specimen. The better understanding of the various conditions has come from the widespread use of a vulvar biopsy procedure, which is a simple procedure performed under total local anesthetic and using either a small scalpel or a Keyes punch biopsy directed by a toluidine blue application. Recent studies suggest that the transition of a vulvar dystrophy into a carcinoma is less common than has been assumed, although it has to be emphasized that the appropriate diagnosis only can be made from a biopsy specimen. The descriptive term leukoplakia does not, on its own, provide a diagnosis.

The most common lesion in an elderly patient is a lichen sclerosus. This is a truly atrophic lesion that leads, in the absence of coitus, to a contraction and shrinkage of the introitus and progressive destruction of the labia minora. The pruritus that accompanies this lesion may be intense and cause much distress. Topical application of testosterone may be helpful, even though in some cases the symptoms are so refractory that a subcutaneous injection of absolute alcohol may be used as a last resort.

A hyperplastic dystrophy varies from lichen sclerosus in that the gross anatomic distortion of the labia minora and introitus is absent, and the lesions may be isolated and not always confluent. Again, this diagnosis is obtained by a biopsy procedure. When an atypia has been ruled out, the intense pruritus is best managed with steroid cream and Eurax (Valisone—7 parts, Eurax—3 parts in a cream base). As with lichen sclerosus, the symptoms may be so intense and disabling that tranquilizers or mild sedatives have been used to modify an individual's response to the symptoms.

Carcinoma in situ is more common in younger females, but it may occur at any age. Atypia may be demonstrated in association with any of the dystrophies, but appears to be more common in the mixed dystrophies. Severe atypia should be treated by eradication (excision or laser therapy) on an individualized basis.

TABLE 18-2   Classification of Leukoplakia

Hyperplastic dystrophy
  Without atypia
  With atypia
Lichen sclerosus
Mixed dystrophy (lichen sclerosus with foci of epithelial hyperplasia)
  Without atypia
  With atypia

Cancer

The peak age for cervical cancer is 40. Widespread, cervical cytologic screening has led to the identification of cancer at earlier stages and in younger patients. Nevertheless, cervical cancer may be detected for the first time in an elderly patient, often in females who have not continued with regular cervical screening; the maximal recommended interval is 3 years. The classic presenting symptom of a carcinoma of the cervix is postmenopausal bleeding, although any unusual discharge (particularly when brown in color) should be regarded with suspicion and investigated.

A carcinoma of the body of the uterus, the most common gynecologic malignancy, occurs in older females. The largest group is found in the 5th decade with the median age being 58.[10] Multiple risk factors have been identified; specifically nulliparity, obesity, and late menopause that is often associated with hypertension and diabetes mellitus. The use of estrogen therapy in postmenopausal patients has been clearly associated with the development of an adenocarcinoma, and it is one of a number of reasons given for the rise in the incidence rate of this disease, which is now twice as common as carcinoma of the ovary and cervix. It is hoped that more careful screening of patients and the introduction of progesterone in addition to estrogen may lead to a reduction in this disease. The endometrial cavity is not as accessible for cytologic screening, as is the cervix. Abnormal Papanicolaou smears are only found in about one third of all patients with endometrial cancer. While some commercial kits are available for cytologic sampling of the cavity, they have not been widely accepted or applied. The most important presenting symptom is postmenopausal bleeding, which is initially investigated where possible (approximately 95% of all cases) by an outpatient sampling of the endometrial cavity. When this does not provide an adequate sample, or when this sample does demonstrate an adenocarcinoma or atypical adenomatous hyperplasia, a fractional curettage is required to exactly locate the lesion with particular reference to the cervical involvement.

The ovary is the least accessible of all female genital organs, and its intraperitoneal location may lead to a delay in diagnosis and treatment. This is a problem regardless of age. However, an enlarged ovary may be found incidentally in a premenopausal female who has more frequent pelvic examinations. This is an opportunity that does not present itself frequently in an elderly patient. The highest number of cases is found in the 6th decade, although the age-specific incidence rate continues to increase to 80 years of age.

Advanced ovarian cancer may present with gastrointestinal symptoms, abdominal distension, and weight loss as the tumor spreads through the peritoneal cavity and ascites develop. The sine qua non of early detection in a postmenopausal patient is the palpable ovary. Within 5 years of the onset of menopause, the ovary has shrunk to 25% of its size during the reproductive years and usually is not palpable. If the ovary is palpable and felt to be larger than a normal postmenopausal ovary, then a laparotomy should be strongly considered where a malignant lesion might be anticipated in about 10% of all cases.

A carcinoma rarely occurs in the fallopian tube, which accounts for less than 0.5% of all gynecologic malignancies with most cases presenting in the 40–60-year-old age group; however, cases sporadically occur in the later years. As with an adenocarcinoma of the uterus, the presenting symptom is a blood-stained discharge, which usually is described as being amber in color rather than the purer color of the blood that extrudes directly from the uterine cavity. A cytologic diagnosis is positive in less than 10% of all cases. A diagnosis only is made at a laparotomy for the presence of a pelvic mass where an ovarian tumor is expected, or when a laparotomy is performed because of persistent uterine bleeding in spite of negative endometrial biopsy specimens.

A genital carcinoma that is most commonly associated with old age is a vulva carcinoma. It accounts for 3–5% of female genital malignancies and occurs beyond 60–70 years of age in 70% of all patients.[11] The presenting symptom in the majority of cases is the development of a lump or an ulcer on the vulva, although attention may be drawn to the mass by the presence of pruritis from an accompanying dystrophy or dermatitis. Other presenting symptoms include bleeding, pain, discharge, or dysuria. In rare cases, the presenting symptom will be the development of a mass in the groin. Squamous cell carcinoma is by far the most common histologic variety, with melanoma, basal cell carcinoma, and adenocarcinoma of the Bartholin's gland occurring much less frequently.

A carcinoma of the vagina is most commonly due to a direct extension from the cervix or an indirect spread from the body of the uterus; it is of the squamous type in 90% of all cases. A primary carcinoma may occur at any age and may be associated with specific carcinogenic stimuli (e.g., diethylstilbestrol [DES] exposure in females born in the 1940s and 1950s). Carcinoma of the vagina is relatively more common in an elderly patient in whom two possible carcinogenic influences are the use of vaginal pessaries to correct prolapse and previous exposure to radiation, usually (but not exclusively) for the treatment of malignancy. This is a history that may make difficult the separation of the primary from the secondary lesion. The presenting symptom is bleeding or a blood-stained discharge.

Many treatment options are available for elderly females with a genital carcinoma. The principles of management should not be compromised by a patient's age, except where her general medical condition may limit anesthesia and restrict surgical opportunity. This problem has largely been overcome by advances in anesthetic techniques in recent years. The principles of management include an early diagnosis, confirmation via biopsy specimen, accurate staging of the disease, and an appropriate selection of treatment according to the natural history of the disease from a particular stage.

Treatment decisions should be made by interdisciplinary teams, which include surgeons and radiologists, whether or not the final decision is the selection a single modality, surgery, or radiotherapy. The goals of treatment are to remove the malignancy, prevent or limit recurrence, and restore maximal functional ability. With an early diagnosis, the number of patients presenting with an advanced disease should be few, and primary palliative surgery rarely is required. The case of a patient with an advanced recurrent disease again requires careful individualization, as the patient with anemia from renal failure caused by an obstruction to the ureters from a carcinoma of the cervix has very different problems than a patient with massive ascites or intestinal obstruction from a carcinoma of the ovary.

In general, the primary treatment should be surgery for the majority of genital malignancies.

In early stages, the surgery should be extensive enough to include the lymphatic drainage of the lesion site, as all female genital cancers (with the exception of those arising in the ovary) spread primarily via the lymphatic system. In later stages or in recurrence, the purpose of surgery may be for debulking, and to aid radiotherapeutic or chemotherapeutic adjuncts. On occasion, palliative surgery to divert the bowel or bladder can help to alleviate some of the discomfort of a widespread disease. Radiotherapy often is used together with surgery in the management of carcinoma of the body of the uterus where careful staging of the disease again is essential before the introduction of any particular treatment plan.

Of all the tumors of the female genital tract, the one best suited for primary radiotherapy is a carcinoma of the cervix. While there may be some continuing disputes as to whether surgery or radiotherapy should be the principal method, there is no doubt that good results have been obtained with radiotherapy. These good results also apply to cancer of the cervical stump, in spite of the absence of the uterus for a good placement of the radium. Subtotal hysterectomy is very rarely performed nowadays, but there are many elderly females who had hysterectomies during the era when subtotal hysterectomies were more common. The treating physician should be careful to confirm the absence of the cervix as well as the uterus in an elderly patient with a history of a hysterectomy.

Chemotherapy has a limited value in female genital cancers, although it is used for advanced ovarian diseases where different drug combinations and regimens are under an ongoing review by organizations such as the Gynecological Oncology Group. Age is not a contraindication to chemotherapy, although frailty or debilitation may require a dose reduction. Apart from the various categories of chemotherapeutic agents used for ovarian cancer, some success has been reported with the use of high doses of progesterone (17 hydroxyprogesterone acetate) in recurrent endometrial tumors in which late recurrences with well-differentiated tumors seem to be particularly responsive.

The management of any patient has, of course, to be individualized with the maximum input from all members of the health care team and a tailoring of the appropriate treatment not only according to the known nature of the tumor, but also to the known circumstances and needs of the individual patient. Preparation for the postoperative circumstances, and help with the adaption to any limitations induced by surgery, chemotherapy, or radiotherapy is as important as selecting the optimum mode of treatment.

A functional, thorough, and interdisciplinary approach should be used in helping an elderly patient adapt to the impact of major surgery, whether or not she is deemed to be terminal or whether or not the surgery was curative or palliative. Elderly persons, in particular, need a continuum of care that extends from the preoperative diagnosis, the hospital treatment, the return to their own environments, help with dealing with the discomforts and disabilities of the treatment, and (hopefully) a return to a comfortable and satisfying existence.

Other Pelvic Pathologies

The aging female pelvis may be prone to disorders that are associated with a hormonal withdrawal and malignancy; but, they are spared the two main benign problems of the reproductive years: endometriosis and pelvic inflammatory disease. Some benign conditions may linger on, such as a fibromyoma of the uterus, which may slightly regress in size after menopause. However, they may also persist (particularly if already calcified) and may later cause symptoms by pressure effects in the bowel or bladder. Alternatively, a submucous fibroid may be responsible for postmenopausal bleeding.

The concern for a palpable ovary has already been alluded to as a precaution in recommending histologic evaluation of any ovarian mass. Still, no more than 50% of postmenopausal tumors will prove to be malignant. Although so-called physiologic cysts become rare as the ovary becomes inactive, epithelial neoplasms of the serous and mucinous varieties are found quite frequently and may reach an enormous size.

Fistula formation in an elderly patient is a distressing and disabling condition. Most gynecologic fistulas are due to obstetric or surgical events and are corrected before menopause. Some unfortunate females, however, may develop recto-vaginal or intestinal-vaginal fistulae many years after radiotherapy for a pelvic malignancy or following radiotherapy to induce menopause, as was the practice in the 1940s.

Pyometra

A rare cause of uterine enlargement is a pyometra caused by an obstruction at the cervix due to atrophic changes or tumor development. Tuberculous pyometra is rare but should be considered, particularly in patients with a relevant history of tuberculosis. The presenting symptom usually is an intermittent discharge and deserves a full investigation.

An elderly patient with gynecologic problems deserves the special consideration of a broad functional approach to these problems without the limitation of a narrow focus on the specific gynecologic disorder. This discussion has been conducted with a tight focus on the specific disorder and the reader is referred elsewhere in this volume for discussions regarding sexuality, hormonal replacement therapy, bladder and bowel disorders, and the care of the terminally ill; all are important areas without which a chapter on gynecologic disorders is incomplete.

References

1. Glik I, Soferman N: Gynecological survey of hospitalized elderly women. *J Am Geriatr Soc* 19(1):61–67, 1971.
2. Emge LA: Correction of genital prolapse of the elderly. *Am J Obstet Gynec* June 1, 1966, pp 362–365.
3. Russell JK: The dangerous vaginal pessary. *Br Med J* 2:1595–1597, Dec 16, 1961.
4. Huffman JW: Gynecologic disorders in the geriatric patient. *Geriatric Gyn* 71(1):38–51, Jan 1982.
5. Robertson EG, Russell JK: Surgical management of prolapse in elderly women. *Br Med J* 2:1420–1423, Dec 10, 1966.
6. Papaloucas A, Mantis C, Zervos S: Vaginal hysterectomy in aged women. *Int Surg* 53(2):144–149, Feb 1970.
7. Ellenbogen A, Agranat A, Grunstein S: The role

of vaginal hysterectomy in the aged woman. *J Am Geriatr Soc* 29:426–428, 1981.

8. Friedrich EG: Major problems in obstetrics and gynecology, in Friedrich EG (ed): *Vulvar Disease*. Philadelphia, WB Saunders & Co, 1976, vol 9, pp 98–146.

9. Friedrich EG: New nomenclature for vulvar disease—report of the committee on terminology. *Obstet Gynec* 47(1):122–124, Jan 1976.

10. DiSaia PJ: *Clinical Gynecologic Oncology*. St. Louis, The CV Mosby Co, 1981, p 140.

11. Morrow CP, Townsend DE: *Synopsis of Gynecologic Oncology*. New York, John Wiley & Son, 1981.

CHAPTER 19

Rheumatology

LOUIS A. HEALEY, M.D.

Arthritis and rheumatism are problems in almost all older people. While osteoarthritis is the most common condition in this age group, other diseases may affect the joints as well. Patients naturally assume that their symptoms are the inevitable result of growing old. It is the physician's initial task to be certain that the symptoms are indeed due to osteoarthritis, and that other more treatable causes of pain and stiffness are not present.

This chapter describes the common joint disease of older patients. Some of them (osteoarthritis, pseudogout, polymyalgia rheumatica, and giant cell arteritis) are, with few exceptions, only seen in an elderly patient. Other diseases (gout, rheumatoid arthritis, and other immune complex diseases) can occur at any age, but they may have a different presentation and progression in elderly persons.

Osteoarthritis

It is safe to say that osteoarthritis is universal in older patients. For many of them, this will mean knobby fingers or some stiffness and creaking of the knees that is accepted as inevitable and usually ignored. However, perhaps 30% of the geriatric population will have symptoms at one time or another; for 10%, osteoarthritis will pose a significant problem. The basic lesion of osteoarthritis is a deterioration and abrasion of articular cartilage. In contrast to rheumatoid arthritis, the inflammation of the synovium is milder and less intense. While there is still some debate, most authorities agree that inflamma-

tion is not the primary process in osteoarthritis, but is secondary to the degenerative changes in the cartilage. Since purists no longer insist that the disease be termed degenerative joint disease rather than osteoarthritis (even though it may not be a true or primary inflammation), patients now can be spared the discouraging connotations many would experience when given the diagnosis of a degenerative disease.

Research has reasonably well established that the basic problem is in the cartilage structure, and that changes in the synovium and bone are secondary. In a minority of all patients, the disease is the result of a previous joint insult, which is either trauma or an inflammatory form of arthritis at a younger age. For most patients, the mystery still remains why these cartilage abnormalities, which might be viewed as the characteristics of aging, should proceed at an accelerated pace in certain patients and certain joints. Some biochemical abnormalities have been detected, but not enough is known to explain the entire sequence or to suggest any therapeutic measures to prevent or reverse the process.

While the basic problem, cartilage deterioration, is the same in all involved joints, it is important to point out to patients that this is not a systemic disease. While they may have osteoarthritis in one area (such as the hands), it is not inevitable and, in fact, it is unlikely that it will spread to other joints. The disease then poses a series of local problems that depend on location. The following locations are susceptible: 1) The proximal interphalangeal, distal interphalangeal, and first carpometacarpal joints in the hands; 2) Hips; 3) Knees; 4) First metatarso-phalangeal or bunion joints in the foot; and 5) The cervical and lower lumbar vertebrae. Os-teoarthritis rarely is seen in the metacarpopha-langeal joints, wrists, elbows, shoulders, and ankles, unless there has been a pre-existing in-flammatory disease, trauma, or an occupation that requires unusual physical stresses on one of these joints. Symptoms usually begin insidi-ously with aches and pain in the involved joint. Initially, this discomfort is experienced with motion, weight-bearing, or activity, although there may be pain at rest in the later stages. Except for the knee, effusions are rare. There are no systemic symptoms, such as fever or weight loss, and stiffness of the affected joint is of a much shorter duration than in rheumatoid arthritis or other forms of inflammatory sy-novitis. Flare-ups in the disease frequently are associated with use of the joints and corre-spondingly are relieved by rest.

A diagnosis of osteoarthritis is suggested by typical symptoms in the usual joints of an older patient and is confirmed on an x-ray film. In the early stage of the disease before changes are apparent on an x-ray film, the diagnosis can be suspected, but it should not be regarded as cer-tain. There are no diagnostic blood tests. The erythrocyte sedimentation rate (ESR) is impor-tant because a low or normal value tends to confirm the impression of osteoarthritis, whereas a rapid ESR should raise a suspicion that another disease process is present.

Treatment essentially is symptomatic, since there are no available measures to prevent or reverse the cartilage damage. Contrary to the prevalent belief of patients, diet plays no part in the pathogenesis or treatment of osteoarthritis. While most patients correctly reject the sugges-tion to use canes or crutches, a sensible modifi-cation of strenuous activities is appropriate and will be helpful. Patients should understand that they need to limit what they do only as the symptoms dictate. In contrast to unusual occu-pations or sports that demand marked, repeti-tive physical stresses, the ordinary activities of daily life do not greatly accelerate a progression of osteoarthritis. It makes no sense for a patient with mild or moderate osteoarthritis to forego enjoyable pursuits and adopt a sedentary life to preserve joint function when the pain really is not that severe or limiting.

Some general principles influence the use and choice of medications in the treatment of osteoarthritis.[1] First, since the goal is a relief of symptoms rather than any prevention of the dis-ease, medicines are more appropriately used episodically to relieve symptoms rather than on a regular schedule. Second, since inflammation is minimal or not present, oral or intramuscular corticosteroids play no role in osteoarthritis and should not be given. Aspirin and non-steroidal drugs, which are prostaglandin inhibitors, have both analgesic and anti-inflammatory properties and may help. It is not possible to predict which patients will benefit from which agent. It often is necessary to try several agents, bearing in mind the likelihood that the initial benefit from any agent probably is a placebo response and it may take several months to determine any drug's true value.

Aspirin and other prostaglandin inhibitors share the same risk of toxicity to the gastric mucosa. Recognizing the limited benefit of such agents, it is not worthwhile to continue them in older patients who develop gastrointestinal symptoms, since the risk of a gastric ulcer and bleeding outweighs their possible benefits in cases of osteoarthritis. Simple analgesic agents such as acetaminophen or propoxyphene, which are not prostaglandin inhibitors and do not injure the gastric mucosa, are better choices. Drugs marketed as analgesics that are prostaglandin inhibitors have the same potential gastric toxicity and should be used with cau-tion. For some elderly patients with severe os-teoarthritis and constant pain, small doses of codeine can provide great relief and make it possible for them to be more active.

Hands

Osteoarthritis typically affects the distal inter-phalangeal joints, which results in a bony en-largement that often is associated with lateral angulation and the small paired dorsal cysts known as Heberden's nodes. The proximal in-terphalangeal joints may be similarly affected. The other common site is the first carpometa-carpal joint, in which an enlargement can lead to a squared appearance of the base of the thumb (see Figure 19-1). Other hand joints are spared. These changes may develop insidiously and painlessly. With osteoarthritis, morning

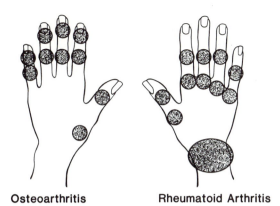

Osteoarthritis   Rheumatoid Arthritis

FIGURE 19-1   The location of involved joints is the most helpful feature in differentiating osteoarthritis of the hands from rheumatoid arthritis.

stiffness is not prolonged and grip strength is well maintained. Hand function remains good, although there may be some loss of dexterity that will particularly be noticed by people such as typists or pianists who use their hands for skilled maneuvers. Osteoarthritis of the hands is more common in females and often will be seen in female members of the same family. This sex predilection is unfortunate, since the knobby appearance frequently is distressing and cannot be prevented. Pain is more likely to occur in the early years of the disease and gradually disappears as time progresses. Some patients may have an acute onset, with several interphalangeal joints showing evidence of inflammation. At this stage, an intra-articular injection of a steroid may be helpful. Based on x-ray films that show considerable joint damage and prominent subchondral cysts, a subset of the disease termed erosive osteoarthritis has been described. Some consider this an inflammatory variant, while others regard it as a more severe form of osteoarthritis. The eventual prognosis for most patients with osteoarthritis of the hands is to have no pain and a nearly normal function, but there will be an altered appearance. If severe damage to the first carpometacarpal joint prevents use of the thumb in opposition, then a fusion or insertion of a prosthesis can be beneficial in restoring function.

Since osteoarthritis may begin in females as early as their mid-40s and frequently involves the proximal interphalangeal joints, its differentiation from the onset of rheumatoid arthritis is a common diagnostic problem. The distribution of involvement provides the most helpful differentiating clue. Osteoarthritis has a predilection for the distal interphalangeal joints and it spares the metacarpophalangeal joints and wrists, which are the two areas characteristic of rheumatoid arthritis. Patients with rheumatoid arthritis also show reflections of the inflammatory nature of the disease: 1) Pronounced morning stiffness; 2) Loss of grip strength; 3) Fluctuant fusiform synovial swelling; and 4) An elevated ESR. The rheumatoid factor, if present, is helpful in confirming the diagnosis. Once rheumatoid arthritis has been excluded, a patient should be strongly advised that this is a limited condition rather than a generalized disease, that the symptoms of discomfort will gradually subside, and that hand function will not be significantly impaired.

Hip

Osteoarthritis of the hip is seen more often in males than in females and may be unilateral or bilateral. The chief symptom is pain on walking, which is experienced in the lateral hip area, the groin, and along the inner aspect of the thigh radiating to the knee. Many patients who complain of "hip pain" or "arthritis of the hip" actually have pain in the iliac crest or buttock, which is referred from the back. As the disease progresses, patients develop a characteristic limp, with the adducted flexed hip producing a functional shortening of the leg. In some patients, the referred pain to the knee is such a prominent feature as to suggest that this joint is the site of the arthritis; however, on examination, the maneuver of internally rotating the hip reproduces the pain and indicates the true diagnosis. This loss of internal rotation is the earliest physical finding of hip arthritis. This diagnosis is confirmed by x-ray films that show a narrowing of the cartilage space and subsequent sclerosis, spur formation, and subchondral cysts. Analgesic anti-inflammatory drugs, particularly indomethacin, may provide considerable relief of the pain. However, in many patients, as the disease progresses and when the pain significantly interferes with daily activities, the patient decides when he or she is a candidate for surgery. A total hip arthroplasty has produced excellent results, particularly in an

TABLE 19-1 Synovial Fluid Analysis

Diagnosis	White Blood Cell Count (mm^3)	Crystals
Osteoarthritis	<2,000	—
Gout	>2,000*	Sodium urate
Pseudogout	>2,000*	Calcium pyrophosphate
Inflammatory rheumatoid arthritis, other	>2,000*	—

* White blood cell counts may range from 2,000–50,000, which depends on the severity and acuity of the inflammation.

older patient who is less likely to wish to pursue strenuous activities that may stress or loosen the prosthesis. Patients find they can comfortably resume activities such as walking, gardening, golfing, and even doubles play in tennis.

Knee

The knee is another frequent site of osteoarthritis, which often is bilateral and occurs equally in males and females. The chief complaint is pain on motion, particularly after sitting, perhaps accompanied by a creaking noise or sensation. These chronic symptoms may be interspersed with acute episodes of increased pain and effusion. Medications are of variable help in the chronic stage; acute flare-ups are appropriately treated with rest, aspiration of fluids, and an injection of a steroid preparation into the joint. A synovial fluid analysis is necessary to differentiate the various causes of an acutely swollen knee, since patients whose x-ray films show evidence of osteoarthritis also may suffer an attack of gout, pseudogout, or another inflammatory disease (see Table 19-1). For patients with progressive osteoarthritis in whom pain or limited motion significantly interferes with ambulation, a total knee arthroplasty can provide great help.

Spine

Radiologic evidence of osteoarthritis of the spine, disc space narrowing, vertebral body sclerosis, and spur formation, is exceedingly common and will be found, to some degree, in all patients over 65 years of age. These x-ray film changes may have little to do with the symptoms of pain and stiffness, which probably arise from the paraspinous ligaments and mus-

cles. Many people with an abnormal x-ray film have no symptoms. The pain and stiffness are more appropriately treated with heat, posture modification, weight loss, and an exercise program, than with anti-inflammatory medications. The sudden onset of a severe, localized, and persistent back pain (particularly in a postmenopausal female or coming on after lifting) should not be attributed to osteoarthritis, but should suggest a collapse of an osteoporotic vertebra. A posterior spurring or bony overgrowth of lumbar vertebrae can produce the condition known as spinal stenosis, which is due to a narrowing of the spinal canal or intervertebral foramina. The typical complaint is one of pain in both thighs that comes with walking and is improved with rest. It is differentiated from the claudication of a vascular insufficiency by palpation of the peripheral pulses. Patients also may experience the same pain on prolonged standing in one position at the sink or stove, and they also may note an ill-defined weakness or paresthesias in the anterior thighs. A neurologic examination may be normal, but the spinal canal narrowing can be demonstrated by a computed tomography (CT scan). If conservative measures do not relieve the symptoms, a decompression laminectomy may be indicated.

Gout

Gout is common in older patients, but with significant differences from the typical picture. In patients with hyperuricemia that is due to either a metabolic overproduction of uric acid or a renal underexcretion, the initial attack of gout usually appears in the 5th decade. Gout in an elderly person almost always is related to hyperuricemia that is secondary to the use of diuretics such as thiazide and furosemide, which partially block urate excretion by the kidney. Thus, it is seen with equal frequency in males and females. The clinical picture may be different as well. Classic podagra with redness, pain, and swelling of the great toe can occur, but an inflammation in the knee, wrist, ankle, and elbow bursa appear as frequently. Often, the attack is not as acute as with primary gout. A low-grade inflammation of the ankle or instep can suggest tendinitis or cellulitis. A diagnosis in these patients depends on suspecting the possibility of gout in any patient taking a diuretic and observing a prompt response to treatment with an anti-inflammatory drug. The response of an acute attack to treatment is a better criterion for a diagnosis than is hyperuricemia, since almost all patients taking a diuretic will have elevated urate serum levels. In patients with a painful swollen knee, gout can be distinguished from other possible causes by the aspiration of fluid and demonstration of birefringent urate crystals via the use of polarizing microscopy. Colchicine, the traditional specific agent for gout, is not the best choice for treatment in older patients because of the attendant nausea and diarrhea. Indomethacin or other non-steroidal anti-inflammatory drugs (NSAIDs) will produce a response within a few days with less toxicity.

Once the initial attack has been diagnosed and treated, there are several satisfactory alternatives for continued management. Since patients with diuretic-induced hyperuricemia do not form renal stones, probably will not develop tophi and face no risk from hyperuricemia per sé; the problem is one of repeated attacks of gouty arthritis. The most simple approach is to stop the diuretic. However, in many patients this is not practicable. Recurrent attacks can be prevented by taking 0.5–1.0 mg of colchicine each day. If recurrences are infrequent, patients may prefer simply to have an anti-inflammatory drug on hand to take at the first sign of an attack. If recurrences are frequent, which rarely is the case, it may be desirable to lower the urate level. This is best accomplished by the uricosuric drugs probenecid or sulfinpyrazone, which neutralize the urate-retaining effect of the diuretics. Allopurinol is not recommended for the reversal of thiazide-induced hyperuricemia, since there may be a greater risk of serious toxicity.[2]

Pseudogout

Gout is the best-known crystal-induced arthritis, but pseudogout—also known as chondrocalcinosis and calcium pyrophosphate deposition disease (CPPD)—occurs almost as frequently in older patients.[3] As the name suggests, pseudogout resembles gout in that there is an acute attack of pain and swelling, usually of one joint, that subsides in several days to 1 week. In contrast to the big toe, which is the hallmark of gout, the knee most often is the site of a pseudogout attack. A diagnosis is made by the aspiration of fluid and a polarized light microscopic examination. In this disease, the crystal that initiates the inflammation is calcium pyrophosphate, which has the appearance of a small rhomboid in contrast to the needle-like urate crystals of true gout (*see* Figure 19-2). Pseudogout attacks respond rapidly to an intra-articular corticosteroid or to a short course of an NSAID, which is predictably more effective than colchicine.

CPPD has a characteristic appearance on the x-ray film known as chondrocalcinosis. Punctate and linear radiodensities can be seen in the hyaline cartilage of the joint as well as in fibrocartilages such as the knee meniscus and symphysis pubis (*see* Figure 19-3). This type of radiographic appearance, either alone or in association with the changes of osteoarthritis, may be seen in many older patients who are not having an acute inflammatory attack. The linear

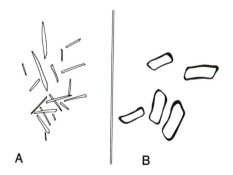

A   B

FIGURE 19-2 (A) Needle-like sodium urate crystals. (B) Rhomboid crystals of calcium pyrophosphate.

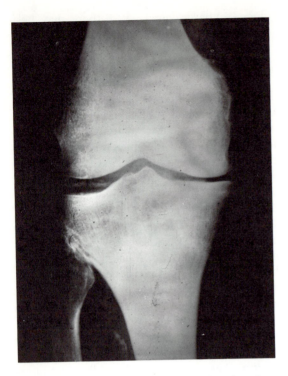

FIGURE 19-3   X-ray film of the knee showing chondrocalcinosis, which is a linear calcification in the meniscus.

calcifications on an x-ray film have been identified as calcium pyrophosphate crystals that are identical to those found in the synovial fluid at the time of an acute attack. The significance of this x-ray film is similar to that of hyperuricemia in that it does not establish a diagnosis, but it identifies those patients who may develop pseudogout. There is no diagnostic blood test for pseudogout, nor is there any predictably effective prophylaxis against recurrent attacks.

Polymyalgia Rheumatica

A rheumatic disease that is unique to older patients is polymyalgia rheumatica. This syndrome consists of pain and stiffness in pelvic and shoulder girdles, a very rapid ESR, and a prompt response to small doses of a corticosteroid drug. For reasons that are unknown, it is not seen in patients younger than 50 years of age and, in fact, the majority are over 60 years of age. Females are affected two to three times as often as males and 99% of all patients are white.

Patients complain of pain in the neck, back, shoulders, upper arms, and thighs. The onset may be gradual, but in approximately one third of all patients it is so abrupt that they go to bed feeling well and awaken in the morning as stiff and sore as though they had chopped wood or shovelled snow. Morning stiffness and jelling after a period of inactivity are essential features of a patient's history. Patients complain of pain in attempting to turn over during the night. They graphically describe how a spouse has to pull them out of bed in the morning or, if they live alone, how it may be necessary to wiggle like a snake to a kneeling position beside the bed and then push themselves erect. In some patients, the symptoms are widespread and they complain that they hurt all over; in other patients, the pain may localize to the shoulders or hips, but it is symmetrical in all. A low-grade fever, malaise, apathy, and weight loss may be present.

Despite the severity of complaints, the examination of these patients is surprising for the lack of findings. Tenderness or pain on moving the shoulders and hips may be detected, but there usually is no joint swelling or synovial thickening. Muscle strength proves to be normal. Radiographs either are normal or show only the changes of osteoarthritis expected in this age group. The clue to a diagnosis is the ESR, which always is elevated, usually is very high, and may exceed 100 mm/hour if measured by the Westergren method. Unless an ESR is performed, a diagnosis of polymyalgia rheumatica may be missed. This is the only abnormal laboratory test, and 95% of all patients have an elevated ESR. There may be a slight anemia, but the white blood cell count usually are normal. The rheumatoid factor and antinuclear antibodies are not present; protein electrophoresis is normal except for a non-specific elevation of α-2 globulins.

Although polymyalgia rheumatica is a distinct clinical entity, there are no specific laboratory or x-ray film findings; to make a diagnosis, it often is necessary to exclude other diseases. An elevated ESR indicates that this is an inflammatory disease and is not osteoarthritis, which is common at this age. When a patient with a pre-existing osteoarthritis gives a history of new symptoms of pain during the night, such as pronounced morning stiffness, difficulty in getting out of bed, or jelling after sitting, then polymyalgia should be suspected. The trouble in getting out of bed or arising from a chair may suggest that this is due to the muscle weakness of polymyositis. However, testing specific muscle groups shows that they are not weak and that strength is maintained. Electromyograms (EMGs) and muscle biopsy specimens are normal, and serum levels of muscle enzymes such as glutamic oxaloacetic acid transaminase (SGOT) and creatinine phosphokinase (CPK) are normal in contrast to polymyositis, in which they are elevated. Despite the term polymyalgia, current opinions hold that the muscles are normal and the symptoms of pain and stiffness may represent a synovitis. Scintigrams have shown a localization of the isotope in and about the shoulder, wrist, and knee joints.

For this reason, the most commonly encountered diagnostic problem is differentiating polymyalgia rheumatica from the onset of rheumatoid arthritis in this age group. Patients with rheumatoid arthritis have more synovitis of the distal joints. An examination may reveal a swelling of the wrists and metacarpophalangeal joints, as well as tenderness of metatarsophalangeal joints. If present, the rheumatoid factor is helpful in making this differentiation. Some patients with apparent polymyalgia rheumatica also may have swelling of the wrists, carpal tunnel syndrome, and effusions in the knees. In such instances, it is not possible to make a definite decision and a diagnosis of polymyalgia or rheumatoid arthritis will depend on the subsequent course of the illness.

The response of the pain and stiffness of polymyalgia rheumatica to low drug doses, such as 10–20 mg of prednisone, may truly be described as dramatic. Many patients are well by the next day, and improvement is so invariable that if it does not appear within 1 week the original diagnosis should be questioned. After 1 month the initial dose can be tapered, and patients remain free of symptoms with 5–7.5 mg/day of prednisone without risk of side effects. This is true even in this older age group, where postmenopausal females are so susceptible to osteoporosis and vertebral collapse. The duration of therapy is uncertain; approximately 30% of all patients can discontinue prednisone after 2 years without a recurrence of symptoms, but other patients will have to continue for a longer

period. The exact duration only can be determined by attempting to stop the steroid and noting whether the pain and stiffness recur. Aspirin and other NSAIDs provide a partial relief of symptoms, but they are not as effective as even small doses of steroids.

When a diagnosis of polymyalgia rheumatica is suspected but uncertain, as in those few patients with a normal ESR, a low steroid dose may be used as a therapeutic trial. The prompt relief of pain and stiffness with 1–2 days would confirm this diagnosis. For those patients in whom a diagnosis lies between polymyalgia rheumatica and seronegative rheumatoid arthritis, a low dose of prednisone also is recommended. If the synovitis clears completely and does not recur, then a diagnosis of polymyalgia rheumatica is favored. Rheumatoid arthritis may be helped by giving a steroid, but some evidence of synovitis will persist.

Giant Cell Arteritis

There is unquestionably a relation between polymyalgia rheumatica and giant cell arteritis, but the exact nature is uncertain. Both are diseases of older white persons, and both frequently coexist in the same patient. Of all patients with giant cell arteritis, 60% experience polymyalgia rheumatica either as a prodromal syndrome or at some time during the course of their illness.[4]

Clinical manifestations of giant cell arteritis may be localized or systemic. An inflammation of the temporal artery produces a severe and persistent headache, which most often is unilateral. The artery may be swollen and tender; because of its superficial location, it was the first recognized presentation of this disease, which led to the initial term temporal arteritis. Since then, it has become apparent that any of the medium or larger arteries may be similarly involved, so the term giant cell arteritis is the preferred designation. A sudden unilateral blindness that is due to an occlusion of the terminal branches of the ophthalmic artery is irreversible and is the most dreaded complication. Inflammation of a facial artery may lead to pain in the masseter muscles on chewing; this jaw claudication is a pathognomonic symptom. Transient diplopia that is due to an ischemia of extraocular muscles is important to recognize since it can lead to an early diagnosis, appropriate treatment, and prevention of blindness. Giant cell arteritis occasionally may involve the aorta and its branches, thus producing an aortic arch syndrome with claudication in the arms, unequal pulses, or aneurysm formation.[5] Less common manifestations of a cranial artery blockage can include scalp gangrene, blanching or necrosis of the tongue, and pain in the throat or ear.

Systemic manifestations may include the polymyalgia rheumatica syndrome and varying degrees of fever, anemia, weight loss, and malaise. In as many as 25% of all patients with a biopsy-proven giant cell arteritis, localized symptoms or polymyalgia rheumatica may be minimal or absent. Thus, the disease may present as a diagnostic problem of a fever of unknown origin or unexplained anemia.[6] A very rapid ESR can provide the clue that leads to a temporal artery biopsy procedure and proper diagnosis. Abnormal liver function tests, particularly an elevation of the serum alkaline phosphatase level, are frequent in cases of giant cell arteritis. When an elevated level is found in an elderly patient with malaise and weight loss, an occult carcinoma is possible. Extensive investigation with radiographs, scans, and biopsy procedures may be avoided by considering the possibility of giant cell arteritis. A diagnosis only is established by a biopsy specimen from the temporal artery and a demonstration of a characteristic inflammatory infiltrate composed of histiocytes, lymphocytes, and giant cells that surround a fragmented, internal, and elastic lamina with intervening segments of a normal artery. When temporal headache, visual symptoms, or the other signs of cranial artery involvement are present, a biopsy specimen usually is positive. However, it has also been positive in some patients with polymyalgia rheumatica, fever, or other systemic symptoms, even when the artery appears clinically normal.

Giant cell arteritis responds very well to steroid treatment, but higher doses are needed to suppress the inflammation than the low doses that suffice for polymyalgia. When cranial arteritis is diagnosed or even suspected, treatment should be started immediately with 50 mg/ day of prednisone to prevent any visual loss. Even if a biopsy procedure cannot be performed for several days, the histology will not be altered by steroid treatment. If a diagnosis is confirmed by a biopsy specimen, this high dose should be continued for 4 weeks before a gradual reduction is instituted. The dose then is gradually reduced over the next few months, primarily following symptoms and only secondarily the ESR, which usually (but not invariably) is a guide to tapering. The goal is to maintain control of the disease and arrive at the same low, safe level as in the long-term treatment of polymyalgia rheumatica. Such a program carries a risk of steroid toxicity, particularly osteoporosis, which must be balanced against the risk of blindness. If a patient has been treated with a high-dose steroid for 1 month, it is better to follow the clinical response as the dose is tapered. The risk of steroid toxicity, due to treating the ESR, is greater than the risk of blindness or other complications of the disease.

The exact relation of polymyalgia rheumatica and giant cell arteritis remains a persistent problem. Even though as many as 10% of all patients with polymyalgia rheumatica and normal-appearing temporal arteries may have a positive biopsy specimen, the great majority run an uncomplicated course and never show evidence of arteritis. For this reason, neither high-dose steroid treatment nor a temporal artery biopsy procedure is recommended as a routine for every patient with a diagnosis of polymyalgia rheumatica. If a history and physical examination reveal no evidence of cranial arteritis, it is preferable to use a low-dose steroid program with both the patient and physician remaining alert to signals that would indicate the need for a higher dose and temporal artery biopsy procedure, such as headache, diplopia, jaw claudication, or visual blurring.

Rheumatoid Arthritis

Rheumatoid arthritis may have its onset at any age. There has been too much emphasis placed on the peak incidence rate in the 3rd and 5th decades so that, at times, the disease has gone unrecognized in an older patient. Epidemiologic surveys are in agreement that the disease may appear at any age, with documented cases beginning in the 9th decade. It is not unusual for a person of 60 or 70 years of age to get rheumatoid arthritis.

Since it rarely is a fatal disease, there are

many patients who will age with proven rheumatoid arthritis since their youth or middle years. For many patients, inflammatory synovitis by that time is either under control or else has run its course. The symptoms these patients experience and the functional problems they face essentially are those of osteoarthritis (i.e., joints are damaged as a result of the preexisting inflammation). Therapeutic decisions cannot be based solely on a diagnosis of rheumatoid arthritis. A physician must decide whether active inflammation is present, in which case anti-inflammatory or disease-controlling drug programs are appropriate, or if such measures are not appropriate; then, the program is the same as that of a patient with osteoarthritis.

Infrequently, an older patient with long-standing, inactive rheumatoid joint disease may shift into the extra-articular or vasculitic form of the disease. A patient may be anemic, systemically ill, have an elevated ESR, but the joints remain without inflammation. Manifestations include a peripheral neuropathy, rash, arteritis of smaller vessels leading to fingertip infarcts or leg ulcers, and (rarely) visceral manifestations such as pleurisy, pericarditis, coronary occlusion, or bowel infarction.

Several studies have focused on rheumatoid arthritis with an onset after 60 years of age. In approximately 75% of these patients, the presentation is no different than rheumatoid arthritis in younger patients. It is marked by a symmetrical synovitis with a predilection for the distal joints, wrists, fingers, and toes. Synovitis of the wrists may lead to carpal tunnel syndrome with nocturnal numbness and paresthesias in the fingers, which not infrequently may be the presenting manifestation and antedate obvious joint swelling by several months. When a patient has a pre-existent osteoarthritis of the fingers, there frequently is both a delay in recognizing that these symptoms may be something different and some difficulty in arriving at a correct diagnosis. Morning stiffness that persists for at least 30 minutes and a diminution in grip strength both suggest the onset of rheumatoid arthritis. The location of the involved joints is of particular importance. The proximal interphalangeal joints may be involved in either osteoarthritis or rheumatoid arthritis, but pain and swelling of the metacarpophalangeal joints are the hallmark of rheumatoid arthritis (see Figure 19-1). As in younger patients, a rheumatoid factor and rheumatoid nodules frequently are present.

For these patients, the treatment program is standard with only those modifications as indicated by a patient's age.[7] For example, aspirin, which is the anti-inflammatory drug prescribed for many younger patients, may not be well tolerated by an elderly person. While a younger patient will note a ringing in the ear or tinnitus as a sign that a toxic dose is being reached, older patients may not have this warning symptom and may simply experience a significant decrease in their already compromised hearing ability. Ill-defined cerebral symptoms, such as confusion, memory loss, and an inability to think clearly, seem to be a unique reaction of older patients to aspirin and other non-steroidal agents. A corticosteroid can be a helpful anti-inflammatory drug for older patients, since it takes effect rapidly and is free of side effects in low doses. The factor that limits its use in this population is the risk of osteoporosis and vertebral collapse. Males can tolerate up to 10 mg/day of prednisone for prolonged periods. In postmenopausal females, who are more susceptible to osteoporosis, the maximum dose for prolonged periods must be limited to 5 mg/day.

In 25% of all older patients, rheumatoid arthritis has a unique onset.[8,9] The features are more involvement of the proximal muscles, a marked morning stiffness, and constitutional symptoms such as fever, weight loss, or malaise. There may be synovitis of the wrists and swelling of the knees, but the physical findings often are more subtle and difficult to detect than in typical rheumatoid arthritis. Anemia often is present and the ESR is very greatly elevated. The rheumatoid factor may not be present. Frequently, a diagnosis of rheumatoid arthritis is not suspected, and these patients are thought to have an occult malignancy or infection. As can be seen from this description, the disease closely resembles polymyalgia rheumatica, and it often is not possible to make an initial differentiation between the two. As in polymyalgia rheumatica, these patients may respond to low doses of prednisone, such as 10–15 mg/day. This subsequently can be tapered to a safe dose of 5 mg/day and the disease can be satisfactorily controlled.[9] Many patients require no additional treatment, other than small doses of aspirin or other non-steroidal drugs. It is worth trying a low-dose steroid in an elderly patient, because a significant number (not only patients with this "benign" pattern of disease, but also many with typical rheumatoid arthritis) will be controlled satisfactorily on this medication alone; they will not require the inconvenience, expense, and risks of gold or other remission-inducing drugs. Even more than younger patients, elderly patients fear a disabling disease that will curtail their ability to fend for themselves. Steroids, in safe doses, may make the difference between a significant dependency and an independent existence.

Of the disease group formerly known as connective tissue or collagen diseases—and now termed "autoimmune disease"—only rheumatoid arthritis is commonly seen in geriatric patients. Ankylosing spondylitis is a disease of young adults. Scleroderma (progressive systemic sclerosis) and polyarteritis (periarteritis nodosa) are rare in this age group. When they do occur, the presentation is the same as in younger patients. Polymyositis is not common, but it is worth describing because it is treatable once recognized. The main symptom that patients note is a weakness of proximal muscles manifested as a difficulty in rising from a chair or commode, climbing stairs, or lifting objects above their heads; pain is not prominent. Elevations in serum levels of the enzymes SGOT or CPK provide the clue to a diagnosis that can be confirmed by a biopsy specimen of an affected muscle. The erythematous rash of dermatomyositis may or may not be present. Most patients respond readily to corticosteroid doses in the range of 50 mg/day of prednisone; first with a reduction in the serum enzyme levels and, subsequently, with a return of strength. The steroid dose then is gradually tapered using the enzymes as a guide. In younger patients, polymyositis shows evidence of an autoimmune disease, such as antinuclear antibodies. In an older age group, it is more likely to be associated with a malignancy; but even here the incidence of cancer is less than 10%, which is considerably lower than has been previously estimated.[10]

Systemic lupus erythematosus occurs in elderly persons and usually is a benign disease.[11] Manifestations include rash, fever, arthritis, pleurisy, and pulmonary infiltrates. A diagnosis is based on demonstrating antinuclear antibodies in the serum; however, a significant titer is required for a diagnosis, since small amounts frequently are found in normal patients with advancing age. Symptoms respond to anti-inflammatory medications such as aspirin, indomethacin, or a corticosteroid in a relatively low dose. A similar limited form of SLE can be induced by the antiarrhythmic drug procainamide or the antihypertensive agent hydralazine. When these drugs are stopped, the symptoms soon clear even though the antibody may persist in the serum for longer periods. In both drug-induced SLE and spontaneous SLE in elderly persons, renal disease is not present and antibodies against native DNA are rare.[12]

References

1. Moskowitz RW: Management of osteoarthritis. *Bull Rheum Dis* 31:31–34, 1981.
2. Healey LA: Management of gouty arthritis induced by thaizide. *Med Times* 105:26–30, 1977.
3. McCarty DJ: Diagnostic mimicry in arthritis—patterns of joint involvement associated with calcium pyrophosphate dihydrate crystal deposits. *Bull Rheum Dis* 25:804–809, 1975.
4. Healey LA, Wilske KR: *The Systemic Manifestations of Temporal Arteritis*. New York, Grune & Stratton, 1978.
5. Klein RG, Hunder GG, Stanson AW, et al: Large artery involvement in giant cell (temporal) arteritis. *Ann Int Med* 83:806–812, 1975.
6. Healey LA, Wilske KR: Presentation of occult giant cell arteritis. *Arthritis Rheum* 23:641–643, 1980.
7. Hunder GG, Bunch TW: Treatment of rheumatoid arthritis. *Bull Rheum Dis* 32:1–7, 1982.
8. Ehrlich GE, Katz WA, Cohen SH: Rheumatoid arthritis in the aged. *Geriatrics* 25:103–113, 1970.
9. Corrigan AB, Robinson RG, Terenty TR, et al: Benign rheumatoid arthritis of the aged. *Br Med J* 1:444–446, 1974.
10. Bohan A, Peter JB, Bowman RL, et al: A computer-assisted analysis of 153 patients with polymyositis and dermatomyositis. *Medicine* 56:255–286, 1977.
11. Baker SB, Rovira JR, Campion EW, et al: Late onset systemic lupus erythematosus. *Am J Med* 66:727–732, 1979.
12. Blomgren SE, Condemi JJ, Vaughn JH: Procainamide-induced lupus erythematosus: clinical and laboratory observations. *Am J Med* 52:338–348, 1972.

Chapter 20

Immunology

JAMES S. GOODWIN, M.D.

Immunologic function declines with age. Indeed, most physiologic functions decline with age. Why, then, has so much attention been given to the study of immunologic changes in elderly humans and laboratory animals? Immunologic function probably is the most intensively studied physiologic process in gerontology. Part of the reason has to do with the rapid growth in all aspects of immunologic research in the past 3 decades. In addition, immunocytes (lymphocytes, monocytes, and polymorphonuclear leukocytes) are the most easily biopsied tissue specimens in humans. A tube of venous blood provides the immunologist with millions of cells with which to study antibody production, cytotoxicity, proliferation, migration, and other characteristics that are necessary for the continued health and survival of an organism.

There are more fundamental reasons, however, why the study of immunology is particularly relevant to gerontology. An understanding of those changes might be important not only in understanding the aging process, but also in developing potential strategies to prevent some of the inevitable changes that occur with age.

Relevance of the Issues

Makinodan[1] has given five reasons why an effort should be devoted to the understanding of the immune system and its changes with age. First, the immune system, which is known to be intimately involved in the adaptation of organisms to environmental stress and change, declines in efficiency with age. Second, associated with this decline is a rise in the susceptibility to viral and fungal infections and cancer. Third, more is known about differentiation, ontogenetic, and phylogenetic processes of the immune system at the cellular, genetic, and molecular levels than about any other system. Fourth, the immune system is amenable to precise cellular and molecular analysis and, therefore, offers a promise of successful manipulation. Finally, there is a reasonable chance that a reversal in the decline of normal immune functions may delay the onset and lessen the severity of diseases of aging.

Evidence that links depressed or disordered immune function in humans to a subsequent morbidity and/or mortality is scarce. Most authorities simply have assumed that a decline in immune function is deleterious, or they have used theoretic arguments to support this belief. One example is the idea of "immune surveillance," which is first conceptualized by Erlich,[2] named by Burnet,[3] and popularized by Thomas,[4] and others. It proposes that the cellular immune system is the first defense against cancer. The most enthusiastic proponents of immune surveillance contended that new malignancies were popping up every day, only to be eliminated by the ever-vigilant immune system. A corollary of this theory is that clinical cancer represents a failure of immune surveillance. Thus, individuals such as elderly persons with a depressed immune function should have a higher incidence rate of malignancy. More recently, the lack of a generalized increase in most malignancies in immunosuppressed humans and experimental animals has thrown this theory into relative disrepute.[5,6]

The question of whether a decreased cellular immune response was a risk factor for the subsequent mortality in an elderly population was addressed by placing a reported series of five delayed-type hypersensitivity skin tests for common antigens on 52 octogenarians and correlating the response to their tests with survival after 2 years.[7] Of those subjects who responded to none or only one antigen (the "anergic" group), 80% were dead within 2 years; 35% of the group that responded to two or more antigens were dead by the 2-year follow-up (see Table 20-1). The octogenarian subjects in this reported series were not well characterized as to the presence of medical illnesses on initial skin testing. While the investigators used their data to suggest that anergy was a risk factor for subsequent mortality, an equally plausible explanation was that whatever the underlying medical condition ultimately responsible for death, it also contributed to the depressed cellular immunity in these individuals. Perhaps, the least controversial conclusion from this study is that octogenarians do not live long, regardless of their immune status. Actually, the overall 65% death rate during the 2-year follow-up in this Australian study contrasted sharply with the mean life expectancy of 8 years for all males and females 80 to 85 years of age in the United States.[8] This again suggests that the population studied had serious underlying illnesses.

The other major body of evidence that links a disordered immune function to disease and death concerns the possible role of autoantibo-dies and circulating immune complexes (CICs) in the etiology of atherosclerosis.[9] While it had been recognized for many years that CICs caused by repeated injections of a foreign antigen could cause an acute arteritis,[10] it only has been within the last decade that evidence has accumulated suggesting that autoimmunity might contribute to atherosclerosis. The combination of injections of foreign proteins and atherogenic diets in rabbits resulted in more atherosclerosis than with an atherogenic diet alone.[11] In addition, the histologic type of atherosclerosis produced in these rabbits closely resembles that found in humans.[12] Similar data were obtained in baboons.[13] Chronic stimuli for CIC formation will lead to atherosclerosis even in animals on a non-atherogenic diet.[14] The most striking evidence that links autoimmunity to atherosclerosis in experimental animals was in a study of the long-term effects of vasectomy on rhesus monkeys.[15,16] Vasectomy can be seen as a mild stimulus for autoantibody and CIC formation. Antisperm antibodies develop in about 50% of all vasectomized human males and experimental animals.[17,18] Alexander and Clarkson demonstrated that vasectomies led to accelerated atherosclerosis in monkeys who were fed a high-fat diet.[16] They then showed that monkeys vasectomized and maintained on a very low-fat no-cholesterol diet (fruit and commercial monkey chow) had an increased incidence rate and degree of atherosclerosis, at autopsy, 9–14 years later than did non-vasectomized control subjects.[15] Thus, a very mild stimulus for autoantibody formation leads to accelerated athero-

TABLE 20-1 Response to Delayed-Type Hypersensitivity Skin Testing and 2 Year Survival Rate in 52 Subjects Over 80 Years of Age

Number of Positive Skin Tests	Number of Subjects	Number Dead After 2 Yrs	Percent (%) Dead at 2 Yrs
0	21	17	80
1	14	11	
2	10	2	
3	3	2	35
4	4	2	
5	0	34	

SOURCE: Adapted from Roberts-Thompson IC, Whittingham S, Youngchaiyud I, et al: Aging, immune response and mortality. *Lancet* 2:368–370, 1974.

sclerosis even without an atherogenic diet. This evidence provides a strong theoretic basis for proposing that autoantibodies and CICs in humans, by causing a low level of chronic irritation in blood vessels, contribute to the development of atherosclerosis.

In addition to the studies in experimental animals, there also is some epidemiologic data in humans that supports a link between autoimmunity and atherosclerosis. Mackey and his colleagues measured a variety of autoantibodies in the sera of most of the adult population of the town of Busselton in western Australia.[19-21] There was an association between the presence of autoantibodies and the presence of cardiovascular diseases in the population. More important, the presence of autoantibodies in 1969 (the time of the comprehensive survey) was associated with an increased risk of death due to vascular disease and cancer during the period 1970–1975. As in the study summarized in Table 20-1, the association of the disordered immune function (in this case autoantibodies) and subsequent mortality rate may have been due to both phenomena being secondary to a serious medical illness that was present when the subjects were first tested.

Specific Changes in Immune Function with Age

Problems of Methodology

There are two major methodologic questions that plague gerontologists. First, do age-related changes found in short-lived species such as mice or guinea pigs have any relevance to age-related changes in humans? Are the processes responsible for making a mouse old at 3 years of age the same as those making a human old at age 75? Second, is a given physiologic change that is found in a majority of aging organisms secondary to the aging process per se, or is it secondary to one of the many diseases whose prevalence increases with age. Concern about the first question would tend to move investigators away from experimental animals to the study of aging humans, while concern about the second question would tend to push investigators in the opposite direction.

The problems raised by these questions are real; many reported investigations on immuno-logic changes with age suffer from a lack of a rigorous approach to dealing with these issues.[22] It is not at all uncommon to see articles on the differences in some immunologic response in young versus old mice based on data obtained in 2-month-old versus 1-year-old animals. These would be analogous to 4-year-old and 25-year-old humans. Even when truly aged experimental animals are used, there are few parallels between the physiologic changes, diseases, and causes of death in these animals and humans. Conversely, few studies of immunologic changes in elderly persons rigorously define their subjects in terms of the underlying disease, medication status, occupational exposure history, and so on. It is surprising how many widely accepted immunologic changes in aging humans were based on studies of hospitalized, potentially malnourished, and psychologically stressed males and females taking a great variety of prescription medications and suffering from a great variety of acute and chronic diseases. A sentence that is commonly encountered in the "Methods and Materials" sections is that "the subjects studied had no diseases or medications known to affect the immune system." This is an empty promise, for most medications have not been studied for their effect on immunologic function. Even experimental animal studies sometimes may be labelled as age-related changes something that in reality is secondary to stress, chronic disease, or diet.

Given all the reservations expressed above, it still is possible to reach a consensus on some changes in immune function that would seem to occur as a function of age. The following sections in this chapter will describe those changes, as well as the mechanisms thought to cause these changes. When possible, the emphasis will be on data from human rather than experimental animal studies.

Changes in Cellular Immunity

The immune system classically has been divided into the cellular and humoral compartments, with monocyte and granulocyte function treated separately. The cellular immune response is responsible for rejecting grafts of foreign tissues, for killing virus-infected cells, for protecting against fungi and some intracellular parasites and bacteria, and (possibly) for defense against the growth of tumors. The function of the humoral immune system is the production of antibodies, which are the main defense against bacteria and other infectious agents that gain entry into an organism. Cells of the monocyte-macrophage series, in addition to ingesting and/or killing foreign material that may or may not have been previously opsonized with antibodies, also play an important regulatory role in both humoral and cellular immune responses.

The depression of cellular immune responses is the most universal and easily demonstrated age-related change in immune function. The incidence of anergy (lack of a delayed-type hypersensitivity response to intradermal testing with a battery of common antigens) increases over 60 years of age.[7,21–24] In a prospective study of 300 healthy males and females over 65 years of age, 33% were anergic versus none of the young control subjects.[23] In this study, only subjects who had no known medical illnesses after a comprehensive physical examination, and who were on no prescription or regular non-prescription medications, were included. Analogous findings have been reported in mice, which manifest a decreased ability to reject foreign skin grafts with age.[1]

The in vitro correlate of delayed-type hypersensitivity skin testing is the proliferative response of lymphocytes that are cultured with specific antigens or non-specific mitogens. Lymphocytes are isolated from the peripheral blood and cultured in media with candida, streptokinase-streptodornase (SKSD) or trichophyton (all specific antigens), or else with phytohemagglutinin (PHA) and concanavalin A (Con A) (mitogens that non-specifically activate most T cells). The degree of a proliferative response then can be quantitated by adding radiolabelled thymidine to the cultures, harvesting the cells, and measuring the amount of radioactivity incorporated into the lymphocyte DNA. Most investigators have reported that antigen or mitogen-stimulated cultures of lymphocytes from persons over 65 years of age incorporate less radiolabelled thymidine,[7,25–28] but there are also conflicting reports.[26,29,30] Czlonkowska and Korlak[26] reported a decreased proliferative response of lymphocytes in 30 study subjects over 60 years of age compared with young subjects to PHA, but not to Con A, candida, or SKSD. Portaro, Glick, and

Zighelboim[29] studied 200 healthy, working persons 21–70 years of age and found no age-related decrease in response to several concentrations of PHA. The authors noted that their group of subjects was better characterized as to their health status than previously reported subjects in whom a decline in the PHA response had been found. Conversely, the oldest subjects in this study were only 70 years of age, and the number of subjects in the two oldest categories (ages 61–65[11] and 66–70[14]) may have been too small to recognize substantial differences in PHA responses. The author's study of 300 healthy elderly people showed a substantial decrease in PHA response with age.[23] The distribution of responses to one dose of PHA of healthy elderly subjects compared to young control subjects is shown in Figure 20-1. The mean response of the elderly subjects was significantly less than the mean response of the young control subjects to all mitogen doses ($p < 0.0001$). An inspection of Figure 20-1 reveals that the distribution of PHA responses are not normal; they are skewed towards higher PHA responses. Thus, there is a population of healthy elderly persons with PHA responses grouped about the mean of the PHA responses for the young control subjects, while the majority of healthy elderly persons have depressed PHA responses. To pursue the distinction between age-related changes in PHA response versus changes due to chronic illnesses or medications that frequently accompany aging, we also measured the PHA responses of 24 chronically ill patients over 65 years of age who had a variety of life-threatening medical conditions and who were on a number of medications. The PHA responses of this chronically ill group was not different from the response of the healthy group. Thus, age per se, and not an accompanying illness, was the major determinant of a depressed cellular immunity in this population. Within the healthy elderly group, there was a significant decrease in PHA response with age ($r = -0.23$, $p < 0.0001$).

Mechanism of Decreased Cellular Immunity

The causes of depressed cellular immune responses with age are most certainly multiple, and they may differ depending on the aspect of the cellular immune function that is examined.

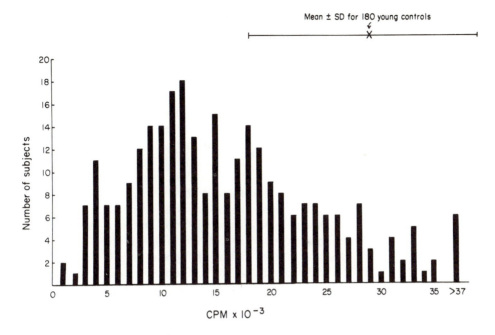

FIGURE 20-1   The distribution of responses of lymphocytes from 279 healthy elderly people to an optimal concentration (4.0 μg/ml) of PHA. The mean ± 1 standard deviation of the response of lymphocytes from 180 young control group persons obtained simultaneously is shown for comparison. (Adapted from Goodwin JS, Searles RP, Tung KSK: Immunological responses of a healthy elderly population. *Clin Exp Immunol* 48:403–410, 1982.)

For example, anergy to delayed-type hypersensitivity skin testing could represent problems with antigen recognition, T-cell proliferation, lymphokine production, lymphocyte or monocyte chemotaxis, vascular response to inflammatory mediators, or a multitude of other steps that are required to produce induration after an intradermal challenge with antigens. Given the complexity of the in vivo system, it is understandable that immunologists who are searching for mechanisms have turned to in vitro assays in which specific cell functions can be more or less studied in isolation. Such investigations have, as expected, resulted in the identification of several, specific age-related lesions in cellular immune functions.

Hyporesponsiveness to PHA of lymphocytes from aging humans has been demonstrated to be a sum of two deficiencies.[31] First, the number of mitogen-responsive cells is reduced in lymphocyte preparations from elderly persons. Second, the mitogen-responsive cells from elderly persons do not proliferate as vigorously after exposure to PHA as do lymphocytes from young persons. Lymphocytes from healthy

males and females over 70 years of age are reported to be significantly more sensitive to inhibition by prostaglandin E_2 (PGE_2) in mitogen-stimulated cultures.[28,32] Because PGE_2 acts as a normal endogenous feedback inhibitor of cellular immune responses in vitro and in vivo,[33] we postulated that an increased sensitivity to this immunomodulator may partially account for the depressed cellular immune responses seen in this group of subjects. Indeed, the addition of drugs that block the production of PGE_2 in PHA stimulated cultures reversed much of the depressed response of lymphocytes from subjects over 70 years of age.[28] The increased sensitivity with age to PGE would not appear to be part of a general increase in sensitivity to all immunomodulators; for example, lymphocytes from subjects over 70 years of age actually are less sensitive to inhibition by histamine and hydrocortisone than are lymphocytes from young control subjects.[32]

The proliferative response of T cells to mitogens is dependent on several earlier steps that involve the secretion of glycopeptides from lymphocytes (lymphokines) and monocytes (monokines). After the exposure of peripheral blood mononuclear cells to a mitogen, the monocytes secrete interleukin I, which stimulates a subset of T cells to produce interleukin II (also called a T-cell growth factor). A second set of T cells becomes sensitive to interleukin II by developing cell surface receptors for this lymphokine. This interleukin II-sensitive subset then proliferates on exposure to interleukin II. This recently described system, which has been used to further dissect the age-related defect in cellular immunity, demonstrated both a decreased production of interleukin II after mitogen stimulus and a decreased responsiveness of T cells to interleukin II.[34] Additional experiments in mice and rats suggest that the picture might be more complex, with specific defects in production of or sensitivity to interleukin II depending on the immunologic stimulus.[35,36]

The most obvious change that is associated with the decline in cellular immunity with age is the involution of the thymus. Thymic lymphatic mass, particularly in the cortical area, decreases with age in humans and experimental animals.[37] Thymic involution starts in adolescence. The thymus mass of an aging human and experimental animal has approximately 10% of the mass of a younger thymus.[37] Associated with a loss of thymic mass is a decreased output of thymic hormones.[38] A thymectomy leads to the acceleration of normal age-related changes in immune function in mice, which suggests that thymic involution may indeed be a central cause of age-related immunodeficiencies.[39] Moreover, the treatment of aging mice with thymic hormone preparations causes a reversal of the immunodeficiencies.[39,40]

Changes in Humoral Immunity with Age

The distinction of cellular and humoral immunity is, in some ways, artificial because both B cells (bone marrow-derived) and T cells (thymus-derived) can participate in each reaction. For example, B cells can act as antigen-presenting cells in cellular immune responses, while T cells are required for the great majority of humoral immune (antibody) responses. Thus, changes in humoral immunity frequently are secondary to alterations in T-cell function, and not to any change in intrinsic B-cell function.

It generally is agreed that changes in humoral immune responses with age are not as marked as are the changes in cellular immunity. The number of circulation B cells in humans[41] and splenic B cells in mice[42] does not change with age. Specific antibody responses after antigenic challenges tend to decrease in aging organisms, and this is more apparent with so-called T-dependent rather than T-independent antigens.[43] The distinction between T-dependent and T-independent antigens, which is more clear in mice than humans, is made on the basis of whether there is an absolute requirement for T-cell help in the antibody response. Some artificially constructed simple antigens as well as some polysaccharide antigens are T-independent, while all others appear to be T-dependent. In a study of the antibody response in subjects of different ages to flagellin,[7] which is a potent antigen in humans, the mean titers of IgG and IgM antibodies were similar for the study subjects over 65 years of age and the young control subjects; but, there was a failure of the older subjects to maintain levels of the IgG antibody over time, which was attributed to a failure of helper T cells. Other investigators have reported normal[44,45] or depressed[46–48] antibody responses in older humans after influenza vaccination and tetanus vaccination. In experimental animals, the decrease in T-dependent antibody responses is more obvious, with an 80% decrease in antibody-forming cells in older animals.[39,49]

Mechanism of Depressed Humoral Immunity

As mentioned earlier, a decrease in humoral immune response could be due to a defect in B-cell function, T-cell function, or both. In addition, a decrease in T-cell helpers (suggested by the experiments outlined in the previous paragraph) might represent a decrease in helper T-cell activity or an increase in suppressor T-cell activity. In other words, the apparent failure of T-cell helper activity with age might actually be an increase in the active suppression of the immune response by suppressor T cells. The past decade has brought an appreciation of the importance of suppressor T cells, which modulate normal immune responses and prevent the development of autoimmunity. For example, normal young persons have circulating B cells that are programmed to differentiate into autoantibody-producing plasma cells (producing antinuclear, antithyroid, and antimitochondrial antibodies, and so on); however, tonic inhibition of this autoimmune response by suppressor T cells prevents such an immunologic aberration.[50] Several studies of human lymphocytes that were cultured in vitro have addressed the question of the mechanism of age-related decreases in humoral immunity. Lymphocytes from old persons that were cultured with pokeweed mitogen (PWM), which is a non-specific stimulus for B-cell differentiation, produced greater amounts of IgG and IgM than did lymphocytes from young control subjects.[51] When the lymphocytes were separated into T-cell and B-cell fractions, and various combinations of old T cells were cultured with old B cells (and old T cells with young B cells, and so on), the old T cells were more capable than the young T cells of supporting the immunoglobulin production via either young or old B cells. This increased helper activity of the old T cells could be due to an actual increase in helper activity, a decrease in suppressor activity, or both. The same investigators addressed this question by studying the effects of the irradiation of T cells in this system, taking advantage of the fact that suppressor T cells are sensitive to low doses of x-irradiation while helper T cells are relatively radioresistant.[52] Thus, the increase in immunoglobin production in cultures of B cells plus T cells after T-cell irradiation is an indication of suppressor cell function. T-cell irradiation was less effective in enhancing the immunoglobulin production in B-cell plus T-cell cultures from elderly persons than it was in young people.[52] This suggests that the overall increase in T-cell help with age actually was due to a failure of suppressor cell function. A decrease in suppressor cell function with age also has been found by other investigators who used another assay system for suppressor cell activity termed the concanavalin A-activated suppressor cell.[53,54] However, it is not clear that this particular assay measures anything relevant to the control of humoral immune responses in humans.[50] Aging humans show a more marked age-related depression of the antigen-specific than of polyclonal (PWM-induced) antibody responses. This depression of antigen-specific immunoglobulin production was attributed to a deficiency in helper T-cell activity.

The dichotomy of an age-related increase in helper T-cell activity in polyclonally (PWM) stimulated cultures, with a decrease in helper cell activity in specific antigen-stimulated cultures, also has been reported by other investigators.[48,55]

With the introduction of monoclonal antibodies that recognize specific suppressor and helper T-cell subsets, it is now possible to physically separate helper and suppressor T cells and to directly assay their activity instead of using the indirect means of differential sensitivity to irradiation or Con A.[50] This methodology demonstrated both an increased helper T-cell activity and decreased suppressor T-cell activity with age.[56] Perhaps more importantly, the intrinsic B-cell function, which is measured by culturing purified B cells with soluble helper factors derived from T cells, was found to decline substantially with age. This latter finding suggested the possibility that the age-related changes in helper and suppressor T-cell function actually represent a homeostatic adjustment of an organism that is attempting to maintain an adequate antibody production in the face of a failing B-cell compartment. The concept of a primary failure of B-cell function with age is supported by functional experiments in mice[57,58] and by data showing age-related structural changes in B cells.[46,59,60]

Increase in Autoimmunity with Age

The classic autoimmune diseases generally are associated with young adults. Systemic lupus erythematosus (SLE), polymyositis, rheumatoid arthritis, all have a higher prevalence in young than older adults. Nevertheless, the serologic manifestations of autoimmunity (autoantibodies and CICs) are greatly increased in prevalence in older healthy adults. The possible role of the autoantibodies and CICs in the pathogenesis of arteriosclerosis already was discussed at the beginning of this chapter; it should be kept in mind if the question arises: "Why worry about autoantibodies and circulating immune complexes if they are asymptomatic?"

Many different investigators have reported an increase in the prevalence of positive tests for various autoantibodies with age (antinuclear antibodies, the rheumatoid factor, antithyroid antibodies, antismooth muscle antibodies, and antilymphocyte antibodies). The rise in prevalence becomes steep around 70 years of age.[23,24,61–63] It should be mentioned that as with the data on age-related decreases in PHA response discussed earlier, there are some studies that did not find an increase in autoantibodies with age; however, the great majority of studies did find such an increase.

The prevalence of an antinuclear antibody, lymphocytotoxic antibody, rheumatoid factor, and CICs in 278 healthy elderly subjects is given in Table 20-2, along with analogous findings in 100 young control subjects. There is a clear increase in the percentage of sera from old subjects that are positive for each test, compared with sera in young control subjects. A given sera, which was positive in one of these tests, did not increase the chance of it being positive in the remaining tests.[23] Of the subjects tested, 50% were positive for at least one test, which is exactly the figure predicted if positivity for each test were distributed independently and not clustered in a subgroup of elderly persons. In another study,[63] there was an association between the presence of CICs and the presence of one or more autoantibodies in 189 healthy subjects 20–70 years of age and older. The positive association between the presence of autoantibodies and CICs makes sense from a theoretic perspective; autoantibodies should lead to CICs. Differences in study designs that might explain the discrepancy in these two investigations include the younger subjects and

the greater number of autoantibodies that were measured in the study by Delespesse.

The reason for the increased prevalence of autoantibodies with age is not completely understood. It is important to remember, as stated earlier, that all humans and experimental animals of any age are fully capable of producing autoantibodies (i.e., we all have B cells programmed to produce all described autoantibodies). Indeed, we all have autoantibodies such as the rheumatoid factor, antinuclear antibodies, antithyroid, and so on in our sera; but, they are at low levels that are not detected by the standard agglutination or immunofluorescence tests. Therefore, autoimmunity in aging is a matter of degree, and it presumably results from a failure of immunoregulation.

The suggestion that the increase in autoantibodies with age was secondary to a loss of the T-cell control of B-cell function was supported by the report of a negative association between PHA response and the presence of autoantibodies in elderly persons,[64] (i.e., the higher the proliferation of T cells to mitogens, the lower was the chance of having autoantibodies). The authors, however, found no association between the measures of T-cell function (PHA response and delayed-type hypersensitivity skin testing) and the measures of autoimmunity (CICs, the rheumatoid factor, antinuclear antibodies, and lymphocytotoxic antibodies).

The most popular explanation for increasing autoantibody production with age is a decrease in suppressor cell function. The evidence for

TABLE 20-2 Autoantibodies and Circulating Immune Complexes in Healthy Elderly Study Subjects

Assay	Old Subject Group		Young Control Group	
	Positive/Total Tested*	% Positive	Positive/Total Tested	% Positive
Antinuclear Ab	50/278	18	4/98	4
Rheumatoid factor	38/278	14	4/98	4
Lymphocytotoxic Ab	27/278	10	3/93	3
Circulating immune complexes	43/197	22	5/100	5

* Positive sera were defined as follows: for antinuclear Ab, a titre of >1:10; for rheumatoid factor, a titre of >1:20; for lymphocytotoxic Ab, >30% killing in >50% of the samples of peripheral blood lymphocytes from 11 normal donors; and for CICs >2 SD above the mean of values of a panel of normal control sera.

SOURCE: Adapted from Goodwin JS, Searles RP, Tung KSK: Immunological responses of a healthy elderly population. *Clin Exp Immunol* 48:403–410, 1982.

such a decrease was cited earlier in this chapter. It is interesting that as the overall suppressor cell function declines with age, there is an age-related increase in the percentage of T cells in the peripheral blood, which carry cell surface antigens that are characteristic of suppressor cells.[56,65]

Helper and suppressor cell function was studied in the production of one autoantibody (IgM rheumatoid factor) in cultures of lymphocytes from elderly subjects and young control subjects.[66] The culture system, which used isolated populations of T-cell helper, suppressor T, and B cells, was analogous to the one described earlier in the study of total immunoglobulin production.[56] In contrast to the earlier studies[52,56] that showed a decreased suppressor cell function with age in the total immunoglobulin production, there was no change with age in suppressor cell function with IgM rheumatoid factor production; but, there was a marked increase in helper cell function. Interestingly, we found a substantial decrease in the intrinsic capacity of isolated B cells from older people to make the rheumatoid factor. Thus, the increased production of the rheumatoid factor with age would appear to be due to an overactivity of T-helper cells in the face of a declining B-cell function. In that situation, the more subtle controls that prevent autoantibody production presumably are lost.

Prospects for Therapeutic Intervention in the Age-Related Decline in Immune Function

It is, perhaps, premature to discuss the potential methods of reversing the age-related decline in immune function when it is not clear that a depressed immune function is an independent risk factor for anything. The few studies that link a disordered immune function with a subsequent morbidity and mortality are suggestive, but are far from conclusive. One of the major purposes of the longitudinal study of 300 healthy elderly subjects is to determine if a healthy male or female 70 years of age or older, on no medications and with no known physical illnesses after a comprehensive medical evaluation, is at a greater risk of death or of developing specific illnesses if they are anergic to skin testing, or if they have high levels of autoanti-

bodies or CICs. The above misgivings not withstanding, this chapter will conclude with a brief discussion of the potential ways to stimulate a failing immune function in elderly persons.

Often, the most intriguing scientific discoveries are those that also are without an obvious practical consequence. A prime example was the discovery by McCay and his colleagues in 1935 that the caloric restriction of experimental animals markedly prolonged their life span.[67] These investigators reported that restricting the total caloric intake to 50–60% of what is required to maintain normal growth in adolescent mice, rats, and guinea pigs, resulted in an approximately 50% prolongation of the total life span of animals that survived the 6–12-month period of starvation. This interesting medical oddity received little attention over the next 3 decades until other investigators showed that the early starvation of experimental animals resulted in a preservation of normal immune function into old age.[68] The possibility that lesser amounts of caloric restriction, supplemented with essential nutrients, might have a similar beneficial effect in humans is now being seriously discussed,[40] although not formally tested.

Because thymic atrophy seems central to the loss of immunocompetence with aging, an obvious group of stategies to reverse the decline involves injecting extracts of young thymic tissue, administering thymic hormones, or transplanting young thymic tissue into aging animals.[40] A variety of in vivo and in vitro experimental procedures have indicated that, in certain situations, any of the above stategies can lead to a restoration of immunocompetence in an aging immune system. The work with the various preparations of thymic hormones is of the greatest potential interest, because these hormones or the active portions of these hormones can be chemically synthesized or produced via recombinant DNA technology, which means that large amounts could be made available if it proved efficacious. It is not yet clear whether thymic hormone administration has any effect on the life span of experimental animals.

Another potential means of preventing age-related declines in immunity is immunopharmacologic-administering drugs that in one way or another stimulate immune function. In this regard, prostaglandin synthetase inhibitors, such as the non-steroidal anti-inflammatory drugs (NSAIDs), have received increasing attention. By reducing the production of the feedback inhibitor PGE_2 NSAIDs, stimulate immune responses in vitro and in vivo.[33] For example, two of four patients with an adult-acquired immunodeficiency who were completely anergic became responsive to delayed-type hypersensitivity skin testing when they were placed on the cyclo-oxygenase inhibitor indomethacin.[69] Such a therapeutic strategy might be especially relevant to elderly persons, because their T cells are more sensitive to inhibition by PGE_2,[28,70,71] which partially accounts for the depressed proliferative response to mitogens.[28] Recent evidence would suggest that prostaglandin synthetase inhibitors also might reduce the increase in autoantibody production that occurs with age,[71,72] while stimulating the primary antibody response to new antigens.[71]

The above examples of the potential methods of immunostimulation are representative of the many therapies that have been proposed and/or tested. All these attempts at immunostimulation violate a basic conservative tenet in medicine of leaving well-enough alone. It is difficult, if not impossible, to justify intervention in a healthy individual with a disordered laboratory parameter (low PHA response or skin test anergy), especially when the intervention is not benign (and no intervention is benign), unless: 1) It has been clearly shown that the disordered laboratory parameter is associated with an increased risk of morbidity and mortality; and 2) That the intervention reduces that risk. Neither criteria has been met for the age-related decline in immune function.

References

1. Makinodan T: Biology of aging: Retrospect and prospect, in Makinodan T, Yunis E (eds): *Immunology and Aging*. New York, Plenum Press, 1977, pp 1–8.
2. Erlich P: Uber den jetzigen stano der karzinomforschung. *Ned Tijoschr Geneesk* 53:273–290, 1909.
3. Burnet FM: The concept of immunological surveillance. *Prog Exp Tumor Res* 13:1–27, 1970.
4. Thomas L: Reactions to homologous tissue antigens in relation to hypersensitivity, in Lawrence HS (ed): *Cellular and Humoral Aspects of the Hypersensitive States*. New York, Hoeber-Harper, 1959, pp 529–532.
5. Prehn RT: Immunological surveillance: pro and con. *Clin Immunol* 2:191–203, 1974.
6. Klein G: Immunological surveillance against neoplasia, in *The Harvey Lectures 1973–1974*. New York, Academic Press, 1974, p 71.
7. Roberts-Thompson IC, Whittingham S, Youngchaiyud U, et al: Aging, immune reponse and mortality. *Lancet* 2:368–370, 1974.
8. Abridged life tables by color and sex: United States, 1977, in *Monthly Vital Statistics Report*, Hyattsville, Maryland. United States Center for Health Statistics, 1974, p 18.
9. Mathews JD, Whittingham S, Mackay IR: Autoimmunity and human vascular disease-hypothesis. *Lancet* 2:1423–1427, 1974.
10. Dixon FJ, Vasquez JJ, Weigle WO, et al: Pathogenesis of serum sickness. *Arch Pathol* 65:18–20, 1958.
11. Lamberson HV, Fritz KE: Immunological enhancement of atherogenesis in rabbits. Persistent susceptibility in atherogenic diet following experimentally induced serum sickness. *Arch Pathol* 98:9–16, 1974.
12. Minick CR, Murphy GE, Campbell WG: Experimental induction of athero-arteriosclerosis by the synergy of allergic injury to arteries and lipid rich diet. *J Exp Med* 124:635–652, 1966.
13. Howard AN, Paterski J, Bowyer DE, et al: Atherosclerosis induced in hypercholesterolemic baboons by immunological injury. *Atherosclerosis* 14:17–29, 1971.
14. Friedman RJ, Moore S, Singal DP: Repeated endothelial injury and induction of atherosclerosis in normolipemic rabbits by human serum. *Lab Invest* 30:404–415, 1975.
15. Clarkson RB, Alexander NJ: Long term vasectomy. Effects on the occurrence and extent of atherosclerosis in rhesus monkeys. *J Clin Invest* 65:15–25, 1980.
16. Alexander NJ, Clarkson TB: Vasectomy increases the severity of diet-induced atherosclerosis in macaca fascicularis. *Science* 201:538–541, 1978.
17. Ansbacher R, Keung-Yeung K, Wurster JC: Sperm antibodies in vasectomized men. *Fertil Steril* 23:640–643, 1972.
18. Alexander MJ, Tung KSK: Immunological and morphological effects of vasectomy in the rabbit. *Anta Rec* 188:339–350, 1977.
19. Whittingham S, Irwin J, Mackay IR, et al: Autoantibodies in healthy subjects. *Austr Ann Med* 18:130–134, 1969.
20. Hooper B, Whittingham S, Mathews JD, et al: Autoimmunity in a rural community. *Clin Exp Immunol* 12:79–87, 1972.

21. Mackay IR, Whittingham SF, Mathews JD: The immunoepidemiology of aging, in Makinodan T, Yunis E (eds): *Immunology and Aging,* New York, Plenum Press, 1977, pp 35–50.

22. Hess EV, Knapp D: The immune system and aging: a case of the cart before the horse. *J Chron Dis* 31:647–649, 1978.

23. Goodwin JS, Searles RP, Tung KSK: Immunological responses of a healthy elderly population. *Clin Exp Immunol* 48:403–410, 1982.

24. Mackay I: Aging and immunological function in man. *Gerontologia* 18:285–296, 1972.

25. Hallgren HM, Kersey JH, Dubuey DP, et al: Lymphocyte subsets and integrated immune function in aging humans. *Clin Immunol Immunopathol* 10:65–78, 1978.

26. Czlonkowska A, Korlak J: The immune response during aging. *J Gerontol* 34:9–14, 1979.

27. Inkeles B, Innes JB, Kuntz MM, et al: Immunological studies of aging. III. Cytokinetic basis for the impaired response of lymphocytes from aged humans to plant lectins. *J Exp Med* 145:1176–1440, 1979.

28. Goodwin JS, Messner RP: Increased sensitivity to prostaglandin E_2 in lymphocytes from subjects over age 70. *J Clin Invest* 64:434–439, 1979.

29. Portaro JK, Glick GI, Zighelboim J: Population immunity: Age and immune cell parameters. *Clin Immunol Immunopathol* 11:339–350, 1978.

30. Ben-Zei A, Galili U, Russel A, et al: Age-associated changes in subpopulations of human lymphocytes. *Clin Immunol Immunopathol* 7:139–149, 1977.

31. Inkeles B, Innes J, Iguntz M, et al: Immunological studies of aging. *J Exp Med* 145:1176–1187, 1977.

32. Goodwin JS: Changes in lymphocyte sensitivity to prostaglandin E, histamine, hydrocortisone, and X-irradiation with age: studies in a healthy elderly population. *Clin Immunol Immunopathol* 25:243–251, 1982.

33. Goodwin JS, Webb DR: Regulation of the immune response by prostaglandins: A critical review. *Clin Immunol Immunopathol* 15:116–132, 1981.

34. Gillis S, Kozak R, Durante M, et al: Immunological studies of aging: Decreased production of and response to T cell growth factor by lymphocytes from aged humans. *J Clin Invest* 67:937–942, 1981.

35. Gilman SC, Rosenberg JS, Feldman JD: T lymphocytes of young and old rats. *J Immunol* 128:644–650, 1982.

36. Thoman ML, Wiegel WO: Cell mediated immunity in aged mice: An underlying lesion in interleukin 2 synthesis. *J Immunol* 128:2358–2361, 1982.

37. Hirokawa K: The thymus and aging, in Makinodan T, Yunis E (eds): *Immunology and Aging.* New York, Plenum Press, 1977, pp 51–72.

38. Lewis V, Twomey J, Bealmear P, et al: Age, thymic function and circulating thymic hormone activity. *J Clin Endocrinol Metab* 47:145–152, 1978.

39. Weksler M, Innes J, Goldstein G: Immunological studies of aging: The contribution of thymic involution to the immune deficiencies of aging mice and reversal with thymopoitin. *J Exp Med* 148:996–1006, 1978.

40. Walford R, Meredith P, Cheney K: Immunoengineering: Prospects for correction of age-related immunodeficiency states, in Makinodan T, Yunis E (eds): *Immunology and Aging.* New York, Plenum Press, 1976, pp 183–201.

41. Diaz-Jouanen E, Williams R, Strickland R: Age-related changes in T and B cells. *Lancet* 1:688–689, 1975.

42. Makinodan T, Adler W: The effects of aging on the differentiation and proliferation potentials of cells of the immune system. *Fed Proc* 34:153–158, 1975.

43. Makinodan T, Good R, Kay M: Cellular basis of immunosenescence, in Makinodan T, Yunis E (eds): *Immunology and Aging.* New York, Plenum Press, 1977, pp 9–22.

44. Feery B, Morrison E, Evered M: Antibody responses to influenza virus sub unit vaccine in the aged. *Med J Austr* 1:540–542, 1976.

45. Solomonova K, Vizey ST: Immunological reactivity of senescent and old people actively immunized with tetanus toxoid. *Z Immuun-Forsch* 146:81–90, 1973.

46. Phair J, Kauffman C, Bjornson A, et al: Failure to respond to influenza vaccine in the aged: correlation with B cell number and function. *J Lab Clin Med* 92:822–828, 1978.

47. Mackenzie JS: Influenza subunit vaccine: Antibody response to one and two doses of vaccine and length of response, with particular reference to the elderly. *Br Med J* 1:200–202, 1977.

48. Kishimoto S, Tomino S, Mitsuya H, et al: Age-related decline in the in vitro and in vivo synthesis of anti-tetanus toxoid antibody in humans. *J Immunol* 125:2347–2352, 1980.

49. Gerbase-DeLima M, Wilkinson J, Smith G, et al: Age related decline in thymic-independent immune function in a long-lived mouse strain. *J Gerontol* 29:261–268, 1974.

50. Goodwin JS: *Suppressor Cells in Human Disease.* New York, Marcel-Dekker, 1981.

51. Kishimoto S, Tomino S, Imomata K, et al: Age-related changes in the subsets and functions of human T lymphocytes. *J Immunol* 121:1773–1779, 1978.

52. Kishimoto S, Tomino S, Mitsuya H, et al: Age-related changes in suppressor functions of human T cells. *J Immunol* 123:1586–1592, 1979.

53. Pahwa S, Pahwa R, Good R: Decreased in vitro humoral immune responses to aged humans. *J Clin Invest* 67:1094–1102, 1981.

54. Hallgren H, Yunis E: Suppressor lymphocytes in young and aged humans. *J Immunol* 118:2004–2009, 1977.

55. Delfraissey J, Galanaud P, Dormont J, et al: Age-related impairment of the in vitro antibody response in the human. *Clin Exp Immunol* 39:208–214, 1980.

56. Ceuppens JL, Goodwin JS: Regulation of immunoglobulin production in pokeweed mitogen-stimulated cultures of lymphocytes from young and old adults. *J Immunol* 128:2429–2434, 1982.

57. Friedman D, Globerson A: Immune reactivity during aging. Analysis of the cellular mechanisms involved in the deficient antibody response in old mice. *Mech Aging Dev* 7:299–310, 1978.

58. Price G, Makinodan T: Immunological deficiencies in senescence. Characterization of intrinsic deficiencies. *J Immunol* 108:403–410, 1972.

59. Callard R, Basten A, Blanden R: Loss of immune competence with age may be due to a qualitative abnormality in lymphocyte membranes. *Nature* 281:218–221, 1979.

60. Woda B, Feldman J: Density of surface immunoglobulin and capping on rat B lymphocytes. Changes with aging. *J Exp Med* 149:416–427, 1979.

61. Cammarata R, Rodman G, Fennell R: Serum antiglobulins and antinuclear factors in the aged. *JAMA* 199:455–459, 1967.

62. Pandey J, Fudenberg H, Ainsworth S, et al: Autoantibodies in healthy subjects of different age groups. *Mech Aging Dev* 10:399–404, 1979.

63. Delespesse G, Gausset PH, Sarfati M, et al: Circulating immune complexes in old people and in diabetics: correlation with autoantibodies. *Clin Exp Immunol* 40:96–102, 1980.

64. Hallgren H, Buckley C, Gilbertson V, et al: Lymphocyte phytohemagglutinin responsiveness, immunoglobulins, and autoantibodies in aging humans. *J Immunol* 111:1101–1107, 1973.

65. Gupta S, Good R: Subpopulations of human T lymphocytes. *J Immunol* 122:1214–1219, 1979.

66. Rodriguez M, Ceuppens J, Goodwin JS: Regulation of IgM rheumatoid factor production in lymphocyte cultures from young and old subjects. *J Immunol* 128:2422–2428, 1982.

67. McCay C, Crowell M, Maynard L: The effect of retarded growth upon the length of life span and upon the ultimate body size. *J Nutrition* 10:63–79, 1935.

68. Fernandez G, Good R, Yunis E: Attempts to correct age-related immunodeficiency and autoimmunity by cellular and dietary manipulation in inbred mice, in Makinodan T, Yunis E (eds): *Immunology and Aging*. New York, Plenum, 1976, pp 183–201.

69. Goodwin JS, Bankhurst A, Murphy S, et al: Partial reversal of the cellular immune defect in common variable immunodeficiency with indomethacin. *J Clin Lab Immunol* 1:197–199, 1978.

70. Ceuppens J, Goodwin JS: Endogenous prostaglandin E2 enhances polyclonal immunoglobulin production by tonically inhibiting T suppressor cell activity. *Cell Immunol* 70:41–54, 1982.

71. Delfraisey J, Galanaud P, Wallon C, et al: Abolished in vitro antibody response in the elderly: Exclusive involvement of prostaglandin-induced T suppressor cells. *Clin Immunol Immunopathol* 24:377–385, 1982.

72. Ceuppens J, Rodriguez M, Goodwin JS: Nonsteroidal anti-inflammatory drugs inhibit the production of IgM rheumatoid factor in vitro. *Lancet* 1:528–531, 1982.

CHAPTER 21

Infectious Diseases and Immunizations

KENT CROSSLEY, M.D.

PATRICK IRVINE, M.D.

Infections are important causes of death and sources of morbidity in elderly persons. Although most elderly patients have several diseases that contribute to death, the importance of infections as a cause of their mortality has been recognized for many years. A recent study found infection to be the second most-frequent identifiable cause of death (after atherosclerosis) in a series of 200 autopsies conducted in persons 85 years of age and older.[1]

While morbidity is more difficult to precisely define, recent studies suggest that infections are the most frequent cause of hospital admissions in institutionalized elderly persons and the second most-frequent reason for admission in ambulatory elderly patients.

Knowledge of the frequency and types of infections in elderly persons, and of the factors that are associated with their occurrence, is limited. More substantial information is needed about the nature and frequency of infections in elderly persons.

Basic Considerations

Infections seen in elderly persons may differ in several ways from those encountered in younger patients. There are a number of examples in which either the site of the infection or the etiologic agent that is implicated are a function of the patient's age.

Some infections occur most often in patients over 65 years of age. Examples include herpes zoster, Mycobacterium tuberculosis, and teta-

nus. Urinary tract infections in males are largely unknown before the age at which prostatic hypertrophy and a resultant partial urinary bladder outlet obstruction develops.

Other infections rarely are seen in elderly patients. Presumably because of the immunity acquired over previous years, the exanthematous diseases (e.g., rubella, rubeola, and so on) are decidedly uncommon. Sexually transmitted diseases and occupationally acquired infections are uncommon in individuals over 65 years of age.

To a large degree, the frequency and nature of infections in elderly persons is a function of the occurrence of other chronic diseases. For example, atherosclerotic cardiovascular diseases are most common in elderly patients.[2] An excessive risk of death due to pneumonia and influenza occurs in patients with a cardiovascular disease.[3] Patients with chronic obstructive pulmonary disease (COPD), which is another age-associated condition, are more likely to suffer from recurrent upper respiratory infections and pneumonia. Demented patients, or those who are otherwise neurologically impaired, are less able to define their symptoms and may develop a serious infection before being recognized as ill. The treatment of certain chronic diseases (e.g., using corticosteroids for diseases such as polymyalgia rheumatica and temporal arteritis) also may predispose a patient to the occurrence of infectious illnesses.

Although data are limited, it is reasonable to expect that nutritional deficiencies in elderly persons may be associated with an increased frequency of infection (see Volume II Chapter

12). Vitamin C, for example, is important for wound healing, but it may be lacking in diets of elderly persons.[4] Other substances that are important in host defense, but that may be deficient in the diet of elderly patients include zinc, pyridoxine, and iron.

Profound effects of aging on the immune system have been defined (see Volume I Chapters 1, 20). Many diseases that are more often seen in an elderly patient appear to be a result of age-associated aberrations in cellular immunity. In addition to both cellular and humoral immunity, non-specific host defenses are documented as being important in the protection from agents that cause infectious diseases. For example, the normal bacterial flora in a number of sites and a variety of ways prevents or modifies the colonization with pathogenic microorganisms. Because of differences in the colonization of sites such as the pharynx and skin of elderly patients, when compared with younger individuals, it seems likely that the normal flora is either functionally or qualitatively altered.

Other mechanisms that often are impaired in elderly persons include simple physical activities without which pulmonary infections and cutaneous lesions, such as decubitus ulcers, are likely to occur more frequently. Adequate hydration is important in the defense against urinary tract and respiratory tract infections. Both physical and mental disability often lead to relative dehydration in elderly persons.

Just as pathologic events and physiologic changes that are associated with aging account for more frequent infections in elderly patients, external factors also are thought to be important in the development of infections. Communal living, institutionalization and frequent admissions to acute care hospitals are undoubtedly determinants of infection in older patients.

Although the data suggests that institutionally acquired infections in residents of nursing homes are relatively common, the quantitative impact of these infections is difficult to estimate. While 20% of all American elderly persons are cared for in a nursing home for some period of their life, at any point in time less than 5% are institutionalized.[5]

Information about the occurrence of infections in patients in long-term care facilities is limited. Current studies suggest that infections are acquired in nursing homes with a frequency that approximates the rate observed in an acute care hospital. At any point in time, the proportion of nursing home patients with an infection acquired within the home varies from 15–20%.[6–8] The most frequent site of infection is the urinary tract.[6,7] One study that defined urinary tract infections in such a way as to exclude asymptomatic infections reported infected pressure sore to be the most common type of infection observed.[8]

In addition to the endemic occurrence of respiratory, cutaneous, and urinary tract infections that are acquired within a nursing home, there are some infections that have caused epidemics within long-term care facilities. Tuberculosis recently has been documented on at least two occasions in nursing homes in the United States; the rapid spread of the infection and the high attack rate have been notable.[9,10] The impact of an institutional outbreak of influenza or gastrointestinal infections (e.g., rotavirus) is obvious to anyone who has worked in a nursing home during an outbreak.[11,12]

It is not known whether or not infections that are acquired in nursing home patients are qualitatively different from those seen in non-institutionalized elderly persons. Studies suggest that colonization of the pharynx or urinary tract with antibiotic-resistant organisms is relatively common in nursing home residents. It is not known whether the organisms that are responsible for infection in elderly nursing home residents differ significantly from those that would be recovered from similar infections in an age-matched, non-institutionalized population.[8,13]

Presentation of Infection in Elderly Patients

There are only a few reported studies of the clinical presentation of infections in elderly patients.[14,15] The signs and symptoms of most infections in elderly patients do not differ much from those in younger individuals. However, based on anecdotal data, certain differences occur often enough so that it is appropriate to comment about them.

Many elderly patients who are hospitalized for treatment of an infection initially come to medical attention because of vague complaints. These patients are seen by a physician after a fall or because of symptoms such as confusion, weakness, or anorexia. On occasion, family or nursing home staff may complain that a patient simply "doesn't look right." Signs as non-specific and subtle as a lessened interest in one's surroundings or a decline in performance in occupational or physical therapy may be the first clues to the presence of infection.

The importance of non-specific presentations of infections in elderly persons should be obvious. **In an acutely ill elderly patient with no evident etiology to account for observed signs and symptoms, the possibility of infection should be considered.**

It is the impression of many experienced physicians that elderly persons tend to have physiologic responses that are blunted in comparison with younger individuals. For example, a fever often appears to be less conspicuous in elderly patients. A recent study reported that 28% of all patients more than 65 years of age with blood cultures positive for Streptococcus pneumoniae were afebrile; in a control group of younger patients, all were febrile.[16] The temperatures recorded on admission averaged 100.9°F in the elderly population versus 102.6°F in the control population.

It is unclear whether this trend is seen with other infections. Thus, an analysis of the records of 100 geriatric patients who were hospitalized because of a community-acquired bacteremia showed that only one patient (who had a marked azotemia) was afebrile.[17] In contrast, a recent study described 25 afebrile geriatric patients with bacteremia seen in one hospital over an 18-month period.[18] While specific data are lacking, studies suggest, as a general rule, that the clinical response to infection in elderly patients is blunted when compared with younger patients.[16,18]

Signs and symptoms that are suggestive of an infection are non-specific and may be caused by other illnesses. Thus, those non-infectious diseases that commonly produce fevers (such as malignancies or collagen vascular diseases) occur more frequently in elderly persons. Many symptoms and findings (e.g., rales, cough, urinary urgency, hematuria, and so on) are caused by both infectious and non-infectious diseases.

In evaluation and treatment of infections in older patients, each patient's functional status may determine special clinical strategies. In an outpatient clinic, this is particularly important. For example, an accurate body temperature measurement may not be available. Older people may not be able to read a thermometer due to their compromised manual dexterity, visual acuity, or mental capacity. Since transportation often is difficult for elderly persons, tests that require follow-up visits, such as a purified protein derivative (PPD), may be difficult to arrange. Post-treatment urine cultures (after therapy for symptomatic urinary tract infections) may be difficult to obtain because of the major effort that transporting patients might require. Proper use of public health nurses in the home, or other resources available at elderly housing units, may obviate the need for many return visits to a clinic.

In a nursing home, other strategies are important for properly detecting and treating infections. A fever is the major heralding event of infections, although it may result from other illnesses or from drug therapy. Even fecal impaction must be entertained in a differential diagnosis of fever among frail nursing home residents. For the most part, physicians need to become involved early in caring for nursing home residents with a fever. Since the risk of dehydration increases in a febrile patient, intake and output may need to be measured and diuretic therapy re-evaluated. Antibiotics may need modifications. Digoxin, anticoagulants, phenytoin, and other drugs may require extra monitoring.

All of these considerations mitigate against "PRN" orders for fever. A fever should be approached individually for each patient. Age, medical problems, mental status, and the patient's own philosophy will all modify this approach. Sometimes a fever will not provoke medical action. This was evident in one nursing home study where fever was associated with a high mortality rate. In this case, not treating fevers represented an intentional decision by care providers for terminally ill nursing home residents.[19] Only when supportive care is the primary goal of treatment should specific therapy be withheld in response to a fever (*see* Volume II Chapters 22, 23).

Important Infections and Their Management in Elderly Persons

This section is intended to provide information about infectious diseases that behave differently in elderly persons. We have limited its content to infections that are especially common in elderly persons, or that are known to differ in significant ways from what is observed in younger patients.

Malignant Otitis Media

Invasive external otitis is a syndrome that occurs principally in elderly diabetic patients. It is characterized by the development of an infection within the external auditory canal, which spreads to adjacent soft tissues and the skull.

In a recent review, the average age of affected patients was 67 years.[20] Of the 21 patients studied, 19 presented because of pain in the ear. An equal number were known to be diabetic. External ear-canal discharge was noted in 17 of the 21 patients. Most patients had granulation tissue present within the wall of the canal. Eight patients had evidence of a cranial nerve palsy on admission. A fever was present in only 3 of the 21 patients. Leukocytosis was uncommon. Cultures in all patients yielded Pseudomonas aeruginosa.

The management requires the same therapy as a serious Pseudomonas infection elsewhere. A therapeutic course of at least 3 weeks of an aminoglycoside (e.g., tobramycin or gentamicin) along with an antipseudomonal penicillin (e.g., ticarcillin, mezlocillin, piperacillin, or azlocillin) is required. All of the patients without cranial nerve abnormalities who were treated in this fashion survived.[20] In patients with cranial nerve palsies, there was a 50% mortality rate.

Respiratory Tract Infections

An increased incidence rate of pneumonia and an increased mortality from this disease in elderly patients has been recognized for many years. At the end of the Nineteenth Century, Osler wrote that "Pneumonia may well be called the friend of the aged. Taken off by it in an acute, short, not often painful illness, the old

escape those 'cold gradations of decay' that make the last stage of all so distressing."[21]

Several studies have shown that pneumonic illnesses occur most frequently in patients over 50 years of age. In one report of 292 cases of pneumonia in a general hospital, 25% occurred in patients more than 70 years of age.[22] About 50% of all cases of pneumonia that require hospital admissions are elderly persons.[23]

Mortality due to pneumonia in elderly persons is substantial. Recently, influenza and pneumonia accounted for 211.1 deaths per 100,000 elderly individuals. These infections were the fourth leading cause of death in persons 65 years of age and older.[24]

A British study of 1,330 patients with pneumonia established that 60% of the fatal cases among hospital patients occurred in persons more than 65 years of age.[25] In another study, the mortality rate increased progressively with age. Patients under 40 years of age had an 8% mortality, while patients between 40–69 years of age had a 26% mortality; in those over 70 years of age, the mortality rate was 39%.[22]

About two thirds of all pneumonic illnesses in hospitalized adults are bacterial.[22,26] Of these, the overwhelming majority are caused by Streptococcus pneumoniae. The remaining one third of these cases is about equally divided between cases in which no etiology is identified and cases in which non-bacterial (i.e., viral and mycoplasmal) etiologies are found.

Several recent studies suggest that the pathogens responsible for pneumonic illnesses in elderly persons may be somewhat different. Thus, in one reported study, 38% of all cases of pneumonia in patients over 70 years of age were caused by gram-negative bacilli; but, in patients less than 40 years of age, only 10% were caused by gram-negative bacilli.[22] In a retrospective study of community-acquired bacterial pneumonia in elderly patients, the proportion of patients with gram-negative pneumonia was about three times as great in elderly than in younger subjects.[27]

The clinical data that suggest an increased incidence of gram-negative bacterial pneumonia in elderly persons correlates nicely with the presumed pathogenesis of bacterial pneumonia. It is thought that most cases of bacterial pneumonia develop after an inoculation of pulmonary tissue with bacteria that is aspirated in minute quantities of saliva from the oropharynx. The aspiration of oral fluids has been shown to occur even in normal individuals during sleep.

Several lines of evidence suggest that this is a usual route preceding the development of bacterial pneumonia. First, most bacteria that cause pneumonia are part of the normal oropharyngeal flora. The prevalence of colonization of an organism correlates with the frequency with which the same organism causes pneumonia. There also are seasonal parallels. For example, both an increase in the incidence rate of pneumococcal oropharynx colonization and pneumococcal pneumonia occur during winter and spring.[28] Several lines of evidence suggest that an oropharyngeal colonization with gram-negative bacilli similarly precedes the development of gram-negative bacillary pneumonia. An oropharyngeal colonization with these organisms has been shown to be most common in elderly debilitated patients.[29]

In a group of 407 adults 65 years of age or older who were cared for in various institutional settings, a direct parallel was found between oropharyngeal colonization and the level of care.[30] Only 9% of independent-living elderly persons had gram-negative bacilli present in their oropharynx compared with 60% of patients on an acute-care hospital ward. Gram-negative pharyngeal colonization also was increasingly common as patients became progressively incapacitated. Several other studies document the development of a respiratory colonization with gram-negative bacilli during hospitalization. In one study, 45% of a group of 213 patients who were admitted to a medical intensive care unit developed respiratory tract colonization with gram-negative bacilli.[31] In 22% of this group, colonization developed on the first hospitalized day. The authors also were able to show that a nosocomial respiratory infection occurred in 23% of the colonized patients, but in only 3% of the patients not colonized with gram-negative bacilli.

In nursing home patients, it might be expected that an excessive proportion of pneumonias would be caused by gram-negative bacilli. This conclusion would follow from studies demonstrating that institutionalization and antibiotic administration are associated with an increased incidence of a gram-negative bacillary

infection.[32] Although most of these studies have been conducted in acute care settings, Klebsiella pneumoniae and Staphylococcus aureus were significantly more often recovered from patients with pneumonia in nursing homes than in a control population of ambulatory elderly persons with pneumonic illnesses.[13]

It seems likely that the excess of gram-negative rod bacterial pneumonia in elderly patients results from an increasing frequency of pharyngeal colonization with these organisms. Studies are in progress to further clarify some remaining issues in this area. For example, it has been pointed out that oropharyngeal colonization in the majority of elderly nursing home patients tends to be transient and, therefore, of uncertain significance.[33]

The clinical evaluation of an elderly patient with possible pneumonia requires special care, because signs and symptoms may not be as evident as in younger individuals. British authors recently suggested that an increased respiratory rate may be a clue to the presence of lower respiratory infections in elderly patients. Tachypnea (defined as a respiratory rate greater than 26/min) was present in eight elderly patients with lower respiratory tract infections, while patients with other acute illnesses had respiratory rates between 16–25 breaths per minute.[34]

Although not unique to elderly persons, it is a useful observation that pneumococcal pneumonia usually is associated with a single chill, while pneumonia caused by other bacteria often is associated with multiple rigors. The rusty-colored sputum of pneumococcal pneumonia also is a suggestive clinical clue to this etiology.

Laboratory tests and x-ray film studies in elderly persons may yield somewhat different results than evaluations in younger patients with pneumonia. It has been shown that pneumococcal pneumonia is uncommonly associated with lobar consolidation in patients over 40 years of age.[35] The resolution of x-ray film findings in pneumococcal pneumonia is delayed in elderly persons.[36] Elderly patients also tend to have less extensive infiltrates than younger individuals.[25] On the basis of limited data, the white blood cell response in elderly patients with bacteremic pneumococcal pneumonia does not appear to differ substantially from the response seen in younger individuals.[16]

Using this information, it is possible to develop a rational therapeutic approach to a pneumonic illness in elderly patients. Elderly persons who are likely to develop pneumonia because of an antecedent pulmonary disease or general debility ought to receive both influenza vaccine and pneumococcal polysaccharide vaccine. While appropriate controversies will continue over the effectiveness and cost-benefit ratio of pneumococcal polysaccharide vaccine, its administration is warranted more often than not in elderly persons.

Appropriate antibiotics for use in the treatment of outpatients with pneumonia include penicillin G, ampicillin, and erythromycin. In most cases, the selection depends on a patient's clinical signs and symptoms and laboratory findings. Thus, a patient with a non-productive cough, a normal white blood cell count, and limited lower lobe infiltrates might be best treated with erythromycin (because Mycoplasma pneumoniae is a likely etiologic agent). A patient with rusty sputum, pleuritic chest pain, and a lobar infiltrate could be treated with penicillin G, because Streptococcus pneumoniae usually is responsible when these findings are present. A similar constellation of signs and symptoms recently has been described in elderly patients with Hemophilus influenzae pneumonia.[37]

Elderly patients with limited infiltrates and adequate pulmonary function may, on occasion, be appropriately treated as outpatients. Because older individuals rapidly may become seriously ill, careful follow-up is needed. If there is any question about the advisability of hospital admission, it is best to err on the side of a short admission to initiate therapy and evaluate its response.

When an elderly patient is hospitalized with pneumonia, therapy also must follow a careful clinical evaluation. Thus, an older person with rusty-colored sputum, pleuritic chest pain, a localized infiltrate, and a single rigor with gram-positive diplococci in the sputum, obviously is most appropriately treated with penicillin G. However, for elderly patients in whom the etiology is less clear, broader spectrum antibiotic therapy usually is indicated. The use of combinations such as an aminoglycoside and a cephalosporin or the use of a broad-spectrum cephalosporin probably is appropriate initial therapy (particularly in institutionalized elderly persons). It is likely that most episodes of pneumonia in elderly persons result from infections due to organisms such as Streptococcus pneumoniae and Hemophilus influenzae, which are susceptible to commonly used antibiotics. However, the relatively common occurrence of gram-negative pneumonia in elderly persons requires broad-spectrum initial therapy, *unless* there is clear evidence that Streptococcus pneumoniae or Hemophilus influenzae is etiologic. Therapy can be changed to more specific antibiotics once the results of blood and sputum cultures are available.[38,39]

Tuberculosis

Several excellent reviews of tuberculosis recently have been published.[40–43] Therefore, only those specific problems of tuberculosis that relate to elderly persons will be considered here.

Most people in the United States who are tuberculin-positive are more than 60 years of age. Although the disease may be quiescent, patients who are tuberculin-positive are infected with Mycobacterium tuberculosis. As non-specific defense mechanisms wane with increasing age, infected patients are at risk for developing clinical tuberculosis. Most cases of tuberculosis in this nation, at present, represent a recrudescence of infection that is acquired in childhood or early adult life. Because most clinical tuberculosis in the United States occurs in elderly persons, the recognition and control of this disease in this population is of considerable importance to public health workers and clinicians.

As described in Volume I Chapter 10 the utility of skin testing as a means of identifying tuberculous infection in elderly persons is not well established. Patients more than 60 years of age tend to have relative anergy to commonly applied skin test materials, which implies that the efficacy of skin testing as a technique for detecting cases of tuberculosis in elderly persons probably is overestimated.[44] However, a negative high-dose PPD with positive controls is probably conclusive.

Tuberculosis in elderly persons may present with protean manifestations. Patients may have obscure hematologic findings as the only clue to disseminated tuberculosis.[45] Localized pulmonary, renal, gastrointestinal, or bone diseases also may occur.[41] Lymph node tuberculosis, which is particularly common in elderly females, usually presents as an insidious cervical mass that spontaneously begins to drain through the skin. Even uncomplicated pulmonary tuberculosis may present with atypical clinical and x-ray film findings in elderly persons.[46] Tuberculosis always should be considered when there is evidence of an obscure infection in elderly patients.

In young individuals less than 35 years of age, preventive therapy for patients with positive tuberculin skin tests is widely administered. It is known that the administration of isoniazid, (INH) 300 mg/day for adults, for a period of 12 months significantly reduces the likelihood of development of clinical tuberculosis in patients who are tuberculin-positive.[47] The preventive administration of INH is limited to younger individuals because of evidence that the risk of hepatitis associated with the administration of this drug increases significantly with advancing age.[48] Although some evidence has been accumulated showing that isoniazid may be less likely to cause hepatitis in elderly persons than was previously believed, it is presently recommended that older persons with positive tuberculin tests simply be followed-up with annual chest x-ray films.[49]

For adults with uncomplicated pulmonary tuberculosis, the daily administration of INH and rifampin for a period of 9 months appears to be acceptable therapy.[50] This is not presently recommended for immunocompromised individuals, nor for clinical situations other than uncomplicated pulmonary tuberculosis.

Although clinical tuberculosis in elderly persons probably occurs predominantly in individuals living within the community, outbreaks within nursing homes are described. One such epidemic in 1978 affected 30% of all residents of an Arkansas nursing home.[46] In this instance, a nursing home resident with pulmonary tuberculosis was misdiagnosed as having advanced lung cancer. By the time a correct diagnosis was made many months later, the spread of tuberculosis was extensive. Of all tuberculin-negative employees of this institution, 15% were infected during this outbreak.

Additional outbreaks have been described

among employees of nursing homes in North Dakota and in Oklahoma. In the North Dakota outbreak, an infection among nursing home employees was acquired from a resident with undiagnosed tuberculosis.[51] In the Oklahoma nursing home, 50% of all employees who were in contact with the index case were found to have positive tuberculin tests.[52] These reports have made it clear that tuberculosis is a significant concern for long-term care facilities.

The recommendations for screening for tuberculosis in employees and residents of nursing homes varies somewhat from state to state. The present rules in one state represent an appropriate approach to the problems of potential tuberculosis in long-term care facilities. Long-term care facilities in Minnesota are required to demonstrate that their *employees* are free from tuberculosis. This requires that an employee must have had a negative Mantoux test within 45 days before employment began. If an individual has a positive tuberculin test or is known to have had a positive reaction to tuberculin skin tests in the past, a chest x-ray film is required.

It is recommended that the screening of employees be done using the two-step tuberculin test with PPD. If the first Mantoux test results in less than 10 mm of induration, a second test should be administered 1 week later. The use of two tests is recommended to induce immunologic recall in previously infected persons.[53] The result of the second test is recorded as an employee's baseline. Retesting each year is not required; the interval between tests depends on the likelihood of exposure to tuberculosis within the nursing home.

If the Mantoux reaction is 10 mm or more, a chest x-ray film is required. Preventive therapy may be appropriate in younger employees. Employees with positive skin tests and normal chest x-ray films who complete either 1 year of preventive therapy or a total of 5 years of annual chest x-ray films are considered free of tuberculosis and are exempt from further screening.

For *residents* of nursing homes and board-and-care facilities, a Mantoux test also is required. As with employees, this enables an identification of current cases of tuberculosis and allows the establishment of a baseline if additional testing is needed. For residents older than 35 years of age, it currently is recommended that both a two-step tuberculin test and a chest x-ray film be done at the time of admission to a long-term care facility. Repetitive skin testing is not presently recommended, unless patients are exposed to tuberculosis. Patients with positive skin tests or x-ray films that are consistent with tuberculosis should be carefully evaluated to rule out active disease.

Influenza

Influenza is another common and important respiratory illness in elderly patients. It has been known for years that most patients who die of influenza infection are elderly. A recent study found that of 38 deaths that were associated with pneumonia and influenza, slightly more than two-thirds occurred in patients over 65 years of age.[54] Not surprisingly, 36 of these 38 patients had one or more chronic disease(s). This study provides information about the relative contribution of aging and debility to the development of pneumonia and influenza, and also of the frequency of certain risk factors in patients with pneumonic illnesses and influenza.[55] The factors studied were those that usually are thought to place a patient at high risk for developing influenza and pneumonia. Examples are rheumatic or ischemic heart disease, hypertension with cardiac or renal complications, cerebrovascular disease, COPD, chronic renal disease, diabetes or cirrhosis, epilepsy, or a malignant disease. In this investigation, the incidence rate of pneumonia and influenza in persons over 45 years of age with no known risk factors was 4 per 100,000 persons. If one high-risk factor was present, the incidence was 157 per 100,000. With two or more high-risk factors, the incidence of pneumonia rose to 615 per 100,000.

Fortunately, influenza is relatively uncommon among elderly persons. The incidence of influenza A peaks in children between 5–10 years of age. The attack rate declines dramatically after 35 years of age. Less information about influenza B is available, and conflicting data about the age-related incidence rate of this serotype of the disease has been reported.

Influenza virus infection usually is manifest as a mild pneumonic illness. In a typical case, the disease begins suddenly with chills, fever, and rhinorrhea. The systemic symptoms usually are more impressive than the respiratory complaints. Gastrointestinal manifestations are uncommon.

Influenza becomes clinically important when it occurs in elderly or debilitated patients, and when it is complicated by a bacterial superinfection. Uncommonly, an influenza virus infection, per se, may progress to development of an overt pneumonia. Although it is a cause of both endemic and epidemic disease in the community, an influenza virus infection also has been shown to be associated with outbreaks in long-term care facilities.[55,56] In one such report, there appears to be a correlation between susceptibility to influenza B and increasing age.[56]

Influenza may be prevented by annual immunization or by the use of an antiviral agent such as amantadine. The protective effects of immunization and amantadine are additive; both are suggested in high-risk groups.[57] Immunization is recommended for virtually all patients over 65 years of age and for younger patients with any of the chronic diseases listed above.

One of the principal limitations of the use of vaccine is the "antigenic drift" that occurs in isolates of influenza virus from the community. Specific virus strains are predicted to be likely causes of disease outbreaks about 9–12 months in advance of the "flu season"; the antigenic nature of the vaccine is determined from these data. Unfortunately, in the time between when a decision is made about vaccine formulation and the point at which the material actually can be administered, it is not uncommon for antigenic changes to occur in the virus that is present in the community. Thus, protection against influenza is limited, because the vaccine was derived from influenza strains that differ from those actually causing the disease.

Another approach to the prevention of influenza infections is the administration of an antiviral drug such as amantadine. Amantadine and its analogues act by blocking the replication of the influenza A virus. These drugs are not active against influenza B.

Although approved since 1966 for the prevention of influenza A, amantadine has enjoyed only a limited use in the United States. Amantadine (and rimantadine) may potentially be used to prevent the development of influenza in elderly patients and other compromised individuals. In healthy adults, amantadine is reported to be 70–100% effective in preventing clinical influenza. A recently reported comparative study of amantadine and rimantadine in a group of 450 volunteers showed that the efficacy of these two agents in preventing influenza was similar; the efficacy rates were 85% for rimantadine and 91% for amantadine.[58]

Unfortunately, the side effects from amantadine are commonly seen in elderly persons. The reactions usually consist of mild but often disturbing central nervous system changes, such as dizziness, headache, interference with sleep patterns, and confusion. Of all subjects in a recent trial of amantadine, 13% withdrew because of these adverse reactions. The incidence of side effects with rimantadine appears to be about 50% that of amantadine.[57]

Either of these drugs can be used appropriately in an influenza outbreak, especially in a long-term care institution, to prevent the development of an infection in susceptible elderly patients. Although it is logical to expect a reduction of both influenza disease and influenza-associated deaths, there are no data that clearly demonstrate the efficacy of these drugs in elderly patients. The recommended adult dosage for both amantadine and rimantadine is 200 mg/day, given in one or two doses. The dose needs to be reduced in patients with impaired renal function.

Amantadine also has been shown to be therapeutically useful in ameliorating the symptoms of influenza after an infection has occurred. It is not known whether or not a reduction in the incidence of secondary pneumonias might also follow amantadine administration.

Urinary Tract Infection

Urinary tract infections increase in incidence with increasing age. This association is due to a number of factors. It is known, for example, that the incidence of asymptomatic urinary tract infections in females increases in a linear fashion with increasing age. The incidence of asymptomatic bacteriuria (i.e., the presence of significant numbers of bacteria, usually defined as $>10^5$ organisms/ml in the urine in the absence of symptoms) is about 1%/decade in females.[59] In adult males, infections are uncommon until urinary tract obstruction results from prostatic enlargement.[60] Furthermore, elderly persons spend a disproportionate amount of time in hospitals and long-term care facilities. The likelihood of having a urinary catheterization and resultant infection is much higher in patients in hospitals or nursing homes than in ambulatory individuals.

A number of studies make it clear that asymptomatic bacteriuria is relatively common in elderly persons. Between 19–46% of all residents in long-term care facilities have significant bacteriuria (i.e., >100,000 colonies/ml).[60–63] All of these investigations excluded patients with in-dwelling catheters or a recent history of instrumentation. Several studies have emphasized that bacteriuria is not a constant phenomenon in elderly patients. Of a group of elderly hospitalized patients with initially sterile urine, 47% developed bacteriuria over the course of 1 year.[63] Bacteriuria was especially common among patients who were incontinent of urine. Spontaneous variation in the bacteriologic flora of the urine has been reported in 44 hospitalized geriatric patients, most of whom had in-dwelling catheters.[64]

Published data indicate a definite association between urinary infection and mortality. There is a significantly shorter survival of bacteriuric elderly patients when compared with elderly patients who are not bacteriuric.[62,65] Although the reason for the association between bacteriuria and an increased mortality rate is unknown, it appears not to be caused by other variables (e.g., weight, hypertension, smoking, or myocardial disease).

The clinician, therefore, is faced with a dilemma in approaching asymptomatic bacteriuria in an elderly patient, because the presence of bacteriuria does not seem to be a constant phenomenon, while the apparent increased mortality rate in patients who are bacteriuric suggests a need for concern. There are, however, no data that indicate that treatment of an elderly bacteriuric patient alters the tendency toward an increased mortality.

Except in pregnant women, it is not known whether bacteriuric patients have a significant risk of developing a serious urinary tract infection. An unpublished retrospective study of bacteriuria in 1,700 elderly clinic patients who were followed for an average of 2.8 years showed that 15 of the 1,700 patients had one or more significant positive blood cultures. The urinary tract was felt to be the source of the bacteremia in six of these patients. Only one individual was in good health; the other five patients were terminally ill. Other studies suggest a comparable incidence of bacteremic urinary tract infection.[66]

To further complicate this issue, many elderly patients with asymptomatic bacteriuria are infected with highly resistant organisms (e.g., Pseudomonas aeruginosa). At present, the treatment for most infections that are caused by resistant gram-negative organisms requires the use of parenteral antibiotics, which also carries a risk of morbidity. Hospitalization usually is necessary for the administration of these drugs; thus, treatment becomes very expensive.

It is recommended that asymptomatic bacteriuria only should be treated in elderly persons under certain conditions. In patients with an underlying genitourinary tract disease and in patients with a neurologic impairment of urinary tract function, attempts at treatment are appropriate. The evidence suggests that the development of chronic renal disease is more apt to occur in bacteriuric patients with abnormal urinary tracts. Eradication of bacteriuria should be attempted before genitourinary tract surgery because of the risk of developing a serious infection.[67]

Efforts to limit the acquisition of bacteriuria should be made. Thus, an elderly patient who is hospitalized should not have an in-dwelling catheter in place. If catheterization is unavoidable, it should be of as brief duration as possible. It is appropriate to obtain a urine culture when the catheter is removed, and to treat bacteriuria if present.

Data about clinically symptomatic urinary tract infections in older persons also is limited. Episodes of symptomatic infections in elderly females are especially difficult to decipher because of the non-specific nature of the complaints.[68] Symptomatic infections are especially common in elderly patients with in-dwelling urinary catheters. While a urinary tract infection is the most frequent source for bacteremia in elderly persons, it is unclear as to exactly how often urinary catheters are present in patients who develop bacteremia. Polymicrobial bacteriuria was common, and urinary pathogens that

were resistant to commonly used antibiotics frequently were recovered in a study of 13 elderly patients with urinary catheter-associated bacteremias.[69] These patients had an obstruction or manipulation of their catheter before hospitalization.

The use of urinary catheters in elderly persons is associated with a high risk of infection. The most important rule about in-dwelling catheters is that, whenever possible, they should be avoided. Even single catheterizations (e.g., to obtain urine for cultures) are associated with a risk of developing an infection. More than 10% of all hospitalized elderly individuals subjected to a single catheterization developed bacteriuria.[70]

Patients with in-dwelling urinary catheters universally develop bacteriuria. Even with well-managed, closed urinary drainage systems (a situation far from common in institutions caring for elderly persons), bacteriuria is present in virtually all patients after several weeks.

Unfortunately for individuals in whom in-dwelling catheters are placed for extended periods of time, little can be done to prevent the development of bacteriuria. There is documented evidence that improper care of the urinary drainage system in acute-care hospitals predisposes one to the development of bacteriuria.[71] In the setting of a short-term use of a urinary catheter, strict adherence to procedures for catheter care may be expected to delay the acquisition of bacteriuria.

Recommendations for care of in-dwelling catheters have been published.[72] Care in dealing with these devices may delay the acquisition of bacteriuria and reduce the incidence of symptomatic urinary tract infections. It is recommended to spatially separate catheterized patients. Although it is convenient to house two patients with in-dwelling catheters in the same room, the temptation for nurses and others to manipulate drainage bags or catheters of both patients without washing their hands is strong. The spread of hospital-associated urinary tract infections may be limited by the geographic dispersal of patients with in-dwelling catheters.[73] There presently is no role for chronic antibiotic prophylaxis for patients with in-dwelling urinary catheters. Long-term antibiotic administration usually results in the selection of highly resistant organisms that prove difficult to treat.[74] Patients in an acute-care hospital who are on antibiotics had a short-term benefit when compared with patients who did not receive antibiotics.[75] In this study, 9 of 100 patients who received a placebo developed bacteriuria during short-term in-dwelling catheterization, while only 3 of 96 patients who were receiving antibiotics developed bacteriuria. However, on discharge from the hospital, both groups had equal numbers of bacteriuric patients. These data confirm the clinical impression that antibiotic prophylaxis is not of value in this setting.

Urinary antiseptics are not useful in patients with in-dwelling catheters. The use of methenamine hippurate apparently does reduce catheter complications, although it does not have an important effect on the bacteriuria.[76] Similarly, the irrigation of closed urinary tract drainage systems has not been demonstrated to be effective in preventing bacteriuria.[77]

For some years, the use of intermittent urinary tract catheterization has been suggested as a way of reducing the incidence of infection. This technique has a number of advantages that include the avoidance of an external drainage bag. The majority of data about the use of intermittent catheterization has resulted from studies of younger patients with a spinal cord injury. In this setting, intermittent catheterization appears to be associated with relatively infrequent urinary tract infections.

In elderly patients, the use of this technique has not been carefully evaluated in a prospective study. It might be anticipated that intermittently catheterized elderly patients, (because of their high risk for developing bacteriuria with single catheterizations and because of frequent anatomic abnormalities) would develop an infection during the procedure more often than younger patients. Nonetheless, intermittent catheterization probably has a role in the management of certain elderly patients with a urinary tract dysfunction. Clinical studies are needed to define those patients in whom this technique is appropriate. A detailed discussion of self-catheterization and its technique appears in Kunin's text.[78]

Although data about condom catheter systems are rather limited, there is evidence that the incidence rate of infections in patients who manipulate the condom-collecting system is extremely high. Thus, in uncooperative individuals, these devices probably are no better than in-dwelling catheters.[79]

A vexing problem is deciding the interval at which a urinary catheter ought to be changed. The general consensus appears to be that a catheter does not need to be changed unless a substantial amount of sediment has accumulated within the lumen of the catheter or drainage tubing. While changing catheters at predefined intervals may decrease the incidence of an obstruction due to these amorphous materials, each catheter change also increases the likelihood of introducing new bacteria into the urinary system.

Dermatologic Infections

A variety of cutaneous infections occur in elderly individuals. Cellulitis, cutaneous abscesses, and infections of the skin and soft tissues after wounding probably occur in elderly persons with a frequency similar to that found in younger individuals. It is reasonable to expect that pressure sores (see Volume I, Chapter 32) and cutaneous infections that are associated with peripheral vascular disease and diabetes mellitus occur more often in elderly than in younger subjects. The third group of cutaneous infections that clearly occur more often in elderly individuals would include postoperative wound infections and herpes zoster.

Cellulitis occurs with a frequency in elderly persons that is similar to that in younger individuals. Patients typically present with edema and erythema of the skin and subcutaneous tissue with varying degrees of systemic manifestations. Occasionally, there is evidence of lymphangitis and regional lymphadenopathy. This is particularly common in infections caused by group A beta-hemolytic streptococci. A fever and leukocytosis occur most often in patients with extensive areas of cellulitis.

In most patients with cellulitis, the etiology is not easily determined. The techniques for collecting tissue fluid for culture (usually by aspirating with a small gauge needle from the advancing edge of the area of cellulitis) have been useful in children, but the experience in adults has been unsuccessful. In patients with cellulitis that is associated with a traumatic wound, ulcer, or abscess, it is likely that the organisms recovered from the open lesion are the same as those responsible for the cellulitis.[80] In most patients with cellulitis, a clear etiology cannot be defined.

Patients with cellulitis are treated with a semisynthetic penicillin (nafcillin or oxacillin if a patient is ill enough to require a parenterally administered drug, or dicloxacillin if an oral antibiotic is used) or a cephalosporin (cefazolin, given parenterally or oral cephalexin). These antibiotics are clinically effective, since cellulitis usually is caused by Staphylococcus aureus or group A beta-hemolytic streptococci.

It should be remembered that certain unusual forms of cellulitis may appear to be identical to streptococcal or staphylococcal infections. The cellulitis that is associated with a cat bite is a good example. In this situation, the infecting organism almost always is Pasteurella multocida, which is a gram-negative organism that responds well to penicillin G but poorly to the semisynthetic penicillins that are active against staphylococci. Another example is the cellulitis seen in association with cutaneous injuries that occur in fresh water. In this situation, Aeromonas hydrophila is particularly common. The penicillins are not effective against this organism, and antibiotic therapy needs to be guided by antimicrobial susceptibility testing.[81]

Hemophilus influenzae cellulitis is, in its classic form, associated with a bluish-purple discoloration of the skin and occurs most commonly in children. Cellulitis that is caused by this organism in patients with Hemophilus bacteremia has been reported in older individuals.[82] This etiology needs to be considered when a cellulitis of the neck, chest, or face is associated with a respiratory tract infection. An appropriate antibiotic therapy usually is ampicillin, unless ampicillin-resistant Hemophilus influenzae has been a problem in your community.

Another distinctive variety of cellulitis is erysipelas, which may be present on the face or around a wound. Erysipelas is an unusual form of cellulitis with sharply demarcated borders, which is characterized by a raised, edematous, "peau d'orange" appearance of the skin. It is best treated with parenteral administered penicillin G, although ampicillin or a semisynthetic penicillin may be used initially if a diagnosis is unclear.

Abscesses that involve the skin usually do not need to be treated with antibiotics. Cultures of 135 cutaneous abscesses in outpatients recovered both anaerobic and aerobic bacteria.[83] An incision and drainage without antibiotic therapy was the best management for these infections. In unusual patients with cutaneous abscesses who are febrile, it probably is appropriate to obtain the culture material from the lesion and to administer an antibiotic.

A clear age-associated increase in the incidence of infection is present in only two dermatologic infections: postoperative wound infection and herpes zoster. Two studies have demonstrated an increased infection rate in elderly patients with surgical wounds. In 38 hospitals in Great Britain, the incidence rate of surgical wound infections was highest in elderly persons (see Figure 21-1).[84] Similar data also was developed by the National Research Council in this nation nearly 20 years ago.[85]

Herpes zoster is the other dermatologic infection that is particularly common in elderly persons. While recognized as a disease of immunocompromised persons, it is especially frequent in elderly individuals. The most extensive data about the epidemiology of herpes zoster was reported in a study conducted in Rochester, Minnesota over a 15-year period.[86] There was a marked age-associated increase in the incidence of herpes zoster demonstrated in this study (see Figure 21-2). The disease clearly is most common in patients more than 75 years of age.

Herpes zoster is caused by a varicella-zoster virus. This also is the cause of varicella

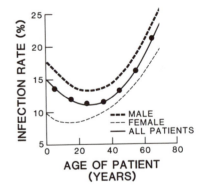

FIGURE 21-1 The relationship between age and the wound infection rate in a group of 2,660 patients in Great Britain. (84) (Ayliffe GAJ: *J Hygiene* 79:299–314, 1977, used by permission.)

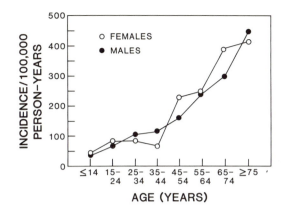

FIGURE 21-2 Incidence rate per 100,000 person-years of herpes zoster among residents of Rochester, Minnesota, 1945–1959, by age and sex. (86) (Ragozzino M. et al: Population-based study of herpes zoster and its sequelae. *Medicine* 61: 310–316, 1982, used by permission.)

("chickenpox"). After a recovery from varicella, patients continue to harbor the varicella-zoster virus, probably in the dorsal route ganglia. Clinical evidence of an infection typically is absent for many years. It is likely that the zoster only results from a reactivation of previous varicella-zoster infections. It does not appear that zoster results from exposure to a patient with varicella.

Factors that control the latency of the virus are unknown; but, in both elderly patients and patients with certain malignancies, a reactivation of the virus and a development of zoster occurs. Cellular immunity against varicella-zoster, as measured by cutaneous delayed-type hypersensitivity, gradually wanes with increasing age beginning at 40 years of age.[87] Antibody levels, however, were present in elderly patients. This suggests that the decline in cellular immunity with increasing age might be causally associated with the reactivation of a varicella-zoster virus.

The cutaneous eruption in herpes zoster involves the trigeminal nerve, with a periocular involvement in approximately 15–20% of affected patients. The remaining patients have an involvement of the neck, trunk, and abdomen. The rash usually is unilateral and characteristically involves 1–3 dermatomes. Patients may have a prodrome of radicular pain before an onset of the rash. The cutaneous lesion is similar to that of varicella, with a vesicle present on an erythematous base. Although all of the vesicles may appear at once, cutaneous lesions may continue to develop over several days following the initial onset of the vesicles. Particularly in patients with a periocular involvement, there often is a confluent erythema with scattered vesicles present on the markedly inflamed skin.

Involvement of the nerves that supply the bladder or the anus may be associated with dysfunction of these organs. Symptoms of bladder involvement (usually those of cystitis or retention) typically occur 1–2 weeks after the onset of a rash.[88] Anal involvement may occur in association with bladder disease or as an isolated event. Most patients with involvement of these organs have a cutaneous perineal zoster. A complete recovery of function is the rule.[89]

The dissemination of herpes zoster occurs in a minority of both immunocompromised patients and normal individuals. Uncommonly, evidence of a central nervous system and hepatic involvement may be seen.[90] The occurrence of herpes zoster is not evidence of an underlying malignancy. Studies in which patients with zoster have been evaluated for evidence of occult malignancies have not been rewarding.[91]

Zoster is of particular importance in an older patient because of the frequent occurrence and disabling nature of postherpetic neuralgias. This complication is uncommon in patients less than 40 years of age.[92] Over 50% of all persons more than 60 years of age develop postherpetic neuralgia that persists for more than 1 year.[86] A dramatic reduction in postherpetic pain has been reported in patients who were treated with corticosteroids.[93,94] Prednisolone in doses of 40 mg/day for 10 days with a stepwise decrease over the next 3 weeks is recommended. When treated with prednisolone, 15% of affected patients had pain lasting for more than 2 months. In the control group, 65% of the patients had postherpetic neuralgia.[94] It is appropriate to question the use of corticosteroids in patients with an active viral infection, but the benefits may outweigh the associated risks. In normal healthy patients more than 50 years of age who develop herpes zoster, the use of glucocorticoids should be considered as a technique for reducing the incidence of a postherpetic neuralgia.

A recent study has evaluated the role of Levodopa (L-Dopa) in 47 patients with herpes zoster.[95] A significant reduction in the occurrence of postherpetic neuralgia was demonstrated 3 weeks after the end of treatment, but not when it was evaluated after 60 days.

Bacterial Endocarditis

Bacterial endocarditis has been excellently reviewed in a Mayo Clinic symposium.[96] A number of papers published earlier in this century suggested that the mortality rate due to bacterial endocarditis was higher in elderly persons and symptoms were less marked. It also was stated that the presence of heart murmurs was less frequent than in younger subjects. A recent review confirms that murmurs may be present less often in the elderly than in younger study subjects.[97] Another recent study of 56 patients with bacterial endocarditis who were 65 years of age and older found that "the clinical features, laboratory manifestations and bacterial etiology of infective endocarditis . . . were similar to those in younger patients."[98] The clinician must consider this diagnosis in any individual who has a fever, heart murmur, stroke, or congestive heart failure that is not explained by another underlying cardiac disease.

Approach to the Acutely Ill Febrile Elderly Patient

Management of a seriously ill, febrile elderly patient should be similar to the approach taken in younger individuals. The unique features of an infection in elderly persons, however, require particular care and promptness in dealing with a seriously ill elderly patient. The blunted nature of physiologic responses that are seen in elderly persons may make both recognition and diagnosis of febrile illnesses more difficult. Older patients, because of underlying diseases or concomitant therapies, often present more complicated problems in therapy than younger individuals.

The distribution of the sites of an initial infection and of infecting organisms in elderly patients who develop bacteremia do not appear to differ substantially from that seen in younger individuals. As with the majority of studies of

bacteremic illness, the urinary tract is the most frequent focus of infection in elderly persons. A recent study of 100 hospital admissions of geriatric patients with community-acquired bacteremia reported that the urinary tract was the primary focus of infection in 34% of the patients.[99] A biliary tract infection was the second most and pneumonia the third most frequent infections responsible for bacteremia. A study of elderly patients in Jerusalem also found the urinary tract to be the most frequent source of bacteremia.[100] A pulmonary infection was the second most and gastrointestinal sources the third most frequent infections. A significant proportion of patients did not have the site of primary infection identified. The bacterial etiology of community-acquired sepsis in elderly persons is poorly defined. About one third of these infections are caused by gram-positive bacteria and the remainder are accounted for by gram-negative organisms. Anaerobic bacteria were associated with a small percentage of cases.

Elderly individuals who suddenly become febrile while hospitalized or living in either a nursing home or community setting, require a careful, intensive evaluation. The initial task is to determine whether or not a patient's illness represents a severe bacterial infection. Not all elderly patients with a serious infection have a fever. In the Israeli study of bacteremic patients, 16% were afebrile.

Other disorders, in addition to a bacterial infection, can result in a fever and chills. For example, it is not uncommon to see an impressive fever due to drugs such as phenytoin, alphamethyldopa, procainamide, and quinidine. Fever also is commonly documented with noninfectious illnesses such as a pulmonary embolism, giant cell arteritis or a variety of malignancies. Bacteremic illnesses in elderly patients may present with a relative paucity of signs and symptoms; also, changes such as malaise, obtundation, or delirium need to be recognized as at least potential clues to the presence of a serious illness.

Laboratory studies that are appropriate for the initial evaluation of a febrile, seriously ill patient include a complete blood count (CBC). A normal white blood cell differential in the presence of a significant bacterial infection is uncommon. The absolute white blood cell count, however, may not be elevated in patients with bacteremic illnesses. Leukocyte counts that are normal or low are not uncommon in bacteremic patients. A chest x-ray film, a gram smear of the sputum and urine, and cultures of blood, sputum, and urine usually are indicated.

Bacteremic illnesses in elderly persons are associated with a greater mortality rate than is seen in younger individuals.[101,102] In one study, the mortality rate with bacteremic illnesses in individuals under 40 years of age was only 4% compared to 40% in persons more than 40 years of age.[101] Therefore, the initial therapy for an elderly patient with a fever and an acute illness needs to be aggressive. In patients with a focus for infection that is shown to be gram-positive in etiology, such as cellulitis or an infected wound in which gram-positive bacteria are seen on a gram smear, nafcillin or oxacillin in doses of 6–12 grams/day may be used.

In patients with bacteremia due to a source that usually is associated with gram-negative organisms such as a urinary tract infection, an aminoglycoside antibiotic such as gentamicin or tobramycin is recommended. In patients from nursing homes or patients who develop a urinary tract infection and fever while in an acute hospital setting, the selection of an antibiotic needs to be guided by the antibiotic susceptibility of organisms recovered from other patients in the same institution. It seems reasonable to expect that isolates from urinary tract infections in patients within nursing homes are more apt to be antibiotic-resistant than isolates from patients living in the community. It is important to gram-stain the urine from patients with an infection because, in many cases, the enterococcus may be present by itself or in conjunction with other gram-negative bacteria. In this case, a drug that is active against enterococci (such as ampicillin) must be added to the aminoglycoside antibiotic.

In situations where the etiology of an infection is not readily apparent (e.g., a patient with intra-abdominal pain and fever, a patient with a pulmonary infiltrate from whom no material can be collected for a gram smear or culture, or a patient who is seriously ill, febrile, and has no obvious focus of infection), the selection of antibiotic therapy is more difficult. Initially, broad-spectrum therapy must be used; once the etiologic agent is recognized and susceptibility

testing is done, therapy can be redirected to use the least toxic antibiotics available. In a setting of an unknown infection, a combination such as tobramycin and nafcillin is recommended. These two antimicrobial agents will be effective against staphylococci, streptococci, and the majority of gram-negative rod bacilli. Since these antibiotics do not have a notable activity against Bacteroides fragilis and some other anaerobes, if the infection appears to be intra-abdominal or involves the gastrointestinal tract, it would be appropriate to use a drug with an activity against anaerobes (such as cefoxitin or clindamycin) along with the aminoglycoside.

We believe in being particularly aggressive in those elderly individuals with a bacteremic infection who are not terminally ill. Because of the debilitating nature of hospitalization in elderly patients, the initial work-up should be prompt and aggressive; subsequent evaluations and therapy should be conducted as rapidly and thoroughly as possible.

Immunizations

Several immunizations are widely recommended for elderly persons. These include tetanus-diphtheria toxoids, influenza vaccine, and pneumococcal polysaccharide vaccine. The role of these immunizations in elderly persons will be reviewed here. Other immunizations occasionally may be needed by older patients. These include immunizations before foreign travel and for persons with certain unusual occupational exposures. Information about these immunizations is available from several sources.[103,104]

Only a small proportion of individuals more than 60 years of age have serum antitoxin levels that are protective against tetanus.[105] Few elderly persons also have significant antibody levels against diphtheria toxin (see Table 21-1). About 50% of all persons more than 80 years of age have protective levels of tetanus and diphtheria antibodies.[106] Nonetheless, a small group of elderly volunteers who were given tetanus-diphtheria toxoid on two occasions 7 months apart had protective levels.

Tetanus is a serious and often fatal disease. Elderly persons are at the greatest risk for this disease. Physicians providing primary care for

TABLE 21-1   Prevalence of Protective Titers* of Tetanus and
Diphtheria Antitoxin in Urban Minnesota Adults

	No (%) of Subjects		
Age (yrs)	Males	Females	Total
Tetanus antitoxin			
>60	11/27(41)	9/31(29)	20/58(34)
40–59	20/23(87)	10/28(36)	30/51(59)
18–39	30/32(94)	36/42(86)	66/74(89)
Total	61/82(74)	55/101(54)	116/183(63)
Diphtheria antitoxin			
>60	6/27(22)	3/31(10)	9/58(16)
40–59	3/23(13)	2/28(7)	5/51(10)
18–39	12/32(38)	16/42(38)	28/74(38)
Total	21/82(26)	21/101(21)	42/183(23)

* More than 0.01 unit/ml.
(Crossley K, Irvine P: *JAMA* 242:2298–2300, 1979, used by permission.)

elderly individuals should remember that tetanus-diphtheria toxoids need to be administered to elderly patients at the same interval that is recommended for other adults (i.e., every 10 years).

Influenza virus vaccine is recommended for "all persons who are at increased risk of adverse consequences from infection of the lower respiratory tract."[107] The Advisory Committee on Immunization Practices of the Centers for Disease Control recommends that influenza vaccine be given to all individuals more than 65 years of age because of the excess mortality rate that is associated with influenza outbreaks in elderly persons. A particular effort should be made to immunize those elderly individuals with heart disease or compromised pulmonary function. There is a reduction in the incidence of pneumonia and hospitalization among immunized elderly persons.[108]

Adverse reactions to influenza immunization include a fever, malaise, myalgia, and (rarely) urticaria and bronchospasm. Guillain-Barré Syndrome has not been seen frequently following influenza immunization, in the years since its association with the "swine flu" vaccine.

Pneumococcal polysaccharide vaccine contains capsular carbohydrates from the 14 pneumococcal types that are most often recovered from patients with bacteremic pneumococcal pneumonia. Although pneumococcal vaccine was available in the late 1940s, the introduction of penicillin resulted in an apathetic response to the vaccine by the medical community. A re-interest in developing an immunization to prevent pneumococcal diseases followed the observation that mortality from pneumococcal pneumonia in the first 5 days of therapy is not affected by administration of antibiotics.[109]

Pneumococcal polysaccharide vaccine is relatively inexpensive and unquestionably efficacious in immunologically normal individuals. Antibody levels occasionally may not be protective against certain pneumococcal serotypes contained in the vaccine. A suboptimal response to immunization has been noted in patients who are asplenic, in patients with sickle-cell disease, in patients with chronic renal failure on dialysis, and in patients with Hodgkin's disease after therapy. Similar observations have been made in patients with multiple myeloma and following a renal transplantation.[110]

The role of pneumococcal vaccine in elderly persons is unclear. There is general agreement that patients with a variety of chronic illnesses are at an increased risk of developing a pneumococcal infection. Cardiac disease, sickle-cell anemia, multiple myeloma, chronic renal failure, splenic dysfunction, and cirrhosis usually are cited as conditions that are associated with an increased risk of pneumococcal infection. Additionally, patients with chronic alcoholism, diabetes mellitus, congestive heart failure, chronic pulmonary diseases, or immunosuppression also are at a particular risk of pneumococcal infection. Individuals, elderly or not, who have these diseases are appropriate candidates for immunization with pneumococcal polysaccharide vaccine.

The effectiveness of a vaccine in healthy elderly persons has been a topic of debate for the better part of a decade. Data are inadequate at present to ascertain benefit from the use of vaccine in healthy, ambulatory, elderly persons. None of the available studies of elderly persons have enrolled large enough numbers of patients to yield meaningful results. Several excellent papers that critically examine these data have been published.[110–112] The American College of Physicians takes the following position:

There is good evidence that the incidence of pneumococcal bacteremia rises with age. But precise data on the rate of pneumococcal infection in the healthy elderly are lacking. Data on the morbidity and mortality of pneumococcal pneumonia and vaccine efficacy among the healthy elderly are inadequate. A strong recommendation for the universal use of the vaccine in healthy elderly persons cannot be made at this time. Nevertheless, in light of the vaccine's safety, cost, length of antibody persistence after vaccination, and the increased incidence of bacteremic infection with advanced age, the vaccine should be offered to those healthy elderly persons who in their physician's judgment might benefit from such vaccination.[113]

The vaccine is widely endorsed for administration to elderly patients with chronic cardiopulmonary disease. Based on these criteria, many elderly persons are appropriate candidates for receiving vaccine.

Pneumococcal polysaccharide vaccine is administered as a single immunization that is effective against the 14 serotypes responsible for about two thirds of all bacteremic pneumococcal infections in the United States. About 50% of all patients immunized with this material develop erythema or mild pain at the site of the injection. Other adverse reactions have been uncommon. Unfortunately, significant local reactions following second doses of vaccine have been reported. For this reason, and because the duration of protection resulting from vaccination is unknown, only a single immunization is recommended for adults at present. Both pneumococcal vaccine and influenza vaccine can be given at the same time without an increased incidence of side effects.[114]

References

1. Kohn RR: Cause of death in very old people. *JAMA* 247:2793–2797, 1982.
2. White NK, Edwards JE, Dry TJ: The relationship of the degree of coronary atherosclerosis with age, in men. *Circulation* 1:645–654, 1950.
3. Louria DB, Blumenfeld HL, Ellis JT, et al: Studies on influenza in the pandemic of 1957–1958. II. Pulmonary complications of influenza. *J Clin Invest* 38:213–265, 1959.
4. O'Hanlon P, Kohrs MB: Dietary studies of older Americans. *Am J Clin Nutr* 31:1257–1269, 1978.
5. Avorn J: Nursing home infections—the context. *N Engl J Med* 305:759–760, 1981.
6. Cohen ED, Hierholzer WJ Jr, Schilling CR, et al: Nosocomial infections in skilled nursing facilities: a preliminary survey. *Public Health Rep* 94:162–165, 1979.
7. Magnussen MH, Robb SS: Nosocomial infections in a long-term care facility. *Am J Infect Control* 8:12–17, 1980.
8. Garibaldi RA, Brodine S, Matsumiya S: Infections among patients in nursing homes. Policies, prevalence, and problems. *N Engl J Med* 305:731–735, 1981.
9. Stead WW: Tuberculosis among elderly persons: an outbreak in a nursing home. *Ann Int Med* 94:606–610, 1981.
10. Center for Disease Control.Tuberculosis—North Dakota. *MMWR* 27:523–525, 1979.
11. Goodman RA, Orenstein WA, Munro TF, et al: Impact of influenza A in a nursing home. *JAMA* 247:1451–1453, 1982.
12. Marrie TJ, Lee SHS, Faulkner RS, et al: Rotavirus infection in a geriatric population. *Arch Int Med* 142:313–316, 1982.
13. Garb JL, Brown RB, Garb JR, et al: Differences in etiology of pneumonias in nursing home and community patients. *JAMA* 240:2169–2172, 1978.
14. Goldman F: Decline in organ function with aging, in Rossman I (ed): *Clinical Geriatrics,* ed 2. Philadelphia, JB Lippincott, 1979, pp 23–59.

15. Finkelstein MS: Unusual features of infections in the aging. *Geriatrics* 37:65–78, 1982.

16. Finkelstein MS, Petkin W, Citrin A, et al: Differences in presentation of pneumococcal bacteremia based on age of patient. *Clin Res* 29:499A, 1981.

17. Esposito AL, Gleckman RA, Cram S, et al: Community-acquired bacteremia in the elderly: analysis of one hundred consecutive episodes. *J Am Geriatr Soc* 28:315–319, 1980.

18. Gleckman R, Hibert D: Afebrile bacteremia. A phenomenon in geriatric patients. *JAMA* 248:1478–1481, 1982.

19. Brown NK, Thompson DJ: Nontreatment of fever in extended-care facilities. *N Engl J Med* 300:1246–1250, 1979.

20. Doroghazi RM, Nadol JB Jr, Hyslop NE Jr, et al: Invasive external otitis. Report of 21 cases and review of literature. *Am J Med* 71:603–613, 1981.

21. Osler W: The Principles and Practice of Medicine, ed 3. New York, D Appleton & Co, 1892.

22. Sullivan RJ Jr, Dowdle WR, Marine WM, et al: Adult pneumonia in a general hospital. *Arch Int Med* 129:935–942, 1972.

23. Hill CD, Stamm WE: Pneumonia in the elderly: the fatal complication. *Geriatrics* 37:40–50, 1982.

24. Siegel JS: Recent and prospective demographic trends for the elderly population and some implications for health care, in Haynes SG, Feinleib M (eds): *Second Conference on the Epidemiology of Aging*. Bethesda, MD, United States Department of Health and Human Services, National Institutes of Health, 1980, p 305.

25. Oswald NC, Simon G, Shooter RA: Pneumonia in hospital practice. *Br J Dis Chest* 55:109–118, 1961.

26. Dorff GJ, Rytel MW, Farmer SG, et al: Etiologies and characteristic features of pneumonias in a municipal hospital. *Am J Med Sci* 266:349–358, 1973.

27. Ebright JR, Rytel MW: Bacterial pneumonia in the elderly. *J Am Geriatr Soc* 28:220–223, 1980.

28. Foy HM, Wentworth B, Kenny GE, et al: Pneumococcal isolations from patients with pneumonia and control subjects in a prepaid medical care group. *Am Rev Respir Dis* 111:595–603, 1975.

29. Johanson WG, Pierce AK, Sanford JP: Changing pharyngeal flora of hospitalized patients: emergence of gram-negative bacilli. *N Engl J Med* 281:1137–1140, 1969.

30. Valenti WM, Trudell RG, Bentley DW: Factors predisposing to oropharyngeal colonization

with gram-negative bacilli in the aged. *N Engl J Med* 298:1108–1111, 1978.

31. Johanson WB, Pierce AK, Sanford JP, et al: Nosocomial respiratory infections with gram-negative bacilli: the significance of colonization of the respiratory tract. *Ann Int Med* 77:701–706, 1972.

32. McCabe WR: Gram-negative bacteremia. *DM*, Dec 1973.

33. Irwin RS, Whitaker S, Pratter MR, et al: The transiency of oropharyngeal colonization with gram-negative bacilli in residents of a skilled nursing facility. *Chest* 81:31–35, 1982.

34. McFadden JP, Price RC, Eastwood HD, et al: Raised respiratory rate in elderly patients: a valuable physical sign. *Br Med J* 284:626–627, 1982.

35. Ziskind MM, Schwarz MI, George RB, et al: Incomplete consolidation in pneumococcal lobar pneumonia complicating pulmonary emphysema. *Ann Int Med* 72:835–839, 1970.

36. Jay SJ, Johanson WG Jr, Pierce AK: The radiographic resolution of Streptococcus pneumoniae pneumonia. *N Engl J Med* 293:798–801, 1975.

37. Berk SL, Holtsclaw SA, Wiener SL, et al: Nontypeable Haemophilus influenzae in the elderly. *Arch Int Med* 142:537–539, 1982.

38. Gerding DN: Etiologic diagnosis of acute pneumonia in adults: a growing challenge. *Postgrad Med* 69:136–150, 1981.

39. Crossley K: The practical use of antibiotics in respiratory infections: when to use, what to use, potential complications, in Drage CW (ed): *Respiratory Medicine for Primary Care Physicians*. New York, Academic Press, 1982, pp 29–37.

40. Khan M, Kovnat DM, Bachus B, et al: Clinical and roentgenographic spectrum of pulmonary tuberculosis in the adult. *Am J Med* 62:31–38, 1977.

41. Farer LS, Lowell AM, Meador MP: Extrapulmonary tuberculosis in the United States. *Am J Epidemiol* 109:205–217, 1979.

42. Glassroth J, Robins AG, Snider DE, Jr: Tuberculosis in the 1980s. *N Engl J Med* 302:1441–1450, 1980.

43. Goldstein RS, Contreras M, Craig GA, et al: Tuberculosis—a review of 498 recent admissions to hospital. *Can Med Assoc J* 126:490–492, 1982.

44. Roberts-Thomson IC, Whittingham S, Youngchaiyud U, et al: Aging, immune response, and mortality. *Lancet* 2:368–370, 1974.

45. Slavin RE, Walsh TJ, Pollack AD: Late generalized tuberculosis: a clinical pathologic analy-

sis and comparison of 100 cases in the preantibiotic and antibiotic eras. *Medicine* 59:352–366, 1980.

46. Stead WW: Tuberculosis among elderly persons: an outbreak in a nursing home. *Ann Int Med* 94:606–610, 1981.

47. Curry FJ: Prophylactic effect of isoniazid in young tuberculin reactors. *N Engl J Med* 277:562–567, 1967.

48. Ad Hoc Committee on Isoniazid and Liver Disease: Isoniazid and liver disease. *Am Rev Respir Dis* 104:454–459, 1971.

49. Barlow PB, Black M, Brummer DL, et al: Preventive therapy of tuberculous infection. *MMWR* 24:71–72, 77–78, 1975.

50. Center for Disease Control: Guidelines for short-course tuberculosis chemotherapy. *MMWR* 29:97–100, 105, 1980.

51. Center for Disease Control: Tuberculosis—North Dakota. *MMWR* 27:523–525, 1979.

52. Center for Disease Control: Tuberculosis in a nursing home—Oklahoma. *MMWR* 29:465–467, 1980.

53. Comstock GW, Daniel TM, Snider DE Jr, et al: The tuberculin skin test. *Am Rev Respir Dis* 124:356–363, 1981.

54. Barker WH, Mullooly JP: Pneumonia and influenza deaths during epidemics. Implications and prevention. *Arch Int Med* 142:85–89, 1982.

55. Mathur U, Bentley DW, Hall CB, et al: Influenza A/Brazil/78(H1N1) infection in the elderly. *Am Rev Respir Dis* 123:633–635, 1981.

56. Hall WN, Goodman RA, Noble GR, et al: An outbreak of influenza B in an elderly population. *J Infect Dis* 144:297–302, 1981.

57. Douglas RG Jr: Amantadine as an antiviral agent in influenza. *N Engl J Med* 307:617–618, 1982.

58. Dolin R, Reichman RC, Madore HP, et al: A controlled trial of amantadine and rimantadine in the prophylaxis of influenza A infection. *N Engl J Med* 307:580–584, 1982.

59. Kunin CM: Epidemiology of bacteriuria and its relation to pyelonephritis. *J Infect Dis* 120:1–9, 1969.

60. Wolfson SA, Kalmanson GM, Rubini ME, et al: Epidemiology of bacteriuria in a predominantly geriatric male population. *Am J Med Sci* 250:168–173, 1965.

61. Gladstone JL, Friedman SA: Bacteriuria in the aged: a study of its prevalence and predisposing lesions in a chronically ill population. *J Urol* 106:745–749, 1971.

62. Dontas AS, Kasviki-Charvati P, Papanayiotou PC, et al: Bacteriuria and survival in old age. *N Engl J Med* 304:939–943, 1981.

63. Brocklehurst JC, Bee P, Jones D, et al: Bacteriuria in geriatric hospital patients. Its correlates and management. *Age Aging* 6:240–245, 1977.

64. Alling B, Brandberg A, Seeberg S, et al: Aerobic and anaerobic microbial flora in the urinary tract of geriatric patients during long-term care. *J Infect Dis* 127:34–39, 1973.

65. Evans DA, Hennekens CH, Miao L, et al: Bacteriuria and subsequent mortality in women. *Lancet* 1:156–158, 1982.

66. Gleckman R, Blagg N, Hibert D, et al: Community-acquired bacteremic urosepsis in the elderly patients: a prospective study of 34 consecutive episodes. *J Urol* 128:79–81, 1982.

67. Sullivan NM, Sutter VL, Mims MM, et al: Clinical aspects of bacteremia after manipulation of the genitourinary tract. *J Infect Dis* 127:49–55, 1973.

68. Dans PE, Klaus B: Dysuria in women. *John Hopkins Med J* 138:13–18, 1976.

69. Gleckman R, Blagg N, Hibert D, et al: Catheter-related urosepsis in the elderly: a prospective study of community-derived infections. *J Am Geriatr Soc* 30:255–257, 1982.

70. Turck M, Goffe G, Petersdorf RG: The urethral catheter and urinary tract infection. *J Urol* 88:834–836, 1962.

71. Garibaldi RA, Burke JP, Dickman ML, et al: Factors predisposing to bacteriuria during indwelling urethral catheterization. *N Engl J Med* 291:215–219, 1974.

72. Stamm WE: Guidelines for prevention of catheter-associated urinary tract infections. *Ann Int Med* 82:386–390, 1975.

73. Maki DG, Hennekens CH, Bennett JV: Prevention of catheter-associated urinary tract infection. An additional measure. *JAMA* 221:1270–1271, 1972.

74. Alling B, Brandberg A, Seeberg S, et al: Effect of consecutive antibacterial therapy on bacteriuria in hospitalized geriatric patients. *Scand J Infect Dis* 7:201–207, 1975.

75. Britt MR, Garibaldi RA, Miller WA, et al: Antimicrobial prophylaxis for catheter-associated bacteriuria. *Antimicrob Agents Chemother* 11:240–243, 1977.

76. Wibell L, Scheynius A, Norrman K: Methenamine-hippurate and bacteriuria in the geriatric patient with a catheter. *Acta Med Scand* 207:469–473, 1980.

77. Dudley MN, Barriere SL: Antimicrobial irrigations in the prevention and treatment of catheter-related urinary tract infections. *Am J Hosp Pharm* 38:59–65, 1981.

78. Kunin CM: *Detection, Prevention and Management of Urinary Tract Infections,* ed 3. Philadelphia, Lea & Febiger, 1979.

79. Hirsch DD, Fainstein V, Musher DM: Do condom catheter collecting systems cause urinary tract infection? *JAMA* 242:340–341, 1979.

80. Ginsberg MB: Cellulitis: analysis of 101 cases and review of the literature. *South Med J* 74:530–533, 1981.

81. Lynch JM, Tilson WR, Hodges GR, et al: Nosocomial Aeromonas hydrophila cellulitis and bacteremia in a nonimmunocompromised patient. *South Med J* 74:901–902, 1981.

82. Drapkin MS, Wilson ME, Shrager SM, et al: Bacteremic Hemophilus influenzae type B cellulitis in the adult. *Am J Med* 63:449–452, 1977.

83. Meislin HW, Lerner SA, Graves MH, et al: Cutaneous abscesses. Anaerobic and aerobic bacteriology and outpatient management. *Ann Int Med* 87:145–149, 1977.

84. Ayliffe GAJ, Brightwell KM, Collins BJ, et al: Surveys of hospital infection in the Birmingham region. I. Effect of age, sex, length of stay and antibiotic use on nasal carriage of tetracycline-resistant Staphylococcus aureus and on postoperative wound infection. *J Hyg (Camb)* 79:299–314, 1977.

85. National Research Council: Postoperative wound infections. *Ann Surg* 160(suppl):1–192, 1964.

86. Ragozzino MW, Melton LJ III, Kurland LT, et al: Population-based study of herpes zoster and its sequelae. *Medicine* 61:310–316, 1982.

87. Burke BL, Steele RW, Beard OW, et al: Immune responses to varicella-zoster in the aged. *Arch Int Med* 142:291–293, 1982.

88. Kent MW, Guerriero WG: Bladder dysfunction secondary to herpes zoster. *South Med J* 68:1043–1045, 1975.

89. Jellinek EH, Tulloch WS: Herpes zoster with dysfunction of bladder and anus. *Lancet* 2:1219–1222, 1976.

90. Mazur MH, Dolin R: Herpes zoster at the NIH: a 20 year experience. *Am J Med* 65:738–744, 1978.

91. Ragozzino MW, Melton LJ III, Kurland LT, et al: Risk of cancer after herpes zoster. A population-based study. *N Engl J Med* 307:393–397, 1982.

92. Burgoon CF Jr, Burgoon JS, Baldridge GD: The natural history of herpes zoster. *JAMA* 164:265–269, 1957.

93. Eaglstein WH, Katz R, Brown JA: The effects of early corticosteroid therapy on the skin eruption and pain of herpes zoster. *JAMA* 211:1681–1683, 1970.

94. Keczkes K, Basheer AM: Do corticosteroids prevent post-herpetic neuralgia? *Br J Dermatol* 102:551–555, 1980.

95. Kernbaum S, Hauchecorne J: Administration of levodopa for relief of herpes zoster pain. *JAMA* 246:132–134, 1981.

96. Multiple Authors: Symposium on infective endocarditis. *Mayo Clin Proc* 57:3–32, 81–114, 145–175, 1982.

97. Thell R, Martin FH, Edwards JE: Bacterial endocarditis in subjects 60 years of age and older. *Circulation* 51:174–182, 1975.

98. Robbins N, DeMaria A, Miller MH: Infective endocarditis in the elderly. *South Med J* 73:1335–1338, 1980.

99. Esposito AL, Gleckman RA, Cram S, et al: Community-acquired bacteremia in the elderly: analysis of one hundred consecutive episodes. *J Am Geriatr Soc* 28:315–319, 1980.

100. van Dijk JM, Rosin AJ, Rudenski B: Septicaemia in the elderly. *Practitioner* 226:1439–1443, 1982.

101. Setia U, Gross PA: Bacteremia in a community hospital. Spectrum and mortality. *Arch Int Med* 137:1698–1701, 1977.

102. Kreger BE, Craven DE, McCabe WR: Gram-negative bacteremia. IV. Re-evaluation of clinical features and treatment in 612 patients. *Am J Med* 68:344–355, 1980.

103. Rimland D, McGowan JE Jr, Shulman JA: Immunization for the internist. *Ann Int Med* 85:622–629, 1976.

104. Center for Disease Control: Health information for international travel. *MMWR* 30(suppl):1–103, 1981.

105. Crossley K, Irvine P, Warren JB, et al: Tetanus and diphtheria immunity in urban Minnesota adults. *JAMA* 242:2298–2300, 1979.

106. Ruben FL, Nagel J, Fireman P: Antitoxin responses in the elderly to tetanus-diphtheria (TD) immunization. *Am J Epidemiol* 108:145–149, 1978.

107. Immunization Practices Advisory Committee: Influenza vaccines 1982–1983. Center for Disease Control. *MMWR* 31:349–353, 1982.

108. Barker WH, Mullooly JP: Influenza vaccination of elderly persons. Reduction in pneumonia and influenza hospitalizations and deaths. *JAMA* 244:2547–2549, 1980.

109. Austrian R, Gold J: Pneumococcal bacteremia with especial reference to bacteremic pneumococcal pneumonia. *Ann Int Med* 60:759–776, 1964.

110. Schwartz JS: Pneumococcal vaccine: clinical efficacy and effectiveness. *Ann Int Med* 96:208–220, 1982.

111. Hirschmann JV, Lipsky BA: Pneumococcal vaccine in the United States. A critical analysis. *JAMA* 246:1428–1432, 1981.

112. Patrick KM, Woolley FR: A cost-benefit analysis of immunization for pneumococcal pneumonia. *JAMA* 245:473–477, 1981.

113. American College of Physicians: Pneumococcal vaccine recommendation. *Ann Int Med* 96:206–207, 1982.

114. Mufson MA, Krause HE, Tarrant CJ, et al: Polyvalent pneumococcal vaccine given alone in combination with bivalent influenza virus vaccine (40804). *Proc Soc Exp Biol Med* 163:498–503, 1980.

CHAPTER 22

Hematology

JOHN R. WALSH, M.D.

Blood disorders are common in elderly persons. The management of blood disorders, particularly in frail elderly persons, often must be weighed in a setting of compromised physiologic reserves and concurrent illnesses. Therefore, judgment regarding treatment of a blood disorder must be balanced between active treatment to help alleviate disabilities from the disorder itself, or from its collusive effect on other physical and mental problems, and the avoidance of harmful effects of therapy. Conversely, a physician who interdicts treatment because of a patient's age unwittingly relegates that patient to inexorable disability, thus denying him or her any opportunity for improvement. Anemia has profound effects in frail elderly persons and will receive more attention, especially since many causes of anemia are eminently treatable. Other disorders that occur more frequently in elderly persons, such as chronic lymphocytic leukemia (CLL), monoclonal gammopathies, and myeloproliferative disorders, will be discussed from the standpoint of diagnostic and management modalities.

Anemia in Elderly Persons

Anemia increases in prevalence and has profound effects in elderly persons. Anemia in adults is characterized by a hemoglobin concentration below 14 grams/dl in males and 12 grams/dl in females. These values are applicable to elderly persons, although a reduction of 1–2 grams/dl in males due to a diminished androgen function is acceptable. Most older people retain standard normal values for red blood cell parameters, and lower values are significant. There is controversy as to what level of hemoglobin concentration signifies anemia. It generally is accepted that the lower the hemoglobin values, the greater the chance for a significant anemia. However, values hovering around the low normal range are an enigma because of an overlap of normal and abnormal values at hemoglobin levels between 10–12 grams/dl in frail elderly females and 11–13 grams/dl in males. A hemoglobin value of 11 grams/dl may represent a normal value for one woman and anemia for another. A clinician should be reluctant to attribute borderline hemoglobin values in this gray zone to old age.[1] In a clinical setting, it cannot be assumed that anemia is due to old age, but rather that old people are anemic because they have a disease.

Nonetheless, there is some justification for the concept of diminished bone marrow function in older people. Some refractory anemias attributed to chronic disease, but with insufficient clinical or laboratory criteria for this type of anemia, may actually be examples of senescent anemia.[2] A recent study of 222 elderly people with no other cause for mild anemia, some with mild neutropenia, supports the concept of an overall reduction in hematopoiesis with a diminished bone marrow reserve capacity in elderly persons.[2] A decreased red blood cell iron uptake in older people suggests either an ineffective erythropoiesis or diminished erythropoietic production.[3] Bone marrow studies have demonstrated a 15% decrease in marrow cellularity in patients over 70 years of age compared to younger adults.[4] The cause of the reduced hematopoiesis is unknown, although a fault in the stem cell has been considered. Bone marrow studies suggest that the defect in aged mice is not in the stem cell, but is an abnormality in the microenvironment.[5] Further research obviously is needed to unravel these issues.

It is difficult to attribute symptoms to anemia in a mileau where aging also affects other organ systems and physiologic functions, multiple interacting diseases produce non-specific or atypical symptoms, and side effects from medication often are misinterpreted as symptoms of disease. Fatigue, weakness, dyspnea, and decreased physical activity are clinical manifestations of anemia, but they also are non-specific disease symptoms and even have been attributed to old age. Because of the marginal physiologic capability of most organs, particularly in frail elderly persons, signs and symptoms of anemia may appear at higher hemoglobin levels than would be expected in younger adults. Indeed, a mild to moderate anemia may aggravate other existing diseases (*see* Figure 22-1). It can cause confusion or worsen a dementia, which in turn increases the likelihood of falls and incontinence. Similarly, syncope, falls, and confusion may develop from postural hypotension that arises from the anemia. Anginal attacks and congestive heart failure frequently are precipitated or intensified by the presence of anemia, and even a myocardial infarction has been an occasional consequence. Weakness and fatigue from anemia may aggravate disability from arthritis, Parkinsonism, or stroke, which consequently increases dependency, dampens motivation for rehabilitative measures, and produces despondency or even depression.

Anemia most often is a sign of another disease and not a diagnosis itself. In elderly persons, it often is due to multiple causes. Nonetheless, iron deficiency anemia and the anemia of chronic disease (ACD) account for over 65%, and macrocytic anemias about 25%, of the anemias in elderly persons. Treatable anemias due to iron, Vitamin B-12, and folate deficiencies should never be overlooked. The initial evaluation of a patient with anemia is straightforward and non-invasive; it embraces a combination of history, physical examination, stool examination for occult blood, study of the peripheral blood smear, reticulocyte count, red blood cell indices, and selected blood tests determined by the results of initial screening tests. Bone marrow studies, which are important for certain indications, are not always necessary.

Successful management stems from decisions that are initially based on the appearance of the erythrocytes and the reticulocyte index, an indirect assessment of bone marrow function. The presence of hypochromic or macrocytic red blood cells reduces the diagnostic possibilities. Conversely, normochromic anemias are caused by a large number of disorders. The

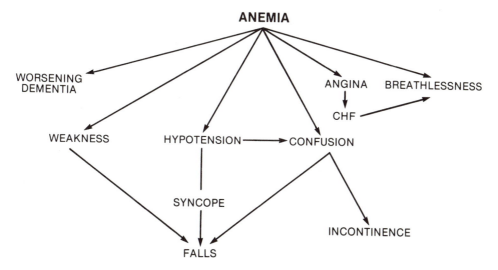

FIGURE 22-1 Major consequences of anemia in elderly persons. CHF = congestive heart failure.

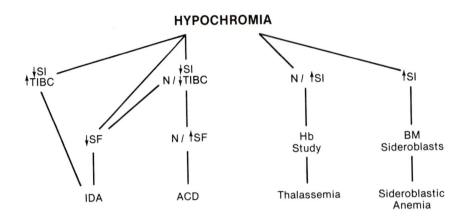

FIGURE 22-2   Laboratory approach to a differential diagnosis of hypochromic anemia.
IDA = iron deficiency anemia, ACD = anemia of chronic disease, SI = Serum iron; SF =
Serum Ferritin; N = Normal; Hb = Hemoglobin; BM = bone marrow.

reticulocyte index classifies the mechanism of
anemia, reticulocytopenia denotes a decreased
marrow erythrocyte production, and conversely, reticulocytosis indicates an enhanced
marrow response to the anemia.

Hypochromia that is observed on a peripheral blood smear is an indicator of defective hemoglobin formation. There are four conditions
characterized by hypochromia: iron deficiency,
anemia of chronic disease, thalassemia syndromes, and sideroblastic anemia. A lack of
available iron to combine with protoporphyrin
leads to a diminished heme formation in iron
deficiency and anemia of chronic disease. In
thalassemia syndromes, globin production is
impaired; in sideroblastic anemia, the production of porphyrin is defective. Standard iron
studies separate these disorders (see Figure
22-2).

Iron Deficiency

Iron deficiency anemia, which is a common
cause of reduced hemoglobin synthesis, is familiar to clinicians who treat elderly people. In
contrast to other types of anemia, its clinical
manifestations are due not only to a diminished
oxygen transfer to tissues because of decreased
quantities of hemoglobin, but also to a shortage
of iron itself.[6,7] A depletion of tissue iron affects
tissue enzymes in ways that contribute to symptoms of iron deficiency anemia. Symptoms may
not be present at rest, but with exercise even a
mild anemia may impair performance. Several

studies provide evidence that iron deficiency
produces impairment in physical activity or
work performance with subsequent improvement after the administration of iron even before the hemoglobin concentration increases.[6,7]
The improvement in activity is attributed to altered cellular function of muscle, especially to
changes in α-glycerophosphate-mediated phosphorylation rather than to concentrations of
muscle cytochromes or myoglobin.[6] Therefore,
for the same level of hemoglobin, symptoms are
more pronounced than with other types of anemia. Clinicians often observe significant clinical
improvement with enhanced physical activity
after iron therapy and before a rise in the hemoglobin level. Minimal decreases in hemoglobin
concentration often have a profound effect on
accompanying disabilities in an elderly patient.
Active treatment can be surprisingly successful
in returning a patient to a more active and independent life.

Sequential changes in iron deficiency begin
with the exhaustion of bone marrow iron stores
that are detected by a serum ferritin below 12
μg/l, followed by a low serum iron and an increase of the total iron-binding capacity (>350
μg/dl), which jointly are responsible for a low
transferrin saturation (<16%); finally, there is
an appearance of hypochromic-microcytic red
blood cells and low red blood cell indices
when the hemoglobin concentration is below 10
grams/dl. The erythrocyte morphology may be
normal in the presence of mild degrees of anemia, but the combination of a low serum iron

and an elevated total iron binding capacity (TIBC) provides a diagnosis of iron deficiency. In elderly persons, however, the presence of chronic disease lowers the transferrin levels and, thus, the TIBC can be low or normal in patients with an iron deficiency. In this setting, a low serum ferritin level establishes the diagnosis (see Figure 22-2). Normally, the concentration of serum ferritin rises with aging, especially with postmenopausal females,[8,9]; therefore, serum ferritin levels sometimes are easier to interpret in elderly persons.

A clinician determines the number and sequence of tests based on the clinical presentation. Hypochromia in a patient with a history of chronic bleeding, tarry stools, or positive tests for occult blood in the stool, obviously is due to an iron deficiency. This is confirmed by a low serum iron and an elevated TIBC. Conversely, if a patient with hypochromia or normochromic anemia has no evident bleeding and negative occult blood stool tests, a diagnosis of iron deficiency will be established with a low serum iron, an elevated TIBC, a transferrin saturation below 16%, or by a reduced serum ferritin below 12 μg/l (see Figure 22-2).

Management mandates not only the treatment of iron deficiency, but also the recognition and correction of the abnormality that is causing the anemia. The assumption that in the United States iron deficiency anemia rarely results from a dietary lack of iron may not always apply to elderly persons. It can be said, however, that poor nutrition rarely is the sole cause, but, it may be a contributing cause of iron deficiency. A normal diet in the United States contains 15–20 mg of food iron, of which 5–10% (0.5–1.5 mg/day) is absorbed. Iron losses in elderly persons are approximately 1 mg/day. It would require up to 3 years to exhaust one's iron stores to allow anemia to develop. Dietary assessment is important, since many elderly people are on surprisingly poor diets because of low income, living alone, dementia, depression, drugs, or diseases that affect the appetite or interfere with swallowing. Caloric intake and the amount of dietary iron are closely associated, usually about 6 mg of elemental iron per 1,000 kcal. Iron is better absorbed from meat than from vegetables. Vegetable sources are high in iron content, but the iron is poorly absorbed unless consumed with meat. Tea inhibits iron absorption. Some elderly persons drink large amounts of tea daily, which may be a contributing factor in iron deficiency (especially if the patient eats little meat).[10] Elderly persons at risk for the development of an iron deficiency should be advised to drink tea between meals rather than with meals.

A clinician must never assume that a poor dietary history explains the anemia until an investigation for a bleeding lesion has been completed. Chronic blood loss from a gastrointestinal lesion is the most common cause of iron deficiency in elderly persons. An examination of multiple stool specimens for occult blood generally will be positive; however, gastrointestinal bleeding may be intermittent, and negative tests for occult blood do not exclude this possibility. Screening tests for stool occult blood enables physicians to detect lesions of the gastrointestinal tract even in asymptomatic patients.[11] A guaiac (hemoccult) test is less sensitive than an orthotolidine (hematest) test, thereby decreasing the rate of false positive tests. Hemoccult tests detect more bleeding lesions in the descending colon and rectosigmoid than in the ascending and transverse colon.[12] Tests for occult blood depend on the reaction of heme proteins as peroxidases. Therefore, these tests are not supposed to give a positive reaction in patients who are receiving iron therapy. However, recent studies show a high percentage of false positive tests with hemoccult or hematest in patients taking ferrous sulfate or ferrous gluconate.[13] This may create a false impression of blood in the stool and lead to unwarranted studies. It, therefore, is prudent to stop iron medication when evaluating for occult blood in patients who have iron in their stool as indicated by dark stools. Gastrointestinal bleeding may occur with drug ingestion, including aspirin, non-steroidal anti-inflammatory (NSAID) medication, alcohol, steroids, phenylbutazone, and indomethacin.[14] Even if a patient has been ingesting one of these drugs, the clinician must not overlook a concomitant lesion. For example, an elderly patient with hypochromic anemia, who was ingesting large doses of aspirin for relief of arthritic pain, had a cecal carcinoma as the cause of his gastrointestinal bleeding. Anemia may be the only clue to a carcinoma of the cecum or ascending colon.

Treatment consists of the replacement of

iron via the oral administration of ferrous sulfate, 300 mg before meals, and gradually increasing the dose from once daily the first week, to twice daily the second week, and to three times daily thereafter. On this regimen, there is less gastrointestinal upset and better compliance. Hemoglobin begins to rise after 10 days and returns to normal levels after 6 weeks of therapy. After correction of the anemia, the amount of iron absorbed decreases, but therapy should be continued for at least 6 months to replenish the iron stores. Iron absorption is no different in elderly than in young persons[3]; therefore, similar responses to therapy should be anticipated. Older people with multiple disorders require several medications and should have the simplest regimen possible. Antacids will prevent the adequate absorption of iron and should not be taken simultaneously. Slow-release iron preparations may simplify the regimen, but they are questionably absorbed. Recently, it has been shown that one iron tablet, containing 105 mg of elemental iron, taken daily is effective in treating iron-deficient elderly patients.[15] This regimen may not suffice for all patients.

Parenteral iron therapy with iron dextran (Imferon) is reserved for patients who are noncompliant with oral therapy, intolerant of oral therapy, or have continuous bleeding from an uncorrected source such as hereditary telangiectasia. Iron dextran may be given intramuscularly, or by intermittent or continuous (total dose) intravenous (IV) infusion. The latter route has been suggested for frail elderly patients with a small muscle mass or hemorrhagic disorders. However, this mode of therapy should be considered only if oral therapy is contraindicated, since severe and even lethal reactions may occur with either IV or intramuscular therapy.[16] Older patients have more adverse reactions to total dose infusions.[17] Immediate life-threatening anaphylactoid reactions that produce hypotension, syncope, purpura, wheezing, dyspnea, respiratory arrest, and cyanosis may occur within the first 5 minutes. Less severe reactions include transient hypotension, malaise, itching, and urticaria that last approximately 5 minutes. Delayed systemic reactions, which are characterized by lymphadenopathy, myalgia, fever, and headaches, typically appear 4–48 hours after injection and persist for 3–7 days. Parenteral therapy, therefore, should be reserved for use only when no other route of administration is feasible.

Anemia of Chronic Disease (ACD)

Anemia of chronic disease (ACD) is a nebulous condition that often is diagnosed in elderly people. An anemia frequently is associated with chronic inflammatory states such as rheumatoid arthritis, infections such as tuberculosis or osteomyelitis, neoplastic diseases, and (occasionally) liver or renal diseases. The anemia is mild to moderate, with hematocrit values ranging from 27–35%, and may be a hypochromic or normochromic anemia. It is further characterized by a low reticulocyte index, low serum iron concentration, and elevated erythrocyte protoporphyrin levels. Laboratory values may resemble those of an iron deficiency anemia.[18,19] An elevated TIBC helps to confirm a diagnosis of iron deficiency; however, many patients with an iron deficiency have a low or normal TIBC, which will therefore not distinguish them. The diagnostic study is a serum ferritin value that is low in iron deficiency, whereas in ACD the value is high normal or elevated (*see* Figure 22-2).

Iron deficiency and inflammatory disease may coexist, especially in elderly persons. In patients with ACD, a serum ferritin below 25 μg/l is highly predictive of an associated iron deficiency and merits a trial of iron therapy. Most studies of patients with a chronic inflammatory disease, liver disease, and malignancy show serum ferritin values over 50 μg/l; values below this level are consistent with iron deficiency in this group, which justifies a trial of iron therapy.[20] Uncertainty exists with values between 50–100 μg/l; most of these patients will have stainable bone marrow iron. Patients with values greater than 100 μg/l practically always have bone marrow iron stores.[20] In patients with chronic renal failure, a serum ferritin below 50 μg/l is highly suggestive of an iron deficiency.[20,21] It has been suggested that patients on maintenance dialysis, with levels below 100 μg/l, should be given 60–100 mg of elemental iron daily monitored by the serum ferritin at 4–6 week intervals.[20] Most iron-deficient patients on maintenance dialysis have serum ferritin values below 50 μg/l.[22]

The anemia is due to a shortening of the erythrocyte life span coupled with a reduced bone marrow response. A block in the release of iron from reticuloendothelial cells results in low plasma iron. The constellation of a chronic inflammatory state, anemia, and iron studies described above are sufficient for a diagnosis of an ACD. However, this diagnosis probably is overused in elderly persons with anemia who lack either a significant inflammatory disorder (although they may have some disabling problem) or sufficient laboratory features. Further clarification must be forthcoming of the heterogeneous disorders that carry the banner of an ACD. With the present state of knowledge, clinicians will continue to use this diagnosis with a considerable degree of uncertainty.

Sideroblastic Anemias

Hypochromia in an anemic elderly patient who is not iron deficient and does not have evidence of a chronic disease is most likely sideroblastic anemia. Hypochromia is due to impaired heme synthesis. Iron that normally incorporates into protoporphyrin to form heme accumulates within the mitochondria of nucleated red blood cells to form the ringed sideroblasts that are characteristic of this disorder. The serum iron level is increased and the iron saturation of transferrin is elevated over 70%. Serum ferritin is elevated, which reflects the increased tissue iron stores.

There are many causes of sideroblastic anemia; alcohol abuse is most common. Megalobastic anemia due to folate and Vitamin B-12 deficiencies sometimes is associated with sideroblastic features. Pyridoxine deficiency, a rare cause, sometimes responds to 200 mg/day of pyridoxine or to intramuscular injections of pyridoxal phosphate. Antituberculous drugs rarely may induce a sideroblastic anemia. Primary sideroblastic anemia is refractory to therapy and may require periodic transfusions. These patients should be closely observed, since sideroblastic anemia may represent a preleukemia, which is an antecedent to acute non-lymphocytic leukemia. A recent study has indicated that a subset of patients with an idiopathic-refractory sideroblastic anemia carry a single allele for hemochromatosis (HLA-A3), which plays a role in increased iron loading in

association with another factor, the sideroblastic factor.[23]

Anemia of Chronic Renal Failure

Anemia is a characteristic concomitant of chronic renal failure. The anemia is hypoproliferative, which is typified by reticulocytopenia with normochromic-normocytic cells on the peripheral blood smear. The level of anemia correlates with the severity of the kidney dysfunction when the creatinine clearance (Ccr) is below 40 ml/minute/1.73 M^2.[24] Above this level, the correlation is poor. Many factors contribute to the anemia of chronic renal disease, but a decreased red blood cell production is its major cause. Associated with deficient marrow erythropoiesis are varying degrees of hemolysis. Furthermore, patients with chronic uremia frequently have gastrointestinal bleeding or, less commonly, bleeding from other sources. An insufficient bone marrow response to either hemolysis or blood loss is considered to be predominantly due to either an insufficient amount of erythropoietin to adequately compensate for the degree of anemia[24] or to the presence of inhibitors of red blood cell production in uremic serum,[25,26] or to both.

The kidney is the main source of erythropoietin. With a progressive kidney disease, there is a loss of both excretory and endocrine function.[24] Recently, erythropoietin levels have been shown to be normal or elevated with anemia of chronic renal failure, but the levels are not comparably elevated, as with similar degrees of anemia due to other causes.

The second factor that is responsible for anemia is the presence of low- and middle-molecular weight substances in uremic serum, which inhibit erythropoiesis.[26,27] These inhibitors are not urea, creatinine, nor guanidinosuccinic acid. Inhibitors to both heme synthesis and bone marrow, erythroid colony-forming cells (i.e., erythroid colony-forming units [CFU-E] and erythroid burst-forming units [BFU-E]) have been reported.[28] The nature of the inhibitor has not been characterized, although it has been shown that a polyamine spermine inhibits erythropoiesis;[26] whether it only is this substance needs further confirmation. Continuous ambulatory peritoneal dialysis removes middle- to low-molecular weight tox-

ins better than hemodialysis, and a normalization of the hematocrit is reported in an increasing number of patients who are undergoing this
method of treatment.[29]

The therapy for the anemia of a chronic renal
disease, therefore, includes dialysis to remove
a dialyzable inhibitor of erythropoiesis. Androgens are effective in some patients who are undergoing dialysis, except in those with bilateral nephrectomy. Daily oral administration of
oxymetholone or weekly intramuscular injections of nandrolone decanoate are commonly
used.[30] Higher hematocrit levels usually are
achieved with parenteral preparations. Erythropoietin replacement is not yet available for therapy; while it is a potentially promising agent, its
effectiveness in the presence of uremic serum
inhibitors remains to be established.

The loss of blood from sources such as the
gastrointestinal tract, laboratory procedures,
and hemodialysis may lead to an iron deficiency
anemia. A diagnosis of iron deficiency anemia
may be difficult to separate from the anemia of
renal disease. However, there is a good correlation between serum ferritin levels and bone
marrow iron stores in patients who are undergoing dialysis; therefore a serum ferritin level less
than 50–55 μg/l provides sufficient evidence of
an iron deficiency and a good indication for iron
therapy.[22] Oral iron therapy is preferable, since
iron absorption has been shown to be normal in
patients with chronic renal failure. Iron absorption is related to the status of iron stores, and
absorption increases with an iron deficiency
that is similar to patients who have no renal
disease.[31] Long-term parenteral therapy has
been responsible for producing hemosiderosis
in some patients with chronic renal disease.
Oral iron therapy does not have to be given
indefinitely. Monitoring the iron stores via serum ferritin levels can aid in management.

Anemia in Thyroid Disease

Anemia frequently occurs with thyroid disease,
especially in association with hypothyroidism.
Several symptoms of anemia and hypothyroidism are similar to changes due to aging, and the
physician may inadvertently attribute them to
aging. Similarly, symptoms of anemia may
cause hypothyroidism to be overlooked.

Thyroid hormones stimulate red blood cell

production, but the mechanism is not entirely
clear. The most plausible explanation is that the
effects of thyroid hormones are mediated by
erythropoietin. Thyroid hormones increase oxygen consumption of peripheral tissues and
increase erythrocyte 2,3 diphosphoglycerate
(DPG) concentrations, which serve to enhance
the delivery of oxygen to tissues. In the absence
of thyroid hormones, anemia frequently develops.[31]

Anemia is found in approximately 23–60% of
all patients with hypothyroidism.[32] Most often,
the anemia is normochromic, but it occasionally
may be a hypochromic or even a macrocytic
anemia. Normochromic anemia usually is mild
with the hemoglobin reduced less than 25% below normal levels. The bone marrow is qualiti-
tatively normal, but there is a diminished marrow volume. The serum iron and total
iron-binding capacity may be low, but iron
stores are normal. There is a decreased iron
turnover rate. The anemia responds to thyroid
hormone treatment, but it often takes several
months for correction.

Hypochromic anemia occurs in 4–15% of all
hypothyroid patients as a result of an increased
blood loss or impairment of gastrointestinal absorption of iron. A careful search for an underlying bleeding lesion must be conducted concomitantly with iron replacement therapy to
correct the anemia.

A folate deficiency has been reported in a
small percentage of patients with hypothyroidism. This anemia responds to folate therapy and
treatment of the hypothyroidism. The mechanism that causes a folate deficiency is unknown,
although in elderly persons it may be due to
poor nutrition, an inadequate intake because of
confusion or depression, alcohol, or drugs.

Pernicious anemia occurs concomitantly in
over 10% of all patients who have hypothyroidism. In a recent study of 162 patients with pernicious anemia, 24% had a clinical thyroid disease, 11.7% were hypothyroid, and 8.6% were
hyperthyroid.[33] In addition, increased thyroid-
stimulating hormone (TSH) levels occurred in
patients with no overt clinical findings of hypothyroidism. There is a strong association between thyroiditis and pernicious anemia; both
have features of an autoimmune disease. Of all
patients with pernicious anemia, 50% have been
shown to have thyroid antibodies, while 25% of

all asymptomatic relatives of patients with thyroiditis have antibodies to parietal cells. Conversely, 50% of all asymptomatic relatives of patients with pernicious anemia have demonstrable antithyroid antibodies. The association of the two disorders occur frequently enough that when one is present the clinician should strongly suspect the other condition.

Anemia and Hyperthyroidism

Anemia is uncommon with hyperthyroidism. Thyroid hormones tend to promote erythropoiesis; therefore, the total red blood cell volume and total blood volume usually are increased in the hyperthyroid patient. When anemia occurs, it is a normocromic anemia. The bone marrow shows a generalized hyperplasia with adequate iron stores, with a picture that is suggestive of ineffective erythropoiesis. The anemic hyperthyroid patient seemingly is unable to use iron efficiently in the formation of erythrocytes. This is reversed with therapy for the hyperthyroidism. As previously mentioned, there is an increased incidence of pernicious anemia in hyperthyroid patients.

Folate and Vitamin B-12 Deficiencies

Folate deficiency is more prevalent than Vitamin B-12 deficiency, because it more commonly has a dietary etiology. Older people who live alone have fewer social contacts and less incentive for preparing meals. Some older people live virtually on tea and toast. A diet that excludes fruit, fruit juices, or fresh vegetables increases the risk of developing a folate deficiency. Likewise, older people with severe anorexia or difficulty in swallowing are predisposed to a folate deficiency. Alcoholics who eat poorly are especially liable to become folate deficient. It occurs frequently among wine and whiskey drinkers, which are beverages that contain practically no folate. There is, however, ample folate in beer.[34] The amount of folate in a normal daily diet is 200–500 μg, with a daily requirement of 100–200 μg. Folates are absorbed in the small intestine, and only small amounts (approximately 10 mg) are stored in the liver.

Vitamin B-12 is found in foods of animal origin but is not available in plant sources. Normal diets contain 5–30 μg of Vitamin B-12 with an absorption rate of 1–5 μg/day. Preliminary binding with a gastric-intrinsic factor is necessary for the absorption of Vitamin B-12, which occurs at specific IF-Vitamin B-12 receptor sites of the terminal ileum (*see* Figure 22-3). Recent studies showing that R-proteins in the stomach have a greater avidity for Vitamin B-12 than for the intrinsic factor complicates this facile explanation.[35] R-protein-Vitamin B-12 complexes, however, are not absorbed by ileal receptors, which have a specificity for IF-Vitamin

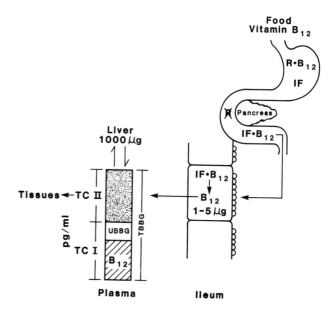

FIGURE 22-3 Simplified scheme of Vitamin B-12 absorption and distribution.

B-12 complexes. Pancreatic enzymes (trypsin and chymotrypsin) in the intestinal tract liberate Vitamin B-12 from R-proteins, thereby making it available to combine with the intrinsic factor.[35] After ingestion of Vitamin B-12, the peak plasma activity is observed in 8–10 hours. After absorption, it binds to a plasma protein (transcobalamin) (*see* Figure 22-3). There are two main transcobalamins (I, II). The turnover rate of Vitamin B-12 that is bound to transcobalamin I is extremely slow (half-life of 9–12 days), while Vitamin B-12 that is bound to transcobalamin II is rapidly released (within hours) for metabolic activity or storage in the liver. Approximately 1,000–3,000 μg of Vitamin B-12 is stored in the liver with a total body storage pool of 3,000–5,000 μg in adults. A dietary deficiency of Vitamin B-12 is extremely rare. The daily requirement of Vitamin B-12 is approximately 2–5 μg/day. Therefore, it would take 2–5 years of a strict vegetarian diet to produce a clinical deficiency.

A Vitamin B-12 deficiency occurs primarily in elderly persons with pernicious anemia, and following a total gastrectomy because of absent gastric-intrinsic factor (*see* Figure 22-4). Histolog achlorhydria is an integral part of a diagnosis of pernicious anemia. A Vitamin B-12 deficiency occasionally occurs in patients with hypo- or achlorhydria after a partial gastrectomy, vagotomy with gastroenterostomy, or chronic gastritis due to insufficient gastric se-

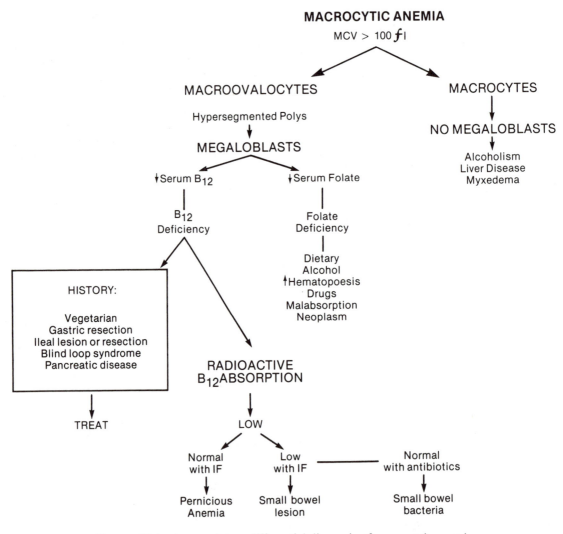

FIGURE 22-4   Approach to a differential diagnosis of macrocytic anemia.

cretions to liberate Vitamin B-12 from food.[36] Under these circumstances, orally administered radioactive Vitamin B-12 normally is absorbed from the gastrointestinal tract, thus yielding a normal Schilling test. Obviously, the removal of ileal receptors through a surgical resection of the ileum or ileal disease (regional ileitis) will cause a malabsorption of Vitamin B-12. Rarely, the absorption of Vitamin B-12 is compromised with severe pancreatic insufficiency due to absent pancreatic enzymes, which are required to liberate Vitamin B-12 from R-protein. Intestinal bacteria in the blind loop syndrome consume Vitamin B-12, thereby producing a deficiency.

Both Folate and Vitamin B-12 share a biochemical relationship that leads to the eventual synthesis of nuclear DNA. The interaction of Vitamin B-12 with 5-methyltetrahydrofolate results in a 5,10 methylene derivative of tetrahydrofolate, which is a coenzyme that with thymidylate synthetase forms thymidylate (an essential component of DNA). A deficiency of either folate or Vitamin B-12 impairs DNA synthesis, thereby producing immature nuclei and larger cells or megaloblasts. Some cells mature to form abnormal macrocytic erythrocytes with a shortened life span. Many megaloblasts hemolyse or die within the bone marrow, which is a condition termed ineffective erythropoiesis. Anemia with reticulocytopenia reflects functionally defective bone marrow.

Several laboratory features are common to Vitamin B-12 and folate deficiencies. Characteristically, macro-ovalocytosis of red blood cells, hypersegmented neutrophils on the peripheral blood smear, a mean corpuscular volume greater than 100 fl, thrombocytopenia, leukopenia, and bone marrow megaloblastosis are all observed. An increased serum lactate dehydrogenase, serum bilirubin, serum iron level, and iron stores are related to an ineffective erythropoiesis. Measurement of serum Vitamin B-12 and folate distinguish these deficiencies (see Figure 22-4).

Several cobalamin (Vitamin B-12) radioassay kits for measuring serum Vitamin B-12 contain non-specific R-proteins, which bind both metabolically active and inactive forms of the vitamin. This yields falsely normal results in patients who are actually Vitamin B-12 deficient.[37–41] Kits that contain only intrinsic factor that specifically bind to active Vitamin B-12 are more reliable. A Schilling test may clarify the issue if the possibility of a Vitamin B-12 deficiency clinically exists despite a normal serum Vitamin B-12 radioassay level. The Schilling test may confirm a Vitamin B-12 deficiency, as well as ascertain the cause of the deficiency (see Figure 22-4). Additionally, some clinical characteristics of a Vitamin B-12 deficiency separate it from a folate deficiency. These include a neuropathy, a family history of pernicious anemia or thyroid disease, and a response to physiologic doses of Vitamin B-12. Conversely, a folate deficiency is observed in elderly people whose diet lacks fresh vegetables and fruit, or in an alcoholic person; it responds to physiologic doses (200–400 μg/day) of folate. A low serum folic-acid level occurs in approximately 2 weeks and a megaloblastic anemia develops in about 4 months, if a subject who receives a normal folate diet is changed to a deficient intake of folic acid. Elderly persons with a loss of appetite due to illness, drugs, or depression often have a low serum folate level (<3 ng/ml) early in their hospitalization. A deficient diet may be too recent an onset to produce anemia, and the red blood cell folate level still will be normal. In this situation, if an adequate diet is administered, the serum folate quickly rises to a normal level. A dietary deficiency of sufficient duration to produce anemia will generate a reduced red blood cell folate level in addition to a low serum folate. Because serum folate levels can quickly become normal with an adequate diet, red blood cell folate is a better index of tissue folate stores. Although the red blood cell folate provides a better assessment of tissue folate coenzymes, most clinicians still rely on the serum folate determination and the clinical setting. When interpreting red blood cell folate levels, a clinician must be aware that Vitamin B-12 facilitates the entry of folic acid into cells. Therefore, in a typical Vitamin B-12 deficiency, the serum Vitamin B-12 level is low, the red blood cell folate is low, but the serum folate is normal or elevated.

Neurologic and psychiatric symptoms are a consequence of a Vitamin B-12 deficiency. The severity of the anemia does not correlate with the gravity of neurologic abnormalities.[42] Neurologic findings occur in about 50% of all patients and include a symmetrical peripheral neuropathy that progresses to posterior and lateral spinal column lesions. Paresthesias, muscle weakness, and impaired vibratory and proprioceptive sensation are all characteristic of a peripheral neuropathy or posterior column spinal cord involvement; spastic movements are the result of lateral column spinal cord lesions. Less well known are the mental changes with irritability, memory disturbance, depression, fluctuations in mood, and psychotic symptoms. Psychiatric symptoms, especially personality changes, dementia, depression, and confusion respond partially or completely to Vitamin B-12 therapy.[43] However, a Vitamin B-12 deficiency may coexist with an Alzheimer's type (SDAT) or multi-infarct dementia. Vitamin B-12 therapy may improve metabolic abnormalities and anemia, which may alleviate some of the manifestations of dementia. However, it cannot be expected to reverse the underlying dementia. All patients with a Vitamin B-12 deficiency must be treated, since it is impossible to predict which neurologic or psychiatric symptoms will respond. A clinician must be aware that neurologic and psychiatric manifestations of a Vitamin B-12 deficiency sometimes occur in patients with normal peripheral blood counts and a normal bone marrow morphology.[44–46] The diagnosis in this unusual circumstance is confirmed by a low serum Vitamin B-12 level and an inability to absorb radiolabelled Vitamin B-12.

Peripheral neuropathy in an alcoholic with a folate deficiency is one condition in which neuropathy and folate deficiency occur together. Folate deficiency itself does not cause neuropathy. The relationship of folate deficiency to psychiatric syndromes is unclear. Folic acid deficiency has been associated with a number of psychiatric syndromes, notably dementia and depression in elderly persons.[42,47,48] It is probable, however, that anorexia and bizarre eating habits of patients with these disorders may cause a folate deficiency. Conversely, insomnia, memory loss, and irritability occur on a folate-deficient diet.[49] Also, folate deficiency has been implicated as a cause of depression by altering the synthesis of dopamine and 5-hydroxytryptamine.[48] This relationship needs further clarification. There is more uncertainty about folate deficiency itself causing dementia. There are a few documented reports of a dramatic improvement of dementia and megaloblastic anemia with folate therapy, but it is so uncommon that a clinician should remain skeptical.

A specific diagnosis is essential for correct treatment. Folic acid therapy that is administered to a patient with a Vitamin B-12 deficiency will produce a hematologic remission, but it may coincidently initiate progressive and often irreversible neuropathy or worsen an existing neuropathy. The progression of the neurologic abnormality is arrested with adequate B-12 treatment. Mild sensory changes usually clear up, severe ones only may improve, symptoms present for several months are less likely to respond, and extensive neurologic disabilities tend to leave residual defects. A response to therapy may require several months; lesions persisting after 10–12 months usually are permanent.[50] A Vitamin B-12 deficiency is treated with either hydroxocobalamin or cyanocobalamin. The initial therapy consists of 1,000 μg injected intramuscularly every 2–3 days for six injections. Hydroxocobalamin maintenance therapy of 500–1,000 μg is administered intramuscularly every 3 months. If cyanocobalamin is used, a maintenance therapy of 500–1,000 μg/month is administered intramuscularly because of the greater urinary excretion of cyanocobalamin than hydroxocobalamin. On occasion, urgent treatment with both folic acid and Vitamin B-12 is indicated before establishing the specific deficiency that is responsible. In this event, a blood specimen is drawn for serum assays of both folate and Vitamin B-12, and the appropriate specific therapy is continued depending on the results of the serum assay. Patients who have had a gastrectomy or ileal resection should receive 1,000 μg of hydroxocobalamin every 3 months as preventive therapy.

An oral dose of 1 mg/day of folic acid is sufficient therapy for a folate deficiency. The length of therapy depends on the underlying cause, but it usually is 4 months. Attention to improving the diet with foods that contain folate often is an important consideration for elderly persons.

The characteristic response to either Vitamin B-12 or folate therapy after the initial reticulocytosis is an increased neutrophil and platelet count within 5–10 days. The bone marrow transforms from a megaloblastic to a normoblastic morphology in 48–72 hours. A reduction in serum iron to a low value occurs in 4–5 days, but there is a subsequent rise to normal levels within a few weeks unless a concomitant iron deficiency exists. Serum bilirubin and serum lactate dehydrogenase levels return to normal in 1–3 weeks. A clinician should anticipate the possibility of hypokalemia after therapy is started. Although it is a rare complication, hypokalemia can be fatal, which is a situation that never should be allowed to occur because it is preventable.

The life expectancy of treated megaloblastic anemia is related to the underlying disorder.[50] The incidence of a gastric carcinoma is two to three times greater in patients with pernicious anemia. Periodic screening studies of patients with pernicious anemia for gastric carcinoma have not yet proved to be effective.[50]

Acute Leukemia

Acute non-lymphocytic leukemia (myeloblastic) is predominantly a disease of elderly persons; 70% of all patients are over 50 years of age. Acute leukemia in older patients once was considered refractory to therapy with a poor prognosis. It was felt that older people fared poorly due to a bone marrow aplasia that complicated therapy. However, evidence is mounting that older patients respond to intensive chemotherapy as well as young adults.[51,52] Recently, complete remissions have been achieved in greater than 60% of all patients. Yet, there still is controversy about elderly patients receiving intensive chemotherapy because of the risk, with these drugs, of bleeding and serious infections that are related to drastic reductions in neutrophils and platelets. However, there also is evidence that patients over 60 years of age are at no greater risk than younger patients of death by infection.[51,53]

Clinical manifestations often differ in elderly persons. An abrupt onset is characteristic in a young adult, whereas a preleukemic phase introduces the disease in 30% of all elderly patients. Elderly patients have non-specific complaints of malaise, anorexia, weight loss, and weakness. Fatigue due to anemia, bleeding and bruising from thrombocytopenia or a dissemi-

nated intravascular coagulopathy, fever due to infection, bone and joint pain, lymphadenopathy, and central nervous system symptoms from a meningeal infiltration, are all part of the clinical inventory of this disorder. Infection is a common serious complication of leukemia and chemotherapy. Neutropenia that is caused by leukemia or its treatment induces a susceptibility to infection. The emergence of an unexplained fever (over 38.5°C) in a patient with less than 1,000 neutrophils/mm^3 must be managed as life threatening.

Anemia, thrombocytopenia, and granulocytopenia with myeloblasts, monoblasts, or both, are typical blood findings. A hypercellular marrow that is composed of myeloblasts, monocytoid features of granulocytic cells, and (occasionally) megaloblastic features of erythroid cells and atypical megakaryocytes, are prominent features.

If untreated, the mean duration from the onset of symptoms to death is less than 6 months. A complete remission in elderly patients occurs less frequently than in younger patients, and there has been no consensus about the treatment of older patients. Recent reports are more encouraging, with remission rates of 60–80% with intensive chemotherapy.[51,52,54,55] One study indicates that older patients have responses similarly to younger patients to intensive chemotherapy.[52] A 76%-remission rate with a 14-month mean remission and 22-month survival rate in patients over 60 years of age was comparable to the results achieved in a younger group.[52] Age, therefore, is not a contraindication to intensive chemotherapy for patients with acute leukemia. There is evidence that patients have remained in remission for 5 years or longer.

Judgment about who shall be treated should not be based on age alone. The guiding premise is that acute leukemia without treatment is uniformly fatal and, therefore, that the patient is entitled to aggressive therapy regardless of age. Yet, a patient with severe physical and mental impairment perhaps should not be exposed to the added risks of chemotherapy. A carefully considered ethical analysis should be made (see Volume II, Chap 11). With older patients, it is as important to know when not to treat as when to treat. Clear examples prevail at either end of the spectrum, but there continues to be a troubling gray zone where better criteria are needed to help a clinician make decisions.

"Smouldering" leukemia in elderly patients is distinguished by mildly elevated white blood cell counts, few myeloblasts, and anemia. There is a risk of infection or hemorrhage. The progression over several years is slow and requires supportive treatment for complications, but no chemotherapy. Eventual progression to an acute stage, however, becomes an indication for antileukemic therapy.

TABLE 22-1   Revised Prognostic Staging of Chronic Lymphocytic Leukemia[57]

Clinical stage A
<3 areas of lymphoid enlargement*
Clinical stage B
3 or >3 areas of lymphoid enlargement*
Clinical stage C
Hb ≤10 g/dl
Thrombocytes ≤100,000/mm^3
Any lymph node enlargement*

* Five areas: liver, spleen, cervical, axillary, and inguinal nodes.

Chronic Lymphocytic Leukemia (CLL)

This is the most common leukemia found in elderly persons, with over 80% of all diagnoses occurring in patients over 50 years of age. It is characterized by the malignant proliferation of monoclonal lymphocytes (usually of B-cell origin) in the bone marrow, peripheral blood, lymph nodes, spleen, liver, and sometimes in other organs. The course of this disease is variable; some patients are asymptomatic with mildly or moderately elevated lymphocyte blood counts that persist for many years, while other patients follow an aggressive course with a lymphocytic replacement of normal marrow cells with a resultant anemia, thrombocytopenia, and neutropenia. Usually, protean symptoms correlate with an adenopathy, splenomegaly, and high lymphocyte counts. Therefore, chronic lymphocytic leukemia (CLL) no longer can be viewed as an indolent disease and ignored by clinicians.

Classification systems have been designed to aid in the prognosis and to allow a better comparison of therapeutic trials. The most widely used is the Rai classification.[56] A new clinical classification system has been proposed[57] to include isolated organomegaly and to simplify the approach to estimating a prognosis of patients (see Table 22-1). A single median survival statistic for a disease with such a varied course is no longer meaningful or useful. Clinical and laboratory abnormalities can be attributed to cytopenia and to immunologic deficiencies.

Susceptibility to infection is due to granulocytopenia, poor cellular immune responses, and hypogammaglobulinemia. Anemia and thrombocytopenia are a consequence of bone marrow replacement with leukemia cells, hypersplenism, or chemotherapy. In those occasional patients who have autoimmune hemolytic anemia and/or thrombocytopenia, corticosteroid therapy achieves good results. The incidence of a second primary neoplasm is high in patients with CLL. These include skin cancers, colorectal cancers, lung cancer, and multiple myelomas.

No therapy is indicated for the asymptomatic patient with the benign form of CLL. This is a very slow, progressive disorder, and patients often die of unrelated causes. However, therapy is used during symptomatic or advancing periods of the illness when infections, anemia, lymphadenopathy, and splenomegaly become part of the clinical picture. Symptomatic patients usually are given alkylating agents such as chlorambucil or cyclophosphamide, which are effective in reducing blood counts and shrinking lymphoadenopathy, splenomegaly, and hepatomegaly. Chlorambucil is the most popular agent used. Prednisone, used with an alkylating agent, is beneficial for cytopenias, but it also is superior to chlorambucil alone. A three-drug regimen that consists of cyclophosphamide, vincristine, and prednisone or a five-drug regimen that adds melphalan and carmustine [(1,3-bis-2-chloroethyl-Imitrosourein)] BCNU, both are being evaluated for a more aggressive disease (stage III or IV). The latter regimen also has been used for treating multiple myeloma, which is another slow-growth lymphoproliferative disorder. Allopurinol and adequate hydration are essential during chemotherapy or radiotherapy to prevent uric acid stones and nephropathy from excessive uric acid that is liberated as a result of cell destruction. Radiation therapy is suitable for bulky adenopathy or is indicated for a localized lymphocytic infiltration that causes a ureteral, bile duct, or bronchial obstruction. Leukapheresis to remove lymphocytes from the circulation is suitable for management of selected patients with significant anemia and thrombocytopenia.[58] None of the present-day treatments cure this disease. Patients with anemia and thrombocytopenia have the worst prognosis, with a median survival of 2 years. Patients with three or more involved areas, but without anemia or thrombocytopenia, have a median survival of approximately 7 years. Those patients with less involvement (clinical stage IV) have survival rates similar to the general population.

Multiple Myeloma

With increasing numbers of older people and better methods of diagnosis, the incidence of plasma cell myeloma is increasing. It usually appears in persons over 50 years of age with over 50% of all cases after age 70. Plasma cell myeloma is the consequence of a selective proliferation of a single clone of plasma cells. The growth rate of malignant plasma cells is slow, with a doubling time of approximately 4 months. A specific immunoglobulin that is produced by these cells is a measure of the size of the myeloma cell mass.[59] When the tumor size reaches 10^{11} cells, this monoclonal protein is seen as a spike on a serum protein electrophoresis. Clinical symptoms usually appear with a cellular mass of approximately 0.5×10^{12} myeloma cells. IgG is the most common myeloma protein; it occurs in 60% of all myeloma patients. Light-chain and IgA myeloma occur with a similar frequency of approximately 20%, and the more uncommon varieties, IgD and IgE, occur with approximately 1% each. A light-chain myeloma produces a diagnostic combination of light chains in the urine and hypogammaglobulinemia.

The major features of a myeloma are: 1) Mature and immature plasma cells in the bone marrow; 2) A monoclonal gammopathy in serum that produces the so-called monoclonal spike on a serum electrophoresis; and 3) Light chains excreted in the urine, osteolytic lesions, hypercalcemia, anemia, and azotemia. A bone marrow examination reveals an increase in plasma cells that are either immature or mature forms, or both. A helpful diagnostic clue is the presence of multinucleated plasma cells. The distri-

bution of these cells is spotty, with sheets of plasma cells appearing only in some areas. Other areas may appear normal; therefore, a single normal marrow study does not rule out a diagnosis. Marrow infiltration by myeloma cells replaces normal cells, which sometimes produces a pancytopenia. Bone pain is the most prominent symptom due to either osteolytic lesions or osteoporosis, or both. Osteoporosis may be the only bone lesion in 25% of all cases. The abnormal plasma cells produce an osteoclastic-activating factor that causes bone resorption and hypercalcemia.[60] Osteoporosis and anemia due to causes other than myeloma are frequent in elderly persons; nonetheless, myeloma should be suspected in an elderly patient with bone pain who has unexplained anemia, particularly with a rouleaux formation on the peripheral blood smear. A diagnosis may be further advanced by an elevated serum protein level on a laboratory screening examination. An elderly patient with renal insufficiency and an elevated serum protein level is likely to have multiple myeloma. Sulfosalicylic acid and p-toluene sulfonic acid are good screening methods for Bence-Jones (light chains) proteinuria. The routine analysis of urine and dip-stick methods will not detect Bence-Jones proteinuria. An electrophoresis and immunoelectrophoresis of concentrated urine will confirm light-chain proteins.

Renal failure is a significant, negative prognostic feature that is second only to infection as a cause of death. Acute renal failure (ARF) due to intravenous pyelography (IVP), hypercalcemia, dehydration, antibiotics, or sepsis is preventable under careful management. Other forms of renal disease in myeloma, such as tubular destruction secondary to light-chain proteinuria, plasma cell infiltration of the kidneys, pyelonephritis, and amyloidosis are discussed in Chapter 16. A urate nephropathy due to hyperuricemia, especially when initiating treatment of a myeloma, should be anticipated and prevented by adequate hydration and allopurinol therapy.

Pneumonia and urinary tract infections are common and should be promptly diagnosed and treated. Decreased levels of normal immunoglobulins with consequent decreased circulating antibody levels, poor antibody responses to antigenic challenges, increased immunoglobulin turnover, cellular anergy, and granulocytopenia with an impaired migration of granulocytes and decreased opsonic activity, are all responsible for an increased susceptibility and poor response to infection.[61]

An untreated plasma cell myeloma pursues an inexorable downhill course with a mean survival of 7 months from the time of diagnosis. Chemotherapy has extended the survival time to 23–40 months in 50–70% of all patients. Elderly patients respond well to melphalan (Alkeran) and prednisone without excessive toxicity. Chemotherapy reduces the tumor cell mass, which can be monitored by a decrease in the amount of monoclonal gammopathy. Prednisone decreases Bence-Jones proteinuria synthesis[62] and inhibits the production of the osteoclast-activating factor, thereby reducing bone loss and ameliorating hypercalcemia. Patients who fail to respond may improve with more aggressive regimens of various combinations of adriamycin and lomustine [CCNU (1-2-chloroethyl 3-cyclohexyl-1-nitrosoureais)], BCNU, cyclophosphamide, melphalan, or vincristine.[63] A more aggressive approach may be effective for patients with a high tumor burden who have the worst prognosis. Several risk factors have been correlated with a poor prognosis, including a high myeloma cell mass, infection, and renal failure. Laboratory indicators that correlate with a high myeloma cell mass are hemoglobin levels <8.5 grams/dl or serum calcium levels >12 grams.[64] Highly significant differences in the survival of patients with low, intermediate, or high tumor cell masses have been shown.

Tumor compression of the spinal cord by an epidural plasmacytoma or a pathologic fracture of a vertebral body constitutes an emergency that requires a prompt diagnosis and treatment.[65] A decompressing laminectomy followed by localized radiotherapy generally has been advocated, although recently localized radiotherapy alone has been observed to be equally effective.[66]

Asymptomatic patients with a low myeloma cell mass have an indolent course. In this case, patients show evidence of a bone marrow plasmacytosis, a monoclonal serum spike, and less than three lytic bone lesions. There usually is a notable absence of bone pain with recurrent infections or hypercalcemia.[67,68] These patients often are diagnosed by screening tests for unrelated disorders and should be followed closely but not treated. Some patients will remain asymptomatic for several years before they eventually require therapy. Localized radiotherapy is effective for the relief of localized pain that is caused by myeloma lesions, and for localized tumors that are composed of plasma cells (plasmacytoma). Over a period of several years (median time 8 years), a localized myeloma usually evolves to a generalized disease with marrow plasmacytosis, monoclonal gammopathy, and osteolytic lesions.[68]

Other Monoclonal Gammopathies

A monoclonal spike on a serum electrophoresis does not always indicate myeloma. An unexplained monoclonal gammopathy (M-spike), noted on an electrophoresis of serum and urine uncovered after a routine examination of an elderly patient, raises possibilities of multiple myeloma, benign monoclonal gammopathy, amyloidosis, lymphoproliferative disorders such as Waldenstrom's macroglobulinemia, CLL heavy-chain diseases, cancer (especially prostate, rectosigmoid, and breast carcinomas), and chronic inflammatory diseases. A benign monoclonal gammopathy is not unusual in an elderly patient; its incidence increases with age and occurs in 1% of all patients over 50 years of age, 3% of all apparently healthy persons over 70 years of age, and up to 19% in persons older than 90 years of age. A benign, idiopathic monoclonal gammopathy is characterized by an M-spike less than 3.0 grams/dl, the absence of Bence-Jones proteinuria, and no apparent lytic bone lesions. There usually is less than a 20% marrow plasmacytosis. A clinician should continue to observe these patients, since some will develop myeloma. Approximately 10% of these cases evolve into a myeloma or other lymphoproliferative disease within 5 years. A progressive increase in the serum monoclonal component usually leads to an ultimate identification of a malignant gammopathy.

Waldenstrom's macroglobulinemia, which is a lymphoproliferative disease of elderly persons, is characterized by a monoclonal component of the IgM type. A hyperviscosity syndrome is a common complication of this disorder and it produces mucosal bleeding, dilation of retinal veins, retinal hemorrhages, loss of vision, impaired hearing, congestive heart failure, headache, dizziness, and coma. Bleeding may occur from the nose, mouth, gums, gastrointestinal tract, or genitourinary tract. Cells with characteristics of both plasma cells and lymphocytes are observed on a bone marrow examination. Most patients are symptomatic at a serum viscosity level greater than 4.[69,70] Plasmapheresis quickly and effectively reverses the symptoms and chemotherapy reduces the cellular infiltrate, which inhibits further production of the monoclonal protein.

Myeloproliferative Disorders

Myeloproliferative disorders encompass several chronic conditions (such as chronic granulocytic leukemia, agnogenic myeloid metaplasia, polycythemia vera, and essential thrombocythemia) as well as acute disorders (such as acute myeloblastic leukemia and erythroleukemia [Di Guglielmo's disease]). Many of the chronic disorders undergo a blast crisis thereby terminating as an acute myeloblastic leukemia. These disorders are characterized by a marrow proliferation of erythroid cells, granulocytes, megakaryocytes, fibroblasts, and osteoblasts. Extramedullary sites such as the spleen, liver or lymph nodes also may contain these cells.

Agnogenic Myeloid Metaplasia (AMM)

This disorder, usually seen in elderly persons, is due to a clonal proliferation of cells in the spleen, liver, and lymph nodes, which produces a characteristic extramedullary hematopoiesis. Cells in these areas resemble bone marrow. A grossly enlarged, firm spleen and abnormal peripheral blood findings are major clues to this diagnosis. The peripheral blood smear shows leukoerythroblastic features, with teardrop-shaped red blood cells, nucleated red blood cells, immature granulocytes, and large bizarre platelets. The white blood cell count frequently is elevated and may suggest chronic granulocytic leukemia. However, it usually is not as high in agnogenic myeloid metaplasia (AMM); it usually is $<30,000/mm^3$ and rarely reaches $100,000/mm^3$. With white blood cell counts $>60,000/mm^3$, the clinician would tend to favor

chronic granulocytic leukemia as a diagnosis. In contrast to chronic granulocytic leukemia with its usually low leukocyte alkaline phosphatase (LAP) scores, LAP is normal or elevated in AMM. Platelet counts may be normal, low, or high. Bone marrow is difficult to obtain and often yields dry taps on aspiration. A bone marrow biopsy specimen shows fibrosis.

Symptoms stem from anemia, thrombocytopenia, an enlarged spleen, or splenic infarcts. Weight loss, sweating, and a low-grade fever are hypermetabolic symptoms of this disorder. Gout occurs from hyperuricemia that is secondary to an increased cell turnover.

The mean life expectancy after diagnosis is 4–5 years. Death usually is due to complications such as infection, hemorrhage, thrombosis, or portal hypertension. AMM may eventuate in a blast crisis which is a transition to acute myeloblastic leukemia. This usually is unresponsive to treatment in elderly persons.

A leukoerythroblastic blood picture also may be found with chronic granulocytic leukemia and metastatic carcinoma. The absence of teardrop poikilocytes, increased basophils and eosinophils on the peripheral blood smear, a low leukocyte alkaline phosphatase score, a hypercellular bone marrow, and the presence of the Ph[1] (Philadelphia) chromosome, all favor chronic granulocytic leukemia. The finding of carcinoma cells on a marrow smear or biopsy specimen ensures that diagnosis.

Anemia associated with AMM may require transfusions. Androgens generally have been ineffective and have many adverse side effects, such as cholestatic hepatitis, edema, and virilization in females. About 29% of all patients on fluoxymesterone therapy have a rise in hemoglobin levels, but their survival expectancy is not changed.[71] Pyridoxine, 250 mg/day, has increased hemoglobin levels in a small number of patients.

Patients with chronic myeloproliferative disorders such as polycythemia vera, chronic granulocytic leukemia, AMM, or an essential thrombocythemia with thrombocytosis (especially platelet counts >1 million/mm^3) are regarded at risk for bleeding or thrombosis. Aspirin and other antiplatelet agents have been used to treat the hypercoagulable state that is due to thrombocytosis.[72] Chemotherapy or ^{32}P decreases platelets and often reduces the splenic size. In a recent study, however, only a few patients with thrombocytosis had bleeding episodes that usually were from the gastrointestinal tract and nearly always with concomitant use of anti-inflammatory agents.[73] Moreover, thrombosis was confined to patients with polycythemia vera who had an associated erythrocytosis. This study, therefore, suggests that aggressive reduction of the platelet count may not be indicated in asymptomatic patients, but it should be reserved for symptomatic patients and possibly for preoperative situations.

Splenectomy is reserved for patients with hemolytic anemia and/or thrombocytopenia that are refractory to medical treatment, splenic infarcts, symptoms due to a massive splenomegaly, and portal hypertension with bleeding.[74]

Chronic Granulocytic Leukemia

Chronic granulocytic leukemia is predominantly a disease of middle age, with the greatest prevalence between the 3rd and 6th decades. However, it recently has been observed that nearly one third of all patients with chronic granulocytic leukemia are over 60 years of age.[75] The incidence sharply diminished after 70 years of age. Some patients are asymptomatic and are discovered inadvertently because of changes in the peripheral blood (i.e., a slightly increased leukocyte count, lymphopenia, a few metamyelocytes and myelocytes, and increased numbers of basophils and eosinophils). Leukocyte alkaline phosphatase (LAP) activity is markedly diminished, and cytogenetic studies reveal the presence of the Ph[1] chromosome. Most patients present with a low-grade fever, fatigue, weight loss, and (occasionally) night sweats. Enlargement of the spleen is prominent in most patients. This is accompanied by laboratory findings of anemia, normal or increased platelets, and a leukocytosis of 20–50,000/mm^3. The peripheral blood smear is characterized by the presence of metamyelocytes, myelocytes, basophilia and (often) eosinophilia. A low or absent LAP is found in the majority of patients, and the Ph[1] chromosome is present in 80–90% of all cases.

Treatment with alkylating agents or ^{32}P have produced remissions in nearly all patients. The length of survival is variable with a median of 3 years. Older patients lacking the Ph[1] chromosome have a shorter survival than Ph[1]-positive patients.[76] Radiotherapy to the spleen is less effective than chemotherapy. Combination chemotherapy with a splenectomy has been attempted to eradicate the Ph[1]-positive clones, but it has not been accepted as a significant improvement in the treatment of chronic granulocytic leukemia.

The transformation from chronic granulocytic leukemia to an acute leukemia (blast crisis) occurs in over 80% of affected patients.[75] It is more common in patients who lack the Ph[1] chromosome.[75] Weakness, fatigue, and an increasing splenomegaly accompanied by anemia, thrombocytopenia, myelofibrosis, and an increasing LAP, are the most prominent features. The blast transformation is most often myeloblastic, but lymphoblastic transformation has been reported. The treatment of a blast crisis generally has been ineffective.

Erythrocytosis

Polycythemia vera, secondary erythrocytosis, and relative erythrocytosis are characterized by an elevated red blood cell count, hemoglobin and hematocrit values. The elevated hematocrit value produces an increased blood viscosity and (consequently) decreased cerebral blood flow, which results in symptoms common to these three groups of disorders (*see* Figure 22-5).[77–80]

In relative erythrocytosis, the elevated hematocrit value is the result of a reduced plasma volume with the red blood cell volume remaining normal. Circumstances that lead to dehydration in an elderly person are most often responsible. The underlying clinical condition that causes the dehydration must be ascertained to resolve the problem.

The demonstration of an increased red blood cell volume with ^{51}Chromium-labelled red blood cells is essential to establish absolute erythrocytosis. Polycythemia vera and erythropoietin-producing disorders (secondary erythrocytosis) are the two major categories of absolute erythrocytosis (*see* Figure 22-6). Secondary types, of which there are many causes, are more common than polycythemia vera and involve only erythropoiesis. Polycythemia vera is believed to be a clonal proliferation of the

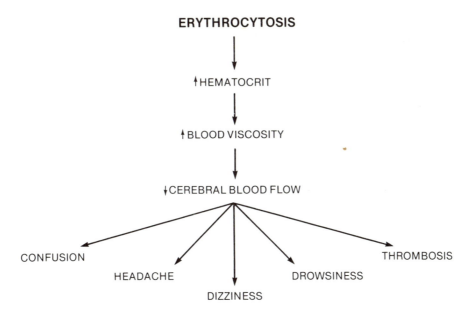

FIGURE 22-5 Symptoms related to erythrocytosis.

pluripotential stem cell,[81] and it is distinguished by hyperplasia of the bone marrow with increased numbers of circulating erythrocytes, granulocytes, and platelets.

Before initiating an extensive diagnostic evaluation to uncover the cause of an increased hematocrit level, a history of cigarette smoking should be sought. In cigarette smokers, the residual carbon monoxide binds to hemoglobin and forms carboxyhemoglobin, which consequently does not bind oxygen. Sequentially, tissue hypoxia stimulates erythropoietin, which ultimately produces an increased hematocrit level. Additionally, cigarette smoking reduces plasma volume, thereby accentuating the increased hematocrit level. If cigarette smoking is not the cause, a logical strategy of study is shown in Figure 22-7. An arterial oxygen saturation <92% warrants an investigation of pulmonary and cardiac causes. If the arterial oxygen saturation is >92%, a search for causes of inappropriately increased erythropoietin is indicated. These are renal parenchymal diseases, tumors, cysts, hydronephrosis, or paraneoplas-

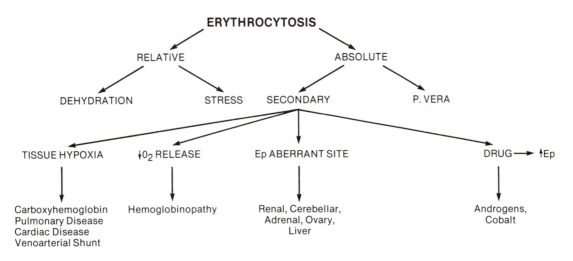

FIGURE 22-6 Causes of erythrocytosis. Ep = erythropoietin.

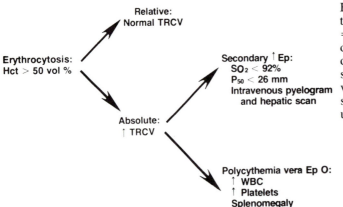

FIGURE 22-7   Evaluation of erythrocytosis. TRCV = total red cell volume; Ep = erythropoietin; SO_2 = arterial blood oxygen saturation; P_{50} = partial pressure of oxygen at which hemoglobin is 50% saturated. (Walsh JR: Polycythemic vera: Diagnosis, treatment and relationship to leukemia. *Geriatrics* 33:61, 1978, used by permission.)

tic syndromes related to the liver, ovaries, adrenal gland, and cerebellar tumors. Rarely, an elderly person may have an abnormal hemoglobin that has an increased affinity for oxygen, which leads to tissue hypoxia, increased erythropoietin production, and (finally) erythrocytosis.

In early stages of polycythemia vera, an erythrocytosis may be the only clinical finding. The erythrocytosis is autonomous and not dependent on erythropoietin; therefore, erythropoietin levels are low to absent in polycythemia vera. Diagnosis is straightforward, if erythrocytosis is accompanied by leukocytosis, thrombocytosis, and/or splenomegaly.

The management of a patient with erythrocytosis is directed at treating the underlying cause. Discontinuation of smoking, oxygen therapy for chronic lung disease, and weight reduction for obesity are important considerations to correct erythrocytosis for these respective disorders. Phlebotomy therapy is considered for all forms of erythrocytosis that have not responded to treatment of the underlying cause, including relative erythrocytosis. There is considerable evidence that the level of the packed cell volume (hematocrit) influences the blood flow through tissue. A high venous hematocrit level produces an increased blood viscosity and, consequently, a reduced cerebral blood flow.[77–80] Cerebral blood flow diminishes in patients with a hematocrit level of 60%, and there is an associated greater risk of a thromboembolism. High hematocrit levels that are associated with a low cerebral blood flow presumably predispose to transient ischemic attacks (TIA) and stroke. Phlebotomy therapy produces a significant reduction of whole blood vis-

cosity when the hematocrit level is reduced to below 45%, thereby allowing the cerebral blood flow to become normal.[77–80,82] This approach is appropriate even for an elderly patient with a modest hematocrit elevation, if the treating clinician is concerned about the risk of cerebrovascular disease.[80] It has been suggested that reduced blood flow from increased blood viscosity that is associated with a high hematocrit level adversely affects the collateral blood flow, thereby increasing the size of the infarct.[83] Interestingly, even patients with relative polycythemia have an increased incidence of vascular disease and, therefore, are good candidates for such therapy.[80] The increase in cerebral blood flow after phlebotomy more than compensates for the calculated decrease in the oxygen-carrying capacity of the blood. This is especially pertinent when considering the effectiveness of this form of therapy in patients with chronic hypoxic lung disease. Until recently, the elevated red blood cell volume has been regarded as a compensatory mechanism designed to raise arterial oxygen capacity and, therefore, therapy to lower it has been considered inappropriate. Nonetheless, at a certain point (approximately 55% Hct), tissue oxygen delivery is compromised more by an increased viscosity; lowering the hematocrit level has been clinically effective in improving the blood flow. Recent studies of patients with erythrocytosis that is secondary to a chronic obstructive lung disease have shown that improving the cerebral blood flow by lowering blood viscosity with phlebotomy therapy results in a resolution of confusion, headaches, dizziness, lethargy, and drowsiness.[78,79] While a reduction of blood viscosity has shown an improved cerebral circulation, a similar reduction of hyperviscosity in the peripheral circulation reveals conflicting results.[84] Further evidence, therefore, is needed before recommending phlebotomy therapy for treating intermittent claudication.

There are three modalities used for the treatment of polycythemia vera: phlebotomy alone, ^{32}P, or chemotherapy. Treatment with ^{32}P or chemotherapy should await a definitive diagnosis. Phlebotomy therapy is initiated early for those patients who have an uncomplicated erythrocytosis. Myelosuppression with ^{32}P or chemotherapy is indicated for patients who require frequent phlebotomies, older patients who tolerate repeated phlebotomies poorly, or patients with platelet counts greater than 1 million/mm[3], patients with intractable pruritis, a symptomatic splenomegaly, or symptoms associated with hypermetabolism. The treatment of choice is ^{32}P since the polycythemia vera study group recently has reported a higher incidence of acute leukemia in chlorambucil-treated patients than in patients treated with phlebotomy or ^{32}P therapy.[85]

References

1. Hto MSH, Kofkoff RL, Freedman ML: Erythrocyte parameters in the elderly: An argument against new geriatric normal values. *J Am Geriatr Soc* 27:547–551, 1979.
2. Lipschitz DA, Mitchell CO, Thompson C: The anemia of senescence. *Am J Hematol* 11:47–54, 1981.
3. Marx JJM: Normal iron absorption and decreased red cell iron uptake in the aged. *Blood* 53:204–211, 1979.
4. Hartsock RJ, Smith EB, Petty CS: Normal variations with aging of the amount of hematopoietic tissue in bone marrow from the anterior iliac crest. *Am J Clin Path* 326–331, 1965.
5. Harrison DE: Defective erythropoietic responses of aged mice not improved by young marrow. *J Gerontol* 30:286–288, 1975.
6. Finch CA, Miller LR, Inamdar AR, et al: Iron deficiency in the rat. Physiological and biochemical studies of muscle dysfunction. *J Clin Invest* 58:447–453, 1976.
7. Ohira Y, Edgerton VR, Gardiner GW, et al: Work capacity, heart rate and blood lactate responses to iron therapy. *Br J Haemat* 41:365–372, 1979.
8. Cook JD, Finch CA, Smith NJ: Evaluation of the iron status of a population. *Blood* 48:449–455, 1976.
9. Casale G, Bonora C, Migliavacca A, et al: Serum ferritin and aging. *Age Ageing* 10:119–122, 1981.
10. Disler PB, Lynch SR, Charlton RW, et al: The effect of tea on iron absorption. *Gut* 16:193–200, 1975.
11. Winawer SJ, Fleisher M: Sensitivity and specificity of the fecal occult blood test for colorectal neoplasia. *Gastroenterology* 82:986–991, 1982.
12. Herzog P, Holtermuller K, Preiss J, et al: Fecal blood loss in patients with colonic polyps: A comparison of measurements with [51]Chromium-labeled erythrocytes and with the hemoccult test. *Gastroenterology* 83:957–962, 1982.
13. Lifton LJ, Kreiser J: False-positive stool occult blood tests caused by iron preparation. *Gastroenterology* 83:860–863, 1982.
14. Jick H, Porter J: Drug-induced gastrointestinal bleeding. *Lancet* 2:87–89, 1978.
15. Fulcher RA, Hyland CM: Effectiveness of once daily oral iron in the elderly. *Age Ageing* 10:44–46, 1981.
16. Hamstra RD, Block MH, Schocket AL: Intravenous iron dextran in clinical medicine. *JAMA* 243:1726–1731, 1980.
17. Shimada A: Adverse reactions to total dose infusion of iron dextran. *Clin Pharm* 1:248–249, 1982.
18. Walsh JR, Fredrickson M: Serum ferritin, free erythrocyte protoporphyrin, and urinary iron excretion in patients with iron disorders. *Am J Med Sci* 273:293–300, 1977.
19. Walsh JR, Cassel CK, Madler JJ: Iron deficiency in the elderly: It's often nondietary. *Geriatrics* 36:121–132, 1981.
20. Cook JD: Clinical evaluations of iron deficiency. *Sem Hematol* 19:6–18, 1982.
21. Cook JD, Skikne BS, Lynch CR: Serum ferritin in the evaluation of anemia, in Albertin (ed): *Radioimmunoassay of Hormones, Protein and Enzymes*. Amsterdam, Excerpta Medica, 1980, pp 239–248.
22. Gokal R, Millard PR, Weatherall DJ, et al: Iron metabolism in haemodialysis patients. *Quart J Med* 48:369–391, 1979.
23. Cartwright GE, Edwards MH, Skolnick RW, et al: Association of HLA-linked hemochromatosis with idiopathic refractory sideroblastic anemia. *J Clin Invest* 65:989–992, 1980.
24. Radtke HW, Claussner A, Erbes PM, et al: Serum erythropoietin concentration in chronic renal failure: Relationship to degree of anemia and excretory renal function. *Blood* 54:877–884, 1979.

25. Wallner SF, Vautrin RM: Evidence that inhibition of erythropoiesis is important in the anemia of chronic renal failure. *J Lab Clin Med* 97:170–178, 1981.

26. Radtke HW, Rege AB, LaMarche MB, et al: Identification of spermine as an inhibitor of erythropoiesis in patients with chronic renal failure. *J Clin Invest* 67:1623–1629, 1981.

27. Rege AB, Moriyama Y, Fisher JW: Characterization of a serum inhibitor of erythropoiesis. *Fed Proc* 1974. 33:597. Abstract.

28. Ohno Y, Rege AB, Fisher JW, et al: Inhibitors of erythroid colony-forming cells (CFU-E and BFU-E) in sera of azotemic patients with anemia of renal disease. *J Lab Clin Med* 92:916–923, 1978.

29. Zappacosta AR, Caro J, Erslev A: Normalization of hematocrit in patients with end-stage renal disease on continuous ambulatory peritoneal dialysis. *Am J Med* 72:53–57, 1982.

30. Neff MS, Goldberg J, Slifkin RF, et al: A comparison of androgens for anemia in patients on hemodialysis. *N Engl J Med* 304:871–875, 1981.

31. Eschback JW, Cook JD, Scribner B, et al: Iron balance in hemodialysis patients. *Ann Int Med* 87:710–713, 1977.

32. Fein HG, Riolin RS: Anemia in thyroid diseases. *Med Clin North Am* 59:1133–1145, 1975.

33. Carmel R, Spencer CA: Clinical and subclinical thyroid disorders associated with pernicious anemia. *Arch Int Med* 142:1465–1469, 1982.

34. Lindenbaum J: Folate and Vitamin B-12 deficiencies in alcoholism. *Semin Hematol* 17:119–129, 1980.

35. Allen RH, Seetharam B, Podell E, et al: Effect of proteolytic enzymes on the binding of cobalamin to R protein and intrinsic factor. *J Clin Invest* 61:47–53, 1978.

36. Lindenbaum J: Aspects of Vitamin B-12 and folate metabolism in malabsorption syndromes. *Am J Med* 67:1037–1048, 1979.

37. Cooper BA, Whitehead VM: Evidence that some patients with pernicious anemia are not recognized by radiodilution assay for cobalamin in serum. *N Engl J Med* 299:816–818, 1978.

38. England JM, Linnell JC: Problems with the serum Vitamin B-12 assay. *Lancet* 2:1072–1074, 1980.

39. Kusbasik NP, Ricotta M, Harrison ES: Commercially-supplied binders for plasma cobalamin (Vitamin B-12) analysis—"purified" intrinsic factor, "cobinamide"—blocked R-protein binder, and non-purified intrinsic factor—R protein binder—compared to microbiological assay. *Clin Chem* 26:598–600, 1980.

40. Mollin DL, Hoffbrand AV, Ward PG, et al: Interlaboratory comparison of serum Vitamin B-12 assay. *J Clin Pathol* 33:243–248, 1980.

41. Dawson DW, Delamore IW, et al: An evaluation of commercial radioisotope methods for the determination of folate and Vitamin B-12. *J Clin Pathol* 33:234–242, 1980.

42. Shorvon SD, Carney MWP, Chanarin I, et al: The neuropsychiatry of megaloblastic anemia. *Br Med J* 281:1036–1038, 1980.

43. Weiger RS: Psychiatric manifestations of hematopoietic system disease, in Levenson AJ, Hall RCW (eds): *Neuropsychiatric Manifestations of Physical Disease in the Elderly (Aging)*. New York, Raven Press, 1981, vol 14, pp 83–92.

44. Victor M, Lear H: Subacute combined degeneration of the spinal cord. Current concepts of the disease process. Value of serum Vitamin B-12 determinations in clarifying some of the common problems. *Am J Med* 20:896–908, 1956.

45. Smith ADM: Megaloblastic madness. *Br Med J* 2:1840–1845, 1960.

46. Strachan RW, Henderson JG: Psychiatric syndromes due to avitaminosis B-12 with normal blood and marrow. *Quart J Med* 34:303–317, 1965.

47. Strachan RW, Henderson JG: Dementia and folate deficiency. *Quart J Med* 36:189–204, 1967.

48. Ghadirian AM, Ananth J, Engelsmann F: Folic acid deficiency and depression. *Psychosomatics* 21:926–929, 1980.

49. Herbert V: Experimental nutritional folate deficiency in man. *Trans Assoc Am Physicians* 75:307–320, 1962.

50. Carmel R: Megaloblastic anemia, in Fries JE, Ehrlich GE (eds): *Prognosis: Contemporary Outcomes of Disease*. Bowie, Maryland, The Charles Press Publishing Co, 1981, pp 165–168.

51. Reiffers J, Raynal F, Boustet A: Acute myeloblastic leukemia in elderly patients. Treatment and prognostic factors. *Cancer* 45:2816–2820, 1980.

52. Foon KA, Zighelboim K, Yale C, et al: Intensive chemotherapy is the treatment of choice for elderly patients with acute myelogenous leukemia. *Blood* 58:467–470, 1981.

53. Smith IE, Powles R, Clink HM, et al: Early deaths in acute myelogenous leukemia. *Cancer* 39:1710–1714, 1977.

54. Gale RP, Cline MJ: High remission-induction rate in acute myeloid leukemia. *Lancet* 1:497–499, 1977.

55. Uzuka Y, Liong SK, Yamagata S: Treatment of acute non-lymphoblastic leukemia using intermittent combination chemotherapy with daunomycin, cytosine arabinoside, 6 mercaptopurine, and prednisolone-DCMP two step therapy. *Tohoku J Exp Med* 118(suppl):217–225, 1976.

56. Rai KR, Sawitsky A, Cronkite EP, et al: Clinical staging of chronic lymphocytic leukemia. *Blood* 46:219–234, 1975.

57. Report from the International Workshop on CLL, Chronic Lymphocytic Leukemia: Proposals for a revised prognostic staging system. *Br J Haematol* 48:365–367, 1981.

58. Cooper IA, Ding JC, Adams PB, et al: Intensive leukapheresis in the management of cytopenias in patients with chronic lymphocytic leukemia (CLL) and lymphocytic lymphoma. *Am J Hematol* 6:387–398, 1979.

59. Salmon SE: Expansion of growth fraction in multiple myeloma with alkylating agents. *Blood* 45:119–129, 1975.

60. Mundy GR, Raisz LG, Cooper RA, et al: Evidence for secretion of an osteoclastic stimulation factor in myeloma. *N Engl J Med* 291:1041–1046, 1974.

61. Norden CW: Infections in patients with multiple myeloma. *Arch Int Med* 140:1150–1151, 1980.

62. Solomon A: Bence Jones proteins and light chains of immunoglobulins: XV Effect of corticosteroids on synthesis and excretion of Bence Jones Proteins. *J Clin Invest* 61:97–108, 1978.

63. Case DC, Lee DJ, Clarkson BD: Improved survival times in multiple myeloma treated with melphalan, prednisone, cyclophosphamide, vincristine and BCNU: M-2 protocol. *Am J Med* 63:897–903, 1977.

64. Durie BG, Salmon SE: A clinical staging system for multiple myeloma. *Cancer* 36:842–854, 1975.

65. Bruckman JE, Blommer WD: Management of spinal cord compression. *Semin Oncol* 5:135–140, 1978.

66. Gilbert RW, Kim JH, Posner JB: Epidural spinal cord compression from metastatic tumor: Diagnosis and treatment. *Ann Neurol* 3:40–51, 1978.

67. Kyle RA, Greipp PR: Smoldering multiple myeloma. *N Engl J Med* 302:1347–1349, 1980.

68. Alexanian R: Localized and indolent myeloma. *Blood* 56:521–525, 1980.

69. Perry MC, Hoagland HC: The hyperviscosity syndrome. *JAMA* 236:392–393, 1976.

70. Crawford J, Cohen JH: An approach to monoclonal gammopathies in the elderly. *Geriatrics* 37:97–112, 1982.

71. Brubaker LH, Briere J, Laszio J, et al: Treatment of anemia in myeloproliferative disorders. *Arch Int Med* 142:1533–1537, 1982.

72. Wu KK: Platelet hyperaggregability and thrombosis in patients with thrombocythemia. *Ann Int Med* 88:7–11, 1978.

73. Kessler CM, Klein HG, Havlik RJ: Uncontrolled thrombocytosis in chronic myeloproliferative disorders. *Br J Haematol* 50:157–167, 1982.

74. Silverstein MN, Remine WH: Splenectomy in myeloid metaplasia. *Blood* 53:515–518, 1979.

75. Maloney WC: Chronic myelogenous leukemia. *Cancer* 865–873, 1978.

76. Kardinal CG, Bateman JR, Weiner J: Chronic granulocytic leukemia. *Arch Int Med* 136:305–313, 1976.

77. Thomas DJ, Marshall J, Ross-Russel RW, et al: Cerebral blood-flow in polycythaemia. *Lancet* 2:161–163, 1977.

78. Wade JPH, Pearson TC, Ross-Russel RW, et al: Cerebral blood flow and blood viscosity in patients with polycythemia secondary to hypoxic lung disease. *Br Med J* 283:689–692, 1981.

79. York EL, Jones RL, Menon D, et al: Effects of secondary polycythemia on cerebral blood flow in chronic obstructive pulmonary disease. *Am Rev Respir Dis* 121:813–818, 1980.

80. Humphrey PRD, Marshall J, Ross-Russel RW, et al: Cerebral blood-flow and viscosity in relative polycythemia. *Lancet* 2:873–876, 1979.

81. Golde DW, Cline MJ: Pathogenesis of polycythemia vera—new concepts. *Am J Hematol* 1:351–355, 1976.

82. Pearson TC, Wetherley-Mein G: Vascular occlusive episodes and venous hematocrit in primary proliferative polycythemia. *Lancet* 2:1219–1222, 1978.

83. Harrison MJG, Kendall BE, Pollock S, et al: Effect of hematocrit on carotid stenosis and cerebral infarction. *Lancet* 2:114–115, 1981.

84. Milligan DW, Tooke JE, Davies JA: Effect of venesection on calf blood flow in polycythemia. *Br Med J* 284:619–620, 1982.

85. Berk PD, Goldberg JD, Silverstein MN, et al: Increased incidence of acute leukemia in polycythemia vera associated with chlorambucil therapy. *N Engl J Med* 304:441–447, 1981.

Chapter 23

Thyroid Disorders

Michael R. McClung, M.D.

Thyroid dysfunction is a frequent medical problem encountered in older individuals; and it may appear in subtle or atypical ways. Physicians must be aware of the various presentations as well as the evaluation and management of these clinical problems. Of particular interest to gerontologists is the relationship between thyroid function and the aging process itself. The thyroid gland and its hormones are major determinants of metabolic activity in humans. Many parameters of thyroid function have been carefully scrutinized by investigators in searching for a link between alterations in thyroid function and the decline in physical, mental, and metabolic activity that is associated with aging.

Thyroid Function

Thyroid Hormone Synthesis and Secretion

The process of the synthesis and secretion of thyroid hormone is dependent on an adequate supply of metabolic substrates (especially iodine), on the appropriate regulation of the thyroid by the pituitary gland, and on the integrity of the thyroid gland itself. The final expression of thyroid function in physiologic processes is additionally dependent on the transport of thyroid hormone to its target tissues, the metabolism of thyroid hormone by peripheral tissues, and the ability of target tissues to respond to the metabolic message conveyed by thyroid hormone. Abnormalities at any of these steps can

result in a clinically significant thyroid dysfunction.

The synthesis of thyroid hormone involves the iodination of tyrosine moieties of thyroglobulin and the subsequent coupling of iodotyrosines to form 3,5,3'-triiodothyronine (T_3) and thyroxine (T_4).[1] Iodine is transported from the plasma across the basal end of the thyroid follicular cell. The enzymatic iodination of thyroglobulin tyrosine residues occurs at the apical membrane of the follicle. Thyroid peroxidase catalyzes both the iodination reaction and the coupling of two iodotyrosine residues to form thyroid hormone. The colloid within the lumen of the thyroid follicles serves as a large extracellular storage site for the thyroid hormone. In response to the thyroid-stimulating hormone (TSH) or other stimulators of thyroid secretion, the colloid is retrieved by endocytosis into the cell, where it undergoes lysosomal hydrolysis. The thyroid hormone released from thyroglobulin by this process diffuses out of the thyroid cell and into the circulation.

Peripheral Metabolism of Thyroid Hormones

The thyroid gland is the sole site of thyroxine synthesis in normal humans. Calculated T_4 production rates average 80–100 μg/day. Much smaller amounts of T_3 also are secreted from the thyroid gland. The primary site of T_3 production is in the extrathyroidal tissues where the outer ring of T_4 is deiodinated to produce T_3.[2] The conversion of T_4 to T_3 is catalyzed by an ubiquitous enzyme, T_4 5'-deiodinase, which is located in the microsomal fraction of virtually all tissues. In healthy individuals, approximately 80% of all T_3 is derived from this peripheral metabolic pathway. Another enzyme, T_4 5-deiodinase, cleaves an inner-ring iodine atom from thyroxine that produces reverse T_3 (3,3′,5′-triiodothyronine), which is a thyronine molecule with essentially no hormonal activity. Very little is known about the regulation of 5-deiodinase activity. However, a number of physiologic and clinical situations are associated with alterations in T_4 to T_3 conversion by 5′-deiodinase (see Figure 23-1). Carbohydrate intake is one of the major determinants of the activity of this enzyme. A decreased carbohydrate intake, even when total calorie intake is maintained, results in a marked decline in T_4 to T_3 conversion. This effect frequently is observed in patients with acute or chronic illnesses that are associated with a decreased intake or with fasting, and it is responsible for some of the changes in the serum thyroid hormone levels in acutely ill patients, which will be discussed subsequently. Increased 5′-deiodinase activity is observed with carbohydrate overfeeding. Frequently used medications, which include some cholecystographic agents, propranolol, and glucocorticoids, also variably decrease 5′-deiodinase activity.

Regulation of Thyroid Function

The regulation of thyroid function involves the stimulation of thyroid hormone synthesis and secretion by TSH (see Figure 23-2). The production of TSH by the anterior pituitary gland is controlled by both the serum concentration of thyroid hormone in a classic negative feedback manner and the thyrotropin-releasing hormone (TRH). In a normal individual, a rise in thyroid hormone concentration decreases TSH secretion, whereas a fall in the serum level of thyroid hormone increases both TSH release and subsequent thyroid hormone secretion until thyroid hormone levels are normalized. The setpoint of the thyroid-pituitary axis, which is the level of thyroid hormone at which TSH secretion is controlled, is determined by TRH. With a hypothalamic TRH deficiency, the control of TSH by thyroid hormones is maintained; but, it occurs at a much lower thyroid hormone level than normal. In addition, the pituitary response to TRH is determined by the thyroid hormone levels. In hypothyroidism, not only is basal TSH concentration elevated, but the response to TRH is exaggerated. However, in hyperthyroidism, both basal and TRH-stimulated levels of TSH are suppressed. This feedback regulatory system is exquisitely sensitive. Alterations

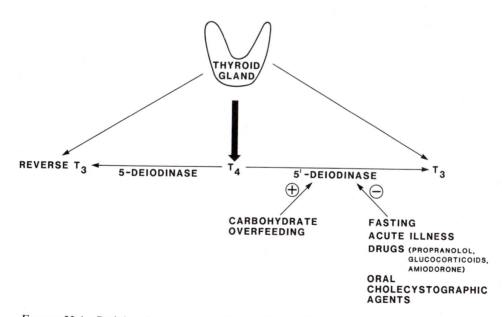

FIGURE 23-1   Peripheral metabolism of T_4 and factors that influence the tissue conversion of T_4 to T_3.

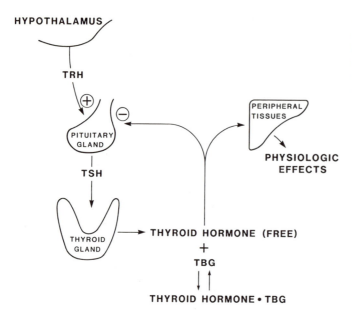

FIGURE 23-2   Regulation of TSH and thyroid hormone secretion. The relationship between bound and free thyroid hormones in the serum is depicted, emphasizing the importance of the free thyroid hormone concentration in the feedback control of TSH release and in peripheral tissues.

in the concentration of TSH can be demonstrated in response to even slight changes in the thyroid hormone levels within the normal range.[3]

In addition to the hypothalamic-pituitary-thyroid axis, thyroid function is modulated by a local control of the response of the thyroid gland to TSH. This autoregulation of thyroid function is predominantly due to the effects of intracellular iodine on several of the steps of thyroid hormone synthesis.[4] In the presence of an abundance of iodine, intracellular iodine levels begin to increase, which results in a partial impairment of thyroid peroxidase activity. This block in the organification of iodine, known as the Wolff-Chaikoff effect, protects the organism from an inappropriate increase in thyroid hormone production during periods of iodine excess. The iodination blockade further increases intracellular iodine levels, which also produces an inhibition of both TSH responsiveness and the efficiency of the iodine transport mechanism. This latter effect ultimately results in a decline of the intracellular iodine level, and normal rates of thyroid hormone synthesis are maintained. Large amounts of iodine also inhibit the secretion of stored thyroid hormone in addition to decreasing hormone synthesis. These autoregulatory events serve to modify the responsiveness of the thyroid gland to TSH stimulation, which depends on the iodine status of the individual.

Serum Transport of Thyroid Hormones

Both T_3 and T_4 circulate in the serum as predominantly bound to transport proteins. Although small amounts of thyroid hormones are bound to thyroxine-binding prealbumin and to albumin, the major transport protein is a thyroxine-binding globulin (TBG).[5] This α-2 globulin is synthesized in the liver, and its rate of production is modulated by sex steroid hormones. Estrogens increase the hepatic production of TBG, while androgens decrease the rate of synthesis. The association constants of T_4 and T_3 binding to TBG are approximately 10^{10} M^{-1} and $10^9\,M^{-1}$, respectively. Because of avid binding, only 0.01% of T_4 and about 0.03% of T_3 is unbound or free in the serum. It is this free fraction of serum thyroid hormones, however, that is in equilibrium with tissue levels of T_3 and T_4 and exerts the metabolic activity of the hormones (see Figure 23-2). The half-life of T_4 in the serum is about 7 days, while that of T_3 is approximately 1 day.

Thyroid Hormone Action

Both T_3 and T_4 enter cells by a passive diffusion and interact with target tissues by binding to specific receptor sites located in the nucleoprotein fraction of the nucleus.[6] Nuclear receptors recognize and bind T_3 much more avidly than they do T_4. Whether T_4 must be converted to T_3

before exerting a metabolic effect has not been clarified. T_4 does have an intrinsic metabolic activity, but whether this is the result of either a direct association of T_4 to nuclear receptors or of a conversion of T_4 to T_3 in the nucleus, as demonstrated in the rat pituitary gland, is not known.[7] The interaction of T_3 with the nuclear receptor results in an increased synthesis of specific messenger RNAs, which result in both quantitative and qualitative changes in the rate of protein synthesis and in subsequent physiologic alterations of cellular function. The metabolic response of a tissue to a thyroid hormone is proportional to the concentration of T_3 nuclear receptors in that tissue. Receptors for thyroid hormones also have been identified in both the mitochondria and the plasma membrane, but the physiologic significance of these extranuclear receptors is not fully understood.

Age-Associated Changes in Thyroid Function

Although the activity of the thyroid gland and serum levels of thyroid hormones now can be carefully quantified, none of these parameters of thyroid function evaluates the physiologic response of the individual to thyroid hormone. Consequently, the ultimate answer regarding the influence of age on thyroid function is not available in spite of a large body of information pertaining to this point.

There is strong evidence that the activity of the thyroid gland diminishes with age. The efficiency and capacity of the thyroid gland to synthesize and secrete thyroid hormones cannot be directly measured, but it can be estimated or inferred from other measurements. The amount of iodine that is assimilated by the thyroid from plasma generally reflects the rate of hormone formation by the thyroid. The absolute rate of iodine accumulation falls about 40% between young adulthood and the 9th decade.[8] The T_4 production rate also can be estimated by measuring the metabolic clearance rate of this hormone, since (in a steady state) the rates of hormone formation and degradation are equivalent. By measuring the metabolic clearance rate of T_4, several studies have demonstrated that the calculated T_4 production rate falls from 80–100 μg/day in young adults to 50–

70 μg/day in patients over the 70 years of age, which is a result consistent with the observed fall in absolute iodine uptake.[9]

The decreased functional activity of an aging thyroid gland also can be inferred from a microscopic examination. The weight of the thyroid gland and the ratio of the follicular elements to connective tissues gradually diminish with age. In addition, the appearance of the follicles suggests a decreased thyroid activity. The follicular cells assume a more cuboidal shape, rather than the columnar appearance that is associated with an active hormone synthesis and secretion. Thus, data from a histologic examination, thyroxine turnover studies, and a measurement of iodine metabolism consistently suggest that the hormone production rate of the thyroid gland is lower in elderly individuals than in young adults.

This decreased activity of the thyroid gland is superficially mirrored by the decline in physical and mental vigor and by the fall in the basal metabolic rate (BMR) that is commonly seen in elderly persons. Measurements of the BMR demonstrate a decrease in oxygen consumption of 15–20% between the 4th and 9th decades.[10–12] However, the cellular response of a thyroid hormone is but one of several determinants of BMR. When the rates of oxygen consumption are expressed as a function of total body water, thereby adjusting for changes in body composition, there is no decline in the metabolic rate. This suggests that cellular metabolic function is well maintained in healthy older adults.[13]

If the decrease in thyroid hormone production indicates a faltering thyroid function in elderly persons, a fall in serum thyroid hormone levels, accompanied by elevated serum TSH levels, would be expected. The results of studies that have examined the influence of age on TSH and thyroid hormone concentration have not been consistent; but, in general, they do not support the notion that elderly people are hypothyroid. T_4 and free T_4 levels in the serum fall only slightly (if at all) with advancing age, and they certainly do not reflect the magnitude of the decrease in T_4 production rates.[14,15] Serum T_3 levels are observed to decline as a function of age in most studies, sometimes to levels that are 50–60% of the normal range in young adults.[16–18] This fall in serum T_3 is predominantly due to a decreased peripheral production of T_3 rather than to a diminished function of the thyroid gland. The initial studies that evaluated the relationship between serum T_3 concentration and age often included elderly patients with a variety of chronic medical problems, which (as previously mentioned) may be associated with a decreased peripheral T_4 deiodination. The question of whether a decreased peripheral conversion of T_4 to T_3 is a necessary accompaniment of aging or is due to age-associated changes in other metabolic parameters has not been clearly answered.

The average basal TSH levels measured in healthy elderly populations are normal, although they may be slightly higher than the mean values of younger patients.[19] A somewhat larger proportion of elderly patients have TSH concentrations that are above the normal range, which reflects the increased prevalence of hypothyroidism in the geriatric population. However, the great majority of older individuals have normal basal TSH levels. It could be argued that the failure to observe a rise in TSH, in the face of decreased thyroid gland activity, signifies that the pituitary gland has lost the ability to respond sensitively and appropriately. Indeed, inadequate TSH secretion is one possible explanation for the decreased thyroid activity. When tested directly via the administration of TRH, older subjects had TSH responses that were variable and described as reduced or more generous than the responses seen in younger people.[20–22] In one study, the age-related decrease in the response to TRH was curiously seen only in males.[23] However, the response to TRH is well maintained in most elderly patients. In some individuals, blunting the response to TRH may reflect the presence of an autonomous thyroid function, which is a frequent occurrence in patients with a non-toxic multinodular goiter, rather than a primary abnormality of pituitary function.[22] The normal TSH content of thyrotrophs from older patients creates an argument against a decreased TSH secretory capacity of the pituitary gland.[24] The well-being of the thyroid-pituitary axis in elderly persons is further demonstrated by the healthy rise in TSH that is seen in older patients who do develop clinical evidence of hypothyroidism.

The autoregulatory control of thyroid function also is well preserved in elderly persons, with the exception of two groups of study subjects. Areas of autonomous thyroid function exist within the glands of patients with a non-toxic multinodular goiter. When exposed to large iodine loads, the autoregulatory system in these patients fails and hyperthyroidism frequently is produced.[25] In addition, individuals with chronic lymphocytic thyroiditis are particularly susceptible to the inhibitory effects of iodine on thyroid function. Thus iodine-induced hypothyroidism may occur when these patients receive iodine.[26] Because both chronic thyroiditis and a non-toxic multinodular goiter occur more frequently in older people, these abnormalities of autoregulatory function are more commonly observed.

Very little information regarding tissue responses to thyroid hormones in aging persons is available. There is a general feeling that elderly persons are more sensitive to the effects of exogenous thyroxine, but this may be explained by its decreased clearance rate. The dramatic clinical improvement resulting from appropriate therapy for hypothyroid elderly patients suggests that the resistance to thyroid hormones is not an important feature of this age group.

These studies do not resolve the question of whether there are changes in thyroid function that are inherently associated with aging. Clearly, several isolated components of the thyroid-pituitary system do change as one ages; however, rather than signifying a failing thyroid function, these changes may be an appropriate integrated response to other metabolic features of aging. The decrease in T_4 to T_3 conversion in older subjects, whether due to aging itself or to associated nutritional changes, is well established and a major factor in the decreased T_4 clearance rate of older persons. An appropriate response of the thyroid-pituitary axis to the decreased T_4 turnover is a slight fall in TSH production and a decrease in both thyroid activity and T_4 synthesis to maintain a normal thyroid hormone balance. Although the incidence rate of thyroid dysfunction is greater in the geriatric population, the vitality and responsiveness of the thyroid-pituitary metabolic system is well maintained throughout an adult life span.[27]

Laboratory Evaluation of Thyroid Function

With the advent of sensitive and practical radioimmunoassay (RIA) techniques to evaluate the thyroid-pituitary system, a diagnosis of a thyroid dysfunction can usually be made in a straightforward manner. Clinicians must, however, be alert to misleading values that are caused by drugs and underlying or concomitant non-thyroidal illnesses.

Serum Concentrations of Thyroid Hormones

Radioimmunoassays (RIAs) for T_4 and T_3 now are routinely available. These assays measure total hormone concentration in the serum, including both the free hormone fraction and the hormone that is bound to proteins. Since only a small fraction of both T_4 and T_3 is unbound, assay levels primarily reflect the bound hormone levels. Major determinants of a total hormone concentration are rates of thyroid hormone secretion and the serum thyroid hormone-binding capacity. Disorders of the thyroid function, which alter thyroid hormone secretory rates, generally result in abnormalities of both the total and free hormone concentrations. Alterations in the thyroid hormone-binding capacity produce abnormal total thyroid hormone levels; but, free hormone values remain in the normal range. Since only a free or unbound hormone diffuses into cells and influences the metabolic processes, individuals who have an abnormal thyroid hormone-binding capacity have a normal thyroid function in spite of the abnormal total thyroid hormone concentrations.

Alterations of TBG levels are the most frequent situations that result in an abnormal thyroid hormone-binding capacity. The serum T_4-binding capacity and TBG concentration increase slightly with age, but not enough to significantly affect total T_4 levels.[28] Common causes for abnormal TBG levels are listed in Table 23-1. Because TBG synthesis is, in part, estrogen-dependent, an elevated TBG is observed in patients receiving exogenous estrogen for postmenopausal symptoms or a prostatic

TABLE 23-1 Clinical Situations Associated with Abnormal Thyroxine-Binding Globulin (TBG) Concentrations

TBG Excess	TBG Deficiency
Estrogen therapy	Androgen therapy
Acute hepatocellular disease	Chronic liver disease
	Severe catabolic illness
	Congenital X-linked

carcinoma. The TBG and, consequently, total serum thyroid hormone levels also may be increased in patients with acute liver diseases. Low concentrations of TBG, which result in depressed serum T_4 levels, are seen in patients with chronic catabolic illnesses (especially chronic liver disease) and in patients who receive large doses of exogenous androgens. A congenital TBG deficiency, which is an X-linked trait, occurs in approximately 1 of every 3,000 males. These individuals have total T_4 levels of 1–2 μg/dl. Females who are heterozygous for this trait have intermediate levels of both TBG and T_4 RIAs. Other conditions that are associated with an abnormal thyroid hormone-binding capacity include patients who have endogenous antibodies to thyroid hormones or elevated total T_4 levels due to the presence of abnormal thyroid hormone-binding proteins.

The RIA for T_4 is the most widely used test for thyroid function. Total T_4 concentrations are between 4–12 μg/dl in normal individuals. These values are constant over an entire adult life span. Clinical situations in which the total T_4 levels are abnormal are listed in Table 23-2. Serum T_4 levels generally are elevated in patients with hyperthyroidism. Because of the

TABLE 23-2 Major Causes of Abnormal Serum T_4 Concentrations in Elderly Patients

Increased T_4	Decreased T_4
Hyperthyroidism	Hypothyroidism
Increased protein binding	TBG deficiency
TBG excess	Serious illness
Anti-T_4 antibodies	
Abnormal binding proteins	
Acute illness (transient)	

* TBG = thyroxine-binding globulin.

wide range of normal T_4 values, however, only about 90% of all elderly patients with hyperthyroidism have T_4 values above the normal range.[29] Total T_4 concentrations can be elevated in euthyroid patients by any one of several mechanisms that lead to an increased thyroid hormone-binding capacity. An acute illness also may result in a mild transient elevation of total T_4, which perhaps is related to the decreased deiodination of T_4 to T_3 seen in that setting. Of all acutely ill elderly patients, 5–8% exhibit increased T_4 levels that normalize following a resolution of the acute illness.[30]

Low T_4 concentrations are observed in patients with a decreased thyroid hormone production, a decreased thyroid hormone-binding capacity, and acquired alterations in the affinity of T_4 binding to TBG. Most hypothyroid patients have low T_4 levels, although a low-to-normal T_4 value does not exclude that diagnosis. The administration of T_3 to a normal person suppresses both TSH and thyroid hormone secretion; also, T_4 concentrations fall to low levels. Euthyroid patients may have low total T_4 levels due to a TBG deficiency. Aspirin, phenytoin, and heparin are capable of displacing T_4 from binding sites on the TBG, which results in lower total T_4 levels. However, the levels rarely will be below the normal range. It recently has been recognized that patients with severe illnesses frequently have low total T_4 concentrations when normal or slightly elevated free T_4 levels are present.[31] The TBG concentrations in these patients usually are normal. This so-called "low T_4 syndrome" may be caused by circulating inhibitors of T_4 that are binding to a TBG associated with a severe illness and tissue necrosis.[32,33] Because both elevated and depressed values of T_4 may be seen in a setting of an acute or severe illness, an evaluation of thyroid function in such patients can be difficult.[34,35]

Interpreting a serum T_4 concentration with regard to a patient's TBG concentration improves the diagnostic accuracy of the test. This can be accomplished by adjusting the total T_4 level via some laboratory measure of TBG. The conventional procedure employs the T_3 resin uptake test (T_3RU), which is an inverse measure of the thyroid hormone-binding capacity in the serum. These T_3RU values decrease as the serum T_4-binding capacity increases. By comparing a patient's T_3RU to the value using normal serum, the T_3 resin ratio is calculated. The product of the total T_4 concentration and the T_3 resin ratio is the free thyroxine index (FTI). It must be emphasized that the T_3RU is not a measure of serum T_3 concentration, is not a thyroid function test, and is only useful in the calculation of the free thyroid hormone index. Since neither the T_3 resin ratio nor T_4 values change appreciably with age, the calculated FTI values do not vary with age either. The FTI is useful in distinguishing between an abnormal thyroid hormone-binding capacity and an altered thyroid secretion as the causes of an abnormal total T_4 level. In patients with normal or only mildly abnormal levels of TBG, there is a good correlation between direct measurements of free T_4 and the FTI.[36] However, when marked changes in TBG levels are present or found with the inhibition of binding that is associated with a severe non-thyroidal illness, the FTI inaccurately reflects the free T_4 concentrations; this may lead to an erroneous diagnosis. In addition, some patients with either hyperthyroidism or hypothyroidism will have normal FTI values. Although the FTI is the best general screening test of thyroid function, a more detailed evaluation of a patient's thyroid status is warranted if the clinical condition and the FTI results are discordant.

Direct measurements of serum T_4-binding capacity or TBG concentration via an RIA have been used in conjunction with total T_4 levels to estimate free T_4 concentrations. Neither of these tests is widely available, nor do they provide a significant advantage over the T_3RU.

Until recently, more direct estimates of free T_4 concentration in serum relied on cumbersome and specialized assay techniques, such as an equilibrium dialysis. Normal free T_4 values generally range between 1–2 ng/dl and do not fluctuate with age.[37] Free T_4 levels are normal in patients with abnormal levels of thyroid hormone-binding proteins and are normal or slightly elevated in patients with a severe non-thyroidal illness and the "low T_4 syndrome." The elevation of free T_4 in some of these patients could be related to the impaired T_4 to T_3 conversion associated with the severe illness. Direct RIAs for free T_4 now have been developed that may provide a practical means of evaluating patients with thyroid abnormalities without interpretative difficulties that are due to changes in the TBG concentration. As more experience is gained with direct assays for free T_4, this test may supplant the FTI as the primary screening test for thyroid dysfunction.

Serum T_3 concentrations are lower than those of T_4 because of the weaker association of T_3 to TBG. The T_3 values in normal young adults range between 80–200 ng/dl. As previously discussed, serum T_3 levels gradually decline with advancing age, although there are no established, age-adjusted normal ranges. The marked influence of T_4 to T_3 conversion rates on the T_3 concentration limits the usefulness of a T_3 RIA as a routine screening test. Serum T_3 levels are of little help in the evaluation of hypothyroidism, since very low values may be seen in severely ill or starving euthyroid patients, and because normal T_3 values frequently are seen in patients with a mild-to-moderate hypothyroidism. However, T_3 assays can be helpful in the differentiation of hyperthyroid and euthyroid elderly patients. In the absence of an increase in the thyroid hormone-binding capacity, a total T_3 value above the normal adult range is strong evidence that a patient has a hyperthyroid condition. Normal T_3 levels may occur in hyperthyroid elderly patients due to the decreased T_4 to T_3 conversion that usually is seen with aging, and to the decreased caloric intake that may accompany this illness. A free T_3 index can be calculated in the same manner as the FTI. The use of this test is not widespread, but it has been used with success to distinguish hyperthyroid patients from euthyroid patients whose T_4 levels are elevated due to illness or fasting.[38,39]

Radioactive Iodine Uptake (RAIU)

A radioactive iodine uptake (RAIU) is performed by measuring the retention of radioiodine in the thyroid gland at a standard interval after the administration of the isotope. Normally, 10–30% of the dose remains in the gland after 24 hours; this range of values does not change appreciably with age.[40] Although this test was a major tool in the diagnosis of a thyroid dysfunction before the availability of RIAs for thyroid hormones and TSH, the RAIU presently is used only occasionally in a diagnosis of either thyrotoxicosis or hypothyroidism. Its

major use now is in a differential diagnosis of hyperthyroidism; it is used to calculate the dose of ^{131}I for the treatment of hyperthyroidism.

Evaluating the Thyroid-Pituitary Axis

The TSH Assays

Serum TSH concentrations reflect the response of the pituitary gland to changes in thyroid function. As such, TSH is the most sensitive laboratory marker of primary hypothyroidism, and it frequently is elevated before serum T_4 concentrations fall below the normal range. In the most sensitive assays available, the normal range for serum TSH in adults is between 0.5–4/μU/ml. Most commercially available TSH assays are somewhat less sensitive and have normal ranges up to 10–12 μU/ml. There is no deviation of the normal range as a function of age, although a larger proportion of elderly individuals will have abnormally high TSH values due to their increased prevalence of hypothyroidism. Theoretically, demonstrating suppressed TSH values should be helpful in establishing a diagnosis of hyperthyroidism. However, routinely used assays currently lack both sensitivity and precision in the lower normal range; also, many euthyroid persons have undetectable TSH concentrations. Consequently, basal TSH concentrations alone are of little practical value in the evaluation of hyperthyroidism.

The TRH Stimulation Test

The TRH stimulation of TSH secretion is a test of the integrity of both the pituitary and thyroid glands. The intravenous (IV) or intramuscular administration of TRH normally produces an increase in the serum TSH concentration, which peaks at 20–30 minutes following a dose and gradually returns to normal over the next hour. In response to this TSH stimulus, serum T_3 rises transiently 2–3 hours after TRH administration. Because of the large circulating pool of serum T_4, the enhanced T_4 secretion following a TRH infusion rarely is evidenced by changes in serum T_4 values.

The TSH response to TRH is dose-related and maximal with IV doses of more than 200 μg. In practice, 400–500 μg of TRH is administered via IV bolus. Serum samples for TSH are collected before and 20–30 minutes following TRH administration. Hyperthyroidism is not induced by a TRH stimulation test, and this diagnostic procedure is used safely in elderly or seriously ill patients.

An increase in the serum TSH concentration of 3–30 uU/ml is normally observed after TRH is administered.[41] The response to TRH may be normal or somewhat depressed, but it is not absent in healthy elderly subjects. Some studies suggest that the response is particularly blunted in elderly males. These findings do not obviate the usefulness of this test, however, because euthyroid elderly patients retain the capacity to increase TSH secretion in response to TRH even though the magnitude of that response may fall with age.

In general, the TSH response to TRH varies directly with basal TSH levels. In patients with primary hypothyroidism, basal TSH concentrations are high and the rise in TSH following TRH is exaggerated. The TRH test rarely is necessary to make a diagnosis of primary hypothyroidism. In hyperthyroidism, basal TSH levels are suppressed and there is no response to a TRH that is due to a negative feedback inhibition via elevated thyroid hormone concentrations on TSH release. The principal clinical use of the TRH test in geriatric practice is found in the evaluation of patients with subtle thyrotoxicosis or with equivocally elevated, routine thyroid function tests. A normal TSH response to TRH excludes a diagnosis of hyperthyroidism, except for those very rare patients with TSH-producing pituitary tumors. The absence of a response suggests that the patient is hyperthyroid, but it is not absolute proof of that diagnosis.

A TRH test also is used to distinguish pituitary from hypothalamic causes of hypothyroidism. Patients with hypopituitarism generally fail to respond to a TRH, while patients with a hypothalamic dysfunction will have a definite, although delayed, response. However, examples exist in which these particular responses are not observed. The TRH stimulation test should be only one of several tests used to localize a hypothalamic or pituitary pathology.

The T_3 Suppression Test

Autonomy of thyroid function is an invariable feature of Graves' disease and toxic nodular goiter. In the occasional patients in whom a clinical question of hyperthyroidism is difficult to answer via routine thyroid function tests, an evaluation of thyroid autonomy with the T_3 suppression test may be useful. After obtaining a baseline 24-hour RAIU, 75–100 μg of L-T_3 (Cytomel) is administered daily in divided doses for 10 days; the 24-hour RAIU is repeated. This dose of L-T_3 suppresses the TSH secretion, and (consequently) the RAIU is then decreased in normal individuals to less than 50% of the baseline values. Patients with autonomous thyroid function exhibit little or no change in the RAIU in response to L-T_3. Demonstrating normal suppression with L-T_3 makes a diagnosis of Graves' disease or a toxic nodular goiter very unlikely. A lack of suppression, while consistent with a diagnosis of hyperthyrodism, also may be seen in euthyroid patients who have a multinodular goiter. In patients who do have autonomous thyroid function, there is a risk of inducing or exacerbating hyperthyroid symptoms. For this reason, then T_3 suppression test is used sparingly and very cautiously in elderly patients with cardiovascular symptoms.

The T_3 suppression test and the TRH stimulation tests are complementary approaches to an evaluation of the thyroid-pituitary axis. The TRH test asks whether a patient's pituitary gland perceives elevated thyroid hormone concentrations; it does not address the issue of autonomy of the thyroid gland. Hyperthyroidism and an abnormal TRH test are observed in patients taking large doses of a thyroid hormone while their endogenous thyroid function is appropriately suppressed. Conversely, the T_3 suppression test simply evaluates the dependence of the thyroid gland on TSH for maintenance of function. An abnormal response does not require that a patient be hyperthyroid, because lack of suppression may be seen in both hyperthyroid patients and individuals with a nontoxic multinodular goiter.

Miscellaneous Tests

Serum Reverse T_3 RIA

Serum reverse T_3 RIAs are commercially available. Normal values of this inactive metabolite of T_4 generally range between 10–15 ng/dl. As with T_3 levels, reverse T_3 concentrations are modified by changes in both the thyroid function and the rate of peripheral T_4 to T_3 conversion. As one of the two major pathways of T_4

deiodination, changes in reverse T_3 levels tend to parallel those of T_4 when the thyroid function is abnormal; but, they vary inversely with serum T_3 concentrations when T_4 5'-deiodinase activity is altered. Reverse T_3 assays rarely are necessary to establish a diagnosis of thyroid dysfunction, but they may be helpful in differentiating hypothyroidism and abnormal T_4 levels that are due to a non-thyroidal illness.[31] Reverse T_3 concentrations generally are low in hypothyroidism, while they are normal or high in situations where T_4 to T_3 conversion is impaired.

In the few studies in which the effect of aging on reverse T_3 values have been assessed, the concentrations tended to be higher as the age of the subjects increased.[17,42] It is not known whether this is a true age-related phenomenon, or if it is due to an impaired T_4 5'-deiodinase activity that is associated with decreased caloric intake or chronic illness.

Serum Thyroglobulin

Thyroglobulin circulates in small amounts in normal individuals and is measured via an RIA. The thyroid gland is the only known source of this protein. Thyroglobulin concentrations are increased in patients with many thyroid disorders, which include hyperthyroidism, inflammatory disorders of the thyroid, and both benign and malignant nodules. A measurement of thyroglobulin can be helpful in differentiating factitious hyperthyroidism from subacute or silent thyroiditis; the values are high in the active inflammatory phase of thyroiditis and normal or low in patients who are ingesting a thyroid hormone. Serum thyroglobulin also is a useful marker of tumor recurrence in patients who have undergone ablative surgical or radioiodine therapy for a thyroid carcinoma.[43]

Antithyroid Antibodies

High levels of serum antibodies to either thyroglobulin or the microsomal fraction of the thyroid gland are found in many patients with an autoimmune thyroid disease. Antimicrosomal antibodies are more specific for an autoimmune thyroid disease, since low levels of antithyroglobulin antibodies are seen in up to 15% of all patients with no evidence of thyroid disease and those with other autoimmune disorders, such as rheumatoid arthritis. The frequency with which antithyroid antibodies are measurable increases with the age of a population and roughly parallels the increased incidence of histologic evidence of chronic thyroiditis that is seen in elderly persons. If present in high titers, antithyroid antibodies can be helpful in both distinguishing Graves' disease from a toxic nodular goiter and confirming a clinical diagnosis of chronic lymphocytic thyroiditis (Hashimoto's disease). In general, however, neither the absolute level of an antibody nor the course of antibody titers influences the management of geriatric patients with thyroid disease. Thyroid-stimulating antibodies are present in the serum of almost all patients who have Graves' disease. At present, practically useful assays of these antibodies are not routinely available.

Clinical Disorders

Clinical thyroid abnormalities in elderly patients include disorders of thyroid function (hyperthyroidism, hypothyroidism) and abnormalities of growth or size of the thyroid gland (goiter, thyroid nodules). Irregularities of both thyroid size and function may coexist, but they frequently are independent disorders. For example, most hyperthyroid patients also have palpably abnormal thyroid glands, but the majority of individuals with a thyroid enlargement are euthyroid.

Nodular Goiter and Thyroid Carcinoma

Thyroid nodularity continues to occur frequently, although better nutrition and the fortification of foods with iodine has virtually eliminated iodine deficiency in the United States. Between 25–50% of all thyroid glands from elderly people that are examined at autopsy are nodular.[44,45] These abnormalities are appreciated less often on a physical examination. In surveys of communities in both North America and Great Britain, palpable thyroid abnormalities were noted in about 5% of all individuals over the 60 years of age.[46,47] As is true with disorders of thyroid function, nodules of the thyroid are much more common in women than in males.[48]

For practical purposes, nodular goiters are categorized as multinodular or as single or solitary nodules. This distinction generally is made by a physical examination of the thyroid gland, although thyroid scanning may also be helpful. The clinical differentiation of the two types of nodular goiters is imperfect, since many patients thought to have solitary nodules on palpation are found to have a multinodular goiter on surgery or autopsy. Nonetheless, this distinction is of practical use, since the predominant issue in patients with solitary nodules is whether the nodule is malignant; therefore, attempts to discern the nature of the nodule are warranted. In contrast, a thyroid carcinoma is of less concern in patients with a multinodular goiter. A determination of thyroid function is a clinician's main objective with these patients.

Solitary Nodules and Thyroid Carcinoma

Malignant lesions of the thyroid gland usually present as isolated areas of enlargement. As a result, both physicians and patients become concerned about the possibility of a malignancy whenever a solitary nodule in the thyroid gland is discovered. Fortunately, only about 10% of such lesions are malignant. Since a diagnosis of thyroid cancer is most common in patients between 20–40 years of age, and because thyroid nodules are more frequent in older patients, the likelihood that a single thyroid nodule is malignant in an elderly patient may be even less than 10%. The task of a clinician evaluating this problem is to differentiate benign from malignant lesions and to select an appropriate therapeutic plan.

Non-malignant lesions of the thyroid gland, which present as solitary nodules, frequently are follicular adenomas and, less commonly, simple cysts. In addition, an asymmetric or localized involvement of the thyroid gland by more generalized benign abnormalities such as a follicular hyperplasia, colloid goiter, or Hashimoto's thyroiditis may clinically mimic thyroid tumors.

The types of malignant thyroid tumors in elderly persons are the same in those found in younger patients. However, whereas well-differentiated tumors predominate in younger adults, tumors in patients over 65 years of age are commonly more poorly differentiated and more aggressive (*see* Figure 23-3).[49] An anaplastic thyroid cancer rapidly invades local structures, has an extremely poor prognosis, and may arise from a transformation of a pre-

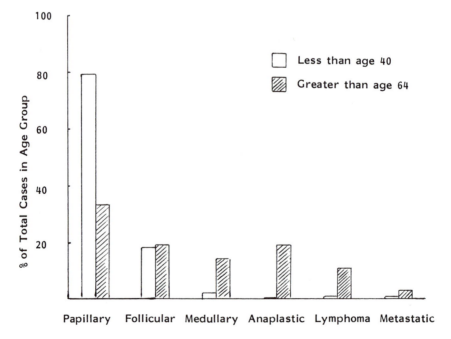

FIGURE 23-3 Relative frequency of histologic types of thyroid carcinomas in young and older populations.[49]

existing well-differentiated carcinoma (in some cases). The thyroid gland often is involved in patients with a widespread lymphoma. Much less commonly, the thyroid gland appears to be the site of origin of a lymphoma; usually, it is in a gland with evidence of chronic lymphocytic thyroiditis. A medullary carcinoma, which is a tumor of the calcitonin-producing parafollicular cells, typically is manifested as a progressively enlarging mass in the upper portion of the thyroid lobes that metastasizes to local lymph nodes early in its course. A metastatic spread to the thyroid via lung, renal, and breast carcinomas and other tumors may occur.

Clinical Presentation

Benign thyroid nodules usually are discovered on a routine examination by a physician rather than by a patient. Occasionally, a hemorrhage into a benign lesion results in a sudden swelling, pain, and tenderness of the thyroid, and even compressive symptoms. Although the suddenness with which this clinical picture develops is characteristic of a hemorrhagic degeneration of a thyroid nodule, it is of little help in predicting the nature of the thyroid enlargement because both benign and malignant lesions may behave similarly. Compressive symptoms that are due to a benign thyroid disorder are more often experienced with diffuse or multinodular goiters than with solitary nodules. However, non-malignant nodules that have slowly enlarged over many years may produce a tracheal deviation and an abnormal sensation on swallowing. Well-differentiated thyroid malignancies often are slow-growing tumors, which usually are firm rather than rock-hard, and they may be impossible to distinguish from benign lesions on the basis of a physical examination. Ipsilateral cervical or supraclavicular adenopathies or fixations of a tumor to the skin and adjacent structures usually is indicative of a malignant process. Both anaplastic carcinomas and lymphomas present as rapidly enlarging thyroid masses, and these tumors often are very firm or hard. Hemoptysis from a tracheal or laryngeal invasion, hoarseness, dysphagia, and tracheal obstructions with dyspnea and stridor often are present at the time a diagnosis of anaplastic carcinoma is made.

Laboratory Evaluation

A variety of diagnostic aids are at the disposal of a clinician attempting to determine the nature of a thyroid nodule.[50–52] In many instances, a diagnosis remains uncertain until or unless the lesion is excised and carefully examined microscopically. It is particularly difficult to distinguish benign from malignant follicular neoplasms since many follicular carcinomas are very well differentiated, and they display their malignant potential only by invading blood vessels or the capsule of the thyroid gland. All of the following laboratory procedures have their limitations, but each may be useful in the assessment of an individual patient. In an attempt to appropriately select patients for a referral to surgery, several diagnostic approaches have been suggested. One such approach to elderly patients with solitary nodules is diagrammed in Figure 23-4.

Thyroid gland function is not an important part of an evaluation of a solitary nodule, except when the nodule has been shown via a thyroid scan to be autonomously functioning. Hyperthyroidism occasionally occurs in patients with a large tumor burden of a follicular carcinoma. Hypothyroidism is not associated with thyroid carcinoma unless the entire gland is replaced with a tumor.

A physical examination may reveal important evidence regarding the nature of the nodule. If, on the basis of the examination, the clinical diagnosis of a thyroid malignancy is made (adherence to underlying structures, cervical adenopathy), a biopsy specimen of the lesion usually can provide a histologic diagnosis on which appropriate decisions can be made regarding the management.

If the features that are characteristic of a malignancy are not present when a patient is initially examined, radionuclide scanning of the thyroid gland is a useful next step. The major use of a thyroid scan is to identify patients with "hot" nodules. These autonomously functioning lesions can produce thyrotoxicosis, although most do not.

If a nodule is hypofunctional or of indeterminant activity, then little diagnostic information is gained. These "cold" nodules may be either benign or malignant, solid, or cystic. The distinction between solid and cystic lesions can be

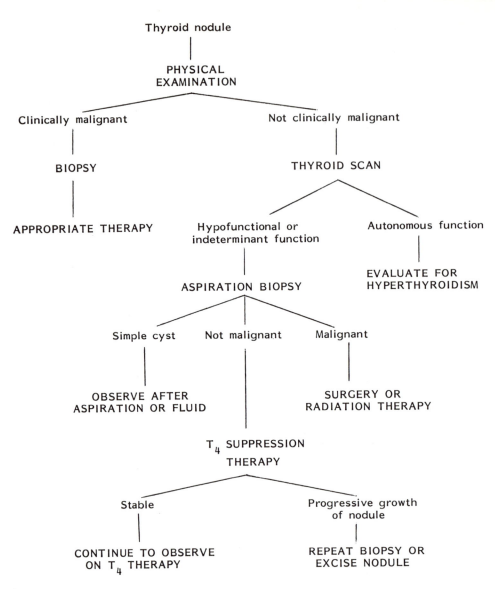

FIGURE 23-4   An approach to a patient with a single thyroid nodule.

made by an ultrasound examination of the nodule. Simple thyroid cysts are sonoluscent, and the fluid-filled cavity on an ultrasonogram corresponds in size to the palpable nodule. Solid thyroid masses include malignant lesions, although the majority are benign. As previously mentioned, a hemorrhagic degeneration of both benign and malignant nodules occurs often. This results in a mixed pattern seen on an ultrasonogram in which one area of an otherwise solid nodule appears cystic. On aspiration of this lesion, serosanguinous fluid generally is obtained. Demonstrating that a nodule has undergone a hemorrhage and cystic degeneration is of little diagnostic help; this lesion should continue to be evaluated as a solid nodule.

A biopsy procedure for a thyroid nodule, using either a fine-needle aspiration or a larger cutting needle, has received renewed interest.[53–55] An excellent correlation with histologic findings via surgery have been obtained using both techniques. Medullary, anaplastic, papillary, and poorly differentiated follicular carcinomas are readily diagnosed by either technique. When these diagnoses are made from a biopsy specimen, plans can be made for appropriate therapy. Neither biopsy procedure, though, satisfactorily distinguishes benign from malignant well-differentiated follicular tumors. Thus, the absence of biopsy specimen evidence of a malignancy is not conclusive proof that a malignant lesion is not present. This is less of a problem in elderly than in younger patients, since a well-differentiated follicular carcinoma occurs relatively infrequently in the geriatric population. However, in patients whose biopsy specimen reveals no malignancy, a further follow-up is necessary. Unless there is a contraindication to thyroid hormone treatment, an attempt to suppress the nodule with L-thyroxine therapy may be useful. Most malignant thyroid tumors do not regress with a suppressive therapy. A decrease in the size of the nodule, while taking 0.15–0.3 mg/day of L-thyroxine suggests that the nodule is either benign or is a hormone-responsive, well-differentiated malignancy. If a suppression of the nodule is observed, a long-term thyroxine therapy in doses that do not render the patient hyperthyroid is indicated. If the nodule continues to increase in size with L-T$_4$ therapy, a repeat biopsy procedure or an excision of the nodule usually is considered.

Simple cysts of the thyroid gland can be both diagnosed and effectively managed with aspiration techniques. These lesions are malignant much less often than solid thyroid nodules. If a cytologic examination of the cyst fluid does not reveal malignant cells, no further evaluation is necessary other than a routine examination of the thyroid at regular intervals.

Management of a Thyroid Carcinoma[56–58]
Surgery followed by L-T$_4$ suppression therapy is the customary treatment of papillary and follicular thyroid carcinomas. Radioiodine ablation of functioning thyroid tissue that remains after surgery will decrease recurrence rates in these patients. A thyroidectomy and regional node dissection is recommended for the management of a medullary carcinoma. The persistence of a medullary thyroid carcinoma following surgery is common and can be demonstrated by measuring the serum calcitonin concentrations. An external radiation of the neck is of some value in these patients. Anaplastic thyroid carcinoma has an extremely poor prognosis and runs a rapid course regardless of the therapy used. Surgery to relieve

compressive symptoms or to decrease the tumor mass before palliative radiotherapy can be considered. The results of chemotherapy in treating thyroid carcinoma have been disappointing. Short-term remissions sometimes are observed, but there is little change in the overall outcome. A lymphoma that involves the thyroid gland responds to external radiation therapy and to systemic chemotherapy, both of which may result in a clinical remission of the disease.

Multinodular Goiter

The pathogenesis of a multinodular goiter is unknown. Chronic autoimmune thyroiditis is present in some patients, but no etiology is apparent in the majority. The gland generally contains: nodules of varying size with areas of small hyperplastic follicles, large follicles filled with colloid, a previous hemorrhagic degeneration, scarring, and calcification. The goiter usually is discovered on a routine examination of the neck. The multinodular gland generally is firm but not hard, non-tender, and moves freely on swallowing. The surface of the gland is granular or lumpy, and discreet nodules frequently are felt. The goiter also may be first noted as a superior mediastinal shadow or as a cause of tracheal deviation on a chest x-ray (*see* Figure 23-5). Less often, a patient will complain of compressive symptoms, which usually is a lump in the throat on swallowing. A hemorrhage into the gland may produce a sudden swelling with a tenderness and pain that is localized to the thyroid lobe or radiates to the angle of the jaw. Rarely, a benign multinodular goiter produces either a venous obstruction and superior vena cava syndrome or compression of the recurrent laryngeal nerve with a vocal cord paresis and hoarseness.

Thyroid scanning occasionally is helpful in evaluating a nodular goiter. Multinodular goiters usually have a patchy or mottled distribution of an isotope, which demonstrates areas of varying functional activity in the gland (*see* Figure 23-6). Thyroid tissue that lies low in the neck or in the superior mediastinum can be correctly identified via thyroid scanning.

Either hypothyroidism or thyrotoxicosis can be associated with a multinodular goiter, and they may be clinically inapparent. Thyroid gland function is best assessed by measuring

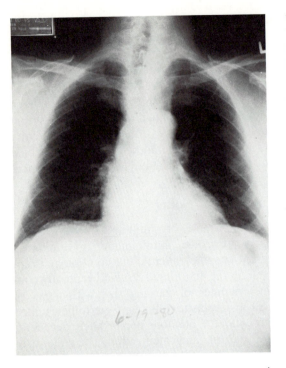

FIGURE 23-5   Tracheal deviation due to a nontoxic multinodular goiter in a 74-year-old male.

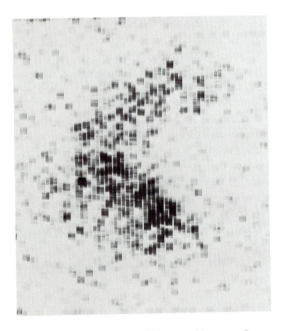

FIGURE 23-6   Rectilinear ^{131}I thyroid scan of a patient with a multinodular goiter that is demonstrating a heterogeneous distribution of uptake. This study is of the same patient whose x-ray film is shown in Figure 23-5.

the serum concentration of thyroid hormone or TSH. Although most patients with a multinodular goiter are euthyroid, many can be shown to have scattered areas of autonomous function within the gland. This is evidenced by a failure of thyroid hormone administration to suppress thyroid activity, as assessed by an RAIU.[59]

If thyroid function is normal, most patients with a multinodular goiter do not require therapy. L-thyroxine occasionally will result in a shrinkage of the goiter, although no change in thyroid size is seen in most patients. In addition, the frequent presence of non-suppressable thyroid function increases the likelihood of iatrogenic hyperthyroidism with thyroid hormone administration. For these reasons, attempts are not routinely made in elderly patients to decrease goiter size with thyroid hormone. If the goiter continues to enlarge, or when evidence of compression of neck structures by the goiter exists, therapy is warranted. If the compressive symptoms are chronic, thyroid hormone may be cautiously administered. External radiation or radioiodine ablation of the thyroid gland usually is not used because of concern that the acute response to radiation would result in a swelling of the thyroid and increased compressive or obstructive problems. A partial thyroidectomy is the most reliable method of relieving obstructive features. If one area of a multinodular goiter progressively enlarges, and if this is not due to a hemorrhage into a nodule, the issue of a malignancy resurfaces. A biopsy procedure or surgical excision of the growing mass should then be considered.

Hyperthyroidism

Hyperthyroidism, or thyrotoxicosis, refers to the clinical state that results from an excess of thyroid hormone from either endogenous or exogenous sources. The clinical expression of thyroid hormone excess may differ markedly among individuals. In general, hyperthyroid older patients present with more subtle and less specific symptoms than do younger thyrotoxic patients. This diagnosis may easily be overlooked as the cause of a geriatric patient's symptoms. A familiarity with the clinical features of hyperthyroidism in an elderly person, a high degree of suspicion of this diagnosis, and the appropriate use of thyroid function tests all are important for the recognition of this clinical problem. Since unrecognized thyrotoxicosis produces serious morbidity, and since effective and safe therapy is readily available, this diagnosis should be aggressively sought in elderly patients.

Prevalence

Clinicians once considered hyperthyroidism to be a disease that primarily affects young adults and is relatively uncommon in elderly patients. Most series reported that only 10–15% of all hyperthyroid patients were over 60 years of age. With an increased interest in geriatric medicine and the availability of more specific screening tests, thyrotoxicosis is being recognized more commonly in this age group. In Denmark, 58% of all hyperthyroid patients seen in a general medicine service were over 60 years old.[60] In an evaluation of 2,000 admissions to a geriatric inpatient unit, 1.1% were found to be thyrotoxic.[61] In recent surveys that were performed in Great Britain and Switzerland, hyperthyroidism occurred in over 2% of all females in the population.[47,62] Males are affected less frequently.

Etiologies

The causes of hyperthyroidism are the same in both young and elderly persons and are outlined in Table 23-3. Graves' disease and toxic nodular goiters account for the majority of cases. However, the uncommon forms of hyperthyroidism always must be considered, since the management of these disorders is much different than that of Graves' disease or toxic nodular goiters.

It is commonly thought that a toxic multinodular goiter is a more common cause of hyperthyroidism in elderly persons than is Graves' disease. This impression is strengthened by the infrequency of an infiltrative ophthalmopathy in hyperthyroid elderly patients. Based on a thyroid imaging or palpation of the gland, however, a diffuse toxic goiter occurs as, or more commonly than, a multinodular toxic goiter in geriatric patients.[29,63] The interpretation of these findings is compromised by both the inability to palpate the thyroid gland in some patients with hyperthyroidism and the in-

TABLE 23-3 Etiologies of Hyperthyroidism in Elderly Patients

Endogenous thyroid hormone production
  Thyroid hormone hypersecretion
    Humoral thyroid stimulators
      Graves' disease (thyroid-stimulating antibodies)*
      Pituitary tumor (TSH)†
    Autonomous thyroid secretion
      Toxic nodular goiter
      Metastatic thyroid follicular carcinoma
      Iodine-induced hyperthyroidism
  Follicular disruption
    Subacute thyroiditis*
    "Silent" lymphocytic thyroiditis*
    Radiation thyroiditis
Exogenous hyperthyroidism
  Factitious hyperthyroidism

* Most important.
† TSH = thyroid-stimulating hormone.
SOURCE: Compiled from the data of DeWind, et al,[67] Davis and Davis,[69] and Kawabe, et al.[70]

accurate prediction of a scan or physical examination of thyroid nodularity on a pathologic examination. Until assays of thyroid-stimulating antibody are routinely available, the clinical distinction between Graves' disease and toxic nodular goiter will continue to be difficult.

Graves' Disease
Graves' disease characteristically includes the triad of hyperthyroidism, a diffuse thyroid enlargement, and an infiltrative ophthalmopathy. Only one or any combination of these findings may be present in an individual patient. The ophthalmopathy of Graves' disease is not caused by a thyroid hormone excess, and it may either precede or follow the development of hyperthyroidism by many years. Pretibial myxedema, which consists of circumscribed plaques of inflammatory and mucopolysaccharide infiltrates occurring over the shin, rarely may accompany Graves' disease.

Graves' disease is a part of the spectrum of autoimmune thyroid diseases, the pathogenesis of which is not known. The hyperthyroidism is currently thought to be related to immunoglobulin stimulators of thyroid function. These thyroid-stimulating antibodies are detectable in the sera of almost all patients with thyrotoxic Graves' disease. There often is a history of

Graves' disease or chronic lymphocytic thyroiditis in other members of a patient's family. The onset of hyperthyroidism may be sudden in Graves' disease, and it usually occurs within a few months of the development of a goiter. The natural history of Graves' disease includes occasional remissions and relapses of hyperthyroidism with an ultimate development of euthyroidism or hypothyroidism in many patients, even in the absence of ablative therapy.

Toxic Nodular Goiter

A toxic nodular goiter differs from Graves' disease in several respects. Infiltrative ophthalmopathy, a dermopathy, and other autoimmune features are not associated with a toxic nodular goiter. A family history of thyroid disease is obtained less frequently than in Graves' disease. Unlike the diffuse hyperfunction of the gland that is observed in Graves' disease, the involvement of the thyroid in a toxic nodular goiter is localized or patchy. Autonomous areas of thyroid function coexist among normal thyroid follicles whose function is suppressed. Solitary hyperfunctioning thyroid nodules, due to a follicular adenoma or adenomatous hyperplasia, account for 10–15% of all hyperthyroidism in young adults and for a somewhat smaller fraction in elderly persons. Even in patients with a euthyroid multinodular goiter, areas of the gland in which the thyroid function is independent of TSH control frequently can be demonstrated with a T_3 suppression test.[59] This autonomous function progressively increases, which leads to the gradual development of hyperthyroidism in some patients with a long history of a multinodular goiter. Both thyroid lobes usually are affected, but occasional involvement is asymmetric. Hyperthyroidism generally is less severe in a toxic nodular goiter than in Graves' disease. However, that impression may reflect both the infrequency with which a toxic nodular goiter is seen in young individuals and the lower tolerance of elderly patients to increased thyroid hormone levels. When serum levels of thyroid hormone were compared in hyperthyroid elderly patients with diffuse and nodular goiters, no differences were observed; the values in thyrotoxic elderly patients were somewhat lower than in young patients with hyperthyroidism.[29]

Iodine-Induced Hyperthyroidism

Patients with multinodular thyroid glands have an abnormal intrathyroidal autoregulatory control, as well as an autonomy from TSH control of the thyroid function. The administration of large quantities of iodine in these patients frequently results in hyperthyroidism.[25] Iodine-induced hyperthyroidism is most often seen with the use of oral iodine solutions as an expectorant in patients with a chronic pulmonary disease, or following the administration of iodinated radio-opaque contrast agents for an angiography, urography, or gall bladder studies. These cases account for only a small fraction of hyperthyroid elderly patients. With the widespread use of iodinated contrast agents for angiography and computed tomography (CT scan), more iatrogenic cases may be seen.

Hyperthyroidism Due to Follicular Disruption

Thyrotoxicosis due to a release of stored thyroid hormones into the circulation occurs with inflammatory or radiation-induced damage to the thyroid gland. Unlike a toxic nodular goiter or Graves' disease, hyperthyroidism due to follicular destruction is not the result of increased thyroid glandular activity. The disrupted follicles cannot trap or store iodine, and the function of any normal follicles that remain is low due to the hyperthyroidism-induced suppression of TSH. Thus, one of the characteristic features of these forms of hyperthyroidism is a very low RAIU. The other important clinical feature is the self-limited nature of these problems. It is important to recognize these patients, since only supportive or symptomatic therapy is necessary.

Subacute thyroiditis often occurs following or during a viral infection, although proof of a viral infection of the thyroid gland rarely has been demonstrated. The clinical features of thyrotoxicosis, which are only mild or moderately severe, may be overshadowed by severe constitutional symptoms such as malaise, fatigue, and arthralgias, as well as by painful and tender thyroid gland. A thyroid biopsy demonstrates a disruption of the follicles and a diffuse inflammatory infiltration with multinucleated giant cells. The hyperthyroidism lasts only a few weeks and permanent hypothyroidism is rare, although a transient period of hypothyroidism may occur during the recovery phase.

Spontaneously resolving lymphocytic thyroiditis or silent (painless) thyroiditis only recently has been recognized, and its etiology is not known. Because of its self-limited nature and low RAIU, it initially was thought to be a variant of subacute thyroiditis. However, thyroid biopsy specimens have revealed a lymphocytic infiltration without giant cell formation. The relationship of silent thyroiditis and chronic lymphocytic thyroiditis (Hashimoto's disease) also is unclear. Antithyroid antibodies and permanent hypothyroidism, which are common in chronic lymphocytic thyroiditis, rarely are seen in patients with silent thyroiditis. As awareness of this form of hyperthyroidism has increased, elderly patients with silent thyroiditis have been described; however, the prevalence of thyrotoxicosis in elderly persons due to this entity has not been defined.[64–65]

Miscellaneous Forms of Hyperthyroidism

Hyperthyroidism can be caused by an ingestion of any form of a thyroid hormone. When this occurs in a patient without an underlying thyroid disease, the thyroid gland is not palpable and RAIU values are low, which make factitious hyperthyroidism difficult to distinguish from silent thyroiditis. Serum thyroglobulin levels may distinguish these two clinical problems; values are very high in the hyperthyroid phase of silent thyroiditis and low in factitious hyperthyroidism. Hyperthyroidism due to L-T$_3$ (Cytomel) ingestion results in low serum T$_4$ and FTI values, as well as a low RAIU. This diagnosis is confirmed by a history or by measuring high T$_3$ RIA concentrations.

Thyroid carcinoma is a very rare cause of hyperthyroidism. When it occurs, it almost always is associated with an obvious, large metastatic tumor burden of a follicular thyroid carcinoma. Uncomplicated hyperthyroidism should not lead to a search for a thyroid malignancy. Hyperthyroidism due to other neoplasms, such as TSH-secreting pituitary tumors, HcG-secreting neoplasms, and ovarian tumors that contain ectopic thyroid tissue (struma ovarii) also is rare.

Clinical Features of Hyperthyroidism

With the exception of an infiltrative ophthalmopathy, dermopathy, and an examination of the thyroid gland, the clinical manifestations of all forms of hyperthyroidism are similar.[63,66–70] Since thyroid hormones affect the function of many tissues, the symptoms and physical features that pertain to multiple organ systems may be observed in a thyrotoxic patient. The overall health and vigor of an individual, as well as underlying physiologic abnormalities, in part determine which symptoms occur in a given patient. Hypermetabolic symptoms, so characteristic of a young patient with Graves' disease, usually are not prominent. Elderly patients with thyrotoxicosis often are described as having apathetic or "masked" hyperthyroidism, because heat intolerance, sweating, nervousness, and hyperactivity are uncommon major manifestations. This clinical presentation was recognized over 50 years ago, and it is now known to be characteristic of hyperthyroidism in elderly persons. Although these metabolic symptoms rarely are a patient's chief complaint, they frequently are present when carefully looked for. The cardiovascular, neuromuscular, and gastrointestinal systems of elderly patients seem to adapt least well to the increased metabolic demand of hyperthyroidism. Consequently, as outlined in Table 23-4, symptoms that are associated with these organ systems predominate. Although elderly patients with hyperthyroidism who presented with predominantly cardiovascular or gastrointestinal features were described many years ago, a diag-

TABLE 23-4 Symptoms of Hyperthyroidism and Their Frequency in Elderly Thyrotoxic Patients

Symptom	% of Patients
Weight loss	70
Nervousness/tremor	63
Palpitations	63
Heat intolerance	63
Dyspnea	59
Increased sweating	52
Weakness	40
Decreased appetite	36
Constipation	26
Increased appetite	11

nosis of hyperthyroidism frequently is overlooked in these patients.

The thyroid gland itself rarely is a source of symptoms. Dyspnea, dysphagia, and hoarseness due to compression by the goiter are uncommon in hyperthyroidism. The absence of a goiter has been described in up to 37% of all hyperthyroid elderly patients. However, abnormalities of texture and consistency, such as firmness or nodularity, can be appreciated in almost all patients in whom the gland can be felt, even when the gland is not perceptibly enlarged.

Cardiovascular and circulatory abnormalities often are the most prominent and most serious features of hyperthyroidism in elderly persons. Thyroid hormones sensitize the myocardium to beta-adrenergic stimulation. Whether T_3 has a direct action on the heart that is independent of catecholamines remains controversial. Cardiac output typically is increased due to a combination of an increased heart rate, increased stroke volume, and decreased peripheral resistance.[71] Cardiac arrhythmia is the most common abnormality noted. Atrial fibrillation occurs with an increasing frequency as the age of the hyperthyroid person advances. A slow ventricular response to atrial fibrillation does not exclude a diagnosis of hyperthyroidism, as it is seen in about one third of all thyrotoxic elderly patients with an atrial fibrillation. The thyroid function in elderly patients who develop atrial fibrillation in the absence of a valvular cardiac disease deserves careful evaluation.[72] Other arrhythmias that are associated with hyperthyroidism include a sinus tachycardia and atrial flutter; a heart block also has been described. Angina may be exacerbated in patients with an underlying coronary artery disease. Dyspnea and peripheral edema commonly occur, although frank congestive heart failure usually is not observed except in patients with a pre-existing myocardial disease or with a very rapid ventricular response to atrial fibrillation. Congestive heart failure that accompanies hyperthyroidism is characterized by a relatively poor response to the usual therapeutic doses of digoxin. This reflects the increased metabolic clearance rate of digoxin in hyperthyroidism, rather than the true cardiac resistance to this medication.[73] Somewhat larger doses of digoxin are required to maintain normal serum digoxin concentrations in hyperthyroid patients.

Gastrointestinal features also may dominate the clinical picture in an thyrotoxic elderly patient.[74] Anorexia and decreased calorie intake are more common than an increased appetite. Consequently, weight loss occurs more often in older than younger hyperthyroid patients. Normal bowel function, increased frequency of bowel movements, and constipation occur about equally. A diagnosis of hyperthyroidism is sometimes delayed by a search for an occult malignancy, which is suggested by anorexia, weight loss, and chronic fatigue. Serum alkaline phosphatase and gamma glutamyl transpeptidase concentrations frequently are elevated, but they normalize after the correction of the hyperthyroidism. More serious hepatic abnormalities rarely are seen.

A variety of neuromuscular features may occur in a hyperthyroid elderly patient; tremulousness is most common. Although the classic thyrotoxic tremor is described as fine and rapid, this may be difficult to distinguish from the coarser tremor that is commonly seen in elderly patients. Muscle weakness, which characteristically involves proximal muscles of both the upper and lower extremities (but often is generalized), is due in large part to a decreased muscle mass that is associated with the patient's weight loss. Anxiousness, irascibility, a shortened concentration span, forgetfulness, and simple confusion are common problems noted by a patient's family. The combination of a tremor and weakness may interfere with a patient's ability to walk or to care for him- or herself. Patients with weakness, weight loss, and cognitive difficulties become apathetic and withdraw from activities and interactions with others, and they unfortunately and mistakenly are labelled as senile. The deep-tendon reflex time is shortened in hyperthyroidism, but this is difficult to quantify clinically, especially in an older patient; also, it is not a reliable diagnostic sign.

Clinically significant hematologic changes usually do not accompany hyperthyroidism. A pernicious anemia more commonly occurs in patients with Graves' disease, as does an autoimmune thrombocytopenia.

Laboratory Evaluation of Hyperthyroidism

The laboratory diagnosis of hyperthyroidism in elderly persons can be difficult. No single test of thyroid function allows a diagnosis to be made with certainty. The serum T_4 level is elevated in about 90% of all hyperthyroid elderly patients. The sensitivity of this test is enhanced when it is used in conjunction with the T_3RU to calculate the FTI. However, 3–4% of all patients admitted to one geriatric department had transient increases in both total T_4 and the FTI, which normalized when the acute medical problem was resolved.[30]

In most hyperthyroid elderly patients, the combination of appropriate clinical features and an elevated FTI is all that is necessary to confirm a diagnosis (see Figure 23-7). When there is a discrepancy between the clinical features and the FTI, then other tests of thyroid function are indicated. In patients who appear to be clinically hyperthyroid, but whose FTI is normal or equivocal, the measurement of a T_3 RIA or the free T_3 index may be useful. Although total T_3 levels are normal in about one third of all hyperthyroid elderly patients, some patients have

"T_3 toxicosis" with elevated T_3 values and normal T_4 levels. Although the T_3 RIA is not a useful primary screening test, for reasons outlined previously, an elevated serum T_3 level in a patient with clinical features of hyperthyroidism will establish that diagnosis.

In patients found to have an elevated T_4 level on routine screening tests, but who do not have cardiovascular, gastrointestinal, or other clinical features of hyperthyroidism, a TRH test is extremely helpful. A normal response to TRH effectively rules out a diagnosis of hyperthyroidism, while a flat response is consistent with (but not positive proof of) hyperthyroidism. If a diagnosis still is in doubt at this point, ancillary tests such as an RAIU or free T_4 levels can be considered. However, note that 41% of all hyperthyroid elderly patients have normal radioiodine uptakes and many ill euthyroid patients have elevated free T_4 values. In some patients, a T_3 suppression test might be considered. Autonomy of the thyroid function is demonstrable in patients with both Graves' disease and a toxic nodular goiter. A normal T_3 suppression test rules out those diagnoses. Alternative considerations include treating the patient symptomatically and carefully re-evaluating thyroid

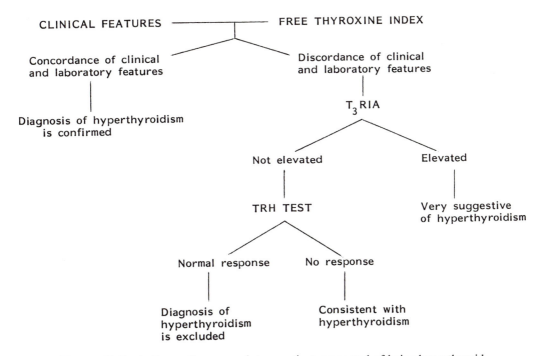

FIGURE 23-7   A diagnostic approach to a patient suspected of being hyperthyroid.

function in 2–4 weeks, or beginning an empiric trial of an antithyroid drug therapy and evaluating this patient's clinical response.

Once it has been determined that the patient is hyperthyroid, the differential diagnosis of thyrotoxicosis must be considered before choosing an appropriate therapeutic regimen. Patients with either subacute and "silent" thyroiditis or iodine-induced and factitious hyperthyroidism must be identified, since neither antithyroid drugs nor radioiodine or surgical therapy has a role in their management. The very low RAIU values that are observed during the thyrotoxic phase of all these disorders distinguishes them from Graves' disease and toxic nodular goiters.

Treatment of Hyperthyroidism

The objectives of managing a hyperthyroid patient are to normalize thyroid function and correct the physiologic abnormalities that are associated with a hyperthyroid state. Thyroid function can be controlled effectively with a variety of therapeutic approaches that include antithyroid drug therapy, radioiodine treatment, and subtotal thyroidectomy following antithyroid drug therapy.[60,70,75] Because each of these modalities requires several weeks before the thyroid function is normalized, the supportive management of patients (especially those with complicating medical problems or severe cardiovascular disease) is an important adjunct to therapy. This includes careful attention to the correction of coexistent medical problems and the provision of adequate nutritional support.

Many of the clinical components of hyperthyroidism can be improved or controlled by the administration of beta-adrenergic-blocking agents. Propranolol is the drug most often used in this setting, but newer beta-blockers also are effective. Neuropsychiatric, gastrointestinal, and cardiovascular features all improve with an adrenergic blockade. This improvement is not the result of a decrease in thyroid function, but rather is due to a blunting of the peripheral effects of thyroid hormone action by beta-blocking agents. The administration of these drugs does not interfere with the subsequent evaluation or management of a patient. Consequently, the therapeutic benefits of beta-blocker therapy can be used during the diagnostic process and

while arrangements are made for a more definitive therapy. The doses of beta-blocking agents that will achieve a therapeutic response are variable, but they generally are somewhat higher than the doses used in the management of other medical problems. As the thyroid function falls following an antithyroid drug or ablative therapy, the dose of beta-blockers can be gradually decreased and then discontinued when the hyperthyroidism has subsided. For patients with subacute or "silent" thyroiditis, this usually is the only form of therapy necessary, and it is used until the hyperthyroid phase of these disorders is resolved spontaneously.

The treatment of congestive heart failure that is associated with hyperthyroidism presents special problems. Even when used in appropriate doses, digitalis and diuretics may not be effective in this setting. For patients who are refractory to the usual treatment for congestive heart failure, a cautious administration of beta-blocking drugs may be effective when heart failure is associated with a tachycardia.

Antithyroid Drugs

The thionamide class of drugs, which include propylthiouracil and methimazole, will effectively control the hyperthyroidism in both Graves' disease and toxic nodular goiters by inhibiting thyroid hormone synthesis. The normalization of the thyroid function usually requires 3–4 months of therapy. Since Graves' disease may undergo a spontaneous remission, some patients may escape the necessity of an ablative antithyroid therapy by controlling the hyperthyroidism with antithyroid drugs until a remission occurs. Most patients, however, ultimately will experience a relapse following a several-month course of antithyroid drug therapy. Since a remission is not a part of the natural history of a toxic nodular goiter, the antithyroid drug therapy for this disorder must continue indefinitely or be followed by ablative therapy.

Antithyroid drugs most often are given in divided doses, but they also are effective when administered as a single daily dose in patients with uncomplicated hyperthyroidism. Initial doses of propylthiouracil are 300–600 mg/day, while methimazole is begun with doses of 30–60 mg/day. Minor side effects such as urticaria, arthralgias, abnormal liver function tests, and gastrointestinal symptoms occur infrequently. Agranulocytosis is the major complication of these drugs and occurs in about 0.1% of all patients treated. This is thought to be an idiosyncratic rather than a dose-related drug reaction. The routine monitoring of leukocyte counts does not help predict the occurrence of this complication. Following the discontinuation of antithyroid drug therapy and aggressive management of infectious complications, granulocyte production returns in several days.

Patients who receive long-term antithyroid drug therapy must be carefully followed to both ensure the adequacy of the therapeutic dose and recognize the development of hypothyroidism due to the drug therapy. If hypothyroidism occurs while a patient is on a maintenance dose of 300 mg of propylthiouracil or 30 mg of methimazole or less, it is more practical to maintain the blockade of thyroid hormone synthesis with this drug dose and add T_4 therapy than to attempt to titrate the dose of the antithyroid drug.

Radioiodine Therapy

In most medical centers, radioiodine therapy is most commonly used in the treatment of an older hyperthyroid patient. The rate of thyroid-cell turnover and, ultimately, the functional capacity of the gland are impaired following radioiodine therapy. Usually, serum thyroid hormone concentrations begin to fall about 6 weeks after therapy, with the full effect of the dose being seen between 3–6 months. There are no absolute contraindications to the use of radioiodine therapy in thyrotoxic elderly patients. The major concerns regarding the use of radioiodine therapy have been the acute exacerbation of hyperthyroidism and the late development of hypothyroidism. Although a few cases of severe hyperthyroidism and thyroid storm following ^{131}I therapy have been reported, patients who have been carefully studied following radioiodine therapy have demonstrated only modest or minimal transient elevations in thyroid hormone levels.[76,77] Patients who were receiving propranolol at the time of their radioiodine therapy experienced no clinical worsening, even when thyroid hormone levels did increase. Pretreatment with antithyroid drugs has been recommended to decrease the likelihood of radiation-induced thyroiditis; however, examples of thyroid storm following ^{131}I therapy in

patients who were pretreated with thionamides have been reported. Hyperthyroid patients with fragile cardiovascular systems can be treated with large doses of antithyroid drugs. After they become euthyroid, the antithyroid drugs can be discontinued for several days to accomplish the radioiodine therapy while the patient receives beta-blocker therapy. The antithyroid drugs can be restarted 3 or 4 days following the administration of radioiodine and can be continued until the therapeutic effect of the radioiodine is observed. Most patients, however, do not require any antithyroid drug preparation before ^{131}I therapy.

The incidence of hypothyroidism within the first year after radioiodine therapy for Graves' disease is dose-related and ranges between 15–30% in most series. Hypothyroidism then continues to develop with an annual incidence rate of 2–3%. This late development of hypothyroidism following radioiodine therapy may represent the natural history of Graves' disease rather than a radiation-induced effect, since this rate is similar to that seen after surgical or antithyroid drug therapy for Graves' disease. Hypothyroidism occurs uncommonly in patients with a toxic nodular goiter after radioiodine therapy. Presumably, the thyroid function is maintained in these patients by the areas of the thyroid gland that were suppressed at the time of therapy and escaped major radiation effects. Since it often is difficult to differentiate Graves' disease from a toxic nodular goiter in elderly patients, all individuals who receive radioiodine therapy need to be followed carefully for the first several months after their dose, and then at regular intervals indefinitely thereafter.

Surgical Therapy

A subtotal resection of the thyroid gland by an experienced surgeon also is an effective means of permanently controlling hyperthyroidism. To minimize the risk of surgical therapy, patients must become euthyroid via preoperative antithyroid drug treatment. They also should receive large doses of iodine for 7–10 days immediately before surgery, while they continue antithyroid drug therapy, to decrease the vascularity of the gland. Because of the ease and safety of using radioiodine therapy, a subtotal thyroidectomy generally is reserved for hyperthyroid patients who also have compressive symptoms or a suspicion of malignancy.

Treatment of Severe Hyperthyroidism

None of the approaches to management previously discussed result in a rapid improvement of thyroid function. For patients with a severe or complicated hyperthyroidism, rapid normalization of thyroid function is indicated. Large doses of antithyroid drugs are administered beginning 3–4 days after a dose of ^{131}I. Within a few hours after the antithyroid drug dose, thyroid hormone biosynthesis is impaired. Advantage then can be taken of the ability of iodine to decrease thyroid hormone secretion. Potassium iodide therapy, either as a supersaturated solution or as Lugol's solution, is begun several hours after the initial antithyroid drug dose. Serum thyroid hormone levels begin to fall rapidly, and the patient may become euthyroid within 1–3 weeks following therapy. Both the iodine and antithyroid drugs are continued until the effects of radioiodine are seen in 2–4 months. Lithium also has been shown to block thyroid hormone secretion and has been used as an adjunctive therapy in the treatment of hyperthyroidism. Side effects are common with lithium therapy. Because it offers no particular advantage compared to iodine therapy, lithium is not often used.

Thyroid Storm

An acute exacerbation of thyrotoxicosis that is associated with hyperthermia and congestive heart failure is known as thyroid storm. This occurs most often when a hyperthyroid patient develops another complicating medical problem or undergoes surgery without an appropriate preoperative control. Thyroid storm is not simply a worsening of the hyperthyroidism, but rather a reflection of the inability of the hyperthyroid patient to tolerate the increased stress that is associated with surgical procedures or infections. The management of thyroid storm includes supportive measures such as controlling body temperature with external cooling, the administration of oxygen, and the treatment of associated medical problems. Propranolol, in either large oral doses or (more usually) IV doses of 1 mg every 5 minutes until a therapeutic response is seen, frequently will control both

the hyperthermia and the cardiovascular manifestations. If beta blockade does not result in a rapid clinical improvement, the administration of large doses of antithyroid drugs followed by iodine, as outlined above, is indicated. Aspirin therapy should not be given as an antipyretic agent, since this may lead to a marked increase in free thyroid hormone levels due to a displacement of T_3 and T_4 from the TBG.

Hypothyroidism

Hypothyroidism occurs frequently, and produces disturbing, if not debilitating, symptoms that can greatly alter the daily activities of an elderly patient; yet, it is readily diagnosed and treated. It is unfortunate that patients often receive thyroid hormone therapy unnecessarily for such non-specific symptoms as obesity and sluggishness, while other patients with neuromuscular or gastrointestinal features of hypothyroidism remain unrecognized for many years before receiving appropriate treatment. It was emphasized several decades ago that hypothyroidism frequently is overlooked as a cause of symptoms, especially in elderly persons.[78]

Prevalence of Hypothyroidism in Elderly Persons

While failing thyroid function is not a universal component of the aging process, the occurrence of hypothyroidism does increase with advancing age. The true prevalence of hypothyroidism in geriatric populations is not known, since different screening methods have been used in various studies and because there is no generally agreed on criteria for this diagnosis. Several estimates have been made showing that hypothyroidism occurs in about 2% of all patients admitted to hospital geriatric units.[61,79,80] In the two large studies in which ambulatory or non-hospitalized populations of elderly patients were screened for a thyroid disease, hypothyroidism was found in 0.5% of all females over 65 years of age (in Whickham, Great Britain) and in 0.94% of all individuals in their 9th decade or older (in a New Zealand community).[47,81] Each of these studies tends to underestimate the true incidence rate of a low thyroid function in the populations surveyed, since low T_4 or FTI levels were a requirement for a diagnosis. However, it is well recognized that a mild or moderate symptomatic hypothyroidism can exist when T_4 levels are in the low-to-normal range. Hypothyroidism in elderly persons, as with most other disorders of the thyroid gland, occurs more commonly in females than males by a ratio of about 5:1.

Etiology

The common causes of hypothyroidism in elderly persons are listed in Table 23-5. Iodine deficiency is no longer an important cause of hypothyroidism in adults in the United States, although it continues to be a major worldwide nutritional problem. At present, chronic autoimmune thyroiditis is the most frequent cause of hypothyroidism. Iatrogenic causes of hypothyroidism are other major considerations. Decreased thyroid function commonly occurs: 1) Following the treatment of hyperthyroidism with radioiodine, surgery, or even antithyroid drugs alone; 2) Following a thyroidectomy for treatment of malignancies of the neck, including a thyroid carcinoma; and 3) Following external radiation to the neck that is used in the management of lymphomas or other tumors of the neck and upper thorax. Some patients who receive iodine solutions for chronic lung disease or lithium carbonate therapy for psychiatric disorders develop a clinical and often profound hypothyroidism. Both lithium and iodine have well-recognized antithyroid effects. Nevertheless, only a small portion of individuals who receive these medications manifest thyroid abnormalities. It is probable that many (if not most) patients who develop hypothyroidism, while receiving iodine or lithium, have a pre-existing defect in thyroid function, which most commonly is chronic lymphocytic thyroiditis.

Hypopituitarism or a hypothalamic deficiency can result in hypothyroidism. This can be caused by a surgical or accidental trauma, radiation therapy or tumors of the pituitary gland and suprasellar region, or (less commonly) a non-malignant involvement of this area by sarcoidosis, tuberculosis, or amyloidosis. Secondary hypothyroidism occurs less commonly in elderly adults than a primary failure of the thyroid gland. An acquired, isolated TSH deficiency is unusual. Patients with secondary hypothyroidism will either submit a history of a previous pituitary or hypothalamic insult, or they will have clinical features that suggest other abnormalities of hypothalamic-pituitary function, such as diabetes insipidus, acromegaly, hypogonadism, or adrenal insufficiency.

Clinical Features of Hypothyroidism in Elderly Persons

A diagnosis of hypothyroidism often can be made on the basis of clinical features alone. A myxedematous patient (one who manifests the features of both hypothyroidism and soft tissue accumulation of mucopolysaccharides) is easily recognized by his or her typical facial appearance, hoarse voice, slowness of speech, and paucity of motion. Although the clinical syndrome of hypothyroidism is characteristic in its totality, none of the individual features is specific. Many of the changes seen with hypothyroidism resemble features of the aging process itself. Consequently, when a patient presents with only one or a few of the manifestations of hypothyroidism, this diagnosis may not come to mind. The difficulty of a clinical diagnosis is further compounded by the gradualness with which hypothyroidism usually develops, even in most patients who become hypothyroid due to iatrogenic causes. Frequently, neither the patient nor his or her family are aware of the impressive changes that occur over a period of several years. Only by observing the resolution

TABLE 23-5 Etiologies of Hypothyroidism in Geriatric Patients

Primary Hypothyroidism
  Chronic lymphocytic thyroiditis
  Iatrogenic
    Radioactive iodine
    External radiation
    Surgical
    Drugs (antithyroid drugs, iodine, lithium)
  Iodine deficiency
Secondary Hypothyroidism
  Hypopituitarism
    Pituitary tumor
    Pituitary destruction
  Hypothalamic failure
    Hypothalamic destruction

of these symptoms following thyroid hormone replacement therapy can the magnitude of those changes become apparent.

The decrease in metabolic activity that is seen with hypothyroidism affects virtually all major physiologic processes. However, the clinical picture in an individual patient often is influenced by underlying medical problems. Cold intolerance and a modest weight gain are common symptoms, although obesity per se very rarely is attributable to hypothyroidism. Changes in one's external appearance often are very striking (*see* Figure 23-8). Decreased sweating and sebaceous gland secretion produce a dryness of the skin. A myxedematous infiltration of the dermis produces an apparent loosening of the connection between the dermal and epidermal layers, which results in a shiny, tissue-paper thin appearance of the skin. Hair loss from the scalp and lateral eyebrows may be noted. A puffiness of the hands and face, especially around the eyes, often is seen.

Proptosis is not a feature of hypothyroidism itself, but it may be present in patients with autoimmune thyroid disease. Some patients with hypothyroidism have thyroid enlargement, but the presence or absence of a goiter is not a reliable index of whether hypothyroidism exists. Females with hypothyroidism due to chronic lymphocytic thyroiditis have an en-

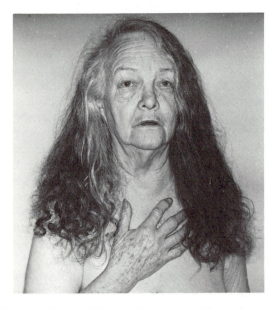

FIGURE 23-8   A 75-year-old woman with a primary hypothyroidism of long duration.

largement of the thyroid gland more frequently than males with the same disease.

Neuromuscular symptoms often dominate the clinical picture. Decreased mental and physical energy is manifested as a loss of motivation, failing memory, confusion, easy fatigability, and somnolence. Individuals may appear depressed, and they may progressively withdraw from social contact and physical activity or become more irritable, hostile, or frankly paranoid. Other patients become garrulous and, combined with their stubborn slowness of speech, may tax the patience of even the most interested interviewer. Positional vertigo and decreased hearing, both reversible with thyroid hormone therapy, can be disturbing symptoms. Cerebellar ataxia, disturbances of gait, and peripheral neuropathies (including carpal tunnel syndrome) are variably present. Muscle cramps and tenderness, and even muscle weakness, may be present. Serum levels of creatinine phosphokinase (CPK) and other muscle enzymes frequently are elevated in hypothyroidism, which is due in part to a decreased clearance of the enzymes from the circulation. A prolongation of the relaxation phase of the deep-tendon reflex is an important and characteristic physical finding. Decreased gastrointestinal motility, sometimes with a true ileus, results in a common complaint of constipation.

Although there are many cardiopulmonary features of hypothyroidism, they infrequently result in symptoms.[82] Bradycardia is a common finding. The cardiac output is decreased because of a reduction in both the stroke volume and pulse rate. Consequently, the glomerular filtration rate (GFR) is decreased and renal retention of both salt and water occurs. Peripheral edema, which occurs more commonly than a true non-pitting myxedema, and hyponatremia both may be present. In spite of the decreased cardiac output, congestive heart failure develops infrequently. Coronary artery disease occurs commonly in hypothyroid elderly patients, although it is not entirely clear that these patients are more prone to atherosclerotic disease than euthyroid patients.[83] An echocardiographic demonstration of asymmetric septal hypertrophy, which is resolved following T_4 therapy, recently was observed in 17 of 19 unselected hypothyroid patients.[84] An increase in the extent of a cardiac dullness on physical examination or in the diameter of the cardiac silhouette on a chest x-ray film may be due to a pericardial effusion or, less commonly, to a true cardiomegaly. The volume of pericardial fluid in a hypothyroid patient may be substantial, although cardiac tamponade or symptoms of constrictive heart disease are not commonly seen.

Compromised respiratory function may occur due to a weakness of the chest wall musculature, to pleural effusions, or (rarely) to an upper airway obstruction that is associated with a swelling of the tongue and pharyngeal tissues. Basal ventilatory rates are low, but usually are proportional to the decrement in oxygen consumption. In addition, the ventilatory response to hypoxemia and hypercarbia may be impaired.[85] The diminished oxygen consumption in hypothyroidism also results in a lower production of erythropoietin; a mild normocytic anemia with a hypoproliferative bone marrow frequently is encountered. Less often, a true pernicious anemia occurs in patients with hypothyroidism due to Hashimoto's thyroiditis.[86]

Laboratory Evaluation of Hypothyroidism

A diagnosis of primary hypothyroidism usually is confirmed easily by demonstrating a low FTI and an elevated TSH level (*see* Figure 23-9).

The TSH concentrations invariably are elevated in primary hypothyroidism unless the patient is receiving drugs such as dopamine, which suppress TSH secretion. Although a normal TSH value effectively rules out primary hypothyroidism, neither a low FTI nor a high serum TSH alone sufficiently confirms that diagnosis. As previously discussed, low FTI levels are seen in situations other than hypothyroidism. Decreased values of T_4 and FTI with a normal TSH may occur in euthyroid patients with a TBG deficiency or abnormal T_4 to TBG binding due to a serious illness. Likewise, an elevated TSH level does not necessarily connote hypothyroidism. An abnormally high serum TSH level and a normal FTI are observed in up to 20% of all elderly patients.[19,87] Some of these patients are symptomatically hypothyroid in spite of FTI levels in the low-to-normal range. These individuals generally have substantially elevated (greater than twice the normal values) TSH values and deserve to be treated. Other patients, generally those with less marked TSH elevations, do not have clinical features of a thyroid hormone deficiency. Whether these patients truly are hypothyroid, or simply require a persistent stimulation of the thyroid to maintain a normal thyroid function (decreased thyroid reserve), cannot be discerned with currently available testing tech-

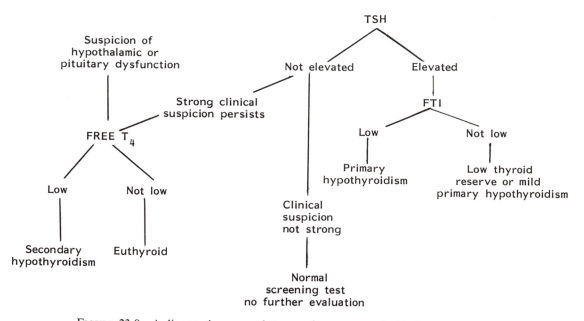

FIGURE 23-9 A diagnostic approach to a patient suspected of being hypothyroid.

niques; whether they should be treated depends on the entire clinical situation.

The TSH response to TRH administration in hypothyroidism is exaggerated; but, this test rarely is necessary to establish a diagnosis of primary hypothyroidism. Serum T_3 concentrations are of little use in the evaluation of a hypothyroid patient. Often, T_3 RIA and FT_3I values are normal in clearly hypothyroid patients; even more often, T_3 concentrations are low in ill euthyroid patients. Radioiodine uptake testing (RAIU) also is of limited help in a diagnosis of hypothyroidism. Value may be low, but they often are in the normal or even the supranormal range (e.g., an iodine deficiency). Since thyroid scans are not a test of thyroid function, they have no role in the determination of whether a patient is hypothyroid. Antithyroid antibodies may provide an insight into a diagnosis of autoimmune thyroiditis, but their presence does not necessarily correlate with thyroid function.

Hypothyroidism that is due to a disturbance of the pituitary or hypothalamus is diagnosed by demonstrating low FTI values in a patient with both hypothyroid symptoms and the presence of, or history of, a hypothalamic-pituitary dysfunction. The TSH levels may be undetectable, normal, or (very rarely) minimally elevated (less than twice the normal levels). It is difficult to exclude a diagnosis of mild secondary hypothyroidism in a patient with known pituitary disease who has symptoms that are compatible with hypothyroidism and low-to-normal FTI levels. Observing the response to a therapeutic trial of thyroid hormone therapy can be helpful in this situation. The TRH test does not reliably distinguish any deficits of pituitary and hypothalamic functions. Localization of the pathology requires a careful radiographic evaluation in addition to a thorough series of pituitary function tests.

Treatment

Regardless of the cause of hypothyroidism, synthetic L-thyroxine is the preferred thyroid hormone preparation for therapeutic use. Serum concentrations of T_4, T_3, and TSH remain constant when fixed doses are given daily.[88] Dessicated thyroid hormones, the mainstay of therapy for many years, contains both T_4 and T_3

in variable proportions; thus, different lots of these preparations may have different potencies. Since adequate amounts of T_3 are produced by a peripheral conversion of exogenous T_4, the combinations of synthetic $L-T_3$ and $L-T_4$ are not necessary. Synthetic $L-T_3$ is a very potent hormone preparation, which produces marked variations in serum T_3 concentrations. For this reason, it is not recommended as a routine maintenance therapy.[88] In addition, it is difficult to monitor the appropriateness of an $L-T_3$ replacement dose with routine laboratory tests, since T_4 levels remain very low and both T_3 and TSH concentrations fluctuate in patients who are receiving $L-T_3$.

The objective of L-thyroxine replacement therapy is to ameliorate the clinical features of hypothyroidism without producing the hypermetabolic symptoms of a thyroid hormone excess.[89] This usually requires L-thyroxine doses of 100–300 μg/day in adults. With advancing age, the average dose that is necessary for the normalization of thyroid function gradually falls to about 120 μg/day in patients over 65 years of age.[90] This decline in the T_4 replacement dose is the pharmacologic counterpart of the fall in endogenous T_4 secretion rates that are noted in elderly patients. It is due, in part, to the decreased body mass of older patients as well as to the decreased rate of T_4 clearance, which was previously discussed. Because of the long serum half-life of T_4, $L-T_4$ can be administered weekly in doses of about 1 mg to patients in whom compliance is a problem.[91]

Patients with asymptomatic hypothyroidism or a low thyroid reserve who are to be treated can be started safely on 100 μg/day of L-thyroxine unless they have a history of angina pectoris. For patients with more severe hypothyroidism, however, doses of 25–50 μg are used initially and then gradually increased in increments of 25–50 μg until euthyroidism is achieved.[92] This is done to minimize the risk of cardiovascular symptoms, which are due to a rapid increase in both the metabolic rate and oxygen demand. It requires several weeks before the full physiologic and clinical responses to a change in the $L-T_4$ dose are seen. Consequently, doses should be increased at intervals of at least 1 month.

The appropriateness of a maintenance dose must be established for each patient. The serum

TSH level is the most sensitive marker of the adequacy of a dose. If serum TSH levels remain elevated 4–6 weeks after the last dose adjustment, the patient is still undertreated. The serum T_4 level is the best index of overtreatment. Although some patients who are clinically euthyroid during L-T_4 therapy may have slightly elevated serum T_4 levels, it is wise (especially in elderly patients) to lower the L-T_4 dose when serum T_4 concentrations are elevated.

Patients with hypothyroidism that is due to a hypothalamic or pituitary dysfunction also are best treated with L-T_4. Before replacement therapy is begun, it is important to recognize and treat a coexisting adrenal insufficiency because thyroid hormone therapy, by increasing rates of cortisol metabolism, can precipitate the development of a symptomatic cortisol deficiency. The dose of L-T_4 that is necessary for euthyroidism in these patients is similar to the dose in individuals with primary hypothyroidism. Since TSH values are not elevated in patients with pituitary abnormalities, the correct dose is determined by a patient's clinical response and serum T_4 levels.

A water diuresis is one of the earliest signs of a response to L-T_4 administration, which begins within a few days of initiating therapy. Gradually the metabolic, neurologic, cardiac, and gastrointestinal features of hypothyroidism resolve over the next few weeks. The anemia and muscle weakness improve more slowly. A normalization of thyroid function may necessitate changes in the doses of medications that a patient receives for other clinical problems. Although this has not been studied extensively, some drugs (notably digoxin) are cleared more quickly in euthyroid patients compared to hypothyroid patients. As the hypothyroidism responds to therapy, the overall medical status of the patient should be re-evaluated.

The coexistence of coronary artery disease and hypothyroidism presents special management problems. The cardiac response to a thyroid hormone therapy is unpredictable in this group of patients. Anginal symptoms in some patients improve as L-thyroxine is cautiously administered, while in many patients the normalization of thyroid function produces no change in their cardiac symptoms.[92,93] In other patients, however, the increased metabolic rate that is associated with an improved thyroid function can result in the aggravation of angina or the development of palpitations and cardiac arrhythmias. These symptoms often can be controlled with beta-adrenergic-blocking agents, which allow gradual and progressive increases in L-T_4 doses and the eventual attainment of euthyroidism. Recently, coronary artery bypass surgery has been used successfully for the relief of angina before the correction of hypothyroidism.[94,95] Coronary angiography is safely performed in hypothyroid patients who are clinically stable. This diagnostic tool can be considered if the patient otherwise is a candidate for a coronary artery revascularization. Regardless of whether thyroid hormone therapy is initiated without or following coronary artery surgery, small initial doses (12.5–25 μgm daily) are indicated that are gradually increased at intervals of about 1 month; the patient's clinical couse must be followed carefully.

Myxedema Coma

Myxedema coma is a serious complication of a long-standing hypothyroidism that principally occurs in elderly patients. The clinical syndrome usually is not due to a sudden worsening of the hypothyroidism. Most often, it occurs after the administration of a sedative drug, after trauma or surgery, or during an infection or another acute medical illness in a chronically myxedematous patient. The sluggish cardiopulmonary system that is associated with severe hypothyroidism is unable to meet the increased metabolic demands imposed by an additional illness. The patient then develops a relatively sudden and progressive neurologic impairment and presents with characteristic features of the syndrome, which include stupor or coma, hypothermia, hypoventilation, hypotension, and bradycardia. Hypoglycemia and hypokalemia may be additional complications. A clinical diagnosis is made by observing these features in an individual with a history or appearance of hypothyroidism. Hypothermia that is due to cold exposure, profound sepsis, or cardiac failure may be difficult to differentiate from a myxedematous coma. If deep-tendon reflexes are present (they often are absent in a hypothermic patient), the delayed-return characteristic of hypothyroidism may be a useful diagnostic sign.

The rapid improvement of thyroid function is an urgent priority. Therapy consists of the IV administration of L-thyroxine, in doses of 0.2–0.5 mg, followed by a maintenance dose of 0.1 mg/day.[96] In addition, both treatment of the underlying infection or illness and general supportive measures are necessary; slow, passive rewarming is recommended. Vasopressors may be necessary to support the blood pressure; but they must be used cautiously, since ventricular arrhythmias are commonly seen as the patient's body temperature approaches normal. Glucocorticoids generally are given, although there is no solid evidence that they improve the outcome. Since myxedema coma that is not treated with thyroid hormone has such a poor prognosis, patients in whom this diagnosis is suspected should receive an appropriate therapy (including the initial dose of L-thyroxine) even before the laboratory confirmation of hypothyroidism is available. The administration of 0.2–0.5 mg of L-T_4 to a patient who is not hypothyroid is associated only with a minimal risk.

References

1. DeGroot LJ, Niepomniszcze H: Biosynthesis of thyroid hormone: basic and clinical aspects. *Metabolism* 26:665–718, 1977.
2. Chopra IJ, Solomon DH, Chopra U, et al: Pathways of metabolism of thyroid hormones. *Recent Prog Horm Res* 34:531–567, 1978.
3. Snyder PJ, Utiger RD: Inhibition of thyrotropin response to thyrotropin-releasing hormone by small quantities of thyroid hormones. *J Clin Invest* 51:2077–2084, 1972.
4. Ingbar SH: Effects of iodine: autoregulation of the thyroid, in Werner SC, Ingbar SH (eds): *The Thyroid*. Hagerstown, Harper & Row Publishers Inc, 1978, pp 206–215.
5. Robbins J, Cheng S-Y, Gershengorn MC, et al: Thyroxine transport proteins of plasma: molecular properties and biosynthesis. *Recent Prog Horm Res* 34:477–519, 1978.
6. Sterling K: Thyroid hormone action at the cell level. *N Engl J Med* 300:117–123, 173–177, 1979.
7. Silva JE, Larsen PR: Pituitary nuclear 3,5,3'-triiodothyronine and thyrotropin secretion: an explanation for the effect of thyroxine. *Sciences* 198:617–620, 1977.
8. Hansen JM, Skovsted L, Siersboek-Neilsen K: Age dependent changes in iodine metabolism and thyroid function. *Acta Endocrinol* 79:60–65, 1975.
9. Gregerman RI, Gaffney GW, Shock NW, et al: Thyroxine turnover in euthyroid man with special reference to changes with age. *J Clin Invest* 41:2565–2574, 1962.
10. Robertson JD, Reid DD: Standards for the basal metabolism of normal people in Britain. *Lancet* 2:687–703, 1952.
11. Shock NW: Metabolism and age. *J Chronic Dis* 2:687–703, 1955.
12. Keys A, Taylor HL, Grande F: Basal metabolism and age of adult man. *Metabolism* 22:579–587, 1973.
13. Shock NW, Watkins DM, Vienst MJ, et al: Age differences in water content of the body as related to basal oxygen consumption in males. *J Gerontol* 18:1–10, 1963.
14. Westgren U, Burger A, Ingemansson S, et al: Blood levels of 3,5,3'-triiodothyronine and thyroxine differences between children, adults and elderly subjects. *Acta Med Scand* 200:1124–1130, 1976.
15. Lipson A, Nickoloff EL, Hsu TH, et al: A study of age-dependent changes in thyroid function tests in adults. *J Nucl Med* 20:1124–1130, 1979.
16. Rubenstein HA, Butler VP Jr, Werner SC: Progressive decrease in serum triiodothyronine concentration with human aging: radioimmunoassay following extraction of serum. *J Clin Endocrinol Metab* 37:247–253, 1973.
17. Caplan RH, Wickus G, Glasser JE, et al: Serum concentration of the iodothyronines in elderly subjects: decreased triiodothyronine (T3) and free T3 index. *J Am Geriatr Soc* 29:19–24, 1981.
18. Olsen T, Laurberg P, Weeke J: Low serum triiodothyronine and high reverse triiodothyronine in old age: an effect of disease not age. *J Clin Endocrinol Metab* 47:1111–1115, 1978.
19. Sawin CT, Chopra D, Azizi F, et al: The aging thyroid: increased prevalence of elevated thyrotropin levels in the elderly. *JAMA* 242:247–250, 1979.
20. Wagner H, Vosberg H, Bockel K, et al: Influence of age on response of TSH to thyrotropin releasing hormone in normal subjects. *Acta Endocrinol Suppl* 184:119, 1974.
21. Ohara H, Kobayashi T, Shiraishi M, et al: Thyroid function of the aged as viewed from the pituitary-thyroid system. *Endocrinol Jpn* 21:377–386, 1974.
22. Croxson MS, Wilson TM, Ballantyne GH: TRH testing, T4 toxicosis and the aging thyroid gland. *NZ Med J* 93:417–420, 1981.
23. Snyder PJ, Utiger RD: Response to thyrotropin releasing hormone (TRH) in normal man. *J Clin Endocrinol Metab* 34:380–385, 1982.

24. Ryan M, Kovaks K, Ezrin C: Thyrotrophs in old age: an immunologic study of human pituitary glands. *Endokrinologie* 73:191–198, 1979.

25. Vagenakis AG, Wang C, Burger A, et al: Iodide-induced thyrotoxicosis in Boston. *N Engl J Med* 287:523–527, 1972.

26. Braverman LE, Ingbar SH, Vagenakis AG, et al: Enhanced susceptibility to iodide myxedema in patients with Hashimoto's disease. *J Clin Endocrinol Metab* 32:515–521, 1971.

27. Ingbar SH: The influence of aging on the human thyroid hormone economy, in Greenblatt R (ed): *Geriatric Endocrinology*. New York, Raven Press, 1978, pp 13–31.

28. Hesch RD, Gatz J, Pape J, et al: Total and free triiodothyronine and thyroid-binding globulin concentration in elderly human persons. *Europ J Clin Invest* 6:139–145, 1976.

29. Caplan RH, Glasser JE, Davis K, et al: Thyroid function tests in elderly hyperthyroid patients. *J Am Geriatr Soc* 26:116–120, 1978.

30. Mankikar GD, Clark ANG: Euthyroid "thyroxine toxicosis." *J Am Geriatr Soc* 29:331–333, 1981.

31. Chopra IJ, Solomon DH, Hepner GW, et al: Misleadingly low free thyroxine index and usefulness of reverse triiodothyronine measurements in nonthyroidal illnesses. *Ann Int Med* 90:905–912, 1979.

32. Chopra W, Solomon DH, Teco GNC, et al: An inhibitor of the binding of thyroid hormones to serum proteins is present in extrathyroidal tissues. *Science* 215:407–409, 1982.

33. Oppenheimer JH, Schwartz HL, Marriash CN, et al: Evidence for a factor in the sera of patients with nothyroidal disease which inhibits iodothyronine binding by solid matrices, serum proteins, and rat hepatocytes. *J Clin Endocrinol Metab* 54:757–766, 1982.

34. Kaplan MM, Larsen PR, Crantz FR, et al: Prevalence of abnormal thyroid function tests in patients with acute medical illnesses. *Am J Med* 72:9–16, 1982.

35. Gooch BR, Isley WL, Utiger RD: Abnormalities in thyroid function tests in patients admitted to a medical service. *Arch Int Med* 142:1801–1805, 1982.

36. Hamada S, Nakagawa T, Mori T, et al: Re-evaluation of thyroxine binding and free thyroxine in human serum by paper electrophoresis and equilibrium dialysis, and a new free thyroxine index. *J Clin Endocrinol* 31:166–179, 1970.

37. Herrmann J, Rusche HJ, Kroll HJ, et al: Free triiodothyronine (T_3) and thyroxine (T_4) serum levels in old age. *Horm Metab Res* 6:239–240, 1974.

38. Gavin LA, Rosenthal M, Cavalieri RR: The diagnostic dilemma of isolated hyperthyroxinemia in acute illness. *JAMA* 242:251–253, 1979.

39. Wiener JD: Value of the free triiodothyronine index in the diagnosis of hyperthyroidism. *Eur J Nucl Med* 5:119–124, 1980.

40. Oddie TH, Myhill J, Pirnique FG, et al: Effect of age and sex on the radioiodine uptake in euthyroid subjects. *J Clin Endocrinol Metab* 28:776–782, 1968.

41. Hershman JH: Clinical application of thyrotropin-releasing-hormone. *N Engl J Med* 290:886–890, 1974.

42. Burrows AW, Cooper E, Shakespear RA, et al: Low serum L-T_3 levels in the elderly sick: protein binding, thyroid and pituitary responsiveness, and reverse T_3 concentrations. *Clin Endocrinol (Oxford)* 7:289–300, 1977.

43. Schneider AB, Ikekubo K: Measurement of thyroglobulin in the circulation: clinical and technical considerations. *Ann Clin Lab Sci* 9:230–235, 1979.

44. Schlesinger MJ, Gargill SL, Saxe IH: Studies in nodular goiter I. Incidence of thyroid nodules in routine necropsies in a nongoitrous region. *JAMA* 110:1638–1641, 1938.

45. Denham MJ, Wills EJ: A clinico-pathological survey of thyroid glands in old age. *Gerontology* 26:160–166, 1980.

46. Vander JB, Gaston EA, Dawber TR: The significance of nontoxic thyroid nodules. *Ann Int Med* 69:537–540, 1968.

47. Tunbridge WMG, Evered DC, Hall R, et al: The spectrum of thyroid disease in a community: the Wickham survey. *Clin Endocrinol* 7:481–493, 1977.

48. Mortensen JD, Woolner LB, Bennett WA: Gross and microscopic findings in clinically normal thyroid glands. *J Clin Endocrinol Metab* 15:1270–1280, 1955.

49. Hamburger JI: The presentation of thyroid malignancy in the geriatric patient. *Henry Ford Hosp Med J* 28:158–160, 1980.

50. Clark OH, Demling R: Management of thyroid nodules in the elderly. *Am J Surg* 132:615–619, 1976.

51. Ashcraft MW, Van Herle AJ: Management of thyroid nodules. I: History and physical examination, blood tests, X-ray tests, and ultrasonography. *Head Neck Surg* 3:216–227, 1981.

52. Ashcraft MW, Van Herle AJ: Management of thyroid nodules. II. Scanning techniques, thyroid suppressive therapy, and fine needle aspiration. *Head Neck Surg* 3:297–322, 1981.

53. Gershengorn MG, McClung MR, Chu EW, et al: Fine-needle aspiration cytology in the preoperative diagnosis of thyroid nodules. *Ann Int Med* 87:265–269, 1977.

54. Miller JM, Hamburger JI, Kini S: Diagnosis of thyroid nodules: use of fine-needle aspiration and needle biopsy. *JAMA* 241:481–484, 1979.

55. Miller TR, Abele JS, Greenspan FS: Fine-needle aspiration biopsy in the management of thyroid nodules. *West J Med* 134:198–205, 1981.

56. Clark OH: Thyroid nodules and thyroid cancer: surgical aspects. *West J Med* 133:1–8, 1980.

57. Mazzaferri EL: Papillary and follicular thyroid cancer: a selective approach to diagnosis and treatment. *Ann Rev Med* 32:73–91, 1981.

58. Simpson WJ: Thyroid malignancy in the elderly. *Geriatrics* 37:119–125, 1982.

59. Miller JM, Block MA: Functional autonomy in multinodular goiter. *JAMA* 214:535–539, 1970.

60. Ronnov-Jessen V, Kirkegaard C: Hyperthyroidism—a disease of old age. *Br Med J* 1:41–43, 1973.

61. Bahemuka M, Hodkinson HM: Screening for hypothyroidism in elderly inpatients. *Br Med J* 2:601–603, 1975.

62. Bürgi H, Geiser J, Rösler H, Studer H: Die vekannte Hyperthyreose beim Spitalpatienten. *Schweiz Med Wochenschr* 108:1257–1262, 1978.

63. Stiel JN, Hales IB, Reeve TS: Thyrotoxicosis in an elderly population. *Med J Aust* 2:986–988, 1972.

64. Gordon M: "Silent" thyroiditis with symptomatic hyperthyroidism in an elderly patient. *J Am Geriatr Soc* 26:375–377, 1978.

65. Gordon M, Gryfe CI: Hyperthyroidism with painless subacute thyroiditis in the elderly. *JAMA* 246:2354–2355, 1981.

66. Seed L, Lindsay AM: Hyperthyroidism in the aged: a review of 100 cases over 60 years of age. *Geriatrics* 4:136–145, 1949.

67. DeWind LT, Commons RR, Starr P: Diagnosis and management of hyperthyroidism in the aged. *Geriatrics* 13:67–74, 1958.

68. Bartels EC: Hyperthyroidism in patients over 65. *Geriatrics* 20:459–462, 1965.

69. Davis PJ, Davis FB: Hyperthyroidism in patients over the age of 60 years. *Medicine* 53:161–181, 1974.

70. Kawabe T, Komiya I, Endo T, et al: Hyperthyroidism in the elderly. *J Am Geriatr Soc* 27:152–155, 1979.

71. Forfar JC, Muir AL, Sawers SA, et al: Abnormal left ventricular function in hyperthyroidism. *N Engl J Med* 307:1165–1170, 1982.

72. Forfar JC, Miller HC, Toft AD: Occult thyrotoxicosis: a correctable cause of "idiopathic" atrial fibrillation. *Am J Cardiol* 44:9–12, 1979.

73. Croxson MS, Ibbertson HK: Serum digoxin in patients with thyroid disease. *Br Med J* 3:566–568, 1975.

74. Scarf M: Gastrointestinal manifestations of hyperthyroidism. *J Lab Clin Med* 21:1253–1258, 1936.

75. McClung MR, Greer MA: Treatment of hyperthyroidism. *Ann Rev Med* 31:385–404, 1980.

76. Shafer RB, Nuttall FQ: Acute changes in thyroid function in patients treated with radioactive iodine. *Lancet* 2:635–637, 1975.

77. Tamagna EI, Levine GA, Hershman JM: Thyroid-hormone concentrations after radioiodine therapy for hyperthyroidism. *J Nucl Med* 20:387–391, 1979.

78. Kimble ST, Stieglitz EJ: Hypothyroidism: a geriatric problem. *Geriatrics* 7:20–31, 1952.

79. Lloyd WH, Goldberg IJL: Incidence of hypothyroidism in the elderly. *Br Med J* 2:1256–1259, 1961.

80. Atkinson RL, Dahms WT, Fisher DA, et al: Occult thyroid disease in an elderly hospitalized population. *J Gerontol* 33:372–376, 1978.

81. Campbell AJ, Reinken J, Allan BC: Thyroid disease in the elderly in the community. *Age Ageing* 10:47–52, 1981.

82. Crowley WF Jr, Ridgway EC, Bough EW, et al: Noninvasive evaluation of cardiac function in hypothyroidism. *N Engl J Med* 296:1–6, 1977.

83. Steinberg AD: Myxedema and coronary artery disease—a comparative autopsy study. *Ann Int Med* 68:338–344, 1968.

84. Santos AD, Miller RP, Mathew PK, et al: Echocardiographic characterization of the reversible cardiomyopathy of hypothyroidism. *Am J Med* 68:675–682, 1980.

85. Zwillich CW, Pierson DJ, Hofeldt FD, et al: Ventilatory control in myxedema and hypothyroidism. *N Engl J Med* 292:662–665, 1975.

86. Means JH, Lerman J, Castle WB: The coexistence of myxedema and pernicious anemia. *Trans Assoc Am Phys* 45:363–374, 1930.

87. Wong ET, Bradley SG, Schultz AL: Elevations of thyroid-stimulating hormone during acute nonthyroidal illness. *Arch Int Med* 141:873–875, 1981.

88. Saberi M, Utiger RD: Serum thyroid hormone and thyrotropin concentrations during thyroxine and triiodothyronine therapy. *J Clin Endocrinol Metab* 39:923–927, 1974.

89. McConahey WM: Diagnosing and treating myxedema and myxedema coma. *Geriatrics* 34:61–66, 1978.

90. Rosenbaum RL, Barzel US: Levothyroxine replacement dose for primary hypothyroidism decreases with age. *Ann Int Med* 96:53–55, 1982.

91. Bernstein RS, Robbins J: Intermittent therapy with thyroxine. *N Engl J Med* 281:1444–1448, 1969.

92. Levine HD: Compromise therapy in the patient with angina pectoris and hypothyroidism. *Am J Med* 69:411–418, 1980.
93. Keating FR Jr, Parkin TW, Selby JB, et al: Treatment of heart disease associated with myxedema. *Prog Cardiovasc Dis* 3:364–381, 1960.
94. Paine TD, Rogers WJ, Baxley WA, et al: Coronary arterial surgery in patients with incapacitating angina pectoris and myxedema. *Am J Cardiol* 40:226–231, 1977.
95. Hay ID, Duick DS, Vlietstra RE, et al: Thyroxine therapy in hypothyroid patients undergoing coronary revascularization: a retrospective analysis. *Ann Int Med* 95:456–457, 1981.
96. Ridgway EC, McCammon JA, Benotti J, et al: Acute metabolic responses in myxedema to large doses of intravenous L-thyroxine. *Ann Int Med* 77:549–555, 1972.

CHAPTER 24

Adrenal Disorders

ITAMAR B. ABRASS, M.D.

Alterations in the regulation of, and responsiveness to, adrenal cortical and medullary hormones in aging could have significant clinical consequences, particularly during stress. Diseases of the adrenal cortex and medulla are uncommon in elderly persons; however, they should not be overlooked, since they may be life-threatening, but treatable. This chapter will address these disorders and the physiologic alterations that are related to adrenal function and hormone responsiveness.

The Adrenal Medulla

Catecholamines are synthesized in the brain, sympathetic nerve endings, and tissue of neural crest origin, such as the adrenal medulla.[1] The major precursor for norepinephrine and epinephrine synthesis is tyrosine. Tyrosine is converted to dihydroxyphenylalanine (dopa) by tyrosine hydroxylase, which is the rate-limiting enzyme in the pathway. In the next step, dopamine is synthesized from dopa by the enzyme amino acid decarboxylase; dopamine then is converted to norepinephrine by dopamine hydroxylase. In the adrenal medulla and organ of Zuckerkandl, norepinephrine is further metabolized to epinephrine by the enzyme N-methyl transferase.

Intraneural regulation of catecholamine synthesis and degradation is complex, but it involves basically two major steps: 1) Newly synthesized norepinephrine demonstrates an end-product inhibition of the rate-limiting enzyme tyrosine hydroxylase; 2) Norepinephrine that enters the neuron by re-uptake regulates a further synthesis of the catecholamine by the same mechanism. Monoamine oxidase is the major intraneuronal degradative enzyme.

Changes of Aging

Circulating catecholamines come from the adrenal medulla or sympathetic nerves. Epinephrine generally reflects adrenal medullary function, while norepinephrine is a parameter of sympathetic nerve activity. There is no apparent alteration in plasma epinephrine with age,[2] which suggests that the adrenal medullary function is not affected by age. However, several groups have demonstrated an age-associated increase in plasma norepinephrine.[2-7] An upright posture and glucose ingestion also result in higher norepinephrine concentrations in elderly persons.[8] Whether these changes reflect a primary hyperactivity of the sympathetic nervous system with age or are compensatory for a decreased catecholamine responsiveness has not been defined.

A decreased catecholamine responsiveness in aging, however, may have important physiologic consequences. The response to both stress and exercise of the cardiovascular system in humans and animals diminishes with advancing age.[9] This decreased responsiveness has been defined as an alteration in the beta-adrenergic pathway of cardiac stimulation. The heart rate response to isoproterenol is decreased in aging humans,[10,11] dogs,[12] and rats.[13] In dogs, despite the decreased isoproterenol responsiveness, there is no age-related deficit in response to electrical pacing.[12] The inotropic response to isoproterenol also is diminished with age in rats, while the contractile response to calcium is unaltered.[14] Taken together, these data demonstrate a decreased myocardial catecholamine responsiveness with aging. The calcium and pacing data, however, suggest that the effector site (contractile elements) is intact in aging, and that the mechanisms of the age difference lie in the sequence of events that mediate the response between the beta-adrenergic receptor and the effector.

The initial site of action of catecholamines is their binding to specific membrane receptors. An alteration in receptor characteristics with age may result in a diminished catecholamine responsiveness. The data, however, demonstrate both unaltered rat myocardium[15–17] and human lymphocyte[18] beta-adrenergic receptor numbers.

In the proposed mechanism of catecholamine action, the step following receptor binding is a stimulation of adenylate cyclase activity, which results in increased intracellular cyclic adenosine monophosphate (cAMP) levels. An age-associated decrease in adenylate cyclase activity has been demonstrated in both rat myocardium[19,20] and human lymphocytes.[21,22] This loss of adenylate cyclase activity may account, at least in part, for the decreased catecholamine responsiveness in senescence. A deficit beyond cAMP generation also has been proposed.[15]

Pheochromocytoma

Pheochromocytoma is rare in elderly persons. Signs and symptoms are (as in young persons) related to the cardiovascular and central nervous systems and to hypermetabolism. However, due to an underlying cardiac or neurologic disease, elderly persons may tolerate the elevated catecholamine levels less well (*see* Table 24-1). Thus, tachyardia, tremor, sleep disorders, and psychic changes, all may be of greater consequence in an older population. A definitive diagnosis is made by demonstrating elevated plasma or urinary catecholamine levels or their metabolites; these need to be age adjusted to take into account the increased catecholamine levels of aging. A localization of the tumor, whenever possible, should be done by

TABLE 24-1 Signs and Symptoms of Pheochromocytoma That May Be of Greater Consequence in Elderly Persons

---

Palpitations and tachycardia
Anorexia and weight loss
Glucose intolerance
Decreased gastrointestinal motility
Postural hypotension
Psychic changes
Sleep disturbances
Tremor

---

non-invasive techniques such as computed tomography (CT scan) or scintigraphy. Medical treatment is with alpha-adrenergic-blocking agents, which should be instituted before any invasive procedure or surgery. The decision for a surgical excision of the tumor must be individualized.

Adrenal Cortex

Adrenal biosynthesis of steroid hormones is complex, with dozens of enzymes in the pathway.[23] The adrenal cortex is able to synthesize cholesterol from acetate or take it up from the circulation. The rate-limiting step in steroid biosynthesis is the conversion of cholesterol to pregnenolone. In the zona fasciculata, pregnenolone is converted to the active glucocorticoid, cortisol. All these steps are regulated by adrenocorticotropin (ACTH).

Aldosterone is synthesized in the zona glomerulosa under the primary regulation of angiotensin. Hyperkalemia and hyponatremia also stimulate aldosterone secretion. Although they do not appear to be necessary for good health, adrenal androgens are quantitatively a major secretory product of the adrenal cortex. Dehydroepiandrosterone is the most important of these, but androstenedione and testosterone also are secreted. The regulation of adrenal androgen secretion other than via ACTH is not well defined.

Pituitary ACTH secretion is regulated by a negative feedback loop. Of the adrenal secretory products, only cortisol has any significant ACTH-suppressing activity, so that low levels of cortisol allow for ACTH secretion while high levels of cortisol suppress the secretion.

Changes of Aging

The changes in cortisol that are associated with aging are similar to those seen with thyroxine (T_4) (*see* Table 24-2). There is a decrease in cortisol secretion,[24] but plasma cortisol levels are normal[25] due to an equivalent reduction in the metabolic clearance rate.[24,26] Urinary cortisol metabolites, such as 17-hydroxy steroids and 17-ketogenic steroids also are decreased, while urinary free cortisol is unaltered.[25] Diurnal variation also is maintained in aging.[25]

Insulin tolerance tests, which assess the integrity of the hypothalamic-pituitary-adrenal axis are normal in aging.[25-27] Metyrapone testing of the pituitary ACTH reserve is normal, as is the cortisol response to surgical stress.[25] The response of the adrenal cortex to exogenous ACTH is maintained,[25,26,28] as is the response to dexamethasone suppression.[27]

Taken as a whole, these data demonstrate a decrease in basal cortisol secretion with aging while there is an intact hypothalamic-pituitary-adrenal axis, which responds normally to stress and the stimulation of any component of the axis. The decrease in the metabolic clearance rate of glucocorticoids will affect exogenously administered steroids; thus, a replacement dosage needs to be adjusted downward. Unfortunately there are no specific guidelines for adjusting the dose. When ACTH assays become more sensitive in the normal and near-normal range, ACTH determinations may become the parameter for assessing appropriate replacement doses.

Aging also is associated with a decreased production of other adrenal steroids, which include pregnenolone,[29] progesterone,[29] 17-hydroxy progesterone,[30] deoxycortisol,[31] corticosterone,[31] and aldosterone.[32-34] Of these, the steroid of greatest consequence is aldosterone. The metabolic clearance rate for aldosterone is decreased, although less than the secretory rate, thus resulting in decreased plasma levels.[32] The plasma renin activity is decreased in aging, as is the aldosterone response to upright posture and sodium restriction.[33,35] The blood pressure response is increased, while the aldosterone response is decreased to a stimulation by angiotensin II.[34] The aldosterone response to ACTH, however, is not decreased.[33] The angiotensin effects might be explained by the effect of angiotensin on its own receptors. Angiotensin down-regulates angiotensin receptors in the vasculature and up-regulates receptors in the adrenal cortex. With a decrease in the plasma renin activity and the concomitant decrease in angiotensin, vascular receptors should be increased and adrenal receptors decreased, which leads to an increased vascular response and a decreased adrenal response.

Although the consequences of decreased ad-

TABLE 24-2   Physiologic Changes of the Aging Adrenal Gland

Steroids	Decreased	Unaltered
Glucocorticoids	Cortisol secretion Metabolic clearance rate of cortisol Urinary 17-hydroxy and 17-ketogenic steroids	Plasma cortisol Urinary free cortisol Diurnal variation of cortisol Insulin tolerance test Metyrapone test Response to surgical stress ACTH* stimulation test Dexamethasone suppression test
Mineralocorticoids	Aldosterone secretion Plasma aldosterone Metabolic clearance rate of aldosterone Response to upright posture and sodium restriction Response to angiotensin II	Response to ACTH
Androgens	Plasma dehydroepiandrosterone and androsterone Urinary 17-ketosteroids	

* ACTH = adrenocorticotropic hormone.

renal androgens with age are not understood, they show the most marked decrease of the adrenal steroids. There is an age-associated decrease in plasma dehydroepiandrosterone, androsterone,[36] and urinary 17-ketosteroids.[37] These changes occur in both sexes and are so marked that plasma adrenal androgens are almost absent by 70 years of age.[36]

Adrenocortical Disease

Addison's Disease

Although adrenal hypofunction is rare in elderly persons, it should not be missed; also, a high level of suspicion should be maintained. Weakness, fatigue, weight loss, hypotension, and hyperpigmentation, which are the common symptoms and signs of Addison's disease, should not be ascribed to aging. The most common etiology is autoimmune disease; but, tuberculosis also is a possible cause, especially in an elderly population with a higher prevalence of this disease. Bleeding into the adrenal cortex that is due to anticoagulation therapy and a discontinuation of glucocorticoid therapy also are etiologic factors.

A diagnosis is made by noting the adrenal response to ACTH. Since the adrenal response to ACTH is unaltered in normal aging, an abnormal response should confirm this diagnosis. If the patient initially is seen during a stress situation such as hypotension, one determination of plasma cortisol and aldosterone (before therapy is instituted) may confirm the diagnosis without further testing. During a hypotensive episode, both cortisol and aldosterone should be elevated if the pituitary-adrenal axis is intact. A low cortisol determination in the presence of a high aldosterone determination would suggest adrenal hypofunction on the basis of an ACTH deficiency. Low levels of both cortisol and aldosterone suggest a primary adrenal disease.

The treatment is with replacement glucocorticoids, but the decrease in the metabolic clearance rate must be considered. Recommendations for replacement therapy in elderly persons have been made based on urinary creatinine levels. The decreased metabolic clearance rate, however, relates to changes in hepatic steroid metabolism rather than to creatinine generation; thus, such recommendations do not seem

to address the issue. When ACTH determinations become sensitive in the normal and near-normal ranges, ACTH levels will be the best parameter for adjusting replacement doses. As in young persons, the dose should be split: two-thirds in the morning and one-third in the afternoon.

Cushing's Syndrome

Hyperfunction of the adrenal glands occasionally occurs in elderly persons. Again, the signs and symptoms (including hypertension, diabetes mellitus, osteoporosis, edema, thin skin, and weakness) should not be overlooked for changes in aging.

Since dexamethasone suppression is unaltered with age, the overnight dexamethasone suppression test constitutes the most useful technique for defining the presence of Cushing's Syndrome. Urinary free cortisols and a diurnal variation also are unaltered with age and may be used in a diagnosis. A determination of the plasma ACTH level may help in differentiating between an adrenal, pituitary, or ectopic disease. Very high ACTH levels are most consistent with an ectopic source, particularly from the lung, pancreas, or thymus. Mild or moderate increases in ACTH should suggest a pituitary source and a direct evaluation to sellar tomography or a CT scan. The ACTH assay is not very sensitive in the normal or mildly elevated ranges, thus, occasionally, a high-dose dexamethasone (8 mg/day) suppression test is indicated to differentiate a pituitary from an adrenal disease. Iodocholesterol scans or a CT scan may assist in localizing an adrenal tumor or in demonstrating a bilateral hypertrophy.

The treatments are a trans-sphenoidal hypophysectomy for a bilateral adrenal hyperplasia and an adrenalectomy for an adrenal tumor. Aminoglutethemide, metyrapone, or o,p'-DDD may be used as a "medical adrenalectomy" in patients who are not surgical candidates.

References

1. Melmon KL: The endocrinologic function of selected autacoids: catecholamines, acetylcholine, serotonin, and histamine, in Williams RH (ed): *Textbook of Endocrinology,* ed 6. Philadelphia, WB Saunders & Co, 1981, pp 515–588.
2. Prinz PN, Halter J, Bennedetti C, et al: Circa-

dian variation of plasma catecholamines in young and old men: relation to rapid eye movement and slow wave sleep. *J Clin Endocrinol Metab* 49:300–304, 1979.

3. Pederson EB, Christensen NJ: Catecholamines in plasma and urine in patients with essential hypertension determined by double-isotope derivative techniques. *Acta Med Scand* 198:373–377, 1975.

4. Ziegler MG, Lake CR, Koin IJ: Plasma noradrenalin increases with age. *Nature* 261:333–335, 1976.

5. Lake CR, Ziegler MC, Coleman MD, et al: Age-adjusted plasma norepinephrine levels are similar in normotensive and hypertensive subjects. *N Eng J Med* 296:208–209, 1977.

6. Brecht HM, Schoeppe W: Relation of plasma noradrenaline to blood pressure, age, sex and sodium balance in patients with stable essential hypertension and in normotensive subjects. *Clin Sci Mol Med* 55:81S–83S, 1978.

7. Jones DH, Hamilton CA, Reid JL: Plasma noradrenaline, age and blood pressure: a population study. *Clin Sci Mol Med* 55:73S–75S, 1978.

8. Young JB, Rowe JW, Pallota JA, et al: Enhanced plasma norepinephrine response to upright posture and oral glucose administration in elderly human subjects. *Metabolism* 29:532–539, 1980.

9. Gerstenblith G, Lakatta EG, Weisfeldt ML: Age changes in myocardial function and exercise response. *Prog Cardiovasc Dis* 19:1–21, 1976.

10. Lakatta EG: Perspectives on the aged myocardium, in Roberts J, Adelman RC, Cristofalo VJ (eds): *Pharmacological Intervention in the Aging Process.* New York, Plenum Press, 1978, pp 147–169.

11. Vestal RE, Wood AJJ, Shand DG: Reduced beta-adrenoreceptor sensitivity in the elderly. *Clin Pharmacol Ther* 26:181–186, 1979.

12. Yin FCP, Spurgeon HA, Green HC, et al: Age-associated decrease in heart rate response to isoproterenol in dogs. *Mech Ageing Dev* 10:17–25, 1979.

13. Abrass IB, Davis JL, Scarpace PJ: Isoproterenol responsiveness and myocardial beta-adrenergic receptors in young and aging rats. *J Gerontol* 37:156–160, 1982.

14. Lakatta EG, Gerstenblith G, Angell CS, et al: Diminished inotropic response of aged myocardium to catecholamines. *Circ Res* 36:262–268, 1975.

15. Guarnieri T, Filburn C, Zitnik G, et al: Contractile and biochemical correlates of beta-adrenergic stimulation of the aged heart. *Amer J Physiol* 230:H501–H508, 1980.

16. Scarpace PJ, Abrass IB: Thyroid hormone regulation of beta-adrenergic receptor number in aging rats. *Endocrinology* 108:1276–1278, 1981.

17. Abrass IB, Davis JL, Scarpace PJ: Isoproterenol responsiveness and myocardial beta-adrenergic receptors in young and old rats. *J Gerontol* 37:156–160, 1982.

18. Abrass IB, Scarpace PJ: Human lymphocyte beta-adrenergic receptors are unaltered with age. *J Gerontol* 36:298–301, 1981.

19. O'Connor SW, Scarpace PJ, Abrass IB: Age-associated decrease of adenylate cyclase activity in rat myocardium. *Mech Ageing Dev* 16:91–95, 1981.

20. Norayanon N, Derby J-A: Alterations in the properties of beta-adrenergic receptors of myocardial membranes in aging: impairments in agonist-receptor interactions and guanine nucleotide regulation accompany diminished catecholamine responsiveness of adenylate cyclase. *Mech Ageing Dev* 19:127–139, 1982.

21. Krall JF, Connelly M, Weisbart R, et al: Age related elevation of plasma catecholamine concentration and reduced responsiveness of lymphocyte adenylate cyclase. *J Clin Endocrinol Metab* 52:863–867, 1981.

22. Abrass IB, Scarpace PJ: Catalythic unit of adenylate cyclase: reduced activity in aged human lymphocytes. *J Clin Endocrinol Metab* 55:1026–1028, 1982.

23. Liddle GW: The adrenals, in Williams RH (ed): *Textbook of Endocrinology,* ed 6. Philadelphia, WB Saunders & Co, 1981, pp 249–292.

24. Romanoff LP, Morris CW, Welch P, et al: The metabolism of cortisol-4-C[14] in young and elderly men. *J Clin Endocrinol Metab* 21:1413–1425, 1961.

25. Blichert-Toft M: The adrenal gland in old age, in Greenblatt RB (ed): *Geriatric Endocrinology.* New York, Raven Press, 1978, pp 81–102.

26. West CD, Brown H, Simons EL, et al: Adrenocortical function and cortisol metabolism in old age. *J Clin Endocrinol Metab* 21:1197–1207, 1961.

27. Friedman M, Green MF, Sharland DE: Assessment of hypothalamic-pituitary-adrenal function in the geriatric age group. *J Gerontol* 24:292–297, 1969.

28. Dubin B, MacLennan WJ, Hamilton JC: Adrenal function and ascorbic acid concentrations in elderly women. *Gerontology* 24:473–476, 1978.

29. Romanoff LP, Grace MP, Baxter MN, et al: Metabolism of pregnenolone-7 alpha-^{3}H and progesterone-4-^{14}C in young and elderly men. *J Clin Endocrinol Metab* 26:1023–1031, 1966.

30. Romanoff LP, Malhotra KK, Baxter MN, et al: Metabolism of 17 alpha-hydroxypregnenolone-7 alpha-^{3}H and 17 alpha-hydroxyprogesterone-4-^{14}C in young and elderly men. *J Clin Endocrinol Metab* 28:836–848, 1968.

31. Romanoff LP, Baxter MN: The secretion rates of deoxycorticosterone and corticosterone in young and elderly men. *J Clin Endocrinol Metab* 41:630–633, 1975.

32. Flood C, Gherondache E, Pincus G, et al: The metabolism and secretion of aldosterone in elderly subjects. *J Clin Invest* 46:961–966, 1967.

33. Weidmann P, De Myttenaere-Bursztein S, Maxwell MH, et al: Effect of aging on plasma renin and aldosterone in normal man. *Kid Int* 8:325–333, 1975.

34. Takeda R, Morimoto S, Uchida K, et al: Effect of age on plasma aldosterone response to exogenons angiotensin II in normotensive subjects. *Acta Endocrinol* 94:552–558, 1980.

35. Crane MG, Harris JM: Effect of aging on renin activity and aldosterone excretion. *J Lab Clin Med* 87:947–959, 1976.

36. Migeon CJ, Keller AR, Lawrence B, et al: Dehydroepiandorosterone and androsterone levels in human plasma. Effect of age and sex; day-to-day and diurnal variations. *J Clin Endocrinol* 17:1051–1062, 1957.

37. Marmorston J, Griffith GC, Geller PJ, et al: Urinary steroids in the measurement of aging and atherosclerosis. *J Am Geriatr Soc* 23:481–492, 1975.

Chapter 25

Diabetes Mellitus

Matthew C. Riddle, M.D.

The Syndrome of Diabetes Mellitus

Diabetes mellitus is not a single disease, but a group of disorders of varying etiologies defined by an elevation of plasma glucose levels. Other abnormalities affecting transport, storage, mobilization, and the use of fuels commonly accompany hyperglycemia. These include high plasma concentrations of free fatty acids, ketones, and triglycerides. With the passage of time, a number of distinctive tissue changes termed the "chronic complications of diabetes" may occur. Hyperglycemia, a disordered fuel metabolism, and these structural changes all have come to be considered as parts of the syndrome of diabetes. However, the defining characteristic of diabetes regardless of the presence of complications or an abnormal lipid metabolism is hyperglycemia.

A new set of criteria for the abnormality of plasma glucose behavior recently has been adopted.[1] Plasma glucose that always is below 140 mg/dl is considered normal. When plasma glucose rises above 140 mg/dl 2 hours after the ingestion of 75 grams of glucose, yet remains below that level in the fasting state, an impaired glucose tolerance (IGT) is believed to be present. Diabetes mellitus is present when the plasma glucose level is greater than 140 mg/dl after an overnight fast. Diabetes itself is further subclassified into insulin-dependent diabetes (IDDM, or type I), non-insulin-dependent diabetes (NIDDM, or type II), and diabetes that is secondary to various causes. The most common type is NIDDM, which is further subdivided into NIDDM in the obese and NIDDM in the non-obese. The glucose tolerance test that has served many years to define diabetes now is rarely used, except for determining the renal threshold for glycosuria and confirming a clinical diagnosis of reactive hypoglycemia.

A diagnosis of diabetes need not imply any specific etiology. Indeed, the etiologies of most forms of this syndrome remain poorly understood. Since this diagnosis rests solely on an abnormality of plasma glucose, diabetes may be said to be transient or reversible in many cases. Not all persons with diabetes are diabetic for life, although a genetically determined vulnerability persists.

Pathogenesis

Most aspects of the metabolism of glucose and other fuels are controlled by the action of insulin. This hormone is secreted by the beta cells of the pancreatic islets into the portal vein and travels to its many sites of action, notably the liver, adipose tissue, and muscle tissue.[2] At the surface of the target cell, insulin is complexed with a specific receptor, thus initiating its cellular actions.[3] It is cleared from the circulation within minutes. Its effects are countered by those of other hormones such as glucagon, norepinephrine and epinephrine, growth hormone, and corticosteroids. Insulin favors both the use or storage of glucose and lipids and the synthesis of proteins, while lowering plasma glucose levels; the "counter-regulatory" hormones[4] favor mobilization of fuels and catabolism of tissue in general, as well as hyperglycemia. The influence of insulin on intermediary metabolism is regulated at several points. Insulin secretion is modulated by: 1) Sympathetic and parasympathetic neural outflow; 2) Glucagon, gastric inhibitory polypeptide, and other hormones of intestinal or pancreatic islet origin; and 3) Plasma concentrations of glucose, amino acids, potassium, and (perhaps) other metabolites.[5] Insulin's interaction with receptors at the surfaces of cells is modulated by factors that alter either the number of receptors or their affinity for the hormone.[6] The cellular response to insulin is further modulated by hormonal and nutritional factors in other ways that still are largely obscure.

The relevance of this review of insulin's physiology lies in its illumination of how diabetes develops and also may wax and wane. When the pathway of action of insulin is obstructed at any point, the plasma glucose level rises and IGT or overt diabetes may ensue. With IDDM, the defect is in the beta cell itself, which is damaged by an acute injury that is believed to have both genetic and environmental components.[7] Some cells die, but some may survive only to be further injured by an ongoing autoimmune process. This type of diabetes is characterized by a severe lack of insulin and a normal efficacy of insulin at the target cell. Diabetes that is secondary to other forms of islet cell injury, such as pancreatitis, tumor invasion, or surgical resection, is quite similar.

The disruption of the insulin pathway in NIDDM is more complex, with all sites possibly affected.[8] Most patients with NIDDM, especially those who are obese, have some interference with actions that are initiated by insulin within target cells beyond the receptor.[9] Studies of receptor function show that fewer receptors are available and the binding of insulin is decreased in NIDDM.[6,10] The rate of secretion and the concentration of insulin in plasma generally are normal or high, but the timing and magnitude of the secretory response following meals may be abnormal.[11] It has been proposed that the islet of NIDDM is "reset" to maintain basal glucose at a higher level than normal.[12] Thus, the secretion, binding, and postreceptor action of insulin all may be altered in NIDDM.

The pathway of insulin action may be transiently interrupted. Severe injuries such as burns or major fractures provoke secretion of catecholamines, which block the release of insulin, and corticosteroids, which decrease the affinity of receptors for insulin and (perhaps) interfere with its action at postreceptor sites. Major medical illnesses and surgery may have the same effects. A syndrome of "alcoholic ketoacidosis" is described,[13] in which an excess of alcohol and lack of food limit glucose production by the liver, while dehydration leads to an inhibition of insulin secretion and a stimulation of fatty acid and ketone production. Finally, several commonly used medications interfere with the secretion of insulin (phenytoin,[14] beta-adrenergic blockers,[15] thiazide diuretics,[16] and possibly calcium channel blockers[17]) or its action (corticosteroids).[18] When a significant impairment is already present, any of these physiologic stresses can lead to metabolic decompensation.

Natural History of IDDM and NIDDM

Both IDDM and NIDDM have characteristic patterns of appearance and progression (see Figure 25-1), which may include exacerbations and remissions. Typically, IDDM develops abruptly in a slender person younger than 40 years of age. After the onset, secretion of insulin may recover to a degree, and the requirement for injected insulin may decline for a time (usually to rise again[7]). Usually (although not invariably), a patient is completely dependent on injected insulin within several years. Although previously referred to as juvenile-onset diabetes, this disorder may develop at any age. In a geriatric population, IDDM is most often encountered as a long-standing illness and usually with significant chronic complications. With improved management, an increasing proportion of persons with IDDM may survive beyond their 7th decade.

In contrast to IDMM, NIDDM develops gradually, with IGT often appearing first during pregnancy or with a weight gain in the 4th or 5th decade. Many persons with IGT never progress to overt NIDDM.[19] Their glycemic control remains constant for years or returns to normal as excess weight or other physiologic stress declines. Other persons progress to a state of se-

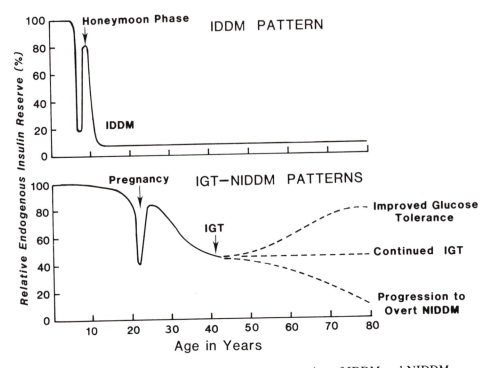

FIGURE 25-1   Patterns of appearance and progression of IDDM and NIDDM.

vere insulin deficiency. Since NIDDM surely is a group of several disorders, it is not surprising that the rate of onset, extent of insulin deficiency, relative effectiveness of insulin, rate of progression, and response to therapy all vary greatly between individuals.

Diabetes in an Older Person

In the population as a whole, glucose tolerance declines with advancing age.[19,20] This decline generally is attributed to a decreased responsiveness of tissues to insulin, which is due in part to reduced physical activity and a lower ratio of lean to adipose tissue. Aging of beta cells also may play a role. The question of whether an age-related change in glucose tolerance should be considered a part of normal aging, or whether it should be considered abnormal (given a diagnosis) and treated, has been much debated.[19,21] Some argue that glucose tolerance should be related to age-adjusted normal values to avoid assigning a diagnosis of diabetes to a very large fraction of our older population.[22] The dilemma is partly resolved if fasting hyperglycemia is accepted as the defining

characteristic of overt diabetes, with the intermediate category of IGT available for lesser abnormalities of glycemia. Although IGT is common among elderly persons, overt diabetes is less common. Fasting hyperglycemia occurs in less than 10% of the population over 60 years of age, while plasma glucose levels over 140 mg/dl following an oral glucose load are found in about one third of all persons over 60 years of age (*see* Table 25-1).[23]

The Relation Between Hyperglycemia and Complications of Diabetes

While most clinicians have assumed that chronic complications of diabetes result from an abnormal regulation of plasma glucose or closely related metabolites, this notion has been challenged.[24] The alternative view offered is that diabetes is a genetically based disorder, with hyperglycemia as one manifestation of the underlying defect and the various tissue changes as separate manifestations. Much experimental evidence argues against this view,

TABLE 25-1   Plasma Glucose Two Hours After a 100 Gram Oral Glucose Load in 1,009 Subjects Without Known Diabetes Studied as Part of a "Diabetes Detection Drive."*

Ages	Over 200 mg/dl %†	Over 140 mg/dl, But Less Than 200 mg/dl %†	Total Over 140 mg/dl %†
20–29	0	15	15
30–39	0	9	9
40–49	0	13	13
50–59	6	14	20
60–69	8	20	28
70–79	14	22	36
80–89	14	21	35

* Persons with fasting plasma glucose levels over 140 mg/dl, representing 2, 4, 2, and 7% of the 6th, 7th, 8th, and 9th decade groups, were excluded from these figures.
† Figures are percentages of total subjects in each category.
SOURCE: Adapted with permission from Mahler RJ, et al: The dilemma of defining diabetes in the aging population. *West J Med* 136:379–383, 1982.

linking hyperglycemia (perhaps in concert with other metabolic abberations) to tissue changes in a variety of ways.[25] However, some evidence does support the concept of a genetically controlled vulnerability or resistance to the damaging effects of a glycemic dysregulation.

While the data support good glycemic control, we do not know at what level of hyperglycemia or variability of glucose the risk of various complications becomes significant, and (thus) which patients with mild glycemic abnormalities should be treated. This question is especially pertinent to the management of persons over 60 years of age. While an acute metabolic decompensation is uncommon in this age group, chronic diabetic complications are very frequent. Moreover, tissue changes that are considered typical of diabetes may be observed in older persons without diabetes at the time of study.[26–28] Such observations suggest that: 1) The lesions may not be limited to persons with glycemic abnormalities; 2) The patient may have had diabetes earlier in life, later experiencing a remission; or 3) Such lesions may, in some cases, result from mild IGT over a span of decades. Choosing between these possibilities is difficult; all may be valid. Better information on the natural history of NIDDM and on the glyce-

mic threshold at which various complications occur is needed to clarify the matter. Meanwhile, we have a clear mandate to seek the best glycemic control attainable in persons with overt diabetes to minimize the extent of chronic diabetic complications. Regarding IGT, the case for intervention is far from clear, although some evidence suggests that rather modest degrees of hyperglycemia may enhance the risk of atherosclerotic events.[29]

Acute Complications of Diabetes

The Spectrum of DKA/HHNKC

The two acute metabolic complications of diabetes mellitus are diabetic ketoacidosis (DKA)[30] and hyperglycemic hyperosmolar nonketotic coma (HHNKC).[31] These are not entirely discrete entities; rather, they are two extreme aspects of the metabolic decompensation of diabetes. While DKA is defined by the metabolic acidosis that results from an excessive production and limited clearance of ketone bodies, HHNKC is defined by the dehydration that commonly results from marked hyperglycemia. Occasionally each exists in pure form, but more often both are present to some degree. In a typical case of diabetic decompensation in a person under 40 years of age, acidosis is a prominent feature. In an older patient, hyperosmolarity usually dominates.

The clinical findings that are characteristic of DKA and HHNKC are somewhat different. The nausea and malaise that results from ketosis are lacking in a patient presenting with HHNKC, in whom thirst and polyuria are more prominent. Since the symptoms of hyperglycemia are less distressing than those of ketosis, patients lacking severe ketosis and presenting because of dehydration generally have been ill for a longer period of time. Weakness, increased urine volume, thirst, decreased appetite, and changes in mental function are the most common symptoms that precede HHNKC. Patients with HHNKC often have significant cardiovascular and renal disease, and a high morbidity and mortality. Fatality rates in the 25–50% range are reported,[32] although perhaps excellent management will improve these figures.

Why ketosis fails to develop in most older patients remains imperfectly explained.[33] Retention of enough endogenous insulin to suppress fatty acid and ketone (but not glucose) production is one proposed factor. An autonomic neuropathy that results in a subnormal rate of lipolysis also may contribute, as may hepatic factors limiting ketone generation. Whatever the mechanism, diabetic decompensation in an older person is characteristically without severe ketosis, is gradual and prolonged in onset, associated with significant underlying complications of diabetes, and attended by risk of further complications or death. It is a major emergency in an older person, more so because it is potentially entirely reversible.

Precipitating Events

The range of precipitating events is the same for both older and younger diabetic patients: omission of insulin or an oral hypoglycemic treatment, an emotional stress or physical trauma, infection, a vascular event, an abdominal crisis, or treatment with drugs that provoke hyperglycemia. However, the frequency with which these various antecedents occur is different among elderly persons. Emotional stress less often precipitates diabetic decompensation in an older patient, while major vascular or enteric illness more commonly does. A myocardial infarction, in particular, must be considered in a patient presenting with an unexplained sudden decompensation. Myocardial ischemia, as well as other internal disorders, may not be announced by typical symptoms in a person with diabetes of long duration, because (perhaps) of an afferent autonomic neuropathy.

Complicating Events

The high morbidity and mortality of HHNKC appear to result from the severity of the metabolic disturbance and from subsequent complications. These include sequelae of coma of any sort (aspiration, atelectasis, and hypostatic pneumonitis). In addition, a vascular thrombosis may occur, either venous (thrombophlebitis with potential for a pulmonary embolism) or arterial (myocardial infarction, stroke). Thrombosis is favored by increased viscosity of blood and aggregability of platelets, and by vascular stasis.[34]

Management

The management of a diabetic decompensation in an older person is similar to that recommended for younger patients; however, it should be more intensive and yet more cautious. The risks are higher and the margin for error narrower. The priorities may be listed as follows:

1. Diagnosis,
2. Initiation of fluid, insulin, and electrolyte treatment,
3. Search for precipitating illness and prevention of complications,
4. Assessment of response to treatment.

Diagnosis

A diagnosis of DKA or HHNKC is based on clinical findings and demonstration of either a metabolic acidosis with significant ketonemia or hyperosmolarity, or both, in the presence of hyperglycemia in excess of 300 mg/dl. Clinical findings commonly include: 1) Lethargy, confusion, stupor, or coma; 2) Dryness of the mucous membranes and a decreased subcutaneous tissue turgor; 3) A fall in blood pressure on sitting; 4) Slow but excessively deep respiration (Kussmaul respiration) if acidosis is present; and 5) A sweet or fruity breath odor if ketosis is present. Since ketosis and acidosis commonly are slight or absent in elderly persons, changes in mental status and dehydration may be the major findings. The concentration of glucose in the urine generally is over 5%, and urinary ketones may be absent to large on Acetest or Ketostix measurement. Values for the concentrations of various electrolytes in a series of patients with an acute decompensation with and without ketosis are shown in Table 25-2. The degree of metabolic acidosis and hyperosmolarity can be assessed by making simple calculations from the initial measurements of both glucose and electrolyte concentrations in plasma.

$$\text{Anion gap} = (Na + K) - (Cl + CO_2)$$

The normal range for an anion gap is 14–20 mEq/l. A value over 20 indicates the presence of an excess of acidic anions. When a prominent ketonuria is present, the excessive anions

TABLE 25-2 Initial Serum Laboratory Values for Groups of Patients with DKA* and HHNKC†

	DKA	HHNKC
Glucose (mg/dl)	733	976
	(400–1,300)	(600–1,800)
Na (mEq/l)	132	142
	(116–144)	(126–165)
K (mEq/l)	6.0	5
	(4.4–8.1)	(2.8–6.6)
Cl (mEq/l)	93	98
	(78–103)	(83–130)
CO$_2$ (mEq/l)	10	22
	(4–15)	(17–28)
BUN†† (mg/dl)	41	65
	(15–75)	(24–141)
Osmolarity (mosm/kg)	331	373
	(317–367)	(327–416)

* 12 patients: 5 males, 7 females; mean age, 43 years; age-range, 20-67.
† 20 patients: 12 males, 8 females; mean age, 57 years; age-range, 28-35.
†† BUN = Blood urea nitrogen.
SOURCE: Reproduced with permission from the American Diabetes Association, Inc, and from the authors, Gerich JE, Martin MM, Recant L: Clinical and metabolic characteristics of hyperosmolar nonketotic coma. *Diabetes* 20:228–238, 1971.

usually are ketone bodies, although nitrogen-containing organic acids (retained due to a reduction of renal perfusion) and lactate (accumulated due to an overproduction and impaired clearance by poorly perfused tissues) are additional possibilities. Fortunately, hydration, insulin, and electrolyte replacement are sufficient remedies for all three types of anion excess in most cases; therefore, a distinction between the contribution from ketones and the other metabolites usually is not necessary.

Plasma/Serum Osmolarity =

$$2(Na + K) + \frac{(Glucose)}{18} + \frac{(BUN)}{3}$$

The normal range is 280–295 mosm/l. Values in excess of 330 mosm/l suggest a dehydration of clinical importance. Values obtained by this calculation correlate well with the less convenient direct measurement of osmolarity. Since mental status correlates better with osmolarity than with pH,[35] most persons with a diabetic decompensation and mental changes will have an elevated calculated osmolarity.

Initiation of Fluid, Insulin, and Electrolyte Treatment

The combination of large volumes of isotonic or half-isotonic saline solutions with low doses of regular insulin given intravenously (IV) has proven safe and effective as an initial treatment for DKA and HHNKC.[36] The initial rate of infusion of insulin that generally is recommended is between 5–10 units/hour, and that of saline is between 0.5–1 liter/hour. The rate of fluid administration must be slowed, and saline concentration decreased, once normal intravascular volume is restored. This is indicated by a return of good urinary output, observations of normal cervical venous pressure, or direct measurements of central venous pressure. Similarly, the rate at which insulin is infused must be reduced to 0.5–2 units/hour, and 5% glucose must be added to the infusion mixture once the plasma glucose level falls to 300 mg/dl. To facilitate a separate manipulation of insulin and fluids, it is convenient to infuse them through separate lines that meet at a Y-connector close to the IV site with separate bottles and pump-driven or manual control systems. If 50 units of insulin are mixed with 500 ml of an isotonic saline solution, and 50–100 ml of this mixture run through the infusion set and discarded, an appropriate delivery of insulin without an undue loss to surfaces of the apparatus is assured.[37]

Regulation of potassium (K) can be the most difficult part of early treatment. Patients who are initially hyperkalemic must not be given parenteral potassium at first, but patients with a low or normal potassium concentration need early replacement. Plasma or serum potassium should be measured repeatedly in the first hours of treatment, and potassium should be added to the given fluids as needed. Typically, about 20 mEq/l is necessary; 50% as potassium chloride and 50% as potassium phosphates. Biocarbonate rarely is necessary for the treatment of DKA in an older patient, and only when a severe acidosis (pH level below 7.1) is present.

Search for Precipitating Illness and Prevention of Complications

Once treatment is underway, infections and cardiovascular and abdominal disorders should actively be sought. A complete physical examination should be done, as well as a blood count, urinalysis, electrocardiogram (ECG), and chest x-ray film. Any suggestive findings should be pursued, since an untreated underlying disorder is likely to both progress rapidly and make the diabetic condition relatively resistant to treatment.

Simultaneously, a patient should be protected against the known complications of DKA and HHNKC. Gastric dilation is common and, if present, should be relieved via placement of a nasogastric tube to reduce the risk of vomiting and aspiration. Patients able to cooperate should be encouraged intermittently to move their legs, sit upright, and breathe deeply. Patients with a severe stupor or coma should be repositioned frequently and given good general nursing care.

Assessment of Response to Treatment

A careful monitoring of vital signs, venous pressure, intake and output of fluids, plasma or serum glucose levels, potassium, phosphate, blood urea nitrogen (BUN), and bicarbonate is mandatory during the first 6–12 hours of treatment. Older patients with diabetes often have poor cardiac or renal function and are easily overloaded with sodium (Na), water, and potassium, which potentially cause either congestive heart failure or a lethal hyperkalemia. These patients also commonly take digitalis preparations; when dehydrated, they may have high concentrations in plasma that enhance the risk of a cardiac arrhythmia attending hypokalemia. Furthermore, overly rapid replacement of water, especially with a rapid reduction of the plasma glucose level below 250 mg/dl, favors cerebral edema.[38] Aggressive treatment, thus, has serious perils. Conversely, casual treatment, which allows dehydration to persist, also carries a substantial risk. Therefore, one must carefully monitor and record responses to treatment and make alterations in the treatment plan as indicated.

Chronic Complications of Diabetes

Biochemical Mechanisms

Our understanding of the biochemical basis of tissue changes of diabetes is limited. However, two attractive molecular mechanisms that are directly related to glucose metabolism have been proposed as models for the harmful effects of hyperglycemia.

Abnormal Glycosylation of Proteins

Many structural and functional proteins normally contain carbohydrates. The carbohydrate groups may be linked to protein either with or without the assistance of enzymes. It has been proposed that high ambient concentrations of glucose enhance the rate of glycosylation. In the case of enzymatic glycosylation,[39] this theory remains unproved even though it is provocative. More certain is the importance of non-enzymatic glycosylation of proteins by an interaction of the aldehyde group of hexoses with exposed amino groups of proteins.[40] The resulting Schiff base rearranges to form a highly stable ketoamine linkage. This reaction has been documented in a number of proteins (hemoglobin, albumin, lens proteins), and it presumably occurs in many others. An altered function of the protein is a likely consequence. In a diabetic state, the proteins that are most affected should be extracellular or within cells that allow an entry of glucose without an insulin action (erythrocytes, nerve, and so on). The glycosylation of hemoglobin is the best-studied example;[41] measurement of its extent serves as a clinical indicator of glycemic control over a span of 1–3 months.[42]

Formation of Sugar Alcohols by Aldose Reductase

Aldose reductase is an enzyme that is present in many types of cells, notably those allowing a free entry of glucose. This enzyme converts glucose to the corresponding sugar-alcohol, sorbitol.[43] The amount of sorbitol that is produced depends on the concentration of glucose. Tissues of hyperglycemic diabetics contain large quantities that may be toxic. Convincing support for this theory comes from studies of the lens of the eye. Lenses suspended in vitro in high concentrations of glucose (or galactose) develop cataracts, which can be prevented by the addition of an inhibitor of aldose reductase.[44] Diabetic cataracts, thus, may derive in part from an accumulation of sorbitol. Applicability of this theory to injuries of other tissues has yet to be proven, although it seems attractive with relation to neuropathies as well.

Pathophysiologic Mechanisms

The biochemical changes of diabetes lead to a functional debility that can be divided into vascular, neural, and direct metabolic mechanisms.

Vascular Mechanisms

Alterations of blood vessels are so common and significant in diabetes as to be considered by some investigators to be an integral part of the diabetic syndrome, and are termed "diabetic angiopathy." However, diabetic angiopathy is not of a single type, and confusion has arisen concerning its nomenclature.

Large arteries often are affected by atherosclerotic changes that are indistinguishable from those in persons without diabetes; but they appear earlier in life and progress more rapidly.[45] Coronary, cerebral, femoral, axillary, renal, mesenteric, and celiac arteries and their major branches all may share in this process. The aorta itself is vulnerable, and an aortic aneurysm and dissection may be more common among persons with glycemic abnormalities.

Small arteries and arterioles are vulnerable to different processes. A cellular proliferation may occur, and extracellular hyaline material may thicken the vascular wall and impinge on the lumen. This arterial and arteriolar sclerosis is not limited to persons with diabetes; however, it seems more prominent in this group,[46] although there has been dispute on this point.[47] Evidence of a greater abnormality of small arteries in the diabetic population includes both the frequency of an occlusion of small cerebral and digital vessels and the well-described arteriolar changes in the heart[48] and kidney[49] of diabetic individuals.

An injury to capillaries is the most distinctive type of diabetic angiopathy, and is termed "diabetic microangiopathy."[50,51] The capillary basement membrane is thickened and functionally abnormal, and it seems structurally weak and overly permeable to macromolecules. A dilation of, or focal leakage from, retinal capillaries is well described (microaneurysms, blot hemorrhages). An abnormal diffuse leakiness of the capillaries has been documented in the retina, glomerulus, and muscle, and it presumably occurs elsewhere. The capillary-supporting cells (pericytes) and endothelial cells may be injured and die, with occlusion and loss of the capillary channel. Thus, areas of tissue may become ischemic. At least in the retina, both leakage from capillaries and focal ischemia are believed to have a major functional impact. Proliferation of the basement membrane certainly is a leading contributor to the morbidity and mortality of diabetic glomerulopathies and renal failure.

The effects of these three kinds of vascular injuries in diabetes seem to be additive; that is, a poor flow through a reduced number of arterioles and capillaries may increase the functional impact of a focal narrowing of a larger vessel (e.g., the coronary circulation). Moreover, surgical correction of a focal atherosclerotic lesion is a greater risk when distal vessels are abnormal since a sluggish flow favors thrombosis and occlusion of a graft or endarterectomy site. Finally, large atherosclerotic plaques may contribute to injuries of smaller vessels by generating thromboemboli that lodge in distal sites. Together, the various types of diabetic angiopathies can lead (through vascular narrowing, thrombosis, or embolism) to ischemia and injury to most organs and tissues.

Neural Mechanisms

The neuropathy of diabetes likewise consists of several types, which are divided according to their pathogenesis or by the portion of the peripheral nervous system affected.

Classification by Pathogenetic Mechanisms

The sudden appearance of a neurologic deficit usually is attributed to an occlusion of a small blood vessel that feeds the affected nerve. Histologic verification of this notion has been obtained in a few cases.[52] The nerve that is distal to the injury shows axonal degeneration. Regeneration of the nerve with at least a partial return of function is usual. A diffuse metabolic injury to the nerves or Schwann cells also occurs and accounts for the symmetric distal sensorimotor and autonomic neuropathies of diabetes.[53] The characteristic histologic lesion is segmental demyelination, which presumably reflects damage to the Schwann cell and is accompanied by a reduced velocity of conduction of neural impulses. From a clinical standpoint, impairment of sensory function appears first, followed by motor impairment and autonomic dysfunction. Physiologically, all types of nerves may be affected simultaneously. A mechanical injury to the nerves, which naturally occurs independent of diabetes, has a special importance in a diabetic person. The metabolically impaired nerve seems to be more susceptible than usual to compression, stretching, or ischemia. Thus, persons with diabetes often have neural symptoms that are related to local trauma. Crossing one leg over the other may induce paresthesias or transient foot-drop. The patient may awaken with a numb arm after a minor compression of the limb during sleep. This nerve compression at the carpal tunnel or the inguinal ligament can cause either dysesthesias or weakness of the hand (carpal tunnel syndrome)[54] or dysesthesias and numbness of the lateral thigh (meralgia paresthetica). A narrowing of the vertebral outlets may cause intermittent pain, paresthesias, or a numbness along the distribution of the affected nerve, which simulates intrathoracic[55] or intra-abdominal disorders.[56] Metabolic and mechanical causes of neural dysfunction both deserve attention, since either the removal of a mechanical stress or the improvement of glycemic control may be rewarded by symptomatic relief.

Classification by the Neural Function Affected Cranial, somatic sensory, somatic motor, and autonomic functions all may be involved.[57] Cranial neuropathies commonly are of a sudden onset and are unilateral; thus, they are likely of vascular origin. Combined sensory and motor lesions that suddenly appear elsewhere also probably are local vascular events. A diffuse sensory neuropathy is insidious at its onset, and is distal, symmetric, and probably metabolic in origin. A patient may be unaware of the deficit, may recognize a loss of function such as numbness or clumsiness, or may describe a distinct tingling, burning, or pain. Unpleasant sensations typically are the worst in the toes or feet and are most bothersome at night. A complete loss of function rarely is reversible; however, paresthesias and dysesthesias often regress with better glycemic control. A diffuse motor neuropathy characteristically follows the sensory neuropathy in time and location. A wasting of foot and leg muscles occurs gradually and often is unrecognized by a patient. A wasting of the intrinsic muscles of the hand is (except when a severe nerve com-

pression in the carpal tunnel is present) a late finding and implies an extensive neuropathy elsewhere. An autonomic neuropathy usually is not recognized until sensory and motor changes are obvious. It is present earlier in many patients, but our present means of recognizing and quantitating it are limited. A significant autonomic neuropathy is suggested by: 1) A history of diminished sweating of the extremities or an increased sweating of the face and neck[58]; 2) An absence of sinus arrhythmia on an ECG[59]; 3) Absence of the postvalsalva overshoot of blood pressure; and 4) Absence of normal pupillary reflexes.[60] Many bodily functions can be affected by a diabetic autonomic injury: 1) Cardiovascular reflexes[61]; 2) Motility of the esophagus, stomach, gallbladder, small and large bowel[62]; 3) Bladder motility and awareness of a need to urinate[63]; and 4) Penile erection.[64] Other important consequences may yet be defined.

Another neural syndrome, about which little is known physiologically, is diabetic amyotrophy or diabetic neuropathic cachexia.[65] This disorder typically occurs in middle-aged or elderly males in the presence of either mild or severe diabetes. It is characterized by a weakness and atrophy of muscles, especially of the hip and upper leg, which sometimes is accompanied by a painful neuropathy that is either distal or in the same distribution as the muscle weakness. The patient often has lost weight recently, may be malnourished and anorexic, often is severely depressed, and may at first be thought to have a malignancy. The prognosis is quite good; a partial or even complete recovery is common, especially with nutritional support and good glycemic control.

Direct Metabolic Mechanisms
Diabetes directly affects many cells and tissues beside the blood vessels and nerves. The following are two prominent examples.

Formed Elements of Blood Erythrocytes, leukocytes, and platelets are, in certain ways, abnormal in persons with diabetes.[66] Erythrocytes are less plastic and less able to negotiate a passage through narrow capillaries. Platelets aggregate and release their contents more readily than normal.[67] In addition, the viscosity of plasma is increased.[68] These changes favor sludging of blood and formation of small and large thrombi. Granulocytes are less able to move toward and kill bacteria.[69] Very likely, the vulnerability of persons with diabetes to an infection by gram-positive organisms results, in part, from the lethargy of these phagocytes. Many abnormalities of diabetic blood are reversible with good glycemic control.[70]

Connective Tissue Persons with diabetes are disposed to palmar fascial thickening and contracture (Dupuytren's contracture),[71] glenohumeral capsulitis with impaired mobility,[72] and possibly dermal thickening.[73] These changes may reflect a general tendency to an excessive accumulation of collagenous tissue. A generalized stiffness and loss of mobility are features of normal aging, and it is tempting to speculate that hyperglycemia in some way accelerates this aspect of the aging process.[74] Alternatively, the possibility that a genetic disposition to premature aging underlies at least some types of diabetes cannot be excluded. It is not known whether glycemic control will retard the aging of connective tissue.

Clinical Impact in Specific Organs

Skin

An inspection of the skin of older persons frequently reveals evidence of diabetes. The most characteristic lesion is diabetic dermopathy (shin spots)[75]. This consists of multiple round or oval, sunken and atrophic, pigmented or depigmented areas on the anterior tibial surface. Patients often attribute these lesions to minor trauma, but they are unlike most traumatic scars in both number and appearance. In size, they range from several millimeters to 1 cm. While unproven, it seems likely that they are a manifestation of occlusions of small dermal blood vessels, which perhaps lead to impaired healing of minor trauma. Necrobiosis lipoidica diabeticorum,[76] which possibly is an inflammatory form of the same sort of lesion, is rare in elderly persons. Palmar fascial thickening with or without an overt Dupuytren's contracture is common. Furunculosis and intertriginal and vaginal moniliasis are more common among persons with diabetes.[77] When diabetes is poorly controlled, the healing of wounds may be delayed.[78]

Brain

The incidence of stroke is increased severalfold among persons with diabetes.[79] In addition, hyperglycemia that is short of overt diabetes also may confer an increased cerebrovascular risk.[80] Whether or not a diffuse small arterial injury that is accelerated by diabetes causes premature organic brain dysfunction in elderly persons is yet to be studied, but this process seems possible.

Eye

Several types of ocular disease accompany diabetes. Diabetic retinopathy[81] is the most characteristic one. Less well known are the vulnerability to cataracts[82] and the disposition to glaucoma[83] of older persons with diabetes.

Heart

The risk of a patient having a myocardial infarction is increased approximately 2-fold by the presence of diabetes.[84] Myocardial infarction also may have a higher mortality when diabetes is present.[85] Recently, a syndrome of diabetic cardiomyopathy has been defined.[86] This provides an explanation for the common finding of congestive heart failure in diabetic persons without any known previous infarction.[87] A partial or complete cardiac denervation by advanced diabetic neuropathy is not rare; a lack of usual symptoms during myocardial ischemia is one consequence of this.[88] Another consequence is a fixed heart rate (which may be slow, normal, or fast) with a limited response to an increased circulatory demand.

Gastrointestinal Tract

Dysphagia and regurgitation may result from a malfunction of the diabetic esophagus.[89] Bloating, fullness, and nausea after eating, all can result from diabetic gastroparesis.[90] The gallbladder may empty poorly, even without stones.[91] Intestinal dyscoordination or atony may lead to either diarrhea or constipation.[92] These abnormalities usually are attributed to an enteric neuropathy; but, other factors may also contribute, which include ischemia and abnormalities of gut hormone regulation.

Genitourinary Tract

Progression of diabetic nephropathy to overt renal failure is less common in older than younger patients.[93] A sudden deterioration of renal function may follow radiologic studies that employ contrast media, but the risk of this complication is minimized by adequate hydration.[94] An abrupt worsening of renal function in an older diabetic person also may signal renal arterial thrombosis. An interstitial renal injury may have more clinical importance than is presently recognized. A syndrome of hyporeninemic hypoaldosteronism[95] accompanies this lesion, with impairment of renin secretion by cells of the juxtaglomerular apparatus and, perhaps, of the distal tubular function as well. These patients have a limited ability to excrete acid and potassium and are vulnerable to metabolic acidosis and hyperkalemia. Persons with a significant renal glomerular injury are more likely to become hypertensive. Any degree of hypertension is hazardous in diabetes, since diabetes and hypertension are additive cardiovascular risk factors. Bladder dysfunction[96] is one of the most under-regarded complications of diabetes. A loss of both sensory and motor innervation allows the bladder easily to become grossly overdistended, atonic, and a reservoir of chronic infection. An older patient with an enlarged prostate or cystocele is at additional risk when bladder function is impaired by diabetes.

Foot

The various mechanisms of tissue injury in diabetes all combine in the foot.[97] A sensory neuropathy prevents warning of an injury to the surface of the foot or to joints of the toes or ankle. A motor neuropathy interferes with the normal coordination of movements. When severe it causes a pull of the tibial extensor muscles to be unopposed by intrinsic muscles of the foot and the peroneal muscles, which leads in time to a deformity that is characteristic of diabetes. Disease of large, medium-sized, and small blood vessels impairs perfusion of the foot so that any injury is slow to heal. Connective tissue repair may be abnormal, and cellular resistance to an infection is limited. When body weight is unevenly distributed on a few vulnerable pressure points, notably over the first and fifth metatarsal heads awareness of an injury to these sites is low; when a breakdown of tissue ensues, the ulcer fails to heal. Serious infection of subcutaneous tissues and bone is common and may lead to gangrene and sepsis. An occlusion of arteries may lead to "dry gangrene." A damaged diabetic foot may mercifully be painless, but nevertheless is a source of chronic aggravation and debility. Amputation often is necessary at the level of the toe, forefoot, ankle, or below or above the knee, which depends largely on the extent of the vascular supply retained.

Management of Diabetes

Evaluation of the Geriatric Patient with Diabetes

Diabetes in an older person usually is relatively asymptomatic, of gradual onset, often of long duration, and frequently is first recognized by laboratory rather than clinical findings. Unlike a younger person with a fasting glucose level in excess of 140 mg/dl, an older diabetic individual may have little or no glycosuria because the renal threshold may be elevated to 250 mg/dl or higher. The classic diagnostic triad of polyuria, polydipsia, and polyphagia, thus, is typically absent. Instead, vague and non-specific symptoms may be the only historic clues present. These include lethargy, easy fatigue, blurring of vision, and itching of the skin. More striking than a patient's immediate complaints may be physical findings that suggest chronic complications of hyperglycemia. When present at diagnosis, these suggest a long-preceding period of IGT or unrecognized diabetes. Physical findings of this sort include diabetic dermopathy, palmar fascial thickening, cataracts, vascular bruits, congestive heart failure, distal muscular weakness and atrophy, and distal sensory loss. The presence of several of these findings on an initial examination should alert a clinician to the possibility of diabetes and other changes that are associated with diabetes.

Confirmation of a suspected diagnosis depends on the measurement of plasma glucose or glycosylated hemoglobin levels, which reflect the mean plasma glucose level of the recent past. Formal testing of glucose tolerance rarely is necessary. The measurement of plasma glucose levels prior to and 2 hours after breakfast usually is sufficient. This procedure will fail to identify some persons with postprandial glucose values below 140 mg/dl whose values after 75 grams of oral glucose would be over 140 mg/dl. However, these are persons with mild IGT in whom an active intervention seldom is necessary. When abnormal values (fasting values over 140 mg/dl suggesting diabetes, or 2-hour postprandial values over 140 mg/dl suggesting IGT) are found in a patient with an acute illness, measurements should be repeated when the patient is in his or her usual state of health before a firm diagnosis is assigned.

Once a diagnosis of diabetes or IGT is made, further studies are advisable. First, the extent of tissue changes that are related to hyperglycemia should be defined. It is most important to consider injuries to the eye, kidney, nervous system, cardiovascular system, and feet. A careful ophthalmologic examination should be performed to identify a treatable retinopathy, glaucoma, or cataract. Renal function should be assessed by a measurement of serum creatinine and urea-nitrogen and daily urinary excretion of protein. Abnormalities of these measurements may alter the choice or dosage of drugs that are used for treating other conditions; specifically, those drugs with renal toxicity or primarily renal excretion. Neurologic examination of a person with diabetes should include testing: 1) Muscle strength in the extremities; 2) Distal tendon reflexes; 3) Distal light touch and position or vibration sensation; and 4) Postural changes in blood pressure or beat-to-beat variation in heart rate as reflections of the integrity of autonomic function. The cardiovascular evaluation should include: 1) An ECG; 2) A search for historical or objective evidence of congestive heart failure; 3) A search for vascular bruits, especially in the carotid and femoral arteries; 4) An assessment of pulse volume at the popliteal, posterior tibial, and dorsalis pedis arteries; and 5) An evaluation of both temperature and the rate of capillary filling in the toes and feet. Finally, the feet should be examined for evidence of deformity, uneven weight bearing, nail dysplasia, ulceration, or infection.

After this search for diabetic complications, attention should be directed to cardiovascular risk factors, which are additive to the risk of diabetes. These include hypertension (over 95 mm Hg diastolic blood pressure), hypercholes-terolemia (over 225 mg/dl), and the use of cigarettes.

Finally, a review of a patient's other medical problems and the drugs being used to treat them is advisable. Often, illnesses or treatments that are likely to exacerbate hyperglycemia can be identified and remedied. For example, a chronic infection (as of carious teeth) or chronic ischemia of the toes or feet can elevate plasma glucose levels. Dental treatment or amputation of ischemic digits may significantly benefit glycemic control. Treatment with even modest doses of corticosteroids for immunologic disorders, or with beta-adrenergic-blocking agents for angina or hypertension, may worsen glycemic control. Elimination of these agents, when possible, can have gratifying results.

Planning the Strategy of Management

Treatment of glycemic abnormalities in older patients involves difficult decisions. Every gradation of abnormality may occur; therefore, the distinction between what is normal, borderline, and clearly abnormal is not straightforward. In addition, the benefits of treatment are not perfectly understood. For example, much information argues that vascular accidents of most types are common among diabetics; however, there is little information defining the possible benefits of lowering blood glucose levels in elderly persons with an established vascular disease. Finally, the risks of various treatments, which include aggressive regimens for weight control, sulfonylureas, and insulin, also are poorly defined. A physician is left with an individual decision for each patient that is based on the nature of the case, the data at hand, and the resources available.

Patients with Fasting Hyperglycemia

Overtly diabetic patients with concentrations of plasma glucose over 140 mg/dl when fasting present the least difficulty. This degree of hyperglycemia, which generally includes postprandial peaks above 250 mg/dl, probably increases the risk of a progressive microvascular disease, neuropathy, vascular thrombosis, and certain pyogenic infections. If fasting hyperglycemia persists after the removal of as many diabetogenic stresses as possible, treatment by diet certainly is indicated. When diet alone fails to reduce fasting glucose levels to below 140 mg/dl, treatment with either a sulfonylurea or insulin also is indicated in most cases.

Patients with Fasting Plasma-Glucose Levels Below 140 mg/dl, but 2-Hour Postprandial Plasma-Glucose Levels over 140 mg/dl or 2-Hour Postglucose Plasma-Glucose Levels Over 200 mg/dl

This group presents more difficulty. It includes persons who, by some standards, should be considered diabetic as they have 2-hour plasma glucose levels after an oral glucose load of over 200 mg/dl, plus another value at 30 minutes or 1 hour over 200 mg/dl. It also includes many persons with an extensive atherosclerotic disease, as well as some with other diabetic complications. Dietary treatment is indicated for all these patients, but intervention with insulin is not justified for most. The use of oral hypoglycemic agents, thus, poses the major decision for this group.

Patients with Fasting Plasma-Glucose Levels Below 140 mg/dl and 2-Hour Postglucose Plasma-Glucose Levels Over 140 mg/dl yet Under 200 mg/dl

Many persons in this large group (*see* Table 25-1) have postprandial values for plasma glucose that always are below 140 mg/dl, and will not be identified unless an oral glucose load is given. Some persons will have what appear to be chronic complications of diabetes; some will go on to become overtly diabetic. Yet in most cases, no intervention other than dietary changes is indicated. Patients with this pattern, yet with a previous decompensation to HHNKC, may represent an exception to this conservative stance, and deserve consideration for treatment with a sulfonylurea.

Treatment with Diet

Our view of the ideal composition of a diet for persons with diabetes has changed in the last few years. Carbohydrates no longer are considered undesirable. Recent evidence even documents benefit from diets that are high in complex carbohydrates and fibers.[98] The beneficial effects of generous portions of unrefined carbohydrates in the diet include both an improvement of glucose tolerance and a tendency to lose weight. The mechanism of these effects is incompletely understood. The American Diabetes Association recently revised its recommendations to state that 50% or more of the calories consumed by persons with diabetes should be from carbohydrates (especially starch), especially in the presence of ample non-absorbable fiber.[99]

A case can be made for the view that all persons regardless of age or illness should follow this type of diet, since another consequence of increasing dietary carbohydrates is a reduction of fat consumption and, thus, of lipid concentrations in plasma. This argument especially applies to persons with IGT or NIDDM because of the additive effects of hyperglycemia and hyperlipidemia as risk factors. Consequently, an effort to evaluate and modify the eating behavior of elderly patients with glycemic abnormalities should be a basic part of management.

An interesting aspect of the relationship between hyperglycemia and nutrition concerns the role of micronutrients in the maintenance of a normal responsiveness of tissues to insulin. A significant amount of information has been collected to argue that a small organic molecule containing chromium is necessary for insulin's action. This so-called "glucose tolerance factor" has been touted outside the medical community as a treatment of diabetes. Its value remains unproven, but it may be the prototype of a group of nutritional factors that affect fuel metabolism, which may be affected by the poor dietary intake of many older persons.

The details of dietary treatment for hyperglycemia in elderly persons are easy to state. Good general nutrition should be provided, with 40–60% or more of all calories from carbohydrates. Refined sugars and saturated fats should be limited, and the consumption of fiber should be encouraged. Calories should be distributed between at least 3 meals. Weight gain that results from an increasing adiposity should be prevented by the restriction of calories to a level that is judged to be appropriate for the patient's age, size, and activity. Conversely, weight gain that results from a restoration of lean tissue in a previously malnourished person is desirable. Hyperglycemia should not be controlled by starvation, which lamentably occurs at times.

In practice, the dietary treatment of an older diabetic person often is ineffective.[100] The eating habits of a life time are not easily changed, and dietary counselling is time-consuming and, therefore, expensive. With the recent renewal of interest in the problems of nutrition in elderly persons, we may see a more effective use of this basic mode of treatment (See Vol. II, Ch. 12). This will require better access to skilled nutritionists, better funding for their services, and more consistent referrals of patients by physicians.

Treatment with Oral Hypoglycemic Agents

All oral hypoglycemic agents that are routinely available in the United States are sulfonylurea derivatives. The last decade has seen much anxiety and confusion regarding their use, which follows reports from the University Group Diabetes Project (UGDP) study.[101] This collaborative study was designed to show whether treatment with oral hypoglycemic drugs (tolbutamide and phenformin, a biguanide which is no longer available because of its toxicity) reduced the long-term complications of diabetes. Under the conditions of this study, in the population examined, no clear amelioration of complications occurred. In addition, cardiovascular mortality was higher in the groups that were treated with either phenformin or tolbutamide. The study however was not designed to deal with the question of toxicity, and it had other methodologic weaknesses. After a decade of debate, no clear resolution of the questions that were raised by the study, concerning the efficacy and safety of tolbutamide and other sulfonylureas, has been achieved.[102] While risk/benefit studies using correct therapeutic methods are badly needed, several practical statements concerning the use of these drugs seem warranted: 1) Sulfonylureas, like all drugs, have adverse effects with a risk that must be justified by clear therapeutic effects; 2) Sulfonylureas are effective in reducing hyperglycemia in some patients, although patients commonly become less responsive with time; 3) Sulfonylureas may cause hypoglycemia, but when used properly they are less likely than insulin to cause an injury through hypoglycemia. Sulfonylureas are still used widely, and

they offer a valuable alternative to insulin for some elderly persons with diabetes.

The mechanism of action of sulfonylureas remains incompletely understood.[103] In short-term studies, the secretion of insulin is clearly increased when a sulfonylurea is taken by a person with NIDDM. Patients with IDDM have been considered to be unresponsive to these agents. Conversely, studies of a longer duration show reduced plasma glucose levels, yet little change in the concentration of insulin in plasma. Recent studies also suggest that sulfonylureas may enhance the sensitivity of cells to insulin by acting either at the receptor, beyond the receptor, or at both sites.

Four drugs of the sulfonylurea family presently are marketed in the United States: tolbutamide (Orinase), acetohexamide (Dymelor), tolazamide (Tolinase), and chlorpropamide (Diabinese).[104] They are roughly comparable in cost, but differ with regard to their duration of action, maximal effectiveness, and side effects. Tolbutamide is a short-acting drug and must be taken at least twice per day; chlorpropamide is a long-acting drug, with a single dose lasting several days. The other drugs are intermediate in their duration of action. Tolbutamide is metabolized largely by the liver and chlorpropamide by the kidney, while the inactivation of acetohexamide and tolazamide depends on both the liver and kidney. Tolbutamide is considered to be the least powerful and tolazamide and chlorpropamide the most powerful, while acetohexamide is intermediate in its effectiveness. All four drugs have a potential for provoking allergy and causing gastrointestinal symptoms. Chlorpropamide, in addition, increases the renal responsiveness to antidiuretic hormone (ADH), which leads in some situations to water intoxication and also causes some persons to have an uncomfortable flushing response to ethanol. Two newer sulfonylureas, glyburide and glipizide, are soon to be released in the United States. They are powerful hypoglycemic agents with properties that are quite similar to the sulfonylureas currently available.

Treatment usually is initiated with a single dose of intermediate or long-acting agents before breakfast (acetohexamide, 250–500 mg; tolazamide, 125–250 mg; chlorpropamide, 125–250 mg), or with doses of tolbutamide (500 mg) before both breakfast and supper. When required, doses can be increased to 750 mg/day of tolazamide and chlorpropamide, 1,500 mg/day of acetohexamide, and 2,000 mg/day of tolbutamide. Doses higher than these may, in some cases, be more effective, but they rarely are indicated and may be hazardous. The effects of these drugs may be potentiated by renal insufficiency (especially chlorpropamide), hepatic insufficiency (especially tolbutamide), and drugs such as salicylates and bishydroxycoumarin, which displace them from binding sites on plasma proteins.

Treatment with Insulin

Insulin is a powerful agent and its use can be hazardous, especially in elderly persons. For this reason, some clinicians advise against its use in older diabetic patients. Conversely, skillful prescription, education of the patient and family, and use of measurement of capillary blood-glucose levels combine to reduce the hazards and improve the outcome. Many geriatric patients are very successfully treated with insulin.

When a decision is made to begin insulin, either the patient or a responsible helper must learn both the mechanics of a subcutaneous injection and the basic actions of insulin. The times of day at which hypoglycemia is most likely should be discussed, and plans for responding to symptoms or signs of hypoglycemia should be outlined. A typical initial dose is 10 units of neutral protamine Hagedorn (NPH) or Lente insulin given before breakfast. Depending on a patient's rate of absorption of depot insulins, the level of physical activity, and the meal pattern, this dose may have a peak action before lunch, in the late afternoon, or in the late evening or early morning. Spry and active persons are more prone to daytime hypoglycemia, while bedridden or sedentary individuals may suffer primarily nocturnal hypoglycemia. The dose should be changed in 2–4-unit increments and not more often than every other day, in most cases. When plasma glucose values at the time of peak insulin action approach the 120–140 mg/dl range (110–125 mg/dl blood glucose), yet glucose remains unacceptably high at other times, a second dose of insulin may be added. This usually is a dose of regular insulin, mixed with the morning dose of intermediate-acting

insulin, or given alone before supper. The addition of regular insulin before breakfast will control morning and early afternoon glucose levels in persons who absorb depot insulin slowly. The addition of regular insulin before supper will improve evening and overnight fasting glucose levels in most older patients in whom a single injection is unsuccessful. A commonly successful regimen includes NPH insulin given before breakfast as about 50% of the total daily dose, with 25% of the total dose as regular insulin in the morning, and 25% regular insulin before supper. An objective evaluation of the outcome of any insulin regimen and an individualization of the prescription is, of course, essential.

Variation of both the rate of absorption and the effectiveness of injected insulin is not just likely; it is inevitable. The absorption of insulin is faster from the abdomen and arm than from the hip and leg,[105] and it is enhanced by warm baths, showers, and room temperature[106] as well as by exercise.[107] The response of tissues to insulin is enhanced by a reduced intake of calories and is impaired by excess calories and many different illnesses. The dose of insulin that is appropriate for a given patient, thus, is certain to vary from time to time, and the patient or persons close to the patient must be both aware of this and prepared to make adjustments.

A severe dependency on injected insulin is uncommon among older persons, but it certainly does occur. Fortunately, persons with IDDM that appears earlier in life who survive to their 8th decade or beyond usually have, by that time, mastered the process of glycemic regulation. These persons require complex insulin regimens with two or more injections daily (as with younger persons with IDDM), and they must continually balance food, insulin, and other factors.

Assessment of Glycemic Control

While the ultimate goal of treatment is to keep a patient feeling well, objective measurements are needed to best achieve this. Glycemic control can be assessed by measuring the glucose level in urine or blood or by the concentration of glycosylated hemoglobin. Tests for urinary glucose (Clinitest, Diastix, and so on) are simple and inexpensive; however, they reveal only excessively high concentrations of glucose in plasma, especially when the renal threshold is high (as often is the case with older persons). For this reason, measurement of capillary blood-glucose levels, is preferable when possible. Reagent strips for this purpose (Chemstrips bG, Visidex) are reliable[108] and not too costly, and they allow the identification of both high (over 240 mg/dl) and low (under 60 mg/dl) blood glucose levels. Nearly painless devices for obtaining a drop of blood from the fingertip are available (Autolet). Simple electronic meters for persons who are unable to read the reagent strips visually can be purchased. The measurement of glycosylated hemoglobin often is helpful, particularly for identifying persons with unsuspected recurrent hypoglycemia that is due to excessive or inappropriately distributed doses of insulin. Glycosylated hemoglobin in the center of the normal range commonly signals recurrent hypoglycemia in persons who are taking insulin.[109] Values at the upper end of the normal range are more safely achievable and within reach for some patients. These correspond to blood-glucose levels largely in the 100–200 mg/dl range. Realistic therapeutic objectives, in terms of desired blood or plasma glucose values, should be established for each individual patient. For older and more fragile patients, these objectives must be especially modest to avoid damage due to hypoglycemia.

The symptoms of hypoglycemia caused by insulin or oral agents often are vague and not recognized by a patient, his or her family, or medical personnel. While a younger person with diabetes is likely to feel sweaty, shaky, anxious, or hungry when plasma-glucose levels fall, an older individual may have none of these sensations.[110] Instead, confusion, change of personality, headache, nausea, or general malaise may be the leading clues. A headache and nausea on awakening in the morning are especially worrisome; these symptoms should draw attention to the possibility of nocturnal hypoglycemia.

Other Illnesses in a Diabetic Patient

Several special concerns arise when an older person with diabetes develops another illness. The patient may be unusually vulnerable to the disorder itself, to the disability and immobilization it causes, or to unwanted effects of diagnostic or therapeutic efforts. For example, both superficial yeast and parenchymal gram-positive bacterial infections tend to be more aggressive in persons with diabetes. Dehydration and electrolyte imbalance due to vomiting or diarrhea may be especially hazardous when a loss of diabetic control ensues. The interruption of food intake by a gastrointestinal illness, depression, or diagnostic studies, brings the hazard of hypoglycemia to persons who are taking insulin. Pressure sores readily develop and slowly heal on the feet of bedridden persons with diabetic neuropathy and vascular injury. A diabetic kidney appears more vulnerable to an injury from hypertonic contrast media that are used for many radiologic tests. Corticosteroids, which are risky enough as therapeutic agents for all older persons, are especially problematic for a diabetic; they will certainly provoke hyperglycemia, and may further impair the limited ability of diabetic tissues to heal and resist infection. Narcotic analgesics and many psychotropic drugs can seriously interfere with autonomic neural functions that already are impaired by diabetic neuropathy. Thus, codeine or amitryptyline may worsen constipation, urinary retention, nausea and gastric retention, and blurred vision, in persons who are already disposed to these prosaic but serious problems.

Major cardiovascular disorders present the most serious dilemmas. Myocardial infarction is common in this population; it often presents with atypical symptoms and may have a higher mortality rate. Cardiac pain, anxiety, and hypotension may provoke a metabolic decompensation. The loss of cardiovascular reflexes due to an autonomic neuropathy may deprive a physician of the usual clinical indicators; the heart rate may not rise and peripheral vasoconstriction may not occur when cardiac output falls. The use of beta-adrenergic-blocking agents (propranolol, metoprolol, and others) after an infarction, or for hypertension, angina, or an arrhythmia, may inhibit the secretion of insulin and reduce the ability to recognize hypoglycemia. Thiazide diuretics also may impair the secretion of insulin, either directly or by causing hypokalemia. With all these factors involved, the management of myocardial infarction, hypertension, angina, or congestive heart failure, becomes especially tricky when a patient has diabetes. A wise clinician remains watchful and cautious with all interventions.

Management of Specific Complications of Diabetes

Several complications of diabetes have specific remedies that are worth mentioning. Proliferative retinopathy can be slowed or arrested by the skillful use of photocoagulation.[111] Some evidence also indicates that good glycemic control retards the progression of retinopathy. A painful neuropathy commonly improves with better glycemic control, especially with the prevention of repeated hypoglycemia. A variety of drugs have been used for treating neuropathic discomfort. Narcotics seem relatively unsuccessful. Phenytoin and carbamazapine are of uncertain value, although they often are used. Fluphenazine and amitrypthyline[112,113] also have been used with some evidence of benefit. Diabetic foot ulcers require meticulous local care that emphasizes debridement, soaks, shoe inserts and special footwear, antibiotics, and various surgical procedures, which depend on individual circumstances. The anticipation and prevention of problems with the feet are far preferable to energetic treatment after serious lesions have developed.

References

1. National Diabetes Data Group: Classification and diagnosis of diabetes mellitus and other categories of glucose intolerance. *Diabetes* 28:1039–1057, 1979.
2. Cahill GH Jr: Physiology of insulin in man. *Diabetes* 20:785–799, 1971.
3. Czech MP: Insulin action. *Am J Med* 70:142–150, 1981.
4. Gerich J, Davis J, Lorenzi M, et al: Hormonal mechanisms of recovery from insulin-induced hypoglycemia in man. *Am J Physiol* 236:E380–E385, 1979.
5. Porte D Jr, Bagdade JD: Human insulin secretion: an integrated approach. *Ann Rev Med* 21:219–240, 1970.
6. Bar RS, Harrison LC, Muggeo M, et al: Regulation of insulin receptors in normal and abnormal physiology in humans. *Adv Int Med* 24:23–52, 1979.
7. Cahill CF Jr, McDevitt HO: Insulin-dependent diabetes mellitus: the initial lesion. *N Engl J Med* 304:1454–1465, 1981.
8. De Fronzo RA, Ferrannini E: The pathogenesis of non-insulin-dependent diabetes: an update. *Medicine* 61:125–140, 1982.
9. Olefsky JM, Kolterman OG: Mechanisms of insulin resistance in obesity and non-insulin-dependent (Type II) diabetes. *Am J Med* 70:151–168, 1981.
10. Kahn CR: Role of insulin receptors in insulin resistant states. *Metabolism* 29:455–466, 1980.
11. Pheiffer MA, Halter JB, Porte D Jr: Insulin secretion in diabetes mellitus. *Am J Med* 70:579–588, 1981.
12. Holman RR, Turner RC: Maintenance of basal plasma glucose and insulin concentrations in maturity-onset diabetes. *Diabetes* 28:227–230, 1979.
13. Cooperman MT, Davidoff F, Spark R, et al: Clinical studies of alcoholic ketoacidosis. *Diabetes* 23:433–439, 1974.
14. Malherbe C, Burrill KC, Leyvin SR, et al: Effect of diphenylhydantoin on insulin secretion in man. *N Engl J Med* 286:339–342, 1972.
15. Cerasi E, Luft R, Efendic S: Effect of adrenergic blocking agents on insulin response to glucose infusion in man. *Acta Endocrinol* 69:335–346, 1972.
16. Fajans SS, Floyd JC Jr, Knopf RF, et al: Benzothiadiazine suppression of insulin release from normal and abnormal islet tissue in man. *J Clin Invest* 45:481–492, 1966.
17. Giugliano D, Torella R, Cacciapuoti, et al: Impairment of insulin secretion in man by nifedipine. *Eur J Pharmacol* 18:395–398, 1980.
18. Baxter J, Forsham P: Tissue effects of glucocorticoids. *Am J Med* 53:573–584, 1972.
19. Davidson MB: The effect of aging on carbohydrate metabolism: a review of the English literature and a practical approach to the diagnosis of diabetes mellitus in the elderly. *Metabolism* 28:688–705, 1979.
20. O'Sullivan JB: Age gradient in blood glucose levels—magnitude and clinical implications. *Diabetes* 23:713–715, 1974.
21. De Fronzo RA: Glucose intolerance and aging. *Diabetes Care* 4:493–501, 1981.
22. Andres R: Aging and diabetes. *Med Clin North Am* 55:835–846, 1971.
23. Mahler R, Romanoff NE, Dunbar A, et al: The dilemma of defining diabetes mellitus in the aging population. *West J Med* 136:379–383, 1982.
24. Siperstein MD: The glucose tolerance test: a pitfall in the diagnosis of diabetes mellitus. *Adv Int Med* 20:297–323, 1975.

25. Skyler JS: Complications of diabetes mellitus: relationship to metabolic dysfunction. *Diabetes Care* 2:499–509, 1979.

26. Winaver J, Teredesai P, Feldman HA, et al: Diabetic nephropathy as the mode of presentation of diabetes mellitus. *Metabolism* 28:1023–1030, 1979.

27. Linner E, Svanborg A, Zelander T: Retinal and renal lesions of diabetic type, without obvious disturbances in glucose metabolism in a patient with family history of diabetes. *Am J Med* 39:298–304, 1965.

28. Danowski TS, Fisher ER, Park EJ, et al: Capillary basement membranes in muscle in glucose intolerance of the chemical diabetes type. *Am J Clin Path* 61:718–723, 1974.

29. Fuller JH, Shipley MJ, Rose G, et al: Coronary-heart disease risk and impaired glucose tolerance. *Lancet* 1:1373–1376, 1980.

30. Kreisberg RA: Diabetic ketoacidosis: new concepts and trends in pathogenesis and treatment. *Ann Int Med* 88:681–695, 1978.

31. Podolsky S: Hyperosmolar nonketotic coma: death can be prevented. *Geriatrics* 34(Mar):29–42, 1979.

32. Arieff AI, Caroll HJ: Nonketotic hyperosmolar coma with hyperglycemia: clinical features, pathophysiology, renal function, acid base balance, plasma-cerebrospinal fluid equilibrium and the effects of therapy in 37 cases. *Medicine* 51:73–94, 1972.

33. Arieff AI, Carroll HJ: Hyperosmolar nonketotic coma with hyperglycemia: abnormalities of lipid and carbohydrate metabolism. *Metabolism* 20:529–538, 1971.

34. Paton RC: Haemostatic changes in diabetic coma. *Diabetologia* 21:172–177, 1981.

35. Fulop M, Rosenblatt A, Kreitzer SM, et al: Hyperosmolar nature of diabetic coma. *Diabetes* 24:594–599, 1975.

36. Johnston DG, Alberti KGMM: Diabetic emergencies: practical aspects of the management of diabetic ketoacidosis and diabetes during surgery. *Clin Endocrinol Metab* 9:437–460, 1980.

37. Peterson L, Caldwell J, Hoffman J: Insulin absorbance to polyvinylchloride surfaces with implication for constant infusion therapy. *Diabetes* 25:72–74, 1976.

38. Arieff AI, Carroll HJ: Cerebral edema and depression of sensorium in nonketotic hyperosmolar coma. *Diabetes* 23:525–531, 1979.

39. Spiro RG: Biochemistry of the renal glomerular basement membrane and its alterations in diabetes mellitus. *N Engl J Med* 288:1337–1342, 1973.

40. Monnier VM, Cerami A: Non-enzymatic glycosylation and browning of proteins in diabetes. *Clin Endocrinol Metab* 11:431–452, 1982.

41. Goldstein DE, Parker KM, England D, et al: Clinical application of glycosylated hemoglobin measurements. *Diabetes* 31(suppl 3):70–78, 1982.

42. Jovanovic L, Peterson CM: The clinical utility of glycosylated hemoglobin. *Am J Med* 70:331–338, 1981.

43. Gabbay KH: Hyperglycemia, ployol metabolism, and complications of diabetes mellitus. *Ann Rev Med* 26:521–536, 1975.

44. Kinoshita JH, Fukushi S, Kador P, et al: Aldose reductase in diabetic complications of the eye. *Metabolism* 28(suppl 1):462–469, 1979.

45. Colwell JA, Lopes-Virella M, Halushka PV: Pathogenesis of atherosclerosis in diabetes mellitus. *Diabetes Care* 4:121–133, 1981.

46. Goldenberg S, Alex M, Joshi RA, et al: Non-atheromatous peripheral vascular disease of the lower extremity in diabetes mellitus. *Diabetes* 8:261–273, 1959.

47. Strandness DE, Priest RE, Gibbons GE: Combined clinical and pathological study of diabetic and nondiabetic peripheral arterial disease. *Diabetes* 13:366–372, 1964.

48. Ledet T: Histological and histochemical changes in the coronary arteries of old diabetic patients. *Diabetologia* 4:268–272, 1968.

49. Mauer SM, Barbosa J, Venier RL, et al: Development of diabetic vascular lesions in normal kidneys transplanted into patients with diabetes mellitus. *N Engl J Med* 295:916–920, 1976.

50. Reddi AS: Diabetic microangiopathy. Current status of the chemistry and metabolism of the glomerular basement membrane. *Metabolism* 27:107–124, 1978.

51. Raskin P: Diabetic regulation and its relationship to microangiopathy. *Metabolism* 27:235–252, 1978.

52. Raff MD, Asbury AK: Ischemic mononeuropathy and mononeuropathy multiplex in diabetes mellitus. *N Engl J Med* 279:17–22, 1968.

53. Clements RS Jr: Diabetic neuropathy—new concepts of its etiology. *Diabetes* 28:604–611, 1979.

54. Jung Y, Hohmann TC, Gerneth JA, et al: Diabetic hand syndrome. *Metabolism* 20:1008–1015, 1971.

55. Ellenberg M: Diabetic truncal mononeuropathy—a new clinical syndrome. *Diabetes Care* 1:10–13, 1978.

56. Longstreth GF, Newcomer AD: Abdominal pain caused by diabetic radiculopathy. *Ann Int Med* 86:166–168, 1977.

57. Ellenberg M: Diabetic neuropathy: Clinical aspects. *Metabolism* 25:1627–1655, 1976.

58. Watkins PJ: Facial sweating after food: a new sign of diabetic autonomic neuropathy. *Br Med J* 1:583–587, 1973.

59. Page MMcB, Watkins PJ: The heart in diabetes: autonomic neuropathy and cardiomyopathy. *Clin Endocrinol Metab* 6:377–388, 1977.

60. Pfeifer MA, Cook D, Brodsky J, et al: Quantitative evaluation of sympathetic and parasympathetic control of iris function. *Diabetes Care* 5:518–528, 1982.

61. Ewing DJ, Campbell IW, Clarke BF: Assessment of cardiovascular effects of diabetic autonomic neuropathy and prognostic implications. *Ann Int Med* 92(part 2):308–311, 1980.

62. McNally EF, Reinhard AE, Schwartz PE: Small bowel motility in diabetes. *Am J Dig Dis* 14:163–169, 1969.

63. Ellenberg M, Weber H: The incipient asymptomatic diabetic bladder. *Diabetes* 16:331–335, 1967.

64. Kolodny RC, Kahn CB, Goldstein HH, et al: Sexual dysfunction in diabetic men. *Diabetes* 23:306–309, 1974.

65. Ellenberg M: Diabetic neuropathic cachexia. *Diabetes* 23:418–423, 1974.

66. Jones RL, Peterson CM: Hematologic alterations in diabetes mellitus. *Am J Med* 70:339–352, 1981.

67. Bern MM: Platelet function in diabetes mellitus. *Diabetes* 27:342–350, 1978.

68. McMillan DE: Plasma protein changes, blood viscosity, and diabetic microangiopathy. *Diabetes* 25(suppl 2):858–864, 1976.

69. Bagdade JD, Root RR, Bulger RS: Impaired leukocyte function in patients with poorly controlled diabetes. *Diabetes* 23:9–15, 1974.

70. Peterson CM, Jones RL, Koenig RJ, et al: Reversible hematologic sequelae of diabetes mellitus. *Ann Int Med* 86:425–429, 1977.

71. Spring M, Fleck H, Cohen BD: Dupuytren's contracture. Warning of diabetes? *NY State J Med* 70:1037–1041, 1970.

72. Bridgeman JF: Periarthritis of the shoulder and diabetes mellitus. *Ann Rheum Dis* 31:69–71, 1972.

73. Rosenbloom AL, Silverstein JH, Lezotte DC, et al: Limited joint mobility in childhood diabetes mellitus indicates increased risk from microvascular diseases. *N Engl J Med* 305:191–194, 1981.

74. Perejda AJ, Vitto J: Nonenzymatic glycosylation of collagen and other proteins: relationship to development of diabetic complications. *Collagen Rel Res* 2:81–88, 1982.

75. Fisher ER, Danowski TS: Histologic, histochemical, and electron microscopic features of the shin spots of diabetes mellitus. *Am J Clin Path* 50:547–554, 1968.

76. Muller SA, Winkleman RK: Necrobiosis lipoidica diabeticorum. *Arch Derm* 93:272–281, 1966.

77. Wheat LJ: Infection and diabetes mellitus. *Diabetes Care* 3:187–197, 1980.

78. Goodson WH, Hunt TK: Wound healing and the diabetic patient. *Surg Gynecol Obstet* 149:600–608, 1979.

79. Kannel WB, McGee DL: Diabetes and cardiovascular disease: The Framingham study. *JAMA* 241:2035–2038, 1979.

80. Riddle MC, Hart J: Hyperglycemia, recognized and unrecognized, as a risk factor for stroke and transient ischemic attacks. *Stroke* 13:356–359, 1982.

81. Kohner EM: Diabetic retinopathy. *Clin Endocrinol Metab* 6:345–375, 1977.

82. Pirie A: Epidemiologic and biochemical studies of cataract and diabetes. *Invest Ophthal* 4:629–637, 1965.

83. Becker B, Bresnick G, Chevrette L, et al: Intraocular pressure and its response to topical corticosteroids in diabetes. *Arch Ophthal* 76:477–483, 1966.

84. Jarrett J: Diabetes and the heart: coronary heart disease. *Clin Endocrinol Metab* 6:389–402, 1979.

85. Czyzk A, Krolewski AS, Szablowska S, et al: Clinical course of myocardial infarction among diabetic patients. *Diabetes Care* 3:526–529, 1980.

86. Rubler S, Dlugash J, Yuceoglu YZ, et al: New type of cardiomyopathy associated with diabetic glomerulosclerosis. *Am J Cardiol* 30:595–602, 1972.

87. Kannel WB, Hjortland M, Castelli WP: Role of diabetes in congestive heart failure: The Framingham Study. *Am J Cardiol* 34:29–34, 1979.

88. Faerman I, Faccio E, Milei J, et al: Autonomic neuropathy and painless myocardial infarction in diabetic patients. *Diabetes* 26:1147–1158, 1977.

89. Scarpello JHB, Sladen GE: Progress report: diabetes and the gut. *Gut* 19:1153–1162, 1978.

90. Kassander P: Asymptomatic gastric retention in diabetes (gastroparesis diabeticorum). *Ann Int Med* 48:797–812, 1958.

91. Grodzki M, Mazurkiewicz-Rozynska E, Czyzk A: Diabetic cholecystopathy. *Diabetologia* 4:345–348, 1968.

92. Malins JM, Magne N: Diabetic diarrhea. *Diabetes* 18:858–866, 1969.

93. Fabre J, Balant LP, Dayer PG, et al: The kidney in maturity onset diabetes mellitus: a clinical study of 510 patients. *Kidney Int* 21:730–738, 1982.

94. Shieh SD, Hirsch SR, Boshell BR, et al: Low risk of contrast media-induced acute renal failure in nonazotemic type 2 diabetes mellitus. *Kidney Int* 21:739–743, 1982.

95. Schambelan M, Sebastian A: Hyporeninemic hypoaldosteronism. *Adv Int Med* 24:385–405, 1979.

96. Frimodt-Moller C: Diabetic cystopathy: a review of the urodynamic and clinical features of neurogenic bladder dysfunction in diabetes mellitus. *Dan Med Bull* 25:49–60, 1978.

97. Levin ME, O'Neal LW: *The Diabetic Foot*. St. Louis, The CV Mosby Co, 1977.

98. Anderson JW: The role of dietary carbohydrate and fiber in the control of diabetes. *Adv Int Med* 26:67–96, 1981.

99. American Diabetes Association: Principles of nutrition and dietary recommendations for individuals with diabetes mellitus: 1979. *Diabetes* 28:1027–1029, 1979.

100. Hadden DR: Food and diabetes: the dietary treatment of insulin-dependent and non-insulin dependent diabetes. *Clin Endocrinol Metab* 11:503–524, 1982.

101. University Group Diabetes Program: A study of the effects of hypoglycemic agents on vascular complications in patients with adult-onset diabetes: III Clinical implications of UGDP results. *JAMA* 218:1400–1410, 1971.

102. American Diabetes Association: The UGDP controversy. *Diabetes* 28:168–170, 1979.

103. Skillman TG, Feldman JM: The pharmacology of sulfonylureas. *Am J Med* 70:361–372, 1981.

104. Shen S-W, Bressler R: Clinical pharmacology of oral antidiabetic agents. *N Engl J Med* 296:493–497, 787–792, 1977.

105. Koivisto VA, Felig P: Alterations in insulin absorption and in blood glucose control that is associated with varying insulin injection sites in diabetic patients. *Ann Int Med* 92:59–61, 1980.

106. Koivisto VA, Fortney S, Hendler R: A rise in ambient temperature augments insulin absorption in diabetic patients. *Metabolism* 30:402–404, 1981.

107. Süsstrunk H, Morell B, Ziegler WH, et al: Insulin absorption from the abdomen and the thigh in healthy subjects during rest and exercise: blood glucose, plasma insulin, growth hormone, adrenaline and nonadrenaline levels. *Diabetologia* 22:171–174, 1982.

108. Shapiro B, Savage PJ, Lomatch D, et al: A comparison of accuracy and estimated cost of methods for home blood glucose monitoring. *Diabetes Care* 4:396–403, 1981.

109. Dorman TL, Peckar CO, Mayor-White VA, et al: Unsuspected hypoglycemia, hemoglobin A_1, and diabetic control. *Quart J Med* 50:31–38, 1981.

110. Balodimos MC, Root HF: Hypoglycemic insulin reactions without symptoms. *JAMA* 171:261–266, 1959.

111. Rand LI: Recent advances in diabetic retinopathy. *Am J Med* 70:895–902, 1981.

112. Davis JL, Lewis SB, Gerich JE, et al: Peripheral diabetic neuropathy treated with amitriptyline and fluphenazine. *JAMA* 238:2291–2292, 1977.

113. Gade GN, Hofeldt FD, Treece GL: Diabetic neuropathic cachexia. Beneficial response to combination therapy with amitryptyline and fluphenazine. *JAMA* 243:1160–1161, 1980.

Chapter 26

Female Reproductive Endocrinology

STANLEY G. KORENMAN, M.D.

SUSAN STANIK, M.D.

In a female, the failure of ovarian function in the 5th or 6th decade is inevitable, and its consequences play an important role in her health and well-being for the remaining 30 years or so of life expectancy. During the postmenopausal years, about 80% of all females will experience symptoms that are due to an ovarian hormone deficiency. Some problems, including sex tissue atrophy and osteoporosis, will become more progressively severe with age.

Ovarian Failure—Menstrual Changes

The length of normal menstrual cycles declines with age due to a shortening of the first (follicular) phase of the cycle.[1] The luteal phase usually is preserved.

As a female approaches the cessation of menses, her cycles become irregular,[2,3] with both long and short intervals between episodes of menstruation. The short cycles usually are ovulatory, with a short follicular phase, a normal luteal phase, and somewhat reduced levels of estrogen secretion. The long cycles typically are associated with a low or absent progesterone secretion, and they are termed luteally inadequate or anovulatory. In both types of cycles, gonadotropin levels (particularly the follicle-stimulating hormone [FSH]) are high due to the lower estrogen levels and reduced production of the follicular peptide, inhibin. Often, the first symptoms of the climacteric period begin to appear at this time. After an average of 5 years of cycle irregularity (varying from 0–8 years and longer in heavier females and in those undergoing a late menopause) menopause occurs. While the establishment of a diagnosis of menopause is not simple, 1 year without menses or, alternatively, the finding of a very low plasma estradiol level (<20 pg/ml) with very high levels of both a luteinizing hormone (LH) and FSH will serve.

Anatomic changes that are observed in an aging ovary correspond to the hormonal aberrations. The disappearance of primordial ova and follicles, a thickening of blood vessel walls, and a generalized fibrosis have been described. The stromal cells appear unchanged or occasionally become hyperplastic.[4,5]

Postmenopausal Hormonal Changes

What are the biologic consequences of ovarian failure? These depend on the remaining production of reproductive steroids and their physiologic activities.

Estrogens

In a premenopausal female, the biologically active estrogens estradiol (E_2) and estrone (E_1) are produced not only by a direct secretion from maturing ovarian follicles, but also by a peripheral conversion of androgenic precursors. Ovarian stromal cells and the adrenal reticularis and fasciculata produce androgens. The stromal tissue is stimulated by LH, so that in any ovulatory female, a mid-cycle increase in androgens

TABLE 26-1 Representative Reproductive Hormone Levels in Females

Hormone	Premenopausal		Postmenopausal		
	Plasma Level	Production Rate	Plasma Level	Production Rate	% Tightly Bound
Androstenedione	150 ng/dl	2.7 mg/day	90 ng/dl	1.6 mg/day	0
Testosterone	35 ng/dl	200 μg/day	25 ng/dl	150 μg/day	>90
Dehydroepiandrosterone	4.5 ng/ml	—	1.8 ng/ml	—	0
Dehydroepiandrosterone sulfate	1,500 ng/ml	—	300 ng/ml	—	0
Estrone	40–200 pg/ml	80–4,000 μg/day	35 pg/ml	55 μg/day	0
Estradiol	40–350 pg/ml	50–500 μg/day	13 pg/ml	12 μg/day	50
Luteinizing (LH)	10–40 ImU/ml	—	70 ImU/ml	—	—
Follicle-stimulating (FSH)	10–40 ImU/ml	—	80 ImU/ml	—	—
Prolactin	10 ng/ml	—	8 ng/ml	—	—

SOURCE: Korenman SG: Menopausal endocrinology and management. *Arch Int Med* 142:1131–1136, 1982.

as well as estrogens is seen. In anovulatory states, where gonadotropin secretion is constant rather than cyclical, thecal (stromal) cells may persist and overproduce the hormone precursor androstenedione (A) and testosterone (T). A peripheral aromatization of androgens to estrogens occurs in fat, muscle, skin, liver, endometrium, and the hypothalamus.[6] Thus, A is converted to E_1 and T to E_2. Although the percentage of A converted to E_1 is small (about 2.8%), the amount of A produced by the ovaries and adrenal gland is large; thus, this accounts for almost one third of the production of E_1 in premenopausal females. In turn, E_1 may be metabolized to E_2. The production of E_2, however, is almost entirely due to a direct ovarian secretion in the premenopausal female.

Circulating estrogens are greatly decreased postmenopausally (*see* Table 26-1). Initially, the ovaries may contribute slightly to plasma estrogen levels; but, at 4 years postmenopause, no significant, direct ovarian secretion of estrogens is seen. The circulating E_2 (*see* Figure 26-1) results from a peripheral conversion of E_1, which in turn is derived almost exclusively from the peripheral aromatization of adrenal androstenedione.[7,8] E_1 levels are higher than those of E_2 after menopause, and neither change consistently with age per se.[9] However, the production rates and serum levels of both estrogens are positively correlated with body weight and surface area (*see* Figure 26-2). Both an increased production of adrenal precursors and an increased rate of peripheral aromatization of androgens to estrogens are reported in cases of

obesity.[10,11] Obese females have a higher incidence of endometrial hyperplasia than their thinner cohorts. Similarly, postmenopausal females with cirrhosis (associated with an increased aromatization of A to E_1) have higher estrogen levels and more endometrial hyperplasias and cancers.[9]

Thus, it is important to take these factors that influence endogenous estrogens into account when evaluating a postmenopausal female for estrogen therapy. Exogenous estrogens do not shut off an endogenous estrogen production, since the feedback inhibition of go-

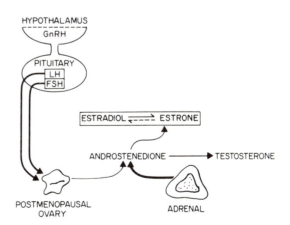

FIGURE 26-1 Alterations of reproductive hormones after menopause. (From Korenman SG: Menopausal endocrinology and management. *Arch Int Med* 142:1131–1136, 1982, used by permission.)

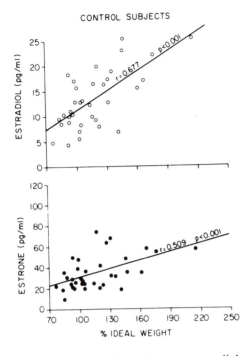

CONTROL SUBJECTS

FIGURE 26-2 Correlations of serum estradiol and estrone levels with percentage of ideal weight in 35 normal postmenopausal females. (From Judd HL, Davidson BJ, Frumar AM, et al: Serum androgens and estrogens in postmenopausal women with and without endometrial cancer. *Am J Obstet Gynecol* 136:859–871, 1980, used by permission.)

nadotropins does not affect the peripheral production of estrogens.

Estrogens may be bound to albumin or a sex hormone-binding globulin (SHBG). The estrogen E_1 is very poorly bound to an SHBG.[12] Since albumin-bound E_2 remains available for entry into cells, but E_2 bound to SNBG does not, only that fraction not bound to SHBG is considered to be metabolically active (i.e., about 60% of E_2 and over 90% of E_1). Recent studies have identified a separate high-affinity serum estrogen-binding protein of uncertain importance.[13] Available estrogens pass freely through the cell membranes and bind to specific high-affinity, low-capacity cytoplasmic receptors, which are present in relatively high concentrations in target cells. The hormone-receptor complex is activated and translocated to the cell nucleus, where it binds to acceptor sites on nuclear chromatin. This process activates transcription at highly selective locations, which results in new messenger RNA and a subse-

quent protein synthesis that is characteristic of the hormonal response.

High concentrations of estrogen receptors are bound in many tissues, which include: 1) Classic reproductive organs such as the endometrium, myometrium, vagina, cervix, fallopian tubes, ovary, placenta, and breast; 2) Involved areas of the brain such as the hypothalamus and pituitary gland; and 3) Less obvious sites such as the liver, skin, heart, pancreas, adrenal gland, kidney, and spinal cord (*see* Table 26-2).

Estrogens generally are associated with growth, development, and a later maintenance of the female reproductive tract. They regulate the menstrual cycles and inhibit gonadotropin production. Both breast ductal and lobulo alveolar development are stimulated, and estrogens with prolactin stimulate lactation. The hepatic effects of estrogens may include increased production of the secreted binding proteins (for thyroid, cortisol, and sex steroid hormones), angiotensinogen, transferrin, hepatic-clotting factors, and the apoproteins for high density lipoproteins (HDL) and very low density lipoproteins (VLDL). Estrogens decrease the excretion of sulfobromopthalein and bile flow, induce many microsomal enzymes, and alter hepatic drug metabolism. Mild anabolic effects are seen that result in nitrogen retention. Estrogen effects on calcium metabolism include an inhibition of bone resorption and an enhance-

TABLE 26-2 Tissues Reported to Contain Estrogen Receptors

Classic Targets	Other
Endometrium	Kidney
Myometrium	Prostate
Oviduct	Adrenal
Vagina	Pancreas
Fallopian tube	Colon
Cervix	Spinal cord
Brain	Eosinophils
Hypothalamus	Heart
Pituitary gland	Skin
Liver	
Placenta	
Leydig's cell	
Ovarian cells	

SOURCE: Korenman SG: Menopausal endocrinology and management. *Arch Int Med* 142:1131–1136, 1982.

ment of gut calcium absorption. Estrogen receptors have not been identified in bone, so that their site of action remains unclear while their protective effect against postmenopausal osteoporosis is accepted.[14]

Estrogens are metabolized largely by a conversion to estrone and estriol and by a hepatic conjugation with glucuronic acid, sulfates, and other inactive conjugates.

Androgens

While the ovary of an aging female undergoes a progressive loss of capacity to produce estrogens, the stromal androgen production continues for some time under a tonic LH stimulation. It is estimated that ovarian secretion accounted for about one half of the circulating T and about one third of A postmenopausally; the remainder was claimed from the adrenal gland secretion.[15]

Postmenopausally, the plasma concentration of A is reduced to about 60% of premenopausal levels. There is disagreement as to whether a continuing decline occurs with age per se. Plasma T levels are much more variable in postmenopausal females. Most investigators found no change in the mean T levels with age after an initial menopausal fall.[16-18] One group found that T and free T concentrations fell from the 3rd to the 6th decades, but they increased again after 60 years of age with great individual variations.[19] Occasionally, postmenopausal LH levels even induce stromal or hilus cell hyperplasias and masculinize a female.

Longcope could not demonstrate a change in the production rate or disposal of androgens with age per se, but the production rates of both A and T were positively correlated with overweight and body surface areas.[11,20]

The target tissue response to these androgens also may vary with aging. The mean levels of plasma and urinary 5α-androstane-3α, 17β-diol glucuronide, 17β-diol (the metabolites of androgens that are felt to reflect androgen activity in target tissues), were decreased in a small number of postmenopausal females compared to younger menstruating women.[21] This suggests decreased androgen effects at the target tissue level.

The clinical importance of androgens in aging females remains to be elucidated, but it may include the maintenance of protein anabolism, bone mass, and other physiologic and behavioral processes. Some studies have suggested that age-related bone loss correlates with declining androgens.[22,23]

Hypothalamic-Pituitary Function

Both gonadotropins continue to rise postmenopausally; they attain an 18-fold FSH elevation 2 years after menopause, and a tripling of LH levels after 3 years.[24] The levels then slowly decrease with advancing age until they level off 30 years after the menopause. The pulsatile secretion of gonadotropins continues after the menopause with peaks of similar frequency (q1–2 hours), but of a much greater amplitude than those in younger females.

Clinical Features

Menopausal symptoms are largely related to estrogen deprivation. They include vasomotor symptoms, sex tissue atrophy, osteoporosis, and emotional alterations.

The most common complaint is the "hot flash" or "flush" that is experienced by 75–85% of all females. While a majority of females experience these disturbing symptoms, a much smaller percentage actually seek medical attention. Patients describe the sensation as occurring in stages. First, a "premonitory" pressure sensation in the head or a headache occurs. This is followed by the flush, which they sense as heart or a burning sensation starting in the face. It progresses to the upper neck, chest, and back, often is visible to others as a splotchy "flush," and concludes with profuse sweating in these areas. Some women also experience weakness, nausea, faintness, or palpitations. "Night sweats" and insomnia also have been related to menopausal hot flashes.[25] The episodes range from moments to 30 minutes and occur several times per day to once a week. They often last more than 1 year and may continue for 5 years or more.

The physiologic study of the hot flash has charted the phases of these episodes. A woman may note the prodromal phase before any physiologic change can be detected. It is thought that during this phase the central thermoregula-

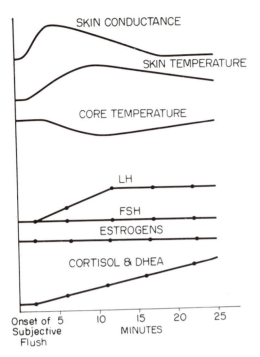

FIGURE 26-3   Physiologic and endocrine features of
menopausal hot flash. LH = luteinizing hormone,
FSH = follicle-stimulating hormone, and DHEA =
dehydroepiandrosterone. (From Korenman SG:
Menopausal endocrinology and management. *Arch
Int Med* 142:1131–1136, 1982, used by permission.)

An atrophy of the estrogen target organs, such as secondary sex tissues, is another distressing consequence of estrogen deprivation. A vaginal atrophy may produce dryness, pain, itching, bleeding, infection, and dyspareunia. The urethral mucosa also may atrophy, which results in symptoms of dysuria. Endometrial atrophy due to an estrogen deficiency could be demonstrated in a biopsy specimen in most postmenopausal females. However, if vaginal bleeding occurs in an older woman, then proliferative or hyperplastic endometrial changes must be suspected; an adenocarcinoma must be ruled out. Hyperplasia suggests the presence of a continuous estrogen stimulation that is unopposed by progesterone. The causes of excess endogenous estrogen in a postmenopausal state may include: 1) Obesity and cirrhosis (via an increased conversion of androgenic precursors to estrogen); 2) Ovarian hyperthecosis or granulosa-theca cell tumors (increased ovarian estrogen production); or 3) Androgen-secreting tumors (increased adrenal or ovarian precursor production).

Osteoporosis (*see* Volume I, Chapter 28), is a major clinical complication in postmenopausal females. In the United States, at least 10% of all females over 50 years of age have a bone loss severe enough to result in hip, vertebra, or long-bone fractures. The incidence rate increases with age, so that at some time 25–30% of all postmenopausal females suffer orthopedic problems.[29] At menopause, a period of accelerated bone loss is initiated, which has been related to the loss of ovarian hormone secretion.

A postmenopausal female has an altered calcium and, perhaps, Vitamin D metabolism, reduced calcium absorption, and an increased overnight urinary calcium excretion.[30] Those postmenopausal females who are likely to develop osteoporosis with fractures often have in common a sex hormone deficiency (no exogenous and little endogenous production), positive family history, caucasian heritage, thinness, sedentary habits, lower initial (premenopause) bone mass, and cigarette smoking. Poor dietary calcium levels with an excessive phosphorus intake, especially in the form of high protein and carbonated drinks, are common. Estrogens inhibit both bone resorption and deposition; which results in a net positive effect on bone density.[31] Despite these find-

tory center misperceives core overheating. The central activation of heat loss mechanisms explains the next changes seen; that is, an increase in skin conductance (measuring perspiration), which is followed by a rise in skin temperature (measuring cutaneous vasodilation). These mechanisms result in a decline to a below-normal core temperature, which returns to normal after about 30 minutes.[26] Preceding the hot flash, there is a pulsatile release of LH, which probably reflects the central origin of the thermal changes.[27,28] The LH rise is not thought to be causal, since hypophysectomized females may experience hot flashes. While plasma catecholamines have not been found to change before, during, or after the event, some investigators believe that a central adrenergic release may initiate the flushing episode; they have noted the similarity to pheochromocytoma symptoms. Hot flashes have been treated successfully with estrogens, progestins, and the central adrenergic agonist, clonidine.

ings, the precise molecular role of a decreased ovarian function and steroid deficiency in the risk of osteoporosis is uncertain. Estrogen receptors have not been demonstrated in bone tissue, so that an indirect action on the skeleton is required, such as an enhanced Vitamin D activation or control of calcium-regulating hormones.

Other symptoms that often are listed as components of the climacteric period include mood changes, irritability, and sexual dysfunction. There is no good evidence that these are specific effects of lack of the estrogen, and they generally have been attributed to the psychosocial changes at menopause. Recent descriptions of the sleep impairment that is associated with hot flashes[25] also may explain some of the disturbances.

Sexual dysfunction is unusual in aging females. A decline in sexual activity is closely related to the availability of an active partner.[32,33] There is no evidence that the libido is affected by menopause. Some women report an increased interest in sex once concerns about late-life pregnancy are past; most others report no change, and a few become disinterested. The available literature attributes these changes largely to cultural expectations. Breast and skin atrophy may alter one's self-image as a sexually desirable mate. A woman also may misinterpret changes in her partner's sexual desires/abilities as a loss of interest in her. Masters and Johnson described physiologic changes in the sexual functioning of aging females.[34] They noted a decreased rate of production and a decreased volume of vaginal lubricating fluid, a loss of elasticity of the vaginal walls, a diminished involuntary vaginal lengthening and diameter changes during sexual stimulation that lead to a fissuring of the mucosa with deep or prolonged penile thrusting. An older female may require more time to reach orgasm and may find that the orgasm itself may be of a decreased duration and diminished intensity. Occasionally, women develop painful uterine muscle cramping during orgasm, which is responsive to estrogen therapy. Vaginismus (an involuntary constriction of the walls of the distal vagina) may occur in response to any painful stimulation. Women may avoid sexual contact if they experience dyspareunia or pruritis vulvae that is related to estrogen deprivation. Estrogen replace-

ment thus may not only reverse the pathology, but it may restore sexual functioning.[35]

Therapy for Postmenopausal Symptoms

Estrogens

Estrogen replacement has been shown to benefit all of the problems discussed above. Since hot flashes and sex tissue atrophy are thought to be caused by estrogen deprivation, the most physiologic therapy would be estrogen administration.

The benefits of their use must be weighed against the possible consequences of estrogen therapy. Known and possible risks include a neoplastic transformation, blood pressure elevation, cardiovascular risks, lipid abnormalities, enhanced liver protein synthesis, altered clotting factors, and gallbladder disease.

The relation between estrogen therapy and endometrial carcinoma has been established in retrospective case-control studies.[36] Postmenopausal estrogens that are unopposed by progestins increase the risk of a carcinoma compared to non-users in a dose- and duration-dependent manner. The administration of a progestin may prevent the development of these lesions.[37] Given an early diagnosis of adenocarcinoma, good results are seen, which mandate medical supervision of females on estrogen therapy and a prompt evaluation of abnormal uterine bleeding.

A relationship between postmenopausal estrogen therapy and breast carcinoma has been proposed but not established. Estrogen-induced benign breast disease may be noted as a nodularity and tenderness by some females, and reversible cystic or dysplastic changes have been noted on a mammogram.[38] Retrospective case control studies disagree on the role of estrogens in malignant changes. A few recent studies report a slightly increased risk,[39–42] although some found no difference[37,43,44] or even a decreased incidence.[45] It is difficult to take into account all the factors that may interact, but Brinton, et al recently made adjustments for age at diagnosis, age at menopause, and type of menopause (natural versus surgical). They determined a relative risk of 1.2 for developing breast cancer in females, who use estrogens following a natural menopause and 1.5 for those with a postbilateral oophorectomy.[46] The risk appeared to be dose-related with Premarin use, and was related to years of use. A hormone-associated risk was especially high in certain subgroups of females who used estrogens after a bilateral oophorectomy, including nulliparous female, those with a positive family history of breast cancer, and those who had previous breast biopsy procedures.

An increase in breast cancer would be expected to appear long after the exposure to estrogen, if one accepts the hypothesis that "unopposed" estrogens promote tumor induction with a long delay before clinical presentation.[47] In the face of these complex relationships and the inconsistent evidence to date, a further evaluation and prospective randomized studies will be required. Current practice dictates that the data regarding the risk of breast cancer be employed only to reject estrogen therapy in females with a strong family or personal history of breast cancer.

While oral contraceptive estrogens constitute a risk for cardiovascular complications, such as myocardial infarction and thromboembolic events, the evidence for such an effect from the smaller doses used to treat postmenopause is thin. Some investigators have reported detrimental effects or increased angina episodes with a difference in the myocardial infarction rate,[48–50] while one found a protective effect of postmenopausal estrogen in the development of a coronary artery disease.[51] Thus, estrogen use still should be viewed with caution in females with other risk factors for ischemic heart disease such as smoking, obesity, or a positive family history.

Estrogens might have adverse effects on the cardiovascular system through indirect effects such as estrogen-mediated blood pressure elevation, increased triglycerides, glucose intolerance, and increased coagulability. While estrogens usually produce only mild elevations of triglycerides, an occasional severe hypertriglyceridemia has occurred in females with a mild pre-existing hyperlipidemia.[52] However, there also is a decrease in low-density lipoprotein (LDL) and an increase in high-density lipoprotein (HDL) cholesterol levels with the use of oral estrogens; a protection against atherosclerosis is believed to be afforded by high levels of the estrogen-inducible subfraction HDL_3.[53]

Susceptible females may develop hypertension while taking birth control pills. Low-dose conjugated estrogens in postmenopausal females are not as likely to cause a blood pressure elevation. Conjugated estrogens may stimulate sodium retention when unopposed by the anti-aldosterone effects of progesterone, and they have been shown to increase plasma renin activity.[54] Postmenopausal estrogen-induced hypertension has been described by some investigators, but it has not been seen by others. When hypertensive changes occur, they usually are reversible once the medication is discontinued. Thus, regular blood pressure measurements should be obtained for patients on an estrogen therapy.

The hypercoagulable effect of estrogens are dose-related, and perhaps a difference exists between the synthetic and natural estrogens. While synthetic estrogens have been shown to increase clotting factors II, VII, X, and fibrinogen and to decrease antithrombin III, there are conflicting studies on coagulation factor changes with the conjugated estrogens. Clinically, no increase in thromboembolic events (such as stroke or thrombophlebitis) has been demonstrated in postmenopausal females who are on conjugated estrogen therapy when other risk factors such as cigarette smoking or diabetes mellitus are controlled.[55] Estrogens are not recommended for women with a pre-existing thrombosis risk.

Women who are receiving estrogen therapy for menopause have a 2.5-fold increase in the risk of requiring gallbladder surgery.[43,56] The mechanism for the increase in gallbladder disease in females on estrogen therapy is unclear, although estrogens reduce bile flow, may increase cholesterol metabolism, and alter the bile salt content of the gallbladder, which results in lithogenic bile.

Dose-related abnormal uterine bleeding may be seen in postmenopausal females on estrogens. An endometrial sampling may be performed to rule out an endometrial adenocarcinoma. Common minor side effects that are seen include nausea and fluid retention with weight gain and edema.

Estrogen Preparations, Route of Administration, Dosage

Synthetic and "natural" estrogens are used in the therapy for a postmenopausal state. A comparison of the therapeutic and adverse effects of the various estrogen preparations has been difficult because of a lack of control for estrogen potency and dosage. All estrogens, if given in sufficient dosage and frequency, will suppress hot flashes and improve sex tissue atrophy. The many unfavorable estrogen effects that are noted above (including hypertension, cardiovascular disease, and neoplasias) one day may be modified by a selection from the variety of estrogens, routes of administration, frequency, and dosages.

Ethinyl estradiol, mestranol, and stilbestrol have been used less frequently in the treatment of menopausal complaints than conjugated equine estrogens. Of these, the most experience has been with ethinyl E_2. Doses as low as 10 μg may control symptoms; but, with its high potency and the oral route of administration, endometrial effects and pharmacologic hepatic effects are seen even at this dose level. The natural estrogens estrone, estradiol and estriol have been widely used. Estrone is the basis of conjugated equine estrogens. Doses of 0.625 mg/day or lower generally are recommended for chronic use, although higher average doses were used in the clinical trials that observed a reduced bone loss in females on estrogens. Studies of vaginal cytology suggest that higher doses may be required to improve the maturation index. Some effects on the liver are seen even in the 0.3 mg/day oral dosage schedule. The ester estradiol valerate and micronized 17-β estradiol also have been used. Estriol is available in a free form or as estriol succinate.

The oral administration of these estrogen preparations delivers estrogens rapidly to the liver, where an action and metabolism occur before they are available to the systemic circulation and other target tissues. Thus, the liver may see a disproportionately supraphysiologic-estrogenic effect with doses that are insufficient to suppress gonadotropins or hot flashes. The portal concentration of estrogen has been reported to be four to five times higher than the systemic concentration.[57] Many side effects of estrogen use, such as hypercoagulability and hypertension, are related to the enhancement of liver protein synthesis by the estrogen induction of clotting factors, angiotensinogen, binding proteins, hepatic enzymes, and so on.

Parenteral, percutaneous vaginal, or subcutaneous pellet implantation routes of estrogen administration bypass the portal circulation and may cause less change in an hepatic synthesis of coagulation factors and renin substrates. Estrogens infrequently are injected, however, because of irregular absorption and plasma levels. Intravaginal administration was used for years, with the belief that local effects would treat atrophic vaginitis/dyspareunia without incurring side effects. Absorption from the vagina is excellent, however, and high plasma estrogen levels are achieved.[58,59] The percutaneous absorption of estradiol is good, thus maintaining elevated plasma levels when used in a daily or alternate-day application[60–62] and in comparison to oral conjugated estrogens and produced estrogen levels that are closer to a physiologic follicular-phase production with less hepatic effects.[63] There has been little experience with the topical route of administration in the United States, but subcutaneously implanted estradiol pellets have been used. Absorption appears relatively stable and a decrease in adverse hepatic effects has been reported.[64] Endometrial stimulation still may occur, when adequate levels are achieved to control symptoms, no matter what route is chosen. Lowering the dosage to reduce this endometrial effect may sacrifice the control of both vasomotor symptoms and genitourinary atrophy and the protective effect on bone. Therefore, alternatives were sought to reduce the adverse effects of estrogens on the endometrium without a further lowering of the dose.

Cyclic estrogen administration to provide an estrogen-free interval has been tried to reduce the likelihood of endometrial hyperplasias and (thus) carcinomas. Estrogens are given for 3 of every 4 weeks, but there is little documentation that this is beneficial. A combination therapy with a progestin has been shown to prevent the adverse endometrial effects.[65]

Progestins

A progestin may be added to estrogen therapy for women who have a uterus to gain protection from an estrogen-induced endometrial hyperplasia. The progestin opposes estrogen effects and causes a secretory endometrium. The mechanisms by which progestins inhibit estrogen effects are believed to occur via a reduction of estrogen receptor production and the increased metabolism of intracellular estradiol to estrone and to estrogen conjugates. Most clinicians administer the estrogen cyclically on the first 3 weeks of the month, abstaining the last week, and they add the progestin for the last 7–10 days of estrogen therapy. Addition of a progestin to an estrogen-stimulated endometrium may cause vaginal bleeding during the last week of the month, which some women will find unacceptable. Progestin use has not been shown to be protective for any other estrogen side effects; therefore, it should be added only for women with a uterus who must take estrogen. The use of a progestin alone, when estrogen therapy is contraindicated, has been tried with a successful control of vasomotor symptoms in 70–80% of all cases.[66]

Medroxyprogesterone acetate, which has few androgenic side effects, is used most often in the United States. A dose of 10 mg/day usually is given during the last 7–10 days of estrogen administration, although lower doses also may be protective. Little data exist on the effects of various other types of progestins, or on the optimal dosage and prescription for their use. It appears that while 7–10 days/month of treatment significantly reduces the incidence of hyperplasia, 13 days may reduce the incidence to 0.[67] The maximal antiestrogenic effects of the 19 nor-testosterone-derived progestins, norethindrone and D/L norgestrel are achieved after 6 continuous days of therapy.[68] Biochemical and histologic evidence support the effectiveness of much lower doses in suppressing the estrogenic stimulation of the endometrium than those commonly used. As little as 1 mg of norethindrone or 150 mg of D/L norgestrel added for 13 days each month were suggested.

The reported side effects of the progestins have included irregular spotting, fluid retention, and depression. However, other potential effects will need a closer investigation if its widespread use is to be recommended. Progesterone itself competitively binds to both glucocorticoid and mineralocorticoid receptors. Progestins bind to androgen receptors, and some have an androgenic activity while others have antiandrogenic effects. The progestin component has been implicated in the impaired glucose tolerance of oral contraceptives. Progesterone binds to β cells in the pancreatic islets and may directly increase insulin secretion. With chronic use, increased insulin levels, decreased insulin receptor numbers, and hyperglycemia may be seen. Progestins also may suppress HDL levels. The potential for enhanced atherosclerosis with long-term use should be considered. A clarification of the role of androgen versus progestin potency in these side effects will be significant to the choice of progestin. A further study to optimize the role of progestins and understand their side effects certainly is warranted to ensure that we do not inflict other disorders in our attempts to prevent an estrogen-induced endometrial stimulation.

Endocrine Replacement Therapy

Therapy must be individualized for any given patient and indication. Estrogen therapy is absolutely contraindicated in the presence of an estrogen-dependent neoplasm, undiagnosed vaginal bleeding, acute or chronic liver disease, or a history of a vascular thrombosis. The use of estrogens must be considered carefully for a patient with hypertension, fibrocystic breast disease, coronary heart disease, familial hyperlipidemias, migraine, epilepsy, endometriosis, diabetes mellitus, gallbladder disease, or a family history of breast or endometrial cancer.

For women with no contraindication to the use of estrogens, disabling vasomotor symptoms are most successfully treated with estrogen replacement. The potential risks must be explained and balanced by a patient's opinion of the benefit (i.e., a relief of hot flashes and, possibly, any coexistent sleep disturbances). For women with a uterus, the protective effects of progestins, as well as offsetting negative effects such as vaginal bleeding and possible metabolic consequences, should be discussed. When cyclic estrogens and a progestin are used, the lowest possible doses are chosen. Most physicians do not require a baseline endometrial biopsy specimen, but will require one if any unscheduled bleeding occurs or every 2 years. The supervision should be similar to that for young women taking oral contraceptive steroids: after 1 month of therapy, then every 6–12 months for a history and physical examination that emphasizes blood pressure, breast, and pelvic examinations. An assessment of the baseline and treated glucose and lipid statuses should be performed. When a woman does not agree to progestin therapy, a baseline endometrial biopsy procedure is performed and repeated every year or if any vaginal bleeding occurs. For a woman with contraindications to estrogen or a hesitancy to use estrogens, a progestin alone or clonidine in a low dose may be tried.

Genitourinary symptoms need to be assessed carefully. If the problem is dyspareunia alone, then vaginal lubricants or a change in sex technique (allowing more time for precoital lubrication) may be advised. When symptoms are more severe, then an estrogen therapy or estrogen/progestin therapy (if there is a uterus) should be recommended; however, unlike the finite period of treatment for vasomotor symptoms, these symptoms do not pass and a lifelong treatment may be required. The same monitoring is involved.

The use of estrogens for the prevention or treatment of osteoporosis is indicated in women who have either suffered a fracture due to osteoporosis or are felt to be at high risk. The optimal dose has not been worked out clinically, but Judd, et al[69] have found that even 0.3 mg/day of conjugated equine estrogens significantly decreased calcium losses. Again, women with a uterus should be advised about cyclic estrogen with an added progestin. Since the discontinuation of estrogen is associated with an acceleration of bone loss, long-term treatment and monitoring would be required. Additions to estrogen replacement, such as exercise, calcium, Vitamin D and fluoride, are discussed in Chapter 28.

While we can correct the estrogen deficiency, we currently do so in unphysiologic ways that create additional risks. The risks versus the benefits always must be considered together with a patient before planning therapy. Fortunately, the close patient monitoring that is required will offer us the opportunity to re-evaluate the state of the art every year.

References

1. Sherman BM, Korenman SG: Hormonal characteristics of the human menstrual cycle throughout reproductive life. *J Clin Invest* 55:699–706, 1975.
2. Treloar AE, Boynton RE, Benn BG, et al: Variation of the human menstrual cycle through the reproductive life. *Int J Fert* 12:77–126, 1967.
3. Sherman BM, West JH, Korenman SG: The menopausal transition: Analysis of LH, FSH, estradiol and progesterone concentrations during menstrual cycles of older women. *J Clin Endocrinol Metab* 42:629–636, 1976.
4. Boss JH, Scully RE, Wegner KH, et al: Structural variations in the adult ovary—clinical significance. *Obstet Gynecol* 25:747–764, 1965.
5. Dennefors BL, Janson PO, Knutson F, et al: Steroid production and responsiveness to gonadotropin in isolated stromal tissue of human postmenopausal ovaries. *J Obstet Gynecol* 136:997–1002, 1980.
6. Siiteri PK, MacDonald PC: Role of extraglandular estrogen in human endocrinology, in Greep RO, Astwood E (eds): *Handbook of Physiology: Endocrinology*. Washington, DC, American Physiological Society, 1973, vol. 2, pp 615–629.
7. Judd HL, Shamonki IM, Frumar AM, et al: Origin of serum estradiol in postmenopausal women. *Obstet Gynecol* 59:680–686, 1982.
8. Korenman SG: Menopausal endocrinology and management. *Arch Int Med* 142:1131–1136, 1982.
9. Judd HL, Davidson BJ, Frumar AM, et al: Serum androgens and estrogens in postmenopausal women with and without endometrial cancer. *Am J Obstet Gynecol* 136:859–871, 1980.
10. MacDonald PC, Edman CD, Hemsell DL, et al: Effect of obesity on conversion of androstenedione to estrone in postmenopausal women with and without endometrial cancer. *Am J Obstet Gynecol* 130:448–455, 1978.
11. Longcope C, Jaffee W, Griffing G: Production rates of androgens and oestrogens in postmenopausal women. *Maturitas* 3:(3-4):215–223, 1981.
12. Anderson DC: Sex-hormone-binding globulin. *Clin Endocrinol (Oxf)* 3:69–96, 1974.
13. O'Brien TJ, Higashi M, Kanasugi H, et al: A plasma serum estrogen-binding protein distinct from testosterone-estradiol-binding globulin. *J Clin Endocrinol Metab* 54:793–797, 1982.
14. Davidson BJ, Ross RK, Paganini-Hill A, et al: Total and free estrogens and androgens in postmenopausal women with hip fractures. *J Clin Endocrinol Metab* 54:115–120, 1982.
15. Vermeulen A: The hormonal activity of the post-

menopausal ovary. *J Clin Endocrinol Metab* 42:247–253, 1976.

16. Roger M, Nahoul K, Scholler R, et al: Evolution with aging of four plasma androgens in postmenopausal women. *Maturitas* 2:171–177, 1980.

17. Vermeulen A, Verdonck L: Factors affecting sex hormone levels in postmenopausal women. *J Steroid Biochem* 11:899–904, 1979.

18. Meldrum DR, Davidson BJ, Tataryn IV, et al: Changes in circulating steroids with aging in postmenopausal women. *Obstet Gynecol* 57:624–628, 1981.

19. Purifoy FE, Koopmans LH, et al: Steroid hormones and aging: free testosterone and androstenedione in normal females aged 20–87 years. *Human Biology* 52:181–191, 1980.

20. Longcope C, Jaffee W, Griffing G: Metabolic clearance rates of androgens and oestrogens in ageing women. *Maturitas* 2:283–290, 1980.

21. Deslypere JP, Sayed A, Punjabi U, et al: Plasma 5α-androstane-3α, 17β-diol and urinary 5α-androstane-3α, 17β-diol glucuronide, parameters of peripheral androgen action: a comparative study. *J Clin Endocrinol Metab* 54:386–391, 1982.

22. Baran DT, Bergfeld MA, Teitelbaum SL, et al: Effect of testosterone therapy on bone formation in an osteoporotic hypogonadal male. *Calcif Tissue Res* 26:103–106, 1978.

23. Hollo I, Szalay F, Szucs J, et al: Osteoporosis and androgens. *Lancet* 1:1357, 1976.

24. Studd-JW, Chakravarti S, Collins WP: Plasma hormone profiles after the menopause and bilateral oophorectomy. *Post Grad Med J* 54(2):25–30, 1978.

25. Erlik Y, Tataryn IV, Meldrum DR, et al: Association of waking episodes with menopausal hot flashes. *JAMA* 245:1741–1744, 1981.

26. Meldrum DR, Shamonki IM, Frumar AM, et al: Elevations in skin temperature of the finger as an objective index of the postmenopausal hot flashes: standardization of the technique. *Am J Obstet Gynecol* 135:713–717, 1979.

27. Tataryn IV, Meldrum DR, Lu KH, et al: LH, FSH and skin temperature during the menopausal hot flash. *J Clin Endocrinol Metab* 49:152–154, 1979.

28. Tataryn IV, Lomax P, Meldrum DR, et al: Objective technique for the assessment of postmenopausal hot flashes. *Obstet Gynecol* 57:340–344, 1981.

29. Avioli LV: Postmenopausal osteoporosis: prevention versus cure. *Federation Proc* 40:2418–2422, 1981.

30. Gallagher JC, Riggs BL, Eisenman J, et al: Intestinal calcium absorption and serum vitamin D metabolites in normal subjects and osteoporotic patients. *J Clin Invest* 64:729–736, 1979.

31. Recker RR, Saville PD, Heaney RP: Effect of estrogens and calcium carbonate on bone loss in postmenopausal women. *Ann Int Med* 87:649–655, 1977.

32. Pfeiffer E, Davis GC: Determinants of sexual behavior in middle and old age. *J Am Geriatr Soc* 20:151–158, 1972.

33. Kinsey AC, Pomeroy WB, Martin CE, et al: *Sexual Behavior in the Human Female*, Philadelphia, WB Saunders & Co, 1953.

34. Masters WH, Johnson VE: *Human Sexual Response*. Boston, Little, Brown & Co, 1966.

35. Lauritzen C, Muller P: Pathology and involution of the genitals in the aging female, in Money J, Musaph H (eds): *Handbook of Sexology*. Elsevier/North-Holland Biomedical Press, 1977, pp 847–857.

36. Hulka BS, Fowler WG Jr, Kaufman DG, et al: Estrogen and endometrial cancer: cases and two control groups from North Carolina. *Am J Obstet Gynecol* 137:92–101, 1980.

37. Hammond CB, Jelovsek FR, Lee KL, et al: Effects of long-term estrogen replacement therapy. II. Neoplasia. *Am J Obstet Gynecol* 133:537–547, 1979.

38. Peck DR, Lowman RM: Estrogen in the postmenopausal breasts. *JAMA* 240:1733–1735, 1978.

39. Hoover R, Gray LA Sr, Cole P, et al: Menopausal estrogens and breast cancer. *N Engl J Med* 295:401–405, 1976.

40. Thomas DB: Role of exogenous female hormones in altering the risk of benign and malignant neoplasms in humans. *Cancer Res* 38:3991, 1978.

41. Ross RK, Paganini-Hill A, Gerkins VR, et al: A case-control study of menopausal estrogen therapy and breast cancer. *JAMA* 243:1635–1639, 1980.

42. Jick H, Watkins RN, Hunter JR, et al: Replacement estrogens and endometrial cancer. *N Engl J Med* 300:218–222, 1979.

43. Boston Collaborative Drug Surveillance Program: Surgically confirmed gallbladder disease, venous thromboembolism and breast tumors in relation to postmenopausal estrogen therapy. *N Engl J Med* 290:15–19, 1974.

44. Bland KI, Buchanan JB, Weisberg BF, et al: The effects of exogenous estrogen replacement therapy of the breast: breast cancer risk and mammographic parenchymal patterns. *Cancer* 45:3027–3033, 1980.

45. Henderson BE, Powell D, Rosario I, et al: An epidemiologic study of breast cancer. *J Natl Cancer Inst* 53:609, 1974.

46. Brinton LA, Williams RR, Hoover RN, et al: Breast cancer risk factors among screening program participants. *J Natl Cancer Inst* 62:37–44, 1979.

47. Korenman SG: The endocrinology of breast cancer. *Cancer* 46:874–878, 1980.

48. Pfeffer RI, Whipple GH, Kurosaki TT, et al: Coronary risk and estrogen use in postmenopausal women. *Am J Epidemiol* 107:479–497, 1978.

49. Gordon T, Kannel WB, Hjortland MC, et al: Menopause and coronary heart disease. *Ann Int Med* 89:157–161, 1978.

50. Rosenberg L, Armstrong B, Jick H: Myocardial infarction and estrogen therapy in postmenopausal women. *N Engl J Med* 294:1256–1259, 1976.

51. Ross RK, Paganini-Hill A, Mack TM, et al: Menopausal oestrogen therapy and prevention from death from ischaemic heart disease. *Lancet* 1:858–860, 1981.

52. Molitch ME, Oill P, Odell WD: Massive hyperlipemia during estrogen therapy. *JAMA* 227:522–525, 1974.

53. Tikkanen MI, Nikkita EA, Vartianen E: Natural estrogen as an effective treatment for type II hyperlipo-proteinemia in postmenopausal women. *Lancet* 2:490–491, 1978.

54. Crane MG, Harris JJ, Windsor W: Hypertension, oral contraceptive agents in conjugated estrogens. *Ann Int Med* 74:13–21, 1971.

55. Pfeffer RI: Estrogen use: hypertension and stroke in postmenopausal women. *J Chron Dis* 31:389–398, 1978.

56. Bennion LJ, Grundy SM: Risk factors for the development of cholelithiasis in man. Part 2. *N Engl J Med* 299:1221–1222, 1978.

57. Mandel FP, Geola FL, Lu JKH, et al: Biologic effects of various doses of ethinyl estradiol in postmenopausal women. *Obstet Gynecol* 59:673–679, 1982.

58. Mishell DR, Moore DE, Roy S, et al: Clinical performance and endocrine profiles with contraceptive vaginal rings containing a combination of estradiol and d-norgestrel. *Am J Obstet Gynecol* 130:55–62, 1978.

59. Rigg LA, Hermann H, Yen SSC: Absorption of estrogens from vaginal creams. *N Engl J Med* 298:195–197, 1978.

60. DeLignières B, Mauvais-Jarvis P: Postmenopausal hormonal therapy, in Scholler R (Ed): *Endocrinology of the Ovary*. Proceedings of the International Symposium Paris—Fresnes (France) October 1976. (Original English language published by Editions SEPE, Paris, France. Copyright 1978) pp 541–562, 1976.

61. Whitehead MI, Townsend PT, Kitchin Y, et al: Plasma steroid and protein hormone profiles in postmenopausal women following topical administration of oestradiol 17β, in P. Mauvais-Jarvis, CFH Vickers, J Wepierre (eds): *Percutaneous Absorption of Steroids*. Academic Press, New York, 1980, pp 231–248.

62. Basdevant A, deLigniéres B: Treatment of menopause by topical administration of oestradiol, in: Mauvais-Jarvis P, Vickers CFH, Wepierre J (eds): *Percutaneous Absorption of Steroids*. New York, Academic Press, 1980, pp 249–258.

63. Elkik F, Gompel A, Mercier-Bodard C, et al: Effects of percutaneous estradiol and conjugated estrogens on the level of plasma proteins and triglycerides in postmenopausal women. *Am J Obstet Gynecol* 143:888–892, 1982.

64. Greenblatt RB, Bryner JR: Estradiol pellet implantation in management of the menopause. *J Repro Med* 18:307–316, 1977.

65. Gambrell RD Jr: The prevention of endometrial cancer in postmenopausal women with progestogens. *Maturitas* 1:107, 1978.

66. Schiff I, Tulchinsky D, Cramer D, et al: Oral medroxyprogesterone in the treatment of postmenopausal symptoms. *JAMA* 244:1443–1445, 1980.

67. Studd JWW, Thom MH, Paterson MEL, et al: The prevention and treatment of endometrial pathology in postmenopausal women receiving exogenous estrogens, in Pasetto N, Paoletti R, Ambrus JL (eds): *The Menopause and Postmenopause*. Lancaster, MTP Press, 1980, p 127.

68. Whitehead MI, Townsend PT, Pryse-Davies J, et al: Effects of estrogens and progestins on the biochemistry and morphology of the postmenopausal endometrium. *N Engl J Med* 305:1599–1605, 1981.

69. Geola FL, Frumar AM, Tataryn IV, et al: Biological effects of various doses of conjugated equine estrogens in postmenopausal women. *J Clin Endocrinol Metab* 51:620–625, 1980.

CHAPTER 27

Male Reproductive Endocrinology

SUSAN STANIK, M.D

STANLEY G. KORENMAN, M.D.

Changes occur in the reproductive systems of both aging males and females, although female menopause always has been in the spotlight in terms of research on its pathophysiology and treatment. In contrast to a female's dramatic cessation of menses and symptoms of estrogen withdrawal, a male's gradual decline in sexual activity and testicular function has been quietly accepted; only recently has research attention shifted to males.

Aside from any obvious cyclicity, male reproductive physiology has all the complexity of the female system and is subject to as many disturbances. The effects of aging on the male reproductive axis appear to be much more varied than a female's inevitable depletion of germ cells and ovarian secretion. Not all males are affected in the same way, degree, or at the same age. The more subtle endocrine changes in a male are not easily detected by our current technology, which is adequate for measuring the more obvious hormonal changes occurring in females.

Physiology of the Male Reproductive Endocrine Axis

There are two functional compartments to the testis: 1) The interstitial or Leydig cell compartment, which is responsible for steroid synthesis and secretion both locally and systemically; and 2) The seminiferous tubule compartment, which is composed of Sertoli cells and developing sperm in the germinal epithelium (*see* Figure 27-1). The regulation of testicular function is accomplished via pulsatile stimulation by the pituitary glycoproteins luteinizing hormone (LH) and follicle-stimulating hormone (FSH). The receptors for LH are found in Leydig cells; in response to a normal pulsatile LH stimulation, the cells increase both the synthesis and release of testosterone and other steroids. The FSH receptors are found in Sertoli cells and stimulate the Sertoli cell production of androgen-binding proteins, so that FSH plays a large role (together with the testosterone released under LH stimulation) in the maturation of the germ cells. A third anterior pituitary hormone, prolactin, may act with LH to regulate testicular steroidogenesis, even though at pathologically high levels prolactin appears to inhibit testosterone production.

Pituitary gonadotropin release is stimulated by a decapeptide, gonadotropin-releasing hormone (GnRH), which is released from the hypothalamus and (possibly) other parts of the brain and is inhibited by plasma testosterone and its metabolites estradiol (E_2) and dihydrotestosterone. An additional feedback inhibition of FHS is achieved by the action of the peptide inhibin which is secreted by the Sertoli cell. There appears to be only one GnRH secreted in pulsatile fashion from the hypothalamus, which promotes both LH and FSH synthesis and release. The 1–2 hour pulsatile pattern of plasma LH levels reflects this stimulation. However, since FSH has a longer half-life (3 hours, compared to a 30-minute half-life of LH), the effect of GnRH pulses on FSH are obscured and FSH

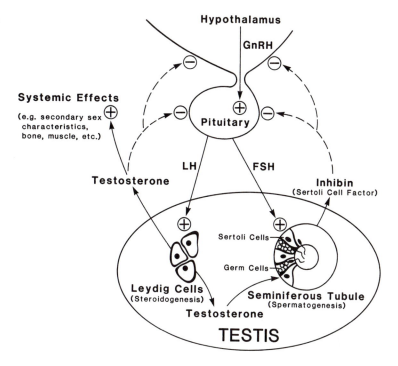

FIGURE 27-1   Hypothalamic—pituitary—testicular axis.

maintains a steady level. Hypothalamic GnRH secretion is inhibited by androgens, estrogens, and possibly by inhibin. Stress, starvation, and temperature also may regulate the hypothalamic center. Dopamine and endogenous opiates may alter the amplitude and frequency of the pulsatile release of gonadotropins, probably through a suppression of GnRH release.

Properly regulated, approximately 7 mg/day of testosterone is produced in an adult male, which results in plasma levels of 300–1,000 ng/dl. Testosterone is bound with a high affinity to the sex hormone-binding globulin (SHBG) and with a low affinity to albumin. In males, approximately 60% of testosterone is bound to SHBG and 38% to albumin. The SHBG produced by the liver is increased by estrogens and thyroid hormone and is decreased by androgens, growth hormones, and obesity. Any of the factors that change the concentration of SHBG may have major effects on the level of metabolically active testosterone.

Androgen-responsive sexual tissues have receptors in their cytoplasm that specifically bind

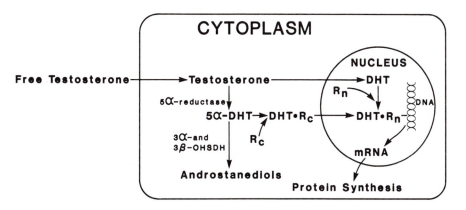

FIGURE 27-2   Androgen-responsive target cell. R_c, R_n = cytosolic and nuclear androgen receptors; 5α-DHT or DHT = 5α-dihydrotestosterone; OHSDH = hydroxysteroid dehydrogenase.

the steroid and transport it to the nucleus, where it initiates a transcription of selected messenger RNAs. Secondary tissues may contain the enzyme 5 α-reductase, which converts testosterone to 5 α-dihydrotestosterone (DHT), the true intracellular androgen (*see* Figure 27-2). 5 α-reduction is critical to maturation of the male fetal genitalia and adult prostate, to accessory sex organ growth, and to hair and sebaceous follicle development. In contrast, testosterone itself regulates bone and muscle growth. In the hypothalamus and pituitary gland, much of testosterone's inhibitory effects are thought to be due to the conversion of testosterone to estradiol.

Testosterone may be metabolized in target tissues by 3 α- or 3 β-hydroxysteroid dehydrogenases to androstanediols. Peripheral tissues such as adipose, muscle, liver, and brain also contain an aromatase enzyme that converts androgens to estrogens, so that testosterone's peripheral conversion to estradiol is the main source of male estrogen production. The bulk of testosterone is metabolized by the liver to become androstenedione and further on to androsterone and etiocholanolone, which are excreted.

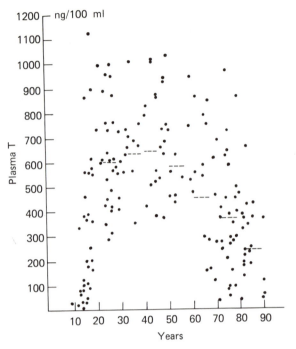

FIGURE 27-3   Distribution of total plasma testosterone in normal males of various ages. (From Vermeulen A, Rubens R, Verdonck L: Testosterone secretion and metabolism in male senescence. *J Clin Endocrinol Metab* 34:731, 1972, used by permission.)

Changes in the Axis with Aging

Testicular Dysfunction

Most studies have demonstrated a decline in average plasma testosterone levels after 50 years of age[1-4] (*see* Figure 27-3). Recent studies, where efforts were made to select extremely healthy elderly male subjects, have raised a controversy about whether the decline is due to aging per se or to age-associated chronic illnesses. Two of these studies reported no change in the testosterone level in their healthy aging males[5,6] while two others noted a decline with age, especially a loss of the normal AM peak serum levels.[7,8] Zumoff confirmed a gradual testosterone decline with age by sampling blood throughout a 24-hour period and observing a 35% decrease in the average testosterone level between 21–85 years of age.[9]

Both gonadotropins (FSH and LH) increase gradually with age and support a primary testic-

ular dysfunction with a central compensation. Aged Leydig cells retain the capacity to respond to exogenous human chorionic gonadotropin (hCG), although the rise may be less than in their younger counterparts.

Corresponding to this testicular endocrine dysfunction, a pathologic examination has shown Leydig cell numbers to be decreased in elderly males.[10,11] This finding has been attributed to a decreased blood flow or vascular lesions in the testis.

Hypothalamic-Pituitary Regulation

A defect in central regulation may be inferred from the observation that gonadotropins are only slightly elevated in elderly males, even in studies that demonstrated decreased testosterone and free testosterone levels. Either an aging pituitary gland has a limited reserve of LH or the hypothalamic input to the gonadotropins is inadequate. Since the measurement of plasma GnRH levels is not available, indirect means were used to look at hypothalamic function. The decreased response to clomiphene, which normally raises gonadotropin levels by blocking the endogenous estrogen inhibition at the hypothalamus, supports either a defect in the hypothalamic feedback regulation and/or an insensitivity of aging pituitary gonadotropins to hypothalamic stimulation. The pituitary gland secretory capacity was studied by administering synthetic GnRH. Most found that LH and FSH levels attained a similar peak in elderly compared to younger males, but, several have reported abnormalities in gonadotropin response, which include a decreased percent increase above baseline levels[3,12] and a delayed peak response.[8,13] Some investigators have found elevated free and total estrogen levels in elderly males.[3,14,15] This suggests that estrogen suppression may limit the compensatory rise of LH that is needed to drive the declining Leydig cells.[16]

Steroid Metabolism and Action

Testosterone production and metabolic clearance rates are decreased in elderly persons. The SHBG levels are increased and more testosterone is bound.[2,16] Increased conversion of androgens to estrogens occurs in the peripheral tissues of elderly males.[17] With this increased production, the amount of free estrogen actually may be greater in elderly than in young males, in spite of the increased SHBG levels.[3,14] Other studies have not confirmed elevated estrogens in elderly males.[5]

Target tissues themselves may play a role in age-related changes in the male reproductive system. Since only androgen target tissues are thought to reduce testosterone to DHT, the measurement of DHT and its metabolites should reflect tissue responsiveness. In aging males, DHT assays have produced conflicting results. A decrease in the excretion of 5α- relative to 5β-reduced metabolites of DHT has been seen with increasing age.[1] A newly described marker of target tissue activity is the measurement of 3α-androstenediol glucuronide, which appears to be derived directly from the DHT metabolism in target tissues. This specific metabolite also is reduced in aging males,[18] which again reflects an altered androgen target-tissue metabolism with age.

Androgen insensitivity with advancing age has been suggested, but it requires further study. Reduced binding of androgen to pubic skin receptors was noted in aging males, but the receptor abnormality was not seen in other biopsied skin sites.[19]

Spermatogenesis

While the retention of fertility and paternity have been reported into very old age, changes in seminiferous tubule function are noted much earlier in life. Testicular volume decreases and the testes may soften.[4] Degenerative changes in the seminiferous tubules have been described that include a thickening of the tubular basement membrane, decreased spermatogenesis, peritubular fibrosis, germ cell arrest, absence of germ cells with a "Sertoli cell only" pattern remaining, narrowing of the tubular lumen, and sclerosis-obliterated tubules.[20] However, areas of normal spermatogenesis still were present at autopsy in over 50% of all males over 70 years of age. While the total number of sperm in an ejaculate may not decrease with age, the number of normally formed and motile sperm is reduced.

Clinical Features of Aging of the Reproductive Endocrine System

Sexual Function

Sexual activity declines progressively in elderly males, (see Figure 27-4) from the teens to old age, with no abrupt reduction even in the highly selected healthy aging populations.[21,22] At 50 years of age, the orgasmic frequency is about 50% what it was at 30 years of age; by 75 years of age, it is less than 20%. Erectile dysfunction has been reported to increase from 18% at 60 years of age to about 50% at age 75 and 75% at age 80.[23]

Physiologic changes have been described in elderly males who remain sexually interested and active. Masters and Johnson worked with relatively few elderly couples, but they described a change in the male sexual response over 50 years of age.[24] An older male requires longer, more intense direct stimulation to

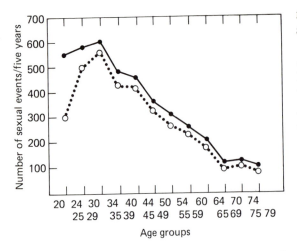

FIGURE 27-4 Mean frequencies of coital (dotted line) and total sexual events (solid line) reported for the last 5-year age interval that preceded interviews. (From Martin CE: Sexual activity in the ageing male, in Money J, Musaph H (eds): *Handbook of Sexology*. New York, Elsevier/North-Holland Biomedical Press, 1977, chap 60, p 815, used by permission.)

may be interpreted as "impotence," thus heralding an end to sexuality and a productive life.

Physiology of the Normal Male Sexual Response

Adequate sexual functioning requires the presence of erotic stimuli, an active libido to translate such stimuli into sexual desire and responses, an interested partner, and intact neurologic, vascular, and endocrine systems. The inter-relationship between these factors is critical but poorly understood.

Various visual, olfactory, auditory, or fantasized cues may be perceived as sexual stimuli. The libido is defined as the threshold for these stimuli to evoke a sexual response. With a low libido (as may be seen with depression or an androgen deficiency), there is a high threshold; stimuli must be intense to be perceived as sexual cues and to elicit an erotic reaction. Minor distractions will alter the response. The mechanism of psychological and environmental facilitation or inhibition of arousal and sexual response is unknown.

Neurologic control of an erection involves the central and peripheral nervous systems. The autonomic control of vascular dilatation and constriction probably is mediated via the release of a neurotransmitter onto receptors of the helical offshoots of the deep penile arteries. A dilatation of the arterial supply increases blood flow into the corporal spaces, which results in an erection through changes in penile volume and rigidity. Erections may be initiated by a variety of stimuli through one of two apparently separate reflex mechanisms. Visual, olfactory, auditory, or fantasy inputs are transmitted from the cortex to the thoracolumbar erection center. The efferent limbs of this reflex pathway are the thoracolumbar sympathetic outflow (T12-L4) and sacral parasympathetic outflow (S2-S4): the nervi erigentes. The other pathway mediates the reflex erectile response to direct genital stimulation. Penile glans and skin receptors transmit sensation to the sacral parasympathetic center via the afferent fibers of the pudendal nerve. The sacral center then reflexively responds via the efferent parasympathetic fibers of the nervi erigentes. These parasympathetic fibers may, in turn, stimulate short adrenergic nerves throughout the corpora to re-

achieve an erection. He has a longer plateau phase, which may end in a resolution without ejaculation or in a brief orgasmic period with a decreased force of ejaculation. Detumescence is rapid, and the refractory period following the resolution phase is lengthened; a recovery time of 12–24 hours may be required before another erection can be achieved. Nocturnal erections that occur in the regular cycles, predominantly during rapid eye movement (REM) sleep, are less full in older than in younger males. In healthy males 30–79 years of age, the peak in the percent of sleep or REM time that was spent in nocturnal tumescence occurred in the teen years, declining sharply by age 30, then more gradually until age 80.[25]

Sexual interest and activity can play an important role in the quality of life, self-image, and sense of well-being in aging couples. For those who were active in their youth and middle years, continued sexual interest and activity are common. The earlier myth of the impotent and sexless elderly person has been replaced by an image demanding that older persons become concerned with sexual performance. Thus, changes with age in the male reproductive system may now be viewed with apprehension or shame. Even a temporary or minor dysfunction lease norepinephrine onto beta receptors; however, the final neurotransmitter that is responsible for the vascular events of erection still is disputed.

Nipple enlargement, skin flushing, and muscle tension also are associated with penile erection in this "excitement phase" of the male sexual response. This state is maintained as a "plateau phase" for a varying length of time. Sympathetic innervation is thought to be responsible for the two phases of orgasm, emission and ejaculation. Smooth muscle contraction in the testis, seminal vesicles, and prostate lead to the expression of both seminal fluid from the vas deferens and secretions from the prostate and seminal vesicles into the urethra. Sympathetic contractions of the internal sphincter of the bladder at this time prevent retrograde ejaculation. The presence of seminal fluid in the urethra triggers the ejaculatory reflex that is carried via the pudendal nerve, which contracts the bulbocavernosus muscles. The final resolution phase of the sexual response, as blood flow to the corpora is decreased and detumescence occurs, also is thought to be mediated by sympathetic nerves.

Given normal neural pathways, penile erection depends on a sufficient arterial inflow. The blood supply to the penis originates from the paired internal pudendal arteries, which then divide into paired bulbourethral arteries and short penile arteries. The penile artery soon divides into the deep penile artery that supplies the corpus cavernosa and the dorsal penile artery. The deep penile and dorsal arteries anastamose throughout their course. The small terminal branches of the penile arteries penetrate the cavernous spaces. A dilatation of these terminal branches, termed the helical arterioles, under neurologic stimulation allows blood to flow into the three spongy erectile tissues (two corpora cavernosa and one corpus spongiosum), which results in an erection. There is no evidence that filling of the vascular spaces with blood requires an impairment of venous return, or valvular penile "polsters" opening the arterial channels.

Endocrine influences on sexual function are diverse. Testosterone plays an important role in male sexual behavior, but its site of action is unknown. Testosterone is necessary for the fetal development of male genitalia, pubertal development, and adult maintenance of the secondary sexual organs. Testosterone also stimulates sexual desire and is necessary for sexual activity. However, the level of testosterone that is needed to maintain the libido and potency has not been determined, nor have the targets for testosterone in erectile tissue been defined. There even are reports of sexual activity persisting for years after castration without testosterone replacement. No consistent correlation has been found between testosterone levels and potency. Certainly, the greater than 50% fall-off of sexual performance between 20–60 years of age cannot be related to the minor decline in testosterone levels that are found over that age range. Conversely hypogonadal males experience a loss of libido and potency and may have hot flashes, which will respond to testosterone treatment. The steroid influence on sexual functioning could be anywhere along the pathway, such as a central enhancement of the libido or a suppression of inhibitory neural impulses, effects on spinal nerves, peripheral nerve endings, penile neurotransmitters, or vascular receptors.

The role of endogenous estrogens on the libido and potency in males is uncertain. Exogenous estrogens produce a gonadotropin suppression via a feedback inhibition, and they diminish testosterone production both as a result of the reduced gonadotropin stimulation of Leydig cells and as a direct inhibition of Leydig cell steroidogenesis.

Prolactin elevation (as in pituitary adenomas) is known to reduce both libido and potency in males above and beyond its effect on the testes to decrease testosterone production. Testosterone replacement alone does not return sexual function, but prolactin levels also must be normalized by administering bromocriptine or by pituitary surgery.

Sexual Dysfunction as a Presenting Complaint in Aging Males

When evaluating males with a complaint of erectile dysfunction, a clinician must keep in mind that any one (and more likely a combination) of these factors (the psychosocial, neural, vascular, or endocrine components of the sexual response) may be affected and may contribute to altered libido, erectile, or ejaculatory functioning. The relative contribution of each has not been assessed, but it is felt that the incidence of organic diseases in older males who are presenting with erectile dysfunctions is much closer to 50%[26] than the previous estimates. While many elderly males accept a declining potency as yet another sign of aging, which perhaps is related to a concomitant depressed desire and arousability,[27] those who seek medical attention for this problem more often are motivated and express a continued desire that is frustrated by an erectile inadequacy. Only this self-selected subpopulation has been evaluated, so that statistics about the incidence rate of various etiologies of erectile dysfunction may not apply to the vast number of affected males in the general population.

The evaluation is directed towards uncovering all the potentially reversible causes of sexual dysfunction. Thus, a careful social/sexual history is obtained, which includes the onset of the disorder and the specific aspects involved (libido, erection, ejaculation), the quality of the relationship(s) with sexual partner(s), prior level of sexual function, fertility, AM or nocturnal erections, response to masturbation, and any previous attempts at therapy. Next, a careful medical history and systems review is performed with an inquiry into occupational exposures, alcohol or recreational drugs, medications, systemic illnesses (e.g., diabetes mellitus, cirrhosis, uremia), neurologic or vascular disease, pelvic surgery, radiation, trauma, changes in secondary sex characteristics, muscle strength and endurance, headaches or visual disturbances, endocrine gland function, and genitourinary infections or obstructions. A physical examination should reveal any abnormalities in body habitus or proportions, secondary sex characteristics, breast development, testes and external genitalia, circulation, or the central or peripheral nervous systems.

Nocturnal penile tumescence monitoring may be used to confirm a patient's report of absent or "soft" erections. Penile systolic blood pressure and a calculation of the penile/brachial pressure index or penile plethysmography are performed as a crude estimate of penile vascular supply by using a small blood pressure cuff around the base of the penis and a doppler ultrasound probe or pulse volume recorder.[28] A further assessment of the autonomic nervous system function is achieved by measuring the bulbocavernosus reflex latency time[29] or by directly documenting abnormalities of either the peripheral sensory nerves (via an electromyogram [EMG] or conduction studies) or bladder function (via cystometry). A screening endocrine assessment is made by obtaining fasting blood samples on 3 mornings for measuring testosterone, E_2 and estrone (E_1), LH, FSH, prolactin, glucose, and thyroid hormones, in addition to routine medical laboratory screening tests. Some form of psychometric testing may be performed, such as the Minnesota Multiphasic Personality Inventory (MMPI) or Derogatis Sexual Functioning Inventory. The finding of one abnormality should not terminate the investigation; often, multiple risk factors coexist in the same patient, and treatment of one or more of these factors may improve sexual functioning.

Psychogenic versus Organic (see Volume II, Chapter 14)

Patients with predominantly psychogenic impotence are believed to have an abrupt onset of this dysfunction, with a preservation of morning erections and orgasms due to masturbation. Nocturnal penile tumescence monitoring will reveal frequent intact erections. When an organic cause is responsible, the onset often is slower, associated with decreased libido, and absent or reduced morning erections or nocturnal tumescence; the dysfunction is independent of the source of stimulation (self, usual partner, new partner).

Masters and Johnson thought that psychological factors were at the base of most male sexual dysfunctioning, even in elderly persons. In their experience, impaired elderly males were frightened by, and unprepared for, the physiologic changes of aging; they could be helped by education-oriented sex therapy. It is very difficult to attribute impotence to psychosocial precipitants—such as monotony, marital disatisfaction, a partner's emotional or physical problem, lack of a partner, lack of privacy, midlife crises, financial or family difficulties—since one or more may be present in every case.

The recent introduction of nocturnal penile tumescence monitoring, to differentiate between organic and psychogenic causes of impotence, is a useful tool. The detection of a normal number, duration, and intensity of erections is an objective measure of the intactness of erectile mechanisms. Most males with a normal nocturnal penile tumescence seemed to respond to behavioral sex therapy, while those with abnormal studies rarely were helped and, thus, were felt to have organic problems. This has been validated primarily in younger groups of males. In older males, where organic factors may play a critical role, it is important not to dismiss the early disturbances, which may present as a change in sexual functioning with frequent erectile failures that are interspersed with occasional normal events (including morning erections). Thus, although the absence of morning erections and abnormal nocturnal penile tumescence may be diagnostic of an organicity, the presence of daytime or nocturnal erections in elderly males does not exclude an organic pathology.

Previously unrecognized organic abnormalities may be detected with newer techniques to evaluate the endocrine, vascular, and neurologic components of sexual function.

Organic-Systemic Illnesses

Elderly males frequently are exposed to the effects of chronic illnesses and medications on their reproductive systems (*see* Table 27-1). Many of the factors that impair the overall health of a male will affect his sexual interest and function at any age, such as systemic diseases, alcoholism, depression, drug abuse, urogenital disease, or extensive pelvic surgery. However, certain chronic diseases increase in elderly persons, such as diabetes, malnutrition, hypertension, coronary disease, emphysema, cancer, arthritis, and sleep disorders. Consequently, the number of medications taken with potential side effects rises greatly as well. Secondary psychological damage may arise from these problems, such as a fear that exertion during sexual activity will aggravate the illness (especially post–myocardial infarction) or an expectation that the illness must cause impotence (a widespread belief in diabetic men and after a transurethral prostatectomy).

There is an increased prevalence of sexual dysfunction among diabetic men that is as high as 60% of all older diabetics.[30] They complain of a gradual loss of erectile competence, but usually maintain a normal libido, tactile sensation, and orgasm. Their sexual dysfunction occasionally may include retrograde ejaculation or premature ejaculation. Current evidence attributes the impotence to diabetic autonomic neuropathy with an involvement of the pelvic parasympathetic nerves (nervi erigentes). An associated autonomic bladder dysfunction and prolonged bulbocavernosus reflex latency times may help to confirm this etiology. Other causes of impotence may contribute to the high incidence rate among diabetics. Diabetics may be subject to greater psychosocial stresses than non-diabetics; there also may be a superimposed psychological element in some men as erections become less firm with early organic disease. A certain number of diabetics have been shown to have normal nocturnal erections, and these men may respond to sex therapy sessions or reassurance.[31] The penile circulation may be impaired in diabetics with arteriosclerosis; however, diagnostic techniques to differentiate neurogenic versus vascular insufficiency etiologies still are being improved and the results of surgical repair are unclear. Implantable penile prostheses may restore sexual function to these men.[32]

Hypertensive males often experience a decrease in sexual activity that is blamed on drug treatment, often without a prior baseline interview or assessment. Untreated hypertensive males of all ages have been reported to have a 15% incidence rate of impotence. Physicians hesitate to elicit a history of a patient's sexual performance for fear of suggesting a dysfunc-

TABLE 27-1 Systemic Organic Disease Resulting in Sexual Dysfunction

Well Established	Less Well Established
Diabetes	COPD*
Uremia	HTN†
Cirrhosis	Epilepsy
Hemochromatosis	
Sickle-cell anemia	
Leprosy	
Myotonia dystrophica	
Paraplegia	
Thyroid disease	
Adrenal disease	
Severe malnutrition, malabsorption	

* COPD = chronic obstructive pulmonary disease.
† HTN = hypertension.

tional state. However, the basal level of sexual functioning should be thoroughly assessed so that the role of the specific therapeutic agent can be clarified, and because patients will attribute their impotence to the drug and often will discontinue medications without informing their physician (especially if that physician ignores or underestimates the problem). Hypertension is associated with an increased incidence rate of other disorders that include diabetes, peripheral vascular diseases, and stroke, which also influence erectile function.

Every antihypertensive agent has been linked to sexual dysfunctioning, but the mechanisms have been poorly studied.[33] The drugs may act through a central nervous system depression, interruption of autonomic neural function, endocrine alteration, or at the target tissue receptor level.

The antihypertensive agents with central and/or peripheral sympatholytic effects most often have been implicated in sexual dysfunction. Up to two thirds of all males who are taking guanethidine or bethanidine have noted problems. Guanethidine depletes neurons of the norepinephrine reserve and results in a state of sympathetic blockage. It is not thought to cross the blood-brain barrier, so that its effect appears to be on the postganglionic adrenergic nerves. Problems with both ejaculation and erection have been noted. Reserpine in low or moderate doses (<0.3 mg/day) (although it also depletes catecholamines in nerve terminals) appears to have much less of an effect on sexual responses that, perhaps, is no different from the placebo. With high doses of reserpine, however, prolactin elevation and gonadotropin depression may occur, which increases sexual dysfunction. Depression of the libido may be the most important effect seen. Methyldopa displaces norepinephrine and causes a false neurotransmission. By producing a limited adrenergic blockage, it also may cause a central depression. The incidence of sexual dysfunctioning with methyldopa is high, ranging from 30% to as high as 50%, in addition to a reduced frequency of intercourse.

Clonidine acts as a partial alpha agonist that binds to presynaptic and postsynaptic alpha adrenoreceptors. The central effect is to decrease sympathetic nerve activity, but an inhibition of the peripheral adrenergic nervous system also is seen; impotence was reported in 24% of all males in one study compared to 8% in the same group of patients during the control period. Erectile dysfunction may be a dose-related effect that especially is common at higher doses, such as >600 ng/day.

Even propranolol, which once was promoted because of its lack of effect on sexual functioning, has been implicated in case reports. Patients on a high-dose therapy (>200 mg/day), usually for control of angina pectoris rather than hypertension, are more likely to report this problem. A beta blockade may directly inhibit arteriolar vasodilatation that is required for an erection; or, by enhancing alpha-adrenergic effects, it may inhibit erections through alpha-adrenergic vasoconstriction.

Hydralazine's antihypertensive action, through the relaxation of vascular smooth muscle (arterioles more than veins), would not obviously be associated with an impairment of sexual function. However, case reports link this drug to impotence, perhaps because large doses may impair the ganglionic transmission.

Spironolactone has been well studied, since patients on this drug complain to their physicians of a painful gynecomastia, which often leads to the discovery of their sexual dysfunction. The drug interferes with both testosterone biosynthesis and androgen action at the target tissue by competing for androgen receptors.

Even the diuretics (hydrochlorothiazide and especially chlorthalidone) have been implicated in sexual dysfunctioning in case reports and small controlled studies.

Other systemic illnesses that are associated with effects on sexual functioning include alcoholism, cirrhosis, and chronic renal failure. Alcoholism may alter sexual responsiveness by inducing an autonomic neuropathy, or through alterations in the sex steroid metabolism. There are both central depressive effects and direct testicular damage. Men with cirrhosis frequently show signs of a decreased androgen effect, such as scanty hair and musculature and atrophic testes, as well as signs of hyperestrogenism, which include spider angiomata, palmar erythema, and gynecomastia. Prolactin elevation has been noted, although the mechanism is unclear and perhaps related to the central effects of alcohol or estrogen-induced prolactin release.

Males of any age who develop chronic renal failure often develop a decreased libido and potency. Studies demonstrate damage to Leydig cells, which is reflected in decreased testosterone and elevated LH levels. Some studies implicate uremic toxins, while others have an elevation of parathyroid hormones or a zinc deficiency in the pathogenesis. Decreased clearance of prolactin levels result in slight elevations of this peptide, which were not correlated with the development of a dysfunction or gynecomastia.

Surgery

Large numbers of elderly men undergo pelvic surgery. While suprapubic or transurethral prostate surgery rarely alter sexual potency directly, a perineal exposure and prostatectomy or other radical resections may interfere with functioning. Most men who do not ejaculate semen from the urethra still experience normal orgasmic sensations. However, without a prior description of the possibility of a retrograde ejaculation, men who experience this problem postoperatively may become depressed, equating a loss of ejaculation with "impotence," and cease sexual activity.

Elderly males are more likely to undergo major abdominal surgery (such as an abdomino-perineal resection of the rectum for cancer) or a vascular repair to the abdominal aorta or iliac arteries, which may disturb pelvic innervation or damage retroperitoneal blood vessels.

A sympathectomy, cordotomy, or bilateral orchiectomy may result in sexual dysfunction at any age. The level of spinal cord trauma determines its effect on sexual functioning. With cervical lesions, reflexogenic erections may still occur; in sacral lesions, some males may retain psychogenic erections (presumably via the thoracolumbar outflow). A total destruction of the sacral parasympathetic nerves is much more likely to result in impotence than lesions of just the sympathetic nerve chains.

Medications

Most elderly males do not have such an obvious source of dysfunction. However, 60% of the population over 60 years of age suffer from conditions that lead to a regular use of prescribed medications. Elderly persons receive an average of 13 prescriptions per year, not including over-the-counter medications. Most elderly persons are on multiple medications, and their combined effects on sexual function are unknown (see Table 27-2).

Psychotropic drugs may be administered to calm an anxious elderly male or help him sleep (phenothiazines, benzodiazepines), or to elevate his mood when depressed (tricyclics, monoamine oxidase [MAO] inhibitors). These are commonly associated with erectile and ejaculatory disorders. The phenothiazines inhibit the central dopaminergic system and may elevate prolactin levels to a mild or moderate degree, usually <100 ng/dl. Peripherally, they have potent alpha-adrenergic a variable cholinergic-blocking activities and block histamine transmission. Thioridazine (Mellaril) especially is known to cause ejaculatory difficulties. Other drugs are more likely to cause erectile difficulties. Those drugs that are more sedating may decrease the libido as well. The tricyclic antidepressants inhibit norepinephrine re-uptake via adrenergic nerve terminals, but they also have prominent atropine-like effects. Both erectile and ejaculatory dysfunctions may be seen. The benzodiazepines have been associated in case reports with a delayed or complete failure of ejaculation and erectile dysfunctions. Even the newer muscle relaxants have been incriminated. As with barbiturates, the central depressant action may be responsible.

Several other drugs that are associated with sexual dysfunctioning have an anticholinergic activity, including gastrointestinal and urinary tract antispasmodics, antivertigo and antinausea medications, the antiarrhythmic disopyramide (Norpace), antiParkinsonism drugs, and many over-the-counter cold remedies. In high doses, the anticholinergic agents act as ganglionic blockers. Erectile dysfunction also has been reported with the use of antiprostaglandin agents, such as indomethacin, although a role for endogenous prostaglandins in erection has not been determined.

Endocrinopathies

Endocrine causes of impotence are uncommon; however, because they often are easily treated, they should be sought even in an elderly male.

TABLE 27-2 Drugs that Affect Sexual Function

Agent	Biologic Effect	Endocrine Effect	Types of Sexual Dysfunction
Antihypertensives:			
Guanethidine	Postganglionic Sympatholytic	—	Erection Ejaculation
Dibenzyline	Alpha-blockers	—	Ejaculation
Reserpine			Libido, erection
Methydopa			Libido, erection, ejaculation
Clonidine	Central alpha antagonist	—	Erection
Chlorthalidone	Diuretic	—	Erection
Hydrochlorthiazide			Ejaculation
Propranolol	Beta-blockers	—	Libido
Metoprolol			Erection
Spironolactone	Antialdosterone	Antiandrogen	Libido, erection
Drugs for Psychiatric Problems:			
Phenothiazines (especially thioridazine)	Anticholinergic dopamine inhibition	↑ prolactin-impaired response to hCG	Libido, erection, ejaculation
Tricylic antidepressants: amitryptyline, imipramine, nortryptyline	Central anticholinergic	—	Libido, erection, ejaculation
Benadryl	Sedative antihistamines	—	Libido, erection
Vistaril	Anticholinergic		
Atarax			
Isocarboxazid	MAO* inhibitors	—	Ejaculation
Phenelzine			
Tranylcypromine			
Barbiturates	Central depression	—	Libido
Benzodiazepines	Gaba facilitation	—	Libido
Miscellaneous Drugs:			
Ethanol	Central nervous system depression, inhibits testes, Steroidogenesis	↓ Testosterone ↓ Estrogens	Libido, erection
Marijuana	—	? ↓ LH†† and FSH† ? ↓ T, ↓ prolactin	?
Opiates	Endorphin agonists	↓ Testosterone ↓ LH ↓ Response to GnRH	Libido, erection Amenorrhea
Cimetidine	H₂ receptor antagonist	Antiandrogen ↑ prolactin	Libido, erection
L-Dopa	Dopamine agonist	—	Ejaculation
Progestogens	—	Antiandrogen	Libido, erection
Digoxin	—	↑ Estrogens ↓ Testosterone & LH	Libido, erection
Estrogens	—	↓ Testosterone ↓ Gonadotropins	Libido, erection

* MAO = monoamine oxidase inhibitors.
† FSH = follicle-stimulating hormones.
†† LH = luteinizing hormones.

Hypogonadism that is due to Klinefelter's (XXY), Kallman's, Reinfenstein's, or male Turner's Syndromes usually is detected at a much earlier age because of a failure to either progress normally through puberty or achieve fertility. Late manifestations of acquired primary hypogonadism may be seen after testicular damage (due to mumps orchitis, infections, irradiation, chemotherapy, and so on) or secondary hypogonadism (due to acquired hypothalamic-pituitary disorders).

Pituitary disorders, which include hormonal excesses in acromegaly, Cushing's disease, prolactinomas, hypopituitarism postablation, tumor metastasis, or infiltrative disorders, will interrupt the function of the reproductive axis. Sexual dysfunction may be the first symptom of a pituitary tumor. Males with hyperprolactinemia that is due to pituitary adenomas commonly present with an advanced disease and visual disturbances, because earlier symptoms of sexual disturbance were ignored. Although most of these males have an associated decrease in testosterone levels, the replacement of testosterone alone will not improve their sexual potency until the prolactin levels are normalized with bromocriptine.[34] The administration of bromocriptine to impotent males without prolactinomas was to no avail.

Hyper- and hypothyroidism, as well as adrenal disorders (Addison's or Cushing's Syndromes), often are associated with male impotence, which may be reversed by a proper treatment of the underlying endocrinopathy.

Other Clinical Changes in an Aging Male

The incidence rate of gynecomastia (i.e., the discovery of palpable breast tissue in a male) increases with aging.[35] Elevated estrogen/androgen ratios are at least partly responsible for the gynecomastia that is associated with testicular dysgenesis, cirrhosis, thyrotoxicosis, neoplasms, refeeding after malnutrition, hemodialysis in uremia, and the administration of certain drugs; such a hormonal basis, however, has not been identified in elderly males with palpable breast tissue. Gonadotropins and estrogen/androgen ratios were elevated in elderly males who presented to a surgical clinic with a substantial gynecomastia.[36]

Benign prostatic hyperplasia (BPH) is un-usual in males under 50 years of age, but it affects the majority of males over 70 years of age. A proliferation of the glands and stroma occurs, and it may lead to urinary outflow obstruction. The relationship of the hormonal changes seen with aging to the development of BPH and prostatic carcinoma is unknown. The presence of estrogen and prolactin, as well as androgen receptors in the prostate, imply a complex endocrine regulation. Estrogens have been implicated in the development of BPH in dogs through the induction of androgen receptors.

Sex hormones affect many anabolic processes, such as protein synthesis, bone and muscle growth, hematopoiesis, cardiovascular functions, and (possibly) immune competence. With aging, a loss of energy and endurance is noted, muscle bulk is decreased even in men still involved in athletic training, bone density declines, and the susceptibility to infection and neoplasms may increase. The role of the reproductive endocrine system in all this is unknown.

Therapy

The management of reproductive endocrine alterations and sexual dysfunction of aging males has been neglected. Investigators still debate whether healthy older men really undergo changes. For those elderly males who experience hypogonadism, gynecomastia, loss of libido, or erectile dysfunctions, the problems are real enough; but, the question of therapy for older men rarely is addressed.

Certainly, subgroups can be identified with remediable disorders. For those men found to have drug-related problems, therapy involves discontinuing the medication. Some patients will be found to have classic endocrine abnormalities that are associated with hypogonadism. The treatment of the underlying hyper- or hypothyroidism, Cushing's disease or Addison's disease, acromegaly, pheochromocytoma, and so on, usually will restore testicular function and potency. A previously undiagnosed primary hypogonadism (with elevated gonadotropins that reflect an androgen deficiency) that is due to a common disorder (such as Klinefelter's Syndrome), a less common acquired problem (such as a residual of adult mumps orchitis, or a long-term chemical exposure), would be an indication for androgen replacement therapy. Secondary hypogonadism (with low or "inappropriately normal" gonadotropins in the face of an androgen deficiency) may be a clue to a pituitary or hypothalamic lesion. Its treatment may involve the surgical removal or irradiation of adenomas or the medical management of hyperprolactinemia with bromocriptine. If a good response is achieved, androgen therapy may not be needed; but, if a gonadotropin and androgen deficiency persists after or secondary to surgery or irradiation, then androgen therapy may be required.

Many other men are found (perhaps not among "super healthy" elderly but those with medical illnesses or other stresses) to have borderline AM testosterone levels in the high 200s or low 300s ng/dl range. While studies have failed to show a good correlation between testosterone levels and sexual activity, clearly androgen deficiency causes loss of libido and sexual ability so that a threshold testosterone level must be necessary to permit normal functioning. No studies of testosterone replacement therapy for elderly males have been published with placebo controls and hormonal measurements. Part of the reluctance may be related to data that is derived from earlier unsuccessful attempts to treat impotence in a younger male population. In such individuals, hormonal therapy (such as testosterone, bromocriptine, clomiphene, or luteinizing hormone releasing hormone [LHRH] was of no greater benefit than a placebo. An uncontrolled study and one controlled case report suggested that testosterone may improve sexual ability and a sense of well-being in older males. Early investigations failed to demonstrate positive anabolic effects, such as improved strength or weight gain, in unselected elderly populations.

The risks of androgen therapy should be considered before recommending it as treatment for other than clearly hypogonadal males; there is a lack of firm evidence of beneficial effects in others. Some side effects are due to the inherent physiologic properties of all androgens, while other adverse actions may vary if males are given androgens with different metabolisms or different routes of administration.[37]

Undesirable androgen actions may include the psychological distress of an increased libido and a stimulation of a BPH or carcinoma. There is hesitation over administering androgens to elderly persons because of possible prostatic hazards; yet, the risk of inducing a prostate carcinoma is unsubstantiated by case studies. The role of androgens in inducing or promoting the growth of a prostate carcinoma in humans has not been investigated.

Sodium retention may be seen during androgen therapy in males with an underlying congestive heart failure or renal disease. An elevation of low-density lipoprotein (LDL) cholesterol and a depression of high-density lipoprotein (HDL) cholesterol levels are reported with androgen therapy. The long-term significance of this effect in increasing the risk of atherosclerosis is unknown.

About 15% of all males who are receiving testosterone preparations are thought to develop gynecomastia, but no studies have determined predictive factors. Males with an increased peripheral aromatization, such as those with obesity, cirrhosis, or elderly males, might be expected to develop these complications with an increased frequency.

A modification of androgens by 17 α-alkylation slows the normally rapid hepatic degradation that is seen after oral testosterone administration, so that reasonable amounts reach the systemic circulation. Absorption from the gut into the portal blood supply delivers pharmacologic doses to the liver; toxic hepatic side effects may be seen. These oral androgens frequently cause bromsulphalein (BSP) retention and an elevation of plasma alkaline phosphatase and conjugated bilirubin levels. Jaundice may be seen, especially in males with an underlying liver disease. The development of blood-filled cysts in the liver (peliosis hepatitis) or a hepatoma has been reported in patients receiving oral androgens. In general, currently available oral preparations are not recommended.

Parenteral testosterone alcohol was absorbed too rapidly, so that esters at the 17 β-hydroxyl site became the preferred form of the hormone. Various durations of effectiveness are seen with different esters, although (in general) the greater the number of carbon molecules in the acid that was esterified, the longer the androgen action. Testosterone enanthate may be injected once every 2–3 weeks, thus maintaining adequate plasma testosterone levels throughout. Abnormalities of the liver function have not been reported with the parenterally administered testosterone esters.

Suspicion of a decreased androgen activity (by low or borderline testosterone levels or elevated gonadotropins) should be the indication for choosing androgen therapy. These known and potential side effects require a careful consideration of an individual patient's predisposing risks, the type of androgen chosen, and the route of administration. After electing to use androgens, a physician must assess the actual benefits achieved after a trial period and continue to monitor benefits and risks throughout the treatment period.

Psychological impotence also may be reversible. Some couples have been helped through a physician's sympathetic listening and educational attempts. Other couples, in whom the relationship appears sound and no major depression or psychiatric disorder is present, may benefit from sensate focus or behavioral modification sex therapy.[24] The couple is encouraged to enjoy non-coital sex play temporarily without the pressure of attempting intercourse. Couples also learn, during this period of retraining, to verbalize sexual desires and improve communication. Couples with troubled marriages, poor interpersonal skills, or psychiatric illness may be referred to mental health professionals.

Vascular and neurologic etiologies of erectile dysfunction may be irreversible. When a vascular insufficiency is suspected from screening doppler tests and a solitary lesion is suspected (rather than a diffuse disease), an arteriography may be diagnostic. Grafts of the inferior epigastric artery to the corpus cavernosum and other corporal revascularization techniques have been attempted; but, the experience is limited and the long-term results have not been studied.[28]

Penile prostheses are offered to males with an irreversible erectile dysfunction, but with a normal libido and ejaculation. Both the permanently erect and inflatable varieties of penile implants will restore the erectile function and allow vaginal penetration and coital ejaculation. The Small-Carrion rigid prosthesis consists of two foam-filled silicone tubes that are pliable yet firm. Vast experience confirms the acceptability of this implant procedure or those using other similar rigid prostheses. The Scott inflatable penile prosthesis works by filling two hollow silicone tubes that are placed in the corpora with fluid from a reservoir inserted in the scrotum. The patient presses the inflate or deflate valve on the scrotal pump/reservoir to achieve an erection or detumescence. The penis looks flaccid when deflated and cannot be detected under clothing or noticed by a sexual partner. This prosthesis is more expensive, more complications are reported with surgery, and late mechanical failures occur. While not all patients accept the idea of a prosthesis, reports of those who have received implants show that satisfaction/improvement rates are high (80–95%)[38,39] (see Volume I, Chapter 17).

The evaluation of a sexual dysfunction is a worthwhile pursuit. Etiologic factors usually will be uncovered and help a patient, his spouse, and his physician to understand the changes he has undergone. Treatment may be offered to most patients and is likely to restore sexual functioning.

References

1. Vermeulen A, Rubens R, Verdonck L: Testosterone secretion and metabolism in male senescence. *J Clin Endocrinol Metab* 34:730–735, 1972.
2. Pirke KM, Doerr P: Age-related changes and interrelationships between plasma testosterone, estradiol and testosterone binding globulin in normal adult males. *Acta Endocrinol* 74:792–800, 1973.
3. Rubens R, Dhont M, Vermeulen A: Further studies on Leydig cell function in old age. *J Clin Endocrinol Metab* 39:40–45, 1974.
4. Stearns EL, MacDonald JA, Kauffman BJ, et al: Declining testicular function with age: hormonal and clinical correlates. *Am J Med* 47:761–766, 1974.
5. Harman SM, Tsitouras PD: Reproductive hormones in aging man. I. Measurement of sex steroids, basal luteinizing hormone, and Leydig cell response to human chorionic gonadotropin. *J Clin Endocrinol Metab* 51:35–40, 1980.
6. Sparrow D, Bosse R, Rowe JW: The influence of age, alcohol consumption and body build on gonadal function in men. *J Clin Endocrinol Metab* 51:508–512, 1980.
7. Bremner WJ, Prinz PN: The diurnal rhythm in testosterone levels is lost with aging in normal men. Proceedings of the 63rd Annual Meeting of the Endocrine Society, (abstract 480), Cincinnati, 1981.
8. Winters SJ, Troen P: Episodic luteinizing hormone (LH) secretion and the response of LH and follicle-stimulating hormone to LH-releasing

hormone in aged men: Evidence for coexistent primary testicular insufficiency and an impairment in gonadotropin secretion. *J Clin Endocrinol Metab* 55:560–565, 1982.

9. Zumoff B, Strain GW, Kream J, et al: Age variation of the 24-hour mean plasma concentrations of androgens, estrogens, and gonadotropins in normal adult men. *J Clin Endocrinol Metab* 54:534–538, 1982.

10. Sarjent JW, McDonald JR: A method for the quantitative estimate of Leydig cells in the human testis. *Mayo Clin Proc* 23:249–254, 1948.

11. Tillenger KG: Testicular morphology. *Acta Endocrinol* 30(suppl):19–36, 1957.

12. Snyder PJ, Reitano JF, Utiger RD: Serum LH and FSH responses to synthetic gonadotropin releasing hormone in normal men. *J Clin Endocrinol Metab* 41:938–945, 1975.

13. Harman SM, Tsitouras PD, Costa PD, et al: Reproductive hormones in aging men. II. Basal pituitary gonadotropins and the gonadotropin responses to luteinizing hormone-releasing hormone. *J Clin Endocrinol Metab* 54:547–551, 1982.

14. Pirke KM, Doerr P: Plasma DHT in normal adult males and its relation to T. *Acta Endocrinol* 79:357–365, 1975.

15. Greenblatt RB, Oettinger M, Bohler CSS: Estrogen-androgen levels in aging men and women: Therapeutic considerations. *J Am Geriatr Soc* 24:173–178, 1976.

16. Kley HK, Nieschlag E, Bidlingmaier F, et al: Possible age dependent influence of estrogens on the binding of testosterone in plasma of adult men. *Horm Metab Res* 6:213–216, 1974.

17. Hemsell DL, Grodin JM, Brenner PF, et al: Plasma precursors of estrogen. II. Correlation of extent of conversion of plasma androstenedione to estrone with age. *J Clin Endocrinol Metab* 38:476–479, 1974.

18. Morimoto I, Edmiston A, Hawks D, et al: Studies on the origin of androstanediol and androstanediol glucuronide in young and elderly men. *J Clin Endocrinol Metab* 52:772–778, 1981.

19. Desleypere JP, Vermeulen A: Aging and tissue androgens. *J Clin Endocrinol Metab* 53:430–434, 1981.

20. Bishop MWH: Aging and reproduction in the male. *J Reprod Fertil* 12(suppl):65–87, 1970.

21. Tsitouras PD, Martin CE, Harman SM: Relationship of serum testosterone to sexual activity in healthy elderly men. *J Gerontol* 37(suppl 3):288–293, 1982.

22. Marin CE: Sexual activity in the ageing male, in Money J, Musaph H (eds): *Handbook of Sexol-* *ogy*. Elsevier/North-Holland Biomedical Press, 1977, chap 60, pp 813–824.

23. Kinsey AC, Pomeroy WB, Martin CE: *Sexual Behavior in the Human Male*. Philadelphia, WB Saunders & Co, 1948.

24. Masters WH, Johnson VE: *Human Sexual Inadequacy*. Boston, Little, Brown & Co, 1970, pp 316–334.

25. Karacan I, Williams RL, Thornby JI, et al: Sleep-related penile tumescence as a function of age. *Am J Psychiatry* 132:932–937, 1975.

26. Montague DK, James RE Jr, DeWolfe VG, et al: Diagnostic evaluation, classification and treatment of men with sexual dysfunction. *Urology* 14(suppl 6):545–548, 1979.

27. Martin CE: Factors affecting sexual function in 60–79 year-old married males. *Arch Sexual Behav* 10(suppl 5):399–420, 1981.

28. Montague DK, James RE Jr, DeWolfe VG: Diagnostic screening for vasculogenic impotence, in Zorgniotti AW, Rossi G (eds): *Vasculogenic Impotence. Proceedings of the First International Conference on Corpus Cavernosum Revascularization*. Charles C. Thomas, Publisher, Springfield, Illinois, 1980, pp 13–21.

29. Siroky MB, Sax DS, Krane RJ: Sacral signal tracing: The electrophysiology of the bulbocavernosus reflex. *J Urol* 122:661–664, 1979.

30. Ellenberg M: Sexual function in diabetic patients. *Ann Int Med* 92(part 2):331–333, 1980.

31. Hosking DJ, Bennet T, Hampton JR, et al: Diabetic impotence: Studies of nocturnal erection during REM sleep. *Br Med J* 2:1394–1396, 1979.

32. Beaser RS, Van Der Hoek C, Jacobson AM, et al: Experience with penile prostheses in the treatment of impotence in diabetic men. *JAMA* 248(suppl 8):943–948, 1982.

33. *Med Lett Drugs Ther,* 22(suppl 25):108, 1980.

34. Franks S, Jacobs HS, Martin N, et al: Hyperprolactinemia and impotence. *Clin Endocrinol* 8:277–287, 1978.

35. Nuttall FQ: Gynecomastia as a physical finding in normal men. *J Clin Endocrinol Metab* 48:338–340, 1979.

36. McFadyen IJ, Bolton AE, Cameron EHD, et al: Gonadal-pituitary hormone levels in gynecomastia. *Clin Endocrinol* 13:77–86, 1980.

37. Wilson JD, Griffin JE: The use and misuse of androgens. *Metabolism* 29:1278–1295, 1980.

38. Narayan P, Lange PH: Semirigid penile prostheses in the management of erectile impotence. *Urol Clin North Am* 8:169–179, 1981.

39. Furlow WL: Use of the inflatable penile prosthesis in erectile dysfunction. *Urol Clin North Am* 8:181–193, 1981.

CHAPTER 28

Disorders of Calcium and Mineral Metabolism

ERIC ORWOLL, M.D.

MICHAEL R. McCLUNG, M.D.

Mineral Physiology

The calcium ion is critical to virtually all biologic systems. In humans, calcium serves important functions in a variety of biochemical processes (such as enzyme function, neuromuscular excitation, membrane integrity, secretory activity), as well as providing structural support in the form of calcium salts in bone tissue. A normal adult human contains approximately 1,000 grams of calcium distributed among skeletal, cellular, and extracellular sites. A human skeleton contains 99% of the total body calcium stores and serves as a reservoir that is available for the maintenance of cellular and extracellular calcium concentrations.

Cellular and extracellular concentrations of calcium are tightly controlled.[1] The concentration of cytosolic calcium is maintained at $10^{-6} - 10^{-7}$ mol, and the ion is distributed among cellular organelles and calcium-binding proteins with a majority present in mitochondria and microsomes. In contrast, extracellular fluid calcium concentrations are $2-3 \times 10^{-3}$ M, which is 1,000 times that of intracellular concentrations. The low cytosolic calcium concentration is maintained partly by membrane-associated, sodium- and potassium-dependent calcium pumps.

Calcium exists in serum in several forms (see Table 28-1). Ionized (free) calcium is available to interact with cells or to exit from the vascular space. It is present in concentrations of 1.0 − 1.5 mmol and represents nearly 50% of the total serum calcium pool. It is the ionized fraction of calcium that is physiologically important

and closely regulated by hormonal mechanisms. Approximately 40% of all serum calcium is bound to circulating proteins (predominantly albumin), and the remainder (10%) is present in the form of complexes with other ions.

Phosphorus concentrations are approximately the same in the intra- and extracellular compartments (10^{-4} mol), and there appear to be no active mechanisms that regulate its transport across cell membranes. Serum phosphorus levels are not as tightly controlled as those of calcium. Extracellular phosphorus levels fluctuate more with changes in diet, age, sex, and endocrine function. The majority is ionized (55%) and the remainder is complexed with other ions (35%) (see Table 28-1).

Magnesium metabolism is not as well delineated as calcium. However, magnesium is clearly essential to a variety of enzyme systems. It exists in intracellular concentrations that are approximately equal to those in the extracellular space ($10^{-3} - 10^{-4}$ mol). As with calcium and phosphorus, extracellular magnesium is present in ionized (physiologically active), protein-bound, and complexed fractions (see Table 28-1). Ionized magnesium concentrations are carefully controlled, primarily by renal mechanisms.

Aging is associated with changes in the serum concentrations of calcium and phosphorus[2,3]; but, serum magnesium concentrations do not appear to change. There is a gradual decline in the total serum calcium concentrations of 0.1 mg/dl per decade after 20–30 years of age in males, yet little change (if any) in females. Ionized calcium levels have not been

TABLE 28-1   Forms of Calcium, Magnesium, and Phosphate in Normal Plasma

	mmol/l	Percentage of Total
Calcium		
Free ions	1.18	47.5
Protein-bound	1.14	46.0
$CaHPO_4$	0.04	1.6
$CaCit^-$	0.04	1.7
Unidentified complexes	0.08	3.2
Total	2.48	100.0
Magnesium		
Free ions	0.53	55
Protein-bound	0.30	32
$MgHPO_4$	0.03	3
$MgCit^-$	0.04	4
Unidentified complexes	0.06	6
Total	0.96	100
Phosphate		
Free HPO_4^{--}	0.50	43
Free H_2PO_4	0.11	10
Protein-bound	0.14	12
$NaHPO_4^-$	0.33	29
$CaHPO_4$	0.04	3
$MgHPO_4$	0.03	3
Total	1.15	100

SOURCE: Walzer, M: Ion association. VI. Interactions between calcium, magnesium, inorganic phosphate, citrate and protein in normal human plasma. *J Clin Invest* 40:723–730, 1961.

studied to define changes with age, but albumin concentrations do not appear to change uniformly. Similarly, phosphorus concentrations decline with age at a rate of 0.2 mg/dl per decade, but they rise again in females after menopause. Aging changes in serum calcium and phosphate levels are thought to be due to a simultaneous decline in renal function and a subsequent alteration in Vitamin D and parathyroid hormone dynamics.

The Control of Mineral Metabolism

The regulation of phosphorus and magnesium homeostasis are intimately related to that of calcium. Several major organs and endocrine systems are involved.

Parathyroid Hormone

In humans, there are two pairs of parathyroid glands; inferior and superior. Uncommonly (<5%), there are one to four supernumery

glands. The parathyroid gland mass increases in size with age until they reach 30–50 mg each in the 3rd decade; thereafter, they maintain that size or decrease slightly with age. The glands are composed of secretory cells (predominantly "chief" cells) and fat. The fat content increases with age and may constitute the majority of parathyroid gland volume in old age.

Parathyroid hormone (PTH) is a single-chain polypeptide of 84 amino acids with a molecular weight of 9,500. The control of PTH secretion is multifactorial, but it is most closely related to extracellular ionized calcium concentrations. A decrease in Ca^{++} results in an increase in PTH secretion within minutes; an increase in Ca^{++} inhibits secretion (*see* Figure 28-1). This relationship is apparent even within the normal range of serum Ca^{++} concentrations. Other factors that appear to modulate PTH release include cyclic adenosine monophosphate (cAMP), beta-adrenergic agonists, histamines, and seratonin, all of which increase PTH release.[4]

Parathyroid hormone has a half-life of approximately 10 minutes and comprises approximately 10% of the serum pool of parathyroid peptides. It is rapidly metabolized, predominantly by the liver and kidney, to amino and

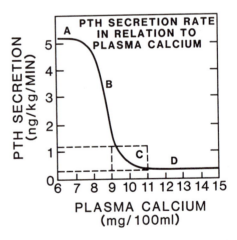

FIGURE 28-1   The relationship of the parathyroid hormone (PTH) secretory rate to plasma calcium concentrations. Parathyroid hormone secretion increases rapidly as plasma calcium falls, and it is suppressed by raising plasma calcium levels. (From Haberner JF, Jacobs JW, Biosynthesis and control of secretion of the calcium-regulating peptides, in Parsons JA (ed): *Endocrinology of Calcium Metabolism.* New York, Raven Press, p. 153, 1982.)

carboxy terminal fragments. Although the amino terminal fragment retains biologic activity, it rapidly clears from plasma and accounts for only a small fraction (less than 10%) of circulating PTH immunoreactivity. The carboxy terminal fragment is biologically inert, but it is cleared slowly (by renal mechanisms) with a long half-life; also, it is the major circulating form of PTH.[5]

The primary role of PTH is the maintenance of the extracellular calcium concentration; hence, the exquisite sensitivity of PTH release to changes in serum Ca^{++} levels. It plays a major role in mineral homeostasis by direct actions on bone metabolism and renal function and by indirect effects on Vitamin D physiology.

The major actions of PTH are to increase the reabsorption of calcium in the distal renal tubule and to decrease the reabsorption of phosphorus in the proximal tubule.[6] Approximately 90% of filtered calcium is reabsorbed in the proximal nephron in a PTH-unresponsive, concentration-dependent, non-saturable process that is intimately linked to that of sodium reabsorption. Sodium and calcium appear to share an active transport system at this proximal site. Thus, the amount of calcium that is reabsorbed depends on the amount of sodium competing for that transport mechanism. Parathyroid hormone exerts its effects to increase calcium absorption in the distal tubule. In the absence of PTH, distal calcium reabsorption virtually ceases and calcium excretion dramatically increases. The average adult filters 10,000 mg/day of calcium, of which 97–99% is reabsorbed. If 10% of that reabsorption (or 1,000 mg) occurs at the distal PTH-dependent site, it is apparent that in the absence of PTH an amount of calcium greater than the total extracellular pool would be lost on a daily basis. Hence, when extracellular Ca^{++} falls, a major effect of the subsequently secreted PTH is an increase in distal tubular calcium reabsorption and, thereby, an increase in serum Ca^{++} levels. PTH also exerts a profound phosphaturic effect. Phosphorus is reabsorbed predominantly (if not solely) from the proximal tubule, and PTH decreases this tubular reabsorption of phosphorus (TRP), which causes a decrease in the serum phosphorus concentration. These effects of PTH on the renal tubule are partly mediated through cAMP. An increase in PTH

action, therefore, is reflected by an increase in the amount of cAMP that is excreted in the urine.

Parathyroid hormone also has major effects on bone tissue, not only in its role as the primary mediator of extracellular calcium concentration, but also as an important coordinator of bone remodeling.[7] When exposed to intact PTH or the N-terminal fragment of PTH, there is an initial rapid and small, transient fall in extracellular calcium. This is due, perhaps, to an influx of calcium into bone cells. It is followed by an efflux of calcium from bone tissue and a resultant increase in extracellular calcium concentrations that persists as long as the exposure to PTH continues. These early effects appear to be due to the effects on existing bone cells. After a delay of hours, PTH also induces the recruitment of new cells (osteoclasts) that effect the dissolution of bone minerals and the release of more calcium. This latter effect, when prolonged, results in a bone rarification that is seen in states of hyperparathyroidism.

PTH affects other tissues as well, including the nervous system, the gastrointestinal system, hematopoietic cells, and granulopoietic cells. Although inconspicuous in a normal individual, these effects may be prominant in states of hyperparathyroidism.

The actions of PTH on kidney and bone tissue provide a rapid calcemic response and comprise the most important mechanisms by which PTH maintains serum calcium concentrations within tight limits on a minute-to-minute basis. The acute effects of PTH seemingly remain intact with advancing age. Nevertheless, some reports indicate that PTH levels are higher in healthy elderly persons, particularly females, than in younger individuals. The interaction of PTH with Vitamin D metabolism does appear to change with aging.

Vitamin D

Vitamin D_3 (cholecalciferol) is obtained by humans from either an endogenous synthesis in the skin or its ingestion in the diet. In most areas of the world, including the United States, the majority of serum Vitamin D activity arises in the epidermis as a result of ultraviolet irradiation and the photolytic conversion of 7-dihydrocholesterol to cholecalciferol. Where sun exposure is minimal, an adequate supply must be obtained from the diet. Cholecalciferol is present in animal tissues, and its equally biopotent isomer ergocalciferol (D_2) is found in plant material. Cholecalciferol and ergocalciferol are fat-soluble compounds that are absorbed via the lymphatics of the duodenum, transported with lipoproteins, and stored in adipose tissue and muscle. The daily requirement in adults for cholecalciferol is 100–400 IU (2.5–10 μg).

Cholecalciferol is relatively inert biologically, and it must be metabolized to achieve full potency. From the skin or intestine, cholecalciferol is transported (by a plasma Vitamin D-binding protein) to the liver, where it is hydroxylated to form 25-hydroxycholecalciferol (25[OH]D). Although somewhat more active than cholecalciferol, 25(OH)D is hydroxylated again in the kidney to form 1-alpha,25(OH)$_2$ cholecalciferol (1,25[OH]$_2$D) (the most active of the cholecalciferols), as well as other metabolites (24,25[OH]$_2$cholecalciferol, and others). The rate-limiting site in this process is the renal 1-hydroxylation step. Parathyroid hormone and hypophosphatemia both exert strong stimulatory influences at that point. Hence, the third major influence of PTH on calcium metabolism is mediated through Vitamin D.[8]

1,25[OH]$_2$D has major effects at two sites; the intestines and bones. In the intestine, 1,25(OH)$_2$D exerts a strong positive influence on calcium and phosphorus absorption, probably through the generation of specific binding proteins. Hence, in response to a prolonged hypocalcemic stimulus (e.g., the assumption of a low calcium diet), PTH release increases and within 12–24 hours 1,25(OH)$_2$D synthesis is stimulated. This results in an increase in gastrointestinal calcium absorption. These actions provide a relatively constant influx of calcium, complement the acute calcemic action of PTH that is mediated through bone calcium efflux and renal tubular calcium reabsorption, and help to maintain a stable serum calcium concentration.

Cholecalciferol also increases phosphorus absorption, but less is known about this process. Phosphorus is more easily absorbed than calcium, and the ubiquitous presence of phosphates in the diet makes a dietary phosphate insufficiency uncommon. Magnesium absorption appears to be similar to calcium absorption in many respects. 1,25[OH]$_2$D may have an effect on gastrointestinal magnesium handling, but the importance of that relationship is unknown.

In young individuals, the institution of a low-calcium diet elicits both a prompt (1–2 days) increase in 1,25(OH)$_2$D levels and a resultant increase in fractional gastrointestinal calcium absorption, which results in preservation of dietary calcium availability.[9] With age, however, and particularly in patients with senile osteoporosis, there seems to be a blunted ability to respond appropriately to this challenge. Elderly individuals do not absorb dietary calcium as well as their younger counterparts, and 1,25(OH)$_2$D levels are lower. 1,25(OH)$_2$D production in response to the institution of a low-calcium diet or to a direct challenge with the administration of PTH is attenuated in older individuals. The biochemical nature of this failure of 1,25(OH)$_2$D synthesis, and whether it is related to the general decline in renal function with aging, is not known. Nevertheless, the potential for a negative calcium balance that is induced by an insufficient intestinal calcium absorption has clear-cut implications on aging and the development of senile osteopenia.[10]

The actions of 1,25(OH)$_2$D on bone tissue are complex and incompletely understood. Normal mineralization is dependent on adequate concentrations of 1,25(OH)$_2$D (and perhaps other metabolites of cholecalciferol such as 25(OH)D, 24,25(OH)$_2$D, etc.), but there also appears to be a release of minerals from bone tissue in response to 1,25(OH)$_2$D.

Calcitonin

Calcitonin, a peptide hormone that is synthesized in the C cells of the thyroid gland, is a hypocalcemic substance.[11] It is released in response to hypercalcemia, and a fall in serum Ca^{++} levels inhibits its secretion. Alpha-adrenergic agents, cAMP, and gastrin stimulate its release. When administered parenterally, calcitonin rapidly decreases bone resorption via osteoclasts and osteocytes, and thus decreases calcium efflux from the bones. Recent studies have suggested that calcitonin may promote bone mineralization. Whereas the hypocalcemic effect of calcitonin is predominantly mediated through its actions on bone tissue, its renal effects result in an increase in calcium excretion. Recent evidence suggests that calcitonin decreases the efflux of phosphorus from bone tissue and promotes its incorporation into bone mineral. Not withstanding these well-demonstrated effects, the physiologic role of calcitonin in humans is not well understood.

Calcitonin concentrations decrease with age, (particularly in females), as does the release of calcitonin in response to secretory stimuli.[12] In view of the inhibitory effects of calcitonin on bone resorption, this age-related fall in calcitonin has been postulated to be important in the pathophysiology of senile osteoporosis.

Hypercalcemia

Calcium concentrations in serum may be measured via several methods. The atomic absorption method of total calcium determination is accurate and reproduceable, but somewhat tedious. More recently, automated methods using dye dilution techniques have become standard and are accurate, except for rare interferences. Since it is the ionized fraction of serum calcium that is physiologically important, it would be ideal to specifically measure that fraction and avoid any confusion that may result from alterations in serum calcium-binding proteins; but, this method is not widely available. Hence, interpretations of total serum calcium concentrations should be made with the knowledge that changes in calcium binding-protein concentrations must be considered. Except in some cases of multiple myeloma where calcium-binding paraproteins may spuriously elevate total calcium concentrations, albumin is quantitatively the most important calcium-binding protein. An approximation of the importance of changes in albumin levels on calcium levels can be made by adjusting the serum calcium concentration by 0.6–0.8 mg/dl for each gram/dl change in the albumin concentration. More elaborate methods of "correcting" serum calcium levels, which make use of albumin levels, pH, and so on, have not proven as accurate as was hoped.

Hypercalcemia occurs when the influx of calcium into the extracellular space exceeds the capacity of the system (predominantly renal) to remove it. It can arise from several mechanisms. Excess calcium may enter the extracellular pool from the bones or gut, and its removal

TABLE 28-2 Major Hypercalcemic Conditions

Hyperparathyroidism
Malignancy
Thyrotoxicosis
Adrenal insufficiency
Pheochromocytoma
Vitamin A or D toxicity
Milk-alkali syndrome
Lithium
Sarcoidosis and other granulomatous diseases
Immobilization
Acute renal failure (ARF)
Familial hypocalciuric hypercalcemia

from that pool can be impaired by changes in renal function. Table 28-2 lists the major hypercalcemic conditions that affect elderly persons.

The symptoms that are caused by elevated serum calcium concentrations are non-specific (malaise, fatigue), neuropsychiatric (memory loss, irritability, lethargy, drowsiness, headache), neuromuscular (myalgia, weakness, arthralgia), gastrointestinal (anorexia, nausea, vomiting, constipation, abdominal pain), or genitourinary (thirst, polyuria, stones). With severe hypercalcemia, mental status changes are prominent and include confusion, disorientation, obtundation, and coma.

The degree of illness does not always correlate with the serum calcium concentration. Some patients are seemingly unaffected by major elevations in serum calcium levels (16–18 mg/dl), whereas others are symptomatic with moderate degrees of hypercalcemia (12 mg/dl). Both the rapidity of the development of the hypercalcemia and the underlying health of the individual play a role in the degree of illness at any particular calcium concentration. In general, elderly individuals are more severely affected by modest elevations in serum calcium concentrations than younger people. A general deterioration in physical functioning, particularly in the mental status (lethargy, confusion), frequently is a result of a relatively mild hypercalcemia (11–13 mg/dl) in old age.

Hyperparathyroidism

Long regarded as a relatively rare disease, primary hyperparathyroidism recently has been recognized as a more common disorder, primarily because of the advent of automated serum calcium analysis. The annual incidence rate of hyperparathyroidism now appears to be approximately 25 cases per 100,000, with a preponderance of new cases being found in elderly persons.[13] Whereas in persons less than 40 years of age the annual incidence rate of primary hyperparathyroidism is approximately 10 cases per 100,000, the incidence rises to 60 cases per 100,000 in males and 100 cases per 100,000 in females at ages 40–60, and to 100 cases per 100,000 in males and 188 cases per 100,000 in females over 60 years of age. Thus, hyperparathyroidism is an important disorder in old age and the most common cause of hypercalcemia in adults.

The manifestations of hyperparathyroidism may be protean, and they include the effects of hypercalcemia as well as those that are apparently due to elevated concentrations of PTH itself. Importantly, however, up to 25% of all hyperparathyroid patients may present with relatively asymptomatic hypercalcemia.

The most frequent symptoms and signs of hyperparathyroidism are neuromyopathic. Weakness and fatigue, predominantly of the proximal muscles, is a prominent complaint; also, physical findings of weakness and muscle atrophy may be present. Fine fasciculations of the tongue have been described as a common sign. These abnormalities are found in both primary and secondary hyperparathyroidism and do not correlate well with serum calcium concentrations, which suggests that PTH itself may have a neuromuscular toxicity. In fact, a PTH-induced neurotoxicity has been demonstrated and apparently is independent of alterations in serum calcium concentrations.[14] A successful parathyroidectomy results in the nearly complete relief of these abnormalities.

Central nervous system complaints frequently accompany hyperparathyroidism and include psychoneurotic syndromes and a global deterioration in mental status. Psychiatric disorders usually are mild and consist of depression, anxiety, irritability, and personality changes. Rarely, psychotic states may be present, but they are difficult to directly ascribe to a parathyroid dysfunction. In spite of the relatively common occurrence of psychiatric complaints in hyperparathyroidism, a favorable response to surgery is unpredictable. The symptoms that are more easily related to hyper-

calcemia (lethargy, confusion, obtundation, and coma) are more amenable to successful surgery. The relief of hypercalcemia usually results in improvement, unless other causes of a central nervous system dysfunction are present. Older individuals and those with concomitant causes of dementia frequently are more affected by changes in their mental status than younger patients with similar degrees of hypercalcemia. Successful therapy may result in a dramatic improvement in mental status.

Although automated calcium screening has increased the number of hyperparathyroid patients who are discovered before nephrolithiasis develops, recent studies continue to illustrate the importance of renal stone disease.[15] Renal stones in cases of primary hyperparathyroidism usually are composed of calcium phosphate or calcium oxalate. Factors that are important in their development include an increase in urine pH induced by the renal tubular effects of PTH, an increase in urine calcium, and other effects on the urinary stone-forming potential (changes in mineral solubility characteristics). There is a subgroup of patients with a primary hyperparathyroidism who have a disproportionate hypercalciuria and are at the greatest risk for nephrolithiasis. Their hypercalciuria appears to be due to higher plasma $1,25(OH)_2D$ concentrations and a consequent gastrointestinal calcium hyperabsorption. In addition to renal stone disease, patients with prolonged or severe hypercalcemia may develop nephrocalcinosis with a resultant decrease in renal function.

Gastrointestinal disturbances have been associated with hyperparathyroidism, particularly peptic ulcer disease and pancreatitis. The significance of initial reports of ulcer disease in association with hyperparathyroidism are clouded by the subsequent recognition of the Zollinger-Ellison Syndrome, which occurs in the context of multiple endocrine neoplasia type I (hyperparathyroidism, islet cell tumors, and pituitary tumors); yet, there still exists evidence that suggests, in cases of sporadic primary hyperparathyroidism, ulcer disease and non-specific abdominal pain unrelated to gastrin-secreting islet cell tumors are more common than would be predicted. Similarly, pancreatitis appears to occur more commonly than expected in hyperparathyroidism. An increase in the incidence of cholelithiasis has been observed, particularly in younger individuals.

Metabolic bone disease once was considered a hallmark of hyperparathyroidism; however, with the increasing identification of patients with milder disease, the incidence rate of clinically demonstrable bone disease in hyperparathyroidism has fallen to 10–15%.[16] Virtually all patients with hyperparathyroidism have a marked acceleration in bone remodeling that is consistent with the effects of PTH on bone metabolism. An uncoupling defect that is induced by PTH allows osteoclastic bone resorption to exceed osteoblastic new bone formation, which in turn leads to osteopenia. The serum alkaline phosphatase elevations of hyperparathyroidism reflect the increase in bone remodeling. Quantitative techniques reveal a fall in bone density with hyperparathyroidism, particularly in postmenopausal women (a group already at risk for the development of osteopenia). The initial clinical result is a generalized loss of bone mass, which presents as osteoporosis. Radiographically, this stage of bone disease is manifested as a dimineralization, specifically subperiosteal and cortical resorption, which is most consistently demonstrable with detailed x-ray films of the hands. Hyperparathyroid bone disease may present as a diffuse osteopenia or as the more dramatic and pathognomonic osteitis fibrosa cystica, which is characterized by bone cysts, brown tumors (composed of osteoclasts and poorly organized bone), and medullary fibrosis. Diffuse osteopenia and osteitis fibrosa cystica probably, but not definitely, represent two stages in a spectrum of bone disease; the osteopenic form represents an early stage and osteitis fibrosa cystica a later stage in the course of hyperparathyroidism. Although bone cysts are not resolved with therapy, brown tumors and medullary fibrosis improve with a successful parathyroidectomy. There also is evidence that osteopenia may improve.

Other features of primary hyperparathyroidism include: 1) Hypertension, which is present in one third to one half of all patients with hyperparathyroidism, (a higher than expected incidence). The pathophysiologic relationship of hypertension to hyperparathyroidism is unknown and the response to successful surgery is unpredictable; 2) Hematologic abnormalities— most commonly a mild, normocytic anemia that probably is due to the direct effects of PTH on erythropoiesis; 3) Skeletal complaints that are unrelated to dimineralization and subsequent fractures. Hyperuricemia and gout, as well as chondrocalcinosis and pseudogout, are more common in hyperparathyroidism. Acute episodes of both have been reported in the immediate postparathyroidectomy period. In view of the frequency with which hyperparathyroidism is found in the geriatric population, a degenerative osteoarthritis may be present and can further aggravate rheumatologic complaints; 4) Finally, the hypercalcemia of hyperparathyroidism may cause cardiac conduction abnormalities (specifically QT shortening and a prolongation of the PR interval), and it can make the myocardium more sensitive to the toxic effects of digitalis preparations. Recent evidence supports a direct adverse effect of PTH on myocardial conduction. Although poorly characterized, this effect may be of particular importance to elderly patients with coexistent ischemic or hypertensive cardiac disease.

Acute hypercalcemia, or "parathyroid crisis," occasionally develops in patients with hyperparathyroidism and clinically presents as severe hypercalcemia, bone disease, and renal impairment. Without a rapid diagnosis and surgical treatment, the outcome has been fatal. A large parathyroid adenoma most frequently is found at surgery, although hyperplasia also may be responsible.

In patients with pronounced hypercalcemia, and particularly in those with a parathyroid mass that is clinically palpable, parathyroid carcinoma should be considered. Carcinomas account for approximately 1% of all cases of primary hyperparathyroidism, occur equally in males and females, and present at a slightly earlier age than benign parathyroid disease. The PTH levels usually are high. In view of the poor life expectancy of patients with a parathyroid carcinoma (approximately 50% survival rate at 5 years after surgery), a successful initial surgery is important. Radiotherapy and chemotherapy for metastatic disease is not particularly effective, and the cause of death usually is due to a sustained or severe hypercalcemia.

Hyperparathyroidism may occur as part of a familial disorder, specifically multiple endocrine neoplasia type I (MEN I), multiple endocrine neoplasia type II (MEN II), or familial hypocalciuric hypercalcemia.[17] All are autosomal dominant disorders in which hypercalcemia occurs as a result of parathyroid hyperplasia. Although the precise prevalence of familial forms of hyperparathyroidism is unknown, they appear frequently enough to prompt their consideration in all patients in whom a diagnosis of hyperparathyroidism is made. However, the onset of symptoms in old age is quite unusual.

Evaluation

The physical examination in patients with hyperparathyroidism rarely is diagnostic, but it does contribute to the evaluation of the metabolic effects of the disease since patients may manifest the physical effects of renal, bone, gastrointestinal, or neuromuscular abnormalities. A band keratopathy may be observed (particularly with a slit lamp) in patients with a prolonged hypercalcemia. The corneal calcification of hypercalcemia is easily confused with that of arcus senilis.

The laboratory evaluation of hyperparathyroidism depends on the demonstration of inappropriately elevated PTH concentrations in the face of hypercalcemia; both criteria must be satisfied. With reliable methods for the measurements of both calcium and PTH, a confident diagnosis usually can be made, particularly in patients with a moderate (11.5–12.5 mg/dl) or more severe (>12.5 mg/dl) hypercalcemia. Fasting hypercalcemia should be verified before the etiology is sought with a PTH determination. Although uncommon, some patients may exhibit elevations only of the ionized calcium fraction with a relatively normal total serum calcium concentration.

Parathyroid hormone immunoassays are intrinsically difficult to interpret, so the characteristics of the assay that are used clinically should be understood. In addition to the vagaries inherent in any immunoassay, those for PTH must consider the presence of multiple molecular forms of PTH in plasma. Assays are available for the detection of amino terminal, carboxy terminal, midregion, and "intact" forms of the hormone. Each type yields similar, but independent, bits of information. Assays for the N-terminal fragment or for intact PTH are good indicators of parathyroid gland secretory activity because of the short half-lives of these forms under virtually all conditions. These assays frequently are used for parathyroid gland localization studies. C-terminal PTH assays detect the C-terminal fragment in addition to the intact hormone. Since the C-terminal fragment has a longer half-life in plasma, C-terminal immunoreactivity tends to be proportionately greater in hyperparathyroidism, which potentially enables a greater discrimination between a normal and hyperparathyroid status. However, because the C-terminal fragment of PTH is cleared by renal mechanisms, a renal insufficiency results in an accumulation of C-terminal immunoreactivity and creates a situation in which C-terminal PTH levels may not reflect parathyroid gland activity. A clinician must be cognizant of these considerations when choosing a PTH assay for an individual patient.[18]

The measurement of urinary cAMP concentrations (nephrogenous cAMP or total cAMP excretion) also are useful in differential diagnosis of hypercalcemia.[19] PTH acts at renal tubular sites, at least in part, via a cAMP-dependent process and, thus, urinary cAMP concentrations can reflect PTH action. The cAMP levels, therefore, are elevated in most patients with hyperparathyroidism. Renal insufficiency, however, reduces cAMP excretion. In some patients with a hypercalcemia of malignancy, cAMP excretion is high (apparently as a result of the presence of a tumor-related, PTH-like substance), which limits diagnostic usefulness of urinary cAMP measurements.

Other laboratory parameters, albeit less specific or sensitive, can be helpful in a differential diagnosis of hypercalcemia. Because of the marked phosphaturic effect of PTH, a fasting hypophosphatemia is found in a majority of hyperparathyroid patients; it may be less pronounced in postmenopausal females and cases of renal insufficiency. An estimation of the tubular reabsorption of phosphorus (TmP/GFR) provides an index of PTH-induced changes in renal phosphorus handling that is corrected for the glomerular filtration rate (GFR). Parathyroid hormone also results in a renal bicarbonate wasting and a subsequent hyperchloremic metabolic acidosis. Hence, hypophosphatemia, mild acidosis, and hyperchloremia are characteristic (but not invariable) features of hyperparathyroidism; also, the serum chloride/phosphorus ratio is elevated (>33) in most patients with a PTH-mediated hypercalcemia. In patients with hyperparathyroid bone disease, the serum alkaline phosphatase may be elevated, although levels are not well correlated with radiographic findings. In addition, there may be a mild anemia, hypokalemia, or hypomagnesemia.

Therapy

Whereas the need for therapy is clear in both moderate-to-severe hypercalcemia or patients with end-organ disease, the role of therapy in patients with mild (serum calcium <11.5 mg/dl) asymptomatic hyperparathyroidism is controversial. Experimental evidence suggests a gradual loss in bone density and renal function in these patients if untreated. The potential for morbidity that is related to worsening hypercalcemia should prompt regular follow-up evaluations. In elderly persons, even mild elevations in serum calcium concentration may result in a disability (particularly a neurologic dysfunction) that is seemingly out of proportion to the hyperparathyroidism and may prompt an early surgical intervention if no contraindications exist.

At present, surgery offers the only hope of a cure. The success of a parathyroidectomy and the incidence of surgical complications (hypoparathyroidism, recurrent laryngial nerve injury) depends heavily on the experience of the surgeon. Medical approaches are not as useful for long-term therapy.[20]

Hypercalcemia of Malignancy

Hypercalcemia is a common concomitant of malignant tumors. In a hospital setting, malignancy is the most common cause of hypercalcemia, which occurs in 10–20% of all patients with cancer. Since hyperparathyroidism and malignancy together account for the great majority of cases of hypercalcemia, and because both disorders occur most commonly in older individuals, hypercalcemia may be considered to be primarily a geriatric disorder.

Although several tumors are particularly associated with hypercalcemia (breast carcinoma, renal cell carcinoma, multiple myeloma, lymphoma, and squamous cell carcinomas of the lung, head, and neck), a wide variety of tumor types have been linked to it.[21] Hypercalcemia in patients with malignancy may be due to one of

several mechanisms, although the factors that result in hypercalcemia most often are mediated by bone resorption. Although once considered the result of bone destruction due to metastases, the presence of bony metastases may have no direct bearing on bone resorption or the occurrence of hypercalcemia. Nevertheless, some tumor cells appear to have direct bone-resorbing properties, and 70–80% of all patients with tumor-related hypercalcemia have bone lesions. In particular breast carcinoma, multiple myeloma, and lymphoma may cause bone resorption in areas that are contiguous with tumor masses. Tumor cells or a local immunologically mediated reaction may produce prostaglandins (particularly prostaglandin E_2 [PGE_2]), which have bone-resorbing capabilities via their effects on osteoclasts.

Humoral factors also may result in hypercalcemia via bone resorption in the absence of direct bone involvement by tumor cells.[21] In addition to its probable local production by tumor cells in the bones, PGE_2 may be present in high concentrations in the plasma and urine of patients with hypercalcemia without bone lesions. In some cases, elevated PGE_2 levels have been shown to be suppressible with prostaglandin synthetase inhibitors, with a resultant improvement in hypercalcemia. The osteoclast-activating factor (OAF) is a peptide substance produced by some lymphoreticular tumor cells (multiple myeloma, lymphoma) that has osteoclast-stimulating, and hence bone-resorbing, and presumably hypercalcemic properties. Other undefined mechanisms also may be responsible for bone resorption and hypercalcemia. Several investigators have identified patients with hypercalcemia and cancer in whom urinary cAMP concentrations were elevated in the face of low or normal levels of immunoreactive PTH. Although a bioassay for PTH has revealed the presence of PTH activity in these patients, presumably as a result of a PTH-like substance, the fact that both 1,25(OH)$_2$ Vitamin D levels and renal tubular calcium reabsorption are low suggests that this substance(s) may have different effects on various tissues. The term "pseudohyperparathyroidism" has been used to describe the hypercalcemia of malignancy. The presence of ectopic hyperparathyroidism has been assumed to occur in that setting. However, PTH production by malignant cells is not well documented. At present, the basis for most tumor-induced hypercalcemias must be assumed to be by means other than the production of PTH itself.

The clinical features of the hypercalcemia of malignancy are attendant on hypercalcemia and the malignant process itself. The anorexia, nausea, vomiting, and immobilization that occur so frequently in malignancy may serve to greatly exacerbate hypercalcemia; conversely, hypercalcemia may aggravate symptoms of a malignancy. A vicious cycle of hypercalcemia, dehydration, immobilization, and worsening hypercalcemia frequently are the terminal events in these patients.

Evaluation
The presence of hypercalcemia always should prompt consideration of a malignancy, but it rarely is necessary to search beyond a complete history, physical, and screening laboratory evaluation (multichemistry screen, complete blood count (CBC), urinalysis (UA), stool guaiac, chest x-ray film) to find the responsible neoplasm. It is rare for hypercalcemia of malignancy to occur before the tumor is clinically obvious. In fact, elevations in serum calcium concentrations frequently reflect the final stages in the course of this disease. In most patients, the diagnosis of a malignancy will antedate that of hypercalcemia. On rare occasions, however, occult neoplasms may cause hypercalcemia. In each patient with hypercalcemia virtually all diagnoses should be clinically evident with the exception of malignancy and hyperparathyroidism. The presence of clearly elevated PTH concentrations is a strong indicator of hyperparathyroidism. In view of its frequency, hyperparathyroidism should be expected to occur at times concurrently with a malignancy. Clear elevations of PTH should suggest that diagnosis, even in the presence of a tumor.

Therapy
The therapy for hypercalcemia of malignancy must be individualized and directed at the specific factors that contribute to the disorder.[21] An effective treatment of the tumor should be sought. In patients with a mild, relatively asymptomatic hypercalcemia, successful surgical, chemotherapeutic, or radiation therapy may be all that is necessary. Rehydration, sodium repletion, and mobilization (important concomitants of any therapeutic approach) often are successful in improving or stabilizing the clinical situation while specific antitumor therapy is undertaken.

With severe hypercalcemia, immediate therapy is necessary. Because virtually all significantly hypercalcemic patients are volume depleted as a result of anorexia, vomiting, and polyuria, rehydration is essential to relieve hemoconcentration and increase renal blood flow and calcium excretion. The administration of saline accomplishes these goals; furthermore, saline diuresis promotes renal calcium excretion by inhibiting proximal renal tubular calcium reabsorption. In a volume-repleted patient, furosemide can further promote sodium and, hence, calcium excretion. Aggressive furosemide-saline therapy may involve as much as 500–750 ml/hour of intravenous (IV) saline solution with 40–80 mg of IV furosemide every 2 hours. In a geriatric patient with diminished cardiac and renal reserve, the volume and electrolyte parameters should be monitored carefully.

Calcitonin has osteoclast-inhibiting properties and may be rapidly effective in lowering serum calcium concentrations within 4–24 hours in doses of 4–8 units/kg per day. Commonly, however, a refractoriness to calcitonin therapy develops within days. The combined use of calcitonin and glucocorticoids may be more effective than either modality alone. Glucocorticoids (usually prednisone in doses of 40–100 mg/day) may decrease serum calcium levels in 24–48 hours by its direct effects on tumor-related bone resorption, by direct effects on tumor cells, and by inhibiting gastrointestinal calcium absorption. Glucocorticoids are most effective in patients with breast carcinoma, multiple myeloma, or hematologic malignancies.

Mithramycin, an antibiotic that initially was used as a chemotherapeutic agent, has potent osteoclast-inhibiting properties and is uniformly effective in lowering serum calcium concentrations. When used in an IV dose of 25 μg/kg, the hypocalcemic effect should be noted within 24 hours. It persists for variable amounts of time, usually approximately 1 week. Toxicity is dose-dependent and consists primarily of thrombocytopenia, nephrotoxicity, and hepatotoxicity.

The toxic effects of mithramycin may compound the effects of other chemotherapeutic agents and may limit its usefulness.

Oral or IV phosphorus administration may lower serum calcium levels by inhibiting bone resorption and by promoting mineralization. Of concern, particularly with the use of IV phosphorus, has been the occurrence of soft tissue mineralization—particularly nephrocalcinosis. Nevertheless, cautious oral phosphorus administration in doses of 1–2 grams/day may be useful in the chronic management of a hypercalcemia in non-azotemic, non-hyperphosphatemic patients.

The management of a chronic hypercalcemia of malignancy in an outpatient setting is more difficult, but it uses similar modalities. Adequate hydration, sodium intake, and mobilization are important. In view of the nearly terminal stage of most tumors that are associated with hypercalcemia, a patient's comfort and quality of life may be more important considerations than vigorous attempts to normalize serum calcium concentrations.

Other Hypercalcemic Conditions

The Milk-Alkali Syndrome
This syndrome occurs in patients who ingest large amounts of calcium and absorbable alkali, most often calcium carbonate (10–60 grams/day).[22] Hypercalcemia, alkalosis, and a renal insufficiency are the hallmarks of this syndrome and are easily reversible in its early stages by discontinuing the intake of calcium and alkali. Later stages of this syndrome are more difficult to treat, since a withdrawal of calcium and alkalis may not result in a resolution of the hypercalcemia; also, renal damage may be severe. The diagnosis is dependent on a history of calcium and alkali ingestion and the exclusion of other causes of hypercalcemia, particularly hyperparathyroidism (which can also present as hypercalcemia with azotemia).

Vitamin Intoxication
Intoxication with either Vitamin A or Vitamin D may result in hypercalcemia. Vitamin A, taken in large amounts (50,000 units/day) for a protracted period of time, or in massive amounts (1 million units/day) for short periods (2 weeks) results in hypercalcemia and osteope-

nia; apparently, this is a result of osteoclastic bone resorption. Vitamin D intoxication may result from the consumption of 100,000 units/day or more, or from biologically similar doses of the newer metabolites 25-hydroxycholecalciferol (25OHD) and 1,25-dihydroxycholecalciferol (1,25[OH]$_2$D). Hypercalcemia may rapidly appear in patients who are chronically treated with cholecalciferol and may persist for months because of the storage of this fat-soluble substance in adipose tissue. The metabolites 25OHD and 1,25(OH)$_2$D may produce hypercalcemia more quickly after therapy is begun; but, a withdrawal of these compounds also results in a more rapid reversal, since they are less extensively stored in fat.

Thiazide Diuretics
These drugs may increase the extracellular calcium pool by renal tubular calcium conservation, gastrointestinal calcium absorption, and bone resorption. Thiazides exacerbate existing hypercalcemic conditions (hyperparathyroidism, Vitamin D intoxication, and so on). However, it is less clear that thiazides can cause hypercalcemia in an otherwise normal individual. The effects of thiazide diuretics should dissipate within 3 days of their withdrawal.

Lithium
This drug is primarily used for manic-depressive illness, and it may be associated with a reversible hypercalcemia. Lithium appears to cause PTH hypersecretion. Before the recognition of these actions, patients who became hypercalcemic while taking lithium and who were noted to have inappropriately elevated PTH concentrations were thought to have a primary hyperparathyroidism. Hypercalcemia that is due to lithium therapy usually is mild (<11.5 mg/dl) and should regress within 1 week after the drug is discontinued.

Thyrotoxicosis
This condition is associated with mild (<11.5 mg/dl) hypercalcemia in 10–20% of all patients; less overt disturbances in calcium metabolism are demonstrable in nearly 50%. The most likely cause of this hypercalcemia is an increased efflux of calcium from the bones. Thyroid hormones induce changes in bone remodeling that are reflected by increases in

osteoblastic and osteoclastic functioning. Bone resorption, however, is proportionately stimulated more than bone accretion, which presumably results in a hypercalcemia and a fall in bone density that is noted in some thyrotoxic patients. Serum alkaline phosphatase levels are increased, as are urinary hydroxyproline excretion rates. The reports of PTH levels in thyrotoxicosis have been inconsistent, but they generally indicate suppressed levels. Urinary cAMP excretion rates are normal and phosphorus excretion is suppressed, which further suggests that PTH secretion is not increased. The 25OH Vitamin D levels are normal, as are both $1,25(OH)_2$ Vitamin D levels and the rates of gastrointestinal calcium absorption. A correction of thyrotoxicosis should relieve the hypercalcemia promptly, and beta-adrenergic blockade has been reported to reduce elevated serum calcium levels in thyrotoxic patients. Alkaline phosphatase levels actually may rise with a resolution of the toxicosis, apparently reflecting an increase in bone-forming activity, but fall to normal levels again within months. This increase in bone formation may reverse the bone loss due to the thyrotoxic state. If hypercalcemia is not reversed with a resolution of the thyrotoxicosis, then hyperparathyroidism (which has been associated with thyrotoxicosis) must be considered.

Adrenal Insufficiency
Particularly when acute, this may be associated with hypercalcemia. Although the pathophysiology is obscure, it may involve hemoconcentration and a decreased urinary calcium excretion as well as a lack of corticosteroid inhibition of gastrointestinal calcium absorption. Hypercalcemia is rapidly corrected with treatment of the adrenal insufficiency.

Pheochromocytoma
Pheochromocytoma is associated with hypercalcemia due to a concomitant hyperparathyroidism in the MEN IIa syndrome; but, it also may be the apparent primary cause of hypercalcemia. Several cases have been reported in which hypercalcemia was resolved with only a surgical removal of a pheochromocytoma.

Immobilization
This leads to an accelerated bone resorption and reduced bone formation. Weight-bearing activity has important trophic effects on bones that are necessary for the maintenance of bone mass. Calcium efflux from the bones during immobilization is commonly associated with hypercalciuria within the first week of confinement. Hypercalcemia may result, particularly in patients with other stimuli to an increased bone turnover (Paget's disease, hyperparathyroidism, malignancy). In geriatric patients with illnesses that demand prolonged bed rest, and in whom other risk factors may exist, hypercalcemia and bone loss can be major problems.

Granulomatous Disease
These diseases, particularly sarcoidosis, but also tuberculosis and fungal infections, may be associated with hypercalcemia. In sarcoidosis, an acceleration in the production of $1,25(OH)_2D$, presumably by the granulomatous tissue itself, has been implicated in the genesis of gastrointestinal calcium hyperabsorption, hypercalciuria, and hypercalcemia.

Hypocalcemia

The development of hypocalcemia represents the failure of one or more of the mechanisms by which serum calcium usually is maintained. Hence, a failure of parathyroid, Vitamin D, bone, or renal function may result in a fall in serum calcium concentrations.

The manifestations of hypocalcemia are primarily neuromuscular in nature. There are a series of symptoms that appear as serum calcium concentrations progressively decrease. Although a patient may tolerate even an impressive hypocalcemia (<7.0 mg/dl) if it has developed gradually, a rapid fall in calcium produces symptoms at a concentration much higher than if the fall is less precipitous. A change in mental functioning is a common symptom of hypocalcemia and includes a decrease in memory and cognitive ability, lassitude, and mood alterations. Although they sometimes are dramatic, these symptoms may develop insidiously and escape recognition by a patient and physician alike. More obvious and physically distressing effects commonly bring patients to the attention of physicians, namely paresthesias and muscle cramps. Paresthesias usually consist of numbness or tingling sensations that may occur anywhere, but most often circumorally and in the hands and feet. The muscle cramps are non-specific, painful, and usually in hand, calf, foot, abdominal, or back muscles. Paresthesias and cramps may be intermittent or persistent and often are precipitated by exercise, hyperventilation, or stress. Unless hypocalcemia is considered, these symptoms are easily disregarded, particularly in elderly persons in whom paresthesias and nocturnal muscle cramps are common.

Tetany, the hallmark of hypocalcemia, occurs relatively rapidly after an acute hypocalcemic stimulus (e.g., parathyroidectomy); however, it also can occur intermittently in patients with a sustained chronic hypocalcemia. Tetany consists of severe muscle cramping, may include seizures, and is precipitated by exercise and stress, as well as by hyperventilation or other causes of alkalosis that further lower ionized calcium levels.

Neuromuscular irritability in hypocalcemia may produce Chvostek's sign, which is a contraction of facial and circumoral muscles in response to tapping the facial nerve in the preauricular area; it also may produce Trousseau's sign, which is elicited by the application of an arm blood pressure cuff at 10–20 mm Hg above systolic pressure for at least 3 minutes. The appearance of carpal and metacarpal flexion with an interphalanged extension and digital abduction constitutes a positive response.

Other manifestations of hypocalcemia include cardiac conduction abnormalities (a lengthening of the QT interval, congestive heart failure, and so on) and, with chronic hypocalcemia, subcapsular cataracts and basal ganglia calcification.

Hypoparathyroidism

The most common cause of hypocalcemia is functional hypoparathyroidism, which can be a result of several processes (see Table 28-3).[23] As previously discussed, PTH plays an integral role in the maintenance of serum calcium and phosphorus levels. In view of its actions, hypoparathyroidism predictably is characterized by hypocalcemia and hyperphosphatemia. Because of the trophic effects of PTH on renal 25(OH)D hydroxylation, hypoparathyroidism is accompanied by low levels of 1,25(OH)$_2$D and an impaired gastrointestinal calcium absorption.

TABLE 28-3   Major Causes of Hypoparathyroidism

Postoperative hypocalcemia and hypopara-
   thyroidism
Idiopathic hypoparathyroidism
   Isolated
   Associated with atrophic polyendocrine failure
Other acquired forms of functional hypoparathy-
   roidism
   Non-surgical parathyroid damage
   Parathyroid infiltration
   Hypomagnesemia
Pseudohypoparathyroidism

Partial or complete parathyroid destruction usually occurs as a result of a surgical procedure (thyroidectomy, parathyroidectomy), but it occasionally may follow radiation exposure (^{131}I therapy), iron deposition in hemochromatosis, or a metastatic disease. A postsurgical hypoparathyroidism may be transient (parathyroid insult) or permanent and may develop immediately after surgery or in the subsequent months.

Idiopathic hypoparathyroidism is an uncommon variety of parathyroid failure that is unassociated with any obvious insult. Although usually first apparent in childhood, it may be present in adults. Parathyroid antibodies are present in a fraction of affected patients, and parathyroid failure may be accompanied by the failure of other endocrine organs as well (pancreatic islets, thyroid gland, adrenal glands, gonads), presumably on an autoimmune basis. Mucocutaneous moniliasis is present in some affected individuals.

Magnesium depletion has been increasingly appreciated as a common cause of hypocalcemia, particularly in hospitalized patients. Parathyroid function is dependent on an adequate magnesium availability; therefore, hypomagnesemia induces a state of functional hypoparathyroidism. In vivo and in vitro studies have shown that the primary mechanism by which magnesium depletion causes hypocalcemia is an inhibition of PTH secretion. Hypocalcemic hypomagnesemic patients, therefore, are characterized by hyperphosphatemia and low PTH levels. Malnutrition, alcoholism, diuretic use, and renal disease are the most common contributing processes toward hypomagnesemia. Geriatric patients in whom these conditions exist are, thus, particularly susceptible to magnesium depletion. This syndrome may occur when serum magnesium concentrations are less than 1.8 mg/dl; but, it is most common when concentrations are less than 1 mg/dl, with a more severe magnesium depletion resulting in a more dramatic hypocalcemia. Since hypomagnesemia causes neuromuscular symptoms that are quite similar to those of hypocalcemia (tetany, seizures), they may be exacerbated when the two occur simultaneously. With magnesium repletion, PTH secretion is rapidly restored, and serum calcium concentrations should be restored to normal within days.

Pseudohypoparathyroidism

Pseudohypoparathyroidism is a heterogenous disorder characterized by partial or complete end-organ resistance to the action of parathyroid hormone. PTH secretion is appropriate and thus PTH levels are normal or high. Approximately half the number of cases are familial, and it may be first noted in adulthood, although most cases are diagnosed in childhood.

Other Causes of Hypocalcemia
These include: 1) Acute pancreatitis, in which hypocalcemia may be severe. It has been ascribed to the deposition of calcium within the pancreatic bed, to pancreatic endocrine effects, or to an inhibition of PTH secretion; 2) Some forms of malignancy that are associated with abnormalities in Vitamin D metabolism; 3) Medications, including mithramycin, citrated blood in large quantities, and phosphates; 4) End-stage renal insufficiency that causes an impaired production of $1,25(OH)_2D$ is commonly associated with hypocalcemia and hyperphosphatemia; 5) Finally, a Vitamin D deficiency of any cause may be associated with hypocalcemia.

Evaluation
In any patient with low serum calcium levels, consideration must be given to protein-binding abnormalities (specifically hypoalbuminemia) as a cause of spuriously low, total calcium concentrations with normal ionized calcium levels. A measurement of serum magnesium levels is important in view of the frequency of hypomag-

nesemia and its simple correction. In patients with hyperphosphatemia or a history of neck surgery, hypoparathyroidism should be considered. It can be documented by demonstrating inappropriately low PTH and urinary cAMP concentrations in the presence of hypocalcemia. Pseudohypoparathyroidism is characterized by ineffectively high PTH levels; when suspected, it can be inferred from low levels of urinary cAMP.

Therapy
The treatment of hypocalcemia depends on its severity and etiology. Acute hypocalcemia is a medical emergency when accompanied by tetany, seizures, or cardiac conduction abnormalities, and it must be treated aggressively to restore normal calcium concentrations regardless of the primary pathophysiology. Intravenous calcium is available in several forms (calcium chloride, 272 mg of elemental calcium per 10 ml; calcium gluconate, 97 mg of elemental calcium per 10 ml) and should be rapidly administered (over 15 min) in 200–400 mg doses when a rapid correction of hypocalcemia is necessary. In view of the large distribution volume for IV-administered calcium (the extracellular space), these doses will only transiently elevate serum concentrations. Repeated administrations may be necessary until the primary abnormality is corrected. It is more effective to use an initial bolus as described above, followed by a constant IV infusion of a calcium-containing solution (1 gram of elemental calcium in 500–1,000 ml) that is titrated to maintain a low-to-normal serum calcium level until more definitive measures are successfully instituted. During this period, the cause of the hypocalcemia should be sought and specific treatment begun (magnesium replacement, Vitamin D, and so on). A less severe hypocalcemia that is unassociated with significant signs or symptoms, frequently can be treated with oral calcium supplementation alone (1–2 grams/day of elemental calcium).

The therapy for chronic hypocalcemia obviously should be directed toward the primary defect (e.g., replenishing magnesium, treatment of pancreatitis, renal failure, or malignancy). Vitamin D repletion in a Vitamin D deficiency is now more easily and rapidly achieved than ever before with the availability of 25(OH)D and

$1,25(OH)_2D.$[24] No practical method exists for administering PTH. Therefore, a control of hypocalcemia in hypoparathyroidism (to maintain serum calcium levels of 8.5–9.0 mg/dl) must be achieved with oral calcium and Vitamin D therapy. Mild forms of hypoparathyroidism may be successfully treated with oral calcium supplementation alone (1–2 grams/day of elemental calcium), but most patients require Vitamin D supplementation as well.

Vitamin D is available as either cholecalciferol (D_3) or ergocalciferol (D_2); they are of equivalent potencies. Doses for hypoparathyroidism average 25,000–100,000 units/day, although occasional higher doses are required. In addition, dihydrotachysterol, which is a derivative of ergosterol with a Vitamin D-like activity, can be useful; commonly, in doses of 0.5–1.0 mg/day. More recently, 25(OH)D has become available and apparently is effective at 50–200 μg/day. The most useful drug for hypoparathyroidism is $1,25(OH)_2D$, which virtually is uniformly effective in doses of 0.5–2.0 μg/day. Although more expensive than other forms, $1,25(OH)_2D$ has the distinct advantages of being rapidly effective (onset of action, 24–48 hours) and easily withdrawn if hypercalcemia occurs. Hypercalcemia is a common and somewhat unpredictable consequence of the supraphysiologic doses of Vitamin D that are used in the treatment of hypoparathyroidism. Whereas D_3 and D_2 are extensively stored in adipose tissue (thus, hypercalcemia dissipates slowly when due to intoxication with these agents), 1,25(OH)D is not particularly stored in fat. Thus, its effects are rapidly reversible (within 2–5 days). When using any form of Vitamin D, serum calcium levels frequently should be checked during the institution of therapy and intermittently checked when a stable regimen is achieved. Finally, in the absence of the renal tubular effects of PTH, urinary calcium excretion may be massive in hypoparathyroid patients who are treated with calcium and Vitamin D, which leaves them at risk for nephrolithiasis. This is particularly true with higher serum calcium concentrations, and levels should be kept on the low side of normal (8.5–9.0 mg/dl). Thiazide diuretics, as previously discussed, have calcemic actions and have been suggested to be useful in the treatment of hypoparathyroidism.

Metabolic Bone Disease

Bone metabolism is a complex phenomenon that is dependent on a variety of local and systemic influences. Because metabolic bone disorders result from alterations in metabolic functions, they usually affect the skeleton in its entirety. The major forms of metabolic bone disease are manifested by a decrease in mineralized bone mass, or osteopenia.

There are two basic types of mature bone: 1) Cortical (compact) bone, which makes up the shafts of long bones and the cortex of other bones; and 2) Trabecular (cancellous) bone, which is found in flat bones and vertebrae. Bone is a metabolically active organ, with the major metabolic functions served by specialized bone cells: osteoclasts, osteoblasts, and osteocytes. Bone resorption is accomplished by osteoclasts, while osteoblasts form new bone matter to replace that removed by osteoclasts. In the process of new bone formation, some osteoblasts become encased within bone to become osteocytes. These remain within osteocytic lacunae in communication both with one another and the systemic circulation, perhaps to participate in the rapid release of minerals on appropriate stimulation. Bone remodeling by osteoclasts and osteoblasts is a continuous process by which old bone is resorbed and replaced by new bone, thus allowing bone to change in size and shape and providing for bone mineral turnover. Bone remodeling is most active in trabecular bone, which has a tremendous surface area, but it occurs in cortical bone as well. Normal bone remodeling accomplishes the orderly and complete replacement of resorbed old bone with lamellar new bone. In an average adult, it affects the turnover of about 10–15% of the skeleton per year. A fundamental concept in bone remodeling is coupling, which is the highly coordinated relationship between osteoclastic bone resorption and osteoblastic new bone formation. If coupling is disrupted and bone resorption exceeds bone formation, bone mass will decline. "Uncoupling," therefore, refers to a disruption in the relationship between osteoclastic and osteoblastic functions and is the basic defect that leads to most forms of metabolic bone disease.

There are several systemic influences on the rate and nature of remodeling and, hence, on

TABLE 28-4 Major Factors
that Influence Bone
Metabolism

Age
Activity/weight bearing
Mineral concentrations
Vitamin D activity
Parathyroid hormone (PTH)
Sex steroids
Thyroid hormones
Glucocorticoids
Growth hormone

the resulting bone structure and mass (*see* Table 28-4). Skeletal maturity, or the attainment of maximum bone mass, occurs at approximately 30 years of age. There is a strong genetic component. Black persons have a greater bone mass than white persons, and maximum bone mass is greater in males than in females. These differences result in lower fracture rates in males and in blacks. The development of an optimum bone mass at maturity is somewhat dependent on dietary elements, with evidence suggesting that individuals in areas of higher calcium and fluoride intake may have more bone mass and a lower incidence of fractures in later life than in other geographic regions. Physical activity affects bone mass and inactivity is detrimental to the maintenance of skeletal integrity. An increase in bone mass has been noted in marathon runners and in those selected areas of the skeleton that are most frequently exercised in tennis players, weight lifters, and ballet dancers. Finally, humoral factors strongly affect bone metabolism and may greatly influence the rate of change of bone mass.

Changes in Bone with Aging

In all races, cultures, and geographic areas, bone mass and bone density increase during childhood and adolescence, are relatively stable during the 3rd decade, and gradually decline thereafter. The loss of bone mass that is associated with aging has been termed "physiologic osteopenia," or when clinically apparent, "senile osteoporosis." Its etiology is multifactorial. Although some responsible factors have been identified, it remains a poorly understood process.

Females lose bone mass more rapidly than males and at an earlier age.[25] Studies show a linear decline in bone density with age in both males and females, with an acceleration of loss in females between 50–70 years of age. This probably corresponds to the endocrine alterations of menopause. The bone mass remaining in elderly persons of both sexes, after years of gradual loss, depends on the skeletal mass at maturity, which is when physiologic bone rarefraction begins. Thus, females, because they begin the process of age-related bone loss with a lower bone density, more frequently become sufficiently osteopenic to fracture than males. Similarly, white persons are more often affected by a clinically significant osteopenia than are black persons.

Whereas the bone loss of aging occurs throughout the skeleton, the rate of loss is clearly non-uniform; it proceeds more rapidly in some areas than others. After middle age (there is a considerable variation between individuals), cortical bone mass is lost at an average rate of 8–10% per decade in females and 3–5% per decade in males. Cortical bone loss primarily is due to an increase in endosteal resorption without a simultaneous periosteal bone apposition, which results in a widening medullary space. Trabecular bone loss begins somewhat earlier than cortical loss. It may proceed more rapidly, perhaps because bone remodeling generally is more active in trabecular bone. For instance, in one study using vertebral dual photon absorptiometry as an index of trabecular bone mass, vertebral density in females fell by 47% between ages 20–80. In the same subjects, cortical bone mass, (assessed by radial photon absorptiometry) fell by only 30%.[26] In males, the decline was much less at either site. In similar studies of iliac crest bone biopsy specimens, trabecular bone volume declined with age in both females (40% decline between ages 20–80) and males (30% decline). The apparent predilection for an age-related loss in trabecular rather than in cortical bone has important consequences in that fractures observed in the geriatric population are more common in the axial skeleton (vertebrae, hip), which is predominantly trabecular, than in the mainly cortical appendicular skeleton.

Physiologic osteopenia results from an uncoupling of the relationship between osteoclastic bone resorption and osteoblastic new bone formation; but, it has been difficult to identify the cellular nature of that defect. Several abnormalities in the function of osteoclasts or osteoblasts, or both, could result in an uncoupling defect and a gradual bone loss. The systematic evaluation of iliac crest bone biopsy specimens using histomorphometric techniques suggests a continued, and perhaps increased, rate of osteoclastic bone resorption in the face of a static or somewhat depressed rate of osteoblastic new bone formation. Poorly defined, age-related changes that affect an elderly patient may be compounded by other factors, which further increase the development rate of a clinically significant osteopenia. The presumed decrease in physical activity that accompanies aging may have a negative impact on bone density. In fact, lean body mass (a rough index of activity) decreases with age in both males and females.[27] Renal function, as assessed by renal blood flow and the GFR, declines progressively after the 3rd decade. Several investigators have suggested that secondary hyperparathyroidism and changes in phosphorus and Vitamin D metabolism, which accompany changes in renal function, may play a part in the pathophysiology of age-related bone loss. Of potential etiologic importance to the age-related decline in renal function may be the relatively high protein intakes that are characteristic of modern cultures. Another effect of increased dietary protein intake is an increase in urinary calcium excretion, which possibly is due either to the titration by bone mineral of the increased fixed-acid production induced by dietary protein or to a direct effect of acid or dietary protein on renal tubular calcium reabsorption. High-protein diets have the capability of inducing a negative calcium balance, even in the presence of adequate dietary calcium; thus, they may well contribute to a progressive bone loss by affecting calcium dynamics directly, as well as indirectly, via their effects on renal function.[28]

Dietary calcium intake is a major concern in the etiology of age-related osteopenia. Although it frequently is stated that geriatric populations ingest inadequate amounts of dietary calcium, and that males and females decrease their intakes of calcium with aging, this has been adequately studied only in females. Mid-dle-aged and elderly females frequently have a negative calcium balance[29], to a small extent when considered on a daily basis but to a sufficient extent over the long term to account for a large part of age-related bone loss. The RDA for dietary calcium has been placed at 800 mg/day. In premenopausal females, however, a positive calcium balance is achieved only with an average intake of 1,000 mg/day.[29] In postmenopausal females who are untreated with estrogen, 1,500 mg/day is necessary. Dietary surveys indicate that, on the average, elderly females consume less than 50% of that amount, which clearly raises the possibility of a nutritional calcium deficiency as an important factor in physiologic osteopenia. In patients with lactose intolerance, calcium intake is low and osteopenia appears more commonly. In addition, considerable evidence indicates that gastrointestinal calcium absorption decreases with age, and that the ability to compensate for a low dietary calcium intake by increasing fractional gastrointestinal absorption is lost in elderly persons. Hence, whereas a young person may maintain calcium balance during a low-calcium diet, an older individual cannot. Recent studies show that the ability to synthesize $1,25(OH)_2$ is impaired in old age. Not only are $1,25(OH)_2D$ levels lower,[30] but provocative maneuvers fail to stimulate $1,25(OH)_2D$ synthesis.[31] When elderly subjects are given $1,25(OH)_2D$ orally, their ability to absorb dietary calcium is normalized, thus incriminating a defect in renal $1,25(OH)D$ production. The observations that dietary calcium intake is low, and that the situation is exacerbated by impairments in Vitamin D metabolism and (in females) menopause, obviously indicate the potential importance of calcium nutrition in the development of physiologic osteopenia. Conversely, epidemiologic studies of correlations between calcium intake and bone density have yielded mixed results. This apparent inconsistency may relate to methodologic difficulties in performing accurate dietary surveys; more likely, however, it reinforces the multifactorial nature of physiologic osteopenia. Finally, some elements in modern diets are particularly rich in phosphates, which raises a concern that a particularly low dietary calcium/phosphate ratio may decrease calcium absorption and/or increase urinary calcium excretion. This aggravates the tendency toward a negative calcium balance. While drastic increases in phosphate intake adversely affect the calcium balance and bone metabolism, clinical studies have failed to support the presumption that modern diets contain detrimentally high phosphate concentrations.[32] Similarly, diets that are low in phosphorus do not appear to increase the risk of osteoporosis, although they may contribute to the development of osteomalacia.

Other humoral substances appear to play a role in the process of bone loss. Menopause is an important event in the evolution of bone mass in females. Bone density falls more rapidly during menopause, but there appears to be a coincidental and dramatic increase in dietary calcium requirements as well. These phenomena have been ascribed, in part, to the effects of estrogen on bone metabolism and Vitamin D physiology. The administration of estrogen to postmenopausal females results in an increase in calcium absorption and an improvement in calcium balance. Recent studies of Vitamin D physiology suggest that the calcium balance improves with estrogen administration because of a stimulation of $1,25(OH)_2D$ synthesis and the resultant effects on gastrointestinal calcium absorption.[33] The mechanism is obscure, but it apparently is not a direct effect of estrogen on the renal Vitamin D hydroxylation system. In addition, estrogen may modulate bone metabolism more directly. There is evidence that bone resorption increases after menopause and that estrogen administration inhibits the resorption. Although efforts to demonstrate estrogen receptors in bone have not been successful, it is possible that estrogen may directly inhibit bone resorption or the response of bone to the stimuli of resorption, such as PTH. Certainly, the effects of estrogens in therapy for postmenopausal osteoporosis appears to be beneficial, not withstanding an incomplete understanding of the mechanisms involved.

Normal males do not experience any dramatic change in sex steroid concentrations similar to that in females at menopause, but the evidence suggests a slow decline in gonadal function with age in males. The effects of a decline in testosterone on the calcium dynamics in males have not been well studied. However, they are presumed to play a role in males similar to that of estrogens in females, particularly in view of the well-described osteopenia seen in hypogonadal males.

Other calcium-regulating hormones change with age and may play a role in physiologic osteopenia. Some studies indicate small increases in PTH levels with aging; a trend that may contribute to the increase in bone resorption.[34] Presently, the role of PTH in the age-related decline of bone mass remains controversial. Calcitonin concentrations decline with age. Because calcitonin inhibits the osteoclastic function, the diminution of its effects may contribute to increased bone resorption with advancing age.[12] Interestingly, estrogen administration recently has been demonstrated to increase calcitonin levels in postmenopausal females, which further stimulates interest in the role of calcitonin in this context.[34]

Osteoporosis

Of all metabolic bone disorders, osteoporosis is the most common in elderly persons. The toll exacted by osteoporosis in the geriatric population is huge, both in terms of individual suffering and the medical resources devoted to its consequences. It is tragic that many forms of osteoporosis are probably preventable if risks are recognized early; but, when established, the disorder is virtually incorrectable. Osteoporosis is defined as a state in which the volume of mineralized bone is inappropriately low for a patient's age, sex, and race, and in which there is no impairment of the mineralization process. Therefore, it must be differentiated from osteomalacia, which is another form of osteopenia where mineralized bone mass is reduced as a result of a defect in mineralization. In fact, osteoporosis is not a disease in itself, but rather a syndrome that may be the result of a variety of processes.

Clinical Characteristics

The development of osteoporosis is gradual, and it is difficult to date the onset of its process. Unlike osteomalacia, osteoporosis rarely causes diffuse bony pain or tenderness. Most patients are asymptomatic until a fracture occurs. Some patients remain without symptoms even after vertebral fractures are radiographically apparent. Most commonly, fractures involve the vertebrae, femoral neck, or distal radius, because these areas bear the brunt of trauma inflicted by weight-bearing and falls. Vertebral fractures present as a pain or deformity, or both. At the time of a fracture, patients may experience sharp severe pain that is localized to the area of the vertebrae, perhaps with an anterior radiation into the chest, abdomen, pelvis, or legs. Movement greatly exacerbates the pain. After days to weeks of pain, relief gradually occurs, presumably as the fracture heals. Alternatively, back pain may be chronic, dull, and midline or paravertebral in character without any obviously inciting event. Paraspinus muscle spasm frequently is demonstrable on a physical examination and may contribute to discomfort. Back pain that is due to vertebral fractures may be intermittent with substantial pain-free intervals. Persistent pain, however, is not uncommon and is frequently aggravated by a degenerative arthritis, which is intensified by the alterations in spinal articulations that are induced by vertebral distortion. Despite an impressive vertebral deformity, there rarely is a direct involvement of spinal nerves.

Spinal fractures may result in a height loss of several inches. In severely afflicted patients, a prominent source of discomfort may be the approximation of the lower ribs with the iliac crest. Dorsal kyphosis ("Dowager's hump") commonly accompanies anterior vertebral crush fractures. A particularly severe fracture may result in a prominent angulation of the spine at that spot.

Osteoporosis represents a major risk factor that contributes to the high incidence of hip fractures in the geriatric population. The rate of hip fractures rises dramatically after 65 years of age, and the complications of the attendant surgery and convalescence result in a mortality rate of at least 10%. The rate of Colle's fractures increases remarkably in elderly persons, but those fractures have less dangerous complications. Females are more commonly affected by serious fractures than males, which reflects the greater rate of osteoporosis in females.

Laboratory testing may be helpful in the search for the pathophysiology of osteoporosis, but there are no characteristic laboratory alterations that are associated with the disorder itself. Unless osteoporosis is present in the context of a specific disorder (hyperparathyroidism, thyrotoxicosis, malignancy, and so on), the serum calcium and phosphorus concentrations are normal. Similarly, the urinary excretion of calcium, phosphorus, and hydroxyproline are not discernible from normal, although immobilization may tend to elevate the urinary calcium excretion if the collection is performed when a patient is hospitalized. Unless an acute fracture has occurred, the alkaline phosphatase level should not be elevated. An increase in alkaline phosphatase suggests osteomalacia or an associated disorder (hyperparathyroidism, thyrotoxicosis, Cushing's Syndrome, and so on). The PTH levels are not abnormal unless there is a coincident stimulus of parathyroid secretion. Similarly, $1,25(OH)_2D$ levels may be low in cases of age-related osteopenia, but there is no clinical use for its measurement in the routine evaluation of the osteoporotic patient. Thus, a diagnosis of osteoporosis is not made on chemical grounds, but laboratory procedures may be useful in the search for a cause.

Radiology

A diagnosis of osteopenia is usually made based on radiographic evidence, but a clinician must be cautious in making the more specific diagnosis of osteoporosis. There are radiographic findings that strongly suggest osteoporosis as the etiology of osteopenia, but none are pathognomonic and none exclude the concomitant presence of other disorders, particularly osteomalacia.

Routine x-ray films are relatively insensitive. It is difficult for even an experienced evaluator to confidently distinguish osteopenia before approximately 30% of the bone mass is lost. Not only is a substantial initial bone loss required before osteopenia is detectable radiographically, but there must be a 5–10% further reduction in bone mass for the change to be clearly documented via these methods. When significant osteopenia has developed, several changes are characteristic of osteoporosis. As osteoporosis progresses in the vertebrae, the horizontal trabeculae in the vertebral bodies are lost because they participate little in weight-bearing; therefore, vertical trabeculae appear more prominent. The vertebral end-plates may appear dense for two reasons: 1) In contrast to the osteopenic vertebral body that has lost considerable amounts of trabecular bone, the cortex may be relatively spared; and 2) As weight-bearing and minor trauma continue, the weakened vertebrae begins to sustain micro-fractures in the region of the end-plates, and a compression and compaction of osteopenic bone creates radiodense zones. As compression worsens, end-plates become concave and intervertebral discs become ballooned, which results in codfish vertebrae (*see* Figure 28-2). Occasionally, the nucleus pulposis may actually break through the weakened end-plate and herniate into the osteopenic vertebral body, thus resulting in the mushroom-shaped Schmorl's node (*see* Figure 28-3). Eventually, a frank compression of the body occurs. Usually, only the anterior portion is involved (wedge fracture), since that area bears the brunt of weight-lifting; but, the entire vertebral body may be compressed to a fraction of its former

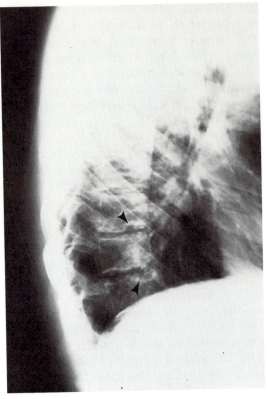

FIGURE 28-3   X-ray film of a 54-year-old patient with osteoporosis and Schmorl's nodes (arrows).

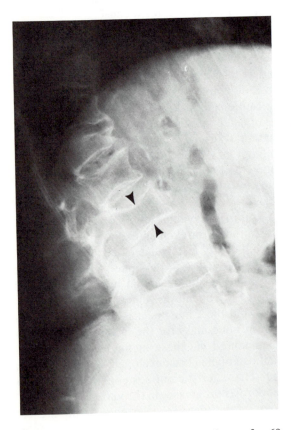

FIGURE 28-2   X-ray film of the vertebrae of a 60-year-old patient with postmenopausal osteoporosis that shows a codfish deformity of the vertebral end-plate (arrows).

size (*see* Figure 28-4). The lower thoracic and upper lumbar vertebrae are most commonly involved, although any area may be affected. Osteomalacia may cause similar changes of biconcavity and fracture, but rarely causes Schmorl's nodes.

The peripheral skeleton also is involved in osteoporosis. A process that is comparable to the one occurring in the vertebral body also affects the proximal femur; non-weight-bearing trabeculae are lost early, which results in an apparent accentuation of trabeculae that do bear weight. These changes of osteoporosis in the upper femur are characteristic and form the basis of the Singh index—a method of quantitating the severity of the disorder. As osteoporosis advances, only the most prominent trabeculae are spared, which results in a relatively consistent x-ray pattern. In long bones, osteoporosis results in a cortical thinning and expansion of the medullary space. These changes (particularly in the metacarpals) form the basis for methods of quantitation of bone

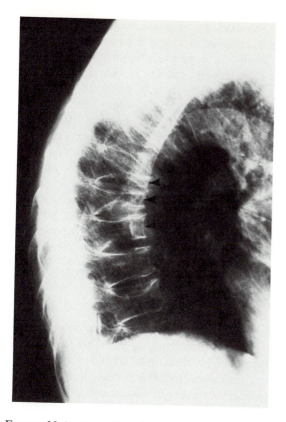

FIGURE 28-4 X-ray film of a 71-year-old female with osteoporosis and crush fractures of the thoracic vertebrae (arrows). Several of the fractures have resulted in a nearly complete vertebral collapse.

loss, which unfortunately are also relatively insensitive.

More sophisticated x-ray methods that were developed to quantitate the degree of bone loss involve the interpretation of x-ray films taken in the presence of a wedge of standard density (so bone density can be assessed more reliably) or methods such as radial photon absorptiometry, in which a penetrance of a collumated beam of photons through the radius is quantitated. This technique is more sensitive than x-ray techniques, since it is capable of detecting 2–3% changes in radial bone density. There is a relatively good correlation between radial density and vertebral x-ray changes. However, to an even greater extent than x-ray techniques, radial photon absorptiometry is a non-specific index of osteopenia (i.e., it is not capable of differentiating between the various causes of bone loss such as osteoporosis, osteomalacia, and so on). The technique of photon absorptiometry

has been refined to allow the use of two photon sources (dual photon absorptiometry), which helps to eliminate soft tissue artifacts and allows the quantitation of vertebral density. Similarly, a computed tomography (CT scan) is being used to quantitate vertebral density. Each of these techniques holds promise as methods that permit sensitive and specific measurements of vertebral bone loss.

Bone Biopsy Procedures and Analysis

Recent developments in procedures used to obtain and analyze bone specimens have increased the use of bone biopsy procedures in the evaluation of metabolic bone disorders. An outpatient percutaneous needle biopsy procedure safely provides a core of bone from near the anterior superior iliac spine; and analysis of the uncalcified specimen may provide a greater understanding of bone remodeling.[35] A bone biopsy analysis includes an estimation of the rate of bone mineralization by using tetracycline antibiotics, which are incorporated into bone as it is mineralized and are fluorescent under ultraviolet light. If a patient is given a 2–3-day course of tetracycline, a linear band of fluorescence is seen at the bone surface, which reflects the mineralization that was occuring during tetracycline administration. If a second 2–3-day course of tetracycline is administered, two bands of fluorescence should be discernible. The distance between the bands is the amount of new bone that was formed during the interval between the two courses of tetracycline. This measurement is critical when considering a diagnosis of osteomalacia, in which the primary defect is one of mineralization and the distance between the bands is reduced or non-existent. A bone biopsy procedure is the most powerful tool presently available to distinguish osteomalacia from osteoporosis.

Classification

Osteoporosis is not a final diagnosis, but rather a condition that is the result of a more fundamental process. There are multiple causes of osteoporosis (see Table 28-5), and each should be considered in evaluating an osteopenic patient. It is common that more than one risk factor will be present.

TABLE 28-5 Major Causes
of Osteoporosis

Aging
Hypogonadism
Hyperparathyroidism
Hyperthyroidism
Cushing's Syndrome
Malignancy
Immobilization
Hepatic insufficiency
Postgastrectomy
Rheumatoid arthritis
Acromegaly
Chronic pulmonary disease
Heparin therapy

Senile Osteoporosis

Bone loss is a universal concomitant of aging, and it is probably a multifactorial process. Approximately 25% of all older females and a smaller fraction of older males have clinically important osteoporosis. A major determinant may be the bone mass that is acquired at maturity; persons with a greater mass at 30 years of age would be protected from the occurrence of significant osteopenia, whereas persons who achieve a lesser bone mass at maturity would be at greater risk. Alternatively, the degree of osteopenia that is present in old age may represent the summation of events encountered during one's life that are detrimental to the skeleton.[36] Thus, persons more frequently exposed to factors that adversely affect bone, such as high dietary protein or acid content, alcohol, tobacco, glucocorticoids, periods of immobilization, gastrectomy, and others[27] would be at a higher risk.

Hypogonadism (Estrogen or Testosterone Deficiency)

The most common hypogonadal state is that found in a postmenopausal female. It generally is accepted that there is an acceleration in the rate of bone loss in the immediate (5–10 years) postmenopausal period. Evidence suggests that the rate of bone loss stabilizes once again thereafter at a rate similar to the rate seen in males or premenopausal females. Premature menopause and an estrogen deficiency due to any cause at any age result in an acceleration in the rate of bone loss that is similar to the one seen at menopause.

The etiology of postmenopausal osteoporosis is multifactorial and depends on changes in calcium and bone metabolism that are caused by an estrogen deficiency, as well as on other factors that contribute to physiologic osteopenia (a dietary calcium deficiency, decreased activity, and so on). Biochemical parameters (urine calcium and hydroxyproline excretion) suggest that bone resorption is a prominent feature, but histomorphometric studies of postmenopausal osteoporosis reveal no consistent pattern of either an increased bone resorption or a decreased bone formation. At present, then, we are left with uncertainty concerning the pathophysiology of postmenopausal osteoporosis.

Therapy for Senile and Postmenopausal Osteoporosis

The prevention of and therapy for osteoporosis is imperfect and controversial. In theory, the treatment of osteoporosis should be effected by using measures that will increase bone mass. In practice, however, this has been a difficult objective to achieve. There are no clearly effective means of inducing a progressive and sustained increase in bone density once a significant loss has occurred in patients with senile osteoporosis. Consequently, the prevention of bone loss is a more promising and realistic goal than the restoration of depleted bone mineral stores.

The importance of weight-bearing in the maintenance of a healthy bone function has been mentioned. While it is well recognized that skeletal immobilization results in an accelerated loss of bone minerals, there is little information regarding the role of exercise and physical activity in human skeletal health. An exercise program of light-to-moderate calisthenics performed three times per week for 1 year decreased the rate of bone mineral loss and increased the calcium balance in two studies.[37,38] Whether one particular form of weight-bearing exercise is more helpful than another or whether any form of exercise decreases the probability or incidence of fractures are questions that have not been answered.

The maintenance of an adequate calcium intake is a basic part of a program to minimize the development of osteoporosis. The effects of an inadequate calcium intake and a decreased efficiency of calcium absorption result in the negative calcium balance that is observed in the majority of postmenopausal females and, presumably, in most elderly males. Calcium supplementation substantially decreases the loss of bone minerals that are measured via bone densitometry or radiogrammetry,[39,40] and it may decrease the likelihood of vertebral compression fractures. Furthermore, the incidence rate of fractures of the proximal femur was higher among elderly residents of a Yugoslavian village where the calcium intake was low when compared to people with a higher calcium diet who lived in another village in the same country.[41] Therefore, providing a total calcium intake of 1,500 mg/day is a reasonable objective for geriatric patients. To accomplish this via dietary means alone requires an increased intake of dairy products with an associated increase in calories and protein, and it frequently is not tolerated by elderly patients. Supplementing the diet with 1,000–1,200 mg/day of elemental calcium is readily achieved with a variety of inexpensive calcium-containing preparations and is associated with minimal complications. In the absence of pre-existing hypercalciuria, these doses of calcium have little effect on renal calcium exertion. Serum and urinary calcium levels should be monitored in patients receiving a calcium supplementation who also receive thiazide diuretics or have an underlying renal disease.

The role of routine Vitamin D supplementation has been less extensively studied. Providing 400 units/day of Vitamin D in the form of a multiple vitamin tablet is both reasonable and safe. Larger doses of Vitamin D have not been useful, except in patients with malabsorption or other abnormalities of Vitamin D metabolism. Because of the risks of hypercalciuria and hypercalcemia, larger doses of Vitamin D are not used routinely as an osteopenic prophylaxis and should not be used unless serum and urine calcium concentrations are carefully monitored.

The use of estrogen therapy in a postmenopausal female continues to be controversial due to uncertainties regarding the potential toxicity of prolonged estrogen use. Recently, several retrospective studies have strongly suggested that estrogen replacement considerably decreases the risk of fractures of the hip and forearm.[42,43] Similar studies demonstrated a protective effect of estrogen on the occurrence of vertebral fractures.[44,45] Direct measurements of bone density using a variety of techniques support these population studies and demonstrate a clear retardation, if not cessation, of bone loss in groups of estrogen-treated females.[39,40,44–48] By most histomorphometric and biochemical parameters, the mechanism involved appears to be an inhibition of bone resorption. This is more likely to be due to an inhibition of PTH-mediated bone resorption by estrogen (possibly mediated by an increase in gastrointestinal calcium absorption) than to a direct effect of estrogen on osteoclastic activity. Although occasional studies suggest a small increase in bone mass with estrogen therapy, this is not a consistent finding.

The timing of estrogen therapy in relation to menopause may be important.[46] Some studies suggest that the initial phase of rapid bone loss that occurs during the first few years following menopause or an oophorectomy can be ameliorated with estrogen therapy, whereas bone loss that occurs several years later is less responsive to estrogen. These findings suggest to some investigators that the most important period for estrogen supplementation is during menopause and the first few years that follow. However, a discontinuation of estrogen therapy that is begun at the time of menopause results in accelerated bone loss, which mimics the bone loss that follows spontaneous menopause or oophorectomy; it also results in a rapid loss of any advantage in bone mass that estrogen supplementation had provided.[49] Thus, it appears that the effect of estrogen on the skeletal mass persists only as long as therapy is continued. The minimal effective dose of conjugated estrogen to prevent bone loss is 0.625 mg per day.[50]

The studies that have compared estrogen and calcium therapy generally demonstrate that estrogen is somewhat more effective than calcium in minimizing a bone density loss.[39,40] In these studies, though, the women may have had a negative calcium balance with both the estrogen and calcium regimens that were used. Whether estrogen therapy is clearly superior to calcium supplementation, and whether the effects of the two forms of therapy are additive, have not been resolved.

The enthusiasm generated by the demonstration that estrogen therapy curtails bone loss is muted to some extent by concern regarding the potential risks of long-term estrogen therapy.[51] The association of endometrial carcinoma with estrogen use has been reported in several studies.[52,53] Although uterine carcinoma that is associated with estrogen use is curable, if diagnosed and treated appropriately, the risk to the patient exists nevertheless. The incidence rate of endometrial hyperplasia and, perhaps, of endometrial carcinoma can be decreased by the cyclic administration of estrogen and a progestational agent, which recapitulates the normal pattern of endometrial proliferation and regression.[54,55] This regimen may result in cyclic withdrawal bleeding, is sometimes not well tolerated by postmenopausal women, and does not obviate the need for careful follow-up.

The data regarding the influence of estrogen therapy on the incidence rate of breast carcinoma is much less clear. While some case-control studies suggest an increased rate of breast cancer that is associated with estrogen use in females with a fibrocystic disease or who have not undergone an oophorectomy, more study is required before the true nature of this possible association is clarified.[56,57]

Given the incomplete data base on which decisions rest with regard to postmenopausal estrogen use, no general recommendations can be made. Estrogen prophylaxis should not be universally recommended nor summarily discounted. The decision must be discussed and made in conjunction with each patient, while considering all aspects of her situation. Perhaps some groups of women at high risk for developing osteoporosis eventually can be identified, as well as those in whom the benefits of estrogen prophylaxis clearly outweigh the potential complications of therapy.

Calcium supplementation and an exercise program form the basis of any regimen of osteopenic prophylaxis. Females who continue to experience a rapid bone loss despite adequate calcium intake and exercise may, in the future, be readily identified via photon densitometry or new measures of bone density and, thus, singled out for a further evaluation and more vigorous management.

Other forms of therapy are being evaluated. Sodium fluoride has long held a promise in the therapy for osteoporosis, and recent studies continue to support a possible role for its use.[58]

As with estrogens, the toxic effects must be considered; further trials are necessary to clearly define its role. Newer regimens with calcitonin, PTH, or cyclical ("pulse") therapies are being evaluated. Cholecalciferol has been uniformly unhelpful and potentially disadvantageous in postmenopausal osteoporosis. However, newer metabolites, particularly 25(OH)D, 24,25(OH)$_2$D, and 1,25(OH)$_2$D, are being studied.

Corticosteroid-induced Osteopenia

Cushing's Syndrome, whether endogenous or exogenous, may result in a rapid bone loss and a virulent form of osteoporosis. Osteopenia can be the major or (occasionally) sole clinical manifestation of glucocorticoid excess, and it results from the direct effects of glucocorticoids on bone as well as the effects on calcium homeostasis. Histomorphometric studies of patients who are taking glucocorticoids reveal both a decrease in bone formation and an increase in resorption; the former is caused, in part, by the effects of glucocorticoids on osteoblastic function and matrix formation, which are consistent with the catabolic and protein-wasting effects of glucocorticoids. This increase in resorption may partly reflect an inhibition of gastrointestinal calcium absorption and a subsequent secondary hyperparathyroidism. In addition, however, glucocorticoids increase the cAMP response of bone to PTH. This suggests a compounding of the effects of the proposed secondary hyperparathyroidism. The degree of osteopenia is time-dependent and, perhaps, even dose-dependent. Alternate-day steroids may afford some protection, and doses of prednisone below 15 mg/day appear to have minor effects in short-term use. When administered with calcium, cholecalciferol (20,000–50,000 units, three to five times per week) or 25OHD (20–50 μg/day) correct calcium malabsorption and prevent the fall in bone mass.[59] Hence, it has been suggested that patients in whom glucocorticoid therapy is necessary should be treated with Vitamin D and calcium to prevent osteoporosis. Whenever therapy with Vitamin D and calcium is undertaken, serum and urine calcium concentrations must be monitored periodically to detect hypervitaminosis D.

Hyperparathyroidism

Parathyroid hormone has potent effects on calcium and bone metabolism. Hyperparathyroidism may result in a form of osteopenia that is characterized by a rapid turnover with excessive osteoclastic and osteocytic bone resorption.

Thyrotoxicosis

As with PTH, thyroid hormones directly affect bone remodeling to result in an increase in bone metabolism and an excess of osteoclastic bone resorption. This is manifested by hypercalciuria, increased hydroxyproline excretion, elevated serum alkaline phosphatase concentrations, and an occasional hypercalcemia. Endogenous or exogenous thyrotoxicosis have similar effects and either can lead to osteopenia. Groups of thyrotoxic patients of all ages have decreased bone densities, but elderly females are most affected. Clinically obvious osteoporosis that is due solely to the effects of thyroid hormones will most often arise in patients with long-standing, severe thyrotoxicosis. Whereas bone accretion occurs in young patients after successful therapy for the thyrotoxic state, this benefit does not occur in older women. Therapy should be directed at the thyroid abnormality, while ensuring adequate calcium and Vitamin D nutrition.

Immobilization

Muscle activity and more importantly weight-bearing are essential for skeletal integrity. It has long been apparent that physical confinement may result in either a generalized or local bone loss accompanied by evidence of bone resorption (hypercalciuria, occasional hypercalcemia, an increase in urinary hydroxyproline, and an increase in resorptive activity that is identified by histomorphometric analysis). The weightlessness that is experienced in spaceflight is associated with a dramatic bone loss that is not preventable by exercise, which emphasizes the importance of gravity itself in skeletal homeostasis. The therapeutic approach should emphasize prevention by avoiding complete bed rest, if possible. Agents that inhibit bone resorption (calcitonin, diphosphates) may be useful and have shown promise in initial studies.

Miscellaneous

Alcoholism, tobacco abuse, and a chronic pulmonary disease have been linked to osteopenia. In view of their prevalence, they may represent important risk factors for the development of osteopenia in elderly patients.[27] Similarly, diabetes mellitus, usually of the juvenile-onset variety is a common disorder that has been associated with a decreased bone density. Insulin affects bone remodeling and perhaps Vitamin D physiology, which may explain osteopenia in insulin-deficient patients. Chronic liver disease and partial gastrectomy have been associated with osteoporosis and osteomalacia. Malignancy, heparin therapy, and rheumatoid arthritis all engender osteoporosis through incompletely understood mechanisms.

Osteomalacia

Osteomalacia also is an osteopenic disorder, but its pathophysiology is distinct from that of osteoporosis. It is caused by an impairment in mineralization. Hence, it is characterized by an excess of unmineralized or poorly mineralized osteoid, the proteinaceous matrix of bone. Although osteomalacia may be associated with several conditions, the major abnormalities that impair mineralization are a Vitamin D deficiency and hypophosphatemia.

Clinical Characteristics

The hallmark of osteomalacia is bone pain, which commonly is manifested as diffuse, poorly localized aches and pains. Patients may complain of localized vertebral, hip, pelvic, rib, or lower extremity pain, particularly when ambulating, exercising, or lifting. The discomfort may be debilitating. Bone tenderness also is present, especially over prominences such as anterior tibial surfaces, clavicles, ribs, and symphysis pubis. Because of its non-specific nature, this syndrome frequently is misdiagnosed or discounted. Deformity is unusual in adults. However, in severe cases, leg bowing, gibbus deformity, or protrusia acetabuli may develop. Fractures occur more frequently, and a vertebral compression that leads to kyphosis and scoliosis may mimic osteoporosis. In fact, osteoporosis and osteomalacia may occur together; differentiating between the two may be challenging. Muscle weakness can be the predominant feature of osteomalacia, and it may cause difficulty in walking or a waddling gait because of hip weakness. Hypophosphatemia, Vitamin D deficiency, and secondary hyperparathyroidism are potentially important in the development of muscle dysfunction.

The serum alkaline phosphatase is elevated in the majority of (but not in all) patients. When the etiology is hypophosphatemic, serum and urine calcium levels are normal. When the etiology is a Vitamin D deficiency, serum calcium and/or phosphorus levels usually are low. In early stages of hypovitaminosis D, however, they may be normal. Secondary hyperparathyroidism accompanies a Vitamin D deficiency and results in a lowered TmP/GFR with an increased urinary cAMP and hydroxyproline excretion. Urinary calcium concentrations usually are low. The assay of 25(OH)D is useful, since it is the major circulating form and is present in low concentrations in a Vitamin D deficiency. Concentrations of 1,25(OH)D frequently are in the low-to-normal range, but nevertheless are inappropriately low in a patient with hypocalcemia and hypophosphatemia.

Radiology
The radiographic osteopenia of osteomalacia is non-specific and difficult to distinguish from that of osteoporosis. When present, vertebral biconcavity and ballooning of the intervertebral discs are more regular throughout the spine than in osteoporosis, but compression fractures occur in both conditions. One x-ray finding that is strongly suggestive of osteomalacia is the pseudofracture (Looser zone, Milkman fracture). These are thin longitudinal bands of radiolucency that occur most commonly in the

ribs, pubic rami, scapula, and long bones. They represent stress fractures that fail to heal because of the defect in mineralization (*see* Figure 28-5). Pseudofractures show an increased uptake of bone-scanning agents.

The histopathology of osteomalacia features an accumulation of unmineralized osteoid, which is a result of the fundamental defect in mineralization. It appears as an increase in both the thickness of osteoid on bone surfaces and the percent of bone surface that is covered by osteoid. Similar findings also occur with normal mineralization during rapid bone turnover, such as in hyperparathyroidism, thyrotoxicosis, or Paget's disease. Therefore, the defect in mineralization of osteomalacia must be demonstrated directly with double tetracycline labelling. Tetracycline uptake is poor and diffuse and the mineralization rate (as measured by the distance between tetracycline bands) is reduced or arrested in osteomalacia, whereas the uptake is good and mineralization rates are normal or accelerated in these other conditions. Finally, with a Vitamin D deficiency that is accompanied by secondary hyperparathyroidism, there may be changes induced by PTH (such as an increase in osteoclast activity and fibrosis).

Classification

In adults, osteomalacia usually is the result of an abnormality in mineral metabolism. In most patients, the failure of normal mineralization is attributable to a Vitamin D insufficiency or to hypophosphatemia.[60]

Vitamin D Insufficiency
Vitamin D activity is essential for normal bone mineralization. Its role is to provide, via the gastrointestinal absorption of calcium and phos-

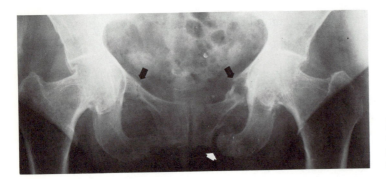

FIGURE 28-5   X-ray film of the pelvis of a 62-year-old female with osteomalacia and pseudofractures in each pelvic ramus (arrows).

phorus, adequate mineral concentrations for the formation of bone. In addition, evidence supports the direct effects of several Vitamin D metabolites (particularly $1,25[OH]_2D$ and $24,25[OH]_2D$) on bone remodeling to permit normal mineralization. An insufficient Vitamin D activity can be the result of an inadequate source of this vitamin, an interruption of its metabolism, or an increase in its excretion.[60]

Vitamin D Deficiency

Since an adequate supply of Vitamin D is obtainable from either the diet or sunlight exposure, a deficiency occurs only when both sources are inadequate. Before the supplementation of several basic foodstuffs with Vitamin D became routine, hypovitaminosis D was a common problem in children. Now the age group at highest risk is elderly shut-in persons without adequate nutrition. Subcultures that adopt dietary and dress codes which minimize Vitamin D availability, also are at risk. Parenteral nutrition has been associated with osteomalacia, but the roles of Vitamin D deficiency (or excess) and hypophosphatemia in that situation are unclear.[61,62]

Malabsorption

Cholecalciferol (Vitamin D_3) and ergocalciferol (Vitamin D_2) apparently are absorbed predominantly in the upper small bowel via a fat-dependent mechanism. Therefore, situations that result in a perturbation of upper small bowel function or fat absorption may be associated with a Vitamin D deficiency.[63] They include a gastrectomy (predominantly Billroth II), intestinal resection, sprue, pancreatic insufficiency, biliary obstructions, bile salt depletion (ileal disease or resection, bile salt-binding resins), and so on. Significantly, patients in whom malabsorption is not obvious (e.g., in sprue when steatorrhea is absent) may develop a Vitamin D malabsorption and osteomalacia because of a relatively selective defect. Malabsorption may result in a Vitamin D deficiency despite adequate sun exposure, which apparently is due to the interruption of an active enterohepatic circulation of Vitamin D metabolites. Vitamin D repletion is necessary in these patients, and it usually is feasible by administering sufficient oral doses of D_3 or D_2 (50,000 units/day); occasionally, large doses (100,000–500,000 units/

day) are necessary. The more polar Vitamin D metabolite 25(OH)D may be more easily absorbed, and hence a more rapid and reliable clinical response may result. Vitamin D doses must be titrated to achieve the desired therapeutic response, essentially by normalizing serum 25(OH)D levels.

Interruption of Vitamin D Metabolism

Hepatic and renal disorders both are associated with an abnormal Vitamin D metabolism.[64] Osteomalacia may be a concomitant of hepatic cirrhosis, apparently on the basis of an impaired 25(OH)D synthesis. The 25-hydroxylating capacity of the liver is large, and a parenchymal dysfunction must be severe to significantly impair it. In hepatic disorders that are accompanied by a reduction in bile salt availability (primary biliary cirrhosis, biliary atresia, and so on), Vitamin D malabsorption may exacerbate a defect in Vitamin D 25-hydroxylation. Therapy with 25(OH)D effectively bypasses the hepatic impairment, restores 25(OH)D levels to normal, and heals osteomalacia.

Renal dysfunction results in metabolic bone disease via its effects on several aspects of bone metabolism, parathyroid function, and Vitamin D metabolism.[65] Of critical importance is a loss of the ability to maintain 25(OH)D-1-hydroxylase activity in the face of renal damage and hyperphosphatemia. Osteomalacia is a prominent lesion in renal osteodystrophy, but the roles of Vitamin D deficiency and other factors in its causation are poorly understood.

Increased Vitamin D Catabolism or Excretion

In several circumstances, the Vitamin D supply insufficiently keeps up with an increased clearance rate. Some medications,[66] particularly anticonvulsants (diphenylhydantoin, phenobarbital), appear to increase the hepatic degradation of 25(OH)D and may result in osteomalacia. This association is well demonstrated in children, but less well in adults. Vitamin D supplementation overcomes the increased requirements. Similarly, some mesenchymal tumors have been associated with low $1,25(OH)_2D$ levels, hypophosphatemia, and osteomalacia, apparently by increasing $1,25(OH)_2D$ degradation or inhibiting its production.[67–69] Finally, in patients with a nephrotic syndrome, the renal losses of Vitamin D can be sufficient to result in osteomalacia.[70]

Hypophosphatemia

Adequate phosphorus concentrations are essential for normal mineralization. In adults, hypophosphatemia may result from renal or gastrointestinal losses.[71,72] The biochemical nature of renal phosphorus wastage is unclear, but it apparently is not due to changes in PTH or Vitamin D dynamics.

Gastrointestinal phosphorus wasting occurs in malabsorptive states, and hypophosphatemia may be due to that direct effect compounded by a Vitamin D deficiency and secondary hyperparathyroidism. When used in large quantities, phosphate-binding antacids may cause hypophosphatemia and osteomalacia.

In hypophosphatemic states, the therapeutic goal is to raise and maintain the serum phosphorus concentrations within normal limits, which usually can be accomplished by the oral administration of a buffered phosphate solution. It is important to maintain serum phosphorus levels throughout the day with a 4–6-hour dose schedule. Compliance may be difficult due to phosphorus-induced diarrhea, but diarrhea can be minimized by gradually increasing the dose until the desired effect is achieved. Vitamin D supplementation is important to correct the hypophosphatemia of malabsorption, but it is less helpful in renal phosphorus wasting. In patients with a frank osteomalacia, hypocalcemia may be a result of rapid phosphorus repletion and the demands of brisk remineralization.

Paget's Disease of the Bones

Paget's disease of the bones, or osteitis deformans, is a chronic localized disorder of bone metabolism that occurs predominantly, although not exclusively, in elderly individuals. Paget's disease, although uncommon, is seen more often in selected populations and occurs in up to 3% of populations of British descent. A positive family history is noted in 20–40% of all patients, although siblings are more often affected than the parents or children of a patient.

Paget's disease is characterized by excessive bone remodeling with an initial increase in osteoclastic activity and bone resorption followed by vigorous, but disordered, new bone formation. The result is an area of distorted and functionally abnormal bone. Although the pagetic lesions are localized, multiple parts of the skeleton may be affected. The involved sites most frequently include the pelvis, skull, proximal long bones, and vertebrae.

The etiology of Paget's disease is not known. Nuclear inclusions in osteoclasts, which are antigenically similar to the measles-RSV family of viruses, suggest that this disorder is an unusual form of a chronic viral illness or another of the "slow virus" diseases.[73,74] This model is an attractive means of explaining the unusual familial and geographic groupings of patients with Paget's disease.

Clinical Manifestations

Many patients with Paget's disease are asymptomatic and discovered accidentally by abnormal x-ray film or biochemical findings. Symptomatic patients probably account for less than 25% of all patients with Paget's disease. Symptoms vary, depending on the activity and location of the pagetic involvement. Musculoskeletal complaints commonly lead to a diagnosis. Pain generally is vague and not severe, unless associated with a fracture. Degenerative joint disease, especially of the hip, knee, and lower spine, is commonly seen in cases of moderate and severe Paget's disease, and it may be difficult to distinguish between pain that arises from an area of bony involvement and pain due to joint discomfort. Headache is a common symptom in patients with a cranial involvement. Pathologic fractures of the pelvis, long bones, or vertebrae may occur through a pagetic lesion. While the healing of most fractures in patients with Paget's disease occurs without any significant delay, the union or surgical correction of fractures of the proximal femur may be complicated by a pagetic deterioration of that area.

Bone deformity, including a bowing of the tibia or femur, acetabular deformation, and enlargement of the skull, may be observed with an extensive involvement. It can produce an entrapment or compression of cranial, spinal, or peripheral nerves that results in a variety of neurologic impairments.[75] A decreased hearing ability that is due to a combined sensory-conductive defect often occurs in patients with a cranial involvement. Angioid streaks may be observed in the retina in up to 15% of affected patients, but they generally are not associated with visual impairment.

Pagetic bone often is vascular, which results in an increased cardiac output in many patients. Cardiovascular abnormalities can be demonstrated in the majority of all patients with symptomatic Paget's disease.[76] It is unusual for Paget's disease alone to be responsible for cardiac symptoms, but the combination of the increased cardiac output that is due to the pagetic lesions and the presence of an underlying heart disease can result in a worsening of cardiac problems.

Hypercalciuria, which is a frequent complication of Paget's disease especially during periods of immobilization, is a result of the marked increase in bone resorption that is seen during the active phase of the disease. Although uncommon, hypercalcemia also may occur when a patient with Paget's disease is immobilized. Hypercalcemia in an ambulatory pagetic patient suggests a coexisting abnormality of calcium metabolism. Primary hyperparathyroidism is seen more frequently in patients with Paget's disease,[77] as are hyperuricemia and clinical gout.

An osteogenic sarcoma that arises in a pagetic lesion is the most serious complication of this disease, but it fortunately occurs in less than 1% of all affected patients. A rapid enlargement of a localized area of bone, an increase in bone pain, progressive elevation of serum alkaline phosphatase, or the development of a pathologic fracture, all may be signals of a malignant degeneration.

Evaluation

A diagnosis of Paget's disease generally is confirmed by the characteristic x-ray features and an elevated alkaline phosphatase level in a patient with suggestive symptoms.[78] Serum alkaline phosphatase and urinary hydroxyproline excretion are elevated in virtually all patients with Paget's disease. Although there is a good correlation between these two biochemical markers, neither test accurately predicts the extent of the pagetic involvement or symptomatology. The serum alkaline phosphatase test most often is used to follow a patient's course.

The characteristic, dense osteoblastic changes on an x-ray film often are the first clues to a diagnosis (see Figure 28-6). Bone scans are more sensitive indicators of the extent and activity than routine x-ray films. Areas of pagetic involvement avidly concentrate bone-scanning agents, and bone scans often are positive in an area that appears to be normal on an x-ray film.

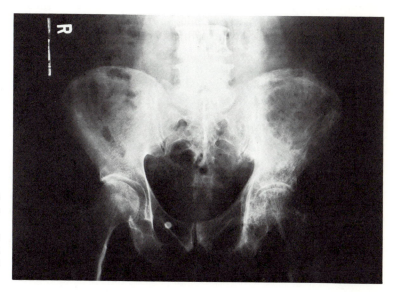

FIGURE 28-6 X-ray film of the pelvis in a 62-year-old male with polyostotic Paget's disease. There are dense sclerotic changes of the left ilium, which involve the areas of the sacroiliac joint and the left acetabulum.

The x-ray film changes of Paget's disease usually are not confused with other bone diseases. On occasion, however, the osteoblastic metastases of a prostatic carcinoma may resemble pagetic lesions, but these two disorders can be distinguished by the elevated acid phosphatase that is seen in prostatic cancer. Isolated lesions, especially when located in the vertebra, also may suggest a malignant process. In such cases, a bone biopsy procedure may be necessary to establish a diagnosis. The histologic pattern of Paget's disease is unique and includes an increased number of multinucleated osteoclasts, which are evidence of an increased bone resorption and the presence of a disordered (woven) bone formation.

Therapy

Pharmaceutical agents that inhibit bone resorption provide useful approaches to the management of Paget's disease.[79] Patients with skeletal, neurologic, and cardiac symptoms are candidates for therapy. Bone pain, headache, and nerve compression syndromes that are not associated with a fracture respond to therapy and cardiac function returns to normal. Unfortunately, a hearing loss rarely improves. Urine calcium excretion decreases with therapy and hypercalciuria can be controlled. Patients who are undergoing elective orthopedic or other surgery should be treated for 3–4 months before surgery to minimize the risk of perioperative complications, such as hypercalcemia and poor bone healing. Therapy also should be considered for asymptomatic patients with an involvement of multiple bones, since the incidence rate of complications and fractures is higher in this group of patients. Both clinical and biochemical responses are observed in patients who receive therapy; but, whether such treatment truly alters the long-term outcome of Paget's disease is not known.

Salmon calcitonin was the first effective therapeutic agent. Although calcitonin from other species (including humans) will inhibit bone resorption, salmon calcitonin is the most potent analogue of this hormone and is now available in synthetic form. It is administered subcutaneously in initial doses ranging from 50 Medical Research Council (MRC) units three times

weekly to 100 MRC units/day. Larger doses are used in patients with extensive disease activity or neurologic complications. About 80% of all patients exhibit a response. Alkaline phosphatase levels typically fall for several weeks and plateau at about 50% of pretreatment levels. Therapy is discontinued after 6–12 months and is reinstituted when evidence of a relapse is observed. The complications of calcitonin therapy consist mainly of mild allergic manifestations. A greater problem is the development in some patients of calcitonin resistance, which is not simply due to anticalcitonin antibody formation. Sometimes, patients regain their responsiveness to calcitonin following a treatment-free interval.

Disodium etidronate is the only member of the diphosphate family of compounds that is approved for the treatment of Paget's disease.[80] This drug inhibits osteoclast activity and decreases both bone resorption and bone turnover. Used in oral doses of 5–20 mg/kg per day, skeletal, neurologic, and cardiac symptoms, as well as alkaline phosphatase and hydroxyproline levels, improve rapidly in most patients. Biochemical parameters stabilize in 3–6 months. After months of therapy, the drug is discontinued. A sustained remission may be seen for many months. Repetitive 6-month courses of therapy separated by treatment-free intervals of at least several weeks are the most common treatment regimen. The larger doses of disodium etidronate also impair bone formation, which results in the development of osteomalacia and increased bone pain when used for several months. For this reason, calcitonin may be preferable to disodium etidronate when a patient is prepared for orthopedic surgery. For other patients, the initial response that is seen with either disodium etidronate or calcitonin is about the same. There are advocates for the use of each drug as a primary therapy in patients with Paget's disease. The effect of calcitonin and disodium etidronate when used together probably is greater than when either drug is used alone.[81]

Mithramycin, which is a potent inhibitor of osteoclastic bone resorption, has been used successfully in patients with Paget's disease. Because it requires IV administration and carries the potential risk of bone marrow suppression, mithramycin generally is not used, except in patients who are unresponsive to calcitonin or disodium etidronate.

Bone resorption can be inhibited by a therapeutic program that suppresses PTH secretion. The careful administration of calcium and Vitamin D has been shown to improve the biochemical parameters of pagetic activity.[82] Although this regimen is attractive in its simplicity, there is little experience with this form of therapy for Paget's disease; therefore, it is not recommended for patients with moderate-to-severe problems.

References

1. Ardaillou R: The endocrinology of renal calcium and phosphate homeostasis, in Parsons A (ed): *Endocrinology of Calcium Metabolism*. New York, Raven Press, 1982, pp 41–85.
2. Kelly A, Munan L, Claude P, et al: Patterns of change in selected serum chemical parameters of middle and later years. *J Gerontol* 34(suppl 1):37–40, 1979.
3. Keating JR Jr, Jones JD, Elveback LR, et al: The relation of age and sex to distribution of values in healthy adults of serum calcium, inorganic phosphorus, magnesium, alkaline phosphatase, total proteins, albumin, and blood urea. *J Lab Clin Med* 73(suppl 5):825–834, 1969.
4. Habener JF: New concepts in the formation, regulation of release, and metabolism of parathyroid hormone, in Ciba Foundation Symposium 41: *Polypeptide Hormones: Molecular and Cellular Aspects*. New York, Elsevier Press, 1976.
5. Slatopolsky E, Martin K, Morrissey J, et al: Current concepts of the metabolism and radioimmunoassay of parathyroid hormone. *J Lab Clin Med* 99(suppl 3):309–316, 1982.
6. Puschett JB: Renal tubular effects of parathyroid hormone: An update. *Clin Orthopaed Rel Res* 135:249–259, 1978.
7. Parfitt AM: The actions of parathyroid hormone on bone: relation to bone remodeling and turnover, calcium homeostasis, and metabolic bone disease. Part I of IV parts: Mechanisms of calcium transfer between blood and bone and their cellular basis: morphological and kinetic approaches to bone turnover, in Clearfield HR, Dinoso VP Jr (eds): *Gastrointestinal Emergencies, 34th Hahnemann Symposium*. New York, Grune & Stratton, 1976, pp 809–844.
8. Norman AW, Roth J, Orci L: The vitamin D endocrine system: steroid metabolism, hormone receptors, and biological response (calcium binding proteins). *Endocr Rev* 3(suppl 4):331, 1982.
9. Mawer EB: Functional control over the metabolic activation of calciferol, in Parsons JA (ed): *Endocrinology of Calcium Metabolism*. New York, Raven Press, 1982, pp 271–295.
10. Johnston CC Jr, Epstein S: The endocrinology of osteoporosis, in Parsons JA (ed): *Endocrinology of Calcium Metabolism*. New York, Raven Press, 1982, pp 467–483.
11. Austin LA, Heath H III: Calcitonin: physiology and pathophysiology. *N Engl J Med* 304(suppl 5):269–278, 1981.
12. Deftos LJ, Weisman MH, Williams GW, et al: Influence of age and sex on plasma calcitonin in human beings. *N Engl J Med* 302(suppl 24):1351–1353, 1980.
13. Heath H III, Hodgson SF, Kennedy MA: Primary hyperparathyroidism. Incidence, morbidity, and potential economic impact in a community. *N Engl J Med* 302(suppl 4):189–193, 1980.
14. Goldstein DA, Massry SG: Parathyroid hormone, uremia, and the nervous system. *Contr Nephrol* 20:73–83, 1980.
15. Broadus AE: Nephrolithiasis in primary hyperparathyroidism, in Coe FL, Brenner BM, Stein JH (eds): *Nephrolithiasis*. New York, Churchill-Livingston Inc., pp 59–85, 1980.
16. Broadus AE: Mineral metabolism, in Felig P, Baxter JD, Broadus AE, Frohman LA (eds): *Endocrinology and Metabolism*. New York, McGraw Hill Book Co, pp 963–969.
17. Marx SJ, Spiegel AM, Levine MA, et al: Familial hypocalciuric hypercalcemia. The relation to primary parathyroid hyperplasia. *N Engl J Med* 307(suppl 7):416–426, 1982.
18. Martin KJ, Hruska K, Freitag J, et al: Clinical utility of radioimmunoassays for parathyroid hormone. *Min Electr Metab* 3:283–290, 1980.
19. Broadus A: Nephrogenous cyclic AMP. *Rec Prog Horm Res* 37:667–701, 1981.
20. Bilezikian JP: The medical management of primary hyperparathyroidism. *Ann Int Med* 96:198–202, 1982.
21. Mundy GR, Martin TJ: The hypercalcemia of malignancy: pathogenesis and management. *Metabolism* 31(suppl 12):1247–1277, 1982.
22. Orwoll ES: The milk-alkali syndrome: current concepts. *Ann Int Med* 97:242–248, 1982.
23. Breslau NA, Pak CYC: Hypoparathyroidism. *Metabolism* 28(suppl 12):1261–1276, 1979.
24. Okano K, Furukawa Y, Morii H, et al: Comparative efficacy of various vitamin D metabolites in the treatment of various types of hypoparathyroidism. *J Clin Endocr Metab* 55(suppl 2):238–243, 1982.

25. Gordon CS: Age-related bone loss with special reference to postmenopausal osteoporosis, in Greenblatt RB (ed): *Geriatric Endocrinology (Aging).* New York, Raven Press, 1978, vol 5, pp 191–199.

26. Riggs BL, Wahner HW, Dunn WL, et al: Differential changes in bone mineral density of the appendicular and axial skeleton with aging. *J Clin Invest* 67:328–335, 1981.

27. Avioli LV: Osteoporosis: pathogenesis and therapy, in Avioli LV, Krane SM (eds): *Metabolic Bone Disease.* New York, Academic Press, 1977, vol I, pp 307–385.

28. Marcus R: The relationship of dietary calcium to the maintenance of skeletal integrity in man—an interface of endocrinology and nutrition. *Metabolism* 31(suppl 1):93–102, 1982.

29. Heaney RP, Recker RR, Saville PD: Menopausal changes in calcium balance performance. *J Lab Clin Med* 92(suppl 6):953–963, 1978.

30. Gallagher JC, Riggs BL, Eisman J, et al: Intestinal calcium absorption and serum vitamin D metabolites in normal subjects and osteoporotic patients. *J Clin Invest* 64:729–736, 1979.

31. Riggs BL, Hamstra A, DeLuca HF: Assessment of 25-hydroxyvitamin D 1-alpha-hydroxylase reserve in postmenopausal osteoporosis by administration of parathyroid extract. *J Clin Endocr Metab* 53(suppl 4):833–835, 1981.

32. Heaney RP, Recker RR: Effects of nitrogen, phosphorus, and caffeine on calcium balance in women. *J Lab Clin Med* 1(suppl 99):46–55, 1982.

33. Gallagher JC, Riggs BL, DeLuca HF: Effect of estrogen on calcium absorption and serum vitamin D metabolites in postmenopausal osteoporosis. *J Clin Endocr Metab* 52(suppl 6):1359–1364, 1980.

34. Stevenson JC, Abeyasekera G, Hillyard CJ, et al: Calcitonin and the calcium-regulating hormones in postmenopausal women: effect of oestrogens. *Lancet* 28:693–695, 1981.

35. Parfitt AM, Oliver I, Villanueva AR: Bone histology in metabolic bone disease: the diagnostic value of bone biopsy. *Ortho Clin North Am* 10(suppl 2):329–345, 1979.

36. Riggs BL: Osteoporosis—a disease of impaired homeostatic regulation. *Min Electr Metab* 5: 265–272, 1981.

37. Aloia JF, Cohn SH, Ostuni JA, et al: Prevention of involutional bone loss by exercise. *Ann Int Med* 89:356–358, 1978.

38. Smith EL, Reddan W: Physical activity—a modality for bone accretion in the aged. *Am J Roentgenol* 126:1297, 1976.

39. Recker RR, Saville PD, Heaney RP: Effect of estrogens and calcium carbonate on bone loss in postmenopausal women. *Ann Int Med* 87(suppl 6):649–655, 1977.

40. Horsman A, Gallagher JC, Simpson M, et al: Prospective trial of oestrogen and calcium in postmenopausal women. *Br Med J* 2:789–792, 1977.

41. Matkovic V, Kostial K, Simonovic I, et al: Bone status and fracture rates in two regions of Yugoslavia. *Am J Clin Nutr* 32:540–549, 1979.

42. Weiss NS, Ure CL, Ballard JH, et al: Decreased risk of fractures of the hip and lower forearm with postmenopausal use of estrogen.*N Engl J Med* 303(suppl 21):1195–1198, 1980.

43. Hutchinson TA, Polansky SM, Feinstein AR: Postmenopausal oestrogens protect against fractures of the hip and distal radius. *Lancet* II:705–709, 1979.

44. Specht EE: Hip fracture, skeletal fragility, osteoporosis and hormonal deprivation in elderly women. *West J Med* 133:297–303, 1980.

45. Paganini-Hill A, Ross RK, Gerkins VR, et al: Menopausal estrogen therapy and hip fractures. *Ann Int Med* 95:28–31, 1981.

46. Lindsay R, Fogelman I, Hart DM: Prevention of postmenopausal bone loss using sex steroids, in DeLuca HF, Frost HM, Jee WSS, et al (eds): *Osteoporosis: Recent Advances in Pathogenesis and Treatment.* Baltimore, University Park Press, 1981, pp 400–406.

47. Heaney RP: Estrogens and postmenopausal osteoporosis. *Clin Obst Gynecol* 19(suppl 4):791–803, 1976.

48. Lindsay R, Hart DM, Aitkeu JM, et al: Long-term prevention of postmenopausal osteoporosis by oestrogen. *Lancet* I:1038–1041, 1976.

49. Lindsay R, Hart DM, MacLean A, et al: Bone response to termination of oestrogen treatment. *Lancet* I:1325–1327, 1978.

50. Genant HK, Cann CE, Ettinger B, et al: Quantitative computed tomography of vertebral spongiosa: a sensitive method for detecting early bone loss after oophorectomy. *Ann Int Med* 97:699–705, 1982.

51. Weinstein MC: Estrogen use in postmenopausal women—costs, risks, and benefits. *N Engl J Med* 303(suppl 6):308–316, 1980.

52. Smith DC, Prentice R, Thompson DJ, et al: Association of exogenous estrogen and endometrial carcinoma. *N Engl J Med* 293(suppl 23):1164–1202, 1975.

53. Antunes CMF, Stolley PD, Rosenshein NB, et al: Endometrial cancer and estrogen use. *N Engl J Med* 300(suppl 1):9–13, 1979.

54. Whitehead MI, Townsend PT, Pryse-Davies J, et al: Effects of estrogens and progestins on the biochemistry and morphology of the postmeno-

pausal endometrium. *N Engl J Med* 305(suppl 27):1599–1605, 1981.

55. Gambrell RD Jr, Massey FM, Castaneda CA, et al: Use of the progestogen challenge test to reduce the risk of endometrial cancer. *Obst Gynecol* 55(suppl 6):732–738, 1980.

56. Hoover R, Gray LA, Cole P, et al: Menopausal estrogens and breast cancer. *New Engl J Med* 295(suppl 8):401–405, 1976.

57. Ross RK, Paganini-Hill A, Gerkins VR, et al: A case-control study of menopausal estrogen therapy and breast cancer. *JAMA* 243(suppl 16): 1635–1639, 1980.

58. Riggs BL, Seeman E, Hodgson SF, et al: Effect of the fluoride/calcium regimen on vertebral fracture occurrence in postmenopausal osteoporosis. *N Engl J Med* 306(suppl 8):446–450, 1982.

59. Hahn TJ, Halstead LR, Teitelbaum SL, et al: Altered mineral metabolism in glucocorticoid-induced osteopenia. *J Clin Invest* 64:655–665, 1979.

60. Frame B, Parfitt AM: Osteomalacia: current concepts. *Ann Int Med* 89:966–982, 1978.

61. Shike M, Harrison JE, Sturtridge WC, et al: Metabolic bone disease in patients receiving long-term total parenteral nutrition. *Ann Int Med* 92(suppl 3):343–350, 1980.

62. Shike M, Sturtridge WC, Tam CS, et al: A possible role of vitamin D in the genesis of parenteral-nutrition-induced metabolic bone disease. *Ann Int Med* 95:560–568, 1981.

63. Meredith SC, Rosenberg IH: Gastrointestinal-hepatic disorders and osteomalacia. *Clin Endocr Metab* 9:131–150, 1980.

64. Stamp TCB: The clinical endocrinology of vitamin D, in Parsons JA (ed): *Endocrinology of Calcium Metabolism.* New York, Raven Press, 1982, pp 363–423.

65. Coburn JW: Renal osteodystrophy. *Kidney Int* 17:677–693, 1980.

66. Hahn TJ: Drug-induced disorders of vitamin D and mineral metabolism. *Clin Endocr Metab* 9: 107–130, 1980.

67. Lyles KW, Berry WR, Haussler M, et al: Hypophosphatemic osteomalacia: association with prostatic carcinoma. *Ann Int Med* 93:275–278, 1980.

68. Drezner MK, Feinglos MN: Osteomalacia due to 1-alpha, 25-dihydroxycholecalciferol deficiency. *J Clin Invest* 60:1046–1053, 1977.

69. Sweet RA, Males JL, Hamstra AJ, et al: Vitamin D metabolite levels in oncogenic osteomalacia. *Ann Int Med* 93(suppl 2):279–280, 1980.

70. Malluche HH, Goldstein DA, Massry SG: Osteomalacia and hyperparathyroid bone disease in patients with nephrotic syndrome. *J Clin Invest* 63:494–500, 1979.

71. Neer R: Clinical disturbances of calcium and inorganic phosphate homeostasis, in Parsons JA (ed): *Endocrinology of Calcium Metabolism.* New York, Raven Press, 1982, pp 1–37.

72. Stoff JS: Phosphate homeostasis and hypophosphatemia. *Am J Med* 72:489–495, 1982.

73. Rebel A, Basle N, Pouplard A, et al: Bone tissue in Paget's disease of bone: ultrastructure and immunocytology. *Arthritis Rheum* 23:1104–1114, 1980.

74. Mills BG, Singer FR, Weiser LP, et al: Cell cultures from bone affected by Paget's disease. *Arthritis Rheum* 23:1115–1120, 1980.

75. Schmidek HH: Neurologic and neurosurgical sequelae of Paget's disease of bone. *Clin Ortho* 127:70–77, 1977.

76. Henley JW, Croxson RS, Ibbertson HK: The cardiovascular system in Paget's disease of bone and the response to therapy with calcitonin and diphosphonate. *Aust NZ J Med* 9:390–397, 1979.

77. Posru S, Clifton-Bligh P, Wilkinson M: Paget's disease of bone and hyperparathyroidism: coincidence or causal relationship? *Calcif Tiss Res* 26:107–109, 1978.

78. Singer FR: *Paget's Disease of Bone.* New York, Plenum Press, 1977.

79. Wallach S: Treatment of Paget's disease. *Adv Int Med* 27:1–43, 1982.

80. Ibberton HK, Henley JW, Fraser TR, et al: Paget's disease of bone—clinical evaluation and treatment with diphosphonate. *Aust NZ J Med* 9:31–35, 1979.

81. Hosking DJ, Bijvoet DLM, vau Akeu J, et al: Paget's bone disease treated with diphosphonate and calcitonin. *Lancet* I:615–617, 1976.

82. Evans RA: A cheap oral therapy for Paget's disease of bone. *Aust NZ J Med* 7:259–261, 1977.

CHAPTER 29

Dyslipoproteinemia and Obesity

WILLIAM R. HAZZARD, M.D.

Dyslipoproteinemia and obesity, which are two often-related disorders of lipid metabolism, both assume a diminishing significance with advancing age. This occurs by virtue of the following considerations:

1. The incidence, prevalence, and severity of both dyslipoproteinemia and obesity appear to decline with age;
2. The association between these phenomena and their complications in the form of a disease also diminishes in old age;
3. Those persons who survive into old age, often in robust health, despite these disorders often do so by virtue of compensating factors (often inherited) that permit such survival;
4. With respect to disorders of cholesterol metabolism, interventions to ameliorate abnormal lipoprotein distributions appear to have no clear benefit except, possibly, in the primary prevention of atherosclerosis and its complications; secondary prevention through lipoprotein manipulation does not seem efficacious at any age, especially in elderly persons;
5. All forms of intervention, both dietary and/or pharmacologic, appear to have an increasing attendant risk in elderly persons;
6. Given the relatively fixed upper limit of a human life span (85 ± 4 years),[1] the potential benefit of preventing complications of atherosclerosis through a correction of dyslipoproteinemia and/or obesity as measured in person-years of healthy life diminishes progressively as that upper limit is approached.

Hence, only in the most unusual circumstances in which short-term relief can be anticipated (e.g., pancreatitis due to chylomicronemia or immobility due to weight-aggravated osteoarthritis) would therapy for either dyslipoproteinemia or obesity be wisely undertaken in an elderly patient.

Dyslipoproteinemia

Lipid Metabolism And Aging

Mean population levels of both cholesterol and triglyceride increase from adolescence through middle age in both sexes (*see* Figure 29-1, Table 29-1).[2,3] From young adulthood through approximately 50 years of age, median levels of both cholesterol and triglyceride in males exceed those in females. Thereafter, median levels for both lipids appear to reach a plateau in males and, most likely, decline in old age, due perhaps to increased removal from the sample of those with high triglyceride and cholesterol who do not survive to old age (most of these studies are cross–sectional). Median levels of triglyceride and cholesterol continue to rise in females until the 7th decade, beyond which a similar decline is seen. While the mechanism of these age-related changes has yet to be determined, their close coincidence with changes in relative body weight has suggested that adiposity may mediate these changes (with the notable exception of the "postmenopausal overshoot" in cholesterol levels in females, which presumably is attributable to diminished estrogen levels) (*see* Figure 29-2).[4] Hence, if hyperlipidemia is defined inde-

FIGURE 29-1 Plasma cholesterol and triglyceride for white males and females who are not taking sex hormones, median values for 5-year age groups. (From The Lipid Research Clinics Program Epidemiology Committee: Plasma lipid distributions in selected North American populations: The Lipid Research Clinic Program Prevalence Study. *Circulation* 60:427–439, 1970, used by permission of the American Heart Association, Inc.)

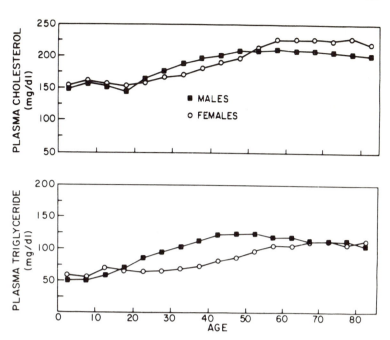

FIGURE 29-2 Plasma cholesterol (chol), triglyceride (TG), and relative body weight as a function of age in free-living populations (From Bierman EL, Glomset JA: Disorders of lipid metabolism, in Williams RH (ed): *Textbook of Endocrinology.* Philadelphia, Saunders, 1974, pp 890–937.)

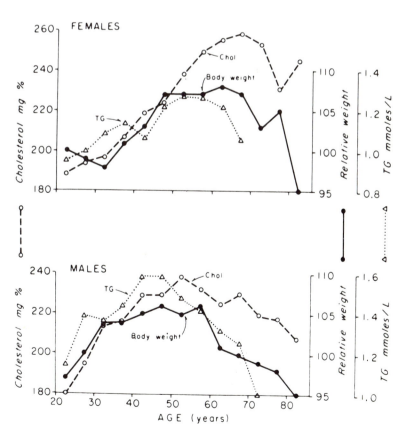

TABLE 29-1   North American Population Plasma Total and Lipoprotein Cholesterol and Triglyceride Values (Means and, in Parentheses Below, 5th and 95th Percentiles) in Adult, Free-Living White Males and Females (not taking hormones)

Sex	Age (yr)	Triglyceride (mg/dl)	Cholesterol (mg/dl)			
			Total	HDL*	LDL	VLDL
Females	20–24	72 (36–131)	164 (122–216)	52	98	12
	25–29	75 (37–145)	171 (128–222)	56 (37–81)	106 (70–151)	12 (2–24)
	30–34	79 (39–151)	175 (130–231)	55 (38–75)	107 (67–150)	11 (0–25)
	35–39	86 (40–176)	184 (140–242)	55 (34–82)	119 (76–172)	14 (1–35)
	40–44	98 (45–191)	194 (147–252)	57 (33–87)	125 (77–174)	14 (3–29)
	45–49	105 (46–214)	203 (152–265)	58 (33–86)	130 (80–187)	17 (2–38)
	50–54	115 (52–233)	218 (162–285)	60 (37–89)	146 (90–215)	16 (0–37)
	55–59	125 (55–262)	231 (173–300)	59 (36–86)	152 (95–213)	21 (2–51)
	60–64	127 (56–239)	231 (172–297)	62 (36–91)	156 (100–234)	18 (1–45)
	65–69	131 (60–243)	233 (171–303)	61 (34–89)	162 (97–223)	18 (0–40)
	70+	132 (60–237)	228 (169–289)	60 (33–91)	149 (96–207)	16 (0–52)
Males	20–24	100 (44–201)	167 (124–218)	45 (30–63)	103 (66–147)	14 (1–28)
	25–29	116 (46–249)	183 (133–244)	45 (31–63)	117 (70–165)	17 (3–36)
	30–34	128 (50–266)	193 (138–254)	46 (28–63)	126 (78–185)	21 (5–48)
	35–39	145 (54–321)	201 (146–270)	43 (29–62)	133 (81–189)	24 (3–56)
	40–44	151 (55–320)	207 (151–268)	44 (27–67)	136 (87–186)	26 (5–56)
	45–49	152 (58–327)	212 (158–276)	45 (30–64)	144 (98–202)	24 (5–51)
	50–54	152 (58–320)	213 (158–277)	44 (28–63)	142 (89–197)	27 (8–62)
	55–59	141 (58–286)	214 (156–276)	48 (28–71)	146 (88–203)	22 (3–49)
	60–64	142 (58–291)	213 (159–276)	52 (30–74)	146 (83–210)	19 (3–44)
	65–69	137 (57–267)	213 (158–274)	51 (30–78)	151 (98–210)	20 (0–45)
	70+	130 (58–258)	207 (151–270)	51 (31–75)	143 (88–186)	17 (0–38)

SOURCE: The Lipid Research Clinics Program Epidemiology Committee: Plasma lipid distributions in selected North American populations: The Lipid Research Clinics Program Prevalence Study. *Circulation* 60:427–439, 1970. Used by permission of the American Heart Association, Inc.
* HDL = high-density lipoprotein; LDL = low-density lipoprotein; VLDL = very low-density lipoprotein.

TABLE 29-2 Likelihood Ratios for Various Lipid Profiles of Coronary
Heart Disease—Framingham Study, Exam 11

Lipid	Males	Females
HDL§ cholesterol	14.03*	21.21*
LDL cholesterol	4.39†	4.53†
Triglyceride	0.51	9.52††
Total cholesterol	1.98	2.26
HDL cholesterol: total cholesterol	17.11*	20.41*
LDL and total cholesterol, triglyceride	8.26†	19.69*
HDL and total cholesterol, triglyceride	19.19*	24.21*
HDL and LDL cholesterol, triglyceride	18.90*	24.73*
HDL and LDL cholesterol	18.66*	23.70*
HDL cholesterol: total cholesterol, LDL cholesterol	17.16*	20.77*

SOURCE: Gordon T, Castelli WP, Hjortland MC, et al: High density lipoprotein as a
protective factor against coronary heart disease. The Framingham Study, *Am J Med*
62:707–714, 1977.
* $p < 0.001$.
† $p < 0.05$.
†† $p < 0.01$.
§ HDL = high-density lipoprotein; LDL = low-density lipoprotein.

pendently of age, its prevalence in old age is reduced, as is its incidence and (presumably) severity.

Since apart from chylomicronemic pancreatitis and the "chylomicronemia syndrome" (*see* below),[5] nearly all of the clinical relevance of plasma lipid and lipoprotein levels stems from their association with atherogenic risk, it is important to note that the correlation between total plasma lipid levels and the risk of atherosclerotic complications is not significant in old age (*see* Table 29-2).[6] This is predominantly attributable to the declining relationship between low-density lipoprotein (LDL) cholesterol levels and the atherogenic risk in this age group. These lipoproteins, which comprise the clear majority of total cholesterol levels at all ages, appear to be most clearly related to the risk of premature atherosclerosis, while their relationship to atherosclerosis with a clinical onset in old age is only marginal. Nevertheless, monogenically determined hypobetalipoproteinemia in old age has been reported as a "longevity syndrome."[7] Conversely, the inverse relationship between high-density lipoprotein (HDL) cholesterol levels and atherogenic risk is, if anything, enhanced in old age; also conversely, median HDL cholesterol levels in very old persons appear to be increased,[8] and hyperalphalipoproteinemia has been reported as another "longevity syndrome" that may be transmitted by a separate major gene.[7] While triglyceride

levels appear to be positively associated with atherosclerotic complications in older females, this appears to be mediated through their inverse relationship with HDL cholesterol levels to the point that on multivariate analysis this association is lost. Thus, the assessment of the atherosclerotic risk profile in an individual elderly patient must address both LDL and HDL cholesterol concentrations, with the ratio between the two being a convenient index.

Physiology of Lipid Transport

The decision whether or not to treat dyslipoproteinemia regardless of a patient's age requires a conceptual framework of the physiology and pathophysiology of lipoprotein metabolism in humans. This can be understood by focusing on the major "control points" of metabolic regulation that control entry into and exit from the plasma compartment. Dietary lipids are absorbed across the small intestinal mucosa (control point 1) and transported to the plasma via the thoracic duct. They enter in the form of the large (approximately 5,000 Å, triglyceride-rich, cholesterol-poor, light-scattering chylomicrons that bear the specific intestinal structural apolipoprotein B-48 on their surface.

Next in order of decreasing size, triglyceride concentration, and (as a consequence) increasing density, are the very low-density lipoproteins (VLDL) of endogenous and primarily hepatic origin. Their triglyceride is synthesized from carbohydrates and fatty acid precursors (control point 2); their cholesterol is synthesized from an intrahepatic pool including some which is synthesized from acetate precursors and tightly regulated by the enzyme hydroxymethyl glutaryl (HMG) CoA reductase (control point 3). These VLDL have the structural apolipoprotein B-100 on their surface, which also is synthesized in the liver (control point 4). Both chylomicrons and VLDL also contain apolipoproteins C-I (of uncertain function), C-II (a necessary cofactor for lipoprotein lipase activity), and C-III (potentially modulating the hepatic uptake of triglyceride-rich lipoproteins in an inhibitory manner), plus apo-E, which serves as the signal apoprotein for hepatic lipoprotein-remnant uptake (*see* below). While the apolipoprotein B is retained on the lipoprotein surface until the entire particle is removed from the plasma, the other, smaller apoproteins appear to exchange between VLDL and HDL (shuttling to VLDL during alimentary lipemia and back to HDL with its resolution). The level and composition of VLDL may vary by virtue of the differential changes in triglyceride, cholesterol, and apolipoprotein B-100 synthesis and release from the liver into the plasma. Triglycerides in both chylomicrons and VLDL appear to serve as the substrate for lipoprotein lipase (control point 5), which is synthesized in adipocytes and muscle cells under the influence of insulin and thyroxine. Lipoprotein lipase migrates to the adjacent capillary endothelium, where chylomicrons and VLDL are transiently bound during the process of selective triglyceride hydrolysis. The surplus lipoprotein surface material that is generated by this selective core triglyceride extraction (consisting primarily of free cholesterol and lecithin) is the substrate for the plasma enzyme (of hepatic origin) lecithin-cholesterol acyltransferase (LCAT) (control point 6), for which the principal HDL apolipoprotein A-I is an essential cofactor. The cholesterol ester thus formed appears to transiently reside in HDL before its transfer (predominantly) to both intermediate-density lipoproteins (IDL) and LDL, where it forms part of the neutral lipid core.

The lipoprotein "remnants" that are formed by the combined actions of lipoprotein lipase and LCAT are relatively enriched in cholesterol ester and apoE, in addition to the residual apoB. These lipoproteins are efficiently recognized by hepatic receptors that are specific for isoapolipoproteins E_3 and E_4, but not for most variants of E_2 (control point 7). The liver-remnant encounter appears to result in the selective removal of apoE and some cholesterol ester (and, possibly, residual triglycerides via the enzyme hepatic triglyceride lipase). The efficiency of this process is reflected in a down-regulation of hepatic cholesterol synthesis via HMG CoA reductase. Estrogens and thyroid hormones appear to enhance this process.

The LDL are generated at the end of this catabolic cascade and retain apoB-100 and a high proportion of total plasma cholesterol esters. The LDL are, in turn, catabolized (control point 8) following their recognition by a specific receptor for apoB (and E), which has been demonstrated (e.g., on fibroblasts, adipocytes, endothelial cells, aortic smooth-muscle cells, and monocyte-derived macrophages) and by certain steroid-producing cells (e.g., adrenal cortex, ovary, placenta, which may also recognize HDL). Whether or not these exist on the hepatocyte of an adult human is currently being debated. The interaction of LDL with its receptor and the chain of subsequent intracellular events have been carefully elucidated by Goldstein and Brown,[9] who describe the following sequence: 1) Binding of the LDL apoB to specific receptors in cytoplasmic membrane areas that are characterized by "coated pits"; 2) Internalization via endocytosis; 3) Transport to primary lysosomes where acid hydrolases cleave cholesterol esters and convert apoB to amino acids; 4) Transport of the free cholesterol to the microsomes, thereby serving to down-regulate both HMG CoA reductase activity and LDL receptor number; 6) Esterification of cholesterol esters with oleate via the enzyme, acyl-cholesterol acyltransferase (ACAT).

An alternative mechanism, termed the "scavenger pathway" (control point 9), which involves monocyte-derived macrophages, appears to clear lipoproteins that either are abnormal de novo or become so in the process of catabolism (e.g. the β-VLDL of type III hyperlipoproteinemia or acetylated LDL in familial hypercholesterolemia).[9]

The removal of cholesterol from cells appears to be accomplished by HDL (with

LCAT). This, in turn, up-regulates HMG CoA reductase activity and the LDL receptor mechanism. Thus, LDL appear to be the primary vehicles for centrifugal cholesterol transport, while HDL appear to mediate centripetal ("reverse") cholesterol transport back to the liver (control point 10); in the liver, cholesterol may be converted to bile acids (control point 11) or secreted as such into the bile (the ratio between the two is a primary determinant of bile lithogenicity and, hence, gallstone formation). Finally, intestinal bile acids normally are efficiently recycled via the portal system (control point 12), and they ultimately are excreted in the feces after manifold enterohepatic recycling.

Pathophysiology of Lipid Transport

Using this conceptual framework, one can address the influences on the lipoprotein metabolism of nutrition (including adiposity and alcohol), heredity, hormones, disease, and age. At control point 1, there is no form of hypertriglyceridemia that is primarily caused by the overingestion of dietary fat. This appears to reflect the exquisite efficiency of lipoprotein lipase and triglyceride clearance mechanisms (which are induced by fat ingestion) and also the compensatory down-regulation of endogenous triglyceride synthesis by such ingestion. Hypercholesterolemia of dietary origin is debatable, but there are clear correlations across populations between dietary cholesterol intake and plasma cholesterol (specifically LDL cholesterol) levels. Carefully controlled metabolic studies have demonstrated increased cholesterol levels with increased intake and vice versa.[10] Moreover, for reasons which remain obscure, the amount of saturated fat in the diet also is a major determinant of plasma (LDL) cholesterol levels. Given the normal distribution of cholesterol levels in all populations, it seems most likely that an individual response to a diet of a given cholesterol-saturated fat content is determined by multiple genes (including those that regulate endogenous synthesis control point 3), as well as by environmental influences. However, it remains to be demonstrated whether or not certain individuals are uniquely predisposed to develop hypercholesterolemia that is solely of dietary origin.

In contrast, high levels of VLDL can proceed from a high triglyceride production rate (control point 2), a high cholesterol synthesis rate (control point 3), and/or a high apoB apoprotein synthesis rate (control point 4). Triglyceride production appears to be enhanced by overfeeding, increased hepatic production due to alcohol precursors, and several conditions that are associated with a high circulating insulin level, which usually reflects a peripheral insulin antagonism as seen in obesity, estrogen (including oral contraceptive) treatment, uremia, and corticosteroid excess. Triglyceride synthesis also appears to be increased in persons with familial hypertriglyceridemia, which is a monogenic disorder that may occur in as many as 1% of the United States population,[11] but, it only is clearly expressed in adulthood (perhaps influenced by growing adiposity). Whether or not familial hypertriglyceridemia increases the risk of atherosclerosis is currently debated. However, the prevailing consensus is that if it is so, it represents a far less atherogenic risk than familial combined hyperlipidemia[12,13] (see below), with which atherosclerosis may be confused in an individual patient.

A high secretion rate of apoB (control point 4) may occur in patients with a nephrotic syndrome or during corticosteroid treatment (e.g., in patients on an immunosuppressive therapy); but, it is most significantly seen in persons with familial combined hyperlipidemia ("multiple lipoprotein phenotype hyperlipoproteinemia," "hyperapobetalipoproteinemia"), who may comprise as much as 1–2% of a general population.[11] It also is seen in up to 10% of patients with a myocardial infarction before age 60[2]. While apoB concentrations appear to segregate into two modes (one normal and one high) in a given family with this disorder, triglyceride and cholesterol levels are variably increased in affected family members. This presumably reflects their relative rates of synthesis of both triglyceride and cholesterol. This gives rise to multiple lipoprotein phenotypes (type IV [increased VLDL alone], type II$_a$, [increased LDL alone], or type II$_b$ [combined elevations of VLDL and LDL]) in a single family, or even in a given patient at different points in time. This depends, in part, on the relative adiposity, which is positively correlated with triglyceride levels, and treatment; a decline in VLDL usually is associated with an increase in LDL cholesterol levels in this disorder.

Defective triglyceride removal (control point 5) may proceed from a deficiency in either lipoprotein lipase or (rarely) apoC-II. A lipoprotein lipase deficiency rarely is attributable to an autosomal recessive disorder, but it is commonly seen in uncontrolled diabetes mellitus. Severe hypertriglyceridemia, however, most commonly reflects the coexistence of two disorders, usually with one that limits lipoprotein lipase activity (e.g., diabetes) and another that is associated with triglyceride overproduction (e.g., familial hypertriglyceridemia, obesity, alcohol excess, or estrogen treatment), which saturates the limited triglyceride removal capacity.[5] Obese persons with type II (non-insulin-requiring) diabetes and a coexisting genetically determined hyperlipidemia are, thus, at a special risk of developing severe hypertriglyceridemia and the attendant consequences of a prolonged and profound chylomicronemia.[5] This variously includes an eruptive xanthomatosis (miliary, pearl-like lesions on an erythematous base, distributed over extensor surfaces), pancreatitis, and other aspects of the "chylomicronemia syndrome," which is characterized by an apparently reduced PO_2 (with hyperpnea) and a reversible mental impairment.

A defective LCAT activity (control point 6) is most clear-cut in a rare autosomal-recessive genetic disorder that is characterized by high concentrations of unesterified cholesterol (reflecting circulating "surface remnants"), hemolytic anemia, and renal failure. It also is present when apo A-I levels are very low (as in Tangier disease, wherein HDL cholesterol virtually is absent and cholesterol accumulates in reticuloendothelial cells, which gives rise to the suggestive pale tonsillar hypertrophy) and, since the enzyme is of hepatic origin, in severe liver disease. In the case of the latter, this often produces a complex pattern of dyslipoproteinemia, given the multiple lipoprotein regulatory roles of the liver.

At control point 7 (remnant removal), the homozygous presence of isoapolipoprotein E_2 (i.e., with an E_3 and E_4 deficiency) produces a defect in hepatic remnant recognition. In this circumstance, an alternative pathway of great efficiency that is not dependent upon E_3 and E_4 appears likely to remove these remnants (per-

haps via the LDL apoB/E receptor). However, the capacity of this pathway is limited. Hence, persons with a normal apoB production and B/E receptors, but who are homozygous for $apoE_2$, have (paradoxically) among the lowest LDL and total cholesterol levels. However, persons with high apoB production rates (most commonly from coinherited familial combined hyperlipidemia) or diminished LDL receptor activity (familial hypercholesterolemia [see below], hypothyroidism, or estrogen deficiency) have extraordinarily high levels of the cholesterol-rich, triglyceride-poor VLDL and chylomicron remnants. These may escape the plasma compartment and form xanthomas of a tuberous configuration over elbows and knees and fill the palmer creases with "xanthoma striatum palmaris," which virtually is pathognomonic of this disorder (type III hyperlipoproteinemia, dysbetalipoproteinemia, or broad-beta disease).

At the level of the LDL receptor (control point 8), individuals homozygous for an LDL (apoB/E) receptor deficiency have extreme LDL cholesterol elevations (averaging four times that of normal) and no demonstrable catabolism of LDL in the peripheral cells.[9] No such person has been known to live into adulthood because of vastly accelerated atherosclerosis. Those persons (approximately 1 in 500 in the population) who are heterozygous for this condition lack approximately 50% of the normal complement of LDL receptors. They compensate for this by virtue of an approximate doubling of LDL cholesterol levels, which is a circumstance detectable in cord blood as well as throughout life. This also is associated with accelerated atherogenesis; these persons are vastly overrepresented among patients with a myocardial infarction before age 60 (approximately 3% of this group). Other factors that cause hypercholesterolemia, presumably via a reduced LDL receptor activity, include a thyroid hormone deficiency.

The fact that cholesterol levels in persons who are totally lacking LDL receptors do not rise to infinity led to the postulation and later demonstration of alternative "scavenger" pathways (control point 9) for the removal of LDL that is altered by virtue of prolonged circulation.[9] The monocyte-derived macrophage appears to be an important mediator of this process and a likely precursor to foam cells in atherosclerotic lesions.

HDL metabolism (control point 10) is less well understood and, hence, mechanisms for alterations in HDL levels only can be postulated at present. Estrogens are associated with increased HDL levels[12] (as is aerobic exercise, alcohol ingestion, and certain drugs such as nicotinic acid, clofibrate, and colestipol), while androgens (notably anabolic steroids) are associated with diminished levels[13] (as are increasing adiposity, cigarette smoking, a high-carbohydrate diet, a high polyunsaturated fatty acid diet, and certain other drugs including probucol). High-density lipoproteins are a heterozygous class of lipoproteins, with a minority subfraction, HDL_2, being the more labile and accounting for almost all of the potent inverse relationship between HDL cholesterol levels and atherogenic risk. Hepatic triglyceride lipase (perhaps activated by apoA-II) has been suggested as relating to HDL catabolism via its activity as a phospholipase, which may destabilize the phospholipid-rich HDL and render them susceptible to apolipoprotein hydrolysis.

A conversion of intrahepatic cholesterol to bile acids (control point 11) involves a series of enzymatically regulated steps, with the rate-limiting being catalyzed by 7-α-hydroxylase. Forces that deplete the bile acid pool, such as a biliary diversion, or those that prevent reabsorption ([control point 12] as with the resins cholestyramine or colestipol, or ileal bypass) increase the rate of such a conversion.

Treatment of Dyslipoproteinemia

The treatment of dyslipoproteinemia can be conveniently considered by reference to this framework of human lipoprotein physiology and pathophysiology.

Secondary disorders are diagnosed by their association with dyslipoproteinemia and the lipoprotein response to their treatment: 1) Hypertriglyceridemia and/or hypercholesterolemia that is associated with obesity to weight reduction; 2) Hypertriglyceridemia of diabetes to hypoglycemic therapy (including weight reduction in an insulin-resistant obese diabetic); 3) Hypertriglyceridemia with estrogen (or oral contraceptive) treatment to its withdrawal; 4) Hypertriglyceridemia with alcohol excess to abstinence; 5) Hyperlipidemia (often hypercholesterolemia and hypertriglyceridemia) of corticosteroid excess to steroid withdrawal (or adrenalectomy with Cushing's disease); 5) Hypercholesterolemia of liver disease to its treatment; and 6) Hypoalphalipoproteinemia of obesity to weight reduction.

Most commonly, however, such secondary conditions exaggerate primary disorders that are determined by single or multiple genes. Hence, their treatment ameliorates, but does not normalize, the lipoprotein levels; therefore, additional treatment may be indicated. This usually is multipronged, consisting of alterations in life style that include diet and (often) drug therapy as well.

Life style alterations should address the larger issue of atherogenic risk (since that attributable to dyslipoproteinemia is mediated almost solely in this manner). Hence, while the cessation of cigarette smoking may raise HDL levels, its major health-related benefit is through a directly reduced atherogenic risk, which interacts with dyslipoproteinemia in a synergistic fashion. Adipose mass reduction through caloric restriction can reduce LDL and increase HDL cholesterol levels; if accomplished through an increased caloric expenditure via aerobic exercise, HDL levels may be further increased (in addition to other benefits of exercise for cardiovascular function).

Apart from a caloric restriction for persons who are overweight (and severe fat reduction for persons with the rare primary lipoprotein lipase deficiency), dietary therapy for all forms of dyslipoproteinemia can be unitary. The degree of modification is tailored to the severity of the disorder, as well as a patient's and his or her supporters' willingness to adhere to it.

The reduction of total fat to about 30–35% of daily calorie intake (from about 40%, which is average among Americans) via isocaloric substitution by carbohydrates is a first step. The carbohydrate that is selected may be simple (sugar) or complex (starch), but the latter provides less intense alimentary hyperglycemia (probably desirable in a diabetic) and is likely to be admixed with fibers (non-absorbable carbohydrates). This is especially desirable in persons with retarded gastrointestinal motility, which includes many elderly persons. Equal distribution of the fat among saturated, mononounsaturated, and polyunsaturated triglycerides reduces the absolute saturated fat intake. Finally, the intake of foods that are relatively concentrated in cholesterol, such as eggs, organ meats (liver, kidney, brain, sweetbreads), and certain shellfish (generally, those that turn orange when cooked, such as lobster, crab, and shrimp), is minimized. This translates into a diet of low cholesterol content (less than 300 mg/day) and a high polyunsaturated/saturated ("P/S") ratio.

In practical terms, this is a diet that is high in complex carbohydrates (pasta, potatoes, bread, vegetables), vegetable oils, poultry, and fish, and low in red meat and high-fat dairy products. Recent surveys indicate that the typical American diet that has evolved over the past 20 years bears many of these characteristics, which resemble the "prudent" diet long espoused by the American Heart Association. Hence, the diet prescribed for most patients with dyslipoproteinemia represents an extension of trends that already are popular among the public at large. Moreover, persons with known hyperlipidemia often assume even more restrictive diets (at least temporarily after a diagnosis of their lipid disorder and/or an atherosclerotic event); hence, little dietary intervention other than reinforcement is commonly required.

The decision to add pharmacologic hypolipidemic treatment is made only when secondary disorders have been treated maximally and dietary intervention has proven inadequate. Even then, the decision must carefully weigh the disadvantages (cost, nuisance side effects, and serious toxicities) versus the advantages of a further lipid reduction. It also must consider both the duration to its maximal effect in plasma lipid alteration and (more important) to a reduction in atherogenesis (or optimally the reversal thereof) versus a patient's estimated remaining life span (including reductions thereto from end-organ damage due to atherosclerotic complications or competing disease processes). As noted previously, only rarely will such consideration result in a decision to treat hyperlipidemia with drugs in an elderly patient.

Hypolipidemic drugs[14] can be grouped broadly into those that reduce triglycerides (often concomitantly raising HDL cholesterol), cholesterol, or both. More rationally, they can be considered via their likely mechanisms of

action at the lipoprotein metabolic control points outlined above.

Non-absorbable drugs, such as neomycin and β-sitosterol, appear to impair cholesterol absorption (control point 1). Nicotinic acid and its analogues and clofibrate and its analogues (e.g., bezafibrate, gemfibrosil, fenofibrate) appear to reduce VLDL production; triglyceride production (control point 2) seems most clearly reduced, but cholesterol (control point 3) and apoB-100 (control point 4) also may be reduced, especially by nicotinic acid. These drugs also appear to facilitate lipoprotein lipase activity and, hence, triglyceride removal (control point 5). A decrease in VLDL with these agents often is met with an increase in LDL, especially during early usage, which perhaps reflects this stimulation of VLDL catabolism. An intriguing possibility is that this especially may be seen in persons with familial combined hyperlipidemia.[15] In addition, these drugs appear disproportionately to ameliorate dysbetalipoproteinemia (type III); since an apoE$_{3,4}$ deficiency remains unchanged, this may reflect a decrease in VLDL flux. This desaturates the putative high-affinity, low-capacity, apoE$_{3,4}$-independent remnant-removal pathway, possibly the LDL (apoB/E) receptor (control point 8), an increase in the capacity of that pathway, or an as yet unknown effect on another alternative remnant-removal mechanism.

Certain drugs that lower LDL cholesterol levels appear to decrease cholesterol synthesis (control point 3). These include nicotinic acid and (probably to a lesser extent) clofibrate and its analogues, as well as others that affect only cholesterol levels (such as probucol). An exciting prospect is the discovery of drugs that are competitive inhibitors of HMG CoA reductase. Currently, two such agents are under investigation, with encouraging preliminary results; ML-236B[15] and mevinolin,[16] which are related compounds synthesized by microorganisms and, hence, of special practical potential.

Other drugs appear to reduce LDL cholesterol levels by mechanisms that enhance LDL receptor activity and, hence, LDL catabolism. These include thyroxine, both L- and D-isomers, and the bile acid-binding resins, cholestyramine and colestipol. The latter work indirectly by causing an increased fecal bile acid loss, which leads, in turn, to an increased conversion of intrahepatic cholesterol to bile acids.

This, in turn, leads to enhanced LDL removal from the plasma.

No agents have been specifically introduced to raise HDL cholesterol levels. However, modest rises often are seen with nicotinic acid, clofibrate, and colestipol. Hence, the theoretic benefit derived from the use of these agents is greater than that reflected in the reduction of total plasma or LDL cholesterol levels. Conversely, since probucol reduces both HDL and LDL, its potential benefit is less than what is predicted on the basis of its reductions in total plasma or LDL cholesterol levels. Estrogens also have been suggested to reduce LDL cholesterol levels in "type II$_a$ hyperlipoproteinemia",[17] and these hormones also raise HDL cholesterol; for reasons that remain unclear, they appear especially specific for dysbetalipoproteinemia.[18]

Placing drug treatment in the perspective of the physiology and pathophysiology of dyslipoproteinemia especially assists in the formulation of a combination therapy. For instance, nicotinic acid appears to overcome the compensatory increase in cholesterol synthesis that accompanies treatment with bile acid sequestrants, thus permitting a normalization of LDL cholesterol levels in persons heterozygous for familial hypercholesterolemia.[19]

While the rationale for, and efficacy of, the use of these hypolipidemic agents are clear, the side effects (both short- and long-term) limit their use. This is especially relevant in geriatric medicine, given both the reduced theoretic benefit of lipid lowering (especially as measured in person-years of reduced morbidity and mortality) and the increased probability of, and susceptibility to, adverse reactions in elderly patients.

Nicotinic acid (niacin) almost universally produces flushing and gastric distress, although these generally abate with continued use; these side effects can be minimized by gradual increases in dosage to the full level of 3–6 grams/day and by taking the drug with meals (especially if preceded by aspirin). Some increase in arrhythmias was reported with this agent in the Coronary Drug Project (CDP), which was a well-designed and executed secondary prevention trial study in middle-aged males. Overall, however, there was a 29%-reduction in non-fatal myocardial infarctions in persons who took niacin in this trial.

Clofibrate is perhaps better tolerated than nicotinic acid and produces only occasional dyspepsia, nausea, and diarrhea. However, no reduction in cardiovascular events was evident with this agent in the CDP.[20] More importantly, in a three-country World Health Organization (WHO)-sponsored, European primary prevention trial of clofibrate in marginally hypercholesterolemic middle-aged males (from the upper one third of the cholesterol distribution), while there was a significant reduction in non-fatal myocardial infarctions, there was an off-setting increase in total mortality in persons taking the active drug.[21] This was largely attributable to increased diseases of the biliary tract and intestine, which perhaps was related to the increased biliary excretion of cholesterol and the enhanced bile lithrogenicity that is associated with clofibrate use. This discouraging report has led to a marked reduction in the use of clofibrate among patients of all ages, and has spurred an investigation of alternative drugs that include several clofibrate analogues.

Thus far, few side effects have been reported with probucol. However, reservations regarding its unknown mechanism of action and associated reduction in HDL cholesterol levels have limited its widespread use.

Estrogens produce the predictable feminizing side effects. Moreover, their use in elderly males with non-invasive prostatic carcinoma was associated with an increased overall death rate attributable to cardiovascular causes.[22] Also (in the CDP), with 5 mg/day of conjugated equine estrogens, there was an increased myocardial infarction and death rate in spite of lower cholesterol levels.[23] However, their effect in postmenopausal females may be quite different, with as much as a 58% reduction in cardiovascular mortality having been reported among elderly users in a retirement community.[24]

D-thyroxine produces a degree of hypermetabolism that may prove to be intolerable. Moreover, its use in the CDP was associated with increased hypertension, arrhythmias, sudden death, and total death, thus essentially eliminating its use in an older population.[25]

The bile acid sequestrants thus far appear to be free of serious systemic effects, perhaps because of their retention in the gastrointestinal tract. For this reason, one such agent, cholestyramine, was selected for the Coronary Primary Prevention Trial of the Lipid Research Clinic in hypercholesterolemic middle-aged males; morbidity and mortality related to coronary disease was decreased in the treatment group.[26] However, the high cost and incidence rate of unpleasant gastrointestinal side effects have limited their use. The associated constipation that is attributable to the binding of bile acids and the consequent reduction in stool water content make these agents especially difficult for elderly persons to tolerate.

Treatment of Dyslipoproteinemia in Old Age

Since the major forms of dyslipoproteinemia are associated with premature atherosclerosis and (hence) a high death rate before to old age, the prevalence of these disorders is likely to be diminished in elderly persons. The reduced caloric intake of elderly persons and the associated diminution in adipose mass also would appear to ameliorate both inherited and acquired disorders of lipoprotein metabolism. The differential survival of females versus males in old age also selects for those among elderly persons who are relatively resistant to atherosclerosis. Thus, only rarely would an intervention to reduce lipid levels be indicated in elderly persons, even if drug treatment was innocuous. Thus, treatment would be indicated only in a patient with a lipoprotein lipase deficiency or another cause for the accumulation of chylomicrons after an overnight fast (with triglyceride levels usually exceeding 1,500 mg/dl). This condition is distinctly rare in old age; it can be managed (as in younger patients) via insulin replacement (for a diabetic), alcohol withdrawal (in one who is alcohol-sensitive), or treatment to reduce triglyceride production (clofibrate, nicotinic acid, androgenic progestins, or anabolic steroids).

Obesity in Elderly Persons

The above argument against an aggressive treatment of dyslipoproteinemia in elderly persons has several parallels in consideration of obesity in elderly persons. However, since the mechanisms that regulate adipose mass are less well understood than those that control plasma lipoproteins, and since formal clinical trials of weight reduction have not been successfully undertaken at any age, the guidelines for selective intervention against obesity in elderly persons require a greater extrapolation than those against intervention for dyslipoproteinemia. The central message is, however, the same; only in extreme cases of obesity that specifically aggravate a functional disability should weight loss therapy be undertaken in an elderly patient.

As with plasma lipid levels (and very likely related thereto, *see* above), relative body weight increases until middle age and appears to decline in both sexes in old age (*see* Figure 29-2). While data from cross-sectional studies might imply that weight reduction in old age could be attributable to a differentially increased mortality rate among the more obese before old age, data from the Framingham Study clearly indicated that this is indeed not the case.[27] Quite the contrary, a recent re-analysis of tables of standard ("ideal," "desirable") body weights by the Metropolitan Life Insurance Company consistently suggest that while both extremes of relative body weight may be associated with increased overall mortality rates in the population at large, especially among elderly persons (e.g., 80-89-year old persons in studies sponsored by the American Cancer Society), those who survive the longest might be characterized as distinctly on the obese side. Moreover, in those studies, it appeared more advantageous to be quite grossly obese than in the lowest weight group in this age interval. Most studies (recently reviewed by Andres[28]) suggest that the minimum mortality rate at all ages is associated with average relative weight rather than "ideal" weight. The nadir of the J-shaped relationship between mortality and relative body weight is some 12–19% over the "desirable" weight according to earlier life insurance table standards. Overall, the many studies that were reviewed suggest no clear relationship between body mass index and all-cause mortality; the relative weights of decedents and survivors in prospective studies virtually are identical, on the average. To some extent, this lack of a relationship between mortality rate and relative body weight may reflect the phenomenon of competing causes for mortality that are not always carefully documented in cause-specific mortality rate tables (e.g., any increase in deaths attributable to coronary heart disease, perhaps positively associated with relative body weight, might be offset by a decrease in mortality attributable to malignancy). Possible confounding factors are the well-known inverse relationship between relative body weight and cigarette smoking, and the increased death rate that is attributable to it. However, a preliminary analysis of available data on this topic suggests that even among cigarette smokers death rates are highest at the lowest body weight. The overall impression one gets from an analysis of the relationship between all-cause or cause-specific mortality rates is that there may be quite a broad range of weights over which relatively little change in mortality can be appreciated, and that this range may extend to as high as 20–30% above the "ideal" reflected in the 1959 Metropolitan Life Insurance Company tables.

Thus, there seems to be little indication for recommending weight loss for reasons of health, except in persons in whom an adverse risk factor profile for an atherosclerotic-cardiovascular disease has been clearly aggravated by excessive weight. While little, if any, direct relationship between excess adiposity and cardiovascular risk can be demonstrated independently of its effect on those risk factors, a reduction in weight is a clear means whereby a risk factor reduction can be accomplished. This lowers blood pressure, raises HDL cholesterol levels, lowers LDL cholesterol levels, lowers triglyceride (if desirable), reduces insulin requirements, and hence improves control of glucose intolerance in an obese diabetic, and so on. This type of intervention could be expected to be as effective in an elderly patient with an obesity-aggravated adverse risk factor profile as in a younger person. However, proceeding from the line of reasoning developed above, the wisdom of a risk factor reduction in an older patient for either the primary or secondary prevention of atherosclerotic cardiovascular disease is debatable; the risks are not trivial. Furthermore, a patient who has survived into old age in spite of obesity is likely to bear some compensating longevity factor that makes intervention, especially measured in person-years of benefit, theoretically less attractive.

Finally, one must consider the cost and risks

of intervention to reduce body weight. These include not only the frustration and depression that is attendant on hypocaloric dietary intervention, but also the increased risk of pharmacologic intervention with, for instance, amphetamines or thyroid hormones in a vulnerable elderly patient. Given that weight reduction regimens frequently meet with (specifically long-term) failure in obese patients regardless of age, an obese elderly patient who has adjusted to his or her adiposity is unlikely to change relative body weight until an ominous cause intervenes (i.e., illness). Thus, even in obese elderly persons, weight loss usually is discouraging to a patient, family, and physician. Weight loss all too often signals a serious illness as it does at any age, but perhaps it has even more significance than in young persons. Considering the multiple causes for weight loss in elderly persons (e.g., depression, social isolation, loss of taste sensation, diminished appetite related to diminished exercise and caloric expenditure, poor dentition, and diminished gastrointestinal efficiency), it is little wonder that the national history of relative body weight is a decline in old age, which perhaps predicts the impending end of the life span. Hence, weight loss should be advised only in an elderly patient immobilized by his or her obesity (perhaps aggravating osteoarthritis, preventing self-care or socialization, or compromising cardiopulmonary function). Even then, if it succeeds, a discerning geriatrician must suspect causes for a "successful" weight loss that are attributable to underlying disease, not simply to voluntary caloric restriction.

References

1. Fries J: Aging, natural death, and the compression of morbidity. *N Engl J Med* 303:130–135, 1980.
2. The Lipid Research Clinics Program Epidemiology Committee: Plasma lipid distributions in selected North American populations: The Lipid Research Clinics Program Prevalence Study. *Circulation* 60:427–439, 1970.
3. Heiss G, Tamir I, Davis CE, et al: Lipoprotein-cholesterol distributions in selected North American populations: The Lipid Research Clinics Program Prevalence Study. *Circulation* 61:302–315, 1980.
4. Bierman EL, Glomset JA: Disorders of lipid me-

tabolism, In Williams RH (ed): *Textbook of Endocrinology.* Philadelphia, Saunders. 1974, pp 890–937.

5. Brunzell JD, Bierman EL: Chylomicronemia syndrome: interaction of genetic and acquired hypertriglyceridemia. *Med Clin N Am* 66:455–468, 1982.

6. Gordon T, Castelli WP, Hjortland MC, et al: High density lipoprotein as a protective factor against coronary heart disease. The Framingham Study. *Am J Med* 62:707–714, 1977.

7. Glueck CJ, Gartside PS, Steiner PM, et al: Hyperalpha- and hypobeta-lipoproteinemia in octogenarian kindreds. *Atherosclerosis* 27:387–406, 1977.

8. Nicholson J, Gartside PS, Siegel M, et al: Lipid and lipoprotein distributions in octo- and nonagenarians. *Metabolism* 28:51–55, 1979.

9. Goldstein JL, Brown MS: The LDL receptor defect in familial hypercholesterolemia: implications for pathogenesis and therapy. *Med Clin N Am* 66:335–362, 1982.

10. Connor WE, Stone DB, Hodges RE: The interrelated effects of dietary cholesterol and fat upon human serum lipid levels. *J Clin Invest* 43:1691–1696, 1964.

11. Boman H, Hazzard WR, Albers JJ, et al: Frequency of monogenic forms of hyperlipidemia in a normal population. *Am J Human Genet* 27:19A, 1975.

12. Albers JJ, Wahl PW, Cabana VG, et al: Quantitation of apolipoprotein A-1 of human plasma high density lipoprotein. *Metabolism* 25:633–644, 1976.

13. Taggart MMcA, Applebaum-Bowden D, Haffner S, et al: Reduction of high density lipoproteins by anabolic steroid (stanozolol) therapy for postmenopausal osteoporosis. *Metabolism* 31:1147–1152, 1982.

14. Levy RI, Fredrickson DS, Shulman R, et al: Dietary and drug treatment of primary hyperlipoproteinemia. *Ann Int Med* 77:267–294, 1972.

15. Mabuchi H, Haba T, Tatami R, et al: Effects of an inhibitor of 3-hydroxy-3-methylglutaryl coenzyme A reductase on serum lipoproteins and ubiquinone-10 levels in patients with familial hypercholesterolemia. *N Engl J Med* 305:478–482, 1981.

16. Tobert JA, Bell GD, Birtwell J, et al: Cholesterol-lowering effect of mevinolin, an inhibitor of 3-hydroxy-3 methylglutaryl coenzyme. A reductase in healthy volunteers. *J Clin Invest* 69:913–919, 1982.

17. Tikkanen JJ, Nikkila EA, Vantiainen E: Natural estrogen as an effective treatment for type II hyperlipoproteinemia in post-menopausal women. *Lancet* 1:490–491, 1978.

18. Kushwaha RS, Hazzard WR, Gagne C, et al: Type III hyperlipoproteinemia: Paradoxical hypolipidemic response to estrogen. *Ann Int Med* 87:517–525, 1977.

19. Kane JP, Malloy MJ, Tim P, et al: Normalization of low-density-lipoprotein levels in heterozygous familial hypercholesterolemia with a combined drug regimen. *N Engl J Med* 304:251–258, 1981.

20. Coronary Drug Project Research Group: Clofibrate and niacin in coronary heart disease. *JAMA* 231:350, 1975.

21. Miller GJ, Miller NE: Plasma high density lipoprotein concentration and development of ischemic heart disease. *Lancet* 1:16–19, 1975.

20. Taggart H, Haffner S, Chesnut C, et al: An anabolic steroid (Stanozolol) markedly reduces high density lipoproteins in postmenopausal women. *Circulation* 62(suppl III):45, 1980.

21. Oliver MF, Heady JA, Morris JH, et al: A cooperative trial in the primary prevention of ischaemic heart disease using clofibrate. Report from the Committee of Principal Investigators. *Br Heart J* 40:1069–1179, 1978.

22. The Veteran Administration Cooperative Urological Research Group. Treatment and survival of patients with cancer of the prostate. *Surg Gyn Obstet* 124:1011, 1967.

23. Coronary Drug Project Research Group. The coronary drug project: Initial findings leading to modifications of research protocol. *JAMA* 214:1303, 1970.

24. Ross RK, Paganini-Hill A, Mack TM, et al: Menopausal oestrogen therapy and protection from death from ischaemic heart disease. *Lancet* 1:858–860, 1981.

25. Coronary Drug Project Research Group. Findings leading to further modifications of its protocol with respect to dextrothyroxine. *Jama* 220:996–1008, 1971.

26. The Lipid Research Clinics Coronary Primary Prevention Trial Results, *JAMA* 251:351–373, 1984.

27. Sorlic P, Gordon T, Kannel WB: Body build and mortality in the Framingham Study. *JAMA* 243:1828–1831, 1980.

28. Andres R: Aging, diabetes and obesity: standards of normality. *Mt Sinai J Med* 48:489–495, 1981.

CHAPTER 30

Hypothermia

JAMES B. REULER, M.D.

In the minds of many health care practitioners, the problem of hypothermia is associated either with a dramatic presentation that is related to severe environmental exposure in the wilderness or military campaigns or a result of alcohol intoxication. Over the past 25 years, however, it has become recognized that a significant segment of the elderly population is at risk for developing this disorder, which may present in a subtle fashion. Although much work has been done in Great Britain to characterize the epidemiology of hypothermia in elderly persons, the magnitude of this problem in the United States remains unknown. However it is likely—given the higher latitudes and the larger elderly population—that this problem represents a major public health issue for the United States, particularly in times of decreasing economic resources. In this chapter, the particular problem of hypothermia in elderly persons will be discussed. For more broadly based treatises on accidental hypothermia, the reader is referred to several recent reviews.[1-4]

Pathophysiology

Defined as a core body temperature lower than 35°C, hypothermia represents the body's inability to maintain a constant body temperature despite changes in environmental temperature. Any influence which tends to lower the core temperature is met by the mobilization of a number of forces to prevent heat loss and increase heat production. The physical laws involved with heat loss, which are important to the understanding of the development and prevention of hypothermia, include: 1) Conduction, the transfer of heat by direct contact; 2) Convection, the transfer of heat by particles of air or water that have been heated by contact with the body; 3) Radiation, the transfer of energy by non-particulate means, such as heat loss from an unprotected head; and 4) Evaporation of water.

With respect to temperature regulation, the body can be viewed as a core that is protected by several outer layers that modulate heat loss and gain. The skin and subcutaneous tissue, with its thermal receptors, represent the superficial zone and are the most important aspects of the heat exchange mechanism. Body temperature at this level varies with blood flow, ambient air temperature, humidity, and air velocity, and it may drop to nearly environmental temperatures in an attempt to conserve heat. The intermediate zone is comprised of the skeletal muscle mass, which ordinarily contributes little to heat production until the core temperature is in danger of falling; at which time, the muscles provide heat by the mechanism of shivering. The preoptic anterior hypothalamus integrates these various components of heat exchange with the neural network and acts by both the autonomic nervous system to provide a rapid control of heat conservation and by the neuroendocrine axis, thus involving a more gradual increase in heat production.

There are multiple consequences for various organ functions as the body temperature begins to drop. Most obvious is a decrease in the basal metabolic rate, which falls to about 50% of normal at 28°C. Blood pressure initially may rise, but it then gradually falls, with hypotension being clinically significant below 25°C. Most important are the hemodynamic effects, which include the frequent development of atrial fibrillation that is seen with mild temperature reductions and more serious high-grade ventricular dysrhythmias and conduction disturbances at temperatures lower than 28°C.

At lower body temperatures depression of the respiratory center, level of consciousness, and cough reflex, all may lead to problems with aspiration and respiratory insufficiency. In profound hypothermia, major alterations in acid-base equilibrium also may be seen, with acidosis resulting from respiratory failure and tissue hypoxia. In addition, urine flow may increase as the temperature decreases secondary to depressed oxidative tubular activities in the kidney and, combined with shifts of fluids to the extracellular spaces, it may render the patient hypovolemic.

Significant effects are manifested in the central nervous system, where the cerebral blood flow decreases by 6–7% per 1°C drop in body temperature. This decreases, along with alterations in the microcirculation that are due to increased viscosity, may cause decreased mentation. These central nervous system alterations, combined with a frequently observed hyporeflexia, impalpable pulse, and unmeasurable blood pressure, may cause a patient to appear dead.

Epidemiology

In 1964, the British Medical Association published a memorandum on accidental hypothermia in elderly persons, which stated:

Hypothermia is a serious though unspectacular condition with a very high mortality rate, and its early recognition in general practice is therefore important. It may arise independently as a spontaneous condition or it may be secondary to organic or endogenous causes.

The term, "accidental hypothermia" is employed as it is in common usage and because it emphasizes the cause of the majority of cases in elderly people in which environmental and endogenous factors play a part either singly or together. A large number of elderly people who are found to be hypothermic die either from the condition itself or from the underlying disease or from complications which supervene.[5]

The same year, Geoffrey Taylor, a general practitioner in Great Britain, studied environmental and body temperatures as he made his rounds.[6] He found that the average minimum temperature of the bedrooms of his patients was only 2–3° above the ambient environmental temperature, with a low bedroom temperature of −14°C; also, the average oral temperature of his patients was 34.4°C (with a range of 31.6°–35.7°C).

In 1966, the Royal College of Physicians surveyed 10 hospitals in England and Scotland during 3 winter months and found that 0.68% of all admissions had core temperatures less than 35°C, and that 47 of 126 hypothermic patients died.[7] Elderly patients made up 11.25% of the total admissions, but they accounted for 28.6% of all hypothermic admissions. Extrapolating those numbers to all hospital admissions during that period, it was estimated that 9,000 persons could have been admitted with hypothermia. There seemed to be a clear relationship between the incidence of hypothermia and the environmental temperature, since during that period ambient air temperatures dropped to as low as −16°C. Other surveys in Great Britain have found variable magnitudes of hypothermia in elderly persons that ranged up to 11.4% of persons monitored at home and 3.6% of all hospital admissions.[8–11] The most detailed study, The National Hypothermia Survey, involved over 1,000 elderly residents who were evaluated at home with questionnaires. The ambient air temperatures and the mouth and urine temperatures were recorded.[12] These data indicated that 0.58% of elderly persons were hypothermic and that 9.6% were "at risk" (35.0–35.5°C). If extrapolated, these figures represented over 700,000 elderly citizens who were "at risk." Because hypothermia rarely is specified as a cause of death, it is likely that the mortality rates identified for hypothermia in elderly persons are underestimations. Information regarding the incidence rate of hypothermia in elderly persons in the United States is lacking. However, an increasingly large elderly population, decreasing economic resources, and increasingly severe winter seasons, combine to make it likely that hypothermia represents a problem of significant proportion in the United States.

Risk Factors

The development of accidental hypothermia in elderly persons requires some exposure to decreased ambient air temperatures. It appears that, for several reasons, elderly persons are more likely to be faced with an environment in which the ambient air temperature is decreased, and that once in this situation they have fewer physiologic resources available to deal with this stress.

The epidemiologic studies from Great Britain cited above would suggest that many elderly people are exposed to environmental conditions in their homes that approximate ambient environmental temperatures. In the 1972 national survey, 75% of all elderly people had morning living room temperatures lower than 18.3°C (the Council on Housing recommended level) when the mean air temperature was 7°C.[12] Those persons who had bedrooms separate from living rooms seemed to be at a greater risk, since the mean bedroom temperatures were significantly lower than the living room temperatures, dropping as low as 5°C.[13] The decreased environmental temperatures within the home seemed to be directly related to the economic resources of the individual, in that the receipt of supplemental benefits was the only predictor from the analysis of socioeconomic factors that correlated with the development of hypothermia.[10,12] These surveys indicated that elderly persons were more likely to distribute their meager economic resources to food and shelter; therefore, they have inadequate resources for fuel. It also was shown that those individuals living within public housing projects with central heating were at much less of a risk of developing hypothermia than those individuals living in individual dwellings, particularly individuals with separate bedroom and living room combinations.

Thermal comfort, which is the condition of the mind that expresses satisfaction with the thermal environment,[14] is influenced by several variables that include the activity level, the thermal resistance of clothing (clo value), air temperature and its components, the mean radiant temperature, the relative air velocity, and the water vapor pressure in the ambient air.[15] Elderly persons differ little from younger persons regarding thermal comfort requirements.[16,17] However, the ability to discriminate peripheral temperature differences seems to deteriorate with age.[17] In general, elderly persons perceive peripheral temperature changes less than do younger persons; when given control over the environment by means of attaining preferred temperatures, elderly persons are less precise.[18,19] Collins, et al, showed that there was a significant difference between young and elderly subjects in their ability to discriminate mean temperature differences by using digital thermal sensation. The young subjects were able to discriminate differences in cold exposure of 0.8 ± 0.2°C, as opposed to elderly subjects whose mean discrimination was 2.3 ± 0.5°C.[20]

Horvath showed that there were no significant changes in heat production, respiratory quotient, or oxygen consumption, when elderly persons were put in an environmental temperature of 10°C; whereas, there were large increases in each of these parameters in the young persons under similar conditions, and the elderly persons did not complain of being cold during the experience.[21] In response to cold exposure, the rectal and mean skin temperatures decrease with age due to a general decrease in the basal metabolic rate and a reduction in heat conductance.[22] When put into a cold environment, young persons have a rapid increase in their metabolic rate and minimize peripheral heat loss by cutaneous vasoconstriction; whereas, elderly persons are not as able to greatly increase their metabolic rate and are less able to maintain body heat stores by cutaneous vasoconstriction. It is suggested that this inability to maintain heat stores by cutaneous vasoconstriction is a reflection of an underlying autonomic insufficiency.

In summary, physiologic alterations in elderly persons may predispose to the development of hypothermia. These include a decreasing body core-shell temperature gradient, decreased resting peripheral blood flow, a non-constrictor pattern of vasomotor response to cold, a higher incidence of orthostatic hypotension, and decreased precision in attaining a preferred temperature.[17,19,20,23] Additional factors that have been incriminated include the use of sedative-hypnotic and other neuroleptic drugs often prescribed for insomnia and agitation, which alter the central and peripheral neuroendocrine aspects of heat generation and inhibit shivering and the prevalence of falls leading to an increased risk of exposure.

Clinical Evaluation

There are numerous clinical settings in which hypothermia may be a consequence.[2] It is important to re-emphasize that extreme environmental conditions are not required to precipitate hypothermia, with factors of wind velocity, moisture, alcohol ingestion, clothing, and duration of exposure, all playing important roles. In addition to the predisposing factors that were already mentioned, hypothermia may be a consequence of underlying disease processes. The most common association is with myxedema, with an insufficient calorigenesis providing the mechanism.[24] Approximately 80% of all patients with myxedema will have low body temperatures. This may explain the increased incidence rate of myxedematous comas in the winter months and the risk of sedative drugs in this setting.[25] A myxedema coma may present a difficult diagnostic problem, because many of the findings of hypothyroidism may be mimicked by hypothermia, including edema, abdominal distress, ileus, and delayed deep-tendon reflexes. Also, hypothermia may be a manifestation of hypoglycemia due to an exclusion of glucose from central nervous system sites.[26] This may be a particular problem in diabetic elderly patients who may have problems with administering insulin due to a visual impairment.

Central nervous system disorders, which include cerebral vascular diseases, may lead to alterations in the hypothalamic temperature regulatory center that predisposes to hypothermia. In addition, hypothermia is a common manifestation of Wernicke's encephalopathy due to a thiamine deficiency, which usually is seen in the setting of chronic alcohol ingestion and inadequate nutrition. The basis for hypothermia in this setting is the predilection for an involvement of the hypothalamic nuclei.

Drug-induced hypothermia may be caused by an interruption at several steps in the thermoregulatory scheme. A depression of the hypothalamic center, inhibition of shivering by a peripheral curarizing affect, and vasodilatation all play a role. This concept is particularly important with respect to elderly persons due to the frequency with which many of the implicated drugs are prescribed.[11] The postoperative setting also is one in which elderly persons may be vulnerable to the development of core temperature depression. The predilection for development of hypothermia postoperatively will be met with a shivering response that may increase postoperative oxygen demands by up to 500%.[27,28] This factor alone may increase the risk of postoperative complications in an elderly patient, particularly with respect to an acute ischemic cardiac disease and metabolic abnormalities. In addition, the decreasing temperature, combined with age-related changes in drug disposition, will lead to an increase in the half-life of many parenterally administered drugs during the perioperative state, thus heightening the possibility of further complications. The use of anesthetic agents with minimal vasodilatory effects, protection of exposed viscera with warmed saline pads, use of warmed irrigation and intravenous (IV) solutions, use of a heating mattress for prolonged surgical procedures, and monitoring temperatures in the postoperative suite, all will aid in minimizing the development of hypothermia.[29]

Because of the major thermoregulatory role played by the skin, patients with exfoliative dermatitis also may be at risk for hypothermia due to increases in skin blood flow and transepidermal water loss, which lead to heat loss via radiation, conduction, and evaporation.[30,31] Therefore, an elderly patient with an erythroderma may be at particular risk for the development of thermal instability.

In addition to the above-mentioned specific disease entities or clinical settings, hypothermia may develop in any acute or chronic disease in an elderly person, particularly when host defenses are overwhelmed (e.g., in the setting of a severe infection). In fact, in the elderly population, the development of hypothermia frequently is a reflection of a combination of several of the above-mentioned factors.

Increased age, complaints of cold hands, a preference for a warmer environment, and the fact that a patient was receiving supplemental benefits, all were characteristics that were associated with hypothermia in British studies. A diagnosis should be considered in any elderly person at risk with findings of a progressing confusion, slurring of speech, ataxia, and involuntary movements. Establishing a diagnosis highlights further problems. Many patients have presented with hypothermia and have not had a diagnosis made until complications supervened. In part, this is due to the fact that standard thermometers record down only to 34.4°C. If the thermometer had not been shaken down to begin with, a hypothermic patient may be missed altogether. Low-reading thermometers should be available in all hospital emergency rooms and intensive care unit areas. As recommended in the Royal College of Physicians report,[5] any person found to have an oral temperature ≤35°C should have the core temperature measured. Although rectal, esophageal, and tympanic temperatures are all excellent reflections of core temperature, they are impractical in many instances. Studies have shown that the measurement of urine temperature correlates well with core temperature, and it may be particularly useful for population screening in the community.[12,32]

Physical examination may disclose a clouding of consciousness, with a coma frequently supervening with temperatures under 27°C. Often, the blood pressure may be unmeasurable, the pulse slow or absent, and respiration shallow and infrequent. When the core temperature is lower than 30°C, shivering will be absent, and the patient may appear to be in rigor mortis because of increased tone. The pupils may be dilated and sluggishly reactive, deep-tendon reflexes may be either absent or delayed, and heart sounds may be absent. All these findings may be combined to lead to a presumptive diagnosis of death at the time of initial evaluation. The above points emphasize the fact that the usual criteria that are used to indicate reversibility are not valid in determining a prognosis in a hypothermic patient. Life may be sustained for long periods after an apparent cardiac arrest because of the decreased oxygen requirements. Few conclusions can be drawn regarding the nature or extent of complicating disorders until the patient is warmed.

Treatment

The management of a hypothermic patient must focus on both general supportive measures and specific rewarming techniques. For patients with mild hypothermia (core temperature higher than 33.3°C), hospitalization may not be required, and management may consist of external rewarming and assuring adequate heating in the living environment. However, a patient with further decrements of core temperature should be hospitalized and monitored more closely, since the lower the core temperature, the more likely the presence of both supervening complications and underlying precipitating disease processes. In addition to a history and physical examination focusing on the identification of precipitating events, laboratory screening should include plasma sugar, amylase, and renal function studies, and coagulation parameters.

In a profoundly hypothermic patient, intensive care unit management and continuous electrocardiographic monitoring is imperative because of the frequency of rhythm disturbances. Atrial flutter and fibrillation will revert once the patient is warmed, and ventricular dysrhythmias generally are abolished with a correction of hypoxia and acidosis. A hypothermic heart, however, is relatively unresponsive to atropine, electrical pacing, and counter-shock. If a ventricular fibrillation occurs and electroshock is not successful, cardiopulmonary resuscitation (CPR) should be instituted and continued until the core temperature is raised, because a successful recovery has been documented after several hours of continued CPR in this setting.[33] The administration of drugs during the period when the patient is profoundly hypothermic may have little therapeutic effect, but it may cause serious problems when the patient is rewarmed; this highlights the hazards of overmedication due to a delayed metabolism of the drugs. In this regard, hyperglycemia should be treated cautiously because of the risk of postwarming hypoglycemia. In the setting of chronic hypothermia, volume depletion may be a particular problem given the tubular dysfunction that is seen, often in association with diuretic therapy and an underlying renal dysfunction in elderly persons. Intravenous fluids may

be warmed via passage through a blood-warm-
ing coil that is maintained at 37°–40°C. Other
details of particular problems that are encountered in a profoundly hypothermic patient may
be found in general review articles.[1-4]

In conjunction with general supportive maneuvers, mechanisms for rewarming should be
instituted. Rewarming methods fall into three
categories: 1) Passive rewarming includes removal from environmental exposure and the
use of insulating materials (e.g., blankets or
sleeping bags); 2) Active external rewarming
techniques would include immersion in heated
water and the use of electric blankets or heated
objects (e.g., hot water bottles); 3) Active core
rewarming would include the use of intragastric
or colonic irrigation, peritoneal dialysis, extra-
corporeal blood rewarming and inhalation rewarming.

The use of particular rewarming methods remains a controversial area within hypothermia
management. Within the available literature,
concern has been raised about the risks of active external rewarming because of inherent
physiologic changes that may aggravate the effect of hypothermia on core tissues, thus leading to what has been termed an "after-drop" of
core temperature after removal of chronic cold
stress. However, most survivors of accidental
hypothermia have been treated with either passive or active external measures without evidence of significant harm. Recent information
from Britain suggests that core rewarming is not
required for the majority of patients with hypothermia.[34] However, the use of core rewarming
techniques should be instituted in patients who
have profound hypothermia and who have evidence of a cardiovascular instability or refractory dysrhythmias. When discussing the use of
more aggressive rewarming techniques, it is important to consider the fact that mortality rates
in cases of accidental hypothermia are not as
related to the degree of temperature depression
per se, as they are correlated with the other
underlying disease processes present.[34-36]

Prevention

As highlighted previously, the problem of hypothermia in elderly persons is in reality a public
health problem of an unclear, but likely, significant magnitude in the United States. The British survey[12] found that a large proportion of elderly persons have cold living conditions; while
most elderly persons maintain reasonable inner
body temperatures, a significant minority fail to
do so and are at risk for developing hypothermia. Of those persons at risk, a small proportion have inner body temperatures below the
hypothermic level, a small but significant proportion of elderly hospital admissions are hypothermic, and an unknown number die from
hypothermia in hospitals, in their own homes,
and elsewhere. The circumstances that surround hypothermia in elderly persons generally
are less dramatic than the more well-known settings that involve outdoor recreationists and the
alcoholic population. Hypothermia usually develops in an indoor setting that involves socially
isolated individuals and is associated with common problems in elderly persons, including immobility and falls. The implications of these
studies have importance for the planners of social service programs, as well as for health care
providers. Policies must focus attention on the
provision of adequate heating in both individual
and multiunit dwellings for elderly persons and
assure frequent social contact—particularly for
the group of elderly persons who live alone in
isolated situations without family support.
Within these policies, priority must be given to
increasing the awareness of the general public
to the scope of the problem. In this regard, the
National Institute of Aging has begun to make
inroads into heightening public awareness by
sponsoring workshops for social service agencies and public policy makers, broadcasting
messages on radio and television, and publishing written materials for the general public.

Within the United States, as compared to
Great Britain, education of health care providers is in its infancy. The increasing focus in
the United States on geriatric care and education in geriatric medicine will help to dissemi-
nate information to this group. In addition, organizations such as the Center for Accidental
Hypothermia in Portland, Maine, have educational programs for health care providers that
address the prevention and detection of accidental hypothermia in elderly persons. It is
hoped that cooperation between government
agencies and private social service and research
organizations will lead to a better understanding

of the epidemiology and magnitude of this problem.

References

1. MacLean D, Emslie-Smith D: *Accidental Hypothermia*. Oxford, England, Blackwell Scientific Publications, 1977.
2. Reuler JB: Hypothermia: pathophysiology, clinical settings, and management. *Ann Int Med* 89:519–527, 1978.
3. Martyn JW: Diagnosing and treating hypothermia. *Canad Med Assoc J* 125:1089–1096, 1981.
4. Fitzgerald FT, Jessop C: Accidental hypothermia: a report of 22 cases and review of the literature. *Adv Int Med* 27:127–150, 1982.
5. Committee on Medical Science, Education, and Research of the British Medical Association: Accidental hypothermia in the elderly. *Br Med J* 2:1255–1258, 1964.
6. Taylor G: The problem of hypothermia in the elderly. *Practitioner* 193:761–767, 1964.
7. Royal College of Physicians: *Report of the Committee on Accidental Hypothermia*. 1966.
8. Hypothermia Subcommittee of the Welfare Group of the Society of Medical Officers of Health: A pilot survey into the occurrence of hypothermia in elderly people living at home. *Public Health* 82:223–229, 1968.
9. Fox RH, MacGibbon R, Davies L, et al: Problem of the old and the cold. *Br Med J* 1:21–24, 1973.
10. Fox RH, Woodward PM, Exton-Smith AN, et al: Body temperatures in the elderly: a national study of physiological, social and environmental conditions. *Br Med J* 1:200–206, 1973.
11. Goldman A, Exton-Smith AN, Francis G, et al: A pilot study of low body temperatures in old people admitted to hospital. *J Coll Physicians* 11:291–306, 1977.
12. Wicks M: *Old and Cold—Hypothermia and Social Policy*. London, Heinemann Educational Books Ltd, 1978.
13. Salvosa CB, Payne PR, Wheeler EF: Environmental conditions and body temperatures of elderly women living alone or in local authority home. *Br Med J* 4:656–659, 1971.
14. Benzinger TH: The physiological basis of thermal comfort, in Fanger PO, Valbjorn O (eds): *Indoor Climate—Effects on Human Comfort, Performance, and Health in Residential, Commercial, and Light-industry Buildings*. Copenhagen, Danish Building Research Institute, 1979, pp 441–476.
15. Fanger PO: *Thermal Comfort-Analysis and Applications in Environmental Engineering*. New York, McGraw-Hill Book Co, 1970.
16. Rohles FH Jr, Johnson MA: Thermal comfort in the elderly. *Trans Am Soc Heat Refrig Air Cond Engineers* 78:131–137, 1972.
17. Collins KJ: Hypothermia and thermal responsiveness in the elderly, in Fanger PO, Valbjorn O (eds): *Indoor Climate—Effects on Human Comfort, Performance, and Health in Residential, Commercial, and Light-industry Buildings*. Copenhagen, Danish Building Research Institute, 1979, pp 819–833.
18. Watts AJ: Hypothermia in the aged: a study of the role of cold-sensitivity. *Environ Res* 5:119–126, 1971.
19. Collins KJ, Exton-Smith AN, Dore C: Urban hypothermia: preferred temperature and thermal perception in old age. *Br Med J* 282:175–177, 1981.
20. Collins KJ, Dore C, Exton-Smith AN, et al: Accidental hypothermia and impaired temperature homeostasis in the elderly. *Br Med J* 1:353–356, 1977.
21. Horvath SM, Radcliffe CE, Hutt BK, et al: Metabolic responses of old people to a cold environment. *J Appl Physiol* 8:145–148, 1955.
22. Wagner JA, Robinson S, Marino RP: Age and temperature regulation of humans in neutral and cold environments. *J Appl Physiol* 37:562–565, 1974.
23. Macmillan AL, Corbett JL, Johnson RH, et al: Temperature regulation in survivors of accidental hypothermia of the elderly. *Lancet* 2:165–169, 1967.
24. Edelman IS: Thyroid thermogenesis. *N Engl J Med* 290:1303–1308, 1974.
25. Angel JH, Sash L: Hypothermic coma in myxoedema. *Br Med J* 1:1855–1859, 1960.
26. Freinkel N, Metzger BE, Harris E, et al: The hypothermia of hypoglycemia. *N Engl J Med* 287:841–845, 1972.
27. Roe CF, Goldberg MH, Blair CS, et al: The influence of body temperature on early postoperative oxygen consumption. *Surgery* 60:85–92, 1966.
28. Vaughan MS, Vaughan RW, Cork RC: Postoperative hypothermia in adults: relationship of age, anesthesia, and shivering to rewarming. *Anesth Analg* 60:746–751, 1981.
29. Heymann AD: The effect of incidental hypothermia in elderly surgical patients. *J Gerontol* 32:46–48, 1977.
30. Grice KA, Bettley FR: Skin water loss and accidental hypothermia in psoriasis, ichthyosis, and erythroderma. *Br Med J* 4:195–198, 1967.
31. Krook G: Hypothermia in patients with exfoliative dermatitis. *Acta Derm Venereol* 40:124–160, 1960.

32. Fox RH, Woodward PM, Fry AJ, et al: Diagnosis of accidental hypothermia of the elderly. *Lancet* 1:424–427, 1971.

33. Southwick FS, Dalglish PH Jr: Recovery after prolonged asystolic cardiac arrest in profound hypothermia—a case report and literature review. *JAMA* 243:1250–1253, 1980.

34. Ledingham I McA, More JG: Treatment of accidental hypothermia: a prospective clinical study. *Br Med J* 2:1102–1105, 1980.

35. Hudson LD, Conn RD: Accidental hypothermia: associated diagnoses and prognosis in a common problem. *JAMA* 227:37–40, 1974.

36. Miller JW, Danzl DF, Thomas DM: Urban accidental hypothermia: 135 cases. *Ann Emerg Med* 9:456–461, 1980.

CHAPTER 31

Dermatology

FRANK PARKER, M.D.

Physiology of Changes in Aging Skin

Alterations in the skin of elderly people seldom can be attributed solely to aging skin; age-related lesions usually are inextricably mixed with changes that are caused by years of exposure to the elements. This is particularly true in fair-skinned, blue-eyed blond or redheaded persons. They are more subject to such changes than dark-haired, brown-eyed persons who have more pigment in their skin; therefore, the latter tan easily when exposed to the sun. Both the life-long cumulative effects of wind and ultraviolet light combine with time to cause the typical changes of thinning, wrinkling, pigmentary changes, and a variety of benign and malignant skin lesions (*see* Figures 31-1, 31-2).

The aging process involves both the epidermis and the dermis, as well as the cutaneous appendages. Table 31-1 outlines these various alterations.[1,2] With advancing age, the proliferative activity of the epidermal cells is diminished and the total thickness of the epidermis is reduced, thus causing the veins to show through the skin surface more readily as well as contributing to dryness of the skin. The pigment-producing cells (melanocytes), which are found in the basal layer of the epidermis, undergo noticeable changes in aging skin that are related to the distribution of pigment and to the proliferation of melanocytes. The number of functioning melanocytes progressively decrease by 10% per decade, resulting in uneven skin pigmentation and graying hair.[1] In some skin regions, especially skin that is exposed to sunlight, there are localized areas of increased pigment formation within the melanocytes and a proliferation of melanocytes that lead to hyperpigmented lentigos (*see* Figure 31-3). The most striking alterations in the skin occur in the dermis, particularly in sun-exposed regions that consist of changes in the collagen, elastic fibers, and ground substance. The organization of the collagen bundles is altered and, chemically, the collagen becomes less "soluble" and "brittle" with age; the fibers also show homogenization and breaking (elastotic changes). Elastic fibers are decreased in number[1,2] with age. Ground substance, glycoaminoglycans, and water content of the dermis, all decrease with age. Taken together, all of these alterations in the dermis are responsible for the wrinkling, sagging, less supple texture, and leathery characteristics of aged skin. Aged skin is flaccid and inelastic, with a poor load extensibility. In infancy, extensibility is 40–60% of its resting length; but, by 65 years of age, extensibility has been reduced to 15–20%.[3] The epidermal-dermal junction, which in young skin is highly convoluted, shows a progressive flattening out of the elaborated undulant ridges and grooves that strengthen the junction zone. This loss of interlocking ridges and grooves between the two layers of the skin weakens the junction, so resistance to shearing forces is diminished. This leads to easy blistering and, possibly, an ease of developing pressure sores. Virtually all the skin appendages' growth and function gradually are impaired and slow down in aged skin. Sebaceous gland activity declines and the decrease

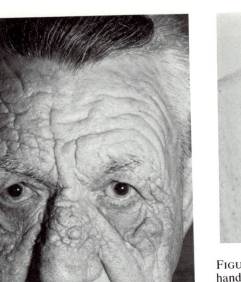

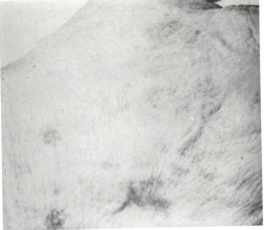

FIGURE 31-3   Senile lentigos on the dorsum of the hand. These flat, light-brown, pigmented areas represent regions of increased melanin accumulation.

FIGURE 31-1   Typical alterations in aged skin. Note the deep wrinkling, sagging, and leathery appearance in sun-exposed areas of the skin, as well as a loss of pigment in the hair.

in oily sebum production may predispose to the dry skin that is so commonly encountered in elderly persons.[1,2] Similarly, eccrine sweat gland numbers and their activity decline, which also contributes to skin dryness.[1] Furthermore, the response to stimuli that ordinarily elicit

sweating is decreased to the point that the primary function of sweating, which is to prevent hyperthermia, is impaired in elderly persons. Hair growth is decreased in some follicles, and the density of follicles is progressively decreased throughout the life span, especially over the scalp and extremities and in the axillae of both males and females.[1] In other follicles, such as those on the face and chest, hairs become larger and more obvious with age. Nails become thinner, longitudinally ridged and brittle, and they grow at a rate that is approximately 50% of that in young adults.[1,2] It is likely that this is the cause of the ineffectiveness of griseofulvin in treating chronic fungal infections of the toenails in elderly patients.

Clinical Conditions in Aged Skin and Their Treatment

Xerosis and Eczema Craquelé

Dry skin (scaling, flaking, fissuring), or xerosis, perhaps is the most common dermatologic problem in persons past middle age.[4] Eccrine sweat and sebaccous gland function, which contribute to hydration and the prevention of water loss through the stratum corneum, are lost with aging and contribute to dryness. Xero-

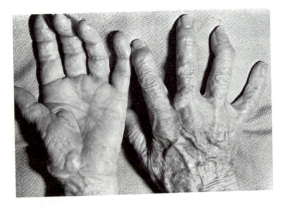

FIGURE 31-2   Wrinkling and thinning of aged skin with a prominence of the cutaneous veins.

TABLE 31-1 Anatomic and Physiologic Changes in Human Skin with Aging

Anatomic Portion of the Skin	Anatomic or Physiologic Change	Clinical Consequence
Epidermis	Decline in epidermal cell proliferation	Mild scaling and fine wrinkling of skin
Melanocytes	Decreased melanocytes, some regions increased pigment formation	Uneven skin pigmentation; gray hair
Dermal	Loss and alteration in collagen and elastic fibers; loss of hyaluronic acid and water content	Deep wrinkling, leathery, loss of elasticity. Sagging skin. Easy bruising (liver spots). Loss of turgor and extensibility
Dermal-epidermal junction	Flattening of normal highly undulated junction	Less resistance to shearing forces and easy blistering, and perhaps an ease of developing pressure sores
Sebaceous glands	Decrease activity with decline of androgen secretion	Decreased sebum lipids on the surface of the skin that predisposes to dryness, xerosis
Eccrine sweat glands	Decline in number of active sweat glands and output per gland	Dryness of skin; less ability to cope with hot environment
Hair	Decrease growth of hair in some follicles, (i.e., scalp and axillary hair)	Male and female pattern baldness and sparsity of hair axillae due to a decline of androgen secretion
	Stimulation of growth of some hair follicles, (i.e., face)	Terminal face hairs on males and females
Nails	Decreased growth	Thickening and irregular shape, especially on the toenails; ridging, splitting, thinning of the fingernails

sis is more prevalent during the winter, when humidity is low. Clinically, the skin is dry, rough, and slightly scaling. When areas of eczematization occur (erythema, accentuation of normal skin lines—lichenification, scaling, fissuring, and itching), the condition is termed dermatitis hiemalis or winter eczema.[4] In xerosis, tiny fissures develop in skin lines. When these linear fissures become widened and inflamed, resembling railroad tracks, the reaction is termed eczema craquelé (see Figure 31-4).[4]

Xerosis responds to the frequent use of emollient creams, to decreased bathing (which tends to dry the skin), to bath oils when the patient does bathe, and to mild topical steroid (1 or 2½% hydrocortisone) ointments that are applied two or three times a day for eczematous eruptions.

Pruritus

Itching of the skin, without xerosis or other obvious skin changes, often occurs for unknown reasons in elderly persons. However, other eti-

ologic factors must be searched for, because generalized or localized pruritus may be a sign of several underlying disease processes. These include drug reactions, internal carcinomas or lymphomas, liver or kidney impairment, thyrotoxicosis, and diabetes. Some elderly people with generalized pruritus have arteriosclerosis that produce "crawling" paresthesias on the extremities. If no underlying cause for the pruritus is found, emollients and low doses of antihistaminics or sedatives will improve the itching. Great care must be used in prescribing antihistaminics and sedatives in elderly persons, as small doses often cause intense soporific effects. Ultraviolet light (given two to three times a week) also may allay pruritus when used for several weeks.

Stucco Keratoses or Stucco Ichthyosis

These lesions occur in about 10% of the population over 40 years of age, with a higher incidence in males. The etiology of these lesions is unknown. They do not occur on sun-exposed

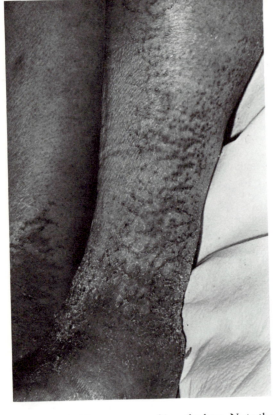

FIGURE 31-4   Eczema craquelé on the legs. Note the criss-crossing, linear fissures within the inflamed dry skin.

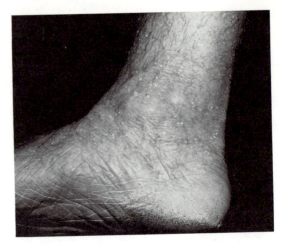

FIGURE 31-5   Stucco keratoses appear as small, round, grayish-white, hard, rough, and hyperkeratotic papules. They frequently appear on the lower legs in varying numbers.

areas, but rather more commonly on the lower legs and, less often, the forearms. Stucco keratoses appear as 1–5 mm, round, grayish-white, hard, rough, and hyperkeratotic papules that number a few to hundreds of lesions that increase with age (*see* Figure 31-5).[4] No treatment is needed for these asymptomatic papules, but they can be removed by simple electrodesiccation or by cryotherapy.

Clinical Conditions Associated with Degenerative Changes of Dermal Collagen

Nodular Cutaneous Elastosis
This is a term given for a clinical picture of dark comedones with patulous openings that are surrounded by cystic follicles engorged with keratinous debris localized around the periorbital and malar areas and the neck (*see* Figure 31-6).[4] Of all people over 40 years of age, 6% develop

these changes, which are brought about by extensive degenerative changes in both collagen and elastic fibers in sun-exposed areas. Treatment is not very effective, although topical Vitamin A acid (retinoic acid) that is applied once or twice a day may remove some of the comedones. A plastic surgical excision of the areas may be necessary if the changes are extensive.

Colloid Milium
This is a term for the degenerative effects of long ultraviolet light exposure on the dermal

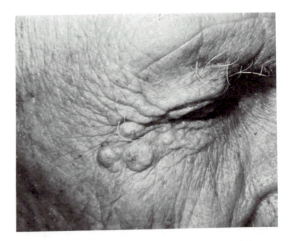

FIGURE 31-6   Extreme elastosis of the dermal collagen leads to nodular cutaneous elastosis (i.e., yellowish nodules with dark comedones and patulous openings).

collagen, which appear as yellow, soft, 2–4-mm papules and plaques on the face and dorsum of the hands.[4] No satisfactory treatment is available.

Cutis Rhomboidalis Nuchae

Extreme effects of degenerative changes in the collagen with aging and chronic sun exposure results in a marked thickening and accentuation of skin lines, which form deep furrows over the nape of the neck and, at times, on the lateral sides of the neck and the anterior chest.[4] The skin is leathery and may become red and hyperpigmented. The changes are irreversible and no treatment is available.

Age-Related Vascular Skin Lesions

Purpuric lesions on the dorsal areas of the forearms—senile purpura—are quite common, particularly in females; they occur in at least 20% of all persons over 70 years of age. These flat, purplish-red, non-blanchable patches are the result of reduced dermal collagen support around the superficial vessels that results from an elastotic degeneration of the collagen. Even minor shearing injuries cause vessel ruptures and purpura, which last from 1–4 weeks. No alteration in blood coagulation parameters are found. Pseudoscars develop on the dorsum of the hands and forearms in conjunction with senile purpura. These flat, white, slightly depressed, and small scars may be linear or starshaped. They persist indefinitely, increase with age, and are painless, although they occasionally may ulcerate.

Cherry or Senile Angioma

These appear in the 3rd or 4th decade, and the lesions become larger and more numerous with age. Virtually all persons in their 8th decade acquire these angiomas. The lesions are flat, red- to reddish-brown in color when small (they often are numerous and confused with petechiae on the trunk); but, then they develop into dome-shaped papules 5 mm or more in diameter and display a purple hue. Even though the lesions are principally found on the trunk, they may be more widespread. Most lesions persist indefinitely, although some regress. Cherry angiomas require no therapy, but they can be lightly fulgurated for cosmetic reasons under lo-

cal anesthesia. They invariably are benign and unrelated to internal conditions or diseases.

Venous Stars

These are formed by dilated veins when venous pressure is increased, and they usually develop on the feet and legs with advancing age.[5] These star-shaped, deep-blue, vascular lesions resemble arterial spiders. However, they are not pulsatile and fill from the periphery rather than the center. Venous stars occasionally can occur in association with cirrhosis of the liver and an obstruction of the vena cava. The stars require no therapy.

Venous Lakes

These are soft, asymptomatic, dark-purple papules that occur most commonly on the ear, lower lip, face, and neck (see Figure 31-7). Although a patient may be alarmed by occasional bleeding from these lesions, their dark-blue to even black color is of greatest concern, as they may be mistaken for a melanoma. These lesions definitely are formed more commonly in older males. Although their precise cause is unknown, ultraviolet light is thought to play a role in their evolution. Venous lakes are not related to cancer or other internal diseases, and they can be treated by shaving off the lesion with a scalpel and fulgurating the area lightly.

Senile Telangiectasis

This is a condition that is characterized by dilated superficial blood vessels, especially over the face and neck, in older people who have had

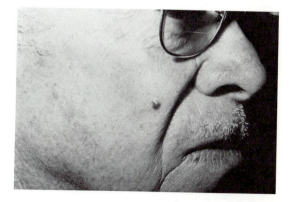

FIGURE 31-7 A small, soft, dark-purple papule on the cheek. Venous lakes commonly occur on the face, lips, and ears.

cumulative extensive sun exposure and actinic skin damage. In fact, senile telangiectases are more common in blond, blue-eyed, and fair-skinned individuals. A better term for this condition is actinic telangiectasis. Such changes are irreversible, but they may be hidden by cosmetics.

Angiokeratomas of Fordyce

These are an extremely common finding in an older male over 50 years of age.[5] Numerous benign, raised, dark-purple, firm, and asymptomatic papules evolve on the scrotal skin and represent dilated cutaneous blood vessels (see Figure 31-8). Treatment is not necessary.

Kaposi's Sarcoma

This is a more serious vascular skin lesion, which represents a sarcomatous vascular tumor that most commonly involves the legs and arms. The typical lesions are large, dark-red or purple nodules and plaques on the extremities, and often are associated with brawny edema.[6] Symptoms are mild, but pain, itching, bleeding, and ulceration can occur. In some instances, the disease seems multifocal; in others it appears to metastasize to the lymph nodes and viscera.

Kaposi's sarcoma occurs twice as frequently in males as in females, with the highest incidence rate during the 6th and 7th decades. The course is similar to that of other neoplasia, with variable survival times that may be as brief as a few months, but more commonly exceeds 20 years. Despite treatment with local radiotherapy (the sarcomatous lesions are extremely radiosensitive) and chemotherapy (vinblastine[7]), a permanent cure is unusual. An increased incidence of Kaposi's sarcoma is found in patients on a chronic immunosuppressive therapy,[8] such as recipients of renal transplants and patients with temporal arteritis or rheumatoid arthritis on a long-term steroid therapy who also have a multiple myeloma.

Angular Cheilitis

This is a common condition in older patients that presents as inflamed, moist, and fissured skin at the angles of the mouth. Several factors may play a role in the cause of this condition, such as a vitamin (riboflavin) deficiency, latent or overt iron deficiency, monilial infection, and changes in the tissues in edentulous persons.[5] The skin of the cheeks loses support, and the additional decrease in skin tone with age leads to overlapping folds at the mouth angles that act as a reservoir for both saliva and (subsequently) monilial infections. Dentures may correct the cheilitis by eliminating the folds, restoring lip contour, and preventing saliva accumulation on the skin. An allergy to denture materials or cleansing agents may be another factor in angular cheilitis. Treatment of this type of cheilitis consists of eliminating the underlying cause and treating the secondary infection. Mild topical steroids (hydrocortisone ointment) applied several times a day will decrease the inflammatory component.

Vulvar Atrophy and Problems of the Genitalia as Common Skin Problems in Elderly Persons

The development of genital atrophy in females is a natural consequence of aging. The loss of subcutaneous tissue occurs with decreased der-

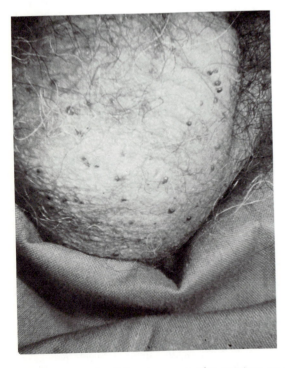

FIGURE 31-8 Angiokeratomas on the scrotum appear as firm, dark-purple-reddish papules. They usually are asymptomatic and require no therapy.

mal and epidermal thickness, and a postmenopausal decrease in secretions causes drying and associated pruritus.[5] An itch-scratch cycle may then result in lichenification. Secondary eczematization due to topical medications, lubricants, soaps, and clothing may occur. Candidal or trichomal vaginitis, dermatophyte infections, diabetes with glucosuria, stress incontinence, and increased heat, sweating, and maceration all may serve to aggravate the pruritus.

Kraurosis Vulva

This is a progressive, inflammatory, and sclerosing vulvar atrophy in middle-aged and elderly females that does not appear to be dependent on hormones. It often is characterized by tenderness, dyspareunia, and dysuria, rather than by pruritus. Kraurosis vulva often causes vaginal stenosis and may progress to leukoplakia.

Lichen Sclerosis et Atrophicus

This is a more severe, sclerosing atrophy of the vulva that occurs in all ages, although more than 50% of all patients are over 45 years of age. Ivory-white, coalescing macules with cigarette-paper wrinkling and atrophy, and a violaceous rim develop in an hourglass pattern around the vaginal and anal orifices (see Figure 31-9).[9] The lesions may be pruritic and may fissure or ulcerate. Leukoplakia (i.e., histologic atypia of the epidermal cells) develops in 50% of all patients, and a carcinoma may follow in 3%. A similar

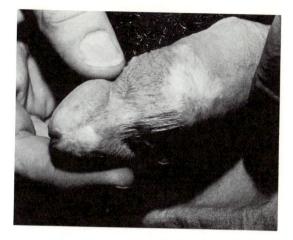

FIGURE 31-10 Balanitis xerotica obliterans is the same sclerosing, atrophic process on male genitalia as lichen sclerosis atrophicus that is found in a female. This process can lead to phimosis and urethral stenosis.

process termed balanitis xerotica obliterans is seen in elderly males, and it may result in phimosis and urethral stenosis (see Figure 31-10).[10]

Treatment of these atrophic lesions is often unsatisfactory. One should aim at using emollients and mild topical steroids (hydrocortisone) to control the itching. The atrophic lesions should be observed carefully for the development of leukoplakia and carcinomas.

Benign and Malignant Skin Tumors

An elderly patient frequently confronts a physician with a variety of benign, premalignant, and malignant skin tumors.[11] Several factors appear to play a role in the etiology of skin malignancies, which include electromagnetic radiation (sunlight, x-ray), chemical carcinogens (arsenic), and genetic predisposition and chronic scarring processes of the skin (i.e., sites of thermal burns and chronic sinus tract). Furthermore, immunosuppressed patients (i.e., kidney allograft recipients) have an increased incidence of certain cancers (squamous cell cancers).[12] Particular concern, therefore, must be given to persistent non-healing ulcers of the skin, to ulcers or tumors that evolve in thermal burn or x-ray scars, and to cutaneous lesions in light-skinned, easily sunburned individuals exposed to a life time of ultraviolet irradiation and moles that are undergoing an unusual growth pattern.

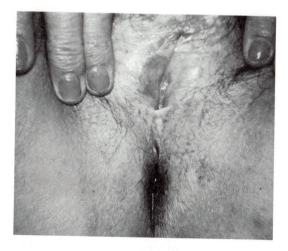

FIGURE 31-9 Lichen sclerosis et atrophicus causes sclerotic atrophy in the perivulvar area and appears as ivory-white, wrinkled areas of the skin.

Various types of benign and malignant tumors can be best differentiated clinically by dividing them into tumors with and without pigmentation.

Non-Pigmented Skin Tumors

Basal Cell Carcinomas These are the most common form of skin cancer originating from the basal cells of the epidermis. They usually are found over sun-exposed areas of the skin, with 93% occurring on the head and neck and 7% on the trunk. These cancers can take several forms. Nodular ulcerative basal cell cancers are the most common form and present as waxy or pearly appearing nodules with a central ulceration (rodent ulcers) and telangiectatic vessels threading across the translucent rolled borders (*see* Figure 31-11). Bleeding due to minor trauma and a lack of healing of ulcerated areas are common clinical features. Superficial basal cell cancers present as sharply marginated plaques with pearly, thread-like borders and a central crust (*see* Figure 31-12). They often are mistaken for eczema patches, but they fail to clear with topical steroid applications. Occasionally, basal cell cancers can be darkly pigmented and, therefore, may be mistaken for melanomas (*see* Figure 31-13). The most subtle and difficult form of basal cell cancer to cure is the morphea or sclerosing type, which appears as a flat, depressed, and scarring patch that slowly enlarges (*see* Figure 31-14). Telangiec-

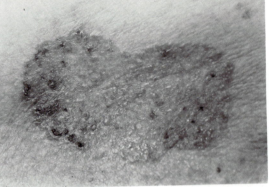

FIGURE 31-12 Superficial spreading basal cell cancers are difficult to identify. Note the sharply marginated plaque with pearly thread-like borders. These can be easily confused with psoriasis or eczema.

tases are present, and there is a shiny, waxy quality to these lesions. All unexplained scarring lesions in sun-exposed areas should be biopsied to aid an early diagnosis.

Benign Hyperplasia of Sebaceous Glands These are particularly common lesions found on the face that evolve with advancing age and frequently are confused with basal cell cancers. The sebaceous hyperplasia appears as solitary or multiple groups of yellow papules that may take on an annular configuration with a central

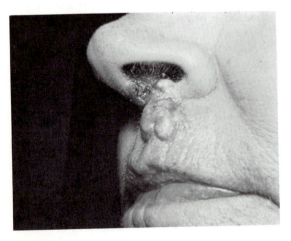

FIGURE 31-11 This nodular, ulcerative, basal cell cancer appears as waxy, pearly nodules with ulceration and (as shown here) some destruction of the nasal mucosa.

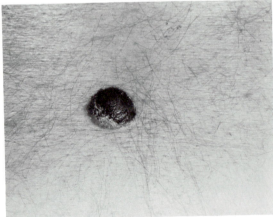

FIGURE 31-13 Pigmented basal cell cancers may be mistaken for melanomas. When the lesion is placed under stretch, it has a characteristic, opalescent, pearly appearance.

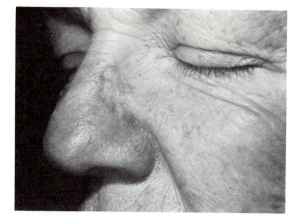

FIGURE 31-14 Sclerosing basal cell cancer appears as a depressed white scar. A clue to the diagnosis is the presence of telangiectasis in the scar and a shiny waxy appearance.

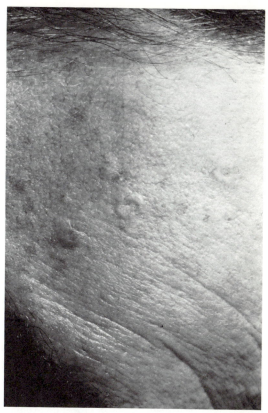

FIGURE 31-15 Benign hyperplasia of the sebaceous glands often are confused with basal cell cancers, because they form groups of papules in annular configurations. This enlargement of sebaceous glands occurs primarily on the face, as shown here on the forehead.

depression (*see* Figure 31-15). The yellow color is an important clue in differentiating these benign lesions from basal cell cancers.

Squamous Cell Carcinomas Fortunately, these occur less frequently than basal cell cancers, as these tumors have a greater propensity to metastasize than basal cell epitheliomas. The clinical appearance of squamous cell cancers (that arise from the keratinizing cells of the epidermis) varies from scaling, ulcerated, and papular lesions to elevated, nodular, and bleeding fungating tumors. They most commonly appear on the face and dorsum of the hands, especially on the lower lip, as indurated, eroded nodules (*see* Figure 31-16).

Squamous cell cancers may arise de novo or from indolent premalignant lesions, such as actinic keratosis, Bowen's disease, and actinic cheilitis, or leukoplakia of the lip. Actinic keratoses are premalignant, erythematous, scaling, and poorly marginated lesions with telangiectatic vessels coursing through them (*see* Figure 31-17). Some lesions become very hyperkeratotic and can assume the appearance of a cutaneous horn. Cutaneous horns also may represent a squamous cell cancer and always should be viewed with concern. Actinic keratoses usually are associated with freckled pigmentation and yellowed furrowing of the skin due to actinic elastosis. A skin biopsy procedure may be necessary to distinguish actinic keratosis from squamous cell tumors. Liquid nitrogen freezing

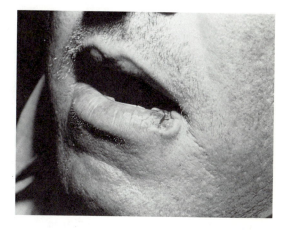

FIGURE 31-16 A typical well-advanced squamous cell carcinoma presenting as a very firm, ulcerated, nodular lesion on the left side of the lower lip.

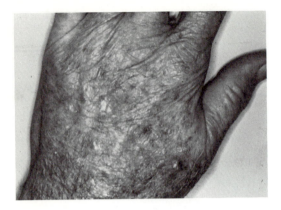

FIGURE 31-17 Actinic keratoses commonly occur on the sun-exposed areas of the hands and face. These red scaling papules may evolve into squamous cell cancers.

or topical 5-Fluorouracil applications for 2–4 weeks are effective forms of therapy.

Bowen's Disease This is an intraepidermal squamous cell cancer in situ. The lesions appear as eczematous or psoriasiform, scaling, and red plaques with a slow enlargement over many years before becoming nodular, invasive, squamous cell cancers (*see* Figure 31-18). The lack of a response to topical steroid applications, which often are mistakenly used to resolve these cancers that mimic the appearance of eczema or psoriasis, should raise a physician's level of suspicion; a skin biopsy speci-

men will provide a correct diagnosis. Bowen's disease should be removed by either excision or curettage and electrocautery. A variant of Bowen's disease, the so-called "erythroplasia of Queyrat" on the glans penis of uncircumcised individuals, appears as red, velvety, and eroded plaques and represents a carcinoma in situ (*see* Figure 31-19).[13] A skin biopsy specimen should be obtained, because a metastasis from these cancers can occur after dermal invasion occurs. Such lesions can be removed by using topical 5-Fluorouracil or by surgical excision under the direction of a urologist.[3]

Keratoacanthoma Of great importance and considerable difficulty in a differential diagnosis in relation to squamous cell cancer is a keratoacanthoma. This rapidly growing, epidermal tumor that is found on sun-exposed areas be-

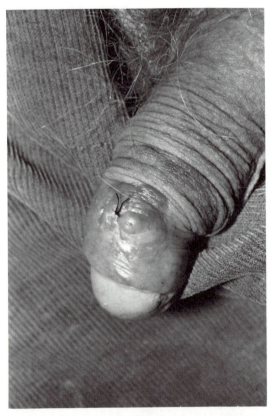

FIGURE 31-19 Erythroplasia of Queyrat appears as velvety red plaques on the penis of uncircumcised males. These patches should be biopsied early to establish a diagnosis of squamous cell cancer in situ before the tumor invades the dermis and metastasizes.

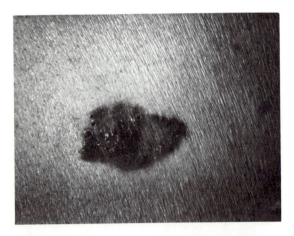

FIGURE 31-18 Bowen's disease, or squamous cell carcinoma in situ, appears as a slightly elevated red scaling patch. Small papules of the carcinoma are evolving in the center of the lesion.

gins as a firm red papule that rapidly enlarges over 4–6 weeks to a 1–2-cm size, which results in a large nodule with a characteristic horny keratotic plug in the center of the lesion (*see* Figure 31-20).[14] These tumors spontaneously resolve over an 8–12-week period, leaving a scar in their wake. They can be large and aggressive, and appear with an ulcerative, central keratotic mass that clinically may be difficult to differentiate from squamous cell cancer. In general, keratoacanthomas evolve more rapidly than squamous cell cancers (although some squamous cell neoplasms also can show rapid growth), have a typical crater-form shape with a keratotic plug, and heal spontaneously. An elliptical incisional biopsy procedure through the center of the entire lesion is required to differentiate keratoacanthomas from squamous cell cancers; but, even then it may not always be possible to pathologically distinguish these lesions so that, as a general rule, it is best to totally excise keratoacanthomas.

Several modes of therapy are available for basal cell and squamous cell cancers, including excisional surgery, curettage and electrodesiccation, or x-ray therapy. Mohs' chemosurgery has a high degree of success in curing difficult, recurrent basal and squamous cell carcinomas. Unless a physician has experience and skill in these modalities, a patient should be referred to therapeutic experts in these various fields.

Pigmented Tumors and Lesions of the Skin
Pigmented lesions of the skin may appear as flat or raised papular or nodular masses. The major clinical concern for a physician is whether the lesion is a melanoma or a benign pigmented growth.[15] It often is difficult to precisely distinguish pigmented malignant conditions from benign conditions, clinically, so that skin biopsy procedures frequently are required. A definitive diagnosis of suspicious pigmented lesions is best confirmed by a total excisional biopsy procedure; but, if the lesion is too large to easily excise, an adequate and representative incisional biopsy procedure may be performed. There is no evidence that the incisional procedure will cause a spread of melanomas.

Benign Senile Lentigos and Lentigo Malignas Flat pigmented lesions may be benign senile lentigos or lentigo malignas (premelano-

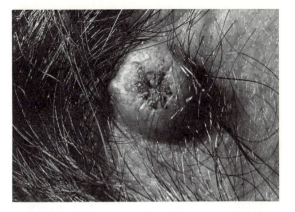

FIGURE 31-20 Keratoacanthomas are rapidly enlarging, epidermal cell tumors that evolve into a 1–2-cm nodule with a horny keratotic plug in the center.

mas). Benign lentigos are flat, uniformly light-brown lesions with discrete borders that are found on the face, arms, and hands, especially in chronically sun-damaged skin (*see* Figure 31-3) (seen with senile purpura, pseudoscars). Lentigo malignas are flat, circumscribed, and preinvasive melanomas with variations in color ranging from tan to darker brown (*see* Figure 31-21). Lentigo malignas gradually enlarge and their color alters with shades of tan, brown, and

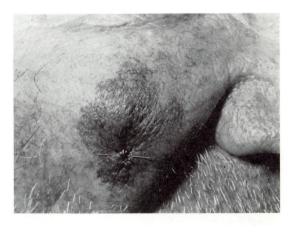

FIGURE 31-21 Lentigo malignas characteristically appear as flat, variably pigmented, and irregularly shaped lesions on the face in older individuals. They remain flat and slowly enlarge for many years (approximately 10–30) before they evolve to dark-brown or black nodules that represent an invasive melanoma. At times, they are clinically impossible to differentiate from senile lentigos, so that a biopsy procedure may be necessary.

black until, after 10–30 years, dark nodules evolve within the macular areas to become lentigo maligna melanomas.

Acral Lentiginous Melanomas Similar-appearing, slow-growing, macular, and pigmented lesions may evolve on the acral areas of the body, which evolve into acral lentiginous melanomas.[16] These lesions on the palms, soles, and phalanges display both variations in color (black, blue, red) and papular and nodular infiltrative areas that herald overt melanoma formation (*see* Figure 31-22). These innocuous-appearing, early melanomas in situ often are overlooked until an invasive melanoma has evolved, so a physician is urged to obtain a biopsy specimen of these lesions early in their course.

Elevated Pigmented Lesions Thickened or elevated pigmented lesions may represent a second form of melanoma, superficial spreading melanoma, or such common benign pigmented lesions as seborrheic keratosis and nevi.

Superficial Spreading Melanomas These melanomas begin as small brown papules that early on are difficult to distinguish from benign pigmented spots. Then, irregular and variegated color within the lesion is seen with hues of light- and dark-brown, black, gray, and even white (*see* Figure 31-23). These variations in color represent a proliferation of malignant mela-

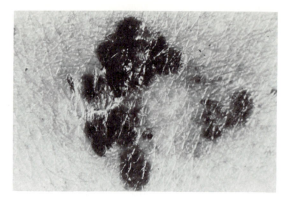

FIGURE 31-23 Superficial spreading melanomas show irregular and variegated colors of browns, blues, and blacks, along with irregular borders with indentations and notching.

noma cells at different depths in the skin. A suspicion of melanoma is raised by the variation in coloration, irregular borders with indentation and notching, and irregularity of skin surface and topography.

Seborrheic Keratoses These can be darkly pigmented and, thus, resemble melanomas; but, certain features of these very common lesions found in an older patient are useful in differentiating them. Their color varies from yellow to brown and black, but there usually is a uniformity of color throughout any given keratosis (*see* Figure 31-24). They are sharply marginated with a "stuck-on" look and a waxy appearance in which comedonal keratin plugs are found on the surface. In doubtful instances, a biopsy specimen of the lesion is needed.

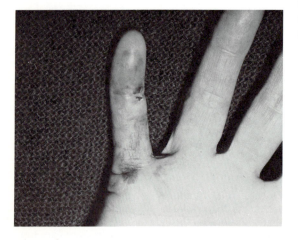

FIGURE 31-22 Acral lentiginous melanomas appear as macular, irregularly pigmented lesions on the hands and feet. These early melanomas display variations in color (brown, blue, red, black) and slowly enlarge.

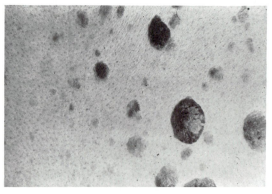

FIGURE 31-24 Multiple seborrheic keratoses on the back. These lesions are sharply marginated with a "stuck-on" and waxy appearance.

Benign Nevi These can be darkly pigmented, thus mimicking melanomas. However, nevi generally show a uniformity of coloration with no irregularity to the borders, and usually the epidermal surface markings are intact. Yet, melanomas can arise from benign nevi (indeed, up to 50% of all melanomas arise from pre-existing nevi). Therefore, a history of changes in size, color, or configuration may be very important in detecting early malignant changes in pre-existing nevi (*see* Figure 31-25).

Nodular Melanoma A third form of malignant melanoma is a nodular melanoma, which consists of dark, blue-black, or brown nodular lesions from the outset, with an early growth deep into the dermis so that metastases occur early in their evolution. The surface of nodular melanomas may be smooth or ulcerated (*see* Figure 31-26).

Blue Nevi and Dermatofibromas Other nodular pigmented skin lesions that can be mistaken for nodular melanomas include blue nevi and dermatofibromas. Blue nevi are small, dark, and blue-black papules that have been present from early life without a change in color or size. Although almost invariably benign, there have been a few reports of melanomatous degeneration. Dermatofibromas are commonly seen, firm, benign, and red-to-brown dermal nodules that often are found on the legs. An important clinical sign is the dimple-like depression over-

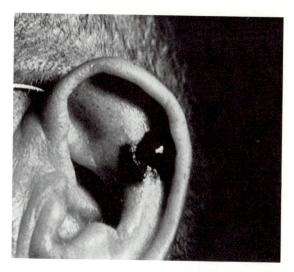

FIGURE 31-26 A dark, black, nodular melanoma with a dark-brown "staining" of the adjacent skin of the ear. These are the most aggressive and difficult melanomas to cure, because they grow vertically into the dermis early in their course.

lying the skin when lateral compression is applied on each side of the lesion (*see* Figure 31-27).

A few additional points should be made with regard to distinguishing melanomas and considering their prognosis. A high index of suspicion of melanoma should be entertained in any individual with a past history of melanoma, a family history of melanoma, and, a celtic ancestry with light-colored skin who sunburns easily and has a history of excessive sun exposure. Certain

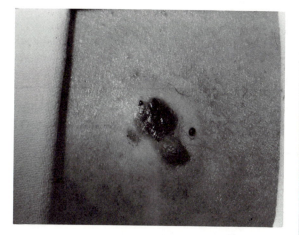

FIGURE 31-25 A darkly pigmented melanoma arising from a more lightly pigmented, benign nevus. One half of all melanomas appear to arise from pre-existing benign nevi.

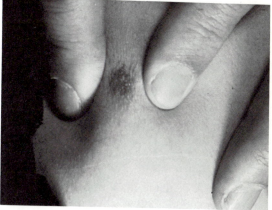

FIGURE 31-27 Dermatofibromas are light or dark-brown nodules that show a "dimpling" of the skin when lateral compression is applied.

clinical signs should alert a physician if they occur in a newly evolving, pigmented lesion or if they are seen with pre-existing nevi: 1) Changes in color, especially red, white, and blue—along with spreading of pigmentation from the periphery into previously normal skin; 2) Changes in size and shape, especially a sudden enlargement and thickening; 3) A change in surface configuration, especially scaling, erosion, oozing, and ulceration; 4) A change in consistency with softening and friability; and 5) A change in the surrounding skin, especially redness or satellite pigmentation.

The depth of malignant melanoma cell growth into the dermis correlates directly with a prognosis. Thus, the deeper the malignant cells penetrate, the more likely a metastasis occurs; therefore, the earlier a physician identifies the melanoma, the less likely the lesion will have penetrated into the dermis. Different forms of melanomas seem to have variable horizontal (along the basal layer of the epidermis) and vertical (cells penetrating into the dermis) growth rates. Thus, lentigo maligna and acral lentiginous melanomas have a long horizontal growth phase before invading the dermis. This means an early diagnosis provides a patient with a better chance of a cure. Nodular melanomas, almost from their inception, invade the dermis and (hence) there is less opportunity for cure. Superficial spreading melanomas have biologic growth characteristics somewhere between lentigo malignas and nodular melanomas.

Skin and Mucous Membrane Changes in Nutritional Diseases

Elderly persons often are subject to poor nutrition because of intercurrent diseases that impair appetite or cause weight loss or malabsorption, as well as an insufficient intake while living alone or under less than ideal conditions. Eccentricity or alcoholism also may contribute to inadequate nutrition. Since the skin and mucosa are among the most rapidly proliferating tissues, a deficiency of major nutrients becomes apparent in these tissues early in the course of an illness.[17] A deficient intake of total nitrogen or essential amino acids results in an impaired protein synthesis. This causes a slowing of cell proliferation as evidenced by thinning hair shafts and the hair becoming brittle and breaking readily. A Vitamin A deficiency causes the skin to roughen, wrinkle, and become hyperkeratotic (especially around the hair follicles) on the anterolateral surface of the thighs and extensor areas of the extremities. Dryness and thickening also occur on the mucosal surfaces with a lack of Vitamin A, thus causing metaplasia of columnar to squamous epithelium, which leads to increased susceptibility to bronchopulmonary infections and xerosis of the conjunctivae and cornea. A niacin deficiency (pellegra) causes red, scaling, and even pustular eruptions of the skin in sun-exposed areas (butterfly rash, Casal's necklace), as well as an atrophy of the mucous membranes of the gastrointestinal tract and tongue. A riboflavin deficiency leads to angular cheilitis and blepharitis, while a Vitamin C deficiency causes the typical skin findings of scurvy; namely, hyperkeratosis of hair follicles with perifollicular hemorrhages and corkscrew growth of hairs on the trunk and extremities.

Skin Surgery in Aging Skin

There seems to be little or no change in healing time or problems with the strength of healed wounds, despite the various alterations in skin structure and function that are imposed by aging.[18] Indeed, one study that evaluated the time required to replicate abraided areas of the skin revealed no difference in the time to full recovery in aged versus young skin.[3] Thus, surgery on aged skin poses no undue problems when surgical procedures are required.

The question arises in respect to dermatosurgical procedures of the value in treating aged skin, particularly in reducing the rate of keratotic and epithelioma occurrence in sun-exposed areas. Dermal planing, or dermabrasion, is one method by which sun-damaged aged skin can be removed with a regeneration of new skin from the deeper adnexal structures that have not been damaged to the same degree by solar irradiation.[19] There is some evidence that, in localized areas, such treatment may decrease the keratotic and neoplastic changes.[19] Chemosurgery or the use of cauterizing chemicals (20% trichloroacetic acid and phenol) have been used for many years to remove keratoses, pigmented lentigos, and to cause peeling and edema to minimize wrinkles. These methods temporarily reverse the processes of aging, but the inevitable invariably continues. Plastic surgery can remove excessive wrinkled skin; with an adequate undermining of residual tissues, a tightening and appropriate cosmetic tailoring of the skin can be obtained.[17] A properly executed face-lift should last from 5–10 years. It is understood that no operation can permanently eliminate aging.

References

1. Carlsen RA: Aging skin: understanding the inevitable. *Geriatrics* 30:51–54, 1975.
2. Stoughton RB: Physiological changes from maturity through senescence. *JAMA* 179:636–638, 1962.
3. Millington PF, Wilkinson R: Changes in skin with age. 4th European Symposium, Basic Research in Gerontology. *Scand J Clin Lab Invest* 25(suppl 14):52–53.
4. Ogawa CM: Generative skin disorders: toll of age and sun. *Geriatrics* 30:65–69, 1973.
5. Fritsch WC: Managing age-related vascular skin lesions. *Geriatrics* 30:45–48, 1975.
6. Reynolds WA, Winkelmann RK, Soule EH: Kaposi's sarcoma: a clinicopathologic study with particular reference to its relationship to the reticuloendothelial system. *Medicine* 44:419–443, 1965.
7. Solan AJ, Greenwald ES, Silvay O: Long-term remissions of Kaposi's sarcoma with vinblastine therapy. *Cancer* 47:637–639, 1981.
8. Gange RW, Wilson-Jones E: Kaposi's sarcoma and immunosuppressive therapy: an appraisal. *Clin Exp Dermatol* 3:135–145, 1978.
9. Panet-Raymond G, Girard C: Lichen sclerosis et atrophicus. *Can Med Assoc J* 106:1332–1334, 1972.
10. Perry HO, Greene LF: Common diseases of the skin of the penis. *Geriatr Pract* 88:87–97, 1966.
11. Lynch PJ: Common malignant and premalignant tumors of the skin. *Ariz Med* 34:90–91, 1977.
12. Walder BK, Robertson MR, Jeremy D: Skin cancer and immunosuppression. *Lancet* 2:1282–1283, 1971.
13. Goette OK: Review of erythroplasia of Queyrat and its treatment. *Urology* 8:311–315, 1976.
14. Schwartz RA: The keratoacanthoma: a review. *J Surg Oncol* 12:305–317, 1979.
15. Sober A, Fitzpatrick TB, Mihm M, et al: Early recognition of cutaneous melanoma. *JAMA* 242:2795–2799, 1979.
16. Coleman WP, Loria PR, Reed RJ, et al: Acral lentiginous melanoma. *Arch Dermatol* 116:773–776, 1980.
17. Bollet AJ: The skin and mucous membranes in nutritional diseases. *Resident and Staff Physician* Dec 1981, pp 101–109.
18. Conley JJ: Management of aging skin by plastic surgery. *Arch Dermatol* 86:407–409, 1962.
19. Epstein E: Dermatologic surgery in aging skin. *Arch Dermatol* 86:399–403, 1962.

CHAPTER 32

Pressure Sores

JAMES B. REULER, M.D.

THOMAS G. COONEY, M.D.

A pressure sore is one of those common clinical problems to which many physicians have been exposed, but about which few possess any knowledge. In part, this is due to the facts that these festering wounds often occur in patients who are deemed "undesirable,"[1] that their management is frustrating and fatiguing for both doctor and patient, and that the topic is viewed as intellectually unattractive by health care providers. This lack of interest has led to inadequate attention to prevention, the institution of ineffective therapeutic measures, increases in health care expenditures, and adverse impacts on patient morbidity and mortality. In this chapter, we will review the salient features of the pathophysiology and management of pressure sores, highlighting issues that are particularly germane to the geriatric population.

The term "decubitus ulcer," which is derived from the Latin word "decub," meaning "lying down," frequently is used to describe this problem. This is a misnomer, however, since the greater proportion of these lesions develop while a patient is in a sitting position. Therefore, the term "pressure sore" is preferred, because it is more accurate and describes the underlying pathophysiology.

Epidemiology

At the turn of this century, pressure sores were most often seen in young persons afflicted with a variety of debilitating diseases, which include tuberculosis, osteomyelitis, and chronic renal disease.[2] At present, the groups that account for the vast majority of pressure sores include those with spinal cord injuries,[3] those with chronic neurologic diseases (such as cerebrovascular disease and multiple sclerosis), and elderly persons.[4,5] In the first group, 25–85% of all afflicted patients develop pressure sores that account for 50% of admissions to specialized cord-injury centers and 7–8% of all related deaths.

A recent survey from Glasgow, Scotland, that involved over 10,000 patients revealed that 8.8% of both the hospitalized and home-care groups had at least one pressure sore, and that those persons 70 years of age and over accounted for 70% of all patients with pressure sores (the proportion of the total population of the area over 70 years of age was 8.4%).[6] Of all elderly patients admitted to a hospital, 10–25% will develop pressure sores, usually within the first 2 weeks[4,5]; these lesions represent the most common site of infection in patients who are residing in skilled-care nursing homes.[7] Factors that were implicated in the high prevalence rate of pressure sores in elderly persons include falls which lead to trauma and immobilization[8,9], incontinence, and a diminution in cognitive function.

Pathophysiology

Of the many factors that contribute to the development of pressure sores, four appear to be critical: pressure, shearing forces, friction, and moisture.[10] Of these factors, pressure, which is the force exerted on a unit area, is the most important; however, the precise mechanism by which pressure produces tissue necrosis remains clinically controversial.

Pressure

Experimental work reveals that, in skin, the capillary arteriolar limb pressure is 32 mm Hg, the midcapillary pressure is 20 mm Hg, and the venous limb pressure is 12 mm Hg.[11] A 70-kg male lying in the supine position with pressure evenly distributed would have an average pressure exerted, at any given point, of 5.7 mm Hg. Unfortunately, pressure is not equally distributed, but is concentrated in focal areas; generally over bony prominences (*see* Figure 32-1).[12,13] Increased pressure over these areas leads to a wide, three-dimensional pressure gradient (*see* Figure 32-2).

Within the tissues, a negative interstitial fluid pressure exists that is balanced by a positive solid tissue pressure, which results in a total tissue pressure of 0.[14] On application of external pressure, interstitial fluid pressure increases and, when pressure in the venous limb is exceeded, a marked increase in total tissue pressure results. This leads to increased capillary arteriolar pressure, filtration of fluid from capillaries, edema, and autolysis.

The occlusion of lymphatic vessels is another consequence of these pressure gradients. An impairment of the active contractility of lymphatics, combined with changes in the blood microvascular system, leads to an accumulation of anaerobic metabolic waste products and, ultimately, tissue necrosis.[15]

Early investigative work by Dinsdale showed that a pressure of 70 mm Hg applied for more than 2 hours produced irreversible tissue damage.[16] However, if pressure was intermittently relieved, a minimal change was seen even to pressures of 240 mm Hg. Kosiak confirmed

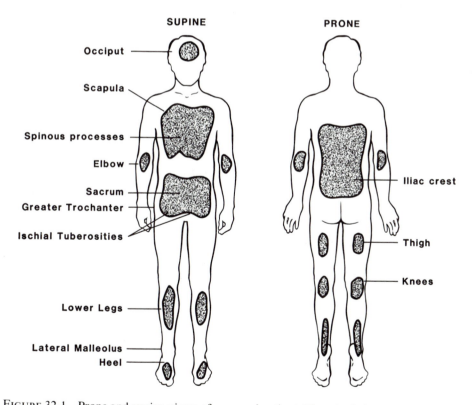

FIGURE 32-1 Prone and supine views of a normal patient. The stippled areas denote areas where pressures equal to or greater than mean capillary pressure are exerted. Common sites of ulceration are identified. (From Reuler JB, Cooney TG: The pressure sore: pathophysiology and principles of management. *Ann Int Med* 94:661–666, 1981, used by permission.)

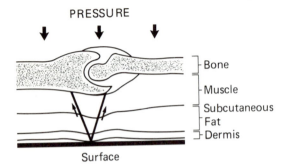

PRESSURE

- Bone
- Muscle
- Subcutaneous Fat
- Dermis

Surface

FIGURE 32-2 Compression of the soft tissues between the underlying surface and the bony prominence leads to a cone-shaped pressure gradient. (From Reuler JB, Cooney TG: The pressure sore: pathophysiology and principles of management. *Ann Int Med* 94:661–666, 1981, used by permission.)

these findings, but noted that if pressure was alternated every 5 minutes few changes were seen.[17] No difference was noted between animals with injured and uninjured spinal cords, thus negating the existence of the hypothesized neurotropic factor that was believed to be responsible for the increased incidence of pressure sores in cord-injured patients. These studies suggest that the critical period of pressure application is less than 2 hours, after which time irreversible changes occur.

Studies of pressure measurements under the buttocks of a person sitting in a wheelchair demonstrated that pressures were greatest (up to 500 mm Hg) under and just lateral to the ischial tuberosities.[11] Pressures at these points remained higher than 150 mm Hg despite the addition of 2 inches of foam padding to the chair. All other points of measurement were greater than the capillary arteriolar pressure.

More recently, the traditional ischemic etiology of pressure sores has been questioned. Using a swine model, Daniel, et al showed that initial pathologic changes occur in muscle and subsequently progress towards the skin with increasing pressure and/or duration.[18] Muscle damage occurred at high pressure of short duration (500 mm Hg, 4 hours), whereas skin destruction required high pressure of long duration (800 mm Hg, 8 hours) and was not evident after 15 hours at 200 mm Hg. This information suggests that normal tissue is much more resistant to a pressure-induced ischemia than earlier studies would suggest, and that the pressure-

duration threshold for the development of pressure sores is lowered significantly by changes in soft tissue coverage.

Shearing Forces

Tangential pressures, or shearing forces, are caused by the sliding of adjacent surfaces of laminar elements, which provides a progressive relative displacement.[19] At high levels of shear pressure, approximating 100 grams/cm^2, the normal pressure that is necessary to produce vascular occlusion is 50% of the pressure required when shear forces are absent.[20] Clinically, these forces are in play when the head of the bed is raised, which causes the torso to slide down, transmitting pressure to the sacrum and deep fascia. At the same time, the posterior sacral skin is fixed secondary to friction with the bed, and shearing forces in the deep part of the superficial fascia lead to the stretching and angulation of vessels, thus causing a thrombosis and undermining of the dermis.[21] The most vulnerable vessels are the posterior branches of the lateral sacral arteries and the superficial branches of the superior gluteal artery, which pass through the posterior sacral foramen to perforate the muscles and deep fascia. In addition, subcutaneous fat, which lacks tensile strength and is particularly susceptible to mechanical forces, accentuates the shearing phenomenon.

Friction

Friction, which is the force created when two surfaces in contact move across each other, is exemplified when a patient is dragged across the bed sheets. The impact of friction is to remove the outer protective stratum corneum, thus accelerating the onset of ulceration. Age-related changes in the skin, including epidermal atrophy, a decreased turnover rate of cells in the stratum corneum, stiffening of dermal collagen, and a decrease in dermal blood vessels, all may combine to amplify the effects of friction and, therefore, increase the risk of pressure sore development in elderly persons.[22]

Moisture

The final critical causative factor is moisture, which is caused by fecal or urinary soilage or perspiration; it substantially increases the risk of pressure sore formation.

Clinical Evaluation

Over 90% of all pressure sores are located in the lower part of the body, with the majority found in the sacral and coccygeal areas and over the ischial tuberosities and greater trochanters.[23] Prominences such as those caused by hypertrophic bone formation or by fixation pins also may serve as foci for pressure sore development.

Of the many classifications of pressure sores to be found in the available literature, the classification devised by Shea is most clinically applicable.[24] A stage 1 sore involves an acute inflammatory response in all layers, with an irregular ill-defined area of soft tissue swelling, induration, and heat. This resembles an abrasion, is confined to the epidermis, and is reversible. A stage 2 ulceration includes an inflammatory and fibroblastic response that extends through the dermis to the subcutaneous fat and also is reversible. A stage 3 ulcer is essentially a full thickness skin defect that extends into the subcutaneous fat with extensive undermining. A stage 4 lesion includes penetration into the deep fascia with involvement of muscle and bone.

A physical examination is essential, particularly for early identification. Early in its development, an ulcer is irregular in shape contrasted with chronic ulcerations, which tend to have regular edges with a thick fibrous ring under the surface. Due to the pressure gradient phenomenon, a small defect at the surface may overlay a large undermining lesion, highlighting the necessity of a palpation of the ulceration. On occasion, bimanual palpation of an ischial ulcer may reveal an extension to the rectum.

Given the usual locations and clinical settings, little concern generally is given to a differential diagnosis of these wounds. Occasionally, however, an incipient pressure sore may be mistaken for an early ischial-rectal abscess. Vasculitis may present as a pressure sore, most notably in a bedridden patient afflicted with rheumatoid arthritis. The presence of pustular lesions at the surface may suggest a deep mycotic infection, and the finding of verrucous margins should raise suspicion of a malignancy.

TABLE 32-1 Pressure Sores—Complications

Sepsis
Osteomyelitis
Pyarthroses
Joint disarticulation
Extension to deep organs
Heterotopic calcifications
Tetanus
Amyloidosis

When these latter diagnoses are entertained, obtaining a biopsy specimen of the area is advisable.

Complications of pressure sores are multiple and often life-threatening (see Table 32-1).[25] A sepsis that is due to pressure sores often is polymicrobial in nature, with obligate anaerobes representing frequently recovered organisms.[26,27] When sepsis from pressure sores is considered, antibiotic coverage should include gram-negative and anaerobic bacteria, and a surgical consultation should be obtained promptly. Extension to a bone frequently is encountered, which leads to osteomyelitis, pyarthroses, and joint disarticulation.[28] In addition to an extension to a bone, pressure sores may extend to any of the deeper structures, including communication with the bowels and bladder. These deep, indolent infections may cause a formation of heterotopic calcifications or may increase the susceptibility to tetanus.[29] Studies suggesting that most older adults have not been appropriately immunized against tetanus, and the high mortality rate, make an awareness of this complication particularly important.[30] The administration of tetanus toxoid should be considered in any patient with a deep pressure sore and inadequate documentation of immunization status.

A re-emphasis of the deceptive nature of these often superficial-appearing wounds is critical. For this reason, radiologic studies are important in the evaluation. Questions to be answered include: 1) Are there bony abnormalities underlying the lesion, particularly osteomyelitis? 2) Is ectopic bone or heterotopic calcification adjacent to the sore? and 3) What is the extent of the wound?[31] Plain x-ray films may demonstrate bony changes or air in the pressure sore, which suggests that the wound may be larger than predicted from a physical examination. A direct magnification x-ray film is useful when plain films raise a question of cortical erosion, which indicates possible osteomyelitis. Because of the high false-positive rate of [99m]Technetium bone scans in the diagnoses of osteomyelitis that is associated with pressure sores, a positive study does not aid in the assessment and a magnification x-ray film is preferred.[28,31] A negative scan may help to exclude osteomyelitis, although a small false-negative rate is reported. When there is clinical uncertainty about the size or extent of the wound, particularly one with undermined margins and sinus tracts, sinography is indicated. This study not only will demonstrate the internal size of the cavity, but it may reveal an extension to the joint space or other structures (*see* Figure 32-3).[31-33] Computed tomography (CT scan) usually is reserved for complicated lesions that are greater than 5 cm and is most useful in the ischial, sacral, and trochanteric sites due to the generous amounts of subcutaneous fat present. A CT scan provides a definition of the external fibrotic margins and aids in predicting the surgical void.

Systemic amyloidosis, which is a frequently reported complication of spinal cord injury

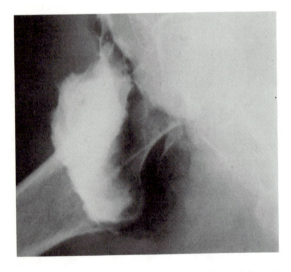

FIGURE 32-3   Sinogram of a patient with a right trochanteric pressure sore that demonstrates a fistulous tract extending into the subcutaneous tissues to the greater trochanter. Destruction of the cortical margin suggests osteomyelitis. (From Reuler JB, Cone TG: The pressure sore: pathophysiology and management. *Ann Int Med* 94:661–666, 1981, used by permission.)

found in the older available literature, may be a consequence of these chronic, suppurative wounds.[34,35]

Prevention

The dictum, "an ounce of prevention is worth a pound of cure," is particularly germane to the management of pressure sores. Due to the morbidity that is associated with these lesions and the limited resources, it is crucial that patients who are at risk are identified, so that preventive measures may be selectively (but intensively) employed. The Norton scale, or a modification thereof, appears to be a clinically applicable and sensitive assessment tool.[5] This system assesses five variables (physical condition, mental condition, activity, mobility, and incontinence), may be scored by nursing personnel, and possesses good inter-rater reliability (*see* Table 32-2). An almost linear relationship exists between the initial score and the incidence rate of pressure sores; the lower the score, the higher the incidence rate. In the original study, 48% of all patients with an initial score of 12 or less developed a pressure sore, whereas those with scores of 18–20 had an incidence rate of only 5%.[5] Of all the sores, 70% developed within the first 2 weeks of hospitalization. Although each individual component was associated to a high degree with the development of early sores, incontinence was the single best indicator of risk. A recent study that used a discriminant function analysis, as applied to the Norton score, suggested that ratings of activity and mobility alone may be as reliable as using all five factors.[36]

Thermography also has been reported to be a useful tool in assessing risk.[37,38] Using a portable heat-sensitive TV camera, this technique is used to define areas of occult tissue damage as evidenced by thermal flares. In the application of this modality to all admissions to a geriatric assessment unit who did not have any clinical evidence of tissue damage, a thermogram appeared to be a better predictor than the Norton score of the development of pressure sores within 10 days of admission.[38] Given the costs and technical factors involved, however, further studies are required to define the use before advocating a universal application of this method.

TABLE 32-2   Method of Scoring for Vulnerability of Developing Pressure Sores

General Physical Condition	Mental Status	Activity	Mobility	Incontinence
4. Good	4. Alert	4. Ambulant	4. Full	4. Not
3. Fair	3. Apathetic	3. Walks with help	3. Slightly limited	3. Occasional
2. Poor	2. Confused	2. Chair-bound	2. Very limited	2. Usually; urinary
1. Very bad	1. Stupor	1. Confined to bed	1. Immobile	1. Urinary and fecal

In prevention, quality nursing care is crucial. To minimize friction, particulate matter (e.g., food) should be removed from the bed, sheets should be loose so that movement is not restricted, and patients should be lifted, not dragged.[19] The skin should be patted dry, not rubbed, and the surface should not be kept too dry or too moist.

Spasticity may interfere with proper positioning and increase the risk of friction. Therapeutic alternatives include medications such as diazepam, baclofen, and dantrolene sodium, intrathecal injections, and neurosurgical ablation.[39]

The head of the bed should not be raised and an upright position should be maintained while sitting in a wheelchair to minimize shearing forces. When it is necessary to tilt the bed, the use of a firm footboard will reduce slippage. Sheepskin pads are useful in this regard due to their shear resistance properties.[40]

Moisture control depends on timely skin care, prevention of soilage, and maintenance of a low-humidity interface. The evaluation and management of urinary incontinence, which is a frequently encountered problem in elderly persons, is extremely important.[41] On occasion, a surgically created fecal diversion may be required. Again, because of its high capacity to absorb water vapor, sheepskin provides an excellent contact surface.

The most important preventive measure is the relief of pressure itself.[5,42] Rotation of the patient is the simplest mechanism to accomplish this goal. Given the previously cited experimental data, rotation should be performed at roughly 2–hour intervals (see Table 32-3). Bridging, using six or more soft pillows placed at strategic locations, also may provide pressure relief.[43] The use of "donuts" is to be avoided, however, due to the resulting undesirable stress distribution and vessel occlusion.

With good nursing care, it is possible to heal most pressure sores without the use of special equipment. In some instances, however, alternate support surfaces may be useful adjuncts. These may include fluid-support systems, in which the body floats and evenly distributes weight over the surface that is in contact with the fluid medium, or air-support systems, which provide a form of levitation.[42,44,45] Alternating pressure mattresses and mud beds also are included in this category of systems.[46] One of these alternatives should be available for the handling of special problems, particularly a patient with multiple sores who cannot be positioned to adequately unload pressure from the sites. It must be cautioned that an inordinate reliance on gadgetry, much of which may malfunction, often diverts attention from good positioning. No substitute exists for vigilance in nursing care.

In the geriatric population, in contrast to the cord-injury group, a wheelchair is a less significant source of pressure ulceration. This issue, however, remains a major problem confronting rehabilitation engineers.[47–49] None of the available cushions are as effective as intermittent, complete unloading of pressure, although appropriate seating combined with flat support boards and thick foam cushions may reduce the risk. Sophisticated pressure and temperature measuring devices are being used to provide for

TABLE 32-3   Schedule of Rotation to Relieve Pressure

Time	Position
8:00 AM/PM	Right side
10:00 AM/PM	Left side
12:00 noon/midnight	Supine
2:00 PM/AM	Right side
4:00 PM/AM	Left side
6:00 PM/AM	Supine

an individual prescription for custom-made or modular seating systems.[50,51]

Management

Once present, the management of a pressure sore is similar to that of other wounds; the primary goal is a promotion of wound healing.[10] General medical care should begin with assessing nutritional status, given the prevalence of protein-calorie malnutrition in hospitalized geriatric patients and its deleterious effect on wound healing.[52,53] A correction may require enteral or intravenous (IV) hyperalimentation to reverse protein catabolism and promote wound healing.[53,54] A correction of edema and anemia, control of hyperglycemia, and improvement in oxygenation and tissue perfusion, all may contribute to more rapid wound healing. Insufficient information exists to recommend Vitamin C or zinc supplementation, as some authors have advocated.[55,56]

The majority of pressure sores are superficial and will heal by secondary intention. The objectives of the management plan include the relief of pressure, wound debridement, the promotion of healing and excision, and the closure of defects, when necessary.

The goals of wound debridement are to remove devitalized tissue that (if allowed to remain) promotes infection, delays granulation, and impedes healing. A variety of topical therapies has been advocated to enhance debridement and accelerate healing; yet, no single agent has been shown to be uniformly useful or superior to simple saline dressings.[3,57,58] The application of these topical preparations requires moving the patient so that the wound is exposed. This relief of pressure may be the most critical factor in studies that report the efficacy of these agents.[59] Some investigators have reported success by using localized hyperbaric oxygen treatments; but again, a relief of pressure that is inherent in the procedure may be the most critical factor.[60]

Our recommendations for initial debridement include wet-to-dry dressings, using fine mesh gauze soaked in normal saline and loosely packed in the wound, with removal every 3–4 hours. Numerous biochemical agents are available to aid in wound debridement, which include enzyme preparations that attack undenatured collagen and liquify necrotic wound debris.[3,61–66] Studies of most of these agents have been uncontrolled or subject to potential methodologic error, so that the precise role of these possibly beneficial agents remains controversial. In the initial management of infected, purulent, and wet wounds, the use of silver sulfadiazine or dextranomer may be beneficial.[67,68] Although a local infection may play a role in the development and maintenance of these ulcers, a systemic antibiotic therapy usually is not effective and should be reserved for lesions that are complicated by sepsis.[67,69]

Stage 1 and stage 2 sores may be managed with local therapy, as described above.[24] Stage 3 and stage 4 ulcerations generally requires surgical intervention. The exact role of surgery, which has been defined extensively in younger spinal cord injury patients, remains problematic in elderly persons because of the poor prognosis of many patients in chronic care facilities and the increased risk of recurrence. Sepsis in association with pressure sores, however, generally requires a wide debridement to gain control of the infection, regardless of age. Fortunately, these deeper sores are not commonly encountered in elderly persons.

Surgical objectives include the excision of ulcerated areas, resection of bony prominences that may delay healing and cause a recurrence of the ulcer if left in place, resurfacing of the defect, formation of large flaps, and the obtainment of additional padding by using muscle flaps.[70] Many surgical techniques have been employed to accomplish these goals.[23,70–72]

References

1. Papper S: The undesirable patient. *J Chronic Dis* 22:777–779, 1970.
2. Shaw TC: On so-called bed-sores in the insane. *St. Bartholemew's Hosp Rep* 8:130–133, 1872.
3. Sather MR, Weber CE, George J: Pressure sores and the spinal cord injury patient. *Drug Intell Clin Pharm* 11:154–169, 1977.
4. Rosin AJ, Boyd RV: Complications of illness in geriatric patients in hospital. *J Chronic Dis* 19:307–313, 1966.
5. Norton D, McLaren R, Exton-Smith AN: *An Investigation of Geriatric Nursing Problems in Hospital (1962, Reissued)*. Edinburgh, Churchill Livingstone, 1975, pp 194–236.

6. Barbenel JC, Jordan MM, Nicol SM, et al: Incidence of pressure-sores in the greater Glasgow health board area. *Lancet* 2:548–550, 1977.

7. Garibaldi RA, Brodine S, Matsumiya S: Infections among patients in nursing homes—policies, prevalence, and problems. *N Engl J Med* 305:731–735, 1981.

8. Steel K, Gertman PM, Crescenzi C, et al: Iatrogenic illness on a general medical service at a university hospital. *N Engl J Med* 304:638–642, 1981.

9. Miller MB, Elliott DF: Accidents in nursing homes: implications for patients and administrators, in Miller MB (ed): *Current Issues in Clinical Geriatrics.* New York, The Tiresias Press, 1979, pp 97–135.

10. Reuler JB, Cooney TG: The pressure sore: pathophysiology and principles of management. *Ann Int Med* 94:661–666, 1981.

11. Kosiak M, Kubicek WG, Olson M, et al: Evaluation of pressure as a factor in the production of ischial ulcers. *Arch Phys Med Rehab* 39:623–629, 1958.

12. Lindan O: Etiology of decubitus ulcers: an experimental study. *Arch Phys Med Rehab* 42:774–783, 1961.

13. Lindan O, Greenway RM, Piazza JM: Pressure distribution on the surface of the human body: 1. Evaluation in lying and sitting positions using a "bed of springs and nails." *Arch Phys Med Rehab* 46:378–385, 1965.

14. Guyton AC, Granger HJ, Taylor AE: Interstitial fluid pressure. *Physiol Rev* 51:527–563, 1971.

15. Krouskop TA, Reddy NP, Spencer WA, et al: Mechanisms of decubitus ulcer formation—an hypothesis. *Med Hypoth* 4:37–39, 1978.

16. Dinsdale SM: Decubitus ulcers: role of pressure and friction in causation. *Arch Phys Med Rehab* 55:147–152, 1974.

17. Kosiak M: Etiology of decubitus ulcers. *Arch Phys Med Rehab* 42:19–29, 1961.

18. Daniel RK, Priest DL, Wheatley DC: Etiologic factors in pressure sores: an experimental model. *Arch Phys Med Rehab* 62:492–498, 1981.

19. Tepperman PS, DeZwirek CS, Chiarcossi AL, et al: Pressure sores: prevention and step-up management. *Postgrad Med* 62:83–89, 1977.

20. Bennett L, Kavner D, Lee BK, et al: Shear vs pressure as causative factors in skin blood flow occlusion. *Arch Phys Med Rehab* 60:309–314, 1979.

21. Reichel SM: Shearing force as a factor in decubitus ulcers in paraplegics. *JAMA* 166:762–763, 1958.

22. Boss GR, Seegmiller JE: Age-related physiological changes and their clinical significance. *West J Med* 135:434–440, 1981.

23. Vasconez LO, Jurkiewicz MJ, Schneider WJ: Pressure sores. *Curr Prob Surg* 14:1–62, 1977.

24. Shea JD: Pressure sores—classification and management. *Clin Orthop* 112:89–100, 1975.

25. Conway H, Stark RB, Weeter JC, et al: Complications of decubitus ulcers in patients with paraplegia. *Plast Reconstr Surg* 7:117–130, 1975.

26. Galpin JE, Chow AW, Bayer AS, et al: Sepsis associated with decubitus ulcers. *Am J Med* 61:346–350, 1976.

27. Rissing JP, Crowder JG, Dunfee T, et al: Bacteroides bacteremia from decubitus ulcers. *South Med J* 67:1179–1182, 1974.

28. Waldvogel FA, Vasey H: Osteomyelitis: the past decade. *N Engl J Med* 303:360–370, 1980.

29. LaForce FM, Young LS, Bennett JV: Tetanus in the United States (1965–1966): epidemiologic and clinical features. *N Engl J Med* 280:569–574, 1969.

30. Crossley K, Irvine P, Warren JB, et al: Tetanus and diphtheria immunity in urban Minnesota adults. *JAMA* 242:2298–2300, 1979.

31. Hendrix RW, Calenoff L, Lederman RB, et al: Radiology of pressure sores. *Radiology* 138:351–356, 1981.

32. Lopez EM, Aranha GV: The value of sinography in the management of decubitus ulcers. *Plast Reconst Surg* 53:208–210, 1974.

33. Putnam T, Calenoff L, Betts HB, et al: Sinography in management of decubitus ulcers. *Arch Phys Med Rehab* 59:243–245, 1978.

34. Newman W, Jacobson AS: Paraplegia and secondary amyloidosis. *Am J Med* 15:216–222, 1953.

35. Dalton JJ, Hackler RH, Bunts RC: Amyloidosis in the paraplegic; incidence and significance. *J Urol* 93:553–555, 1965.

36. Goldstone LA, Roberts BV: A preliminary discriminant function analysis of elderly orthopaedic patients who will or will not contract a pressure sore. *Int J Nurs Stud* 17:17–23, 1980.

37. Barton A, Barton B: *The Management and Prevention of Pressure Sores.* Boston, Faber & Faber, 1981, pp 46–59.

38. Newman P, Davis NH: Thermography as a predictor of sacral pressure sores. *Age Ageing* 10:14–18, 1981.

39. Young RR, Delwaide PJ: Spasticity. *N Engl J Med* 304:28–33, 96–99, 1981.

40. Denne WA: An objective assessment of the sheepskins used for decubitus sore prophylaxis. *Rheumatol Rehab* 18:23–29, 1979.

41. Ouslander JG: Urinary incontinence in the elderly. *West J Med* 135:482–491, 1981.

42. Anonymous: Sore afflicted. *Lancet* 2:21–22, 1981.

43. Stewart P, Wharton GW: Bridging: an effective and practical method of preventive skin care for the immobilized person. *South Med J* 69:1469–1473, 1976.

44. Weinstein JD, Davidson BA: Fluid support in the prevention and treatment of decubitus ulcers. *Am J Phys Med* 45:283–290, 1966.

45. Scales JT, Lunn HF, Jeneid PA, et al: The prevention and treatment of pressure sores using air-support systems. *Paraplegia* 12:118–131, 1974.

46. Reswick JB, Rogers JE: Experience at Rancho Los Amigos Hospital with devices and techniques to prevent pressure sores, In Kenedi RM, Cowden JM, Scales JT (eds): *Bedsore Biomechanics*. Baltimore, University Park Press, 1976, pp 301–310.

47. Houle RJ: Evaluation of seat devices designed to prevent ischemic ulcers in paraplegic patients. *Arch Phys Med Rehab* 50:587–594, 1969.

48. Mooney V, Einbund MJ, Rogers JE, et al: Comparison of pressure distribution qualities in seat cushions. *Bull Prosthet Res* Veterans Administration, Washington DC, 10–15:129–143, 1971.

49. Cochran GVB, Palmieri V: Development of test methods for evaluation of wheelchair cushions. *Bull Prosthet Res* 17:9–30, 1980.

50. Ferguson-Pell MW, Wilkie IC, Reswick JB, et al: Pressure sore prevention for the wheelchair-bound spinal injury patient. *Paraplegia* 18:42–51, 1980.

51. Brand PW: Comments on the article "Development of test methods for evaluation of wheelchair cushions." *Bull Prosthet Res* 17:3–4, 1980.

52. Barrocas A, Giardina MA: Nutritional assessment in the community hospital. *South Med J* 73:55–58, 1980.

53. Cashman MD: Geriatric malnutrition—recognition and correction. *Postgrad Med* 71:185–194, 1982.

54. Heymsfield SB, Bethel RA, Ansley JD, et al: Enteral hyperalimentation: an alternative to central venous hyperalimentation. *Ann Int Med* 90:63–71, 1979.

55. Taylor TV, Rimmer S, Day B, et al: Ascorbic acid supplementation in the treatment of pressure sores. *Lancet* 2:544–546, 1974.

56. Hallbook T, Lanner E: Serum-zinc and healing of venous leg ulcers. *Lancet* 2:780–782, 1972.

57. Anonymous: Preparations for pressure sores. *Drug Ther Bull* 15:69–71, 1977.

58. Morgan JE: Topical therapy of pressure ulcers. *Surg Gynecol Obstet* 141:945–947, 1974.

59. Fernie GR, Dornan J: The problems of clinical trials with new systems for preventing or healing decubiti, in: Kenedi RM, Cowden JM, Scales JT (eds): *Bedsore Biomechanics*. Baltimore, University Park Press, 1976, pp 315–320.

60. Rosenthal AM, Schurman A: Hyperbaric treatment of pressure sores. *Arch Phys Med Rehab* 52:413–415, 1971.

61. Constantin MB, Jackson HS: Biology and care of the pressure wound, in Constantin MB (ed): *Pressure Ulcers—Principles and Techniques of Management*. Boston, Little Brown & Co, 1980, pp 69–100.

62. Vetra H, Whittaker D: Hydrotherapy and topical collagenase for decubitus ulcers. *Geriatrics* 30:53–58, 1975.

63. Rao DB, Sane PG, Georgiev EL: Collagenase in the treatment of dermal and decubitus ulcers. *J Am Geriatr Soc* 23:22–30, 1975.

64. Boxer AM, Gottesman N, Bernstein H, et al: Debridement of dermal ulcers and decubiti with collagenase. *Geriatrics* 24:75–86, 1969.

65. Lee LK, Ambrus JL: Collagenase therapy for decubitus ulcers. *Geriatrics* 30:91–98, 1975.

66. Varma AO, Bugatch E, German FM: Debridement of dermal ulcers with collagenase. *Surg Gynecol Obstet* 136:281–282, 1973.

67. Kucan JO, Robson MC, Heggers JP, et al: Comparison of silver sulfadiazine, povidone—iodine and physiologic saline in the treatment of chronic pressure ulcers. *J Am Geriatr Soc* 29:232–235, 1981.

68. Floden CH, Wikstrom K: Controlled clinical trial with dextranomer (Debrisan®) on venous leg ulcers. *Curr Ther Res* 24:753–760, 1978.

69. Robson MC, Krizek TJ: The role of infection in chronic pressure ulcerations, in *Symposium on Neurological Aspects of Plastic Surgery*. St. Louis, The CV Mosby Co, 1978, pp 242–246.

70. Campbell RM, Delgado JP: The pressure sore, in Converse JM (ed): *Reconstructive Plastic Surgery*, ed 2. Philadelphia, WB Saunders & Co, 1977, pp 3763–3799.

71. Constantin MB, Jackson HS: The ischial ulcer, in Constantin MB (ed): *Pressure Ulcers—Principles and Techniques of Management*. Boston, Little Brown & Co, 1980, pp 215–246.

72. Herceg SJ, Harding RL: Surgical treatment of pressure sores. *Arch Phys Med Rehab* 59:193–200, 1978.

Chapter 33

Orthopedic and Foot Disorders

Elmer E. Specht, M.D.

Fractures

Elderly males and females are subjected to the same kinds of fracture-producing traumas as are their younger counterparts; however, there is a superimposed skeletal fragility from osteoporosis[1] that is particularly apparent in postmenopausal females and greatly increases the risk of fracture. Areas that are particularly prone to fracture, as a consequence of skeletal fragility due to hormonal deprivation and osteoporosis, are the hip, the distal radius, and the vertebral column.[2]

Hip Fracture

Fractures of the hip, in particular, have been shown to have very significant personal and social consequences for elderly persons. Every effort must be made to implement prophylactic measures to prevent this process, which has become an increasingly greater burden on the health care system as the population ages. In a survey of Medicare data in 1967, the rate of femur fracture was 909/100,000 white females over 65 years of age.[3] This represents an annual incidence rate of almost 1%. The rate doubled in both males and females 80–84 years of age. All reported series show a consistent ratio of females to males of 3 : 1 in the overall risk of hip fracture. In Sweden (1955),[4] the annual fracture rate for the femoral neck was estimated as 220/100,000 females between 65–69 years of age; this increased to 11% over age 80. Other investigators have published similar data.[5–7] Females

who had previously sustained a fracture of the distal radius (Colles') were at an even greater risk, as their age advanced, than their cohorts who had not sustained such a fracture.[7] Additional epidemiologic and clinical studies have demonstrated the association between fractures of the neck of the femur, the distal radius, the vertebrae, and osteoporosis. As early as 1824, Sir Astley Cooper in his *Treatise on Dislocations and on Fractures of the Joints*[8] made the following observations:

. . . the fracture of the neck of the thigh bone within the capsular ligament seldom happens but at an advanced period of life;

That regular decay of nature which is called old age is attended with the changes which are easily detected in the dead body; and one of the principal of these is found in the bones, for they become thin in their shell and spongy in their texture;

Women are much more liable to this species of fracture than men . . .

It is not the purpose of this chapter to discuss treatment in detail; however, it must be noted that treatment of fractures of the hip involves an operative procedure whose magnitude varies with the location and extent of the fracture. This inevitably carries with it an attendant morbidity and mortality. Intracapsular fractures usually are treated either by open reduction and insertion of pins[9] or a replacement by a metallic hemiprosthesis (*see* Figures 33-1, 33-2, 33-3).[10] There have been several studies of fracture mortality. A retrospective study of subcapital femoral fractures in Great Britain showed that 24% of 1,618 reported cases died before the results of their treatment could be fully evalu-

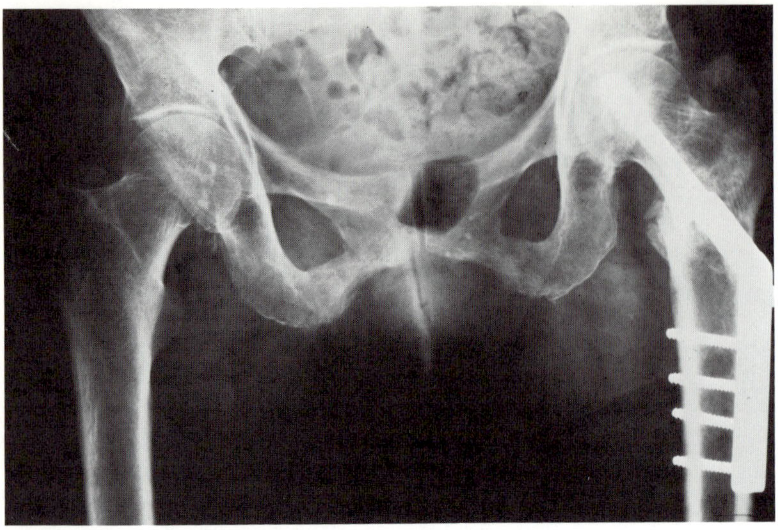

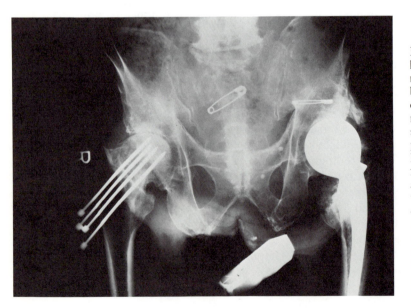

FIGURE 33-1 Intertrochanteric fracture of the left hip in a 79-year-old female who sustained a Colle's fracture of the left distal radius during the same fall. The fixation device is a sliding nail-plate. While recuperating from this surgery, she fell in the hospital and sustained an impacted fracture of the left proximal humeral surgical neck. Note the osteoporotic trabecular pattern in the right hip. All three of these fractures are indices of skeletal fragility that are due to osteoporosis.

ated.[11] Of the females, 7.4% and 13.3% of the males died within 1 month postoperatively. In addition, approximately one third of the displaced fractures failed to unite, presumably with an increased likelihood of additional surgery. The probability of non-union was noted to increase with age. Late segmental collapse, no doubt on a vascular basis, developed in 24% of the females, 15% of the males, and was physically disabling in 29% of this subset. A peak incidence rate of hip fracture has been found in persons 78 years of age; 8.5% of the cases already had sustained one previous hip fracture. At the end of 1 year following the fracture, only 50% remained alive.[6] After 4 years, only 15% of the males and 41% of the females over 75 years of age were still alive.

Distal Radius Fracture

A fracture of the distal radius,[12] is not accompanied by a similar mortality risk, but morbidity may be substantial.[13] Falls on an out-stretched arm are the cause of this fracture, which causes a shortening of the radius and may be intra-articular in a significant number of cases. Plaster immobilization with or without internal fixation is regularly required, but it frequently

FIGURE 33-2 An intracapsular fracture of the femoral neck in a 73-year-old male has been fixed with multiple pins on the right. Resorption of the neck has occurred and resulted in a backing out of the pins into the soft tissues. The left hip had been previously fractured and was replaced by a Thompson hemiprosthesis, which has been surrounded by considerable heterotropic new bone. The joint space has narrowed as well. Also note the degenerative changes in the lumbar spine. (Used by permission of Marvin H. Bloom, M.D.)

FIGURE 33-3 A Cathcart type hemiprosthesis inserted for an intracapsular fracture of the right hip. Notice the loss of joint space, a bad long-term prognostic sign. Also note the increased prominence of the primary trabecular pattern and the loss of density in the center (Ward's triangle) of the left femoral neck, which indicates a significant osteoporosis and a hip at risk for fracture. Of all hip fractures, 8% occur in individuals with a previous hip fracture.

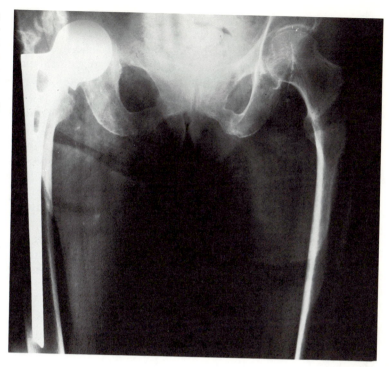

results in stiffness of the radiocarpal joint. There may be some cosmetic deformity due to the shortening of the distal radius, with some tendency to radial deviation of the radiocarpal joint. Vigorous postimmobilization rehabilitation is important in the management of this fracture. Some orthopedic surgeons believe that this fracture should be immobilized only for a minimal period of time (approximately 3 weeks), thus accepting some residual cosmetic deformity in the belief that the earliest possible institution of the rehabilitation process following control of pain is more important than good cosmetics. Obviously a loss of hand function distal to a fracture of the radius may significantly impair the ability of an elderly person to care for himself. This is the most significant social consideration in managing this common fracture.

Vertebral Fracture

Fractures of the vertebrae,[1,14] usually compression or wedge types, also are common in association with postmenopausal osteoporosis. These produce acute pain, often from very minor trauma such as attempting to lift a bag of groceries, and frequently are disabling for days to weeks. Vertebral fractures often are multiple, and cause a diminution in axial height. This is demonstrated by measuring the span and comparing it to the height. These two measurements are roughly equal, but with vertebral collapse, span measurement exceeds height. Vertebral collapse accounts for the so-called "dowager's hump" of the spine seen in elderly females, which is an excessive kyphotic appearance of the upper thoracic area. It is important to recognize that either vertebral fractures and/or distal radial fractures in an elderly person constitutes an index event that must be associated in the treating physician's mind with the potential for hip fracture and its attendant disastrous complications. It is incumbent on physicians to pursue vigorous prophylactic measures in this age group.

Pathologic Fracture

A pathologic fracture[15] also must be dealt with on occasion. Such fractures occur through a metastasis, most commonly from either a breast or prostate carcinoma, but they also are seen in association with pulmonary, renal, and thyroid carcinomatosis. These can occur in any bone, but are most commonly seen in the proximal bones of the extremities, pelvis, and vertebral column. Those fractures in the extremities may require internal fixation, which in recent years has been supplemented by the use of polymethylmethacrylate cement in the area of metastasis. This creates a more stable and immediate fixation and enables the patient to regain his or her previous activity level as soon as possible. The radiation treatment of metastases is regularly indicated. Vertebral fractures do not lend themselves to this kind of management, but require bracing and appropriate administration of analgesics.

In an individual who has skeletal carcinomatosis, an increase in pain (particularly in the proximal femoral area) may represent a stress fracture through a weakened area of bone. When such areas are identified, prophylactic internal fixation with or without polymethylmethacrylate is indicated to prevent the pain and psychological trauma of a fracture, which will almost certainly ensue and require a surgical procedure under less ideal circumstances. Even if no fracture is identified at the time of the first examination, it is important to monitor these areas carefully as the incidence of subsequent fractures is high.

Arthritis

The term "arthritis" encompasses a large and increasing number of diseases that have, as one part of their spectrum, inflammatory and degenerative changes of varying severity in the axial and appendicular joints. These conditions represent a major challenge to an orthopedic surgeon, as well as an internist and rheumatologist. Although they occur at all ages, arthritic diseases are distinctly more common with advancing age. This chapter will not deal with the medical management, which is the primary basis of therapeutic intervention in these processes, but will be limited to the surgical and rehabilitative aspects of these conditions. All individuals with arthritis should be managed with anti-inflammatory medications and appropriate assistant devices such as canes, crutches, and orthotic measures in the shoes. (*See* Volume I, Chapter 19.)

Total Hip Replacement

The introduction in the 1960s of total hip replacement procedures, which use a high-density polyethylene acetabular cup with a metallic femoral prosthesis, and the use of polymethylmethacrylate bone cement[16–18] has ushered in a new era in the management of arthritis, especially in end-stage diseases (*see* Figure 33-4). An orthopedic surgeon has a legitimate role to play in the team approach that is required in the management of more severe forms of arthritis. An internist or rheumatologist, physical therapist, occupational therapist, and medical social worker are key members of the team as well. Joint replacement is indicated in the intermediate and late stages of rheumatoid arthritis when there has been a loss of the cartilage space, often accompanied by bone erosion, joint contractures, and angular deformities, such as those that occur commonly in the knee. The complete destruction of the joint that is manifested by subluxation, frank dislocation, and/or ankylosis also is an indication for joint replacement in appropriately selected individuals.

Nearly two decades of experience with total hip replacement procedures has clearly demonstrated that the vast majority of patients, particularly those with disabling pain who have been unable to maintain a satisfactory quality of life by the use of anti-inflammatory medications and a cane or crutch, will be greatly benefited by hip replacement. Good or excellent results can be reliably expected in over 90% of these individuals, and the pain relief that is obtained is gratifying to both the patient and surgeon. Before surgery, however, a patient must be apprised of risks and complications of any major surgical procedure, which include anesthetic complications, pulmonary embolus, and cardiorespiratory problems. The most serious threat is an infection of the prosthetic implant itself.[19] The use of prophylactic antibiotics along with a better understanding of the surgical techniques that are required has progressively helped to diminish the frequency of this disastrous complication. Infection rates are on the order of magnitude of 1% in nearly all reported series. Although late developing infections have been a concern, they are not as frequent as had initially been feared. When an infection does occur,

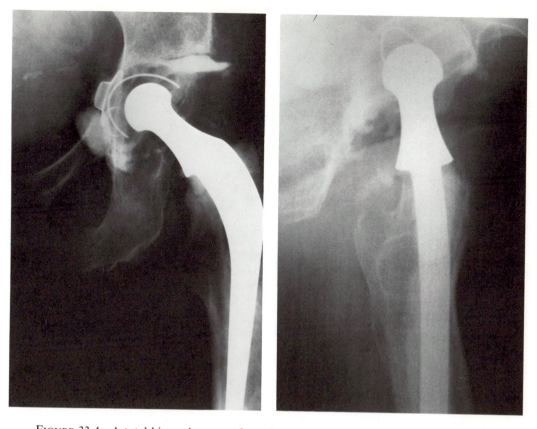

FIGURE 33-4   A total hip replacement for a degenerative joint disease. This was done at age 84 and still was serving the patient 4 years later. A total hip replacement significantly increases the quality of remaining life for many elderly persons with either a degenerative or rheumatoid disease with a joint surface disruption.

however, a patient must be aware that it will be necessary to remove the prosthesis in a second operation and institute vigorous treatment. It may be possible to reimplant the prosthesis at some later date, but at present this procedure must be considered controversial if not, in fact, experimental.

Following a total hip replacement, postoperative rehabilitation always is required. This partly entails teaching a patient that the prosthesis is not as stable as a normal hip and can become dislocated with excessive flexion and adduction of the hip. Dislocation ordinarily requires a subsequent anesthetic for reduction. The patient also must understand that there are late complications with this procedure, such as the loosening of one or both components of the prosthesis as time goes on. In spite of initial fears, "wearing out" the polyethylene acetabular cup has not been a significant problem as the

years have elapsed. Fractures of the femoral prosthetic stem have occurred on occasion, but these often are related to inadequate positioning of the component. If the greater trochanter is osteotomized in the process of exposing the joint, there also may be a subsequent pull-off related to inadequate fixation.

Total Knee Replacement

When it became evident that a total hip replacement procedure offered a dramatic relief of the pain and disability of arthritis, it was inevitable that total knee replacement procedures[20] would be developed (Figure 33-5); in fact, experimental replacement prostheses for nearly every joint in the body have been designed. With regard to total knee replacement procedures, however, it can be said that the results (although not quite

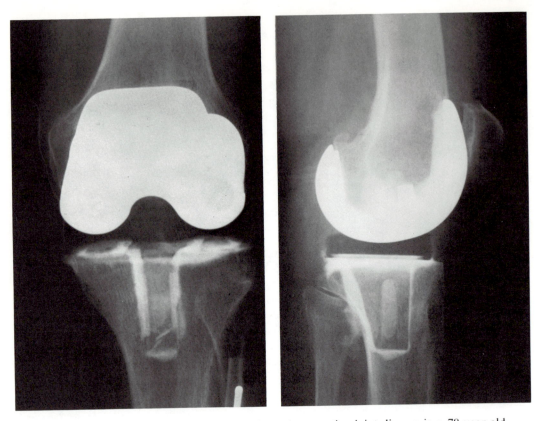

FIGURE 33-5   A total knee replacement for a degenerative joint disease in a 78-year-old female. Rheumatoid arthritis with erosive destruction of articular cartilage also responds well to joint replacement.

as reliable as those obtained with a total hip replacement) are none the less good or excellent in 85–95% of all patients treated with up-to-date techniques. In the early years of total knee implant development, certain considerations regarding both prosthetic design and alignment of the prosthesis in relationship to the weight-bearing axis of the tibia and femur were not fully understood. This resulted in an unacceptable incidence rate of failure, as high as 20–25%. At present, however, the reoperation rate is very much lower.

Patients can be offered this option when their disease is sufficiently advanced to warrant its consideration with a considerable confidence of pain relief and amelioration of disability. Again, this procedure should be reserved for those patients who have a loss of joint space with or without angular deformities and flexion contractures, which can be dealt with by surgery. Before such surgery, however, conservative management always must be given priority for a

period of some months. The knee joint is subjected to considerably higher stresses than the hip joint because of its relatively more constrained nature; therefore, eccentric loading and alignment considerations become more important. The complications of loosening components and a postoperative infection always must be considered in knee replacement, as well as in hip replacement. In addition, an obese patient becomes a serious consideration. Although this is also a matter of concern in the hip replacement, it is doubly so in the knee replacement. Many surgeons will not operate on a patient who weighs over 200 pounds.

A postoperative regimen following total knee replacement is more stringent than following hip replacement. The usual hospital time for regaining function is between 2–3 weeks. Following this, additional time must be spent, particularly in regaining flexion, for a period of some weeks and months after discharge from the hospital. It can be stated that a patient with an unusually good range of motion prior to surgery may lose some motion as a trade-off for symptomatic relief. In contrast, a patient who has very poor motion preoperatively probably will gain motion in both the flexion and extension portions of his or her range. This, however, requires an intensive physical therapy program.

Synovectomy

Aside from joint replacements, which probably are the procedures most commonly performed for patients with rheumatoid arthritis, additional procedures are occasionally indicated. Synovectomy of the knee[21] sometimes is helpful, and at least one study had demonstrated this procedure to have prophylactic value in knees that are enlarged with persistant medically refractory synovial hypertrophy.[22] This probably is the only joint in which this procedure can be reasonably expected to provide significant prophylactic benefits.

Arthrodesis of certain joints may be helpful at times, particularly in the wrist,[23] which commonly becomes subluxed in a volar direction during end-stage diseases. In this instance, flexor tendon function also is compromised and grasp becomes weak, unstable, and painful. Stabilization of the wrist in this manner will provide relief of pain and improve grasp strength in the majority of patients. When properly selected, most of these patients already have a loss of wrist motion, and the specific postoperative loss does not create an additional disability. A synovectomy of the wrist[24] may be helpful when synovial hypertrophy has occurred in spite of adequate medical management. Extensor tendon rupture, particularly of the extensors to the ring and middle fingers, commonly occurs in association with synovial hypertrophy and a dorsal dislocation of the distal ulna: the so-called caput ulnae syndrome.

A synovectomy and radial head excision of the elbow[25] also may benefit selected individuals who have been refractory to medical management. Silastic metacarpophalangeal joint replacements[26] are helpful for those patients who have lost function due to an involvement of these joints with volar subluxation and ulnar deviation, as commonly occurs. Cosmetic improvement can regularly be expected from this procedure, and the majority of patients (although not all) will obtain a functional benefit as well. It should be noted, in this regard however, that if a patient's hand function is adequate to meet their needs and they are not particularly concerned by the cosmetic aspects of the disease process, this procedure remains entirely elective and should not be urged on a hesitant individual. Although the infection rate is very low, a late fracture of the implants may occur and improvement in the range of motion may be disappointing in spite of vigorous—and always necessary—occupational therapy that is instituted as soon as possible in the postoperative period.

In the foot, subtalar arthrodesis, on rare occasion, may be helpful when there is a collapse of the hindfoot. However, a procedure performed more commonly that many patients find to be of great benefit is the so-called "forefoot resection"[27] in which the commonly prominent and painful metatarsal heads are resected. In addition, a hallux valgus can be corrected by means of a hemiarthroplasty of the first metatarsophalangeal joint.

Certain other procedures have been found to be helpful in dealing with rheumatoid arthritis. An excision of prominent and painful subcutaneous nodules, division of the flexor tendon sheath in the trigger finger, and surgical decompression of the carpal tunnel may be of considerable benefit to selected patients when symptoms warrant them.

Degenerative Joint Disease

Osteoarthritis, or degenerative joint disease, in elderly persons may occur throughout the axial skeleton and, in fact, is quite common in the cervical and lumbar areas. With the exception of the carpometacarpal joint of the thumb, it is not common in the upper extremities. The hip joints are commonly affected, and a total hip replacement, either unilateral or bilateral, may give marked relief. Indications and complications are similar to those discussed above in rheumatoid arthritis. At one time, osteotomies for a degenerative joint disease of the hip were recommended, but this procedure is no longer believed to be sufficiently beneficial to justify its use in other than very rare cases. In a degenerative joint disease of the knee however, there still may be a use for a high tibial osteotomy[28] when there is a unicompartmental disease, particularly in association with a varus deformity of the knee. However, this is probably only a temporary procedure, and many patients will go on to a correction of bicompartmental disease with a total knee replacement procedure.

Total Shoulder Replacement

At the time of this writing, a total shoulder arthroplasty procedure[29] has yet to reach the stage of general clinical acceptance; however, there are several recent studies that indicate good functional results following this procedure. As is always the case following the introduction of a new surgical procedure, early enthusiastic results must be confirmed by other observers and final results cannot be assessed for several years.

Initial favorable reports regarding total elbow and (particularly) total ankle arthroplasty procedures have proved disappointing, with a high incidence of subsequent failures.[30] The more constrained the joint (the less the freedom of motion), the more likely are increased stresses on the adjacent bone-cement interfaces, with subsequent mechanical failure. Both the ankle and elbow are such joints, and late complication rates have been high in all series in which a replacement arthroplasty procedure has been attempted in these two areas. Ankle arthrodesis remains a time-tested and useful procedure, when indicated.[31]

Osteomyelitis

In contrast to pyogenic osteomyelitis in childhood, which localizes in the metaphyseal regions of the long bones, adults seem to be particularly prone to the development of pyogenic vertebral osteomyelitis.[32] Less than 5% of all cases of osteomyelitis occur in the vertebral bodies, and an occurrence is more common in persons over 50 years of age. Because it is not common, it represents a serious diagnostic pitfall. Like the more common pyogenic osteomyelitis of the extremities that is found in young persons, a blood-borne infection probably is the most common predisposing factor. A direct in-

noculation by means of an open wound, or a postoperative infection that produces osteomyelitis, also can occur. There is some debate about the blood-borne mechanism of onset, with opinion being divided between those who adhere to the Batson's view theory of retrograde filling of the vertebral veins from the pelvic organs, and those who believe with Trueta that an infection probably is arterially induced in this area just as it is in the extremities. In any case, there is a clear association with other systemic and urologic diseases. Diabetes mellitus is a commonly associated condition.

Symptoms include those caused by the associated bacteremia or septicemia and localized signs or symptoms, which occasionally are accompanied by a demonstrable radiculopathy. When a patient complains of back pain, percussion of the spine is critical and extremely painful. Early in the course of this infection, there may be an elevated white blood cell count and erythrocyte sedimentation rate (ESR), more commonly the latter. However, after the acute phase, only the ESR will remain elevated. Blood cultures are positive only in the early stages. An additional diagnostic pitfall is the absence of radiologic changes for approximately the first 6 weeks. It may be misdiagnosed as either an osteoporotic vertebral fracture or an osteolytic metastasis. Early signs include an erosion of the subchondral bone, and these are best delineated by a computed tomography (CT scan). Later, changes include a progressive loss of vertebral body height, and there occasionally is a spread to an adjacent vertebra. This characteristically occurs anteriorly; in the thoracic spine, the pleural space may become involved. In the lumbar spine, psoas and perinephritic abscesses may develop. In the cervical spine, a retropharyngeal abscess may occur. Abscesses also may occur posteriorly, which produce epidural compression and long tract signs. A myelography and/or gallium^{-67} scan are indicated if there is a diagnostic doubt. During the healing stages, there may be a reactive sclerosis and spontaneous fusion of the vertebral bodies.

A definitive diagnosis often can be made via a needle biopsy procedure for the purpose of a histologic examination and culture. The most common organism that is encountered in the available literature has been Staphylococcus aureas; but, all species of bacteria that have been described as producing osteomyelitis elsewhere also have been isolated from the vertebral bodies. Treatment consists of antibiotics determined by sensitivity studies, bed rest, and the use of a brace or cast. Frank abscesses, especially those that produce neurologic signs or symptoms, must be drained.

Pyarthrosis

Bacterial (suppurative) arthritis in elderly persons also is an insidious infection in which an early diagnosis may be difficult. In one series[33] the duration of symptoms before an accurate diagnosis exceeded 1 month in more than 50% of the patients studied. Any anemic elderly patient with joint pain and an ESR must be evaluated for pyarthrosis. This is particularly true when there is an associated disease such as rheumatoid arthritis, osteoarthritis, trauma, or a history of corticosteroid administration, which either follow an intra-articular injection or are orally administered. A pre-existing infection elsewhere in the body, diabetes mellitus, and malignant diseases, all seem to increase the risk. The knee, hip, and glenohumeral joints are the most commonly involved, in that order of frequency. The most common organisms involved are Staphylococcus aureus, followed by gram-negative bacilli, streptococcus, and diplococcus. The sedimentation rate usually is elevated, but not always. An accurate aspiration of the joint is essential to a diagnosis. Unless frank pus is aspirated with ease, it is better to obtain an arthrogram by injecting a water-soluble contrast medium into those joints (especially the hip and shoulder) where the aspirate is thought to be negative. This serves to delineate the joint surfaces, and also to prove that the needle actually entered the synovial cavity. Antibiotic treatment should be based on sensitivities that are obtained by a culture of the synovial fluid aspirate. This always should be done both anaerobically as well as aerobically, and adequate drainage of the infected joint is critical. This is a serious infection; in the series cited above, the mortality rate was approximately 15%. The morbidity that is associated with joint destruction also is substantial, and it can result in a permanent impairment of the ability to live independently.

Tuberculosis of Bones and Joints

Although there is a peak incidence rate of tuberculosis during the first 4 decades, there is an appreciable incidence among elderly persons. An involvement may occur in any part of the body, but the greatest frequency in all series is in the thoracic and lumbosacral spines.[34] The hip, knee, ribs, manubrium, and sternum also are involved with some regularity. One must maintain a high index of suspicion, particularly because of the chronic and often low-grade nature of this infection. Typically, a patient complains of back pain that restricts spinal movement. All motions are guarded and a protective gait can be detected. As the destruction of bone progresses, there may be a development of a sharp angular deformity of the spine, which is termed a gibbus. Complications of the tuberculous process include psoas abscess, Pott's paraplegia, and tuberculous meningitis.

Modern therapy primarily is chemotherapy, which is described in Chapter 21. It must be noted, however, that surgery frequently is indicated, particularly when a so-called "cold abscess" develops and produces local neurologic symptoms and signs. Anterior surgical decompression and fusion frequently is helpful in the management of Pott's paraplegia[35], in which both the gibbus and the neurologic impairment usually respond very gratifyingly to surgical intervention. Similarly, in the management of tuberculosis of the hip joint, surgical arthrodesis may be required for both the control of infection and relief of pain. In the knee joint, immobilization and chemotherapy is indicated, but authorities vary in their recommendations as to whether or not an excision of the synovial membrane (synovectomy) is indicated. With severe cartilage and bone destruction, surgical arthrodesis is frequently helpful. However, a disease of such severity is rarely seen in developed countries.

Hand Problems

Dupuytren's contracture[36] occurs with considerable frequency among elderly persons and is more common in males than females. The essential pathology is a nodular thickening of the pretendinous bands of the palmar fascia. It often is associated with similar changes in the plantar fascia and the corpus cavernosum (Peyronie's disease). In addition, associations with a greater than expected frequency have been described with liver disease, alcoholism, gout, diabetes, and epilepsy. There most commonly are contractures of the fourth and fifth fingers as well as the thumb. For reasons that are not clear, the index and ring fingers frequently escape involvement. The process is a gradually progressive one with an ultimate clawing of the fingers, which suggests a neurologic disease and/or involvement of the flexor tendons to the digits. The pathologic process, however, is limited to the palmar fascia. In those cases that warrant surgical intervention, an excision of the thickened tissue via limited incisions, which sometimes require skin grafting, is the method chosen by most surgeons. Complications are considerably higher using the method of complete palmar fasciectomy, which was formerly practiced.

Trapeziometacarpal (Carpometacarpal) Degenerative Joint Disease

Degenerative changes in the basal joint of the thumb are common. Although they initially may be asymptomatic, the repeated use of a "sprain" may direct attention to the process that has frequently been going on for some time. A patient complains of pain, usually well localized to the area of the trapeziometacarpal articulation, that is painful to palpation and on motion. X-ray films will confirm the diagnosis by demonstrating a characteristic loss of the joint space and marginal osteophytes. There often is some tendency to instability and subluxation of the joint as well. There is no agreement on treatment, and both arthrodesis[37] and silastic interposition arthroplasty[38] have their proponents. Thumb function, especially of the dominant hand, is critical to many aspects of life; therefore, treatment is warranted. Neither of these procedures carries a substantial morbidity, and symptomatic relief usually is gratifying.

Stenosing Tenosynovitis of the Wrist (deQuervains' Disease)

Stenosing tenosynovitis of the tendons that pass over the radial styloid[39] (i.e., the extensor pollicis brevis and the abductor pollicis longus) is a common condition at all ages. The presenting complaint frequently is of wrist pain or "arthritis." A physical examination reveals tenderness specifically limited to the radial styloid area, and Finkelstein's test produces exquisite pain in the area. This test is performed by having a patient grasp his or her thumb in the palm with the other fingers of the same hand, and then forcefully deviating the wrist to the ulnar side. In sufficiently symptomatic patients, surgical intervention is indicated. The procedure itself is a relatively minor one, but a skilled surgeon is necessary because a common complication is an iatrogenic neuroma of the sensory branch of the radial nerve that crosses over this area.

Trigger Finger (Stenosing Tenosynovitis)

The so-called "trigger finger"[40] is a common condition in which there is a painful blocking of free movement of the tendon to one of the digits; most commonly the fourth, at the level of the metacarpal neck just proximal to the metacarpophalangeal joint. Frequently, a patient finds that he is unable to extend this joint once the triggering has occurred, and it is necessary to use the other hand to correct the flexed position that persists. Occasionally, the symptoms are entirely referred to the proximal interphalangeal joint. In most instances, the patient can demonstrate the phenomenon, although he or she frequently is reluctant to do so. Tenderness over the proximal flexor pulley in the palm will be demonstrable. A disproportion in the size of the pulley and the tendon produces an excessive snugness and causes the entrapment in flexion or "triggering." Treatment consists of an incision in the pulley under local or regional anesthesia. This frequently can be done as an outpatient procedure, although tourniquet ischemia is essential to a surgeon for a proper identification of the anatomic structures. There is no need for subsequent immobilization, and immediate motion is encouraged. Properly done, the complication rate is negligible.

Carpal Tunnel Syndrome

Carpal tunnel syndrome[41] is a peripheral entrapment neuropathy that produces symptoms of compression of the median nerve at the wrist, beneath the flexor retinaculum. The etiology often is obscure, but it is seen with considerable frequency in rheumatoid arthritis, following Colles' fracture, during pregnancy, and (rarely) in association with acromegaly and myxedema or any condition that causes an increase in the hydrostatic pressure in this closed space. One recent study[42] demonstrated that carpal canal pressures were of an order of magnitude 10 times that of normal in carpal tunnel syndrome.

Patients usually complain of painful paresthesias in the cutaneous distribution of the median nerve; typically, the index and long fingers. These symptoms frequently are disturbing at night. The typical history is one of an elderly female who awakes at night with pain, and then arises to massage her hands and/or run them under water. On occasion, pain may radiate proximally into the forearm as well. Typically, only sensory symptoms occur in the early stages of this disease, but there subsequently may be a wasting of the muscles of the thenar eminence with weakness of thumb opposition. A careful differential diagnosis from cervical spondylosis is necessary. The Tinel's sign, which is produced by tapping on the median nerve in the carpal canal, may be positive. However, a higher incidence rate of success on clinical examination is produced by the Phalen test, in which the wrists are forcefully palmarflexed maximally for a period of 60 seconds. This frequently will produce painful paresthesias in the hand. A definitive diagnosis, however, should be made by the use of electrical studies that demonstrate a slowing of conduction through the carpal tunnel in both the motor and sensory components of the median nerve. Sensory delay is a more sensitive and reliable finding.

Treatment may be either conservative or operative. Mild symptoms sometimes respond to the wearing of a splint at night to immobilize the wrist. Injections of steroids into the carpal tunnel may give temporary relief, but definitive treatment consists of a surgical section of the flexor retinaculum through a volar wrist incision. There is disagreement on which incisions render the best results; transverse incisions are cosmetically desirable. However, one of the common complications of this procedure is the production of a painful neuroma in the palmar cutaneous branch of the median nerve. A curved incision probably is best. It runs longitudinally along the ulnar side of the hand with no part of the incision extending radially beyond a line drawn from the base of the ring finger to the center of the wrist, as delineated by the palmaris longus tendon. Properly performed, good results occur in over 95% of all cases.

Supraspinatus Syndrome (Rotator Cuff Lesions)

A number of structures may be involved with inflammatory or degenerative processes, thus causing shoulder pain (see Table 33-1 and Figure 33-6). In contrast to the hip, where chronic pain most frequently is an indication of inflammatory or degenerative processes of the articular surface itself, the glenohumeral joint, (although it may be involved as part of any systemic arthritis) seldom is involved with a degenerative process of the joint surface. The musculotendinous cuff commonly is involved, however, as are the adjacent biceps tendon and the subacromial bursa. The terms "bursitis" and "painful arc syndrome" sometimes are used to describe the symptom complex in the shoulder area.

Among the lesions seen in elderly persons are incomplete or complete tendon ruptures, especially of an insertion of the supraspinatus tendon, calcific deposits, subacromial (subdeltoid) bursitis, bicipital tenosynovitis, biceps tendon rupture, and adhesive capsulitis. It frequently is difficult to distinguish between these afflictions. Fortunately, from a therapeutic standpoint, it is not always necessary; many physicians simply diagnose a "supraspinatus syndrome"[43] or "rotator cuff lesion, type undetermined." The term "bursitis" infers a localized inflammation of the subacromial bursa, which may indeed be the case; but, such an inflammation may be secondary to an underlying lesion.

Rotator Cuff Tear

Minor trauma (or occasionally no trauma) in older patients may produce tears of varying extents of any of the tendons of the rotator cuff. Probably, most shoulder pain of sudden onset is of this variety. There is pain, muscle spasm, and a limitation of both active and passive motion. Physical examination frequently demonstrates tenderness that is located throughout the

TABLE 33-1 Supraspinatus Syndrome—Degenerative Conditions of the Rotator Cuff

Condition	History	Physical Findings	Lab/X-ray Film Studies
Rotator cuff tear	Shoulder pain, sometimes of sudden onset, followed by transitory pain—free interval	"Pseudoparalysis," painful arc of motion, "drop-arm" sign	Arthrogram* shows extravasation of contrast material into subacromial bursa; inferior acromial facet formation
Calcific tendinitis of supraspinatus; "bursitis" of subacromial bursa	Often asymptomatic, sometimes acutely painful	Localized tenderness, painful arc of motion	Amorphous calcium in supraspinatus tendon over humeral head
Bicipital tenosynovitis	Anterior shoulder pain, especially when flexing elbow to lift	Anterior shoulder tenderness, pain in anterior proximal arm (bicipital groove) with resisted elbow flexion	—
Biceps origin rupture (long head)	Sudden onset of pain in anterior shoulder, weakness of elbow flexion	Tenderness over bicipital groove, abnormal shape of biceps belly ("balled up")	—
Adhesive capsulitis "frozen shoulder"	Pain and marked loss of motion	All motions diminished	Arthrogram* will show a shrunken capsule

* Gordan GS, Vaughan C: *Clinical Management of the Osteoporoses*. Acton, MA, Heyden Publishers 1976.

area of the rotator cuff. The supraspinatus tendon that lies on the superior surface of the humeral head and inserts into the uppermost facet on the greater tuberosity most commonly is involved. There is a discrepancy between the frequency with which rotator cuff tears are diagnosed clinically and the incidence occurring as a routine postmortem finding. In autopsies of persons over 60 years of age, there is a 20–30% incidence rate of such tears.[44] If a large rotator cuff tear has occurred, a patient may experience a sudden sharp pain in the shoulder that is

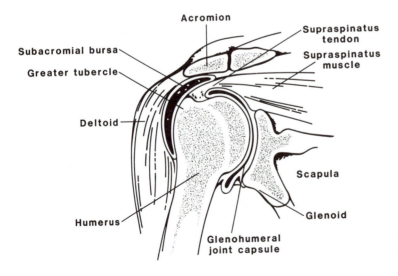

FIGURE 33-6 Anatomy of the shoulder.

followed by a period of a few hours during which the pain subsides before its reappearance in a persistent form. A patient usually is not seen during this painless period, but a history is helpful. A patient then presents with a "pseudoparalysis" in which he is unable to maintain abduction of the arm, even though it can be put through a full passive range of motion. The first 20–30% of abduction from the side also may be possible, but the arc between 30–60% of abduction is very painful. If the shoulder is passively placed in that position by the examiner, a patient will immediately let the arm fall to the side, which is the so-called "drop arm sign." After several weeks, it also may be possible in a thinly muscled individual to palpate a defect in the rotator cuff. It must be remembered, however, that the deltoid muscle overlies the rotator cuff, making palpation difficult.

In a younger individual who sustains a significant acute tear during athletic activity, these tears frequently are repaired via surgery.[45] Some surgeons believe that this is a necessity in elderly persons as well, if function does not return within 5 or 6 weeks. However, approximately 90% of all individuals will show a good return of spontaneous function with conservative management alone. The added trauma of surgical repair in an elderly person must be considered as well.

A routine x-ray film examination of the shoulder in an early rotator cuff tear will be unremarkable. However, as the condition becomes chronic, the humeral head may come to lie in a relatively superior position, so that there is a diminution of the space between the underside of the acromion process and the superior surface of the humeral head.[46] On occasion, pseudofacet formation may be seen on the underside of the acromion, with a corresponding lesion on the humeral head. A definitive diagnosis is made by an arthrogram.[47] The contrast material normally is contained within the glenohumeral joint, but if there is a tear through the full thickness of the rotator cuff, the dye will be seen in the subacromial bursa as well.

Management consists of placing the arm in a sling. The use of cold applications frequently gives symptomatic relief. Analgesics and anti-inflammatory medications also may be useful, as with any self-limited painful state. As pain subsides, active motion should be instituted gradually.

Supraspinatus Calcific Tendinitis[48]

Although amorphous calcium deposits may be seen in the rotator cuff of asymptomatic people (2.7% of one large series), such deposits also may be associated with acute shoulder pain and exquisite tenderness over the area of the deposit. These calcium deposits occur most frequently during middle age. It is believed that both vascular and mechanical factors may predispose to the laying down of calcium, which most commonly is deposited near the insertion of the supraspinatus tendon. Vascular perfusion studies of the rotator cuff indicate that this area has the least an abundant blood supply, perhaps because here it is stretched tautly across the head of the humerus. It is likely that the acutely painful stage is associated with an inflammation of the overlying subdeltoid bursa. This diagnosis can be made by taking an anteroposterior x-ray film of the shoulder, using a soft-tissue technique in which the bone is underpenetrated even though the calcium deposit (which may not be very dense) is more likely to appear. This acute stage may progress to a more indolent symptom complex in which the "painful arc syndrome," mentioned above, may supervene. The patient then may have discomfort only when the arm is held in the abducted position, or when lying on it during sleep.

Treatment consists of analgesics and anti-inflammatory medications; in addition, ice packs applied to the shoulder may be helpful. Some physicians treat the calcium deposit by "needling"; in this technique, an 18-gauge needle is repeatedly placed into the calcium deposit (under x-ray control) with the intent of releasing the amorphous calcium, which is of toothpaste consistency, into the subacromial bursa from which it becomes phagocytized. If conservative management fails, it may (on rare occasion) be necessary to perform a surgical excision of the calcium.

Adhesive Capsulitis

Following any pathologic process of the shoulder, there may be a significant loss of motion. The shoulder is the most mobile joint in the body; its function is to allow positioning of the hand; consequently, a loss of motion may be quite disabling. Adhesive capsulitis[49], or "frozen shoulder," frequently has an insidious onset following immobilization for a fracture of the arm or forearm, following rotator cuff pathology (such as a relatively minor cuff tear), or in association with calcific supraspinatus tendinitis for which the shoulder is immobilized. It also has been seen following a radical mastectomy, myocardial infarction, and chest surgery. In order for the humerus to be raised into an overhead position in abduction, it is necessary that there be a pouch of redundant capsule and synovial tissue, inferiorly. It is this tissue that becomes adherent with the result that this slack area becomes effectively obliterated, thus limiting motion in the glenohumeral joint. It frequently is possible for these patients to abduct their arm to approximately 40–50°, but a careful examination will reveal that all of this motion has occurred in the scapulothoracic joint. X-ray films usually are negative.

The treatment of a frozen shoulder involves eliminating any predisposing conditions, when present. The patient must always be advised that the treatment process probably will require months of management, because it essentially consists of stretching out and redeveloping the normal laxity of the infraglenoid capsular pouch. Analgesic medication may be helpful, but the essential treatment is the institution of a supervised progressive range of motion exercises.

Bicipital Tendinitis[50]
and Biceps Tendon Rupture

Pain in the anterior aspect of the shoulder that is accompanied by localized tenderness overlying the bicipital groove and pain in the anterior shoulder that is precipitated by attempting to lift an object or push up against the examiner's hand with the forearm supinated, are both an indication of an inflammation of the tenosynovial sheath of the long head of the biceps in the bicipital groove. This inflammatory process probably is, in most instances, a part of the overall syndrome of rotator cuff problems. Its greatest incidence is after the 45 years of age. Its onset may be either acute or gradual, and it also may be complicated by adhesive capsulitis.

Treatment consists of rest and the administration of analgesics and anti-inflammatory medications. Steroid injections in the area of the biceps tendon is a limited number (i.e., not more than three) may be helpful. Occasionally, a patient who does not respond to conservative management of this type may require surgical intervention, at which time the biceps tendon is permanently affixed in the bicipital groove in such a manner as to prevent its excursion up and down the inflamed tenosynovial sheath. This does not appear to interfere significantly with either forearm flexion, supination, or shoulder motion.

The long head of the biceps tendon may rupture, usually acutely and following stressful activity. When this happens, the normal elongated configuration of a spindle is lost, and the bulk of the biceps belly will be found to become more prominent and spheroid in the distal forearm. The insertion of the biceps muscle on the bicipital tuberosity of the radius also may rupture, in which instance the muscle belly retracts proximally. This less common rupture requires surgical management, whereas a rupture of the proximal tendon in the groove (at least in the elderly persons) is not associated with a significant disability. There initially may be weakness of elbow flexion and supination. However, in a period of weeks or months, there appears to be adequate compensation when one compares strength with the opposite unaffected biceps. Therefore, surgical intervention ordinarily is not required in elderly persons, unless it is desired for cosmetic reasons.

Foot Problems
in Elderly Persons

Problems that affect the forefoot occur more commonly in elderly persons than those that affect the hindfoot. The major exception would be a neuropathic arthropathy, which affects the midtarsal joints in diabetes mellitus. Such conditions of the forefoot as hammertoes, claw toes, painful calluses (metatarsalgia), hallux valgus, hallux rigidus, and interdigital neuralgia all are common. These problems may be seen in association with rheumatoid arthritis, and the reader also is referred to the section dealing with that subject. (*See* Volume I, Chapter 19.)

Metatarsalgia (Painful Plantar Callosities)

Painful forefoot calluses frequently are seen in association with claw toes.[51] There is some argument about terminology; however, for the purposes of this discussion a clawing of the toes will be defined as a hyperextension deformity of the metatarsophalangeal joint, usually with contracture of the extensor tendons across this joint as well as flexion deformities of the interphalangeal joints. When this occurs, the normal fibrofatty pad that underlies the metatarsal heads is drawn distally, so that the soft tissue cushioning beneath the weight-bearing areas of the metatarsal heads is thinner than normal. This condition, in association with the normal thinning of skin and subcutaneous tissues that occurs as age advances and collagen declines throughout the body results in calluses in this area. Patients complain of pain in the forefoot, which is accentuated by excessive walking. Although any metatarsal head may be involved, the most frequent ones are the second, third, and fourth.

Pain in the forefoot also may occur with interdigital neuroma; the differentiation must be made. In metatarsalgia, there are obvious calluses that correspond to the overlying metatarsal heads. Pain can be easily reproduced by direct pressure over these heads. A further distinction must be made with plantar warts. These can be distinguished by paring away the superficial keratin surface of the lesion and observing the structure underneath. In a wart, a sharply marginated lesion appears with many bleeding capillary ends, which rise perpendicularly to the surface of the skin. In contrast, a callus merges imperceptibly into the surface of the skin at its edges and the capillary structure is not present.

Conservative treatment of metatarsalgia consists of a metatarsal pad that can be placed within the shoe in such a manner as to relieve pressure on the affected areas of the bone. A well-placed metatarsal bar on the sole may accomplish the same purpose. Calluses should be trimmed on a regular basis, and preparations that consist of a mild acid can be obtained for this purpose at any pharmacy. When they are placed on the callus overnight beneath a piece of tape, they will soften the horny skin so that the patient can pare away the surface pain-

lessly. If these measures fail, osteotomies of the necks of the metatarsals themselves and/or the phalanges can be done. This ordinarily affords gratifying relief and most patients who have a bilateral disease return to have the second foot done, which is a measure of subjective approval.

Hallux Valgus (Bunion)[52]

Although bunions may occur at any age, they are distinctly more common in elderly persons and usually are bilateral. In most instances, the great toe is angulated laterally at the metatarsophalangeal joint, which results in subluxation of the joint. Once this process begins, the flexor and extensor tendons become displaced to the lateral side of the center of the joint and, therefore, begin to bowstring across it, thus maintaining the deformity against efforts to correct it by conservative means. This condition frequently is seen in rheumatoid arthritis, but it also is seen in relatively normal feet. It is believed that wearing pointed or poorly fitting shoes or high heels may be causative factors. It occurs more commonly in females. In addition to the lateral angulation, an exostosis or bony enlargement occurs on the medial side of the first metatarsal head. Because of pressure between the shoe and this bony prominence, a bursa frequently develops. On occasion, these bursas may become acutely inflamed and may suggest gout of the metatarsophalangeal joint. In some feet, a bunion seems to consist almost entirely of this exostosis and its accompanying bursa, and the lateral deviation of the toe is not nearly as striking. In these feet, management sometimes can be accomplished by the simple expedient of wearing larger shoes or having the shoes stretched by a shoemaker's swan in an orthopedic shop. Felt pads and other devices to alleviate pressure also may be useful. If these measures fail, surgical intervention for removal of the exostosis is indicated.

In those toes where there is a marked lateral subluxation of the first metatarsophalangeal joint, the second toe may be found to overlap or underlap the great toe. A degenerative joint disease of the metatarsophalangeal joint also may occur. It is important to distinguish intra-articular symptoms from those related entirely to pressure over the metatarsal head. Numerous surgical procedures for bunions have been described, but the operation that most benefits those patients who have an intra-articular pathology is the so-called "Keller bunionectomy" in which the base of the proximal phalanx is resected for a distance of approximately 1 cm. Under no circumstances should the first metatarsal head be resected, as this severely interferes with the weight-bearing pedestal of the forefoot.

Hallux Rigidus[53,54]

The term "hallux rigidus" is used to describe a painful stiffness of the first metatarsophalangeal joint. In normal gait, the first metatarsophalangeal joint dorsiflexes to approximately 60°; when this is not possible because of rigidity of the joint, a patient tends to limp in such a manner as to avoid pressure on the forefoot. This is a painful and tiring gait. The essential nature of this process is a degenerative joint disease, although it occasionally may represent a post-traumatic arthritis. On an x-ray film, a narrowing of the joint space and marginal osteophytes will be seen, as with any degenerative joint condition. Treatment consists of the use of an anterior heel or rocker to alleviate the pressure on this area. If this is not satisfactory, either arthrodesis of the joint or a resection arthroplasty (Keller operation) may be helpful.

Hammertoe[55,56]

Hammertoes usually are distinguished from claw toes (in which there is an extension contracture of the metatarsophalangeal joint and flexion contractures of the interphalangeal joints) by the fact that the distal interphalangeal joint in a hammertoe is not flexed; ordinarily, the extension deformity at the metatarsophalangeal joint is not as striking. This results in a toe that may develop a painful callus on the tip, because the normal and necessary flexibility at the proximal interphalangeal joint is lost. This may respond to conservative measures, such as a passive manual stretching of the proximal interphalangeal joint and regular trimming of the terminal callus (*see* the section on "Metatarsalgia"). If symptoms persist, however, a partial phalangectomy or interphalangeal joint arthrodesis is helpful.

Bunionette (Tailor's Bunion)[57]

A bunionette is a bony enlargement of the lateral side of the fifth metatarsal head at the level of the metatarsophalangeal joint. As with the similar condition in the great toe, there frequently is an associated overlying bursa. There may or may not be a medial deviation of the fifth toe. Conservative treatment with stretching the shoe and the use of felt pads usually is sufficient. Occasionally, an excision of the bony prominence may be required.

Interdigital Neuroma (Morton's Neuralgia/Morton's Toe)[58]

Anterior foot pain that is due to a plantar interdigital "neuroma," usually between the third and fourth toes, is a relatively common condition. It may be distinguished from metatarsalgia that is associated with metatarsal head prominence and painful callosities, which are absent or slight in this condition. An interdigital neuroma is more prevalent in females than males by a ratio of approximately 4:1. It commonly occurs beginning in middle age and extends into advanced age. It usually is unilateral, but about 15% of the time it may occur bilaterally. The usual complaint is of a burning sensation in the forefoot, which is aggravated by activity and relieved by rest. Often, these patients will remove their shoes and rub their feet to obtain symptomatic relief.

A diagnosis can be made by pressing firmly in the interdigital space on the plantar surface of the foot at the level of the metatarsal necks. This frequently will be painful in the area that is affected by the neuroma, but not in the adjacent toes. Similarly, side-to-side compression of the metatarsal heads between the examiners interlocked hands may reproduce symptoms. A further check is to perform an interdigital block with 1%-lidocaine or a similar local anesthetic. This must be done during a symptomatic period, and a positive response is the temporary relief of the pain.

The pathology in this condition, in spite of the usual terminology of "neuroma," is not neoplastic. This probably represents an entrapment neuroma, in which there is a proliferation of the fibrous tissue surrounding the nerve. A histologic examination of these swellings on the nerves reveals dense fibrous and hyaline tissues, that sometimes are accompanied by an edema. The findings, however, are not specific. Also, nerves removed from asymptomatic feet may appear very similar.

Symptomatic relief often can be achieved by the use of a slightly convex pad that is placed on the inside of the shoe in such a position as to allow the metatarsal necks to spread over the dome, thus allowing more space for passage of the neurovascular bundles. Metatarsal bars placed on the outside of the sole also may give some relief. In instances where relief is insufficient, an excision of the interdigital nerve through a dorsal incision at the level of the metatarsal necks gives symptomatic relief in the vast majority of patients. Although it would appear that this would produce a disturbing numbness in the area that is distal to the excision, this (in fact) does not occur in the majority of cases. This probably is attributable to an overlap of the nerve supply in this area. A recurrence of the neuroma is reported in a relatively small percentage.

Surgery for the foot in elderly persons always must be undertaken with considerable caution and only following a careful evaluation of the vascular status. Ischemic pain must be carefully excluded; evaluation of capillary pulses and a Doppler evaluation of blood flow are mandatory if there is any question about the adequacy of perfusion before surgical intervention. Diabetic or other polyneuropathies may present as foot pain, and this must be carefully excluded.

Sore Heel Syndrome
(Calcaneal Spur, Plantar Fasciitis)[59]

Pain in the heel with weight-bearing, and particularly following vigorous exercise, is common at all ages. As the pursuit of physical fitness has been taken up by elderly persons, a geriatric physician must be prepared to deal with various "overuse" complaints. Characteristically, pain is centered in the heel pad without physical findings other than a well-localized, pressure-sensitive area on the plantar surface. Although this pain frequently is attributed to a "calcaneal spur," which may be seen on an x-ray film, this spur actually represents a normal variant and consists of an in-growth of osseous tissue into

the attachment of the plantar fascia into the calcaneus. This bony metaplasia of the fascia, in itself, is not painful. It appears that the problem in a painful heel syndrome is one of repetitive microtrauma to the soft tissues in this area. A loading of the foot causes repetitive pronation of the arch, which places the plantar fascia under an excessive stretch.

Steroid and local anesthetic injections into the area of maximum tenderness may produce some relief, but it is the author's experience that this tends to be temporary. The problem may be persistent and may necessitate some modification of activities. A useful device is the University of California Biomechanics Laboratory shoe insert, which must be custom-made to an individual's foot and holds the heel in a position of relative supination. In this position, the plantar fascia is more relaxed and subjected to less stretching. The patient must be advised, however, that symptoms may persist for months and that the need for exercise can be met by swimming, if such facilities are available. The use of the so-called SACH heel, which originally was developed for use in lower-extremity prostheses, also may provide a better cushioning for these patients. An orthopedic shop can supply these devices.

Tarsal Tunnel Syndrome[60]

Tarsal tunnel syndrome is a form of entrapment neuropathy that affects the posterior tibial nerve as it deeply passes behind the medial malleolus to the flexor retinaculum in that area. It produces symptoms that are related to the medial and lateral plantar nerves, both of which are terminal branches of the posterior tibial nerve. Burning paresthesias occur on the plantar surface of the foot and sometimes on the heel. On occasion, pain may radiate proximally toward the knee. This may follow an injury that produces a deformity and encroachment on the tarsal tunnel, such as a fracture, sprain, or crush injury; however, many cases are idiopathic. This condition should be suspected whenever there is a burning forefoot pain, especially in the plantar surface. It frequently is present both at rest and following activity. Tinel's sign, which is elicited by a tapping over the posterior tibial nerve behind the medial malleolus, may be positive; but, the most reliable diagnostic findings are derived from electrical conduction studies as the nerve passes through the tunnel.

Treatment consists of a surgical release of the flexor retinaculum in this area. This procedure is analogous to the carpal tunnel release. Unfortunately, however, the results of surgical intervention do not seem to be as consistently beneficial. Nonetheless, it should be undertaken, because conservative management rarely is of any significant benefit.

References

1. Gordan GS, Vaughn C: *Clinical Management of the Osteoporoses.* Acton, MA, Heyden Publishers, 1976.

2. Specht E: Hip fracture, skeletal fragility, osteoporosis and hormonal deprivation in elderly women. *West J Med* 133:297–303, 1980.

3. Wylie CM: Hospitalization for fractures and bone loss in adults. *Public Health Rep* 92:33–38, 1977.

4. Bauer GCH: Epidemiology of fracture in aged persons. A preliminary investigation in fracture etiology. *Clin Orthop* 17:219–225, 1960.

5. Morgan B: *Osteomalacia, Renal Osteodystrophy and Osteoporosis.* Springfield, Ill, Charles C Thomas Publisher, 1973.

6. Beals RK: Survival following hip fracture, long-term follow-up of 607 patients. *J Chron Dis* 25:235–244, 1972.

7. Alffram PA: An epidemiological study of cervical and trochanteric fractures of the femur in an urban population. *Acta Orthop Scand* 65 (supp):1–109, 1964.

8. Cooper A: *Treatise on Dislocations and on Fractures of the Joints,* ed 4. London, Longman, 1824.

9. Edmonson AS, Crenshaw AH (eds): *Campbell's Operative Orthopaedics,* ed 6. St. Louis, Mosby, 1980, p 635ff.

10. Edmonson AS, Crenshaw AH (eds): *Campbell's Operative Orthopaedics,* ed 6. St. Louis, Mosby, 1980, p 656ff.

11. Barnes R, Brown JT, Garden P, et al: Subcapital fractures of the femur: A prospective review. *J Bone Joint Surg* 58B:2–24, 1976.

12. Ure CL, et al: Decreased risk of fractures of the hip and lower forearm with postmenopausal use of estrogen. *N Engl J Med* 303:1195–1198, 1980.

13. Cooney WP, et al: Complications of Colles' fractures. *J Bone Joint Surg* 62A:613–619, 1980.

14. Gordan GS, et al: Antifracture efficacy of long-term estrogens for osteoporosis. *Trans Assoc Am Physicians* 86:326–332, 1973.

15. Harrington KD, Sim FH, Enis JE, et al: Methylmethacrylate as adjunct in internal fixation of pathologic fractures: Experience with 375 cases. *J Bone Joint Surg* 58A:1047–1055, 1976.

16. Charnley J: Total hip replacement by low-friction arthroplasty. *Clin Orthop* 72:7–21, 1970.

17. Charnley J, Cupic Z: The nine and ten year results of the low-friction arthroplasty of the hip. *Clin Orthop* 95:9–25, 1973.

18. Wilcock GK: A comparison of total hip replacement in patients aged 69 years or less and 70 years or over. *Gerontology* 27:85–88, 1981.

19. Edmonson AS, Crenshaw AH (eds): *Campbell's Operative Orthopaedics,* ed 6. St. Louis, Mosby, 1980, p 2333ff.

20. Pritchard RW: Total knee replacement in the elderly. *J Maine Med Assoc* 71:378–379, 1980.

21. Laurin CA, Desmarchais J, Daziano L, et al: Long-term results of synovectomy of the knee in rheumatoid patients. *J Bone Joint Surg* 56A:521–531, 1974.

22. Taylor AR, Hill AGS: Synovectomy. *Clin Rheum Dis* 4(suppl 2):287–309, 1978.

23. Millender LH, Nalebuff BA: Arthrodesis of the rheumatoid wrist. *J Bone Joint Surg* 55A:1026–1034, 1973.

24. Eiken O, Haga T, Salgeback S: Assessment of surgery of the rheumatoid wrist. *Scand J Plast Reconstruct Surg* 9:207–215, 1975.

25. Copeland SA, Taylor JG: Synovectomy of the elbow in rheumatoid arthritis: The place of excision of the head of the radius. *J Bone Joint Surg* 61B:69–73, 1979.

26. Beckenbaugh RD, Dobyns JH, Linscheid RL, et al: Review and analysis of silicone rubber metacarpophalangeal implants. *J Bone Joint Surg* 58A:483–487, 1976.

27. Watson MS: A long-term follow-up of forefoot arthroplasty. *J Bone Joint Surg* 56B:527–533, 1974.

28. Coventry MB: Osteotomy about the knee for degenerative and rheumatoid arthritis: Indications, operative technique and results. *J Bone Joint Surg* 55A:23–48, 1973.

29. Cofield RH: Total joint arthroplasty: Shoulder. *Mayo Clin Proc* 54:500–506, 1979.

30. Stauffer RN, Segal NM: Total ankle arthroplasty: Four years' experience. *Clin Orthop* 160:217–221, 1981.

31. Boobbyer GN: The long-term results of ankle arthrodesis. *Acta Orthop Scand* 52:679–682, 1981.

32. Collert S: Osteomyelitis of the spine. *Acta Orthop Scand* 48:283–290, 1977.

33. Kelly PJ, Coventry MB, Martin WJ: Bacterial arthritis. *J Bone Joint Surg* 52A:819–820, 1970.

34. Moula T, et al: Pott's paraplegia: A clinical re-

view of operative and conservative treatment in 63 adults and children. *Int Orthop* 5:23–29, 1981.

35. Hodgson AR, Yau A, Kwon JS, et al: A clinical study of 100 consecutive cases of Pott's paraplegia. *Clin Orthop* 36:128–150, 1964.

36. Mikkelsen OA: Dupuytren's disease—initial symptoms, age of onset and spontaneous course. *Hand* 9:11–15, 1977.

37. Eaton RG, Littler JW: A study of the basal joint of the thumb. Treatment of its disabilities by fusion. *J Bone Joint Surg* 51A:661–668, 1969.

38. Swanson AB: Disabling arthritis at the base of the thumb. Treatment by resection of the trapezium and flexible (silicone) implant arthroplasty. *J Bone Joint Surg* 54A:456–471, 1972.

39. Pick RY: DeQuervain's disease. A clinical triad. *Clin Orthop* 143:165–166, 1979.

40. Graham WP: Non-specific inflammatory and constrictive conditions. in the hand, in Kilgore ES, Graham WP (eds): *Surgical and Non-Surgical Management*. Philadelphia, Lea & Febriger, 1977, p 101.

41. Phalen GS: The carpal tunnel syndrome. Seventeen years' experience in diagnosis and treatment of 654 hands. *J Bone Joint Surg* 48A:211–228, 1966.

42. Gelberman RH, Hergenroeder PT, Hargens AR, et al: The carpal tunnel syndrome. A study of carpal canal pressures. *J Bone Joint Surg* 63A:380–383, 1981.

43. Bosworth DM: Supraspinatus syndrome: Symptomatology, pathology and repair. *JAMA* 117:422–428, 1941.

44. Macnab I: Degenerative changes in the rotator cuff of the shoulder: A pathological and clinical study. *Jefferson Orthop J* 4:7, 1974.

45. Wolfgang GL: Surgical repair of tears of the rotator cuff of the shoulder: Factors influencing the result. *J Bone Joint Surg* 56A:14–26, 1974.

46. Weiner DS, Macnab I: Superior migration of the humeral head: A radiological aid in the diagnosis of tears of the rotator cuff. *J Bone Joint Surg* 52B:524–527, 1970.

47. Neviaser TJ: Arthrography of the shoulder joint. *Orthop Clin North Am* 11:205–217, 1980.

48. DePalma AF, Kruper JS: Longterm study of shoulder joints afflicted with and treated for calcific tendinitis. *Clin Orthop* 20:61, 1961.

49. McLaughlin HL: On the "frozen" shoulder. *Bull Hosp Joint Dis* 12:383, 1951.

50. Neviaser RJ: Lesions of the biceps and tendinitis of the shoulder. *Orthop Clin North Am* 11:343–348, 1980.

51. Scranton PE Jr: Metatarsalgia: Diagnosis and treatment. *J Bone Joint Surg* 62:723–732, 1980.

52. Mann RA, et al: Hallux valgus-etiology, anatomy, treatment and surgical considerations. *Clin Orthop* 157:31–41, 1981.

53. McMaster MJ: The pathogenesis of hallux rigidus. *J Bone Joint Surg* 60:82–87, 1978.

54. Mann RA, et al: Hallux rigidus: A review of the literature and a method of treatment. *Clin Orthop* 142:57–63, 1979.

55. Scheck M: Etiology of acquired hammertoe deformity. *Clin Orthop* 123:63–69, 1977.

56. Newman RJ, et al: An evaluation of operative procedures in the treatment of hammertoe. *Acta Orthop Scand* 50:709–712, 1979.

57. Mann RA, DuVries HL: Acquired nontraumatic deformities of the foot, in Mann RA (ed): *DuVries' Surgery of the Foot*, ed 4. C. V. Mosby Co., St. Louis, 1978, pp 273–277.

58. Mann RA (ed): Diseases of the nerves of the foot, in *DuVries' Surgery of the Foot*, ed 4. C. V. Mosby Co., St. Louis, 1978, pp 463–468.

59. Mann RA (ed): Acquired non-traumatic deformities of the foot, in *DuVries' Surgery of the Foot*, ed 4. C. V. Mosby Co., St. Louis, 1978, pp 287–290.

60. Mann RA: The tarsal tunnel syndrome. *Orthop Clin North Am* 5:109–115, 1974.

CHAPTER 34

Oral Diseases

JAMES S. BENNETT, D.M.D., M.S.

HOWARD R. CREAMER, Ph.D.

This chapter will focus on perspectives and problems of oral health maintenance, disease prevention, and disease management, with which providers of health services should be familiar. For elderly persons, the major diseases of the teeth and gums are addressed similarly to other chronic diseases (i.e., they usually are managed, controlled, and/or contained rather than totally prevented).

A physician and nurse should be aware that: 1) The etiologic basis and methods of control of the major oral disease—dental caries and periodontitis—have been established; and 2) Significant advances in preventive dentistry enable more people to maintain more of their natural teeth in a reasonably functional state.[1] The care of elderly persons needs to be customized for an individual patient, and should not necessarily be oriented toward technical ideals. Dental care modalities that are ideal for younger adults may represent overtreatment for elderly people.

The health professions are now faced with approximately 23 million persons over 65 years of age who have various combinations of full dentures, partial dentures, crowns/bridges, silver fillings, plastic fillings, implants, and so on. The issues of dental management primarily concern: 1) Ill-fitting dentures—60% or more of all elderly people have full or partial dentures, which probably will require relining or remaking; 2) Periodontitis (pyorrhea) of moderate-to-severe proportions will afflict about 80% of all elderly people who have their remaining natural teeth[1]; 3) Dental caries will afflict the roots or recur around restorations in most elderly peo-ple who have their remaining teeth; and 4) Oral cancers will occur in about 4% of the elderly population, particularly in males and in persons who smoke heavily and/or use alcohol.

Etiologies

Dental plaque probably causes up to 95% of the oral problems found in elderly persons, including the necessity for prostheses. The chief problems are dental caries (decay) and periodontitis (pyorrhea) and their multiple sequelae. Systemic problems attributable to dental plaque arise from bacteremias resulting from infections of the periodontium, dental pulp and/or alveolar bone (see the section on *Plaque-Related Infectious Diseases* and *The Progressive Oral Dysfunction Syndrome*). The rapid progression of the plaque-caused diseases can be clinically silent, even to the point where decay cleaves off the entire tooth crown and the patient has been unaware of the preceding events. The cascade of plaque-related processes may finally result in masticatory dysfunction through the loss of adequate numbers of tooth units and chewing surfaces (see the section on *Masticatory Dysfunction*).

Pathophysiologic dynamics of oral aging represent interactions of genetics, metabolism, nutritional status, effects of medications, and specific disease entities.[2-5] There is little valid information regarding oral aging and a tendency to stereotype as age-caused the common oral changes and problems found in older persons.[6] Vigorous elderly people may show little clinical evidence of a significant physiologic change. Atrophic and degenerative changes of mucosa, alveolar bone, teeth, and muscles often are found in a very old person. Clinical observations may reveal:

1. Atrophy of epithelium with a decreased tolerance for dentures or local trauma;
2. Loss of tooth support (alveolar bone) that is related to periodontitis and/or, possibly, to osteoporosis;
3. Alteration of chewing function and efficiency (*see* the section on "Masticatory Dysfunction"), particularly from a loss of coronal enamel;
4. Functional changes in the temporomandibular joint that are related to bone changes of the condyle and articular fossae, changes in the ligaments and discs that influence masticatory function, and changes in the muscles of mastication or the nerves that control them; and
5. The teeth may be more deeply stained, the enamel crazed (or cracked), and the dental pulp regressed (or absent) because of a laying down of secondary dentin.

There often is decline in oral sensory motor functions, particularly in people who have suffered a stroke or dementia that leads to:

1. A general decline in taste that may discriminate more toward sweet and sour stimuli[6];
2. Odor perception that declines in discrimination; and
3. An apparent loss of neuromuscular discrimination and control in chewing, especially in denture wearers.

Adequate maintenance of the oral environment in an elderly population includes preventive and restorative care. Dentists must plan to provide dental care to persons of retirement age who will need to maintain a reasonable dental function for another 10–25 years. Primary care professionals should be able to assess and monitor the mouth for:

1. Significant variations from normal structure and functioning such as swellings, caries, periodontitis, fistulae, loose or broken teeth, and so on;

2. The presence or absence of adequate oral hygiene;
3. Possible oral cancer and/or premalignant situations; and
4. Significant oral dysfunction (e.g., a patient's inability to chew, talk, or maintain his or her mouth).

Nursing staffs should be able to provide instruction and supervision in the maintenance of oral health.[7] Acute and chronic health care systems should insure that the principles of oral health maintenance become a recognized and accepted standard of a health care facility, group, or practice. Significant oral problems too often are without symptoms and are ignored by both a patient and health care providers until they reach an advanced stage. A progressive oral dysfunction syndrome may develop insidiously in some elderly people when they are beset by multiple medical and social problems.

Historical Perspective

Although few individuals expect to lose a hand or foot due to aging, past generations have expected to lose their teeth and to be fitted with full dentures. George Washington and his dentures may have helped to popularize (and equate) the concept of successful aging with full denture replacement. Today, many elderly people have lived their earlier years in a cultural environment where the edentulous state was accepted. During the early 1900s, wholesale extractions of teeth often were recommended to combat focal infections, arthritis, and other medical disorders. It was expected that many adults would obtain full dentures as they grew older. Such expectations for a "normal" aging process still are ingrained in some professionals and families.

By the 1950s and 1960s, antibiotics and fluorides, among other advances, offered new possibilities for the maintenance of natural teeth. Dental research made significant progress in understanding caries through the use of germ-free animals,[8] while the caries-preventing effect of fluorides that occur naturally in water supplies had been described earlier.[9] The use of fluorides in mouth washes, toothpastes, and topical applications is a part of our current culture, although documented benefits apply primarily to younger persons. For certain older persons with specific oral conditions, the use of fluorides on a daily basis becomes a virtual necessity.[10,11]

During the 1960's and 1970's various preventive and clinical approaches to improve dental disease control began to appear. Educational programs in dental hygiene expanded when the need for individuals trained in applied preventive dentistry became apparent. The behavioral sciences have been recognized more recently as being relevant to further improvement in the preventive dental management of elderly people;[12] new terminologies deal with techniques of behavior modification, patient compliance, cognition and stress management.

Dentures

Although the ultimate goal of dentistry is to conserve natural dentition for the entire life span,[13] dentures are a part of our current culture and, to some extent, will remain so. The major dilemma regarding dentures is deciding which teeth or tooth roots are salvageable; these decisions are based on such factors as existing disease conditions, the natural teeth involved, the biomechanical conditions for denture retention, and a patient's desire to cope with various forms of prosthetic replacement. The asthetic requirements of many people have resulted in the development of immediate dentures; when the natural teeth are removed, false teeth are inserted during the same procedure. The maintenance of dignity for many elderly people is achieved by having at least a maxillary denture with which to smile and talk, even if it is non-functional. Currently, many modes of both fixed and removable prostheses are being employed; the degree of sophistication is limited mainly by finances. Implants of various kinds are being tried. There is a current treatment mode that favors maintaining key natural teeth to use as abutments for fixed bridges and partial dentures whenever possible.

An important dilemma in prosthetic dentistry has been the question of whether exodontia followed by full dentures should be recommended early for an individual (while there is still signifi-

cant alveolar bone available to function as denture base), rather than later in life after further loss of teeth and alveolar bone has occurred due to periodontitis. Preventive dentistry fosters attempts to motivate a patient toward the maintenance of natural teeth and supporting structures as long as possible. Studies indicate that cultural trends and attitudes towards oral health and dental care probably will modulate with each generation; however, there remains the potential for most persons to choose the level of health maintenance desired.[14]

Assessment

Important issues to be considered and managed by a dentist are: 1) Physical/medical status; 2) Attitudinal and emotional factors; 3) Social issues; and 4) Financial perspectives.

Staging and planning dental care for elderly people is influenced by the medical status of a patient, particularly when precautions are to be taken or medications are to be prescribed. A dental staff becomes anxious when an elderly patient is taking several different drugs, has several significant chronic diseases, and is not particularly compliant in health maintenance. Although dental offices are expected to be prepared for the emergency and high-risk patient situations, such events are uncommon; also, many dentists feel uncomfortable with even a moderately risky elderly patient. Many dental offices are geared for a well-placed active flow of patients. Elderly patients using walkers, wheelchairs, crutches, or canes, require extra time and help. Unfortunately, for home-bound or institutionalized elderly patients, many dentists do not feel they can provide quality care outside of a private office.

Given all the attributes of emotional and attitudinal expression, the face and mouth are a major basis of personality and communication. Facial aging and tooth loss can significantly change a person's attitude and actions. Psychosomatic reactions may center in the mouth when a person is under heavy stress (e.g., acute gingivitis during bereavement and grief). Similarly, emotional problems may be projected through oral disorders, such as the dentures that are "never comfortable" and the clenching and grinding of the teeth (bruxism). Although visiting a dental office may be the social event of the week for some elderly persons, others have had traumatic experiences with dentists when they were younger, which fosters continued anxiety. To cope with such attitudes and feelings (e.g., anxiety, fear), dentists often employ relaxation and suggestion techniques before turning to tranquilizers, nitrous oxide (N_2O), sedation, or general anesthesia.

Most elderly persons strive to maintain independence and personal responsibility, but relatives, trustees, ministers, and others, may become the responsible party or guiding force. The more common problems that dentists experience are: 1) Lack of clarity among the patient, relatives, and others as to who is financially and legally responsible; 2) Disagreement in the extent, mode, and goals of dental therapies; 3) Issues involving transportation, supervision, and reassurance while obtaining dental care; and 4) Difficulty in gaining support for compliance and follow-through with oral health maintenance.

Although the demographic figures on poverty seem to indicate that about 25% of all elderly people are below the poverty level, a realistic appraisal of the fixed-income status of elderly individuals and the costs of dental care probably would place 50–65% of them in the category of being dentally indigent. Even though many elderly dental patients require some complex, advanced, and costly forms of therapy, the financial and economic realities are that: 1) Few can afford private dental insurance; 2) Medicare presently does not cover the costs of general dental care; 3) Medicaid usually funds treatment of the urgent dental emergencies; and 4) Most elderly patients have to fund dental costs from out-of-pocket funds.[15]

Nutrition

Dentists are particularly interested in promoting balanced diets that are low in sugars, rich in calcium and proteins, and possess the variety of nutrients considered basic to the maintenance of oral tissues, immunocompetency, and so on.[16–18] For frail elderly people, the use of soups that contain basic nutrients have been advo-

cated. Hospitals and long-term care facilities may serve prepared foods that contain high levels of sugar. A related concern is the amount of sugars in liquid medications.[19] For a homebound and/or isolated patient, hollow calories in low-cost carbohydrates, low-protein or no-protein foods, poor variation in food selection, and poor eating habits are problems. Whereas dessert and candy may be the only sweet things in an elderly person's existence, they may be devastating to the remaining natural teeth in patients who are unable to adequately care for the mouth. Cariogenic effects of sugar are enhanced, especially in patients with a decreased salivary flow and decreased neuromuscular activity of the tongue, cheeks, and so, in cleaning the mouth of foods and fluids. Occasionally, persons will even compress a soft dessert into the palatal vault and slowly ingest it over the next several hours.

Medications

Dentists are concerned about patients who have valvular defects, implanted prostheses, and tissue grafts. Close coordination is required with the primary physician for antibiotic premedication when oral tissue manipulation occurs, and/or for the management of bleeding/clotting factors when oral bleeding results in patients taking anticoagulants. Few professionals fully appreciate the severe oral discomfort and alteration of eating habits that may result from the chronic long-term use of medications that cause stomatitis and/or xerostomia. Diuretics, phenothiazines, and tricyclic antidepressants are examples of drugs that can cause these problems; their benefits must be weighted against their risks. They may be reduced in dosage or a different medication substituted. Certain drugs, held in the mouth, may produce chemical burns of the soft tissues, which can mimic oral cancers.

Dental Plaque Management

Dental plaque control consists of a daily routine of mechanical, chemical, and nutritional principles. Even though everyone cannot be induced to practice habits of self-care, significant numbers can be motivated if given the basic facts. Experience suggests that even less than the optimal oral disease-preventive habits will decrease the rate of tooth loss. Prevailing rates of decay in the dentulous population in the United States have dropped dramatically during the last decade[20] (mostly in children). It is conceivable that within a single generation enamel caries can be eliminated as a serious burden to a society.

These considerations, coupled with the increasing average life span and the demographic shifts expected in the United States during the next 50 years, lead to the conclusion that an increasing number of people will reach their later years with much of their natural dentition intact. However, these teeth and their supporting tissues will remain at risk for disease. If preventive and maintenance care is not provided, especially for those with declining potentials for self-care, a significant increase in dental diseases will occur. Such an occurrence would detract significantly from the quality of life during the final years, and would add significantly to the personal and societal costs that are associated with aging.

The Progressive Oral Dysfunction Syndrome

It is easy for health care providers, relatives, and a patient to lose track of silent, painless, and progressing oral problems when acute medical and social problems must be given high priority. The mouth may be relatively unattended for days, weeks, or even months. A predictable outcome of continued oral neglect in patients with severe medical and/or psychological problems may be termed the progressive oral dysfunction syndrome. The syndrome is related primarily to the uninterrupted presence of dental plaque over extended periods of time; in the later stages of oral neglect, severe masticatory dysfunctioning may occur. In the early stages, the teeth may be relatively intact (see Figure 34-1A). However, with the passage of time, inappropriate nutrition, and oral hygiene, the situation progresses to a loss of tooth crowns (see Figure 34-1B). Periodically, an acute episode

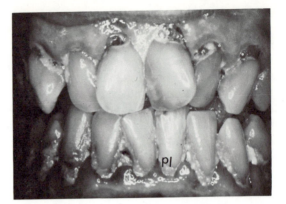

FIGURE 34-1A The progressive oral dysfunction syndrome. In the early stages, the syndrome is marked by very little or no plaque control for weeks or months. Globular formations of dental plaque (PL) in the interdental areas of the teeth may result in rampant caries and advanced periodontitis.

will occur that brings attention to the situation. Non-institutionalized elderly persons who display several of these characteristics may be heavily dependent on relatives and often are in poor compliance with diet and medication regimens. The patient may present with:

Heavy deposits of dental plaque on natural teeth, denture, and tissue surfaces, and calculus on teeth and dentures (see Figure 34-1B).

Rampant dental caries, especially on roots, interproximal spaces, and around dental restorations. These may rapidly progress to tooth crown fractures and pulp necrosis with fur-

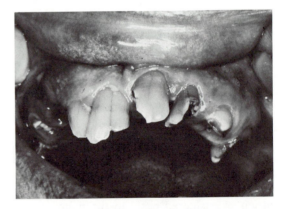

FIGURE 34-1B Later stages of the progressive oral dysfunction syndrome. A progressive loss of coronal tooth structure with possible multiple sequelae (see text). Fractures in caries-undermined enamel are evident.

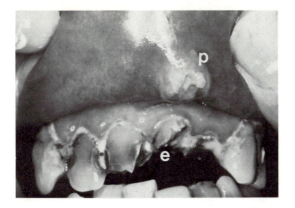

FIGURE 34-2   Fungating, ulcerated tissue (p) in the vestibule of the upper lip. A sharp fragment of tooth enamel (e) was responsible, and the lesion cleared up when the tooth was removed.

ther sequelae of acute/chronic inflammation of the periapical area of bone. Fistulae from periapical abscesses may be present in vestibular areas or even to external skin areas. Sharp enamel edges on abraded teeth may lacerate soft tissues of the tongue, cheek, or lips (Figure 34-2).

Inflammation and infection of the gingiva and periodontium with a "flooding" of blood with gentle probing or tooth brushing. Purulent exudates may be expressed from chronic periodontal pockets and fistulae that appear in the gingiva or adjacent mucosa.

Ill-fitting and/or poorly maintained dentures (when present).

Cognitive dysfunction or dementia.

Poor functioning in daily personal upkeep.

One or more sequelae of arteriosclerotic diseases (e.g., stroke, myocardial infarction).

Depression.

Muscle weakness (asthenia) with slow coordination of movement.

Embarrassment by "bad breath" and the "horrible" appearance of their mouths.

Poor chewing ability (masticatory dysfunction) because of loose teeth, missing teeth, chronic pain of the periodontium and jawbones, or loss of normal tooth anatomy due to attrition (or bruxism).

Generalized or regional stomatitis and/or glossodynia that are related to mucosal atrophy, malnutrition, medications, xerostomia, allergies, moniliasis, anemia, or combinations of such factors.

It is unclear to what degree there may be a causal relationship between such a neglected mouth and the status of the other bodily systems. It can be speculated that the extra antigenic and toxic burden to the system that is posed by the heavy dental plaque and bacterial products (supplemented by foci of chronic and granulomatous inflammation) may be partially responsible for systemic immune abnormalities.

The progressive oral dysfunction syndrome probably occurs most frequently in low-income elderly people; however, it has been seen in well-to-do elderly persons in long-term care facilities when responsible persons have refused to authorize basic oral care. The syndrome is destined to increase in incidence as the members of this fast-growing population continue to maintain increasing numbers of their natural teeth while experiencing an increasing morbidity in other systems.

Health practitioners should be especially cognizant of the potential development of this syndrome when:

1. A patient is becoming increasingly dependent, anxious, and cognitively dysfunctional;
2. There is a chronic lack of oral hygiene (heavy accumulations of dental plaque have an easily recognizable odor); and
3. There is increasing disinterest in personal oral hygiene and/or an increasing inability to perform effective oral hygiene.

Plaque-Related Infectious Diseases

The vast majority of tooth loss is caused by two categories of infectious disease processes (*see* Figure 34-3): 1) Those that attack tooth structure directly (caries); and 2) Those that slowly destroy the tooth-supporting periodontal tissues (gingiva, attachment epithelium, periodontal ligament, and alveolar process). Neither is due to a natural aging process. Dental function can be retained throughout life via extremely cost-effective preventive practices. The tremendous cost of dental disease, in terms of pain, disfigurement, and dollars, reflects the relative neglect of known effective preventive habits.

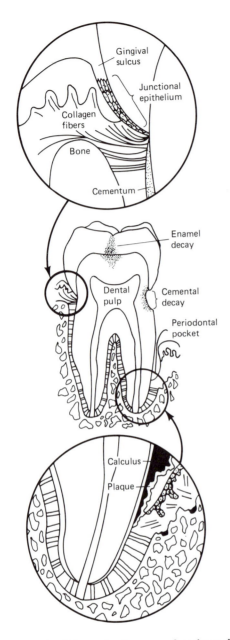

surfaces and reach densities similar to that found in feces (10^{11} organisms per gram-wet weight). Multiple kinds and high numbers of microorganisms are present that include bacteria belonging to at least 30 genera and to species and serotypes approaching 10 times that number. Socransky, et al[21] have estimated that 50–100 bacterial species make up a core group that is regularly found at different concentrations in different states of oral health and disease. Protozoa and fungi may be present in low numbers.

Dental plaques are living communities of microorganisms that affect and are affected by the nature and environment of the colonized surface. Salivary access, frictional forces, available nutrients, pH and oxidation reduction potentials vary considerably at different colonization sites (e.g., occlusal pits and fissures versus periodontal pockets). Differences among these factors determine the kinds of bacterial communities that can develop; in addition, the environment is altered continuously by the ongoing microbial metabolism. The nature of plaque varies not only from site to site within the mouth, but also in microenvironments within the same plaque.

Plaque development represents the first stages of the infectious process (i.e., colonization of the susceptible host and replication of the infectious agent). Unlike the situation in most other infectious diseases, however, the microbial invasion of host tissue is not an early required step in the infectious processes that result in caries or in inflammatory periodontal diseases. Rather, metabolic products of plaque microorganisms gain access to and affect sound, undamaged tissue at plaque-tissue interfaces. The subsequent alteration of those surfaces allows a more efficient ingress of plaque products, which (in turn) triggers the continued and advancing destruction of the tissues.

FIGURE 34-3 Schematic diagram of early and advanced plaque-caused dental disease. The junctional epithelium is the key structure in the maintenance of the integrity of the supporting apparatus (collagen fibers and alveolar bone).

Both caries and chronic inflammatory periodontal disease are infectious diseases that are caused by microorganisms parasitic to the host. The microorganisms exist in highly organized floras that develop after colonization of ecologically different sites of the oral cavity. Complex bacterial communities develop rapidly on tooth

Caries

In coronal caries, the initial lesion is the result of a demineralization of tooth structure by organic acids that are formed during the metabolism of dietary carbohydrates by acidogenic plaque bacteria. The microorganisms thought to be most directly involved in enamel caries are Streptococcus mutans and the oral lactobacilli. S. mutans depends on hard structures for oral colonization sites, is acidogenic and aciduric (resists the effects of high-acid environments), and appears to be selected by an environment resulting from the frequent consumption of readily fermented carbohydrates (glucose, fructose, sucrose, and so on), or by the retention of less readily fermentable starches.

In addition to its fermentative mode of metabolism, in which lactic acid is produced as the major waste product, S. mutans—through exoenzymes—converts a portion of dietary sucrose into at least two homopolymers of glucose (dextran and mutan) and one of fructose (levan). The relatively insoluble and stable glucose polymers form a significant part of the intermicrobial matrix of dental plaque when sucrose is in the diet. Glucose polymers render plaques less permeable to saliva, thus reducing its protective effects of dilution, buffering, and remineralization.[22] The lactobacilli are the most acidogenic and aciduric of the oral microorganisms, and they appear to preferentially colonize and replicate in sites with low pHs.

Mechanisms of damage that lead to cemental caries (root decay, senile caries) are less well understood and may involve arthrobacteria and actinomyces, as well as S. mutans and lactobacilli. A prerequisite of root surface colonization and decay is the exposure of that cemental surface to the oral environment. Since this most commonly occurs as a result of pocket formation in chronic inflammatory periodontal disease, cemental caries is age-associated. Preventive measures that consist of plaque control, fluoride applications, and reductions in the frequency of fermentable carbohydrate consumption are effective in preventing both enamel and root surface decay.

Chronic Inflammatory Periodontal Disease

More teeth are lost in our society because of chronic inflammatory periodontal disease than to any other cause. The disease is painless, insidious, chronic, and involves the destruction of the integrity of the tooth-supporting structures. Again, an invasion of gingival tissue or alveolar bone rarely is seen; when seen, it is a late phenomenon in the disease process.

A junctional epithelium at the base of a shallow gingival sulcus is tightly opposed to the surface of the tooth (see Figure 34-3). Collagen fibers within the gingival connective tissue form an interwoven matrix that maintains an attachment of the gingiva to the cementum and the alveolar crest. The epithelium of the shallow sulcus that surrounds the tooth is a few cell layers deep and, like the junctional epithelium, is non-keratinized. The supporting tissues have a rich blood supply and a well-developed lymphatic drainage. Although saliva contains secretory IgA, which bathes exposed surfaces, secretory IgA is not synthesized by gingival tissues. Sulcular fluid is most like plasma in composition, and its presence is primarily the result of inflammatory reactions in the gingival tissues.

When crevicular plaque is allowed to develop, microbial products penetrate the junctional and sulcular epithelium and engender inflammatory responses in the supporting structures. These chronically triggered responses are ineffective in removing the source of the insult, since plaque is external to the system, and chronic inflammatory damage of host tissue occurs (gingivitis). The junctional and sulcular epithelium is ulcerated and eventually destroyed, the attachment fibers are degraded, attachment is lost, the sulcus deepens, plaque extends into the pocket (see Figure 34-3). Continued inflammatory responses lead to a deepening of the pocket and to a resorption of alveolar bone in that area (periodontitis).

Periodontitis usually is a slowly progressing disease; but, rates of loss of periodontal attachment appear to vary, with alternating periods of active and quiescent disease. Longitudinal studies[23] have revealed attachment losses averaging 0.10 mm/year and 0.30 mm/year in two populations that practiced relatively good and poor oral hygiene, respectively. By 40 years of age, one third of the total periodontal support had been lost in the latter group.

Although dental plaque is the primary etiologic agent of chronic inflammatory periodontal disease, numerous factors can modulate the amount of tissue damage by affecting host responses and/or the microbial component. For example, dental fillings with poorly designed margins ("overhangs") enhance plaque formation and retention, patients with neutrophil defects experience exaggerated periodontal bone loss, and an increased incidence of gingivitis and atrophy may be seen during menopause. It is unknown whether a particular microorganism, or a unique set of organisms, is required for the generation or maintenance of gingivitis or periodontitis. Chronic inflammatory periodontal diseases may be diseases that are initiated by a variety of plaque products (endotoxins, leukotoxins, exoenzymes, chemotactic materials, antigens, polyclonal activators of B cells and possibly T cells, and so on) that trigger a variety of host inflammatory responses.

Invasive Oral Infections

Few invasive infectious diseases of oral tissues are caused by a single pathogenic agent. Examples of these infections, which also have a relatively low incidence rate, include herpes stomatitis, candidiasis and syphilitic chancres. In cervicofacial actinomycosis, *Actinomyces israelii* may be the sole opportunistic invader of devitalized tissue, or it may be accompanied by other anaerobic and facultative organisms. Mixed opportunistic infections[24] that develop subsequent to caries, periodontitis, trauma, stress (acute necrotizing ulcerative gingivitis), or severe protein malnutrition, are more frequent. Periapical abscesses and other invasive lesions of the gingiva, cheeks, palate, and bone most often are mixed infections that consist of gram-negative anaerobic rods in association with other anaerobic and facultative organisms.

Laboratory reporting of "mixed flora" may confuse a diagnosis and delay treatment. Reports, at least, should list isolates to the genus level and give an estimate of the relative numbers of each. Oral strains of neisseria rarely are involved in invasive infections, but they are routinely found when salivary contamination of a sample has occurred.

Systemic Aspects of Caries and Inflammatory Periodontal Disease

Accessible tooth surfaces are bathed in saliva that: 1) Removes loosely adhering microorganisms and, therefore, inhibits colonization efforts; 2) Penetrates plaque, thereby diluting and buffering organic acids formed by fermentation; 3) Provides a source of ions for remineralization of damaged surfaces; and 4) Contains a variety of potential inhibitors of microbial function that include lysozyme, the lactoperoxidase system, and secretory IgA antibodies.

Rampant dental caries progressing to pulpal abscesses are expected if salivary flow is markedly reduced. Less dramatic reductions in salivary flow, or the loss of a salivary gland or its function in one area, results in modest increases in overall or local susceptibility. Evidence is accumulating that a secretory antibody protects against caries. Persons with a secretory IgA deficiency, in whom IgM compensation had not occurred, revealed higher caries rates than normal controls or IgM-compensated patients.[25]

The inflammatory response, which is a major non-specific mechanism of resistance, also is elicited by antibody and cell-mediated immunologic signals. Inflammatory responses to plaque products are thought to be the fundamental cause of chronic inflammatory periodontal disease. In this context, then, the resistance mechanisms become the mechanisms of pathogenesis. Since the source of phlogistic products is external, and since the microorganisms replicate, the insult cannot be effectively cleared by the inflammatory and phagocytic defenses. Tissue damage results, and cumulative effects over long periods of time can be large. That inflammatory responses, which cause the local tissue damage, are at the same time protective is indicated by the rarity of a significant invasive oral disease, even though a non-oral invasive disease in damaged tissues following bite wounds is common.

The potential systemic effects of caries and inflammatory periodontal disease are well recognized. Caries may progress to pulpal abscesses, cellulitis, and osteomyelitis. The ubiquitous showering of the blood stream by oral bacteria in individuals with gingivitis and periodontitis is a recognized risk to systemic health in those compromised patients who are subject to the colonization of damaged heart valves or implanted prostheses. Less well documented are other potential risks related to the systemic burden that pocket plaque might represent in an individual. It generally is not appreciated that such a tremendous area of connective tissue is exposed to pocket plaque. Pockets of 7–10 mm in depth are not uncommon (*see* Figure 34-2), and the exposed connective tissue has either an ulcerated epithelium or none at all. To visualize the antigenic and toxic burden that periodontitis might represent, it should be appreciated that approximately 20 cm^2 of connective tissue is exposed to plaque products if two thirds of the teeth are present, if an average pocket depth of only 4 mm surrounds each tooth, and if plaque is not controlled.

It is evident that individuals become routinely immunized to a variety of plaque antigens.[26] In addition, levels of serum IgA have been reported to be positively correlated with the severity of periodontal disease in adult patients.[27] It has been reported that not only the percentage of IgD-bearing peripheral blood lymphocytes is increased in patients with periodontal disease, but also that the percentage drops after treatment of the condition.[28] Other potentially important effects are conceivable, which include the generation of circulating soluble immune complexes or the production of immunosuppressive effects as a result of the antigenic burden.

Great numbers of inflammatory cells migrate into the oral cavity via gingival sulci and pockets. The traffic of neutrophils out of the blood vessels, through the connective tissues, and into the gingival sulcus or periodontal pocket, has been estimated in subjects with different levels of periodontal disease.[29] Neutrophils were collected from washings of the oral cavity every 30 seconds for a period of 25 minutes from a patient with mild, chronic gingivitis. The rate of appearance of cells in the oral cavity stabilized after the first six collections and then averaged 4.95×10^6/30 seconds for the next 22 minutes. Over a 24-hour period, this would yield 1.43×10^9 neutrophils that—given a blood count of 7,000 white blood cells/mm^3 and a differential of 55%—would equate to the number of polymorphonuclear neutrophils in 370 ml of blood. Similar calculations for a patient with severe periodontitis indicate that 1.4×10^{10} neutrophils emigrated into the oral cavity in 24 hours (equivalent to the number in over 3,600 ml of blood), while in a patient with excellent oral health, only 4×10^8 neutrophils per day emigrated into the oral cavity (equivalent to 105 ml of blood). These findings imply that the antigenic and toxic burden that is associated with inflammatory periodontal disease may be a systemically significant one.

Age-Correlated Versus Age-Induced Changes

A major distinction must be made between age-correlated and age-induced changes in the prevalence, incidence, or severity of caries and inflammatory periodontal diseases. Enamel caries has been a disease of young persons and cemental caries and periodontitis are diseases of adulthood. Are these associations age-induced? Are the periodontal structures more susceptible to, or less able to repair the damage caused by, a standard increment of insult in elderly persons? Are enamel surfaces more resistant to acid attack in elderly persons while cemental surfaces are more susceptible to attack?

Cemental caries cannot occur until cementum is exposed. Although some physiologic and traumatic gingival recession may come about with age, it appears that recession is primarily due to the apical migration of the attachment apparatus that is due to periodontitis. Enamel caries decrease with age in the average population, because those surfaces that are most susceptible to attack have been destroyed by caries at an early age. The decline in enamel caries in adulthood that has been seen classically is dependent on the earlier removal of the most susceptible surfaces; not on the increased resistance in older persons. As more tooth surfaces are retained, a greater number will be at risk and susceptible to attack in older adults if preventive practices cannot be maintained.

The correlation between inflammatory periodontal disease and age is so strong[30] and so obvious that many patients believe that tooth loss is a natural consequence of aging. The lack of knowledge of the specific mechanism(s) that cause periodontitis makes it difficult to evaluate the physiologic effect of aging on the generation of the disease. It does appear that gingival tissue may under-respond to 3 weeks of plaque accumulation[31] in prepubertal children and over-respond in elderly persons as compared with young adults.[32] However, it cannot be concluded that age-related physiologic effects accounted for the differences in gingivitis that were seen, since the amount and nature of the insult delivered to the tissues cannot be accurately quantified. In the latter study, plaque did (in fact) accumulate at a more rapid rate and to a higher level in the elderly population than in the young adult population.

The implications from cross-sectional and prospective studies are that: 1) Periodontal damage is cumulative; 2) There is a fairly constant long-term rate of destruction after puberty for a particular level of oral hygiene; and 3) The destruction continues and progresses with time only if plaque is allowed to remain in association with the periodontal structures.[33]

Soft-Tissue Problems

The oral soft tissues of elderly persons may be relatively atrophic and prone to damage from ill-fitting prostheses, sharp teeth/fillings, harsh foods, and so on. Chronic irritation commonly leads to erosions, abrasion, and/or the development of redundant granulomatous formations (see Figure 34-2). Benign inflammatory lesions cannot be clinically differentiated from premalignant or malignant entities. Therefore, it is wise to periodically monitor and obtain a biopsy specimen of any lesion exhibiting changes that could be cancer: pemphigus, lichen planus, leukemic infiltrates of gingiva, moniliasis, focal keratoses, and so on.

The most important oral soft-tissue problem of elderly persons is a squamous cell carcinoma. This affects about 4% of all adults. The median age of occurrence is 60 years, and it occurs more frequently in males who report a long history of smoking and alcohol intake.[34] The most common sites are the lower lip, floor of the mouth, and the lateral border of the tongue. Premalignant formations, carcinoma-in-situ, and early invasive malignant lesions, cannot be clinically differentiated from reactive lesions. A biopsy procedure is recommended for lesions that fail to respond to the removal of oral irritants within about 2 weeks.

Xerostomia

Xerostomia or dry mouth is caused by a reduction or cessation in salivary flow and may be reversible or irreversible. Severe xerostomia usually is extremely uncomfortable, is conducive to rampant tooth decay, and can create problems with denture retention. Artificial saliva is now available, although some patients accept it poorly. Other remedies are cold water or ice water, glycerin (with lemon), sugar-free carbonated beverages, papase (papain), and Vitamin E (oil form).

The loss of salivary glandular units and their replacement by fat cells is said to cause age-associated xerostomia. Following head and neck radiation, the function of damaged glands may or may not return, which depends on radiation dosage. Medications (especially anticholinergic-type drugs or diuretics) are common causes of xerostomia. When possible, medication levels should be reduced and/or changed to test whether or not salivation can be increased.

Sjogren's Syndrome is an age-associated entity that is related to the autoimmune diseases. Antibodies develop against salivary gland tissues, thus leading to glandular tissue loss and subsequent xerostomia. A biopsy specimen of a lip gland may be diagnostic.

Bruxism

This condition is an unconscious, usually nocturnal, grinding of teeth. It is proposed that bruxism is most likely related to psychophysiologic processes that are influenced by stress.[35] Bruxing may lead to a moderate-to-severe loss of coronal tooth enamel and dentin, a loss of vertical dimension, and a loss of normal anatomic features, which in turn are related to decreased chewing efficiency and increased stress to the periodontium. Plastic splints (night guards) may be required to keep the teeth separated during sleep or even during waking hours.

Masticatory Dysfunction

The inability to chew food effectively or efficiently can be related to causes such as broken or missing teeth, smooth chewing surfaces, ill-fitting dentures, or neuromuscular chewing deficits. Dysfunctions that are related to missing teeth usually involve those used for chewing, (e.g., molars and bicuspids). The molars often are at higher risk of being lost because they have multiple roots (periodontal disease and caries) and are difficult to keep clean. Many elderly people can chew adequately with just the bicuspids, if they take small bites, chew slowly, and prepare foods that are easiest to masticate. Smooth, faceted teeth provide very little trituration of the food. The usual patient complaint is that they cannot chew such foods such as lettuce or meats. A patient who has dentures with smooth anatomically flattened molars is particularly prone to masticatory problems.

Ill-fitting dentures often become a major factor in masticatory dysfunctioning. The denture problem usually is part of a multifactorial complex that may include nutritional imbalance, low-fluid intake, xerostomia, medications that create stomatitis and/or decreased salivation, atrophy of denture-bearing mucosa and bone, and/or systemic diseases that influence tissue hydration (such as diabetes, renal disease, chronic heart failure, and so on). There also is a behavioral component to ill-fitting dentures, because such patients often will avoid talking and socializing.

Neuromuscular chewing deficits that result from strokes, medications, and so on, lead to problems in mastication and swallowing. Some elderly people function best in a totally edentulous state. If the dysfunction is related to a marked tooth crown loss, it often is best either to smooth down the crown towards the gingiva or to remove the remaining crown and root if there is a progressive disease.

Iatrogenic Problems

Because dental care is so often an intense restorative and prosthetic undertaking, iatrogenic problems are prone to occur; fortunately, such problems may be resolvable and adequately managed. Common examples are defective tooth fillings that lead to an entrapment of food and debris, or rough and/or slightly distorted dentures that lead to sores and ulcerated oral mucosa. Many simple restorative/prosthetic defects may lead to larger problems over long periods of time if not corrected. The natural teeth used to support fixed bridges and partial dentures require special monitoring and management.

Oral Health Maintenance

Debridement of the Mouth and Dentures

In many older individuals, oral hygiene has been ignored. The teeth and dentures may be difficult to inspect because of heavy accumulations of plaque, calculus, and debris. An initial removal of debris/plaque is required for a preliminary examination or assessment. Oral debridement is accomplished by moistening a 4 × 4-inch gauze sponge (or washcloth) and by scrubbing all oral tissues, teeth, and denture surfaces with mild toothpaste. This should be continued until full and partial dentures can be removed, then shifting to a soft toothbrush to clean all tooth and tissue surfaces. Calculus formations, which sometimes hold teeth in place, should be left for a hygienist and dentist to manage. Dentures can be cleaned with a denture brush in warm soapy water. A washcloth should be placed in the bottom of the wash basin, so that the denture is protected if dropped. For a comatose or very debilitated patient, oral debridement should be carried out as needed (but at least once a day) by the nursing staff.

Assessing the Mouth

Oral assessment should be practiced by all health care professionals.[36] Oral assessment is appropriate during physical examinations and during initial and recall dental appointments. For an institutionalized elderly person, daily or weekly assessment should be based on a patient's ability to perform personal hygiene. Therefore, three general types of assessments should be within the scope of competency of physicians, nurses, and certain allied health professionals. These are: 1) The initial oral assessment, which should be a thorough visual and mechanical examination using a tongue blade and light; mouth mirrors are preferable if available. The tongue blade can be used to check both tooth mobility and the fit of partial denture clasps. Bimanual palpation of the salivary glands and lymph nodes in the submandibular and submental areas is recommended. Using a finger cot, palpate the soft tissues of the mouth, including the tongue. A gauze sponge can be used to grasp the extruded tongue, so that the lateral borders and dorsum can be visualized and palpated; 2) Periodic assessment, which should take place when there are oral problems that need to be monitored; and 3) Daily assessment, if a patient has difficulty with dentures, oral hygiene, or has an acute oral condition.

Routine Oral Hygiene

The routine assessment of a patient's compliance and ability to follow oral hygiene procedures is basic to oral health maintenance. Poor compliance will require dental visits every 2–3 months. Patients who are unable to perform hygiene protocols should have assistance from relatives, nursing staff, occupational therapists, physical therapists, or aides. Instructions should be clear with regard to the intake of sugars in the regular diet, desserts, candies, medication, supplements, and so on. The use of sugar candies to make the breath smell better should be avoided.

Mechanical devices, such as toothbrushes and toothpicks, must be used judiciously. There should be a physical removal of plaque and debris without damage to the teeth, gingiva, or mucosa. Toothbrushes should meet such physical standards as having soft polished bristles; the handle can be modified to better fit a patient's hands. Cheap stiff brushes can damage the gingiva and decrease a patient's compliance with appropriate oral hygiene. Interproximal cleaning devices, such as floss, toothpicks, and small brushes, may help considerably when the interdental space is open and prone to the trapping of food. A patient usually requires training and assistance to insure the proper use of such devices. Fluoridated toothpastes and/or topical fluorides are recommended, especially in patients who have received radiation to head and neck regions.[10,11] However, once periodontal pockets have become greater than 4–5 mm in depth, these measures are usually no longer adequate.

Denture Maintenance

Dentures require routine care and assessment; a timely relining or remaking of dentures is important to patient comfort and oral function. Denture adhesives may be helpful for loose dentures until dental care can be obtained. Soft-lining plastics can be used to adjust dentures and to condition the soft tissues for patients whose mouths are in a constant state of change because of medications (e.g., diuretics), metabolic diseases (e.g., diabetes), or generalized stomatitis.

Dentures should be cleaned daily or rinsed after eating. When not in the mouth, they should be kept in clean water. Identification marks can be made on any oral prosthesis, especially those that contain plastics. Short-term identification can be made with a laundry pen and clear plastic (nail polish), while long-term identification is done by embedding an I.D. tag of paper under clear acrylic in the denture flange.

Medical Management of Oral Problems

Medical personnel often provide preliminary oral care or participate in the assessment and care of emergency or urgent oral/dental problems. It is recommended that the majority of urgent oral problems ultimately be managed by a general dentist (with oral surgery when acute). Some of the more common events that are likely to involve medical personnel are:

1. Acute infections of the dental apparatus that result in abscesses, fistulae, cellulitis, and so on. Pain, fever, and malaise that is associated with the problem may require appropriate medications (e.g., analgesics and antibacterial therapies). Penicillin and related antibiotics remain the agents of choice for the more common mixed dental infections; antibiotic sensitivity cultures are recommended when deep abscesses or cellulitis is present. An incision and drainage can be initiated if the process has localized sufficiently.

2. Generalized stomatitis that is associated with allergies, moniliasis, or heavy medications (e.g., phenothiazines). Combination mouth rinses that contain nystatin, hydrocortisone, tetracycline, and benadryl may be helpful in some situations; close patient monitoring is required.

3. Excessively loose teeth, crowns, bridges, and dentures that may enter the oropharynx

or be swallowed or aspirated. Excessively loose teeth often can be removed with a gauze sponge if there is no dental care immediately available.

4. Chronic irritation and/or laceration of tissues by sharp teeth or appliances, which are common problems in elderly persons that occasionally cause a perforation of the lip or tongue mucosa (*see* Figure 34-3). Protection of the area with sponges should be provided until dental care is obtained.

5. Systemic diseases, nutritional problems, and/or effects of medications that may be first noted in the mouth. Diuretics can be associated with dry mouths, thus resulting in a discomfort in chewing, talking, and swallowing. The tissues may have the appearance and texture of dry leather and a parotitis may result from a retrograde infection of the salivary ducts. A physician must seriously consider the dilemma of balancing medications with a patient's oral discomfort, because severe xerostomia may affect a patient's ability and willingness to take fluids, chew food, or use dentures.

6. Infective endocarditis, infection of prosthetic cardiac valves, or infections of vascular grafts that are not uncommon in older patients.[37,38] The mouth always should be considered as a potential source of blood-borne organisms, especially if natural teeth are present and if oral hygiene is poor. A patient's mouth should be rendered free of caries and significant periodontitis before prosthetic devices or grafts that are subject to infection are implanted. Furthermore, a physician should educate high-risk patients about good oral hygiene under dental direction, and about when prophylactic antibiotics should be used for dental or other procedures that are likely to induce bacteremias.

Elderly people will be best served when a genuine, cost-effective, and multidisciplinary delivery system has become a common mode of health care. The development of such a system will bring with it many benefits, not the least of which will be the prevention of an otherwise certain epidemic of oral disease in compromised elderly individuals.

References

1. Bureau of Economic Research and Statistics, American Dental Association: *Utilization of Dental Service by the Elderly Population.* Chicago, 1979.
2. Franks AST, Hedegard B: *Geriatric Dentistry.* Oxford, England, Blackwell Scientific Publications, 1973.
3. Davidoff A, Winkler S, Lee MHM: *Dentistry for the Special Patient: The Aged, Chronically Ill and Handicapped.* Philadelphia, WB Saunders & Co, 1972.
4. Freedman KA: *Management of the Geriatric Dental Patient.* Chicago, Quintessence Publishing Co, 1979.
5. Swoope CC, Smith HE, Lukers EM: Geriatric dentistry, in Clark JW (ed): *Clinical Dentistry.* Hagerstown, MD, Harper & Row, 1:34, 1–14, 1979.
6. Baum B: Research on aging and oral health: An assessment of current status and future needs. *Spec Care Dent* 1:156–165, 1981.
7. Bennett J: in Carnevelli D, Patrick M (eds): Oral health maintenance in nursing management for the elderly, in *Nursing Management for the Elderly.* Philadelphia, JB Lippincott, 1979, pp 111–136.
8. Orland FJ, et al: Use of germ-free animal technic in the study of experimental dental caries. I. Basic observations on rats reared free of all microorganisms. *J Dent Res* 33:147–174, 1954.
9. McKay FS: The establishment of a definite relation between enamel that is defective in its structure, as mottled enamel, and liability to decay. *Pac Dent Gaz* 37:599–610, 1929.
10. Wescott WB, et al: Chemical protection against post irradiation caries. *Oral Surg* 40:709–719, 1975.
11. Shannon IL, Edwards EJ: Reaction of tooth surface to three fluoride gels. *N Y S Dent J* 1980, pp 426–429.
12. Barkley RF: A preventive philosophy of restorative dentistry. *Dent Clin North Am* 15:569–575, 1971.
13. Kiyak HA, Bennett J: Special problems of the geriatric patient, in Ingersoll B (ed): *Behavioral Aspects in Dentistry.* New York, Appleton-Century-Crofts, 1982, pp 135–150.
14. Ettinger RL, Beck JD: The new elderly: What can the dental profession expect? *Spec Care Dent* 2(suppl 2):62–69, 1982.
15. Gift HO: The seventh age of man: Oral health and the elderly. *Am Coll Dent J* 46:204–207, 1979.
16. Slavkin HC: The aging process and nutrition:

Conception to senescence. *J Spec Care Dent* 1:31–36, 1981.

17. Nizel HE: Role of nutrition in the oral health of the aging patient. *Dent Clin North Am* 20:569–584, 1976.

18. Massler M: Geriatric nutrition. I: Osteoporosis. *J Prosthet Dent* 42:252–254, 1979.

19. Feigal RJ, Jensen ME: The cariogenic potential of liquid medications: A concern for the handicapped patient. *Spec Care Dent* 2:20–24, 1982.

20. National Caries Program, National Institute of Dental Research: *The Prevalence of Dental Caries in United States Children 1979–1980. The National Dental Caries Prevalence Survey.* Bethesda, Md, National Institutes of Health, 1981. (NIH Publication No. 82–2245).

21. Socransky SS, Tanner ACR, Haffajee AD, et al: Present status of studies on the microbial etiology of periodontal disease, in Genco RJ, Mergenhagen SE (eds): *Host-Parasite Interactions in Periodontal Disease.* Washington, DC, American Society for Microbiology, 1982, pp 1–12.

22. Gugenheim B, Regolat B, Schmid R, et al: Effects of topical application of mutanase on rat caries. *Caries Res* 14:128–135, 1980.

23. Loe H, Anerud A, Boysen H, et al: The natural history of periodontal disease in man. The rate of periodontal destruction before 40 years of age. *J Periodontol* 49:607–620, 1978.

24. Finegold SM: *Anaerobic Bacteria in Human Disease.* New York, Academic Press, 1977, chap 4, pp 78–104.

25. McGhee JR, Michalek SM: Immunobiology of dental caries: microbial aspects and local immunity. *Ann Rev Microbiol* 35:595–638, 1981.

26. Tolo K, Brandtzaeg P: Relation between periodontal disease activity and serum antibody titers to oral bacteria, in Genco RJ, Mergenhagen SE (eds): *Host-Parasite Interactions in Periodontal Disease.* Washington, DC, American Society for Microbiology, 1982, pp 270–282.

27. Shillitoe EJ: Immunoglobulins and complement in crevicular fluid, in MacPhee T (ed): *Host Resistance to Commensal Bacteria.* Edinburgh and London, Churchill Livingstone, 1972, pp 110–115.

28. Pazandak DP, Rogers RS III, Reeve CM: T and B lymphocyte distribution in periodontal disease. *J Periodontal* 49:625–630, 1978.

29. Klinkhamer JM: Quantitative evaluation of gingivitis and periodontal disease. I—The orogranulocytic migratory rate. *Periodontics* 6(suppl 5):207–211, 1968.

30. Russell AL: International nutrition surveys: A summary of preliminary dental findings. *J Dent Res* 42:233–244, 1963.

31. Mackler SB, Crawford JJ: Plaque development and gingivitis in the primary dentition. *J Periodontol* 44:18–24, 1973.

32. Holm-Pedersen R, Agerbaek N, Theilade E: Experimental gingivitis in young and elderly individuals. *J Clin Periodontol* 2:14–24, 1975.

33. Axelsson P, Lindhe J: Effect of controlled oral hygiene procedures on caries and periodontal disease in adults. *J Clin Periodontol* 8:239–248, 1981.

34. *National Cancer Institute Cancer Patient Survival Report No. 5, 1976.* DHEW Publication No. 77-992. Bethesda, Md, National Institutes of Health, 1976.

35. Kreisburg MK: Alternative view of the bruxism phenomenon. *Gen Dent* 30:121–123, 1982.

36. Bennett J, Creamer H, Fontana-Smith D: Dentistry, in O'Hara-Deveraux, Andrus LH, et al (eds): *Eldercare: A Practical Guide to Clinical Geriatrics.* New York, Grune & Stratton, 1981, pp 103–114.

37. Barry J, Gump DW: Endocarditis: An overview. *Heart Lung* 11:138–143, 1982.

38. Kluge RM: Infections of prosthetic cardiac valves and arterial grafts. *Heart Lung* 11:146–151, 1982.

PART III

Psychiatric Disorders in the Geriatric Patient

CHAPTER 35

Organic Disorders
RICHARD C. U'REN, M.D.

Psychiatric Disorders in Elderly Persons

In old age the balance of forces that enable a person to live independently and enjoy a sense of well-being is more fragile than in younger persons. Physical integrity, self-esteem, satisfying personal relationships, and some measure of financial security are prerequisites for good health at all ages; but each is particularly liable to disruption in old age: physical health deteriorates, self-esteem slips, relationships are broken by death, and financial security often wanes, especially after retirement.

Personality assets and personal bonds will buffer individuals from many troubles, at least for awhile. For instance, a moderately demented male can continue to live happily in his community if he has the help of a healthy wife. However, sooner or later, a decline sets in as resources and strengths diminish. It is, in fact, unusual for most people over 85 years of age to live on their own in the community without substantial outside help. Since this decline is set in motion by many factors, and rarely by just one, physicians should never confine their attention to physical status alone when they evaluate older people. A patient's personal relationships, self-esteem, feelings, financial status, and home environment always should be assessed as well.

The diagnostic spectrum for psychiatric conditions in older people is narrower than in younger patients. Conditions such as substance abuse, alcoholism, personality disorders, acute anxiety states, and schizophrenia occur less frequently in elderly than in younger patients. Depression and dementia are the major psychiatric illnesses found in a geriatric population. The classification of psychiatric disorders in old age is shown in Table 35-1.

The majority of older people do not suffer from a psychiatric illness. Estimates of the prevalence of mental illness among elderly persons vary widely, but a reasonable judgment would put the figure between 15–25%.[1]

In one of the best-known American studies, the point prevalence (the number of people with a particular diagnosis at a specific point in time) of major depression was found to be 3.7% in a group of older patients living in the community, while the point prevalence of minor depression was found to be 4.5%—a total of 8.2%.[2] Other investigations have estimated the prevalence of depression that "warrants intervention" to be 13% and the prevalence of transient depression to be 30% or more.[1]

The prevalence of confirmed dementia in people over 65 years of age is 5%; the prevalence of mild dementia may be as much as 15%.[1] At least 20% of all people over 80 years of age suffer from moderate-to-severe dementia. About 60% of all patients in nursing homes are diagnosed as being demented, although fewer than 5% of elderly persons, mentally ill or not, live in nursing homes or other institutions.[3] The incidence rate of delirium in elderly persons is unknown.

The prevalence of minor psychiatric disorders and personality disorders is 5–10%. The prevalence of paranoid disorders is estimated to

TABLE 35-1 Classification of Psychiatric Disorders
in Elderly Persons

Organic brain syndromes
  Delirium
  Dementia
  Other organic brain syndromes
    Amnestic syndrome
    Organic hallucinosis
    Organic delusional syndrome
    Organic affective syndrome
    Organic personality syndrome
Affective disorders
  Major depressive disorder, single episode or
    recurrent bipolar affective disorder mixed,
    manic, or depressive dysthymic disorder (de-
    pressive personality or chronic depression);
    cyclothymic disorder (mood swings)
  Adjustment disorder with depressed mood (reac-
    tive depression)
Neuroses
  Anxiety
  Hypochondriasis
  Obsessive-compulsive disorder
  Hysteria
  Phobias
Paranoid disorders
Personality and behavioral disorders

---

be 1–3%, but most patients in this category are life-long schizophrenics.[1] Less than 1% of all paranoid patients develop symptoms after 65 years of age.

There are seven parts of a psychiatric evaluation that should be included in the medical work-up of every geriatric patient:

A brief survey of relevant psychiatric symptoms;

A patient's past history of psychiatric illness, diagnosis, treatment, and response to treatment;

Family history of psychiatric illness;

Description of a patient's personality before illness;

Recent personal upheavals;

Descriptions of a patient's social network and important personal relationships; and

A standard mental status examination.

Since depression and dementia are the major psychiatric problems in old age, all elderly patients should be asked about their mood, their level of interest and/or pleasure in their usual activities, their sleep patterns, their appetite, and whether they have lost or gained weight

recently. A persistently low mood and a decrease of interest in daily activities should alert a physician to the possibility of depression. A patient (or a person who knows the patient well) also should be asked about changes in memory, periods of disorientation, and alterations in behavior or personality, which are all symptoms of dementia.

Different episodes of a particular psychiatric illness tend to resemble each other over time. The signs and symptoms of one episode of depression, for example, usually will be similar to an earlier episode. A patient's past history can be a valuable clue to a diagnosis. A favorable response to a particular form of treatment in the past may be a reliable guide to the most effective treatment in the present, especially in the case of depression or a paranoid illness.

Many psychiatric illnesses show some tendency to run in families. This is true of dementia and depression. A positive family history of a particular psychiatric illness also may be an important clue to a diagnosis.

A marked change in a patient's personality should alert a clinician to the possibility of an organic illness. A patient's premorbid personality also may give a clinician some idea of the limits of treatment. A characterologically depressed female, for example, will usually not be buoyant and optimistic after treatment of a superimposed, major depressive episode; her personality will remain much as it was before treatment. In addition, clinicians who are sensitive to differences in personality will be able to manage their patients more effectively than those who ignore personality differences. Patients with dependent personalities, for example, often require nurturance and advice, while patients with paranoid personalities need more personal distance, more explanation, and more sense of control.

An inquiry into recent personal upheavals, such as retirement or the death of a spouse, and their meaning to a patient often will shed light on the precipitants of the current illness or disability. A knowledge of a patient's social and personal relationships may help a physician to appreciate both sources of stress (a bad marriage, which may have precipitated or complicated the current medical or psychiatric problem, and the sources of emotional and material support (strong family cohesiveness), which help to maintain well-being. It has been suggested that elderly people who lack a confiding relationship with another person are more vulnerable to depression than people who have at least one intimate relationship.[4]

The traditional psychiatric mental status examination is far too unwieldy for a general physician to use. Fortunately, some good short questionnaires have been validated for use in assessing an older patient's mental state.

The first is the Short Portable Mental Status Questionnaire (SPMSQ).[5] It consists of 10 questions and is scored in the following manner:

0–2 errors: normal mental functioning
3–4 errors: mild cognitive impairment
5–7 errors: moderate cognitive impairment
8 or more errors: severe cognitive impairment

In each category, one more error is allowed in the scoring if a patient has had a grade school education or less. One less error is allowed if the patient has had education beyond the high school level.

The 10 questions in the SPMSQ are:

1. What is the date, month, year?
2. What is the day of the week?
3. What is the name of this place?
4. What is your phone number? (or, What is your address?)
5. How old are you?
6. When were you born?
7. Who is the current president?
8. Who is the past president?
9. What was your mother's maiden name?
10. Can you count backwards from 20 by 3s?

The SPMSQ, which primarily assesses memory and orientation, has both good validity (i.e., it detects organic mental impairment accurately and reliably) and a high degree of inter-rater and test-retest reliability. Performance on the SPMSQ correlates highly with the degree of brain failure, regardless of the cause. It is not always sensitive to the earliest stages of memory loss in dementia, but one study showed that even one or two incorrect answers (usually considered to be normal) correlated significantly with an impaired performance on memory testing, which indicated that the SPMSQ may be more sensitive to early impairment than previously thought.[6]

The second questionnaire is the Mini Mental State Examination (MMS) (see Table 35-2).[7]

This examination, which takes slightly longer to administer than the SPMSQ and assesses a wider range of functions. It taps immediate and delayed recall as well as language and visuographic ability. The highest possible score on the MMS is 30. Scores of 24 or below are indic-

TABLE 35-2 Mini-Mental State Examination

Maximum Score	Score	
		Orientation
5	( )	What is the (year) (season) (day) (month)?
5	( )	Where are we: (state) (county) (town) (hospital) (floor)?
		Registration
3	( )	Name 3 objects: 1 second to say each. Then ask the patient all 3 after you have said them. Give 1 point for each correct answer. Then repeat them until he or she learns all 3. Count trials and record. (trials: _____)
		Attention and Calculation
5	( )	Serial 7's (begin with 100 and count backwards by 7). 1 point for each correct. Stop after 5 answers. Alternatively, spell "world" backwards.
		Recall
3	( )	Ask for the 3 objects repeated above. Give 1 point for each correct.
		Language
9	( )	Name a pencil, and watch (2 points). Repeat the following: "No ifs, ands, or buts" (1 point). Follow a 3-stage command. "Take a paper in your right hand, fold it in half, and put it on the floor." (3 points) Read and obey the following: Close your eyes (1 point). Write a sentence (1 point) Copy design (1 point)
_____	_____	Total score
		Assess level of consciousness along a continuum:

Alert Drowsy Stupor Coma

SOURCE: Folstein MF, Folstein SE, McHugh PR: "Mini-mental state: A practical method of grading the cognitive state of patients for the clinician." *J. Psychiatr Res* 12:189–198, 1975. Used with permission.

ative of cognitive impairment. The mean scores for four different groups of subjects tested in the original study were:

Normal individuals: 27.6
Depressed patients without cognitive deficits: 25.1
Depressed patients with cognitive deficits: 19.0
Demented patients: 9.6

In everyday practice, the SPMSQ should be administered to every older person and supplemented by selected items from the MMS, especially the questions that test delayed recall (the ability to recall three words after 2–5 minutes) and constructional ability (the ability to copy a design, such as a half-circle intersecting a square). The questions that pertain to language in the MMS are, of course, designed to detect dysphasia and will be useful for selected patients.

Both the SPMSQ and the MMS are designed to help a physician detect organicity. It can be hard to distinguish between organic and functional signs and symptoms. However, a history of previous neurologic events (a stroke, a subarachnoid hemorrhage, meningitis, or a head injury) should raise one's index of suspicion of an organicity; so should neurologic symptoms such as headaches, seizures, or incontinence. A possible organic basis of symptoms also should be suggested by a history of: 1) A medical illness (emphysema, kidney problems, thyroid abnormalities, diabetes, alcoholism, myocardial infarction, and cancer); 2) Almost any kind of medication or drug use; and 3) Surgery with postanesthetic complications.

The major psychiatric symptoms that point to organicity are the individual signs and symptoms of delirium and dementia: clouding of consciousness, impaired concentration and attention, poor memory, disorientation, and deterioration of intellect and personality.

Localizing signs and symptoms also point to organicity. Dysphasia and hemiparesis are obvious examples, but more subtle lesions in major areas of the brain each give rise to characteristic clinical pictures. Frontal lobe lesions often lead to personality changes. Lesions in the parietal lobe cause visuo-spatial difficulties, topographic disorientation, dysphasia, apraxia, and agnosias. Temporal lobe pathology produces disturbance of intellectual functioning, as well as dysphasia, amnestic syndromes, and personality disturbances—especially emotional instability and aggressiveness.[8]

Whatever the roots of their illness—organic, functional, or in many cases, both—patients will feel better understood by their physicians if their feelings are given attention. A feeling of being understood increases confidence in a physician, enhances morale, and promotes cooperation. Patients inevitably have strong feelings about: 1) Their medical conditions; 2) Their wives, husbands, children, and friends; 3) Their hospitals and clinics; 4) Their physicians; 5) Their financial situations; and 6) Their futures. Intense feelings that are negative, embarrassing, or socially unacceptable are apt to cause friction and a lack of understanding between physician and patient if they are not attended to. Unfortunately, attention to the more subjective aspects of a patient's life has not always been part of medical training. In terms of its consequences, however, a strong feeling is as important as a low potassium level or an abnormal electrocardiogram (ECG). Without attention to a patient's feelings and the interpersonal events that generate them, many clinical problems will not make sense, as the following example shows:

An 84-year-old married male became the source of frustration, anger, and perplexity to the house staff because he had made five visits to an emergency room (and was admitted several times to a hospital) in the past 10 months for anginal-like chest pain. Several evaluations revealed no evidence of an organic heart disease. When the patient was questioned closely about his home life, it was discovered that he had assumed increasing responsibility throughout the year for both the care of his seriously ill wife and the management of the household. He reluctantly admitted that, at times, these jobs became so overwhelming that he wished that both he and his wife were dead. The couple's only daughter, somewhat undependable because of her own emotional problems, at least could be counted on to come over to her parents' home and take care of her mother when her father was admitted to the hospital. It appeared as if the patient's cardiac symptoms represented a request for his own respite care. Once this was understood, the house staff felt less frustrated with him and went ahead with plans to get him some help for his wife.

In geriatric psychiatry, as in geriatric medicine, an attitude of fatalism and pessimism toward the diagnosis and treatment of older patients is still too prevalent. However, we rarely understand a condition or a situation so well that we can afford to be pessimistic about it; and the treatment of psychiatric problems in elderly persons can be very rewarding. Delirious states usually clear up once the underlying causes have been detected and treated. Major depressive episodes and paranoid illnesses in older patients respond well to specific medications and supportive psychotherapy. It is true that most dementias in the elderly persons are irreversible, but irreversibility does not mean untreatability. Much can be done to help demented patients live more comfortably with their impairments, and to help relatives cope with the emotional and behavioral problems that so often accompany this unhappy illness.

Organic Brain Syndromes

Organic brain syndromes are psychiatric signs and symptoms that are caused by metabolic derangements in the body or structural damage of the brain. In the current classification system of psychiatric disorders there are seven organic brain syndromes, excluding intoxication and withdrawal syndromes (*see* Table 35-1).[9] Of these seven, the two most important are delirium and dementia.

Delirium

Delirium, which also is referred to as an acute confusional state, is a disorder that is characterized by an impairment of higher mental functions in a patient who shows a clouding of consciousness. A clinical picture of delirium reflects a widespread dysfunction of brain tissue. It frequently is due to disease processes outside of the central nervous system, is not associated with neuropathologic changes in such cases, and often is reversible once its causes are identified and corrected.[10]

The hallmark of delirium is a clouding of consciousness that fluctuates in intensity during the day or from day to day. Clouding of consciousness refers to changes in the level of alertness and disturbances of awareness. It varies from the mildest impairment of thinking, attending, perceiving, and remembering to the extreme of coma. Four stages of consciousness usually are distinguished: full alertness, lethargy, semicoma, and coma; however, some patients with delirium will show hyperalertness. The state of a patient's consciousness can be determined by observing the intensity of stimulation needed to arouse the patient, the patient's response, and the patient's behavior after the stimulation has ceased. Delirium is probably the most common organic mental syndrome that physicians will confront in their work with older patients.[11]

Clinical Features

The onset of an acute delirium is rapid and leads from normality to a gross disturbance in a matter of hours to days. Early signs and symptoms are non-specific and may include anxiety, depression, irritability, insomnia, and sometimes vivid nightmares. Patients may seem absentminded and may complain of difficulty in concentrating. As the condition develops, patients may lose the thread of their conversation or be unduly distracted by noises outside the room. A disorientation to place and (especially) for time, as well as a loss of recent memory, are constant features and vary in degree from mild to severe. Perceptual disturbances are common, such as misinterpretations, illusions, delusions, hallucinations, and paranoid thoughts and feelings. Speech may be rambling or incoherent at times. Restlessness and agitation or lethargy, one or the other, will be present. A fluctuating course (so that a patient may appear relatively normal at one time of the day and extremely confused at another) is another common feature. Insight may vary with the fluctuating level of consciousness; a wide range of emotional reactions (anxiety, depression, fear, irritability, or panic) can be seen, although apathy probably is the most common.

There are noisy and quiet forms of delirium. The noisy form, which is marked by restlessness, agitation, fear, anxiety, illusions, and hallucinations, is usually associated with alcohol or drug intoxication or withdrawal; but it may occur with almost any medical illness. The quiet form of delirium is more common among elderly patients and presents as drowsiness or lethargy, poor concentration, and distractibility. The form of delirium may also alternate between the noisy and quiet varieties in any one patient.

Subacute delirious states come on more gradually and follow a more protracted course. Often associated with medical conditions such as anoxia, uremia, hepatic failure, subdural hematomas, and hypothyroidism, they possess clinical features of both delirium and dementia and may be hard to distinguish from dementia.

Etiology

In most cases of delirium, one should look for multiple causes rather than a single cause (*see* Table 35-3).[11–14] Conditions that predispose to the development of delirium in older patients are sensory deprivation, previous brain damage, drug addiction or a history of such, and dementia. In a number of cases, the first symptom of an undetected dementia is delirium that is precipitated by a seemingly trivial event. It may be, however, that even in the absence of dementia, the aging brain is particularly vulnerable to the development of delirium.

An enormous variety of physical illnesses can cause delirium. Cardiovascular conditions, infections, and drugs are responsible for the majority of delirious states in elderly persons. Congestive heart failure, myocardial infarction, various arrhythmias, pneumonia, chronic obstructive pulmonary disease, and urinary infections, as well as major strokes or transient ischemic episodes, are among the many examples. Digitalis, steroids, L-Dopa, anti-hypertensive agents, and oral antidiabetic agents, as well as the tricyclics and benzodiazepines, all may produce delirious states. Also, in elderly persons, dehydration and electrolyte disturbances, hypothermia, carcinomatosis, and severe pain that is caused by herpes zoster, glaucoma, a toothache, or fecal impaction, may cause confusional states, particularly if dementia is already present.[15]

Evaluation

Delirium as a presenting symptom occupies a central place in geriatric medicine. Its importance can hardly be overemphasized, since delirium is a more common early symptom of physical illness in older patients than fever, pain, or tachycardia.[16] If unrecognized or untreated, several of the disease processes that underlie delirium may lead to permanent cognitive impairment in normal older persons and hasten intellectual decline in those with dementia.

Underlying physical causes, therefore, always should be searched for. Whenever an older patient develops psychiatric symptoms in a short period of time (hours to days), delirium is the prime diagnostic consideration. An older person with serious physical problems who is taking several medications is at risk for delirium. Minor degrees of renal impairment and/or anemia often contribute to, although they may not cause, delirium.

A careful physical and neurologic examination is mandatory, of course, as is a mental status examination (MSE). Physically, the patient almost always is ill—seriously in many acute delirious states. Asterixis and multifocal myoclonus are two neurologic signs that are virtually pathognomonic for delirium, but they often are absent in older patients. Particular abnormalities on a mental status examination that should alert a clinician to the presence of delirium are lethargy or hyperalertness, diminished awareness, distractibility, disorientation, an inability to remember recent events, and a fluctuating clinical picture (so that a patient is almost normal at certain times and quite confused at others). On the MSE or MMS, a patient may show an inability to subtract serial 3s from 20, to spell "world" backwards (and sometimes forwards), to remember three words after a distraction, and to remember the date, the day of the week, or the time of day. Necessary laboratory examinations include a complete blood count (CBC) and erythrocyte sedimentation rate (ESR), urinalysis and culture, chest x-ray film, PO_2 and PCO_2, ECG, serum electrolytes, blood urea nitrogen, blood sugar, tests of liver function, a qualitative VDRL, thyroid-stimulating hormone (TSH) and free Thyroxine (T_4) levels, serum Vitamin B-12 levels, and a test for occult blood in the stool. If these tests are negative, a drug screen, an electroencephalogram (EEG), computerized tomography (CT scan), and a lumbar puncture should be carried out. An EEG can be very helpful in a diagnosis of delirium. The most common pattern in the early stages is a reduction of the dominant alpha rhythm from 10–11 cps to 8–9 cps, along with a decrease of voltage. In later stages of delirium, theta and delta rhythms, particularly high-voltage rhythmic delta activity in the frontal re-

TABLE 35-3   Causes of Delirium in Elderly Persons

Cardiovascular
   Congestive heart failure
   Myocardial infarction
   Transient ischemic episodes and major strokes
   Arrhythmias: Atrial fibrillation, heart block
   Pulmonary embolism
   Hypertensive crises
   Aortic stenosis
   Subdural hematoma
   Temporal arteritis
Infections
   Pneumonia
   Urinary tract infections
   Cellulitis
   Subacute bacterial endocarditis
   Neurosyphilis
   Cerebral abscess
Drugs
   Digitalis
   Sedatives
   Antidepressants
   Steroids
   Alcohol
   Barbiturates
   Anticonvulsants
   Neuroleptics
   Antihistamines
   Diuretics
   AntiParkinson agents, including L-Dopa and amantadine
   Antihypertensive agents (propranolol, methyldopa, guanethidine, clonidine, hydralazine)
   Cimetidine
Fluid, electrolyte, and metabolic disturbances
   Dehydration
   Hypo- and hyperglycemia
   Kidney disease (uremia)
   Liver disease
   Chronic diarrhea
Endocrinopathies—under or over activity of
   Thyroid
   Beta cells of pancreas
   Parathyroid glands
   Adrenal glands
   Pituitary
Other
   Neoplasm, primary and metastatic, particularly from lung, breast, or bowel
   Respiratory insufficiency (e.g., COPD,* asthma)
   Fractures (fat embolism)
   Surgery (e.g., black patch delirium, complications of anesthesia)
   Hypothermia
   Severe pain (e.g., shingles, glaucoma)
   Epilepsy
   Alteration in sensory environment (e.g., intensive care unit)
   Vitamin deficiency: thiamine, nicotinic acid, Vitamin B-12
   Functional psychiatric conditions: depression, mania, and paranoid states

* COPD = chronic obstructive pulmonary disease.
SOURCE: References 8, 11–14.

gions, are prominent.[8] However, it is the degree of slowing rather than the absolute frequency that is significant.[17] An ECG always should be ordered, because delirium often has a cardiovascular cause, such as a painless myocardial infarction. Digitalis and tricyclic blood levels also should be requested when delirious patients have been receiving these medications.

In most cases, a thorough investigation will reveal the probable causes of the delirium. There are a small number of patients, however, in whom it will be hard to discern an exact etiology.

Differential Diagnosis

The most important disorder from which delirium needs to be distinguished is dementia. The alteration in the level of consciousness is the main distinguishing point. Delirium is marked by a change in the level of consciousness, whereas dementia is characterized by a change in the content of consciousness. Fluctuations in the level of awareness and alertness, insomnia, illusions, visual hallucinations, and vivid subjective experiences always favor a diagnosis of delirium. The onset and length of illness also are distinguishing points between the two conditions. If signs and symptoms have developed rather suddenly, within hours or days, a diagnosis has to be delirium; dementia invariably has a longer history. When a delirium is superimposed on a previously undiagnosed dementia, it may be hard to tell the two conditions apart on clinical grounds alone. However, careful questioning usually will elicit a story of increasing forgetfulness or minor episodes of disorientation or personality changes that point toward an underlying dementia.

Both manic and depressive episodes can initially present as delirium. After a few days, however, the delirious features usually subside and the more typical picture of mania or depression becomes apparent. A past history of mania or depression should raise the possibility of these psychiatric diagnoses. To complicate matters, serious physical illnesses can precipitate mania (as well as depression) in predisposed patients.

Clinical Points

Tricyclic antidepressants may cause not only an acute delirious episode with peripheral autonomic signs, but also a more subtle subacute delirious state that is marked by various degrees of disorientation, forgetfulness, a protracted course, and even intermittent episodes of urinary or bowel incontinence. Acute confusional episodes should not be attributed too quickly to transient ischemic episodes if the patient does not have neurologic signs and symptoms, although the occurrence of confusion without paresis following infarction in the territory of the right middle cerebral artery is not uncommon.[18] Mild episodes of acute confusion may occur in the course of senile dementia, but other causes of delirium should be conscientiously sought before dementia is accepted as the explanation. If a delirious state persists after a stroke, an EEG should be requested to rule out an epileptic confusional state that is caused by overlying brain damage.[19]

Course and Prognosis

Once the responsible medical conditions are identified and corrected, delirium usually subsides within 1 to 4 weeks. However, a great variation in the clinical course can be seen. Some patients recover very quickly, while others take a protracted fluctuating course, especially after a stroke, that may last weeks to months and ends in recovery or leaves the patient with residual brain damage. When delirium is superimposed on a dementia, the dementia often becomes permanently worse. Following recovery from a delirium, patients may pass through a transitional period lasting 1 or 2 weeks in which they show abnormalities of thought (paranoid thoughts), mood (depression or anxiety), behavior (restlessness or lethargy), or memory (amnesia) without clouding of consciousness.[20]

Delirium is a serious condition in elderly persons. For the first month of illness, mortality rates range from 17–25%. Mortality may be as high as 30% within 2 years of the initial episode.[21–23] Medically ill patients who are diagnosed as delirious during their first admission have significantly higher mortality rates than patients who are demented, depressed, or cognitively intact.[24] Recovery from a delirious episode is inversely related to both age and the duration of the episode. In one study, 76% of all patients whose delirium had lasted less than 7 days had recovered by the time of discharge, whereas only 12% of all patients whose delirium had lasted over 7 days had recovered by the time of discharge.[25] The presence of delirium in the course of a medical illness should serve to alert a clinician to a high-risk group of patients.

Management

The first step in management is the diagnosis and treatment of any underlying medical conditions. Myocardial infarction, pneumonia, urinary tract infection, drugs, and fluid and electrolyte disturbances are the most common causes of delerium in the elderly. While evaluation is proceeding, supportive measures are mandatory and can be divided into three categories: physiologic support, environmental support, and medications.[11] Physiologically, a patient needs nourishment and rest. An adequate intake of fluid is essential. This must be given intravenously if a patient will not or cannot take liquids orally. Attention also should be paid to urinary output and bowel function. A urine output of less than 1 liter/day should suggest either inadequate fluid replacement or a urinary obstruction. A fecal impaction can be very uncomfortable and will increase confusion, as will any kind of pain.

Delirium is a bewildering and frightening experience for a patient. Noises, voices, and sights often are distorted in an unusual and sometimes threatening way. A picture on a wall may look like a misshapen face or a physician's hypodermic needle may look like a knife. Because of these perceptual distortions, which may be severe, a patient should be placed in a quiet room that is well lit throughout the day and night and is near a nursing station. A patient should be neither sensorily isolated nor overstimulated. The use of a bedside radio or a TV may help with orientation.

The most important aspect of environmental support, however, is played by the staff and relatives. A special duty nurse (and sometimes a relative) should stay with a delirious patient during the worst stages of confusion, if possible, to provide companionship, reassurance, and frequent orientation to time, place, and what is happening around the patient. Quiet, competent, and caring people probably are the best antidote for the confusion and disorganized behavior that afflicts delirious patients. Physical restraints should be avoided if at all possible, as they actually may aggravate disorganized behavior. Some medications have an important place in the treatment of delirium, while other medications have a propensity to cause it. As a general rule, all medications that a patient has been receiving should be discontinued. Many delirious states will clear up with this measure alone.

Sedation should be used sparingly, but it may be necessary when a patient is restless, agitated, fearful, if exhaustion is a risk, or when belligerence makes proper management impossible. The benzodiazepines, especially chlordiazepoxide and diazepam, often are the drugs of choice in the treatment of delirium in younger and middle-aged patients; but, they should not be the drugs of choice in the treatment of older patients because of their long half-lives, their subsequent tendency to accumulate in the body, and their propensity to increase a patient's confusion. Haloperidol is better in this situation and can be given by mouth (0.5–5 mg every 1–2 hours until restlessness subsides) or by intramuscular injection (0.5–5 mg repeated every 2 hours as needed). Haloperidol produces sedation without excessive drowsiness, and it has fewer hypotensive and anticholinergic effects than phenothiazines such as chlorpromazine or thioridazine. The most common side effects are a drug-induced Parkinson's Syndrome or a subjective feeling of restlessness—akisthisia.

There is no evidence that any of the drugs alter the basic course of a delirious episode, but they do relieve symptoms effectively in most cases while the delirium runs its (in most cases) time-limited course.

Dementia

Dementia is an acquired impairment of intellect, memory, and personality in an alert patient.[26] Put operationally, "Dementia is the global impairment of higher cortical functions including memory, the capacity to solve the problems of day-to-day living, the performance of learned perceptuo-motor skills, the correct use of social skills and control of emotional reactions in the absence of gross clouding of consciousness."[27] Put emotionally, dementia is a devastating illness for patients and relatives alike.

Dementia is the most common psychiatric disorder in persons over 70 years of age. Its prevalence increases with age to the extent that 20% of the population in the United States over 80 years of age are estimated to be suffering from moderate to severe dementia.[1] The number of demented patients in the population will grow, not only because the relative and absolute numbers of older people are increasing, but also because older demented patients are living longer than they used to. How to care for this large number of incapacitated people will be one of the major medical and social problems in the coming decade.

Clinical Picture

The usual case of dementia is not hard to diagnose. There is a history of increasing forgetfulness over a 1–2-year period that is accompanied by other evidence of impaired intellectual functioning. If a patient has been working, there will be a history of errors, loss of efficiency, or forgetfulness on the job. A relative usually will report that (at home) a patient shows an increasing reliance on lists, forgets appointments and faces, and misplaces bills, household objects, and personal articles. A patient may start to fail at interests and skills that he or she was previously good at, will have trouble with card games, will show an inability to follow directions or read a map, will neglect to balance the checkbook, and will ask the same question repeatedly. A patient's ability to plan and put plans into action also wanes. In addition, the loss of ability to add and subtract easily (which means that bills go unpaid), lapses in judgment, surprising but temporary periods of disorientation, and personality changes (irritability, insecurity, egotism, and apathy or inertia) are all familiar parts of a clinical history.

A patient's emotional response to the bewilderment and confusion that cognitive loss brings always colors the clinical picture of dementia. Anxiety and depression are common in the early stages, while bland denial and sudden outbursts of tears or anger (catastrophic reactions) characterize the later stages.

Dementia may be impossible to diagnose in its earliest stages. Anxiety and depression, mild obsessiveness, irritability, and subjective forgetfulness or vague physical complaints may be the only symptoms. In the early stages of senile dementia, a diagnostic work-up will not be very much help. Older patients who complain of memory loss always should be evaluated for depression. It is a fairly reliable clinical axiom that patients who complain of memory loss are more likely to be depressed than demented. Relatives—not the patients—complain of the memory loss that is associated with dementia. Patients with a subjective memory loss only should be re-examined every 6 months.

Reisberg and others have suggested that the most common form of dementia—primary degenerative dementia or senile dementia, Alzheimer's type—can be divided into three phases.[28] Phase I, termed the "forgetfulness phase," consists of subjective memory impairment and concern about it. Only careful psychological testing can reveal deficits on memory tests. Phase II, "the confusional phase," is characterized by the first appearance of clear-cut clinical deficits, which include difficulty recalling words, names, and reading material, displacing objects of value, disorientation in familiar surroundings, and problems with concentration and attention. In the early stage of this phase, however, patients still may answer all the questions on the SPMSQ correctly. Phase III, "the dementia stage," is characterized by a severe disorientation, marked memory loss, and the first manifestations of behavioral problems such as restlessness, delusions, hallucinations, and paranoid ideation. Patients in the early stages of this phase cannot live without outside assistance; in the later stages, they usually require institutionalization.

Etiology

Dementia is a syndrome and not an etiological diagnosis (*see also* Volume I, Chapter 4). There are as many medical causes of dementia as there are of delirium.[8,29–31]

Senile dementia—also called senile dementia, Alzheimer's type (SDAT); dementia, Alzheimer's type (DAT); Alzheimer's disease; or primary degenerative dementia (PDD)—accounts for at least 50–80% of all cases of dementia in patients over 65 years of age.[32,33] It is a disease of unknown etiology that is characterized histopathologically by neurofibrillary tangles and neuritic plaques in the neocortex and hippocampus and by granulovacuolar degeneration in the hippocampus. The concentration of these lesions is strongly correlated with the degree of dementia. The brain is not necessarily atrophied in senile dementias when compared to age-matched normal controls.[34] A deficiency of acetylcholine (ACh) has been implicated in senile dementia, as well as deficiencies of norepinephrine and dopamine.[35-38] Alzheimer's disease (previously considered to be a dementia coming on before 65 years of age) and senile dementia are thought to be the same disease, because their histopathology is identical and their clinical pictures are similar.

Multi-infarct dementia is less common than senile dementia, but it still accounts for 10–15% of all cases of dementia among elderly persons. As many as 20% of all demented older patients unluckily suffer from both conditions.[32,33] It can be difficult to distinguish between the two conditions on clinical grounds, because many patients with multi-infarct dementia do not present with the typical picture of step-wise deterioration. However, an abrupt onset of symptoms, a fluctuating course, a history of strokes and step-wise deterioration, relative preservation of personality, depression, emotional incontinence, a history of hypertension, and the presence of focal neurologic signs and symptoms all favor a diagnosis of multi-infarct dementia.[39]

Normal pressure hydrocephalus is characterized by the triad of dementia, gait disturbances, and incontinence. Gait disturbance or incontinence that comes on early in the course of a mild dementia should alert a clinician to this diagnosis; so should a history of meningitis, head trauma, or a subarachnoid hemorrhage (SAH). The CT scan will show ventricular dilatation out of proportion to cerebral atrophy.

Myxedema can present as a dementia that is characterized by a progressive loss of interest and initiative, easy fatigue, slowness in comprehension and movement, and general intellectual deterioration. Patients often say they feel as if there is a thickness, a heaviness, or a fogginess in their heads. Physical signs such as coarse hair, absence of the outer third of the eyebrows, hoarse voice, and a puffy appearance should suggest this diagnosis.

A major depression occasionally can mimic dementia, and depression can be misdiagnosed as dementia if a clinician gives too much weight to a patient's subjective complaints of memory loss and inability to concentrate (and attributes them to dementia) or fails to recall that physical slowing and sluggishness of thought are common symptoms of depression.

Alcoholism, which can produce a primary dementia even without Wernicke's or Korsakoff's Syndromes, should be suspected when a patient has many vague symptoms (gastrointestinal symptoms, malaise, dizziness, falls, depression, and cognitive impairment) for which there is no obvious cause. A history of heavy drinking is more frequently elicited from a relative than from the patient. Alcoholism probably has been underestimated as a cause of intellectual deterioration. Many other drugs can cause alterations in the mental state; in particular, the benzodiazepines and some of the antihypertensive agents can cause a picture of mental dullness and psychomotor slowing that may resemble dementia. A chronic overdose of barbiturates and bromides also can cause a state that resembles dementia.

Dementia is a frequent accompaniment of Parkinson's disease; many Parkinsonian patients with cognitive impairment show Alzheimer's pathologic changes in their brains on autopsy.[40] Tremor, rigidity, hypokinesis, and postural abnormalities are the cardinal neurologic signs. The degree of dementia often correlates with the severity of the akinesis and rigidity in this disease; unfortunately, however, the improvement in motor function that follows the administration of L-Dopa is often not associated with an improvement in cognitive performance.

Evaluation

The assessment of a suspected case of dementia first requires a careful history, which should be recorded with the major causes of the dementia syndrome in mind. This should be obtained from family members as well as from the patient. Senile dementia, Alzheimer's type, usually presents with progressive forgetfulness over months to years. As memory decline accelerates, changes in personality and intellect become apparent, although personality and social skills may remain remarkably well preserved even in the face of advanced intellectual impairment.

The relatively long history of increasing forgetfulness that is typical of senile dementia implies a pathology in the temporal lobe. The occasional case of late-onset Alzheimer's disease may present with parietal lobe symptoms instead (dysphasia, dyspraxia, loss of visuo-spatial ability), and insight may be well preserved. In most cases of senile dementia, insight into the reality of one's condition seems to be mercifully lost along with memory.

A history of brief episodes of difficulty in speaking, weakness of an arm or a leg, transient numbness of the face or an arm, hemianopia or temporary blindness in one eye, diplopia, vertigo, tinnitus, or drop attacks, all should lead one to think of the transient ischemic attacks (TIAs) that often precede an established case of multi-infarct dementia. A history of head trauma, a subarachnoid hemorrhage, or meningitis should lead one in the direction of a normal pressure hydrocephalus. A depression that resembles dementia usually has a shorter history than senile dementia, and there often is a story of earlier depressive episodes. The history of a previous thyroidectomy should alert one to the possibility of hypothyroidism. A history of heavy drinking points to alcoholism as the cause of intellectual impairment, while various cancers (particularly of the lung, breast, or bowel) may cause a dementia syndrome that is associated with an encephalopathy. A slow-growing frontal lobe meningioma may cause dementia without focal neurologic signs, but this condition is rare. A history of syphilis or of a recent fall, which may have caused a subdural hematoma, will suggest other arrestable if not reversible causes of dementia. Repeated episodes of hypoxia, which often are associated with a cardiac arrhythmia or hypoglycemia, also may result in a dementia syndrome.

A careful physical examination, which includes a neurologic and MSE, is indicated in each and every case. Attention deficits that are associated with delirium and language disorders render the accurate evaluation of higher cognitive functions (e.g., memory, learning, and abstract thinking) almost impossible. In the presence of those disorders, a diagnosis of dementia should be avoided, except when there is a clear and documented prior history. When a history of increasing forgetfulness is elicited, and there is no deficit in the SPMSQ, a referral for psychological testing of intellectual function is indicated to establish a baseline for later evaluations.

Laboratory investigations of dementia should include[31]:

CBC and ESR
Urinalysis
Chest x-ray film
VDRL and/or Fluorescent treponemal antibody absorption (FTA-ABS)
SMAC-18 (chemistry screening examination that includes an estimation of blood creatinine, blood urea nitrogen (BUN), alkaline phosphatase, bilirubin, glucose, electrolytes, calcium, phosphorus, and so on)
Serum Vitamin B-12 and folate
TSH and free T_4 estimates
CT scan

The above battery of ancillary examinations combined with the history and physical examination will enable a clinician to diagnose the great majority of treatable causes of dementia. A lumbar puncture has been discarded as a routine examination in many centers since the advent of the CT scan, but it can be helpful in selected instances, such as when chronic (e.g., cryptococcal) meningitis is suspected or when there is reason to think a case of syphilis may have been inadequately treated. An EEG usually is not routinely done either, but it also may be helpful in certain cases. The EEG changes in senile dementia often are identical to the EEG changes of normal aging, although the dominant rhythm may be in the low alpha or even the theta range. The presence of a more conspicuous abnormality is a point against a diagnosis of senile dementia.[41] A tracing that is marked by high-voltage delta activity is characteristic of delirium. Prolonged delirious states, some of them bearing a close resemblance to dementia, may be caused by epileptic foci. In those cases, an EEG has great value.

A CT scan is not good for helping a clinician to make a positive diagnosis of senile dementia. Most cases of advanced senile dementia will show a mild-to-moderate cerebral atrophy and ventricular dilatation. However, a substantial number of normal elderly persons have those same findings (16% in one study), and as many as 25% of all patients with senile dementia by clinical criteria have normal CT scans.[42,43] A CT scan is most useful in a diagnosis of normal pressure hydrocephalus, tumors, subdural hematomas, infarcts, and intracerebral hemorrhages.

A decision about how far to pursue an evaluation of dementia in an older person depends on the history and clinical features that suggest potentially treatable conditions, the age of the patient (the older a patient, the less likely a reversible cause will be found), physical status, the presence or absence of neurologic signs and symptoms, and the family's as well as the clinician's wish to know the exact diagnosis. The younger the patient, the shorter the history, and the more atypical the presentation for senile dementia, the more vigorously should the search for treatable conditions be pursued.

The percentage of potentially reversible causes of dementia that will be discovered in the course of a complete evaluation varies widely, depending on the setting. At a neuropsychiatric institute where the cases of presumed dementia were well screened before referral, only 3.8% of the dementias had a treatable cause. Fifty-five patients over 65 years of age were evaluated. Three of these had reversible conditions: one had a normal pressure hydrocephalus, another had hypothyroidism, and a third had depressive pseudodementia.[44]

In another study, however, 111 selected nursing home residents were completely evaluated for dementia; 53% had either SDAT or multi-infarct dementia. Another 23% had irreversible dementia on the same bases, but (in addition) had medical conditions (e.g., hypothyroidism or Vitamin B-12 deficiencies) that contributed to the loss of function. The final 23% of the patients, who were previously diagnosed as demented, showed no evidence of senile or multi-infarct dementia; instead, they suffered from clinical problems that were potentially reversible, such as pseudodementia, hypothyroidism, and so on.[45] In a study of 35 patients referred for an evaluation of dementia who were admitted to a medical psychiatric unit of a private teaching hospital, 13 (37%) were discovered to be suffering from either delirium or pseudodementia instead; in other words, they had been misdiagnosed. Of 44 patients who, in fact, had a dementia syndrome, 18 (41%) had medical conditions that probably had caused the dementia and were potentially reversible.[46] More conservatively, other studies have suggested that the rate of reversible conditions causing a dementia is between 10–20%.[31]

It may be that the issue of "reversible" dementia has been somewhat overstated, perhaps, in reaction to the older and mistaken concept that dementia was a more or less homogeneous syndrome. Most clinicians only rarely will discover a distinctly reversible cause of dementia in the great majority of patients they evaluate for dementia. Furthermore, many patients who are found to have a potentially reversible condition do not improve when that condition is treated.[47] Nevertheless, each and every case of dementia should be evaluated conscientiously. A patient's cognitive function may improve, sometimes dramatically, if an unrecognized medical illness is brought to light. The diagnosis and treatment of unrecognized medical problems (e.g., congestive heart failure, urinary tract infections, Parkinson's disease, iron deficiency anemia, and so on) is as important as the search for "reversible" causes of dementia and is statistically much more rewarding. The treatment of medical conditions also may result in an improvement of a patient's mental function, even when dementia is already established.

Differential Diagnosis

The major conditions to be distinguished from senile dementia are delirium, benign senescent forgetfulness, the amnestic syndrome, depression, and dysphasia.

A clouding of consciousness, a fluctuating level of awareness, disorientation, and memory disturbances usually coming on within a short period of time, all are typical signs of delirium—even when they are superimposed on dementia. Their presence should prompt a vigorous search for physical causes. Benign senescent forgetfulness refers to minor difficulties with memory that are presumed to be part of normal aging. In contrast to malignant forgetfulness, which is progressive and probably part of senile dementia, benign forgetfulness shows minimal progression. Also, in this condition, recent or past events will be remembered, but some details will be forgotten and recalled at another time. Individuals with benign forgetfulness show an awareness of their shortcomings and may apologize for them.[48] In contrast, patients with malignant forgetfulness cannot remember certain recent or past experiences at all, much less the details. If the details are recalled at a later time, they usually will be distorted. These patients deny they have any problem with their memory and may excuse any mistakes they make by saying that they do not wish to clutter up their memories.

The existence of other types of memory disorders in elderly persons should at least draw attention to the fact that by no means are all memory disturbances in old age due to dementia. It is impossible, in fact, to predict which patients with a mild cognitive impairment will go on to develop dementia. In one English study, one third of all patients with a mild cognitive impairment had dementia on follow-up 4 years later. An additional one-third had shown no progression of their impairment, while the final one-third were shown to have been misclassified as cognitively impaired in the first place.[49]

An organic amnestic syndrome may be mislabelled as dementia. In this condition, immediate memory is retained (e.g., the ability to repeat digits forwards and backwards or to remember three words immediately after hearing them), but there is a marked impairment for learning new material (e.g., as measured by the ability to recall three words after 3–10 minutes). Long-term memory also is impaired, but less than short-term memory. Both forms of memory impairment are out of proportion to the degree of intellectual and personality impairment. The amnestic syndrome is most commonly associated with the Wernicke-Korsakoff Syndrome. However, other causes include cerebrovascular accidents, carbon monoxide poisoning, subarachnoid hemorrhage with basal organization, trauma to the base of the brain, bilateral hippocampal infarction, transient global amnesia, and early Alzheimer's disease.[26]

A severe depression may occasionally be confused with dementia, a condition known as depressive pseudodementia. A history of recent onset, signs and symptoms that are typical of depression, accentuation of disability, a past history of depression, and negativism all favor a diagnosis of depression, not dementia.[50] Furthermore, the cognitive impairment tends to appear when the depression is most severe, so there often is a history of typical depressive signs and symptoms up until the point when cognitive impairment becomes prominent. Occasionally, it can be impossible to tell the two conditions apart; then, it is advisable to administer a trial of antidepressants, particularly if the patient has a past history of depression or if depressive signs or symptoms figure prominently in the clinical picture. Patients can die of depression, so it is especially tragic when it is misdiagnosed as dementia. One should be cautious about diagnosing dementia in the presence of depressive symptoms. The great majority of depressed patients with a cognitive impairment will, in fact, have a depression that is superimposed on a dementia. Only 15% of all patients will have a cognitive impairment because of depression alone.[51] In cases where depression is superimposed on a pre-existing dementia, the depression should, of course, be treated.

The various dysphasias also should be differentiated from the dementia syndrome. A history of a stroke should alert a clinician to this diagnosis. The inability to use language correctly—dysphasia—does not imply dementia. It clearly means damage to the centers of speech, but other cognitive functions may be left intact even though hard to test because of the language difficulties. In some cases of senile dementia, a Wernicke's dysphasia that is a result of early parietal lobe involvement may be an early manifestation of the disease, but this is unusual. Problems with language usually occur late in the course of senile dementia.

Course and Prognosis

The average age of onset of SDAT is 74 years.[52] Most patients live between 5–10 years after the onset of symptoms.[53] Patients with senile dementia may be living longer today than they did 25 years ago, probably because they receive better nutrition in institutions, have broken hips that are pinned early, and get more vigorous antibiotic treatment for infections.[54]

The rate of progression of senile dementia can be predicted by the state of the disease. Patients with a very mild or mild cognitive impairment (Reisberg's stages 2 or 3) show no decline over the next 2–3-year period. Patients with a moderate cognitive impairment (stage 4) fare less well; over 50% show a notable decrease of mental functioning and a few are dead after 27 months. Patients with a moderately severe cognitive impairment (stage 5) have a bad prognosis; 50% are institutionalized or dead between 2–3 years, and the rest have noticeably deteriorated even if they remain in the community.[55]

Management

Once a clinical diagnosis of dementia has been made, any reversible causes of dementia or medical conditions that contribute to the impairment should be ruled out. A comprehensive program of management for patients with a dementing illness is outlined in Table 35-4.[56] The following discussion will focus on psychopharmacologic management and the ways in which a physician can help relatives to manage a patient with senile dementia.

The overall goal in the management of senile dementia is to enable patients to remain at home with some measure of independence without an undue risk to themselves and without overburdening their families. A diagnosis of dementia means a deterioration of memory, intellect, and personality. These disabilities portend an increasing inability to cope with the tasks of everyday life and an increasing dependence on other people. There often are behavioral and emotional problems, which are associated with senile dementia, that make independent living for a patient and attentive caregiving on the part of others even more difficult than it needs to be.

There are three pharmacologic approaches to the treatment of senile dementia: rational, empirical, and conventional.[57] Rational approaches are based on the hypothesis that senile dementia may be caused by a deficiency of a specific neurochemical. Acetylcholine is the leading contender at the moment. Experimental studies are underway that aim to increase the level of ACh in the brain and to follow the effects on the course of senile dementia. The evidence that it is effective in reversing or significantly improving senile dementia is meager, thus far.[58]

The empirical approach to the treatment of senile dementia consists of the use of drugs that seem to help in some way, but whose mecha-

TABLE 35-4   Comprehensive Management Program for Irreversible Dementing Illnesses

Treatment of specific causes
    Treat reversible causes of dementia and/or contributing medical illnesses
Environmental therapy
    Maintain social, physical, and mental stimulation and expectations
    Stabilize patient's life; limit change while avoiding deprivation
Counselling
    Help patients adapt to dysfunction and build self-esteem
    Teach family tolerance and understanding of the disorder (realistic prognosis, tips on management, and so on)
    Referral to community agencies for help with patient
Increase patient understanding
    Repetition, clarity, slower pace
    Written instructions, charts on medication times, and so on
    Prepare patient for changes, procedures, moves, and so on
    Increase orienting cues: night lights, calendars, clocks, signs, and so on
General health care
    Nutrition, hydration, physical activity, rest
    Active treatment of other ailments; provide glasses, braces, wheelchairs, hearing aids, and so on
Pharmacotherapy

Metabolic	Dihydrogenated ergot alkaloids; possibly effective, give at least a 2-month trial; the most likely beneficial non-specific therapy
Multiple vitamins	Given empirically, doubtful efficacy unless diet is inadequate
Antidepressants	For depressive illness; watch toxicity closely; consider tricyclics, tetracyclics, and MAO-inhibitors*; ECT† is another option
Neuroleptics	For management of behavioral or psychotic symptoms

* MAO = monoamine oxidase inhibitors.
† ECT = electroconvulsive therapy.
SOURCE: Lippmann S: The treatment of dementia. *Res Staff Physician* 28:86–96, 1982.

nism of action has an unclear relationship to the neurochemistry of the disease. The results here have not been overwhelming either.

One of these drugs is the ergot alkaloid, dihydroergotoxine mesylate (Hydergine). In several studies, this drug has proved to be superior to a placebo in the treatment of senile dementia. However, the magnitude of the therapeutic effect, while significant, has been small. Patients who are administered the drug may show improvement in mental alertness, orientation, confusion, emotional lability, anxiety, and, (particularly) depression.[59] It may be that Hydergine is helpful for some patients, particularly in the early stages of senile dementia. The starting dose is 1 mg three times per day. If there is no effect after 2 weeks, the dose should be increased to 2 mg three times per day and continued for at least 3 months. Improvement may be seen only after many weeks have passed. The drug is safe and has almost no side effects, with the occasional exception of nausea.

Methylphenidate (Ritalin) is another pharmacologic agent that has been used empirically in the treatment of senile dementia. Methylphenidate is a psychostimulant that has received mixed notices. It does not appear to significantly improve cognitive functioning in demented patients in doses up to 30 mg/day.[60] However, it has been reported to be effective in demented patients with depression,[61] and it may be useful in depressed older patients who are unable to tolerate tricyclic antidepressants or who have a medical illness that contraindicates tricyclic therapy.[62] The starting dose usually is

5 mg twice per day. Doses higher than 40 mg/day are not advised.

Conventional pharmacology refers to the use of well-known psychiatric medications to control particular symptoms and behaviors that are associated with senile dementia (see Table 35-5).

Neuroleptics are the most commonly used drugs in the treatment of behavioral and emotional problems that are associated with senile dementia. The range of drugs from which to choose is broad. All of the neuroleptics are equally effective in controlling disordered behavior, but they differ significantly in side effects. As the milligram potency of a neuroleptic increases, the frequency and severity of sedation, orthostatic hypotension, and anticholinergic effects decrease, while the frequency and severity of extrapyramidal symptoms increase. Table 35-6 lists the common neuroleptics that are used in elderly persons, as well as the dose equivalent for each drug.[63] Because elderly patients metabolize and excrete drugs more slowly than younger patients, the starting doses of neuroleptics should be low and the dosage should be increased only in small increments.

Agitation, restlessness, paranoia, hostility, and catastrophic reactions all may respond to neuroleptics. A starting dose for haloperidol would be 0.5 mg/day; for thioridazine, 10 mg once or twice per day. Haloperidol should be increased in 0.5-mg increments every third or fourth day until the desired effect is achieved; 10-mg increments are advisable for thioridazine.

TABLE 35-5   Behavioral and Emotional Problems Associated with Senile Dementia and Recommended Psychotropic Agents

Problem	Psychotropic Agents
Restlessness, agitation Hostility, paranoia Sundowning Hallucinations, delusions Catastrophic reactions	Neuroleptics (e.g., thioridazine, haloperidol)
Depression Emotional lability	Antidepressants
Anxiety	Anxiolytic drugs (e.g., oxazapam, alprazolam, lorazepam)
Sleeplessness	Chloral hydrate, temazepam

TABLE 35-6 Common Neuroleptics and
Their Dose Equivalents

Generic Name	Trade Name	Dose Equivalent (mg)
Chlorpromazine	Thorazine	100
Thioridazine	Mellaril	95
Perphenazine	Trilafon	10
Trifluoperazine	Stelazine	5
Fluphenazine	Prolixin	2
Haloperidol	Haldol	2
Thiothixene	Navane	5
Loxapine	Loxitane	15

"Sundowning" refers to the syndrome of confusion, restlessness, agitation, and hallucinations that a demented patient sometimes shows at night. It is thought to be caused by a loss of external orienting cues that are associated with darkness. Behavioral-environmental management should be tried before medications are used. A gentle night-light and a softly playing radio may provide reassurance and orientation to a confused patient. Sundowning also occurs when patients sleep during the day or do not have enough stimulation during waking hours. Keeping them awake and encouraging activity during the day often are helpful measures. If medications are needed, thioridazine (25–50 mg at bedtime) or haloperidol (1–5 mg at bedtime) can be prescribed. Neuroleptics, however, also may exacerbate sundowning if they increase sedation during the day and, therefore, aggravate insomnia at night. When this happens, the proper course of action is to discontinue the neuroleptic.

The major side effects of the neuroleptics include oversedation, orthostatic hypotension, and various extrapyramidal symptoms. Oversedation, which commonly occurs with thioridazine or chlorpromazine, can be corrected by reducing or stopping the medication. Patients who are receiving low-milligram potency neuroleptics should be advised to get up slowly from bed in the morning to avoid hypotension; supportive stockings also may be recommended.

It has been estimated that as many as 50% of all patients between 60–80 years of age who receive neuroleptics develop extrapyramidal symptoms.[64] The most susceptible patients are those with brain damage, dementia, and Parkin-

son's disease. Drug-induced Parkinsonism, akithisia, and the Pisa syndrome (a marked tilt of the body toward one side or the other) are the symptoms most troubling to older patients and usually are caused by the high-milligram potency drugs such as haloperidol or trifluoperazine. The best treatment of neurologic symptoms is to stop the neuroleptic. Anticholinergic medications can be prescribed, particularly in the case of drug-induced Parkinsonism; but, they have their own side effects, which may increase confusion and discomfort. Amantadine (100–300 mg/day) is recommended because it is the least anticholinergic of the antiParkinsonism drugs.

Tardive dyskinesia is a neurologic syndrome that usually develops in older patients who have been taking neuroleptic medications for months to years. The term refers to a chronic syndrome of hyperkinetic involuntary movements that most frequently are limited to the face, lips, tongue, jaw, and neck, but also can involve the trunk, arms, and hands. The most common type of this syndrome is referred to as the "Buccolingual-masticatory" syndrome. It is characterized by frequent lateral movements of the jaw, together with a puckering and pouting of the lips, and tongue movements that distend the cheek. The best treatment of tardive dyskinesia is preventive; neuroleptics should be prescribed in the lowest doses possible for a limited period of time. Once the syndrome has developed, many patients will improve after months or years when the offending medication is discontinued. Sometimes, however, tardive dyskinesia is truly irreversible.

The emotional lability and depression that sometime accompany dementia can be helped by low doses of a tricyclic drug (e.g., imipramine, 10 mg three times per day). Sleeplessness should be approached first through behavioral methods: not allowing the patient to sleep during the day, encouraging some activity, giving instructions to go to the bathroom before bedtime, discouraging the drinking of fluids after 5 o'clock in the evening, and so on. Chloral hydrate (1 gram at bedtime) or temazepam (15 mg at bedtime) may be useful in selected cases.

In every case of a behavioral or emotional problem for which neuroleptics or other medications are being considered, careful inquiry should be made into the environmental and psychological factors that may either exacerbate or relieve the problem. For example, a patient who presented as a sundowner turned out to be cold at night; an extra blanket solved the problem. Another patient, whose restlessness and hostility was marked at night in a nursing home, turned out to have a roommate who got up in the middle of the night and rummaged through her own and the patient's bureau. Catastrophic reactions (over-reactions in the form of anger or crying in response to seemingly trivial events) often are brought on when patients feel suddenly overwhelmed. These reactions can be greatly reduced by simplifying instructions or specific tasks for a demented person.

We cannot know what it feels like to experience a deterioration of intellect and personality, but it surely is, at least, a bewildering, threatening, frightening, and depressing experience for a person who is affected; especially in the early stages before insight has been lost. The realization that one cannot make sense out of normal experiences and cannot cope with situations that previously were handled with ease surely provokes severe apprehension and insecurity.

Patients respond in their own unique ways to their decline. Several forms of reaction have been described that include "dependent decline," in which patients react with a greater than necessary dependence on those around them and abdicate responsibility prematurely; others react with "defensive limitation": a restriction of their activities, hoarding of material assets, isolation, and suspiciousness. Still, other patients overcompensate by becoming interfering and dogmatic, while others show a "projective decline," which is typified by the tendency to blame others for mistakes and errors. Other forms of response include egocentricity, depression, and hypochondriasis.[65]

In the early stages of a dementing illness, supportive psychotherapy can be helpful to a patient. A positive confiding relationship with a physician may do much to bring reassurance and to relieve distress. Regular short appointments should be made, so that the patient will not feel abandoned. Occasionally, a physician may have a part in influencing a patient to give up certain activities (driving, social activities), which no longer are pleasurable but are instead anxiety producing. This should be done without, in any way, lowering the patient's self-esteem.

The burden of worry, if not of care, inevitably falls on a patient's family. Early in the course of the illness, families experience anxiety and confusion about the meaning of particular symptoms, such as forgetfulness and apathy. A thorough assessment and diagnosis often clears up much of this apprehension. As the disease inexorably progresses and the burden of care grows heavier, other common feelings are anger, fatigue, depression, grief, and frustration. When a husband or wife discovers that his or her spouse is becoming demented, depression and anger comes from the realization that one's way of life has been altered and, in many ways, destroyed by the patient's illness.[55] Spouses are forced to take on responsibilities that they have never had to face before. For example, husbands must learn to do domestic work and wives often must learn to handle finances and other practical matters. At the same time, unhappily, friends and other sources of support may become less available because of their own feelings of vulnerability and helplessness when confronted by a friend with senile dementia.

When one partner develops senile dementia, the loss of communication may be especially hard for the other partner. The loss of dreams and hopes for the future also is difficult. As one wife said: "We were always talking about where we would go and what we'd do when we got old." Responsibility, especially for decision making, rests heavily on many people. Isolation, which develops when friends do not come around and when the unaffected spouse discovers it is increasingly hard to get out of the house, is another difficulty that greatly narrows the unaffected spouse's range of activities and limits his or her life. Personality changes in the dementing patient also can be very troublesome. Increased egocentricity, thoughtlessness, and selfishness can be hard symptoms to cope with. One wife, when asked how her husband had changed, said: "The less attractive parts of his personality have become more prominent." Simple fatigue, which is brought on by a patient's awakening at night, frequent demands, and needs for care, is another common problem for a spouse.

Since most elderly females are widowed (70% at age 75[3]), the burden of care, for a dementing female often falls on her children, who must adapt to a role reversal in which they become the care-givers. This always provokes strong feelings (sadness, anger, sometimes resentment), which can be especially intense if the prior relationship between them was conflicted in the first place.

In all cases, relatives—whether they be husbands, wives, or grown children—need help. From physicians, they should expect an explanation of the illness and what is likely to happen as time goes on. They should expect availability on the part of the physician and a willingness to listen to the problems the family is having. They should expect appropriate suggestions and considered advice about patient management and relevant community resources.

It is important for family members to know that the constellation of symptoms about which they have been apprehensive has a name, and that physicians know something about it. Its occurrence is neither a fault of the patient nor the relative. Genetic factors are not major determinants of occurrence most of the time. If a male or female comes down with senile dementia after 70 years of age, there is little chance that a close relative also will come down with it. It is only when the disease occurs in patients below 65 years of age, and when another relative in the family has had the disease, that the risk for other relatives is substantial.[66]

Relatives often ask how rapidly the condition will progress. The answer is that the course often is unpredictable and variable. On the average, patients live 5–10 years after the symptoms have begun, but, some patients die within 2–3 years, while others will live over 10 years.[67] It may be that cases that develop before 65 years of age have a more malignant course than those occurring after 75 years of age. The course, as mentioned earlier, also depends on the stage of the illness. If, for example, a patient has only a very mild or mild cognitive impairment, there will not be much deterioration over the subsequent 2 years.

Physicians should make themselves available not only by setting up regular appointments with the patients and families, but also by making themselves available on the telephone.

Relatives should be invited to call regularly or as needed, which depends on the situation. The invitation rarely is abused and relatives usually are very grateful for it. Taking care of a patient with senile dementia can be a very lonely job.

In terms of general management, relatives should be told that patients with senile dementia need stimulation and security. Relatives often ask physicians and care-givers when to encourage or discourage social functions, family obligations, and hobbies. The general rule is that a patient should withdraw from particular activities when they become a source of anxiety rather than a source of satisfaction.[55] Some relatives believe that forcing patients to get out and keep busy will prevent a further deterioration. This reflects an underestimation of the meaning of brain damage. Although withdrawal is advisable in certain situations, activities that are meaningful and satisfying should still be encouraged.

The need of patients with senile dementia for consistency of their surroundings and routines should be stressed. Structure and predictability give security. Consistency can be provided by:

Keeping the furniture in the same place in the house, apartment, or room;

Trying to schedule activities such as waking, eating, exercise, medications, and going to bed at the same time each day;

Having a clock and a calendar within easy view; and

Labelling the various rooms, sometimes with pictures instead of words, when forgetfulness and disorientation become prominent.

To have the patience and energy to take care of a dementing person, care-givers have to take care of themselves too. Relatives should be urged to let other family members share the burden of care, to seek additional help from community agencies, to take periodic breaks for themselves, and to maintain as much of their own lives as possible.

To share the care for a dementing relative and to maintain one's own life with some degree of satisfaction are infinitely easier if community services for elderly persons and their families are well developed. The availability of these services varies widely throughout the United

States, but there is a general agreement that there is much room for improvement.

The major behavioral problems reported by relatives of patients with senile dementia are listed in Table 35-7.[68] The management of these problems require a combination of imagination and common sense. There now are manuals available that are designed to help families cope with demented relatives.[69,70] They contain a great deal of information, and both relatives and physicians who care for demented patients should own them.

In coping with memory problems, for example, relatives should remember that dementing patients are not responsible for their memory loss; it is a result of brain damage. The success of memory aids depends on the degree of dementia. In mild cases, lists, written instructions, and reminder notes can be helpful. In later stages, when a patient cannot read or write, such aids may be frustrating and make matters worse. Instead, pictures may be more useful than words, and such aids as strips of reflector tapes on the wall from the bedroom to the bathroom may be worthwhile.

For catastrophic reactions, the avoidance of the situations that cause them is the key to management. Catastrophic reactions reflect not just stubbornness or nastiness, but a response that a patient with senile dementia cannot help. They are brought on when patients feel overwhelmed. Speaking calmly, giving simple instructions, not rushing a patient, simplifying tasks, and removing a patient calmly from the situation if a catastrophic reaction occurs, all are advised. Relatives also are well advised to join their local Alzheimer's Disease Society, if one exists in their community. This group usually becomes an invaluable source of information and support for family members. Most spouses feel that they are capable of managing the emotional, social, and practical problems that occur early in the course of senile dementia, but then they invariably come to appreciate the resources of the group as the disease progresses.

In most cases, institutionalization has to be considered sooner or later. This usually becomes necessary when patients require assistance with almost all activities of their daily life,

TABLE 35-7   Behavioral Problems of Patients Cited by Families[68]

	Families Reporting as Occurring (%)	Occurrences as a Problem (%)
Memory disturbance	100	92
Catastrophic reactions	87	89
Demanding/critical behavior	71	73
Night waking	69	59
Hiding things	69	71
Communication difficulties	68	74
Suspiciousness	63	79
Making accusations	60	82
Problems with meals	60	55
Wandering	59	70
Bathing	53	74
Hallucinations	49	42
Delusions	47	83
Physical violence	47	94
Incontinence	40	86
Cooking	33	44
Hitting	32	83
Driving	20	73
Smoking	11	67
Inappropriate sexual behavior	2	—

SOURCE: Rabins PV, Mace NL, Lucas MJ: The impact of dementia on the family. *JAMA* 248:334, 1984. Used with permission.

when patients become management problems—either because of their sheer incapacity or because of behavioral or emotional problems, when a family is near exhaustion, when the price of care is too high for a family, or when community resources are not extensive enough or intensive enough to cover a patient's needs.

It is best to bring up the possibility of institutionalization earlier rather than later. It may take time to find a good nursing home. Also, plans made in the midst of a crisis often are not the best plans.

Guilt, denial, or unrealistic hopes may lead families to keep patients with senile dementia at home beyond either party's best interest. The decision to send relatives to a nursing home often is an agonizing one, particularly if they have said all their lives that they would rather die than go to one. However, a couple of considerations may be worth keeping in mind. Placing a person in a good nursing home may relieve an intolerable burden on a family and enable them to show their love toward the patient better than they were able to do when he or she lived at home. Also, in many cases, a patient really is better off. A good nursing home also provides the constant structure and care that demented patients need.

Other Organic Brain Syndromes

Both delirium and dementia denote a global impairment of higher mental processes. In contrast, the other organic brain syndromes denote a more limited impairment of mental function without the clouding of consciousness of delirium or the generalized intellectual impairment of dementia. For example, the amnestic syndrome is characterized by a disorder of memory (especially for recent events) that is out of proportion to any intellectual and personality impairment that may exist. The organic delusional syndrome consists of delusions caused by an organic factor that is not associated with an impairment of intellect, memory, or consciousness.

It is important to make a distinction between the various organic brain syndromes, because the implications for etiology, course, and treatment are different. By definition, a specific organic factor has to be identified as the etiologic factor in each of the organic brain syndromes.

The amnestic syndrome is commonly associated with a vitamin deficiency and chronic alcohol abuse, but any pathologic process that causes bilateral damage to certain diencephalic and medial temporal structures can be responsible (hypoxia, trauma, infarction, infection, and so on). Related clinical features are disorientation, denial problem, apathy, lack of initiative, emotional blandness, and (when the amnesia is marked) confabulation. When the amnestic syndrome is caused by chronic alcoholism and a vitamin deficiency, the signs and symptoms of a Wernicke-Korsakoff Syndrome usually are present, (i.e., ataxia, peripheral neuropathy, and paralysis of extraocular movements).

Delusions in a setting of clear consciousness are the essential feature of the organic delusional syndrome. Persecutory delusions are the most common type, but sometimes nihilistic delusions (e.g., the belief that part of one's body is missing) also are seen, particularly in subacute delirious states. Amphetamines and alcohol may cause this syndrome, which also is often seen after major surgery and myocardial infarctions. Temporal lobe epilepsy, Huntington's chorea, infarctions, and lesions of the non-dominant cerebral hemisphere (infarcts and mass lesions) also may be responsible. The appearance of delusions for the first time in any older person with no history of schizophrenia or paranoia should alert a clinician to the high probability of an organic etiology. Associated clinical features may include a mild cognitive impairment, mild perplexity, rambling speech, hyperactivity or immobility, and mild depression.

In organic hallucinosis, hallucinations also occur in clear consciousness and a patient shows no significant loss of intellectual ability. The hallucinations can be simple (e.g., noises or single voices) or very complex (e.g., multiple voices talking). Alcohol typically causes auditory hallucinations only after prolonged and excessive use. The voices usually are accusatory or threatening and often charge females with heterosexual offenses and males with homosexual ones. This syndrome usually appears after alcohol reduction or abstinence, but it may occur when a person is still drinking. The hallucinations may be accompanied by great fear. The risk of suicide for alcoholics with hallucinations is increased. Hallucinations last from 1 week to 1 month after a patient stops drinking, are apt to recur if drinking starts again, and may last months to years in some cases.[71]

There often are other organic causes of hallucinations. For example, amphetamines are associated with visual hallucinations. Patients who are blind because of cataracts may suffer from chronic visual hallucinations. Deaf patients may suffer from auditory hallucinations. In fact, any kind of sensory deprivation may be the cause of hallucinations, which may become chronic if the deficits go uncorrected. Seizure foci in the temporal and occipital lobes or syphilis also may cause hallucinations.

The essential feature of the organic personality syndrome is a marked change in personality. The particular personality change depends on the location of the pathology. Two types of personality change may occur with frontal lobe lesions: pseudodepressed and pseudopsychopathic.[72] The first type is associated with indifference, apathy, lack of initiative, and slowness. In the second type, a lack of tact and restraint, coarseness, a lack of social grace, irritability, hyperactivity, sudden temper outbursts, emotional lability, and lapses in social judgment are prominent. Admixtures of the two types also are seen.

Personality changes that are identical with those seen in frontal lobe lesions may occur in patients with temporal lobe lesions; but, intellectual and neurologic deficits (e.g., a contralateral, homonomous, upper-quadrant visual field defect) are more common. Irritability, aggressiveness, and a deepening of emotional responses also are associated with chronic temporal lobe lesions. Suspiciousness and paranoia also can develop.

Frontal lobe personality changes, especially of the pseudodepressed type, are particularly apt to be mislabelled as mild depression or dementia. The tip-off of this diagnosis is a striking disparity between the history and how a patient performs on an MSE. A relative or case worker will report that a patient is unable or unwilling to take care of his or her home or apartment, is apathetic and indifferent, and is unable to carry out the tasks of normal everyday living. Incontinence, which is a common occurrence with frontal lobe problems, is reported as well. Yet the patient looks well, denies all problems, and performs pretty well on the MSE.

A bilateral pathology of the frontal lobes

probably is necessary to produce personality changes. The etiology is varied. In elderly persons, strokes, head trauma, and tumors (e.g., a frontal lobe meningioma) probably are the most common causes of this syndrome. Syphilis, Huntington's chorea, Pick's disease, multiple sclerosis, and previous psychosurgery also may produce it.

The essence of the organic affective syndrome is a mood disturbance, which is either a manic episode or a major depressive episode, that ranges from mild to severe in intensity. The syndrome usually is caused by drugs or specific medical illnesses. Reserpine, methyldopa, propranolol, guanethidine, clonidine, cortisone, L-Dopa, and many other drugs have been implicated. Endocrinopathies of the thyroid or adrenal glands also may cause organic affective syndromes, as do several cancers (most notably, cancer of the pancreas). A mild cognitive impairment sometimes is an associated feature, as are any of the signs and symptoms that go with depression or mania (irritability, lability, sadness, hypochondriasis, anxiety, feelings of worthlessness, euphoria, hyperkinesis, and so on).

The treatment of these organic syndromes is the treatment of underlying organic factors. However, symptomatic treatment of an organic affective syndrome with antidepressants, or of an organic hallucinatory syndrome or delusional syndrome with neuroleptics, often is necessary and important. There is no specific treatment for the frontal lobe personality, but it has been asserted that patients with the pseudodemented type should not be allowed to vegetate; it is implied that rehabilitative efforts through a modality such as occupational therapy may be useful.[72]

References

1. Gurland BJ, Cross PS: Epidemiology of psychopathology in old age: Some implications for clinical services, in Jarvik L, Small, G (eds): *The Psychiatric Clinics of North America.* 1982, pp 11–26.
2. Blazer D: The epidemiology of late life depression. *J Am Geriatr Soc* 30:587–592, 1982.
3. Solda BJ: America's elderly in the 1980s. *Popul Bull* 35:1–50, 1980.
4. Murphy E: Social origins of depression in old age. *Br J Psychiatr* 141:135–142, 1982.

5. Pfeiffer E: A short portable mental status questionnaire for the assessment of organic brain deficit in elderly patients. *J Am Geriatr Soc* 23:433–441, 1975.

6. Zarit SH, Miller NE, Kahn RL: Brain function, intellectual impairment, and education in the aged. *J Am Geriatr Soc* 26:58–67, 1978.

7. Folstein MF, Folstein SE, McHugh PR: "Mini-mental state": A practical method of grading the cognitive state of patients for the clinician. *J Psychiatr Res* 12:189–198, 1975.

8. Lishman WA: *Organic Psychiatry*. Oxford, England, Blackwell Scientific Publications, 1978.

9. *Diagnostic and Statistical Manual of Mental Disorders,* ed 3. Washington, DC, American Psychiatric Association, 1980, pp 101–102.

10. Wells CE: Geriatric organic psychoses. *Psychiatr Ann* 8:57–73, 1978.

11. Liston EH: Delirium in the aged, in Jarvik L, Small G (eds): *The Psychiatric Clinics of North America*. 1982, pp 49–66.

12. Varsamis J: Clinical management of delirium, in Hendrie HC (ed): *The Psychiatric Clinics of North America*. 1978, vol 1, pp 71–80.

13. DeVaul RA, Hall RCW: Hallucinations, in Hall RCW (ed): *Psychiatric Manifestations of Medical Illness*. New York, Spectrum, 1980, pp 91–103.

14. Wells CE: The organic brain syndromes, in Strain JJ (ed): *The Psychiatric Clinics of North America*. 1981, vol 4, pp 319–331.

15. Pitt B: *Psychogeriatrics: An Introduction to the Psychiatry of Old Age*. Edinburgh, Churchill Livingstone, 1982.

16. Hodkinson HM: *Common Symptoms of Disease in the Elderly*. Oxford, England, Blackwell Scientific Publishers, 1976.

17. Engel GL, Romano J: Delirium, a syndrome of cerebral insufficiency. *J Chron Dis* 1959, 12:260–277.

18. Mesulam MM, Waxman SG, Geschwind M, et al: Acute confusional states with right middle cerebral artery infarctions. *J Neurol Neurosurg Psychiatry* 39:84–89, 1976.

19. Ellis JM, Lee SI: Acute prolonged confusion in later life as an ictal state. *Epilepsia* 19:119–128, 1978.

20. Lipowski ZJ: *Delirium: Acute Brain Failure in Man*. Springfield, Ill, Charles C Thomas Publisher, 1980.

21. Epstein LJ, Simon A: Organic brain syndrome in the elderly. *Geriatrics* 22:145–150, 1967.

22. Hodkinson HM: Mental impairment in the elderly. *J R Coll Physicians Lond* 7:305–317, 1973.

23. Simon A, Cahan RB: The acute brain syndrome in geriatric patients. *Psychiatr Res Rep* 16:8–21, 1963.

24. Rabins PV, Folstein MF: Delirium and dementia: Diagnostic criteria and fatality rates. *Br J Psychiatr* 140:149–153, 1982.

25. Morse RM, Litin EN: The anatomy of a delirium. *Am J Psychiatry* 128:111–116, 1971.

26. Marsden CD: The diagnosis of dementia, in Isaacs AD, Post F (eds): *Studies in Geriatric Psychiatry*. New York, John Wiley & Sons, 1978, pp 95–118.

27. Royal College of Physicians, Committee on Geriatrics: Organic mental impairment in the elderly: Implications for research, education and the provision of services. *J R Coll Physicians Lond* 15:141–167, 1981.

28. Reisberg B, Ferris SH, De Leon MJ, et al: The global deterioration scale for assessment of primary degenerative dementia. *Am J Psychiatry* 139:1136–1139, 1982.

29. Small GW, Jarvik LF: The dementia syndrome. *Lancet* 2:1443–1446, 1982.

30. Roth M: The management of dementia, *The Psychiatric Clinics of North America*. 1978, vol 1, pp 81–99.

31. Wells CE: Chronic brain disease: An overview. *Am J Psychiatry* 135:1–12, 1978.

32. Blessed G, Tomlinson BE, Roth M: The association between quantitative measures of dementia and of senile change in the cerebral gray matter of elderly subjects. *Br J Psychiatr* 114:797–811, 1968.

33. Tomlinson BE, Blessed G, Roth M: Observations on the brains of demented old people. *J Neurol Sci* 11:205–242, 1970.

34. Terry RD, Davies P: Dementia of the Alzheimer type. *Ann Rev Neurol Sci* 3:77–95, 1980.

35. Davies P, Maloney AJ: Selective loss of central cholinergic neurons in Alzheimer's disease. *Lancet* 2:1403, 1976.

36. Perry EK, Terry RH, Blessed G, et al: Necropsy evidence of central cholinergic deficits in senile dementia. *Lancet* 1:189, 1977.

37. Cross AJ, Crow TJ, Perry EK, et al: Reduced dopamine-B-hydroxylase activity in Alzheimer's disease. *Br Med J* 282:93–94, 1981.

38. Winblad V, Adolfsson R, Carlsson A, et al: Biogenic amines in brains of patients with Alzheimer's disease, in Corkin S, Davis KL, Growden JH, et al (eds): *Alzheimer's Disease: A Report of Progress in Research (Aging)*. New York, Raven Press, 1982, vol XIX, pp 25–33.

39. Hachinski BC, Lassen NA, Marshall J: Multi-infarct dementia: A cause of mental deterioration in the elderly. *Lancet* 2:207–210, 1974.

40. Hakim AM, Malhreson G: Dementia in Parkin-

son's Disease: A neuropathological study. *Neurology* 29:1209–1214, 1979.

41. Slater E, Roth M: *Clinical Psychiatry*. Baltimore, Williams & Wilkins, 1969, p 557.

42. Jacoby RJ, Levy R, Dawson JM: Computed tomography in the elderly. 1. The normal population. *Br J Psychiatr* 136:249–255, 1980.

43. Jacoby RJ, Levy R: Computed tomography in the elderly. 2. Senile dementia: Diagnosis and functional impairment. *Br J Psychiatr* 136:256–269, 1980.

44. Smith JS, Kiloh LG: The investigation of dementia: Results in 200 consecutive admissions. *Lancet* 1:824–827, 1981.

45. Sabin TB, Vitug AJ, Mark VH: Are nursing home diagnosis and treatment adequate? *JAMA* 248:321–322, 1982.

46. Hoffman RS: Diagnostic errors in the evaluation of behavioral disorders. *JAMA* 248:964–967, 1982.

47. Reifler BF, Larson E, Cox G, et al: Treatment results at a multi-specialty clinic for the impaired elderly and their families. *J Am Geriatr Soc* 19:579–582, 1981.

48. Kral VA: Senescent forgetfulness: benign and malignant. *Canad Med Assoc J* 86:257–260, 1962.

49. Bergmann K, et al: *Psychiatry (Part II)*. (*Med. Int. Congr. Ser. No. 274*). Amsterdam, Excerpta Medica, 1971.

50. Wells CE: Pseudodementia. *Am J Psychiatry* 136:895–900, 1979.

51. Reifler BF, Larson E, Hanley R: Co-existing cognitive impairment and depression in geriatric outpatients. *Am J Psychiatry* 139:623–626, 1982.

52. Reisberg B, Ferris SH, DeLeone MJ, et al: The global deterioration scale for assessment of primary degenitive dementia. *Am J Psychiatry* 139:1136–1139, 1982.

53. Taskforce of the National Institute on Aging. Senility reconsidered: Treatment possibilities for impairment in the elderly. *JAMA* 244:259–263, 1980.

54. Blessed G, Wilson ID: The contemporary natural history of mental disorders in old age. *Br J Psychiatr* 141:59–67, 1982.

55. Reisberg B: Office management and treatment of primary degenerative dementia. *Psychiatr Ann* 12:631–637, 1982.

56. Lippmann S: The treatment of dementia. *Res Staff Physician* 28:86–96, 1982.

57. Sparr JE: Dementia in the aged, in Jarvik L, Small G (eds): *The Psychiatric Clinics of North America*. 1982, pp 67–86.

58. Reisberg B, Ferris SH, Gershon S: An overview of pharmacologic treatment of cognitive decline in the aged. *Am J Psychiatry* 138:583–600, 1981.

59. Reisberg B, Ferris SH, Gershon S: Pharmacotherapy of senile dementia, in Cole JO, Barrett JE (eds): *Psychopathology in the Aged*. New York, Raven Press, 1980, pp 233–261.

60. Gilbert JG, Donnelly JJ, Zimmer LE, et al: Effect of magnesium pemoline and methylphenidate on memory improvement and mood in normal aging subjects. *Int J Aging Hum Dev* 4:35–51, 1973.

61. Kaplitz SE: Withdrawn apathic geriatric patients responsive to methylphenidate. *J Am Geriatr Soc* 23:271–276, 1975.

62. Katon W, Raskind M: Treatment of depression in the medically ill elderly with methylphenidate. *Am J Psychiatry* 137:963–965, 1980.

63. Baldessarini RJ: Chemotherapy, in Nicholi AM (ed): *The Harvard Guide to Modern Psychiatry*. Cambridge, MA, Harvard University Press, 1978, pp 387–432.

64. Ayd F: A survey of drug induced extrapyramidal reactions. *JAMA* 175:1054–1060, 1961.

65. Kennedy A: Psychological factors in confusional states in the elderly. *Gerontologia Clinica* I:71–82, 1959.

66. Harris R: Genetics of Alzheimer's disease. *Br Med J* 284:1065–1066, 1982.

67. Heston LL, Mastri AR, Anderson BE, et al: Dementia of the Alzheimer type: Clinical genetics, natural history, and associated conditions. *Arch Gen Psychiatry* 38:1085–1090, 1981.

68. Rabins PV, Mace NL, Lucas MJ: The impact of dementia on the family. *JAMA* 248:333–335, 1982.

69. Mace NL, Rabins PV: The 36-hour day; A family guide to caring for persons with Alzheimer's disease, related dementing illnesses and memory loss in later life. Baltimore, Johns Hopkins University Press, 1982.

70. McDowell FH (ed): *Managing the Person with Intellectual Loss at Home*. White Plains, NY, Burke Rehabilitation Center, 1980.

71. Kolb LC, Brodie HKH: *Modern Clinical Psychiatry*, ed 10. Philadelphia, WB Saunders & Co, 1982, pp 633–634.

72. Blumer D, Benson DF: Personality changes with frontal and temporal lobe lesions, in Benson DF, Blumer D (eds): *Psychiatric Aspects of Neurological Disease*. New York, Grune & Stratton, 1975, pp 151–170.

CHAPTER 36

Affective Disorders

RICHARD C. U'REN, M.D.

Terminology

Major affective disorders are of two kinds: bipolar disorder and major depression.

An affective disorder is termed bipolar if there is any history of a manic episode. A patient who has suffered only manic episodes without depression is classified as suffering from a bipolar affective disorder, manic type. Major or unipolar depressions are classified as either a single or a recurrent episode.

Minor depressions—states of dysphoria in which the symptoms of depression are not of sufficient severity or intensity to meet the criteria of a major depression—are termed dysthymic disorders if there is no history of hypomanic episodes, (in which a person is less than manic, but still high), and are cyclothymic disorders if there is such a history. Patients who were previously diagnosed as suffering from a "depressive neurosis" or a "depressive personality" now would be placed in this category. Patients who react to an identifiable life stress with a depression that develops within 3 months of the stress are considered to have an adjustment disorder with a depressed mood. If a patient meets the criteria for a major depression, however, he or she should be classified that way and not as having an adjustment disorder, even if there is a clear precipitating cause.

Patients who react with depression (major or minor) or mania following a serious medical or neurologic illness, or in response to a drug or medication, are considered to have an organic depressive syndrome.[1]

All types of affective disorders are common in later life. Depressive symptoms are more common in older people than among individuals in younger age groups, but the rate of major and minor depressive syndromes are no higher than at other stages of the life cycle.[2] Prevalence rates for depression in older people vary widely, depending on the type of investigation and the setting in which it is done. A community study that was carried out in North Carolina, using strict diagnostic criteria, showed that the prevalence rate of depression was 8.2/100 individuals, with major depression accounting for 3.7% and minor depression accounting for 4.8% of the cases studied. Another 14.7% of all individuals in the study had significant dysphoric symptoms.[2] When symptom checklists (instead of psychiatric interviews) are used to identify depressive symptoms in the community, the rates are much higher—from 11–45%. The prevalence of depression among older people who are attending psychiatric outpatient clinics is about 33%; in medical settings, the figure is about the same.[3]

Depression in elderly persons is often underdiagnosed. A study of three general practices in Edinburgh, Scotland, in 1964 showed that 76% of the cases of depression were unknown to the practitioners.[4] Another study discovered that 90% of elderly men who had committed suicide had visited their physicians within 3 months of doing so.[5]

Clinical Picture

Depression as a symptom refers to a low mood. As a syndrome, however, depression refers to a constellation of signs and symptoms that includes not only low mood, but also joyless-ness, a loss of interest, lack of energy, fatigue, sadness, gloominess, crying spells, suicidal thoughts, feelings of pessimism and hopeless-ness, social withdrawal, low self-esteem, inse-curity, physical symptoms, and either a feeling of listlessness or anxiety and agitation.

Vegetative symptoms, such as insomnia (of-ten with bad dreams), a loss of appetite, weight loss, constipation, and loss of sexual interest all may be prominent. Complaints of memory loss, trouble in concentrating, difficulty in making decisions, trouble in thinking quickly, and a fear of losing one's mind are frequent. The more severe the depression, the more frequent and intense are symptoms such as low mood (which improves later in the day), early morn-ing awakening, marked weight loss, retardation or agitation, obsessiveness, self-reproach, hos-tility, and even delusions. Milder depressions are characterized by trouble in getting to sleep, low mood that gets worse as the day wears on, preservation of a sense of humor, stable weight, and the absence of marked retardation or agita-tion, self-blame, or delusions. All depressions exist on a spectrum between mild and severe. Intermediate grades, which combine the fea-tures of both types, are common.

Patients with depression look tired, care-worn, or worried. A single glance often is enough to make a diagnosis.[6] Depressed pa-tients often appear miserable and evoke sad-ness in a physician. If psychomotor slowing dominates the picture, a patient will be rela-tively immobile, retarded in all movements, and slow to answer questions. If agitation is pre-dominant, then restlessness, rocking move-ments of the body, pacing, ceaseless complain-ing, anxious demands for reassurance, and protestations of hopelessness are common. Hostility, irritability, and emotional lability also may be marked.

In severe depression, self-reproach may be extreme. The depression may be viewed as punishment for past sins, and patients may be-lieve that they are giving off a foul odor, that food is rotting in their stomachs, and even that their internal organs have disappeared.

Depression is a very painful emotional expe-rience—perhaps the most painful there is—and the suffering that is caused by the conviction that the future is hopeless, the present is mean-ingless, and the past has been wasted can be profound.

Severe depression usually can be divided into agitated and retarded subtypes, with the agitated form being more common. Of the milder depressions, apathetic and hypochondri-acal presentations are frequent.[7] A lack of inter-est, lack of initiative, social withdrawal, and the complaint that any activity requires too great an effort all distinguish the apathetic type; com-plaints of dizziness, ringing in the ears, burning in the throat and abdomen, diarrhea, constipa-tion, vague pains or headaches, hyperesthesias, numbness, or tingling of the skin define the hy-pochondriacal presentation.

The milder forms of depression are apt to be missed by a physician. Their frequent associa-tion with a genuine physical illness may be eas-ily overlooked. Also, patients may deny a feel-ing of low mood or may not know what the word "depression" means. A careful inquiry into the other symptoms in these patients, spe-cifically a loss of interest and enjoyment, sleep and appetite disturbances, and weight loss is particularly important. Relatives and friends also should be queried.

Atypical or "masked" depressions may also throw a clinician off the track. Depression can masquerade as alcoholism, drug abuse, or a be-havioral disturbance, such as shoplifting. Ideas of persecution and reference may mistakenly lead a clinician to a diagnosis of a paranoid dis-order or schizophrenia when depression is the real problem. Paranoid thoughts are quite com-mon in severe depression. Complaints of mem-ory loss and a lack of concentration may sug-gest dementia. However, in general, patients who complain of a memory loss are much more likely to be suffering from depression than de-mentia. Demented patients frequently deny the presence of any deficits. In all cases, a careful history and examination is imperative. A past history of depression or depressive symptoms always should cause physicians to keep this di-agnosis high on their list. It is worth remember-ing that depression in one form or another is the most common psychiatric disorder of old age.

Major (unipolar) depressions are more com-mon than bipolar affective disorders.[8] Attacks of mania or hypomania constitute 5–10% of all affective disorders later in life. In 50% of these cases, the manic episode appears for the first time after 65 years of age.[9] The attacks typically begin abruptly, sometimes after a few days of mild depression. Patients are overtalkative, euphoric, irritable, and hyperactive. Insomnia, grandiosity, poor judgment, distractibility, and a flight of ideas or a sensation of racing thoughts in the head all may be related features.

Instead of the infectious gaiety that marks the elevated mood of younger patients, older patients often show an "empty euphoria," which is not at all contagious to an examiner. Irritability is more common than real euphoria in older patients, and the hostility and resentment that results when extravagant plans are thwarted can be quite marked. The typical flight of ideas that so often is seen in younger patients is apt to be replaced in older patients by repetitious utterances, long-windedness, and talking around the point.

Etiology

Depressive illnesses in most patients are associated with multiple factors. Genetic, biochemical, medical, pharmacologic, personal, and social factors all need to be assessed in every case. Not only depression itself, but the type of depression that occurs, tends to run in families. Bipolar patients commonly have relatives with bipolar affective disorders, whereas patients with a unipolar more frequently have relatives with unipolar illness.[10] Biochemically, it has been postulated that a relative or absolute deficiency of norepinephrine or serotonin at the synaptic endings may be responsible for depression; but, the matter undoubtedly is more complicated.[11]

Losses of various kinds (financial security, physical health, a spouse) can precipitate depression. Physical illness frequently is linked with depression in elderly persons.[12] Many conditions have been implicated (see Table 36-1).[13–16]

Table 36-1 shows that most of the common medical conditions of old age, and quite a few uncommon ones, can cause or exacerbate depression. These "organic" or secondary depressions fall, in most cases, on the more mild rather than the more severe end of the depressive spectrum, but there are many exceptions.

TABLE 36-1 Medical Illnesses Implicated in Depression

Endocrine causes
  Hyper- and hypothyroidism
  Hyper- and hypoadrenalism
  Hyper- and hypoparathyroidism
  Hypopituitarism
  Hyperinsulinism (of any cause)
  Diabetes mellitus
  Menopause
Neurologic causes
  Cerebrovascular accidents and cerebral ischemia of any cause
  Early- and late-onset Alzheimer's disease
  Parkinson's disease
  Subdural hematoma
  Multiple sclerosis
  Huntington's chorea
Cardiovascular causes
  Postmyocardial infarction
  Congestive heart failure
  Cardiomyopathy
Neoplasms
  Primary brain tumors, metastases, and carcinomatoses
  Chronic myelogenous leukemia
  Pancreatic carcinoma
  Oat cell carcinoma of the lung
Vitamin and mineral disorders
  Deficiencies of Vitamins B-1, B-3, B-6, and B-12
  Folic and ascorbic acid deficiency
  Protein and iron deficiencies
Infections
  Influenza
  Pneumonia (particularly viral)
  Hepatitis
  Mononucleosis
  Encephalitis
  Syphilis
  Tuberculosis
Electrolyte disorders
  Hypo- and hyperkalemia
  Hyponatremia
  Hypomagnesemia
  Hypocalcemia
  Increased or decreased plasma bicarbonate
Systemic diseases
  Gout
  Psoriasis
  Osteo- and rheumatoid arthritis
  Uremia
  Temporal arteritis
Undernutrition

TABLE 36-2   Medications Implicated in the Genesis of Depression

Psychotropics
  Neuroleptics
  Benzodiazepines (especially higher doses of
    diazepam)
Antihypertensives
  Propranolol
  Methyldopa
  Hydralazine
  Clonidine
  Guanethidine
  Reserpine
  Diuretics (leading to dehydration or electrolyte
    imbalance)
Hormones
  Corticosteroids
  Estrogen
  Progesterone
Antiparkinson agents
  L-Dopa
  Amantadine
Analgesics
  Morphine
  Codeine
  Meperidine
  Pentazocine
  Propoxyphene
  Indomethacin
Other drugs
  Digitalis
  Alcohol
  Cancer chemotherapeutic agents
  Disulfiram
  Sulphonamides
  Cimetidine
  Tyrosine decarboxylase inhibitor

A Vitamin B-12 deficiency, hypokalemia, hypomagnesemia, and Huntington's chorea, as well as several drugs (reserpine, methyldopa, steroids, and cycloserine), may cause severe depression. Many pharmacologic agents also are responsible for a depressive syndrome.[17-20] Table 36-2 lists the major ones. Most drugs that cause delirium also cause depression.

Diagnosis

A diagnosis of depression is made on the basis of the characteristic signs and symptoms. A history should be obtained from both a patient and his or her relative. All medical patients should be screened for the presence of depression by being asked about their mood, level of interest in usual activities, sleep, appetite, and weight. A past history of depressive or manic episodes, a family history of depression, significant medical conditions, medications, and recent upheavals also will (of course) be asked about.

To qualify for a diagnosis of a major depressive disorder, a patient should[21]:

A. Show a dysphoric (depressed) mood or loss of interest in most, if not all, usual activities and pastimes.
B. Have four of the following symptoms, each of which has been present nearly every day for 2 weeks:
  1. Poor appetite or significant weight loss, or increased appetite and significant weight gain;
  2. Insomnia or hypersomnia;
  3. Psychomotor agitation or retardation;
  4. Loss of energy, fatigue;
  5. Feelings of worthlessness, self-reproach and excessive or inappropriate guilt;
  6. Complaints or evidence of a diminished ability to think or concentrate, (e.g., slowed thinking or indecisiveness); and
  7. Suicidal thoughts, desire to die, recurrent thoughts of death, or suicide attempts.

To receive a diagnosis of a bipolar affective illness, a patient must have had a manic episode, which occurs for the first time in most people between 20–40 years of age. Elderly males who develop mania for the first time after 60 years of age often have a history of a stroke or head injury.[22]

The major clinical features that are necessary to make a diagnosis of mania are an elevated, expansive, or irritable mood, an increase in activity or physical restlessness, increased talkativeness or repetitiveness, flight of ideas, inflated self-esteem (which may pass into grandiosity), a diminished need for sleep, distractibility, and evidence of poor judgment (manifested by activities such as foolish investments, buying sprees, or reckless driving).

In older persons, a delirious state may be present at the beginning of a manic episode. In fact, the more severe the mania, the more likely that delirious features will occur. A past history of an affective disorder and the absence of medical causes of delirium help to distinguish mania from delirium. Also, paranoia may be marked in manic states and depression can occur with mania—aptly termed "miserable mania." The depressive episodes that so often occur with a bipolar illness are diagnosed by the same criteria as those used for a major depressive disorder.

To warrant a diagnosis of a dysthymic disorder, a patient must show either a depressed mood or loss of interest (or pleasure) in almost all activities for a period of at least 2 years. The other signs and symptoms of depression inevitably are present, but their intensity or duration does not meet the criteria of a major depressive disorder. A cyclothymic disorder has numerous periods of depressive and manic symptoms which are less severe than major bipolar illness.

Many (if not most) older patients experience periods of depression that are marked by a low mood, loss of interest, hopelessness, and fatigue, which last hours to days to weeks and do not qualify as major depressive episodes. When this occurs in response to an identifiable stress, it is termed an adjustment disorder with a depressed mood. If this same condition, or even a major depressive episode, occurs because of a medical illness or a pharmacologic agent, it is termed an organic affective disorder. However, not all depressions in elderly persons can be classified easily. In a study of normal aging males in a community that was conducted over a 17-year period, it was found that 70% of them had experienced relatively short periods of depression for no obvious medical, psychological, or pharmacologic reason.[23]

The place of biochemical tests in a diagnosis of depression in elderly persons is not yet firmly established; there certainly is no evidence, thus far, that any biochemical test is superior to clinical judgment in deciding whether a patient is apt to respond to an antidepressant drug. The dexamethasone suppression test consists of administering a 1-mg dose of dexamethasone at 11 PM at night and drawing blood cortisol levels at 8 AM, 4 PM, and 11 PM the next day. The test is considered to be positive if any of the three plasma cortisol levels is 5 μg/dl or higher. An abnormal result is obtained in at least 50% of all patients with a clinical or research diagnosis of endogenous depression.[24] Dexamethasone resistance is even more frequent in patients with bipolar depression, in patients with delusional depression, and in patients with a family history of depression. Patients with Alzheimer's disease, a serious physical illness, any disease that causes severe weight loss, and in patients who are taking estrogens, reserpine, opiates, and barbiturates, often show a false-positive result on the test.[25] Unfortunately, these conditions preclude using the dexamethasone suppression test on many patients in whom a diagnosis is most problematic.

The thyrotropin-releasing hormone (TRH) test involves an intravenous (IV) injection of 500 ng of TRH between 8:30 AM and 9:30 AM following an overnight fast. Blood samples for a thyroid-stimulating hormone (TSH) are obtained at the baseline (before injection) and at 30 minutes postinjection. Patients with a major depression show a blunted TSH response to TRH, which is defined as a change between baseline and 30 minutes of less than 7 μU/ml. The sensitivity of this test is about 50%. It seems to be positive on a different population of depressive persons than on those who show non-suppression in response to dexamethasone; therefore, the TRH test may extend the range of biochemical tests that are available to a clinician for a diagnosis of major depressive disorders. Renal failure, alcoholism, and starvation also give blunted TSH responses and, therefore, are the cause of false-positive results.[26]

Considerations in a Differential Diagnosis

Physical illness and pharmacologic agents always should be sought as causes of, or contributors to, depression (see Tables 36-1, 36-2). Given the large number of medical illnesses that occur in later life, and the wide range of medications that are prescribed, it is (perhaps) surprising that the prevalence of depression in elderly persons is not higher than present figures show. Medical illnesses should, of course, be treated and pharmacologic agents curtailed when a depression is present; unfortunately, however, there is no guarantee that the depression will then improve. In many cases, the depression—once set off—pursues its own independent course and must be treated on its own. A major depression that is brought on by cancer or steroids, for example, should be treated with supportive psychotherapy and antidepressants. The results of treatment often are gratifying, even when the etiology is obviously organic.

Subjective memory loss, poor concentration, and apathy in a depressed patient may tempt a clinician to label the person demented. However, a diagnosis of dementia should be made with caution in the presence of depressive symptoms. Points of difference between dementia and depression are discussed in Chapter 35. A depression frequently occurs with dementia (memory loss is a discouraging experience), as it does with so many organic conditions.

A generalized anxiety disorder may rarely be mistaken for depression, not only because somatic symptoms are prominent in anxiety disorders, but also because anxiety often is a prominent part of depression. A generalized anxiety disorder should be diagnosed when a patient shows symptoms from three of the following categories for at least 1 month[27]:

1. Motor tension: shakiness, jitteriness, muscle aches, fatigue, inability to relax, restlessness;
2. Autonomic hyperactivity: sweating, palpitations, dry mouth, clammy hands, dizziness, light-headedness, tingling in hands and feet, upset stomach, frequent urination, diarrhea, lump in the throat, high resting pulse, and so on,
3. Apprehension: worry, fear, anticipation of misfortune; and
4. Vigilance and scanning: hyperattentiveness, distractibility, trouble in concentrating, insomnia, irritability, and impatience.

The relative absence of depressive symptoms should help to rule out a depression, but a secondary depression may occur after a generalized anxiety disorder has been present for a period of time. A history of the onset of symptoms usually will help a clinician to decide which disorder came first. The distinction is important, because generalized anxiety disorders may respond poorly to antidepressants. Benzodiazepines and, occasionally, neuroleptics are more useful.

Hypochondriasis, which is an objectively unwarranted preoccupation with body parts and (mal)functions, may be confused with depression. Many patients who present with hypochondriasis will have a long history of physical complaints. When the onset of hypochondriasis is recent, however, a clinician should pay heed. Hypochondriacal complaints that occur in late life for the first time always should be considered to be a manifestation of a depression or a serious and often undetected medical illness until proven otherwise.

Alcoholism or heavy drinking always should be included in a differential diagnosis of depression. Heavy drinking itself causes many physical as well as depressive symptoms, and many alcoholics drink in an attempt to relieve depression.

Apathy, which consists of a blunted affective response and an indifference to the environment, may be difficult to distinguish from a mild depression. The presence or absence of other affective symptoms should help to differentiate between the two. An interview with a patient's relatives usually provides useful information. If they say that a patient, at home, complains of a low mood, hopelessness, sadness, or wishes for death, then depression is the more likely diagnosis. Apathy is associated with a wide range of conditions that include strokes in the non-dominant parietal lobe, the frontal lobe syndrome, senile dementia, the use of pharmacologic agents (particularly psychotropic drugs and antihypertensives), electrolyte abnormalities (low potassium or sodium), hypothermia, undernutrition, loneliness, and boredom.

Grief should be distinguished from depression. Although depression always is part of grief and the two conditions often overlap, a distinction is important because of the implications for management. Many patients who are bereaved have all the symptoms of depression. This is a normal response. Proper management consists of encouraging a patient to express his or her feelings. If the depressive symptoms persist for several months, if the yearning for the lost person continues to be intense and continuous, if there is pronounced guilt or bitterness, and if the symptoms are unusually severe and handicapping, this augers a bad outcome for the grieving process. Intensive psychotherapy and, in some cases, antidepressant medications are indicated.

Suicide

Suicide rates increase steadily in males after 40 years of age. The suicide rate for males over 85 years of age—50/100,000 of the population—is higher than that for any other age group. This is not true for females, who show the highest suicide rates between 50–54 years of age; the rates of suicide decline to a low of 4/100,000 in the female age group over 85 years of age.[28]

The reasons for this marked difference between men and women are only conjectural. It may be that women are better prepared to cope with the practical tasks of everyday living, which makes it easier for them to live alone once they are widowed. It may be that men have more of their self-esteem tied up in work, status, and control, so that retirement brings a greater feeling of uselessness than it does with women. It may be that many women are better at forming intimate bonds with friends outside marriage and have more to fall back on once their husbands die.

Older people make relatively fewer suicide gestures. They are more successful at killing themselves than younger people. Depression is the principal psychiatric diagnosis in at least 70% of all people who commit suicide; alcoholism is a distant second.[29] Men are more likely to kill themselves violently, with guns or by hanging, whereas women take overdoses, especially barbiturates.

All patients suffering from depression and alcoholism should be evaluated for suicidal potential. Physicians should be straightforward about their interest. There is no evidence that questions about suicidal thoughts and feelings make a patient worse. On the contrary, many patients feel relieved when they are asked about their feelings. A series of questions like this can be helpful[30]:

Are you so depressed that life looks hopeless?
Do you ever wish it would end?
Have you thought about ending it?
Have you ever thought about how you would do it?
How close have you come?
Do you have a gun (or drugs) at home?
How do you feel now?

When evaluating a patient for his or her risk of suicide, the risk factors (*see* Table 36-3) should be kept in mind.[31,32] The more risk factors that a patient has, the more likely he or she will be to attempt suicide. Some people with few risk factors will try to kill themselves under the right combination of stressful circum-

TABLE 36-3   Risk Factors for Suicide

Age over 55 years
Male
Presence of a painful or disabling physical illness, especially in a male who was robust and energetic
Alone
History of prior suicide attempts
Family history of suicide
History of drugs or alcohol abuse
Depression, especially associated with agitation, hypochondriasis, excessive guilt or self-reproach, and insomnia
Downward economic mobility
Bereavement
Suicidal preoccupation and talk
Toward the end of the depressive illness, when energy returns but low mood persists

stances, however, and the depressive symptoms that precede suicide are not inevitably severe.

Most suicides are potentially avoidable. An older patient who makes a suicide attempt and who shows many risk factors always is a medical emergency and should be hospitalized immediately. A psychiatric consultation or referral is mandatory. Most depressions remit, as do the suicidal thoughts and feelings that go with them.

Management of Depression

There are good reasons to recognize depression and to treat it vigorously. A major depression is a distressing state of mind and carries an increased risk of suicide. Depressed elderly persons who are misdiagnosed as demented may be prematurely relegated to nursing home care. If their homes and possessions are sold, their chances of being independent after recovery are practically non-existent. Also, patients may die of depression not only because of suicide, but also because of inanition and the vulnerability to fatal infections that depression brings with it.

There are five steps in the management of depression. The first step is to identify the depression by recognizing its characteristic signs and symptoms. The second step is to classify the disorder as a major depression, a bipolar affective illness, an adjustment reaction with depression, an organic depression, or a chronic (characterologic) depression. The third step is to search for medical or pharmacologic causes of the depression. The fourth is to inquire into psychological and social factors, such as recent personal losses or family conflicts, that may have contributed to it. The fifth step is to treat the depression.

Medications and supportive psychotherapy are the mainstays in the management of a major depression and bipolar affective illness. There are three major categories of medications that are used in the treatment of depression: tricyclic antidepressants, monoamine oxidase (MAO) inhibitors, and the newer antidepressants. Lithium carbonate might be included as a fourth type. The tricyclics are represented by tertiary compounds—doxepin (Sinequan), amitriptyline (Elavil), and imipramine (Tofranil)—and by secondary compounds—nortriptyline (Pamelor), desipramine (Norpramin), and protriptyline (Vivactil). The MAO inhibitors are tranylcypromine (Parnate), phenelzine (Nardil), and isocarboxazid (Marplan). The newer antidepressants are maprotiline (Ludiomil), amoxapine (Asendin), and trazodone (Desyrel) (see Table 36-4).[33-35]

Depressed patients should seriously be considered for pharmacologic treatment when their subjective distress is great and when the depression interferes with normal everyday functioning. In general, the more severe the depression and more prominent the vegetative symptoms, the more likely the patient will profit from antidepressant treatment.[36] Hypochondriasis, multiple depressive episodes in the past, and delusions, may predict a poor response to antidepressants in many patients.[37]

The tricyclic antidepressants and the newer antidepressants are equally effective in their ability to relieve depression. The differences in action and side effects may help a clinician to choose one drug over another for a particular depressed patient. Orthostatic hypotension, sedation, tremulousness, anticholinergic symptoms, and cardiovascular effects are the main side effects of tricyclic antidepressants. A blurring of vision, constipation, dry mouth, and urinary retention are the most common and bothersome anticholinergic effects. The most common cardiovascular side effects are hypotension and tachycardia, but conduction abnormalities and non-specific reversible ST-T wave changes also are seen. An electrocardiogram (ECG) should be requested before an elderly patient is placed on a tricyclic antidepressant. However, there is recent evidence to show that,

TABLE 36-4   Tricyclic and Tetracyclic Antidepressants

Structural Class	Trade Name	Usual Elderly Dose (mg/day)	Sedative Properties	Anticholinergic Properties	Neurotransmitter Blocking Activity*
Tricyclic					
Tertiary Amine					
Amitriptyline	Elavil	25–150	+++	++++	5HT
Imipramine	Tofranil	25–150	++	+++	5HT, NE
Doxepin	Sinequan	25–150	+++	++++	5HT
Secondary Amine					
Nortriptyline	Pamelor	10–60	+	+++	NE
Desipramine	Norpramin	25–150	0	++	NE
Protriptyline	Vivactil	5–30	0	+++	?
Dibenzoxazepine					
Amoxapine	Asendin	25–150	++	+++	NE
Triazolopyridine					
Trazodone	Desyrel	50–300	+++	+	5HT
Tetracyclic					
Maprotiline	Ludiomil	25–150	++	+++	NE

* Drug blocks reuptake of serotonin (5HT) or norepinephrine (NE)
SOURCE: Veith RC: Depression in the elderly: Pharmacologic considerations in treatment. *J Am Geriatr Soc* 30:583, 1982. Used with permission.

in the absence of a severe impairment of myocardial performance, patients can be treated safely with these drugs without undue risk.[38] Tricyclic antidepressants should be used cautiously with type 1 antiarrhythmic agents (e.g., quinidine, procainamide) because of their additive effects on the conduction system of the heart.

If restlessness, agitation, or insomnia dominate a clinical picture of depression, then doxepin or trazodone probably are the best medical choices because of their sedative effects. Trazadone may well become the drug of choice in cases of agitated depressions because it has almost no anticholinergic and cardiovascular effects. However, the disadvantage of trazadone is its short half—life (about 7 hours), which means that it has to be given in divided doses during the day, at least for the first 2 weeks of administration. The only significant side effect of trazadone is sedation, although a patient occasionally will complain of dizziness or lightheadedness. Doxepin can be prescribed as a 25-mg tablet at night and increased by 25 mg, in divided doses, every fifth day. A total daily dose of 25–150 mg usually is sufficient. Trazodone also can be started with 25–50 mg at night and increased every fifth day by 50 mg. The effective dosage range probably is 50–300 mg in most older patients.

If a patient is more apathetic, then imipramine, desipramine, or nortriptyline are recommended. Desipramine is the least anticholinergic of the three, but nortriptyline produces the least hypotension. Nortriptyline also has a therapeutic window of effect, which means that the drug may not be effective below or above certain plasma levels.[39] Imipramine can be prescribed in a dose of 10 mg twice per day and increased by 10 mg every fifth day, if a patient tolerates it. Both desipramine and nortriptyline should be started with a dose of 10–25 mg at bedtime and increased by 10–25 mg every fifth day until a therapeutic effect is achieved, severe side effects occur, or the maximum recommended doses are reached.

If a patient has experienced a previous episode of depression, he or she should be asked what tricyclics or neuroleptics were prescribed before and what his or her response to them was. A history of a good response to a particular drug in the past often means a good response

to the same drug in the future. Good or bad responses to pharmacologic agents also run in families. If a mother or a brother of a patient has shown a good response to an antidepressant, the same drug is more likely to be effective for that patient.

Patients and their relatives should be told about the side effects of these drugs, the rationale for prescribing them, and when they can expect to feel better. Patients should be warned of the sedative and anticholinergic effects of the antidepressants. The side effects often are the worst at the beginning; if patients can tolerate them for 1 or 2 weeks, the side effects often diminish. If a particular antidepressant is going to work, most patients will experience a relief of some symptoms within 1 or 2 weeks,[40] but there are exceptions to this.

The only absolute contraindication to prescribing tricyclic antidepressants (because of their negative inotropic effect) is a recent history of a myocardial infarction (within the last 6 weeks); however, extreme care should be exercised if a patient has a history of urinary obstruction or closed-angle glaucoma. Tricyclics can be given without complications in the presence of open-angle glaucoma, which is the most common type. It is wise to give all of the antidepressants in divided doses during the day, because one large dose at night may cause hypotension, a fall, and a possible hip fracture. A patient and a family member should be given oral and written instructions about how the patient should take the drug. Patients or relatives should be asked to call their physicians on the telephone after 3–4 days (sooner if necessary) to report any side effects. Reassurance can be very helpful to a patient at that point. It is extremely important to prescribe the medication in limited amounts if there is any risk of suicide. Any more than 1 gram of a tricyclic that is ingested at one time may be fatal in an older patient. There may be a larger margin of safety with the newer antidepressants, but they still should be prescribed in limited amounts when the possibility of suicide exists.

Depressions usually begin to lift within 2 or 3 weeks of starting the antidepressant, although positive responses occur both sooner and later than this. Some patients may respond well to doses as low as 25–50 mg of imipramine or its equivalent, while other patients require 200 mg or more. When a patient does not have a good response on 150 mg of imipramine or an equivalent dose of another antidepressant, a psychiatrist should be consulted.

Certain pharmacologic agents interact poorly with tricyclic antidepressants. Antacids such as aluminum hydroxide inhibit the absorption of tricyclic antidepressants and should not be taken at the same time as the antidepressant. Tricyclic antidepressants and L-Dopa together may cause a marked hypotension. Tricyclics and antihypertensive agents such as guanethidine or clonidine should not be prescribed together. The tricyclics antagonize the antihypertensive effects of clonidine and block the nerve uptake of guanethidine. If the tricyclic is stopped, a dramatic hypotension may then ensue. When tricyclics and neuroleptics are prescribed together, raised blood levels of both drugs result because of a competition for the same microsomal liver enzymes. Tricyclics and benzodiazepines together may lead to sedation and confusion. The same is true for tricyclic and sedative-hypnotic drugs. Tricyclics alone can produce either an acute or subacute delirium, which is reversible if the drug is discontinued.

When a tricyclic or a newer antidepressant is used in the treatment of a major depression, the drug should be continued for 6 months at a therapeutic dose after a patient feels better; then it should be slowly tapered and stopped over a 3-month period. It always is unwise to terminate tricyclics abruptly; not only because some patients will experience flu-like symptoms (e.g., nausea and malaise), but also because depressive symptoms will return if the depression has not yet run its course. Patients who have had more than two major depressive episodes in a 2-year period should be considered candidates for a long-term drug maintenance therapy. For major recurrent depressive episodes, either tricyclics or one of the newer antidepressants probably are the drugs of choice. In a bipolar affective illness, lithium carbonate is the drug of choice.

There are other drugs that are used in the treatment of depression (e.g., the MAO inhibitors). These also are effective drugs, but they are not the first choice in treatment because of their unfortunate tendency to produce hypertensive crisis when taken with food that contain tyramine. This reaction, in fact, is quite rare, but one still has to be careful. Fermented cheeses, pickled herring, sardines, anchovies, chicken livers, canned or processed meat, canned figs, chianti wine, chocolate, and avocados should not be eaten while taking this class of drugs. The MAO inhibitors usually are prescribed when patients have either refractory or atypical depressions, which are characterized by such symptoms as hypersomnia, anxiety, phobias, and hypochondriasis. A psychiatrist should usually be consulted before any of these agents are prescribed.

Electroconvulsive therapy (ECT), although rarely the first choice of treatment for a major depression, still is the most effective treatment. Improvement rates in selected cases range from 85–90%. Electroconvulsive therapy usually is prescribed when other methods of treatment fail. However, it occasionally may be the first choice of treatment in patients who are severely agitated, suicidal, or in danger of death from inanition. Delusional depressions often do not respond well to tricyclic antidepressants. Neuroleptics alone or neuroleptics that are combined with tricyclics are usually prescribed as the first choice of drugs in such cases, but ECT is a close second. Confusion and memory loss following the treatment are reduced when the electrodes are placed unilaterally on the non-dominant hemisphere.[41]

A psychotherapeutic approach that is characterized by support and encouragement is crucial for depressed patients. They should be told that effective methods of treatment exist, that they will recover from their depression, and that some of their symptoms (such as insomnia) may improve almost immediately. Sometimes, it can be helpful to ask patients to fill out a mood chart. They are requested to keep track of their mood twice a day, at 8 AM and 8 PM, on a scale from 1–10, with 1 representing the worst mood they have ever experienced and 10 representing the highest mood they can recall. This allows patients to keep track of their own improvement and it may serve as a morale booster in itself.

Depressed patients can be very difficult to live with. Their irritability, sense of hopelessness, apathy, difficulty in making decisions, crying spells, suicidal thoughts, hostility, and tendency to criticize can be bewildering and annoying. Family members should be told that these symptoms are part of a depressive illness and will pass as the depression lifts. Spouses, adult children, or friends can be helpful to patients who are caught in the grip of depression by showing patience (not always an easy task), by listening openly, by offering warmth and steady support, by making attempts to engage a patient in family and social activities, by providing plenty of simple non-sexual physical affection (such as fondling, hugging, and holding), by being prepared for anger and rejection, and by encouraging a patient to stay on medications and to follow the prescribed medical regimen.

Major interpersonal problems should not be neglected. There is no question that personal frictions not only contribute to the genesis of a depression, but also to its maintenance. Major conflicts between a husband and wife (which existed prior to the depression) or conflicts with children in the family are common examples. While marital therapy is rarely successful when one partner is suffering from a severe depression, it can be useful later. Family conferences are advised when family difficulties are prominent.

The major fact of both unipolar and bipolar affective disorders is that they are recurrent. The great majority of patients (80%) have more than one attack, and it may be that the older the patient is at the age of onset, the greater the likelihood of a relapse.[42] Over the course of years, attacks may become more frequent.[43] The average length of a depression in both types of major affective disorders is 6–9 months,[43] but it can last much longer even with treatment.[44] There is some evidence to show that as females get older, their depressions last longer; that as males age, their depressive episodes become more frequent. However, there is no good evidence to show that depressive episodes actually become more severe with age.[2,43]

In view of these facts, it is not surprising to hear that a major affective illness in old age often is characterized by frequent and prolonged relapses.[45] After following 92 depressed inpatients for 3 years, Post found that even with treatment only 26% had made a sustained recovery, 37% had a recurrence with subsequent recovery, 25% had recurrent attacks in a setting of a mild chronic depression, and 12% had

failed to respond to anything.[46] A more recent study of 124 depressed older patients who were followed for 1 year after treatment for a depressive episode revealed that by the end of the year, 35% were well, 19% had relapsed, 29% were continuously ill, 3% turned out to be demented, and 14% were dead. The mortality rate for males, but not for females, was significantly higher than expected. Patients with the most severe depressions, with the most chronic physical problems that had become worse over the course of the year, and with the highest frequency of undesirable life events during the year, had the worst prognosis.[45]

Because affective disorders so often are recurrent and sometimes chronic, the care of a depressed patient means a long-term commitment on the part of a physician. While the figures cited above are hardly a cause for rejoicing, it is important to remember that a significant number of depressed patients are helped by treatment, even if the results are not as enduring as one might like.

Management of Other Types of Depression

Manic attacks, which usually develop suddenly, are not uncommon in elderly persons. The vast majority of manic older patients have had past episodes of mania. Hospitalization usually is required and psychiatric consultation is strongly advised. Haloperidol, taken in 1–2-mg doses orally or intramuscularly every 1–2 hours until the attack subsides, is the medication of choice for an acute episode. For long-range prevention, lithium carbonate is required. Because of the reduced renal clearance, elderly patients may only require one small dose of lithium per day (e.g., 300 mg). Regular monitoring of serum lithium levels is essential.

Patients who suffer from adjustment disorders with a depressed mood require, most of all, the opportunity to talk about their feelings. Reassurance that their depressed feelings will pass, encouragement to engage in whatever activities they obtain even a little pleasure from, judicious advice, and practical problem solving also may be helpful. Patients whose depression is associated with a physical illness should have their medical problems corrected, if possible.

Pharmacologic agents that are responsible for depression also should be discontinued whenever feasible. Many cases of depression will improve with those measures alone, but there is no guarantee of it. Medical illnesses or pharmacologic agents may precipitate a depression, which then runs its own course independent of the condition that was originally responsible for it, as mentioned earlier.

When a depression coexists with dementia, the depression should be treated if it is persistent and distressing. For example, desipramine can be prescribed with a starting dose of 10 mg twice per day and increased by 10–20 mg every fourth day. Total daily doses in the 50–75-mg range may be enough to produce a good response.

Often, it is difficult to know what the best treatment is for both dysthymic disorders (chronic depressions) and the milder long-lasting depressions that so often are associated with chronic medical problems. Patients with a life-long depressive personality are unlikely to respond to any treatment however well designed. In many cases of mild depression, however, boredom and loneliness are the real problems behind the depression. A skillful and interested community social worker can be an invaluable catalyst for the social rehabilitation of such patients. In other patients with a mild depression, a course of antidepressant therapy is worth trying.

Grief

To lose a person one loves is, perhaps, the most painful experience that one can know. It is not only the sheer absence of the other person, but also the reconstruction of a new life that makes it so difficult.

People who are grieving show all the signs and symptoms of depression, such as insomnia, a loss of interest in life's activities, little energy, restlessness, agitation, poor appetite, and crying spells. Also, guilt, regret, yearning, searching, anger, and a preoccupation with the deceased often are prominent. Bowlby has suggested that mourning can be divided into four phases[47]:

1. A phase of numbing, which often is interrupted by outbursts of intense distress or anger, that lasts from a few hours to 1 week.

2. A phase of yearning and searching for the lost person that lasts months to years.
3. A phase of disorganization and despair.
4. A phase of reorganization.

The course of normal grief varies, but in most cases it lasts months to years. Physicians and relatives often have unrealistic expectations of the speed and completeness with which they expect a bereaved person to recover from a major loss. Mourning and grieving should be considered to be proceeding normally when an individual shows the various signs and symptoms that constitute the four stages of grieving outlined above and does not seem to be stuck in any one of them. A decreasing preoccupation with the dead person as time goes by and the resumption of normal activities, such as working, socializing, and making use of leisure time, all are indicative of a normal course of mourning. Equally important, the following features should be absent[47]:

Prolonged numbness or inhibition of grief;
Chronic depression;
Persistent anger that is directed against the dead person, oneself, relatives, or physicians;
A disconnection of the emotional response to loss from the event that caused the emotional response—the death itself;
Disturbed personal relationships, which are marked by either excessive demands and clinging or compulsive independence; and
A mislocation of the dead person within another person, in the bereaved person him- or herself (often manifested by physical symptoms that are identical to those the deceased person complained of), in a physical object, or even within an animal.

There are two major variants of disordered mourning. Both lead to many forms of physical and mental ill health. Both impair a bereaved person's capability to make and maintain relationships, and both interfere with a bereaved individual's ability to organize the rest of his or her life. They range in intensity from very mild to very severe and, in their lesser degrees, they may be hard to distinguish from healthy mourning.

The first and more common variant is termed chronic mourning. It is an abnormal extension of Bowlby's second and third phases of mourning. Depression is the main symptom and often is combined with anxiety, agoraphobia, hypochondriasis, or alcoholism. The initial response to the loss is intense and prolonged; anger and self-reproach are dominant, sorrow often is absent. Individuals in a state of chronic mourning are unable to restructure their lives, which remain sadly disorganized.

The second variant, termed inhibited mourning, is distinguished by a prolonged absence of conscious grieving. It seems to be a prolongation of Bowlby's first phase of mourning. An individual seems to carry on with life much as before, seemingly untouched by his or her loss. Nevertheless, people in this state are apt to suffer a variety of psychological and medical illnesses (often chronic) and are vulnerable to acute depressions, which often are precipitated by events such as the anniversary of the death of the loved one, by the death of someone else, or by reaching the same age as the deceased person at the time of death. Even chronic mourners who do not suffer an overt breakdown may experience a dramatic change in their lives for the worse that is marked by a chronic dissatisfaction with empty personal relationships, an absence of warm feelings, and a sense that they are acting in a play and are not engaged in their lives.

The particular course of mourning that an older person follows depends (as it does with younger people) on the circumstances of the death, especially its expectedness or unexpectedness, the type of relationship that the bereaved had with the deceased, the personality of the bereaved person, and the presence or absence of relatives or others who encourage the bereaved person to mourn.

Individuals may respond abnormally to a loss at any age, but there is evidence that the younger a female is when she is widowed and the more unexpected the death, the more intense the mourning is likely to be. The more direct the knowledge of a death, the less likely is the tendency to deny it. Faulty or false information about the death of a loved one supports denial and disbelief, which seem to be major determinants of inhibited mourning. A death preceded by a quarrel or angry words is very distressing and often contributes to abnormal mourning. Partners whose relationship is characterized by insecurity, anxiety, and ambivalence, or by compulsive care-giving on the part

of one partner, are prone to experience chronic mourning upon the death of one of them. Individuals who make these "anxious attachments" often show personality traits of overdependence, anxiety, and emotional instability. By way of contrast, people who are prone to inhibit mourning are described as overly self-sufficient and reliant.

Family members and friends play a critical role in the outcome of grief.[48] Most people with a good outcome to their mourning report that they knew at least one person with whom it was easy to cry and express feelings freely. People with a bad outcome said that at least some of the people they had talked to had made grieving difficult by urging them to pull themselves together, by telling them not to think of the deceased one, by exhorting them to keep busy, or by pushing them to make plans for the future instead of just allowing them to express their feelings of grief, anger, and sadness. This, in fact, turned out to be bad advice.

Management of Grief

For many older people and their relatives, there is an anticipatory period that lasts from weeks to years before death occurs. Relatives should be invited to meet with a physician during this time and to be given accurate information about the probable course of the illness of their loved one. They also should be encouraged to express whatever feelings they have and be invited to ask any questions they wish. Couples and families who can be together before death, who have practical and financial affairs as well as emotional conflicts under control (if not settled), who are able to share thoughts and feelings about the coming separation, and who have said goodbye to each other, may find that the separation and loss (while always saddening) is easier to accept than it otherwise might be. In any case, such couples will be in a far better position to cope with the bereavement than those who have not prepared. Comments by a physician that serve to free family members from guilt and unnecessary responsibility—"No, there was nothing you could have done sooner; this condition is very hard to diagnose at an earlier stage"—may be greatly appreciated. A physician's willingness to provide information, to show interest, to be available, and to encourage the expression of feelings usually are much appreciated by bereaved family members.

While death often brings relief for all involved, it also can bring a feeling of shock when it actually occurs, however well prepared the relatives have been. Physicians should not hesitate to write a note of condolence, to make a telephone call, or to visit the family after the death. A follow-up note or telephone call within 1 or 2 months of the funeral also is appreciated.

It may be a good idea to offer an appointment to some recently bereaved individuals within 1 month of the loss. A physician will have the opportunity to assess how bereavement is being handled. If the course of grieving is following a normal course, if the person is able to express feelings openly and thoroughly, and if relatives and friends are facilitating the expression of grief, there is reason to be optimistic about the outcome of the mourning. If the bereaved person shows the symptoms that are associated with an abnormal outcome, however, the intervention is called for.

Grief work is necessary to achieve a healthy resolution and readjustment after the loss. Unfortunately, this simple fact often is not appreciated by those who deal with bereaved people. Physicians can facilitate the mourning process by encouraging a bereaved person to talk freely about the experiences leading to the death, the feelings experienced after it, the personality of the deceased, and about the marriage (if it is the death of a spouse). It often helps to ask a bereaved person to bring in and talk about photographs, keepsakes, momentos, or anything else that is connected with the deceased. Memories and experiences that are painful should be elicited tactfully. Regular appointments should be set aside for grief work; four to six sessions often suffice. A referral of a bereaved person to a psychiatrist or clinical psychologist is mandatory for physicians who choose not to do this kind of work themselves.

The first rule in the management of grief is not to hinder the expression of mourning, but to encourage it. It has long been recognized that unobstructed grieving often brings its own resolution. The Beatitude from St. Matthew, "Blessed are they that mourn: for they shall be comforted," expresses very well this basic psychological truth.

References

1. *Diagnostic and Statistical Manual of Mental Disorders,* ed 3. Washington, DC, American Psychiatric Association, 1980, pp 118–119, 205–224.
2. Blazer D: Epidemiology of late life depression. *J Am Geriatr Soc* 30:587–592, 1982.
3. Blazer D: *Depression in Late Life.* St. Louis, The CV Mosby Co, 1982, pp 103–117.
4. Williamson J, et al: Old people at home: Their unreported needs. *Lancet* i:1117–1120, 1964.
5. Barraclough B: Suicide in the elderly. *Br J Psychiatr* (spec publ 6) 1972, pp 87–97.
6. Slater E, Roth M: *Clinical Psychiatry,* ed 3. Baltimore, Williams & Wilkins, 1969, p 207.
7. Pitt B: *Psychogeriatrics: An Introduction to the Psychiatry of Old Age.* London, Churchill Livingstone, 1982.
8. Winokur G: Unipolar depression: Is it divisible into autonomous sub-types? *Arch Gen Psychiatry* 36:47–52, 1979.
9. Slater E, Roth M: *Clinical Psychiatry.* Baltimore, Williams & Wilkins, 1969, p 571.
10. Perris C: A study of bipolar and unipolar recurrent depressive psychoses. *Acta Psychiatr Scand* (suppl) 194:1–188, 1966.
11. Schildkraut JJ: The biochemistry of affective disorders: A brief summary, in Nicholi AM (ed): *The Harvard Guide to Modern Psychiatry.* Cambridge, MA, Harvard University Press, 1978, pp 81–91.
12. Gurland BJ, Cross PS: Epidemiology of psychopathology in old age: Some implications for clinical services, in Jarvik LF, Small GW (eds): *The Psychiatric Clinics of North America.* Philadelphia, W.B. Saunders Co, 1982, vol 5, pp 11–26.
13. Hall RCW: Depression, in Hall RCW (ed): *Psychiatric Presentations of Medical Illness: Somatopsychic Disorders.* New York, Spectrum, 1980, pp 37–63.
14. Berger P: Management of depression and anxiety in primary care medicine, in Freeman AN, Sack RL, Berger PA (eds): *Psychiatry for the Primary Care Physician.* Baltimore, Williams & Wilkins, 1979, pp 157–179.
15. Lehmann H: Affective disorders in the aged, in Jarvik LF, Small GW (eds): *The Psychiatric Clinics of North America.* 1982, vol 5, pp 27–44.
16. Klerman GL: Depression in the medically ill, in Strain JJ (ed): *The Psychiatric Clinics of North America.* Philadelphia, WB Saunders Co, 1982, vol 4, pp 301–317.
17. Editorial: Drug induced depression. *Lancet* ii:1333–1334, 1977.
18. Klerman GL: Depression in the medically ill, in

Strain JJ (ed): *The Psychiatric Clinics of North America*. Philadelphia, WB Saunders Co, 1982, vol 4, p 312.

19. Ouslander JG: Physical illness and depression in the elderly. *J Am Geriatr Soc* 30:593–599, 1982.

20. Hall RCW (ed): *Psychiatric Presentations of Medical Illness: Somatopsychic Disorders*. New York, Spectrum, 1980, pp 353–406.

21. *Diagnostic and Statistical Manual of Mental Disorders,* ed 3. Washington DC, American Psychiatric Association, 1980, pp 210–215.

22. Shulman K, Post F: Bipolar affective disorder in old age. *Br J Psychiatr* 136:26–32, 1980.

23. Gianturco DT, Busse EW: Psychiatric problems encountered during a long-term study of normal ageing volunteers, in Isaacs AD, Post F (eds): *Studies in Geriatric Psychiatry*. New York, John Wiley & Sons, 1978, pp 1–16.

24. Carroll BJ, et al: A specific laboratory test for the diagnosis of melancholia. *Arch Gen Psychiatry* 38:15–22, 1981.

25. Gelenberg AJ (ed): The DST in even greater perspective. Massachusetts General Hospital Newsletter: *Biological Therapies in Psychiatry*. 7:1, 1984.

26. Loosen PT, Prange AJ: Serum thyrotropin response to thyrotropin-releasing hormones in psychiatric patients: A review. *Am J Psychiatry* 139:405–416, 1982.

27. *Diagnostic and Statistical Manual of Mental Disorders,* ed 3. Washington, DC, American Psychiatric Association, 1980, pp 232–233.

28. Blazer D: *Depression in Late Life*. St. Louis, The CV Mosby Co, 1982, pp 34–36.

29. Sainsbury P: Suicide and depression. *Br J Psychiatr* (spec publ 2) 1968, pp 1–13.

30. Beebe JE: Evaluation of the suicidal patient, in Rosenbaum CP, Beebe JE (eds): *Psychiatric Treatment*. New York, McGraw-Hill Book Co, 1975, pp 19–41.

31. Blazer D: *Depression in Late Life*. St. Louis, The CV Mosby Co, 1982, pp 35–37.

32. Stengel E: *Suicide and Attempted Suicide*. London, Penguin, 1964.

33. Veith RC: Depression in the elderly: Pharmacologic considerations in treatment. *J Am Geriatr Soc* 30:581–586, 1982.

34. Donlon PT: Cardiac effects of antidepressants. *Geriatrics* 37:53–60, 1982.

35. Ayd FJ (ed): New antidepressants. *Psychiatr Ann* 11:370–401, 1981.

36. Berger PA: Antidepressant medications in the treatment of depressions, in Barchas JD, Berger PA, Ciaranello RD, et al (eds): *Psychopharmacology: From Theory to Practice*. New York, Oxford University Press, 1977, pp 174–207.

37. Bielski RJ, Friedel RO: Prediction of tricyclic antidepressant response. *Arch Gen Psychiatry* 33:1479–1489, 1976.

38. Veith RC, et al: Cardiovascular effects of tricyclic antidepressants in depressed patients with chronic heart disease. *N Engl J Med* 306:954–959, 1982.

39. Hollister L: Plasma concentrations of tricyclic antidepressants in clinical practice. *J Clin Psychiatry* 43:66–70, 1982.

40. Jarvik LF, Mintz J, Steuer J, et al: Treating geriatric depression: A 26-week interim analysis. *J Am Geriatr Soc* 30:713–717, 1982.

41. Weiner RD: The role of electroconvulsive therapy in the treatment of depression in the elderly. *J Am Geriatr Soc* 30:710–712, 1982.

42. Zis AP, Goodwin FK: Major affective disorder as a recurrent illness. *Arch Gen Psychiatry* 36(spec issue):835–839, 1979.

43. Winokur G: *Depression: The Facts*. Oxford, England, Oxford University Press, 1981, pp 54–56.

44. Stengel E: Attempted suicides, in Resnick HLP (ed): *Suicidal Behavior*. Boston, Little Brown & Co, 1968, pp 171–197.

45. Murphy E: The prognosis of depression in old age. *Br J Psychiatry* 142:111–119, 1983.

46. Post F: The management and nature of depressive illnesses in late life: A follow-through study. *Br J Psychiatry* 121:393–404, 1972.

47. Bowlby J: *Loss: Sadness and Depression*. London, Hogarth Press, 1980.

48. Raphael B: Preventive intervention with the recently bereaved. *Arch Gen Psychiatry* 34:1450–1454, 1977.

Chapter 37

Anxiety, Paranoia, and Personality Disorders

Richard C. U'Ren, M.D.

Anxiety and the Other Neuroses

The collective term "neuroses" refers descriptively to five conditions: anxiety, hypochondriasis, phobias, obsessive-compulsive disorders, and hysterical conversion reactions. Neurotic disorders are common throughout life and their prevalence does not diminish much with advancing age. The prevalence rate of isolated neurotic symptoms in individuals over 65 years of age may be as high as 50%, but the prevalence rate for the more carefully defined neurotic syndromes is approximately 5–10%.[1] Relatively few older people with neuroses are referred for psychiatric treatment, possibly because older people minimize certain symptoms for fear that they may be interpreted as evidence of senility. Also, general practitioners may discount neurotic symptoms because older people often have a "reason" to be anxious or hypochondriacal. Possibly, many elderly people are reluctant to be referred to a psychiatrist because they feel it would stigmatize them.

A neurotic disorder in old age, whether it arises for the first time after 60 years of age or represents a worsening of a life-long condition, is always caused by a combination of personal predisposition, life experience, and stress. In old age, there are as many things to be anxious about as there are to be depressed over—or obsessive or hypochondriacal about, depending on one's life-long defensive style. A decrease in strength and stamina, an increase in the amount and severity of physical illness, isolation, lone- liness, loss of independence, forced dependence because of medical illness, loss of a spouse, relocation, and retirement, are all common stressors. Neurotic symptoms are indicative of anxiety-producing situations that are unsettling to an elderly patient.[2]

The different kinds of neuroses rarely present as pure types. Mixtures of neurotic symptoms are common. An elderly patient may present with anxiety, obsessiveness, hypochondriasis, and depression; or one single syndrome—hypochondriasis—may be prominent at another time. Depression is an almost invariable feature of a late-onset neurosis and always makes other neurotic symptoms worse.

Patients over 65 years of age who suffer from neurotic symptoms can be classified into two groups: those whose neurotic symptoms developed much earlier in life and those whose symptoms have developed after 65 years of age. The two groups differ from each other in some significant ways. Individuals with late-onset neurotic disorders report more feelings of loneliness, have more trouble in caring for themselves, and have fewer hobbies than either patients with long-standing neurotic symptoms or normal older people. Individuals with late-onset neuroses have a history of relatively happy childhoods and no evidence of earlier neurotic traits, which is in contrast to individuals whose neuroses have developed earlier in life. Compared to normal individuals and patients with an earlier onset of neuroses, patients with a late-onset neurosis suffer from more actual physical illnesses. This finding underlines the importance of searching for an unrecognized medical illness when a neurosis appears for the first time late in life.[3]

Not much is known about the long-term course of neurotic disorders that begin earlier in life. In one review, 40% of all neurotic patients improved as they got older and another 30% showed a slight improvement with age. It has been suggested that neurotic illness may become less intense with the passage of time.[4]

Anxiety

Anxiety presents in different ways. A patient may have symptoms of anxiety, but the symptoms may not be of a sufficient intensity or number to warrant a formal diagnosis of an anxiety disorder. Common symptoms of anxiety are nervousness, tension, apprehensiveness, hypervigilance, fears of losing one's mind, and a variety of somatic complaints (dyspnea, palpitations, chest pain, hyperventilation, dizziness, light-headedness, sweating, trembling, diarrhea, and abdominal pain). If there are distinct episodes of these symptoms, the condition is termed an acute anxiety state or a panic disorder. If the symptoms are chronic and continuous, the condition is referred to as a chronic or generalized anxiety disorder.

Anxiety symptoms, especially feelings of tension and apprehension, are common in old age. The loss or threatened loss of economic or personal security, the fear of dependency, pain, and failing health, all can create a state of anxiety. As the Reverend Sidney Smith once said: "The evil in old age is that as your time has come, you think every little illness is the beginning of the end. When a man expects to be arrested, every knock at the door is an alarm."[5] An underlying medical cause always should be sought when episodes of anxiety occur for the first time in old age, since a physical illness probably is the most common precipitant of anxiety among older people. The most common form of anxiety in elderly persons is a cardiac neurosis, which is an anxious over-reaction to cardiovascular symptoms. Table 37-1 lists the major organic causes of anxiety in old age.[6,7]

Anxiety also may be a prominent feature of other psychiatric conditions such as delirium, dementia, and (particularly) depression. There are no pathognomonic signs or symptoms in psychiatry; the meaning of any one symptom is

TABLE 37-1 Somatic Causes of Anxiety

Cardiopulmonary
  Coronary insufficiency
  Cardiac arrhythmias
  Mitral valve prolapse
  Recurrent pulmonary emboli
Endocrine
  Hyperthyroidism
  Hypoparathyroidism
  Hypoglycemia
  Pheochromocytoma
  Cushing's Syndrome
Neurologic
  Early primary degenerative dementia (senile dementia)
  Transient ischemic attacks
  Syphilis
Toxic metabolic
  Medications/drugs (caffeine, thyroid preparations, barbiturates, cortisone, psychostimulants, propranolol, vasodilators, and so on)
  Withdrawal states (from benzodiazepines, alcohol, barbiturates, neuroleptics, tricyclic antidepressants)
Other
  Chronic pulmonary disease
  Chronic pain from any source
  Anemia
  Neuroleptic-induced akisthisia

known only by the company of the other symptoms it keeps. The anxiety that occurs with delirium is associated with changes in alertness and awareness. The anxiety that is associated with dementia occurs early in the illness, when a patient is aware of memory loss, and later in the disease whenever threats to routine and security occur. Anxiety symptoms with agitation and restlessness are especially prominent in major (unipolar) depressive episodes. Associated depressive symptoms, such as a low mood, loss of energy and interest, sleep and appetite disturbances, with a history of previous depressive episodes make this diagnosis likely.

The management of anxiety depends on its causes. A careful history, a physical examination, and a laboratory investigation that is relevant to the particular symptoms of the patient, all are imperative—particularly when the anxiety is of a recent onset. Caffeine intake in excess of 250 mg/day is one criterion for a diagnosis of caffeinism, which often is an overlooked cause of anxiety; the figure may be lower for older adults (a 5-ounce cup of brewed coffee contains 90–120 mg of caffeine; a 5-ounce cup of instant coffee or tea contains 70 mg).[7] A withdrawal from neuroleptics and tricyclic antidepressants may cause gastrointestinal symptoms as well as anxiety. Also, rebound anxiety may occur when benzodiazepines, even in relatively low doses, are withdrawn abruptly.

The anxiety that accompanies delirium or depression usually is alleviated when the underlying illness is treated. The anxiety that occurs with dementia diminishes when the disease progresses (and insight is lost) or when measures are taken that lessen threats to security (e.g., when provisions are made so that a demented person is not left alone at home).

When anxiety symptoms are more psychogenic, a physician should pay careful attention to a patient's history to understand the concerns that cause anxiety. Simply listening to a patient's worries may be very therapeutic. Giving the condition a name ("From your symptoms, it sounds to me that you are having anxiety symptoms") and making suggestions about ways to deal with the situation that may be responsible for the symptoms may be helpful. If a great deal of stress has caused the symptoms, a physician should encourage a patient to talk to friends or relatives about his or her feelings. Regular, but limited, appointments during the time of stress also are advised.

Antianxiety drugs should be used with caution and only when the symptoms are intense and disruptive. Drugs with a short half-life, such as oxazepam (10 mg taken once to three times per day) or alprazolam (0.25 mg taken once to three times per day), are favored and should be prescribed for not longer than 2 or 3 weeks. Occasionally, patients with a disruptive chronic anxiety may require benzodiazepines over a longer period of time for control of their symptoms.

Hypochondriasis

Hypochondriasis, which is a persistent obsessional preoccupation with body organs and their function, is common in elderly persons, particularly among older females. Hypochondriasis was, in fact, the most common of the severe neuroses in one study.[8]

Hypochondriacal symptoms are remarkably diverse, but cardiovascular and gastrointestinal symptoms predominate; palpitations, chest or abdominal pains, dyspnea, dyspepsia, diarrhea, and constipation, all are common, as are headaches. The degree of concern can be quite remarkable and a patient's persistent "organ recital" quite taxing. Why hypochondriacal symptoms arise and what they mean is a matter of conjecture. They may represent insecurity, which usually is precipitated by an actual episode of physical illness in an anxious person in difficult personal circumstances,[9] or it may be that hypochondriasis serves the purpose of shifting anxiety away from personal concerns to less threatening concerns with bodily functions.[10] As with the other neuroses, hypochondriasis often is precipitated by a combination of stress, pre-existing personality factors, and an actual physical illness.

There are chronic hypochondriacs (patients who have had their symptoms for a long time) and hypochondriacs whose symptoms have developed later in life. Individuals with a longstanding hypochondriasis differ little from normal older people with the exception of their persistent physical complaints. In contrast, late-onset hypochondriacs more often have an actual physical illness and experience more loneliness and difficulty with self-care than normal elderly persons or chronic hypochondriacs.[3]

As a rule, it is wise to assume that all late-onset hypochondriacs have a depression or a serious (and sometimes undiscovered) physical illness until proven otherwise. Somatic symptoms often are associated with major and minor depressions. Mood and energy disturbances, sleep and appetite problems, or feelings of hopelessness and low self-esteem point to the diagnosis. Hypochondriacal complaints are associated with an increased risk of suicide in depressed older patients.[11] Serious cardiovascular disease, undetected cancer, and early cerebral degeneration all are examples of a physical illness that may underlie late-onset hypochondriasis.

In a number of instances, however, late-onset hypochondriasis will not portend a serious emotional or physical illness, but it will instead serve as a signal of conflict or insecurity produced by the same stressors that cause anxiety. Hypochondriasis should be viewed, then, as an abnormal adjustment reaction to stress. The same techniques that a physician uses to alleviate anxiety (careful listening, advice and reassurance) can be used.

The management of chronic hypochondriacs can be a very taxing proposition, and physicians are advised not to fill up their case loads with such patients. However, management can also be rewarding in some cases, not only because proper management can prevent a patient from undergoing unnecessary diagnostic and surgical procedures, but also because the symptoms will come under a degree of control if physicians are persistent and patient. The principles of management include[12]:

Attentive, but not excessive, medical evaluation and laboratory procedures;

Pharmacologic treatment of any associated or underlying depression;

Explaining to a patient that symptoms are real, but unexplained, and that many medical symptoms fall into such a category;

Avoidance of a confrontation (''the symptoms are in your head''), since that will only spur a patient on in an attempt to prove the existence of symptoms to a physician;

Scheduling regular limited appointments and asking about the rest of a patient's life as well as the symptoms; and

Prescription of vitamins and, occasionally, placebos as non-specific medicines.

This kind of program, while not dramatic, serves to provide hypochondriacal patients with support and consistency. The goal is to reeducate a patient in such a way that somatic concerns can be dealt with on a regular basis and not at the whim of the patient. The management plan also frees patients from having to constantly prove to their physicians that their symptoms are real.

Phobias

Phobic episodes in old age may represent a recrudescence of earlier episodes or may develop for the first time. Phobias that begin late in life are not uncommon and are precipitated by events such as a myocardial infarction or cataract surgery. They usually represent a displacement of anxiety, with all its varied etiologies, into concrete situations that then cause anxiety and are (thus) avoided (phobia = fear). Situations that are most commonly avoided are those of traveling, shopping in crowded stores, riding in elevators, or leaving home at all (agoraphobia). The management starts with an assessment of the possible causes of insecurity and anxiety. A conflict within the family is common, as are physical or economic threats to continued self-care and independence. A depression, if present, should be treated. A referral to a psychiatrist is recommended for longstanding persistent cases that do not respond to simpler approaches. A course of gradual desensitization to the feared situation is the treatment of choice, as it is in younger people, but this treatment is hard to administer outside of specialized psychiatric units.

Obsessive-Compulsive Disorders

Severe obsessive states rarely begin in old age. Obsessive symptoms, however, (repetitive, irrational, unwanted thoughts) are not uncommon and usually are associated with a depression or threats to personal security or physical integrity. Individuals who have suffered from an obsessive-compulsive disorder earlier in life may experience a serious worsening of their condition in old age, especially if depression intervenes. The treatment of late-onset obsessional symptoms usually is the treatment of a depression.

Hysterical Disorders

Hysterical conversion reactions (paralysis, blindness, hyperesthesias, ataxias) and hysterical dissociative stages (fugues, wandering, memory loss) almost never begin in old age. If they do appear abruptly, they usually are indications of a depressive illness or of a rapidly developing organic disease. Three older patients who were diagnosed as suffering from either dissociative states or a conversion reaction were found, on a follow-up examination, to be suffering from cerebral metastases from bronchogenic carcinomas (two of three) and from a cerebral embolus (one of three) that probably followed a myocardial infarction.[13] In the first two cases, the psychiatric illness manifested itself several months before neurologic signs became evident. One author asserts, "It is best to assert dogmatically that primary hysterical illness does not begin in old age."[3]

Paranoid Disorders

The word "paranoia" refers to experiences in which an individual falsely, or to an exaggerated extent, believes him- or herself to be the object of attention of others. These beliefs usu-

TABLE 37-2   Conditions in Which Paranoid Symptoms Occur in Elderly Persons

Organic conditions
　Delirium (any cause)
　Dementia (any cause)
　Drugs
　　ACTH* and cortisone
　　L-Dopa
　　Psychotropics (e.g., imipramine, benzhexol
　　　　[Artane], monoamine oxidase inhibitors)
　　Phenytoin
　　Psychostimulants
　　Alcohol
　　Barbiturates
　　Bromides
　　Withdrawal from alcohol, minor tranquilizers, barbiturates, and hypnotics
　Sensory deprivation; auditory and visual
　Other conditions
　　Hypothyroidism and hypoparathyroidism
　　Head injury
　　Chronic temporal lobe epilepsy
　　Multiple sclerosis
　　Vitamin B-12 deficiency and pernicious anemia
　　Syphilis
　　Brain tumors
Paranoid symptoms with functional psychiatric conditions
　Affective illness (depression, mania)
　Paranoid personality disorders
Functional paranoid states
　Acute paranoid states secondary to
　　Any major procedure in hospital
　　Psychological stress (e.g., bereavement, loneliness, isolation)
　Paraphrenia (late-onset schizophrenia)
　Schizophrenics who have grown old
　Monosymptomatic hypochondriacal delusions
　　(e.g., parasitosis)

*ACTH = adrenocorticotropic hormone.

ally are persecutory in nature; patients believe that others are hounding or harassing them.

Paranoid symptoms are very common in elderly persons. Their diagnostic significance varies greatly.[14] Table 37-2 shows the conditions in which paranoid symptoms occur.

Clinical Considerations

The sudden onset of a paranoid disorder always should suggest the possibility of a delirious state in older people, which is caused by a physical illness and drugs. A misinterpretation of sounds and actions, ideas of reference, and persecutory delusions are common in delirium, but they fluctuate in intensity and usually are poorly organized. Persecutory symptoms are common in demented patients, who deny their forgetfulness, misplace things, and accuse others of stealing their clothing and jewelry. A very wide assortment of pharmacologic agents may precipitate paranoid symptoms and states, which usually—but not invariably—are associated with features of delirium.

The majority of deaf older people are not paranoid, but there is firm evidence to show that a hearing loss predisposes one to paranoia.[15] Persecutory feelings and auditory hallucinations of noises, music, and voices are common. Poor vision and blindness can be associated with visual illusions and hallucinations.

Paranoid symptoms commonly occur in both depression and mania. In the course of a severe depressive episode, patients may begin to accuse others of talking about them, plotting against them, withholding medications, trying to poison them, and so on. Paranoia often is prominent in mania. In fact, delusions of persecution may be the presenting feature, along with great irritability and even auditory hallucinations. Overactivity, overtalkativeness with circumstantiality and repetitiveness, and (in most instances) a past history of manic or depressive episodes should enable a physician to make a correct diagnosis.

Individuals with life-long traits of suspiciousness, mistrustfulness, sensitivity to criticism, argumentativeness, humorlessness, emotional coldness, and guardedness are referred to as having paranoid personalities. Their personality traits are accentuated if dementia, depression, physical illness, or emotional stress are super-imposed; a frank paranoid psychosis may occur in a certain proportion of these individuals.

Acute paranoid reactions may occur in response to great stress among predisposed individuals, and they are not uncommon in medical and surgical wards where a wide range of stressors are operative, such as sensory deprivation, immobility, apprehension, exhaustion, unfamiliar surroundings, lack of knowledge, major medical or surgical procedures, electrolyte imbalance, and drugs.

Of all schizophrenics seen in old age, over 90% are those whose illnesses have developed earlier in life. Many of them have a history of long periods of hospitalization throughout their lives and show a combination of residual schizophrenic defects, institutional deficits, and (in many cases) tardive dyskinesia. Schizophrenia can begin after 65 years of age, however, and it constitutes 10% of all elderly cases of schizophrenia found in a general psychiatry clinic.[1] This condition is known as "late-onset schizophrenia" or "paraphrenia." Paraphrenia differs from early-onset schizophrenia in that patients' personalities and affects are well preserved and do not deteriorate; also, thought disorder is rare. Most paraphrenics present with hallucinations and delusions, but about 20% present with delusions alone.

Paraphrenic patients typically are female, solitary, and eccentric. There often is a history of a hearing loss, of long-standing interpersonal difficulties (such as failure to marry, early divorce without remarriage, or a late and troubled marriage), and of a paranoid or schizoid type of personality.[13] In most cases, there is no history of a previous breakdown—a contrast to depressed elderly persons, most of whom have had depressive episodes before 65 years of age.

A paraphrenic illness usually starts with an accentuation of previous personality traits, such as increased suspiciousness, withdrawal, and depression. Irritability, hypochondriasis, insomnia, weakness, and anxiety may be prominent. The suspiciousness usually is directed at neighbors or young people in the neighborhood; they are accused of stealing mail, pounding on the house at night, shining headlights into the windows or (in one case) putting lint into the clothes dryer. Paraphrenics also may believe that their neighbors are talking about them criti-

cally. Frequent telephone calls to the police, in which an individual complains of harassment by the neighbors, finally may exhaust a police officer's patience and lead to a trip to the emergency room for psychiatric evaluation.

The illness may remain at this phase, or the delusions may become more firmly held and extensive, so that a patient may believe that a conspiracy of people exists who are out to do him or her harm (often for undefined reasons). Relatives or jealous neighbors often are implicated. Patients may believe that they are being spied on, that their house is being broken into in their absence and things are stolen, that poisonous gas is being wafted through the house, that their water is poisoned, or that they are being attacked by ray guns from outside (one woman explained the presence of seborrheic keratosis on the back of her hands that way). In most cases, auditory hallucinations that often develop suddenly also are prominent. They consist of "threatening, demanding, commanding, accusing, or cajoling voices, jeering commentaries, screams, or shouts for help. The patient may hear obscene words spoken and songs performed; loud bangs, rappings, shots, or explosions may be complained of."[16] Hallucinations usually are more intense at night. A visual hallucination may be unusually vivid (e.g, people or animals coming into the room). Fear, anxiety, hostility, and depression are the dominant emotional states.

Post believes that there are three different forms of paraphrenia.[17] The first form is marked by delusions that certain people, usually neighbors, are interfering with a patient's property (breaking in, misplacing, or stealing articles of worth). The second form is less frequent than the first, but the patient is more disturbed. It consists of delusions of persecution that are more widespread. A patient believes that the house is bugged, that people in the street are talking with criticism about this patient, that obscene remarks are being made, and that there is a conspiracy to harass this patient.

The third form closely resembles schizophrenia in younger persons in that a patient manifests first-rank symptoms of schizophrenia: 1) Voices are heard that talk about a patient in the third person singular, comment on his or her activities, or repeat and anticipate a patient's thoughts, feelings, and sensations; 2) Movements are produced in a patient's body by telepathy; and 3) Others are inserting or withdrawing thoughts from a patient's head. The first and second types comprise two thirds of all cases of paraphrenia, while the third type makes up the remaining one-third.

Monosymptomatic hypochondriacal delusions probably are a form of paranoia.[18] This is not a common disorder, but it occurs perhaps more frequently than alleged. In older people, it takes either of two forms: A delusion of parasitosis or a delusion that one is emitting a foul smell. The average age of onset of delusions of parasitosis is 56 years of age. The patient usually is a married female who presents to a dermatologist with complaints of itching, tickling, or prickling sensations on or under her skin, which she ascribes to an infestation by insects such as lice, fleas, beetles, or bees.

Other unusual preoccupations with bodily parts or functions (e.g., the delusion that one's bowels are blocked or a sensation of a persistent burning feeling in the perineal area) usually are associated with a major depression and are alleviated once the depression is treated. Patients with monosymptomatic hypochondriacal delusions may show little or no depressive symptomatology, however, and the condition is chronic and difficult to treat. Reports from Canada indicate that a particular neuroleptic, pimozide (which still is unavailable in the United States), represents a promising treatment for a certain proportion of patients who suffer from parasitosis.[18]

Management of Paranoid States

The treatment of paranoid symptoms that are secondary to delirium, a medical illness, and pharmacologic agents, is the treatment of the underlying illness or a withdrawal of the drug. However, if persecutory symptoms are disruptive and a patient is overly fearful, agitated, or belligerent, then haloperidol may be prescribed orally in doses of 1–5 mg taken twice per day. Paranoid symptoms that accompany dementia may be treated in the same fashion or with thioridazine (25 mg taken twice or three times per day). Attempts to distract a patient and to provide a highly structured environment also may be useful and, in some cases, may make psychopharmacology unnecessary.

Paranoid symptoms that are associated with an affective illness often require the addition of neuroleptics to the antidepressant regimen; but, most of the cases should be referred to a psychiatrist, as should cases of paraphrenia. The treatment of paraphrenia is a combination of drug therapy and social intervention. The correction of hearing or visual deficits is imperative, of course, and relocation sometimes is necessary.

The outcome of therapy for paraphrenia (which untreated is a very chronic illness) is surprisingly good, provided that patients stay on the medication. Post found that of 71 patients with this condition, 61% had a complete remission of symptoms with treatment while another 31% had a social recovery, but with residual symptoms such as mild delusions. Only 8% of these paraphrenics failed to respond at all to treatment.[17] Neuroleptic agents that were used to control symptoms range from haloperidol (1–6 mg/day taken orally) to thioridazine (50 mg/day to begin with, increasing to a total dose of 150–200 mg/day in divided doses after several weeks).[19,20] The maintenance dose of medication that is needed to control the symptoms is about one quarter of the dose that is needed to suppress the symptoms. Only in occasional cases are intramuscular depot injections of fluphenazine (Prolixin) necessary.

The Personality and Behavior Disorders

When long-standing personality traits are exaggerated beyond normal and are associated with rigidity, inflexibility, a pattern of difficulty in getting along with other people, isolation, and personal distress, then they are referred to as personality disorders. The major personality disorders that are seen in old age are well depicted by their descriptive adjectives (see Table 37-3).[21–23]

While most personality disorders tend to increase an individual's vulnerability to the stresses of advancing age, this is not always true. For example, schizoid personalities may fare relatively well in old age because their lack of personal relationships leaves them untouched by the deaths that cause so much grief

TABLE 37-3 Personality Disorders in Old Age

Type of Disorder	Traits	Response to Age-Related Stress
Paranoid	Suspicious Mistrustful, rigid Lack of warmth Critical, argumentative	Increased suspiciousness Paranoid symptoms Reclusiveness
Compulsive	Perfectionism Excessive devotion to work Personal stiffness, formality Preoccupation with rules, procedures, details Insistence on conformity and control	Pervasive anxiety Major depression Hypochondriasis Paranoid symptoms
Narcissistic	Need for constant attention and admiration Grandiose sense of importance Lack of empathy Manipulative	Depression Suicide Drug or alcohol abuse
Dependent	Lack of confidence Passivity Wants others to assume responsibility Subordinates needs Unwillingness to make demands	Depression
Schizoid	Lack of social involvement Lack of warmth Aloofness Indifference to criticism, praise, feelings Reserved, withdrawn, seclusive	Reclusiveness
Histrionic	Lively, dramatic, colorful Exaggerates feelings, thoughts, reactions Excitable, egocentric, vain Charming but superficial	Depression Hypochondriasis Exaggeration of physical illnesses
Passive-Aggressive	Resentment of demands manifested by procrastination, obstructionism, stubbornness, inefficiency	Increased aggressiveness at first Helpless dependency Regression

to more normal people. Many dependent personalities also cope well with old age, because their life-long wish to be taken care of finally is fulfilled. Paranoid personalities, who are constantly at odds with other people, always have a struggle on their hands that provides meaning to life and leaves them with little time for fear, anxiety, and depression.[3]

Patients present themselves to physicians with symptoms, not with personality disorders, but a patient's personality colors every clinical presentation. The physical and emotional stresses of advancing age cause pre-existing personality traits to be exaggerated. Old age, to paraphrase Felix Post, is the ultimate personality test. This means that the ordeals to which an aging personality is put will reveal clearly its assets and vulnerabilities.

Patients with paranoid and compulsive personalities are apt to cause the most trouble for the staff on a geriatric medical ward. These patients cause frustration and irritation to the staff, because their need to gain control over any threatening situation increases when they feel insecure. Compulsive individuals become more fastidious and demanding, while paranoid patients become more mistrustful, negativistic, and oppositional, thereby obstructing the orderly medical work-up to which physicians are accustomed.

The management of personality disorders by physicians can be facilitated by first recognizing and treating any associated physical illness, depression, or sensory deficits, all of which exacerbate troublesome personality traits. Second, a physician should make an effort to dampen the feelings of irritation and frustration that non-compliant patients arouse, to not react with anger and threats, and instead to try to understand the situation through a patient's eyes. This means spending some time alone with a patient, sitting and talking, and getting to know him or her. When becoming tense in the presence of an irritating patient, it may be useful (instead of expressing anger) to relax the muscles of one's shoulders and say to the patient, "Tell me more."

Hospitalization may, in fact, be the ultimate personality test. For paranoid personalities especially—who are mistrustful, prickly, independent, and controlling—a hospital routine, which demands dependency as well as frequent intrusions, is threatening and annoying. After gaining an understanding of a patient's feelings, it often is advisable to assign one member of the treatment team—the person who gets along best with the patient—to serve as a liaison between a patient and the medical personnel. Procedures and their rationales should be explained patiently. Allowing a patient to decide when he or she wants to undergo a certain procedure, which thereby increases a sense of control, is worthwhile. Only a couple of people should go into a patient's room at any time, since a cluster of people may be viewed as overwhelming and more threatening. The same guidelines that are useful in the management of paranoid personalities (correction of associated physical and psychiatric problems, avoidance of overreactions on the part of physicians, and a willingness to spend extra time with a patient and to understand his or her feelings) are, in fact, useful with all personality disorders; in most cases, they can be managed satisfactorily by an understanding physician. A psychiatric consultation will, of course, be warranted when these guidelines do not work.

Behavior Disorders

The term "behavior disorders" is borrowed from child psychiatry and refers to antisocial acts that are not the result of mental illness and do not obviously rise from a patient's previous personality. In most cases, however, a careful history reveals that behavior disorders can be traced back to slight personality defects that have emerged in old age. Hoarding, miserliness, stubbornness, extreme dependency, set and irritating habits, social disinhibition (e.g., tactless outspokenness, sexual offenses), milder forms of aggressiveness, apathy, and an occasional case of urinary incontinence all constitute the list.

Urinary incontinence is not inevitably a manifestation only of infection, local mechanical faults, or dementia. Sometimes, it represents an older dependent patient's way of showing resentment and anger.

Sexual misbehavior, which is much more common earlier in life than after 65 years of age, has been falsely attributed in older males to early dementia. It is, in fact, a relatively rare problem in older males and most often occurs in individuals who are becoming impotent. There rarely is a history of previous psychiatric or legal problems. It is believed that children are selected for sexual activities that range from exhibitionism to masturbation (but rarely intercourse), because older males feel unable to attract females and because children tend to be submissive to them. Sexual offenses, once they have brought satisfaction, tend to recur in spite of threats and actual punishment if a patient is not provided with supervision and support.[20] A psychiatric consultation is advisable, and if the sexual urges persistently interfere with the quality of the patient's life, stilbesterol (1–3 mg/day) can be helpful.

The senile squalor syndrome, also termed the Diogenes Syndrome after the reclusive Cynic philosopher who ended up living in an earthenware jar,[9] describes withdrawn older people who live in socially unacceptable disorder and filth. About 40% of them turn out to be schizophrenic; however, the majority are not psychiatrically ill or demented, although the prevalence of alcoholism in this group may be higher than previously reported.[24] Many have never married and have sometimes shared their isolated existence with a sibling. They tend to be quarrelsome, independent, domineering, and reject help. If forced to enter a hospital, they inevitably resume their old way of life once they return home.

Most behavior disorders, as with personality disorders, must be accepted. However, the correction of associated physical and psychiatric conditions and attempts to understand the feelings (e.g., powerlessness, resentment, anger, frustration, and so on) that lie behind troublesome behaviors always should be undertaken, and may be useful, in at least ameliorating the more troublesome problems.

Aggressive and violent behavior occurs among older people, but it almost always is associated with a major psychiatric illness. In a survey of 220 consecutive admissions to a geriatric unit in a state hospital, it was found that 18 (8.1%) of the patients had used guns or knives in acts of violence. Another 121 patients, who were referred to as the aggressive group and comprised 63% of all these patients, had manifested a history of physical violence without weapons or had verbally threatened violence.

The violent and aggressive groups differed from each other. In the violent group, almost one third of the patients were diagnosed as suffering from paraphrenia. Atypical organic states (e.g., associated with normal pressure hydrocephalus or brain tumors) and the manic phase of a bipolar affective illness each accounted for another 17% of the cases, while senile dementia, alcoholic dementia, and schizophrenia accounted for 11% each.

In contrast, one third of the aggressive patients earned a diagnosis of senile dementia; in another 28%, the diagnosis was schizophrenia. Atypical organic states, alcoholic dementia, mania, and multi-infarct dementia accounted for anywhere from 6–10% each of the remaining cases. Paraphrenia was the least common diagnosis in this group, which was in contrast to the violent group in whom paraphrenia was the most common diagnosis.

The geriatric patients who used a weapon owned their own homes in most cases (i.e., they were not transients and had no history of a previous assault). Most of the aggressive patients were disoriented to time and place and were likely to have hit reflexively at attendants when bothered.

While one must be cautious about generalizing these findings in applying them to geriatric patients in the community, several points deserve attention. Violent behavior seems more likely to occur in patients with paraphrenia, who direct their violence toward their imagined prosecutors, than in patients with any other psychiatric disorder. Patients with senile dementia are more likely to be aggressive than violent. Serious violence may be a problem with some older patients. Almost all of these patients have responded well to treatment. Neuroleptics were used successfully in the violent group, but the aggressive patients responded to a highly structured ward environment and neuroleptics often were not necessary.[25]

References

1. Gurland BJ, Cross PS: Epidemiology of psychopathology in old age: Some implications for clinical services. In Jarvik LF, Small GW (eds): *The Psychiatric Clinics of North America.* Philadelphia, WB Saunders Co, 1982, vol 5, pp 11–26.
2. Simon A: The neuroses, personality disorders, alcoholism, drug use and misuse, and crime in the aged, in Birren JE, Sloane RB (eds): *Handbook of Mental Health and Aging.* Englewood Cliffs, NJ, Prentice-Hall, 1980, pp 653–670.
3. Bergmann K: Neurosis and personality disorder in old age, in Isaacs AD, Post F (eds): *Studies in Geriatric Psychiatry.* New York, John Wiley & Sons, 1978, pp 41–75.
4. Mueller C cited in Brocklehurst JC (ed): *Textbook of Geriatric Medicine and Gerontology,* ed 2. Edinburgh, Churchill Livingstone, 1978, p 188.
5. Pearson H: *The Smith of Smiths.* New York, Harper & Bros, 1934, p 314.
6. Hall RCW: Anxiety, in Hall RCW (ed): *Psychiatric Presentations of Medical Illness; Somatopsychic Disorders.* New York, Spectrum, 1980, pp 13–35.
7. Dietch JT: Diagnosis of organic anxiety disorders. *Psychosomatics* 22:661–669, 1981.
8. Busse EW, Dovenmuehle RH, Brown RG: Psychoneurotic reactions in the aged. *Geriatrics* 15:97–105, 1960.
9. Pitt B: *Psychogeriatrics: An Introduction to Psychiatry of Old Age,* ed 2. London, Churchill Livingstone, 1982, pp 113, 121.

10. Gianturco DT, Busse EW: Psychiatric problems encountered during a long-term study of normal ageing volunteers, in Isaacs AD, Post F (eds): *Studies in Geriatric Psychiatry.* New York, John Wiley & Sons, 1978, pp 1–16.

11. Stengel E: *Suicide and Attempted Suicide.* London, Penguin, 1964, p 61.

12. Busse EW, Blazer D: Disorders related to biological functioning, in Busse EW, Blazer D (eds): *Handbook of Geriatric Psychiatry.* New York, Van Nostrand Reinhold Co, 1980, pp 390–414.

13. Slater E, Roth M: *Clinical Psychiatry,* ed 3. Baltimore, Williams & Wilkins, 1969, pp 578–579.

14. Manschreck TC, Petri M: The paranoid syndrome. *Lancet* ii:251–253, 1978.

15. Post F: *The Clinical Psychiatry of Late Life.* Oxford, England, Pergamon Press, 1965, p 112.

16. Slater E, Roth M: *Clinical Psychiatry.* Baltimore, Williams & Wilkins, 1969, p 583.

17. Post F: The Functional Psychosis, in Isaacs AD, Post F (eds): *Studies in Geriatric Psychiatry.* New York, John Wiley & Sons, 1978, pp 77–94.

18. Munro A: Paranoia revisited. *Br J Psychiatr* 141:344–349, 1982.

19. Varner RB, Gaitz CM: Schizophrenic and paranoid disorders in the aged, in Jarvik LF, Small GW (eds): *The Psychiatric Clinics of North America.* Philadelphia, WB Saunders Co, 1982, vol 5, pp 107–118.

20. Post F: Psychiatric disorders, in Brocklehurst JC (ed): *Textbook of Geriatric Medicine and Gerontology.* Edinburgh, Churchill Livingstone, 1978, pp 185–200.

21. Straker M: Adjustment disorders and personality disorders in the aged, in Jarvik LF, Small GW (eds): *The Psychiatric Clinics of North America.* 1982, vol 5, pp 121–129.

22. Verwoerdt A: Anxiety, dissociative and personality disorders in the elderly, in Busse EW, Blazer D (eds): *Handbook of Geriatric Psychiatry.* New York, Van Nostrand Reinhold Co, 1980, pp 368–380.

23. *Diagnostic and Statistical Manual of Mental Disorders,* ed 3. Washington DC, American Psychiatric Association, 1980.

24. Kafetz KK, Cox M: Alcohol excess and the senile squalor syndrome. *J Am Geriatr Soc* 30:706, 1982.

25. Petrie WM, Lawson EC, Hollender MH: Violence in geriatric patients. *JAMA* 248:443–444, 1982.

PART IV

Pharmacology

CHAPTER 38

General Principles

MICHAEL MYERS, R.PH.
DIANE E. MEIER, M.D.
JOHN R. WALSH, M.D.

Of all people over 65 years of age, 85% have one or more chronic diseases that may require medications for proper management. The judicious use of drugs in elderly persons can improve their well-being and quality of life, and the benefit of appropriate medication should not be withheld simply because of old age. Nonetheless, a clinician must prescribe drugs sensibly and cautiously, with the realization that every problem cannot be solved with drug therapy, that no drug will successfully reverse the aging process, and that adverse drug reactions are more common in elderly persons. A good rule in prescribing for an older patient is to use the minimal number of drugs and the simplest regimen.

Elderly persons have more illnesses, take more than 25% of all prescription medications, and have a higher incidence of side effects than their younger counterparts. Elderly persons with multiple concurrent problems receive from 3–12 drugs per day, which do not include over-the-counter preparations such as analgesics, laxatives and antacids. There is a 2–7-fold higher incidence rate of adverse drug reactions in elderly persons as compared to young adults.[1,2] The rate of adverse drug reactions progressively increases with each decade. Adverse drug effects are twice as common in a 70–80-year-old patient population compared to a 40–50-year-old patient population (12–25% versus 7.5–12%).[1] About 5% of hospital admissions are a consequence of adverse drug reactions.[3] Complications due to drugs are a frequent occurrence in the hospital setting, with a significantly greater number occurring in pa-

tients over 60 years of age.[4–6] Approximately 75% of all drug reactions are predictable and preventable. A clinician must anticipate problems with drugs, especially those that cause syncope, depression, or anticholinergic side effects. Medication problems especially must be anticipated in nursing homes where residents have three or more concurrent problems for which they are receiving between four to seven different drugs each day.[7–9] This frail elderly group with borderline physiological reserves are ingesting large doses of potent medications that cause problems that often are mistakenly attributed to the degenerative effects of age.

Cardiovascular drugs (e.g., digitalis, diuretics, antihypertensives), psychotropic drugs (e.g., sedatives, antidepressants, antipsychotics), and antiarthritic drugs (e.g., aspirin, nonsteroidal anti-inflammatory drugs [NSAID's]) frequently are used by elderly persons and are more likely to produce adverse reactions; therefore, they will be discussed in detail in the following chapters.

Drug Compliance in Elderly Persons

Clinicians often assume that most patients adhere to their prescribed medication schedule. Actually, up to 50% of all patients fail to take their medicine as prescribed. Over 50% of elderly outpatients make at least one drug error, and over 25% make potentially serious medication errors.[10–13] Patients who err make an average of 2.6 medication errors per patient.[10] The consequences of non-adherence to prescribed drug regimens are poorer health for an older patient and a waste of human and fiscal resources as doctors prescribe pointlessly, medicines are bought and not used, and hospital beds are filled with patients with drug-related difficulties.[14]

Non-compliance with therapy usually indicates an error of omission (not taking enough of a drug), but the overuse of a medication, incorrect use of a medication, or the use of drugs not prescribed by a physician, also are included in this definition. It may be intentional or unintentional.

The causes of poor compliance with medical regimens are multiple and complex. Once suspected or determined, the various causes must be explored in an attempt to correct the problem. Discontinuation of a medication is the most common problem that accounts for about 50% of non-compliance.[10] Certain types of illness are more likely to engender non-adherence to a regimen, particularly chronic diseases such as hypertension and tuberculosis in which an omission of therapy leads to no symptomatic change in a patient's state of well-being. Conversely, medications whose discontinuation leads to undesirable symptoms such as shortness of breath, or pedal edema in a patient with congestive heart failure, are associated with higher rates of compliance. Psychiatric illnesses or a memory loss may limit a patient's ability to take responsibility for a drug regimen. Multiple chronic disease processes may limit the ability of a person to take medication properly.[15] For example, decreased vision and severe arthritis may inhibit compliance through simple inability to read instructions and to open pill bottles. Conversely, a patient may be unwilling to become dependent on medications, may be confused about the indications for the drug, may deny the disease process and need for treatment, and have high levels of fear or anxiety about the illness.[16] Loneliness and a sense of isolation and helplessness in relation to the health care providers sometimes encourage a rejection of the proffered assistance.[17]

Economic and social factors may hinder compliance in obvious ways. Elderly patients with fixed incomes often cannot afford drug regimens that are prescribed for them.[18] They may try to stretch their medicines by decreasing the dose or frequency. Older people may not have safe access or transportation to a pharmacy.[18] Differing values and cultural mores may discourage reliance on the technology of modern medicine and lead to non-compliance. An unstable or non-supportive living situation also impairs an elderly person's ability to adhere to a medication schedule.[16]

The drug regimen itself may be prohibitively complicated (e.g., many drugs and frequent doses) and result in a partial or complete non-adherence to the prescriptions.[15,16] This is particularly true in patients who are taking more than three types of medicines, on varying schedules, and for different indications. Regimens that require more than three drugs, or drugs given more frequently than twice per day, have been associated with poor compliance.[19] The similarity in appearance of the pills sometimes leads to mistakes. Unpleasant effects that are associated with medications lead to poor compliance.[15,16] For instance, confusion, drowsiness, and a blurring of vision that result from psychotropic or cardiovascular medication will discourage patients from continuing to take the medication.[20]

About 20% of all non-compliance is due to a lack of knowledge about the reasons for, and uses of, the drug.[10] For example, older patients may take their digoxin ("heart pill") whenever they have angina or increased ankle swelling.[20] A failure of communication about the indications for the drug, and inadequate instruction regarding its use and side effects,[15] are responsible for these misconceptions. The physician-patient relationship affects compliance through such variables as trust, reassurance, physician optimism, and belief in the efficacy of the treatment.[15,16] Thus, patients who are cared for in a clinical setting by several different doctors are at greater risk for inconsistent, confusing, and (possibly) dangerous prescribing. Adequate communication between a patient's physicians is essential.[21] Intentional non-adherence to a drug regimen usually is due to a patient's perception that the drug is not needed in the dosage prescribed,[22] or it may be due to intolerable side effects. In either case, intentional non-compliance should suggest to a physician that a different drug or dosage is more appropriate, or that further patient education is needed. Other patients who do not adhere to their medication regimen may be expressing a desire for greater autonomy and initiative, which is a behavior that precludes reliance on just one source of information or advice.[23] Such persons often use several physicians and several pharmacies. A careful non-judgmental drug history is necessary to elicit this information.

Other sources of error include the use of old medications that are no longer indicated and the practice of obtaining drugs from friends or over the counter. Under these circumstances, there is a risk of a serious drug interaction. A physician must specifically question a patient about all medicines, including those that are purchased over the counter. When changes in the regimen are prescribed, a patient should be advised to destroy the medications that will no longer be used.[22] Drug labels often are unreadable and incomprehensible, and child-proof or tamper-proof containers frequently are impossible for an elderly patient to open.[11]

Verbal, written, and telephone instructions, with frequent repetition have been effective measures in improving compliance in elderly persons.[15-20] Positive reinforcement occurs by written schedules that specify the drug and time of day for it to be taken, color coding (e.g., a red dot on a digoxin bottle and one next to the word "digoxin" on the written medication schedule), and also having a sample pill taped to the schedule with explanatory information (e.g., the words "to prevent chest pain" next to isosorbide dinitrate).[24-29] A copy of the medication schedule that is given to a family member or neighbor may be helpful. Color-coded weekly pill trays also have been useful.[28] In addition, large-print labels that state a drug's purpose and are affixed to a pill bottle (e.g., "water pill" on the furosemide container) may improve compliance.[21] Educating the family, care-giver or neighbors, if a patient is agreeable, may assist in reinforcing the correct uses for the drugs.[24-29] A simplification of the schedule, with minimum numbers of medicines at minimal frequency, contributes to accurate and safe drug taking.[10-16] Inpatients benefit from a practice period of drug self-administration before being discharged from a hospital.[24]

Eliciting a medication history aids in the identification of persons who may need more teaching or assistance at home.[10] Specific inquiries into the use of other physicians, pharmacies, over-the-counter drugs, and old prescriptions should be made. Verbal and written explanations of the purpose, side effects, and duration of therapy all must be given and repeated at frequent intervals. Reassurance about the safety of the medicine when taken correctly is crucial, because many older patients harbor significant and justifiable anxieties and concerns about the modern pharmacopoiea.[22] The time spent talking to a patient will improve the chances that he or she actually will swallow the medicines that the physician has prescribed. Thus time often is the rate-limiting step in the therapeutic process.[15,16]

The term "non-compliance" has a distinctly negative connotation that implies fault and blame. Both physicians and their patients must take responsibility for the provision of optimal health care. A sense of guilt and personal failure on the part of either party does not contribute to an effective physician-patient relationship, which is a prerequisite to successful drug therapy.[10,22]

Efforts to improve compliance require, foremost, a heightened level of concern about the problem with health care providers. Elderly persons, as a group, are particularly susceptible to problems with their medications; also, poverty, sensory deprivation, and isolation are additive risk factors. An awareness of these issues and a willingness to address them openly will reward a physician's diagnostic and therapeutic efforts with healthier patients. The pharmacy service of the American Association of Retired Persons (AARP) have shown leadership by preparing and distributing specially written drug information pamphlets for elderly persons who use medications (see Figure 38-1).

Pharmacokinetic Principles

The aging process produces physiologic changes that may affect drug distribution and kinetics. Ideally, the effects of aging on drug pharmacokinetics should be determined by longitudinal studies, which monitor individual subjects over long periods of time. Unfortunately, time and expense preclude this approach. Consequently, most age-related kinetic studies are cross-sectional; they compare groups of elderly subjects to young subjects. While this approach

Important Information about You and your Medication...

Digoxin

Name of your medication: Digoxin

Other names: Lanoxin

What is it? A heart pill

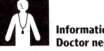 **What is it for?**

It may be used to:
- Strengthen your heart beat.
- Regulate your heart beat (if beat is too fast or irregular).

How long will you have to take it?
- At one time it was believed that once started, you would take it for the rest of your life. This may not be true.
- Every six months ask your doctor if you still need Digoxin.

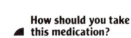 **How should you take this medication?**
- Take your Digoxin according to directions.
- Do not take more than prescribed.
- Take your Digoxin *at the same time each day*.
- If you forget to take a dose, take it as soon as you remember.
- If you do not remember until the next day, do not take two doses.
- Take only the dose or doses scheduled for that day.

 Provided by AARP Pharmacy Service with the assistance and cooperation of the U.S. Food and Drug Administration and experts in geriatric medicine and pharmacy.

Things to remember:
- Do *NOT* change brands of Digoxin.
- This is a necessary drug but there is a narrow range between helpful and harmful amounts of Digoxin in your body.
- You must be particularly careful if you also take diuretics or water pills.
- Your doctor may suggest you eat foods rich in potassium, such as bananas, oranges, or tomato juice.
- You may urinate (pass water) more often than usual for the first day or two after you start taking Digoxin.
- Do not stop taking this medication if you feel better.

Information your Doctor needs:
Do you have or have you ever had:
- Kidney or liver disease?
- Thyroid disorders?

Are you taking:
- Antacids?
- Antibiotics?
- Cortisone-like steroid drugs?
- Cough and cold preparations?
- Laxatives or drugs for diarrhea?
- Quinidine?
- Water pills?

Possible side effects:
Call your doctor immediately if you notice:
- Weakness, fatigue, depression, apathy, or mental confusion. You may not notice. Ask the help of family, friends, and neighbors.

(Continued)

- Loss of appetite, nausea, vomiting, stomach ache, or diarrhea.
- Colored vision (especially green or yellow), blurred or dimmed vision, halos (rings) or spots.
- A change in your usual heart rate — a marked increase, decrease, or irregular heart beat.
- Muscle pains, leg cramps.

If these or other side effects bother you, call your doctor.

Please remember:
- If you want more information about this drug, ask your doctor for a more technical leaflet, the professional label.
- Tell your doctor *all* medications you are currently taking, whether they are prescription or non-prescription drugs.
- Keep this and all drugs out of reach of children.
- If there is a chance you are or will become pregnant or breast-feed a child, please contact your doctor before taking this drug.

3.82 55M ©1982 Retired Persons Services, Inc.

FIGURE 38-1   An example of a drug information leaflet for elderly persons. (Prepared by the American Association of Retired Persons (AARP) with the assistance and cooperation of the United States Food and Drug Administration and experts in geriatric medicine and pharmacology, used by permission.)

is more practical than the longitudinal study, it also presents problems in study design, data analysis, and interpretation.

There are other problems that complicate the design and interpretation of drug kinetic studies in elderly persons. The presence of underlying diseases in study subjects raises the question about whether the kinetic change is due to aging or to disease. In addition, a wide variation may exist between biologic and chronologic aging. A group of elderly persons of similar age will contain individuals at widely varying points on the continuum of physiologic aging. Even if study subjects are as free as possible of concomitant disease, it is unlikely that the elderly subjects will be as homogeneous as the control group. Study subjects must be screened for the drug interactions that are so common in this group, which may alter the kinetics of the drug being studied.

Drug Absorption

The effects of aging on drug absorption have not been systematically studied. Most information currently available on drug absorption in elderly persons either is extrapolated from animal data, based on inferences from studies on the absorption of sugars, vitamins, and minerals, or gathered from kinetic studies that look primarily at distribution or elimination. Few studies have been designed to specifically determine the absorption characteristics of elderly persons.

Several physiologic consequences of aging may influence drug absorption.[30] The rate of gastric emptying is delayed and gastrointestinal motility is decreased. Thus, the rate or extent of drug absorption may be changed due to an altered gastrointestinal transport. Gastric pH levels rise and may alter drug absorption by changing the degree of ionization and solubility. Regional blood flow changes result in a decreased splanchnic blood flow, which may decrease or delay drug absorption.

The aging process also appears to affect active transport absorption systems. The absorption of galactose, thiamine, calcium, and dextrose is reduced in elderly persons.[30] Most drugs, however, are absorbed by passive diffusion; differences in absorption between young and old persons via this route are variable. The rate and extent of absorption are similar for acetaminophen, phenylbutazone, and sulphamethazole.[31] The rate of digoxin absorption was delayed slightly in a group of elderly subjects, but the fraction that was absorbed was unchanged compared to a young control group.[32] In contrast, xylose absorption, which reflects the passive transport ability, shows a 40–50% reduction with age in the amount that is absorbed. In a group of seven elderly males 66–78 years of age, the absorption of prazosin was reduced by 30%.[33]

The absorption of a number of benzodiazepines has been examined. Elderly patients have lower blood levels of the active metabolite desmethyldiazepam after receiving 20 mg of chlorazepate dipotassium.[34] While not conclusively proven, the authors suggest that this decrease was due to the increased volume of distribution in elderly persons rather than to decreased absorption. The absorption of lorazepam and clobazam is unaffected by age or sex.[36,37] The absorption half-life was prolonged in elderly subjects who were receiving prazepam, but the increase was statistically significant only in male subjects.[35] The time to a peak concentration of desalkylflurazepam, which is the active metabolite of flurazepam, also showed sex- and age-related differences.[38] The mean time to a peak concentration for young males was 4.1 hours compared to 23.3 hours, 28.5 hours, and 17.6 hours for young females, elderly males, and elderly females, respectively.

In summary, the physiologic changes of aging may affect drug absorption; but the limited data that is available suggests that aging is not the major cause of altered drug absorption. More studies that are specifically designed to assess the impact of aging on drug absorption are needed.

Drug Distribution

The degree to which a drug is distributed within a biologic system depends on the physiochemical characteristics of the drug and the physiologic functioning of the subject. Age-related changes in body composition that influence drug distribution include an altered regional blood flow, body composition, and protein binding.

Cardiac output declines and blood flow to the liver and kidney decreases with aging. Cerebral, coronary, and skeletal muscle circulations are minimally influenced by the decreased cardiac output, although arteriosclerotic changes may reduce the blood flow in these areas. An altered blood flow has a major impact on drug elimination by the liver and kidney; however, it also may produce an altered tissue distribution, which depends on the drug involved and the areas affected by the altered circulation.

Changes in body composition may influence drug distribution. Elderly persons have both a decreased lean body mass and total body water

(TBW). In males, the decreased TBW is due to decreased intracellular fluid with little change in extracellular fluid (ECF).[39] The percentage of the total body composition that is fat increases with age in both males and females. Between 18–85 years of age, body fat increases from 18–36% of the total weight in males and from 33–48% in females.[40]

These changes may influence the distribution of drugs, which depends on the solubility of the drug. Drugs that distribute through the TBW, such as ethanol, have a decreased volume of distribution.[41] Gentamicin and tobramycin, which are primarily distributed through the ECF show little change in their volume of distribution with increasing age.[42,43] In contrast, lipid-soluble drugs (e.g., the benzodiazepines) have larger volumes of distribution due to the greater percentage of fat in elderly persons.[34,37] The volume of distribution of lorazepam, which is a less lipid-soluble benzodiazepine, is not significantly different in elderly persons.[36] Table 38-1 illustrates the effects of aging on the volume of distribution of a variety of drugs.

The binding of drugs by plasma proteins is potentially altered in elderly persons due to decreases in the plasma albumin level. Some decrease in the serum albumin level may occur with aging itself, but more significant changes occur with underlying diseases. An increase in the free fraction of a drug due to decreased plasma protein binding may: 1) Enhance the pharmacologic effect, since only the unbound drug is active; 2) Increase the volume of distribution by making more of the drug available for distribution; and 3) Alter the elimination rate, since the free drug is available for metabolism or excretion. These factors are most critical with highly protein-bound drugs that have a narrow therapeutic index, such as warfarin or phenytoin. Decreased plasma protein binding in elderly persons exists for phenytoin, warfarin, temazepam, clobazam, and tolbutamide; but, no effect was found on the protein binding of prazepam, isoproterenol, or propranolol (see Table 38-1).

Drug Metabolism

The liver is the major site of drug metabolism, and the effects of aging on hepatic functioning are difficult to quantify. Unlike renal function-

ing, there is no simple test to directly measure the metabolic ability of the liver. Therefore, most studies determine the hepatic function indirectly by measuring the elimination rate of drugs that are metabolized by the liver. Antipyrine often is used, because it is rapidly and completely absorbed from the gastrointestinal tract, is distributed in TBW with little protein binding, is almost completely metabolized by the liver with a low hepatic extraction ratio, and has negligible renal elimination. Studies that use antipyrine have provided information about the environmental effects on drug distribution; nonetheless, the results of antipyrine tests cannot be extrapolated quantitatively to all other drugs.[44]

Factors that enhance metabolic activity include: 1) Drugs such as barbiturates, disulfram, rifampin, and ascorbic acid; 2) Disease states such as hyperthyroidism and osteomalacia; and 3) Exogenous factors such as bed rest, cigarette smoking, and certain diets. Conversely, decreases in the rate of hepatic metabolism may be caused by: 1) Drugs such as cimetidine, allopurinol, delta-9-tetrahydrocannabinol, oral contraceptives, and amitriptyline; 2) Diseases such as hypothyroidism and lead poisoning; and 3) Certain environmental and dietary factors.[44] The multitude of factors that affect liver metabolism result in a wide spectrum of metabolic activity within any given study population.

Aside from the external factors that influence the liver function, the hepatic clearance of drugs is determined by both the intrinsic metabolic ability of the liver and the volume of the hepatic blood flow. Liver mass decreases with age, which results in fewer cells being available to metabolize drugs. The volume of hepatic blood flow decreases 40–45% by 65 years of age.

Characteristics of the drug itself are important in determining the effects of age on liver metabolism. The hepatic clearance of drugs with an intrinsic total clearance that is small relative to total liver blood flow is independent of the blood flow and is determined by the amount and efficacy of the liver enzymes available.[45] Antipyrine has a low extraction ratio and would be affected more by changes in liver mass than by a decreased liver blood flow. In contrast, the hepatic clearance of drugs with intrinsic total clearance, which is high compared to liver blood flow, is limited by the rate of hepatic blood flow.[45] The hepatic clearance of indocyanine green is reduced with age, which reflects a decrease in hepatic blood flow.[46]

The complex interaction of the above factors make it difficult to accurately predict the impact of aging on the drug-metabolizing ability of a given individual. However, there are a few general guidelines. The rate of hepatic drug metabolism declines in elderly persons. This occurs with antipyrine,[47] prazepam,[35] flurazepam,[38] and theophylline.[48] Cigarette smoking, which increases the hepatic metabolism in young subjects, only has a minor effect on elderly persons due to their decreased capacity for microsomal enzyme induction.[46] This suggests that the dosage of drugs with low extraction ratios should not be arbitrarily increased in elderly cigarette smokers. The metabolism of compounds that have high extraction ratios, such as indocyanine green,[47] propranolol,[49] and labetalol,[50] is decreased in elderly persons, possibly due to a decreased "first-pass" effect. These changes are not affected by smoking and reflect the impact of a decreased hepatic blood flow.[46]

In summary, the clearance of drugs that undergo hepatic metabolism is likely to be reduced in elderly persons. The extent to which the clearance is reduced is unpredictable and will depend on a complex interaction between the drug, the environment, and the physiologic changes in each person.

Renal Excretion

The kidney is the primary organ for eliminating drugs and their metabolites. The renal blood flow and, therefore, the glomerular filtration rate (GFR), decrease with increasing age (see Table 38-2).[51] The "normal" serum creatinine in elderly persons is due to a decreased creatinine production from a decreased lean body mass. The discrepancy between serum creatinine and creatinine clearance (Ccr) in elderly persons clearly supports the importance of basing decisions about the dosage for renally excreted drugs on the Ccr rather than on the serum creatinine value (see Volume I, Chapter 16).

Drugs excreted primarily by the kidney have a reduced renal clearance with aging. The aminoglycoside antibiotics are eliminated almost exclusively by glomerular filtration. The mean renal clearance of gentamicin falls from 88 ml/hour/kg in subjects 21–40 years of age to 53 ml/hour/kg in subjects older than 80 years of age.[42] Similarly, the clearance of digoxin is reduced by 52% in elderly persons.[32] Tubular secretion also appears to decline with increasing age. The clearance of procainamide in young subjects is four to five times that of their Ccr, which indicates an excretion by tubular secretion and glomerular filtration. This ratio falls to one to two times the Ccr in elderly persons.[52] A similar, but less dramatic, fall occurs in the ratio of N-acetylprocainamide clearance to Ccr in elderly persons.[52]

There are many other drugs excreted by the kidney that have not been studied in elderly persons. In a survey of 139 drugs used in impaired renal function, 37% (52) need dosage adjustments for Ccr rates less than 50 ml/minute, which will include most elderly patients with a "normal" renal function.[53]

Pharmacodynamics

The pharmacologic action of a drug is determined by the interaction of the drug and its receptor. Pharmacokinetic changes in an elderly person results in an increased or decreased quantity of the drug reaching the receptor and, hence, an increased or decreased response. An essentially unstudied aspect of the aging process is the impact of age on drug receptors. It is reasonable to assume that drug receptors are as dynamic as other living systems; however, demonstrating that changes occur is extremely difficult.

A single dose of nitrazepam impaired the psychomotor function in elderly persons to a greater extent than young subjects.[54] The mean dose of warfarin that is required to produce anticoagulation decreases with each decade of life.[55] Authors of these studies feel that increased receptor sensitivity is a possible explanation. Decreasing beta-adrenoceptor sensitivity to both an agonist (isoproterenol) and antagonist (propranolol) has been demonstrated with increasing age.[56] These findings suggest that pharmacodynamic changes exist, and they show the need for further study.

TABLE 38-1   Pharmacokinetics in Elderly Persons—A Summary of Selected Literature

Drug	Study Population	Population Size	Age Range (yrs)	Sex	Reference (see reference section)	Absorption
Gentamicin	Patients	1,640	1–97	Both	42	
Tobramycin	Patients	77	20–79	Both	43	
Cefuroxime	Patients	18	71–92	Both	60	
Sulphamethazole	Volunteer	13	22–91	Not stated	31	NE
Isoproterenol	Volunteer	27	21–73	Male	56	
Digoxin	Patients	13	34–91	Both	32	NE
Propranolol	Volunteer	27	21–73	Male	56	
Propranolol	Volunteer	27	21–73	Male	49	
Labetalol	Patients	10	28–75	Not stated	50	Increased bioavailability 3-fold in elderly
Prazosin	Volunteer	14	22–78	Male	33	Decreased 29%
Acetaminophen	Volunteer	32	23–78	Both	61	
Acetaminophen	Volunteer	13	22–91	Not stated	31	NE
Phenylbutazone	Volunteer	15	22–91	Not stated	31	NE
Phenytoin	Patients	44	18–87	Both	62	
Phenytoin	Patients	92	21–78	Both	63	
Phenytoin	Volunteer	28	28–82	Both	64	
Clorazepate	Volunteer	24	20–75	Both	34	Decreased (less likely)
Prazepam	Volunteer	29	22–85	Both	35	Rate decreased 296%
Flurazepam	Volunteer	26	19–85	Both	38	Delayed in males. NSS in females
Lorazepam	Volunteer	30	19–80	Both	36	
Temazepam	Volunteer	32	24–84	Both	65	

Volume of Distribution	Protein Binding	Half-Life	Total Body Clearance	Miscellaneous
NE		NE	Decreased in elderly NE Decreased with creatinine clearance	
NE		Increased 72%	Decreased 46%*	
	NE			Decreased chronotropic effect
Decreased 42%		Increased 186%	Decreased 52%	
	NE			Decreased response to given blood level
NE	NE	Increased 120%	Decreased	Greater decrease in smokers
NE		Increased		Increased bioavailability due to ↓ first-pass
Increased 141%		Increased 157%	NE	Increased T1/2 due to increased volume distribution
Decreased 16–18%		NE	Decreased 10%	
NE		Increased 20%	NE	
NE		NE		
	Unbound fraction increased 15%			
				V_{max} 20% decrease km = no change
Free drug Vd decreased 39%	Unbound fraction increased 50%	NE	Decreased 50%	
Increased (more likely)				†
Male = 160% increase. Female = NSS increase	NE	Male = 205% increase. Female = NSS increase Male = 210% increase. Female = NSS increase	Males decreased but NSS	Effects more marked in males
Decreased 11%			Decreased 22%	Little difference in non-smoker
NE	Decreased slightly	NE	NE	

(Continued)

TABLE 38-1   (Continued)

Drug	Study Population	Population Size	Age Range (yrs)	Sex	Reference (see reference section)	Absorption
Clobazam	Volunteer	29	18–72	Both	37	NE
Azapropazone	Patients	18	19–96	Not stated	66	
Tolbutamide	Volunteer	44	23–87	Male	67	
Levothyroxine	Patients	67	24–88	Both	68	
Theophylline	Volunteer	28	19–85	Both	48	
Theophylline	Patients	59	22–81	Both	69	
Cimetidine	Patients	35	20–86	Both	70	

Legend: Blank square = Not examined; NE = No effect seen or difference was not significant; NSS = Not statistically significant; Vd = volume of distribution; * = Clearance correlates with creatinine clearance. † = Decreased serum level of desmethyldiazepam compared to young group.

Drug-Induced Anticholinergic Effects

Drugs with anticholinergic effects are used extensively in elderly persons. Major classes of drugs with anticholinergic effects are belladonna alkaloids, antiparkinson drugs, tricyclic antidepressants, antipsychotics, antihistamines, and some antiarrhythmics. The concurrent use of these agents is common in elderly persons; therefore, they are at a high risk for developing anticholinergic side effects. Adverse side effects include not only the usual anticholinergic actions, but often unanticipated effects. The clinical picture is variable and ranges from dry mouth, constipation, blurred vision, tachycardia, hyperthermia, and flushed faces to urinary retention, confusion, visual hallucinations, picking at bedclothes, grasping at imaginary objects, agitation, somnolence, and even coma.[57] Some older people do not have classic symptoms and may be treated for delirium, dementia, or psychosis, without a consideration of the possible relationship of these disorders to anticholinergic medications.[57] In fact, elderly patients with a bladder outlet obstruction from prostatic enlargement, who previously have been able to cope with the frequency and nocturia, may have a worsening of urinary retention or even may develop overflow incontinence after receiving an anticholinergic drug. Patients who are receiving combinations of drugs with anticholinergic properties more often develop severe complications. For example, a patient who is taking a phenothiazine preparation for

TABLE 38-2   Average Creatinine Clearance (Ccr) in Males with Normal Serum Creatinine by Decade

Age (yr)	Serum Creatinine (mg/100 ml)	Clearance (ml/min per 1.73 m^2)
20–29	0.99 + 0.16	110
30–39	1.14 + 0.22	97
40–49	1.10 + 0.20	88
50–59	1.16 + 0.17	81
60–69	1.15 + 0.14	72
70–79	1.03 + 0.22	64
80–89	1.06 + 0.25	47
90–99	1.20 + 0.16	34

Volume of Distribution	Protein Binding	Half-Life	Total Body Clearance	Miscellaneous
Male = 60% increase. Female = 33% increase NE	Unbound increased male = 6%, female = 12%	Male = 187% increase. Female = 58% increase Increased 172% (wide variation)	Male = 42% decrease. Female = NSS Decreased 47%	
	Unbound fraction increased slightly			
				Dose needed decreased by 25%
Decreased 37% for unbound drug	Increased for unbound drug		Decreased 30% for unbound drug NE Renal clearance decreased 3–4 fold	

agitation develops extrapyramidal symptoms for which an antiparkinson drug (trihexphenydyl, denztropine, procyclidine, or biperiden) is administered. The additive anticholinergic effect will predictably aggravate urinary retention, constipation, glaucoma, or even cause mental confusion. The simultaneous use of neuroleptic, tricyclic, and antiparkinson drugs is not uncommon. Thirteen percent of all patients taking tricyclics and 35% of all patients over 40 years of age who are treated with phenothiazines plus antiparkinson drugs develop toxic confusional states.[59] Older people who are troubled with constipation may notice a worsening of symptoms when taking a drug with anticholinergic properties. A clinician must anticipate the possibility of fecal impaction in this setting. A diminished salivary flow and dry mouth may cause poor dietary intake and malnutrition. Poor motor coordination with falls, ataxia, dysarthria, and muscular weakness may suggest neurologic disease. Hyperthermia and heat stroke or heat exhaustion may be induced by anticholinergic drugs. Drugs with anticholinergic effects that often are used in surgical procedures may impair cognitive functioning and produce delirium. High serum levels of an anticholinergic drug usually accompanies the delirium.[58]

The management of adverse effects due to anticholinergic drugs simply requires a discontinuation of the offending medication. For serious side effects, physostigmine (1–2 mg administered-intramuscularly) may produce a dramatic improvement, thereby confirming this diagnosis.[59] Physostigmine inhibits acetyl cholinesterase and enhances the action of acetylcholine; however, it is short acting and improvement may be brief. It may be given every 30–60 minutes, which depends on the severity of the problem and the clinical course.

References

1. Vestal RE: Drug use in the elderly: A review of problems and special considerations. *Drugs* 16:358–382, 1978.
2. Hurwitz N: Predisposing factors in adverse reaction to drugs. *Br Med J* 1:536–539, 1969.
3. Melmon KL: Preventable drug reactions—

causes and cures. *N Engl J Med* 284:1361–1368, 1974.

4. Hurwitz N, Wade OL: Intensive hospital monitoring of adverse reaction to drugs. *Br Med J* 1:539, 1969.

5. Steel K, Gertman P, Crescenzi BS, et al: Iatrogenic illness on a general medical service at a university hospital. *N Engl J Med* 304:638–642, 1981.

6. Jahnigen D, Hannon C, Laxson L, et al: Iatrogenic disease in hospitalized elderly veterans. *J Am Geriatr Soc* 30:387–390, 1982.

7. Hamilton SF: Therapeutic problems and nursing home patients. *Drug Intell Clin Pharm* 10:703–707, 1976.

8. Kalchthaler T, Corcaro E, Lichtiger S: Incidence of polypharmacy in a long-term care facility. *J Am Geriatr Soc* 25:308–313, 1977.

9. Howard JB, Strong KE, Facnha SR, et al: Medication procedures in a nursing home: Abuse of PRN orders. *J Am Geriatr Soc* 25:83–84, 1977.

10. Schwartz D, Wang M, Geitz L, et al: Medication errors made by elderly chronically ill patients. *Am J Pub Health* 52:2018–2029, 1962.

11. Blackwell B: The drug defaulter. *Clin Pharm & Ther* 13:84–88, 1972.

12. Neely E, Patric ML: Problems of aged persons taking medications at home. *Nurs Res* 17:52–55, 1968.

13. Parkin DM, Henney CR, Quirk J, et al: Deviation from prescribed drug treatment after discharge from hospital. *Br Med J* 2:686–688, 1976.

14. Lundin DV, Dros A, Melloh J, et al: Education of independent elderly in the responsible use of prescription medications. *Drug Intell Clin Pharm* 335:342, 1980.

15. Blackwell B: Patient compliance. *N Engl J Med* 289:249–252, 1973.

16. Billum RF, Barsky AJ: Diagnosis and management of patient noncompliance. *JAMA* 228:1563–1567, 1974.

17. Purtilo R: Loneliness, the need for solitude, and compliance, in Withersty DJ (ed): *Communication and Compliance in a Hospital Setting.* Springfield, Ill, Charles C Thomas Publisher, 1979.

18. Brand FN, Smith RT, Brand PA: Effect of economic barriers to medical area on patients' noncompliance. *Pub Health Rep* 92:72–78, 1977.

19. Bergman U, Wilholm BE: Patient medication on admission to a medical clinic. *Eur J Clin Pharm* 20:85, 1981.

20. Smith R: Use of drugs in the aged. *Johns Hopkins Med J* 145:61–64, 1979.

21. Ramsay LE, Tucker GT: Drugs and the elderly. *Br Med J* 282:125–126, 1981.

22. Swift CG: Clinical pharmacology in the elderly. *Scot Med J* 1981:221–225, 1979.

23. Cooper JK, Lowe DW, Raffoul PR: Intentional prescription nonadherence (noncompliance) by the elderly. *J Am Geriatr Soc* 30:329–333, 1982.

24. Wandless I, Davie JW: Can drug compliance in the elderly be improved? *Br Med J* 1:359–361, 1977.

25. Libow LS, Mehl B: Self-administration of medications by patients in hospitals or extended care facilities. *J Am Geriatr Soc* 18:81–85, 1970.

26. Garnett WR, David LJ, McKenney JM, et al: Effect of telephone follow-up on medication compliance. *Am J Hosp Pharm* 38:676–679, 1981.

27. Crichton EF, Smith DL, Demanuele F: Patient recall of medication information. *Drug Intell Clin Pharm* 12:591–599, 1978.

28. Martin DC, Mead K: Reducing medication errors in a geriatric population. *J Am Geriatr Soc* 30:258–260, 1982.

29. Atkinson L, Gibson I, Andrews J: An investigation into the ability of elderly patients to take prescribed drugs after discharge from hospital and recommendations concerning improving the situation. *Gerontology* 24:225–234, 1978.

30. Bender AD: Effect of age on intestinal absorption: Implications for drug absorption in the elderly. *J Am Geriatr Soc* 16:1331–1339, 1968.

31. Triggs EJ, Nation RL, Long A, et al: Pharmacokinetics in the elderly. *Eur J Clin Pharmacol* 8:55–62, 1975.

32. Cusack B, Kelly J, O'Malley K, et al: Digoxin in the elderly: Pharmacokinetic consequences of old age. *Clin Pharmacol Ther* 25:772–776, 1979.

33. Rubin PC, Scott PJW, Reid JL: Prazosin distribution in young and elderly subjects. *Br J Clin Pharmacol* 12:401–404, 1981.

34. Ochs HR, Greenblatt DJ, Allen MD, et al: Effect of age and bilroth gastrectomy on absorption of desmethyldiazepan from clorazepate. *Clin Pharmacol Ther* 26:449–456, 1979.

35. Allen MD, Greenblatt DJ, Harmatz JS, et al: Desmethyldiazepam kinetics in the elderly after oral prazepam. *Clin Pharmacol Ther* 28:196–202, 1980.

36. Greenblatt DJ, Allen MD, Locniskar A, et al: Lorazepam kinetics in the elderly. *Clin Pharmacol Ther* 26:103–113, 1979.

37. Greenblatt DJ, Divoll M, Surendra KP, et al: Clobazam kinetics in the elderly. *Br J Clin Pharmacol* 12:631–636, 1981.

38. Greenblatt DJ, Divoll M, Harmatz JS, et al: Kinetics and clinical effects of flurazepam in young and elderly noninsomniacs. *Clin Pharmacol Ther* 30:475–486, 1981.

39. Shock NW, Watkin DM, Yiengst MJ, et al: Age

differences in the water content of the body as related to basal oxygen consumption in males. *J Gerontol* 18:1–8, 1963.

40. Novak LP: Aging, total body potassium, fat free mass and cell mass in inalesand females between the ages 18 and 85 years. *J Gerontol* 27:438–443, 1972.

41. Vestal RE, McGuire EA, Tobin JD, et al: Aging and ethanol metabolism. *Clin Pharmacol Ther* 21:343–354, 1977.

42. Zaske DE, Cipolle RJ, Rotschafer JC, et al: Gentamicin pharmacokinetics in 1,640 patients: Method for control of serum concentrations. *Antimicrob Agents Chemother* 21:407–411, 1982.

43. Bauer LA, Blouin RA: Influence of age on tobramycin pharmacokinetics in patients with normal renal function. *Antimicrob Agents Chemother* 20:587–589, 1981.

44. Vesell ES: The antipyrine test in clinical pharmacology: Conceptions and misconceptions. *Clin Pharmacol Ther* 26:275–286, 1979.

45. Wilkinson GR: Influence of liver in pharmacokinetic, in Evans W, Schentag JJ, Jusko W (eds): *Applied Pharmacokinetics: Principles of Therapeutic Drug Monitoring*. San Francisco, Applied Therapeutics, Inc, 1980, pp 57–59.

46. Vestal RE, Wood AJJ: Influence of age and smoking on drug kinetics in man. *Clin Pharmacokinet* 5:309–319, 1980.

47. Wood AJJ, Vestal RE, Wilkinson GR, et al: Effect of aging and cigarette smoking on antipyrine and indocyanine green elimination. *Clin Pharmacol Ther* 26:16–20, 1979.

48. Antal EJ, Kramer PA, Merick SA, et al: Theophylline pharmacokinetics in advanced age. *Br J Clin Pharmacol* 12:637–645, 1981.

49. Vestal RE, Wood AJJ, Branch RA, et al: Effects of age and cigarette smoking on propranolol disposition. *Clin Pharmacol Ther* 26(suppl 1):8–15, 1979.

50. Kelly JG, McGarry K, O'Malley K, et al: Bioavailability of labetalol increases with age. *Br J Clin Pharmacol* 14:304–305, 1982.

51. Friedman SA, Raizner AE, Rosen H, et al: Functional defects in the aging kidney. *Ann Int Med* 76:41–45, 1972.

52. Reidenberg NM, Camacho M, Kluger J, et al: Aging and renal clearance of procainamide and acetylprocainamide. *Clin Pharmacol Ther* 28:732–735, 1980.

53. Bennett WM, Muther RS, Parker RA, et al: Drug therapy in renal failure: Dosing guidelines for adults. *Ann Int Med* 93(part 1) 62–89, (part 2) 286–325, 1980.

54. Castleden CM, George CF, Marcer D, et al: In-

creased sensitivity to nitrazepam in old age. *Br Med J* 1:10–12, 1977.

55. Routledge PA, Chapman PH, Davies DM, et al: Factors affecting warfarin requirements. *Eur J Clin Pharmacol* 15:319–322, 1979.

56. Vestal RE, Wood AJJ, Shand DG: Reduced B-adrenoceptor sensitivity in the elderly. *Clin Pharmacol Ther* 26:181–186, 1979.

57. Blazer DG, Federspicel CF, Ray WA, et al: The risk of anticholinergic toxicity in the elderly: A study of prescribing practices in two populations. *J Gerontol* 38:31–35, 1983.

58. Tune LE, Holland A, Feldstein MJ, et al: Association of postoperative delirium with raised serum levels of anticholinergic drugs. *Lancet* 2:651–653, 1981.

59. Hall RCW, Feinsilver DL, Hott RE: Anticholinergic psychosis: Differential diagnosis and management, *Psychosomatics* 22:581–587, 1981.

60. Broekhuysen J, Deyer F, Douchamps J, et al: Pharmacokinetic study of cefuroxime in the elderly. *Br J Clin Pharmac* 12:801–805, 1981.

61. Divoll M, Abernathy DR, Ameer B, et al: Acetaminophen kinetics in the elderly. *Clin Pharmacol Ther* 31:151–156, 1982.

62. Patterson M, Heazelwood R, Smithurst B, et al: Plasma protein binding of phenytoin in the aged: In vitro studies. *Br J Clin Pharmac* 13:423–425, 1982.

63. Bauer L, Blouin R: Age and phenytoin kinetics in adult epileptics. *Clin Pharmacol Ther* 31:301–304, 1982.

64. Bach B, Hansen JM, Kampmann JP, et al: Disposition of antipyrine and phenytoin correlated with age and liver volume in man. *Clin Pharmacokinet* 6:389–396, 1981.

65. Divoll M, Greenblatt DJ, Harmatz JS, et al: Effects of age and gender on the disposition of temazepam. *J Clin Pharmacol* 22:5A, 1982.

66. Ritch AES, Perera WNR, Jones CJ: Pharmacokinetics of azapropazone in the elderly. *Br J Clin Pharmac* 14:116–119, 1982.

67. Adir J, Miller AK, Vestal RE: Effects of total plasma concentration and age on tolbutamide plasma protein binding. *Clin Pharmacol Ther* 31:488–493, 1982.

68. Rosenbaum RL, Barzel US: Levothyroxine replacement dose for primary hypothyroidism decreases with age. *Ann Int Med* 96:53–55, 1982.

69. Bauer LA, Blouin RA: Influence of age on theophylline clearance in patients with chronic obstructive pulmonary disease. *Clin Pharmacokinet* 6:469–474, 1981.

70. Drayer DE, Romankiewicz J, Lorenzo B, et al: Age and renal clearance of cimetidine. *Clin Pharmacol Ther* 31:45–50, 1982.

CHAPTER 39

Cardiovascular Drugs

DIANE E. MEIER, M.D.

Digoxin

The effect of aging on drug disposition is particularly relevant when using medication with a narrow therapeutic ratio, as exemplified by digoxin.[1] Digitalis glycosides function as inotropic agents by inhibiting the sodium-potassium-ATPase-dependent pump of the sarcolemma. This effect is linear and dose-related in animal studies indicating that there is no threshold for the contractile effects of digitalis.[2] Digitalis induced electrophysiologic changes in the action potential lead to an increased automaticity, decreased conduction velocity, and decreased effective refractory period. Autonomic nervous system alterations lead to an increased vagal tone and decreased sympathetic tone at lower doses; but, at higher doses, there is an increase in the sympathetic outflow that is secondary to hypothalamic and brainstem stimulation.[3,4] These effects combine to cause a shortening of the atrial effective refractory period, a prolonged atrioventricular effective refractory period, and a slowed atrioventricular conduction (manifested as a lengthened PR-interval) or a slowing of the ventricular rate in atrial flutter or fibrillation. The Purkinje system and atrioventricular function undergo an enhanced diastolic depolarization and have an increased automaticity. In a failing heart, digitalis increases myocardial contractility and cardiac output, reverses sympathetically mediated vasoconstriction, and leads to both a net decrease in vascular tone and a net reduction in myocardial oxygen consumption.[4]

Pharmacokinetics

Digoxin normally is absorbed in the upper small intestine. The oral bioavailability of digoxin in tablet form is about 70% because of incomplete gastrointestinal tract absorption.[4] Gastrointestinal tract dysfunction, other than a jejunal-ileal bypass or extensive small bowel resection, does not appear to significantly affect digoxin bioavailability.[5] In about 10% of all patients taking digoxin, a gastrointestinal tract conversion to cardioinactive metabolites by gut flora may occur, which leads to decreased bioavailability of digoxin for absorption.[6] Therapy with antibiotics may markedly alter the rate of digitalization and dosing requirements in these patients.[6] Drugs such as metoclopramide, magnesium-containing antacids, kaolin-pectin antidiarrheal compounds, neomycin, sulphasalazine, cholestyramine, and increased dietary fiber, may inhibit digoxin absorption by diverse mechanisms.[4,7] Drugs that retard gastrointestinal motility, such as anticholinergics, may increase absorption (see Table 39-1). Meals delay, but do not decrease, digoxin absorption.[7] The distribution of digoxin occurs in plasma and extracellular fluid (ECF) space where a rapid equilibrium is attained, and peripherally in tissues such as muscle and skin where a slower steady state is achieved.[4]

TABLE 39-1 Factors That Alter Digitalis Effect

Decreased	Increased
Supraventricular tachycardias (especially if secondary to pericarditis, pulmonary embolism, or thoracotomy)	Electrolyte abnormalities
	Hypokalemia
Hyponatremia (decreased digitalis binding)	Hypomagnesemia
Hyperkalemia (decreased digitalis binding)	Hypercalcemia
Hyperthyroidism	Diuretic therapy
Hypocalcemia	Decreased renal function
Metoclopramide (decreased gastrointestinal absorption)	Ischemic heart disease
	Decreased lean body mass
Magnesium-containing antacids (decreased gastrointestinal absorption)	Hypoxia
	Chronic lung disease
Kaolin-pectin compounds (decreased gastrointestinal absorption)	Acute myocardial infarction
	Hypothyroidism
Cholestyramine (decreased gastrointestinal absorption)	Antibiotic therapy (increased bioavailability)
	Anticholinergic drugs (increased absorption)
Colestipol (decreased gastrointestinal absorption)	Quinidine therapy (increased conduction delay, increased digoxin level)
Sulphasalazine (decreased gastrointestinal absorption)	Verapamil (increased conduction delay, increased digoxin level)
High-dietary fiber (decreased gastrointestinal absorption)	Nifedipine (increased conduction delay, increased digoxin level)
Barbiturates (increased hepatic metabolism)	Bretylium (increased risk arrhythmia)
Phenylbutazone (increased hepatic metabolism)	Procainamide (increased conduction delay)
Phenytoin (increased hepatic metabolism)	Propranolol (increased conduction delay)
	Beta and Alpha-Adrenergic Drugs (increased risk arrhythmia)
	Spironolactone (increased digoxin level)

Decreases in renal function—the glomerular filtration rate (GFR)—and lean body mass that are seen with aging cause a decreased volume of distribution in elderly persons, which leads to decreased loading dose requirements.[7,8] The most important age-related change in digoxin pharmacokinetics is the reduction in the GFR, since digoxin is primarily (75%) eliminated from the body by this route. This age-related decrease in renal function often is associated with a normal serum creatinine level as a result of the decreased lean body mass with age.[8,9] The same dose of digoxin given to elderly and young adult subjects results in blood concentrations that are nearly twice as high in elderly persons,[10] secondary to a decreased lean body mass and a diminished renal excretion of digoxin. Tissue binding is decreased in severe renal failure, which results in further decreases in the volume of distribution.[7] An extrarenal (hepatobiliary) clearance of digoxin normally accounts for about 25% of its excretion, with increasing dependence on this route as renal function declines.[1] Whether normal aging compromises the hepatobiliary clearance of digoxin and contributes to an increase in digoxin's half-

life in elderly persons is not known.[9] As a result of these age-related alterations in digoxin pharmacokinetics, the average half-life of digoxin for patients in their 8th and 9th decades is approximately 70 hours, which is almost twice the 36-hour serum half-life that is seen in younger adults.[8–10] Since four to five serum half-lives are necessary to arrive at steady-state concentrations (in the absence of a loading dose), an elderly patient may require as long as 2 weeks to reach a stable serum digoxin concentration, as opposed to the 1 week that usually is needed in younger patients.[9] However, these effects are subject to wide variation, and their magnitude cannot be accurately predicted in any individual person.[9]

Other factors may contribute to increased digitalis toxicity in elderly persons, including a theoretic increase in both cardiac and central nervous system sensitivity to digitalis,[9] hypokalemia (leading to increased digitalis binding to the Na-K ATPase sites*), hypothyroidism, frequent medication errors,[11] and drug interactions (see Table 39-1).

---

* Na = sodium; K = potassium.

Given these pharmacokinetic changes with age, it is reasonable to use lower doses of digoxin in elderly persons. The use of currently available nomograms for digoxin dosing may overestimate the dose requirements; they are no better than a physician's intuition if these physiologic alterations are kept in mind.[12,13] If a loading dose is necessary, a dose of 5–10 μg/kg in two to three divided doses over a 24-hour period should be given (a 50% reduction from usual recommended loading doses in younger adults).[14] Patients with atrial fibrillation and a rapid ventricular response may require larger loading doses.[9] Maintenance digoxin doses are easily determined by using the estimated creatinine clearance (Ccr):

$$\text{Creatinine clearance (Ccr)} = \frac{(140 - \text{age}) \times \text{weight}}{72 \times \text{Serum creatinine}}$$

Dosage calculations in obese patients should use lean body mass, not total body weight. For instance, elderly patients in the high weight ranges with a Ccr in the 40–80-cc/minute ranges may require 0.1875–0.25 mg/day, whereas a smaller older person with a Ccr in the 20–40-cc/minute range would receive smaller maintenance doses in the 0.125–0.1875-mg/day dosage range.[9] The wide interpatient variation in digoxin pharmacokinetics coupled with a frequent non-compliance is an indication for measuring serum steady-state concentrations (after 2 weeks of therapy if no loading dose is given). A serum level between 0.8–2.0 mg/ml that is correlated with the clinical response probably is indicative of a lowered risk for digoxin toxicity, compared to patients with higher levels.[9]

Toxicity

Digoxin is a major cause of adverse drug reactions in elderly persons; it affects 11.5–20% of all hospitalized geriatric patients.[15] Digoxin toxicity is manifested differently in this age group. Thus, extracardiac manifestations of toxicity may precede cardiac toxicity. Also, non-specific common complaints such as anorexia, gastrointestinal discomfort, hazy vision, restlessness, weakness, fatigue, depression, bad dreams, and delirium, all may predominate—as opposed to the nausea, vomiting, and color vision changes that usually are seen in younger adults.[16] Life-threatening arrhythmias may be

the earliest and sole manifestation of digoxin poisoning in elderly persons.[17] Premature ventricular contractions, bigeminy, and trigeminy are the most common and earliest digoxin-toxic arrhythmias. Almost any dysrhythmia may be precipitated by digoxin toxicity, with the exception of atrial fibrillation or flutter with a rapid ventricular response. A depressed sinus node and atrioventricular node function may lead to an arrhythmia and heart block; thus, bradycardia, the regularization of a previously irregular heart rate, and atrioventricular node conduction abnormalities, are all clues to digoxin toxicity. Of all patients with digoxin-induced arrhythmias, 25% may be asymptomatic and require an electrocardiogram (ECG) for a diagnosis.[17] The treatment of digoxin-induced arrhythmias includes a withdrawal of the drug, cardiac monitoring, potassium replacement (with caution if a high-degree atrioventricular block is present), avoidance of calcium replacement, and treatment of life-threatening arrhythmias that lead to a hemodynamic compromise. Digoxin-induced arrhythmias may be treated with lidocaine or diphenylhydantoin. A heart block with bradyarrhythmias that does not respond to atropine may require temporary pacemaker therapy. Quinidine and calcium antagonists should not be used to treat arrhythmias that are induced by digoxin toxicity, because they decrease digoxin excretion and may cause additive conduction delays. Propranolol and procainamide may cause additive conduction delays and should only be tried if other measures prove to be ineffective.

A clinician should suspect digoxin toxicity in an elderly person with any change in rhythm, worsening renal function, electrolyte abnormalities, hypothyroidism, recent myocardial infarction, visual, gastrointestinal, or central nervous system complaints, and pulmonary decompensation. Digoxin toxicity may cause delirium, pseudodementia, acute psychosis and hallucinations; it should be considered in the differential diagnosis of altered mental status in an elderly person.[18] Normal serum digoxin levels may be seen in incontestable cases of digoxin toxicity and should not dissuade a clinician from considering this diagnosis.[7]

Patients with a significant pulmonary disease may be more susceptible to the toxic effects of digoxin in association with hypoxia, electrolyte and acid-base disturbances, drug interactions, and other mechanisms. Only if there are clear and persistent indications for its use should digoxin be prescribed on a long-term basis in these patients.[19] The use of digoxin in the setting of an acute myocardial infarction remains controversial.[20] However, if the usual indications for its use are present and other modalities have proved to be inadequate, its cautious use in lowered doses can be helpful.[20,21] Patients who are treated with diuretic therapy are particularly susceptible to digoxin toxicity because of concomitant hypokalemia with increased sensitivity to the effects of the drug. Potassium replacement is often necessary in patients taking both diuretics and digoxin. Hypercalcemia and hypomagnesemia increase the sensitivity to digoxin and may enhance its toxicity.

Drug Interactions

Adverse drug interactions are another cause of digoxin toxicity in elderly persons who frequently are treated with multiple medications. Concomitant digoxin and quinidine therapy results in a rapid 2-fold increase in digoxin levels, with considerable individual variation. A peak increase in the serum digoxin level is reached 4–5 days after the initiation of quinidine therapy. The mechanisms of this effect are complex and include decreases in the renal and non-renal clearance of digoxin and a displacement from tissue-binding sites. This increase in the serum digoxin level may lead to toxicity. Since both drugs are commonly taken by elderly persons, the risk is theoretically high in this age group. Quinidine clearance has been reported to diminish with age, and it may contribute to even higher digoxin levels.[9,22,23] The digoxin dose should be reduced by 50% when initiating quinidine therapy, and serum levels should be checked 5 days later to insure proper dose adjustments.[22] Other drugs such as verapamil[23] and nifedipine[24] (increases serum digoxin levels and causes depression of cardiac conduction), spironolactone[7] (which decrease the renal clearance of digoxin), alpha or beta agonists such as terbutaline or ephedrine (causing a further depression of cardiac conduction), propranolol and procainamide (causing a further depression of cardiac conduction), and calcium or Vitamin D supplements[25] (which in-

crease the sensitivity to digoxin), also may precipitate digoxin toxicity (*see* Table 39-1).

Indications for Digoxin Therapy

Digoxin is the seventh most frequently prescribed drug in the United States. It is useful in the treatment of a left-ventricular failure, in the rate control of a chronic atrial fibrillation, and in the prevention of some supraventricular tachyarrhythmias. These problems are commonly encountered in the elderly population, with an incidence that increases with age. Thus, more than 80% of all patients taking digoxin in Great Britain are over 60 years of age, and more than 60% are over 70 years of age.[1] The narrow margin between therapeutic and toxic doses of digoxin requires a careful justification of its use in elderly persons.

Left Ventricular Failure

The clinical use of digoxin in left ventricular failure with sinus rhythm is controversial, especially in elderly persons whose risk of toxicity is high. Some clinicians feel that only those patients who fail to respond to an adequate diet, rest, and diuretic therapy should be treated with digoxin,[26–28] whereas others have demonstrated a long-term improvement in cardiac performance in digitalized patients with left ventricular failure and sinus rhythm.[29,30] Many studies document the safe withdrawal of digoxin from elderly patients with sinus rhythm[31–34]; 60–94% of these patients did not deteriorate over a 3–6-month period of follow-up examinations. These figures are controversial and may result from: 1) An incorrect initial diagnosis of congestive heart failure; 2) Subtherapeutic digoxin levels before drug withdrawal, 3) A resolution of the initial event leading to heart failure and obviating the need for digoxin; or 4) No significant benefit from longterm digoxin use in a left ventricular failure with sinus rhythm.[33]

In view of the uncertain benefit of digoxin in the subgroup of patients with left ventricular failure and sinus rhythm, a high risk of toxicity, and an absence of prospective parameters that identify patients likely to respond, it is justifiable to use diuretics alone if adequate control of symptoms can be maintained. If careful diuretic therapy proves inadequate, it is reasonable to begin digoxin after securing a diagnosis of left ventricular failure, and after treating exacerbating conditions such as thyrotoxicosis, valvular heart disease, anemia, infections, and arrhythmias.[9] Heart failure that is characterized by a high cardiac output (as in thyrotoxicosis, beriberi, atrioventricular fistulae, and anemia) generally does not respond well to digoxin. Digoxin is particularly toxic and contraindicated in patients with amyloid heart disease.

Atrial Fibrillation

Digoxin slows atrioventricular nodal conduction and controls the ventricular rate in atrial fibrillation. The ventricular response rate that is measured at rest and with exercise is the clinical guide to the adequacy of digitalization, unless the doses that are needed appear to be unusually high and toxicity, non-compliance, or thyrotoxicosis are suspected. In such cases, serum digoxin levels may be useful. Beta blockade or calcium channel blockers may be necessary to provide adequate rate control if higher digoxin doses lead to toxicity without slowing the ventricular response. They may be used in combination with digoxin or as a substitute for it. As many as 30% of all elderly patients with chronic atrial fibrillation have slower ventricular response rates (less than 90–100 beats per minute) because of coexisting conduction disease in the atrioventricular node. These patients do not require digoxin therapy and may develop symptomatic bradyarrhythmias if they are given digoxin.[9]

The common clinical settings in which digoxin should be used with extra caution include an acute myocardial infarction (increased risk of arrhythmias and increased myocardial oxygen requirements), sick sinus syndrome (risk of bradyarrhythmia), and electric cardioversion (increased incidence of ventricular arrhythmias, especially with concomitant digoxin toxicity).[4]

Once digoxin therapy has begun, an assessment of the clinical response and a reassessment of the indication for its use should be undertaken. If no clinically measurable improvement has occurred and drug levels are therapeutic, then consideration should be given

to discontinuing digoxin. If a clinical response is observed, the patient should be given the drug for at least 3 months and then re-evaluated. If the precipitating cause of the heart failure or arrhythmia has resolved, or if the serum digoxin level is less than 0.8 ng/ml, a trial without digoxin may be reasonable.[32,33] If the clinician is confronted with a patient who has been treated with long-term maintenance digoxin, has no clear and present justification for its use, and/or serum levels less than 0.8 ng/ml, the drug usually can be safely withdrawn—assuming an early and careful follow-up is possible.[32,33]

Serum Digoxin Levels

The measurement of serum digoxin levels is useful in monitoring therapy, but should not be relied on in isolation from the clinical situation.[34] Many studies have documented a significant difference between the mean values of plasma digoxin concentrations in patients with and without digoxin toxicity but an overlap exists between the two groups.[7] If digoxin toxicity is suspected on clinical grounds, a serum level may be used as confirmatory evidence especially if it is greater than 3.0 ng/ml, or to reject this diagnosis if it is less than 0.5 ng/ml. A normal digoxin level does not rule out digoxin toxicity. Hypokalemia, hypomagnesemia, decreased renal function, hypothyroidism, age greater than 60 years, or a maintenance dose greater than 6 μg/kg/day, are equally important parameters for digoxin toxicity. If under-digitalization is suspected because of an inadequate clinical response to therapy, a serum level less than 0.8 ng/ml suggests that higher doses are appropriate, or that the patient is not taking the medication correctly. If there is a question about the need for continued digoxin therapy in a patient whose indications for its initiation are either unknown or resolved, a serum level of less than 0.8 ng/ml supports a trial without the drug.[7,9,33,34] If drugs that are known to affect digoxin kinetics are begun (such as antacids, quinidine, and calcium channel blockers), serum levels are helpful in altering the dose. Finally, after estimating the correct maintenance dose using age, estimated Ccr values, and the drug regimen, it is appropriate to confirm normal drug levels after a steady state is achieved. The time of collection of the specimen influences the result, and levels should not be drawn until 8 hours after the oral administration of the drug or 4 hours after intravenous (IV) digoxin is given. Other isotopes in the serum from nuclear medicine studies may lead to falsely low serum digoxin levels.[34]

Diuretics

Diuretics are commonly used in the elderly population for treating hypertension and congestive heart failure. Although their therapeutic efficacy depends on their ability to produce a negative sodium balance, they also affect osmolality, acid-base regulation, calcium and potassium balance, renal perfusion, glucose tolerance, uric acid handling, and the effects of hormones on the kidney. An understanding of the mechanism of action, and location in the kidney of the diuretic effect assists in the proper choice of agents.[35,36]

Thiazides

The major site of action of thiazide diuretics is the distal convoluted tubule, involve a direct inhibition of active sodium reabsorption. They cause decreased urinary dilution, have no effect on urinary concentration, and cause increased potassium loss.[36] As the GFR falls, diuretics that act on the distal nephron become progressively less effective because of an increased proximal sodium reabsorption.[35] Information regarding the altered pharmacokinetics of diuretic agents with age is not available. The initial diuretic response to thiazides may be quite brisk, with an eventual decrease in effect, as a compensatory increase in proximal reabsorption of sodium occurs. Mild congestive heart failure and hypercalciuria-associated nephrolithiasis are other indications for the use of thiazide diuretics.

The toxicity of thiazides in elderly persons includes hypokalemia, glucose intolerance, dehydration with azotemia, urinary incontinence or retention (in association with underlying urologic disorders such as a benign prostatic hypertrophy), hypercalcemia due to decreased renal calcium losses, hyperuricemia, and alkalosis. Other less common problems include bone marrow toxicity, vasculitis, and pancreatitis.[35] Hyperuricemia associated with dehydration may precipitate an acute gouty attack. Hypokalemia (less than 3.0–3.5 mmol/liter) should be treated with potassium replacement, especially in patients taking digoxin. Elderly persons have a decreased dietary intake of potassium and a high risk of non-compliance with potassium supplements[37] which are unpalatable and cause gastrointestinal irritation. Potassium-sparing diuretics such as triamterene or spironolactone may be used in a hypokalemic patient who is refractory to standard dietary (see Table 39-2) and pharmacologic potassium supplementation; however, the risk of unpredictable and life-threatening hyperkalemia must be kept in mind.[37] The presence of renal insufficiency, or simply the decrease in Ccr values with normal aging, and the combined use of potassium-sparing agents with oral potassium supplements increase the risk of hyperkalemia.[37] Routine potassium replacement is not necessary unless a patient is receiving concomitant digoxin therapy, demonstrates symptoms of hypokalemia or has laboratory evidence of severe potassium depletion. Thiazides may be used in combination with other diuretics that act at different sites along the kidney tubule, if single-agent therapy proves to be inadequate. Additive toxicity may accompany enhanced therapeutic efficacy.[35] Hypertension in elderly persons may be treated initially with small doses of hydrochlorothiazide, given in the morning to avoid nocturia and its attendant risks of falling and injury after getting out of bed in a dark room.

TABLE 39-2 Foods High in Potassium Content

Banana	Winter squash
Cantaloupe	Milk
Honeydew melon	Apples
Prunes and raisins	Peaches
Grapefruit, orange	Peanuts
Tomatoes	Apricot nectar
White potatoes	Avocado
Molasses	Chocolate
Sweet potato	Mustard greens
Green lima beans	Green vegetables

The dose should be initiated with 25 mg/day and may be gradually increased to 100 mg/day.

Furosemide

Furosemide is a potent diuretic agent with a rapid onset and short duration of action. Its site of action is the ascending loop of Henle via inhibition of active chloride transport. In contrast to thiazides, furosemide diminishes urinary-concentrating mechanisms, leaving partially intact urinary-diluting mechanisms. A decreased GFR with an increased proximal reabsorption of sodium may block the diuretic effect of furosemide, but to a lesser extent than the thiazide diuretics. Thus, furosemide is preferred in patients who have renal failure. The "braking phenomenon," described earlier for thiazides, also occurs using loop diuretics; that is, salt excretion increases initially, but is followed by a restoration of sodium balance as losses decrease to levels equalling intake.[37] Furosemide increases calcium excretion in the urine and may be used in the therapy of hypercalcemia. Intravenous furosemide is useful in the therapy of acute pulmonary edema, because it causes a rapid onset of venodilation and decreased venous return. These effects may cause life-threatening hypotension. Its use in elderly persons is generally restricted to the treatment of congestive heart failure, although it also is indicated in the treatment of hypertension with renal insufficiency.

Initially, even small doses of furosemide may cause transient hypotension and/or a significant diuresis. It is wise to begin with small doses (5–10 mg/day orally or intravenously) and to adjust the medication upward as tolerated. Toxic side effects of furosemide are similar to those caused by the thiazide diuretics, although they are more severe and include dehydration, hypotension, azotemia, electrolyte disturbances (hypokalemia, hypochloremia, hypomagnesemia, and hyponatremia), alkaloşis, hyperuricemia, hyperglycemia, ototoxicity (after high-dose parenteral therapy), allergic reactions, and hepatic coma.[38] Adverse reactions were noted in 10% of hospitalized patients on the drug,[38] with a dose-dependent increase in incidence. Severe hyponatremia or alkalosis may require a temporary decrease in dose or a discontinuation of furosemide. Non-steroidal anti-inflammatory agents (NSAIDs) may antagonize the effects of furosemide by inhibiting intrarenal prostaglandins, especially in patients with underlying renal insufficiency.[39,40]

Beta-Adrenergic Antagonists

The adrenergic receptors are classified into alpha (α) and beta (β) types. Alpha-receptor stimulation leads to the vasoconstriction of arterioles and venules; beta-receptor stimulation increases the rate and force of contraction of the heart, dilates peripheral arterioles, stimulates insulin release, glycogenolysis, and lipolysis, and causes bronchodilation. The beta receptors are further subdivided into β-1 (cardiac, intestinal, and adipocyte) and β-2 (bronchial and vascular smooth muscle) classifications. The beta-adrenergic antagonists work by competitive inhibition of catecholamine agonists.[41,42] The beta-adrenoceptor number (in membrane fractions of lymphocytes) correlates inversely with age and the chronotropic response to isoproterenol diminishes with age. This suggests a decreased sensitivity to beta-adrenoceptor antagonists in older persons. There is some evidence that demonstrates a decrease in beta-receptor affinity for propranolol with age as well.[42] These observations may explain the diminished control of both heart rate and cardiac output after exercise that is seen with the same free drug levels in elderly persons.[42–44]

Propranolol and timolol are non-selective short-acting agents.[41,45,46] Metoprolol and atenolol are β-1 (cardioselective) antagonists. Metoprolol is short-acting, while atenolol may be given in a once-a-day dosage regimen. Cardioselectivity persists at low-to-moderate doses of the β-1 antagonists and thus offers a diminished risk of bronchospasm, hypoglycemia (particularly in insulin-dependent diabetics), and peripheral vasospasm.[41]

Propranolol is cleared by the liver; its half-life in plasma lengthens with age, from about 3 hours in young adults to 6–8 hours in elderly persons.[42,43] Other aspects of propranolol kinetics, such as decreased intrinsic total clearance and the relationship of weight to steady-state serum concentration, are age-dependent only in smokers.[43] Distribution of the drug to the tissues appears to be slowed in elderly persons, and an increase in bioavailability secondary to the decreased rate of metabolism has been noted.[47] The first-pass effect, whereby a high proportion of the absorbed drug is metabolized presystematically by the liver, also diminishes with age; thus, lower doses will provide the same bioavailability in elderly persons.[48] Active metabolites of propranolol are excreted by the kidneys and renal insufficiency therefore may prolong the biologic half-life.

Metoprolol also undergoes first-pass metabolism that decreases with age, which leads to increased bioavailability.[49] The half-life of metoprolol has not been shown to increase with age, nor does the accumulation of metabolites in association with renal dysfunction have any clinical significance.[45] The metabolism of timolol is similar, but severe hypotension has been reported after its use in patients with end-stage renal disease (ESRD) who are undergoing hemodialysis.[45,46] Atenolol, in contrast, undergoes little or no hepatic metabolism and is excreted primarily by the kidneys. Doses must be decreased with impaired renal function. Metoprolol, timolol, and atenolol do not have active metabolites. Nadolol is excreted by the kidneys and has a half-life of 24 hours in normal young adults. Its half-life may be as long as 72 hours in elderly persons with diminished renal function, and its use is relatively contraindicated in this age group.

The dosage of beta-adrenoceptor antagonists is dependent on the clinical response and is best begun at low doses in elderly persons. It should be slowly titrated upwards to achieve the desired clinical effect, while monitoring for evidence of toxicity (*see* Table 39-3). Side effects in the geriatric population are significant and the risk increases with age, renal insufficiency (for propranolol and atenolol), IV route of administration, and length of hospitalization of inpatients.[44] Higher plasma concentrations, extensive cardiovascular disease, multiple organ illness, and adverse drug interactions may explain the susceptibility of elderly patients to complications of therapy with beta-blockers.[42,43] Adverse reactions include bradyarrhythmias, hypotension, pulmonary edema, heart block, angina, neurologic disturbances (e.g., fatigue, bad dreams, lethargy, sexual dys-

function, depression, drowsiness, and confusion), hypoglycemia in diabetics, bronchospasm, and a peripheral vascular insufficiency with claudication or Raynaud's phenomenon.[50] Atenolol has a low lipid solubility and does not cross the blood-brain barrier; thus, it may be a more appropriate drug for patients who suffer depression, fatigue, or altered mental status when treated with beta-receptor antagonists.[45,46] Beta-blocker therapy causes hyperkalemia through uncertain mechanisms. In patients with renal insufficiency, this effect is of particular concern.[51-54] The side effects of β-2-receptor antagonists, such as bronchospasm and claudication, are often seen even with low doses of non-selective agents (propranolol, timolol). However, these side effects may not emerge until moderate-to-high doses of cardioselective β-1 antagonists (metoprolol, atenolol) are used. The rapid discontinuation of beta-blockers may precipitate life-threatening arrhythmias, angina, or infarction. Therefore, the drug should be tapered slowly before withdrawal.[42]

Indications for propranolol include supraventricular and some ventricular arrhythmias, angina pectoris, hypertension, asymmetric septal hypertrophy, migraine headache, benign essential tremor and the symptomatic relief of thyrotoxicosis. The efficacy of beta-receptor antagonists in the prevention of recurrent myocardial infarction has been demonstrated using timolol, metoprolol, and propranolol.[51-54] Beta blockade is contraindicated in patients with a severe reactive airway disease or chronic obstructive pulmonary disease (COPD), second- and third-degree heart block, symptomatic bradyarrhythmias, and a significant congestive heart failure. The coexistent use of drugs that affect cardiac conduction or inotropy, such as digoxin, nifedipine, verapamil, quinidine, or procainamide, may lead to heart block, arrhythmia, or congestive heart failure. Beta-blockers should be initiated at lowered dosages in elderly persons (*see* Table 39-3).

Calcium Channel Blockers

The calcium channel blockers have recently been introduced in the therapy of supraventricular arrhythmias, angina, and hypertrophic car-

TABLE 39-3   Beta-Blocking Agents

Available Agents	Trade Name	Half-Life	Cardio-vascular Selectivity	Cross Blood-Brain Barrier	Active Metab-olites	Route of Excretion	Starting Dose in the Elderly
Propranolol	Inderal	3 hr (young adults) 6–8 hr (elderly)*	No	Yes	Yes	Hepatic and renal	10 mg BID/QID
Metoprolol	Lopressor	3–6 hr	Yes	Yes	No	Hepatic	25 mg BID
Timolol	Blocadren	3–4 hr	No	Yes	No	Hepatic	5 mg BID
Nadolol	Corgard	24 hr (young adults) 30–72 hr (elderly)*	No	No	No	Renal	20 mg QD
Atenolol	Tenormin	6–9 hr (young adult) 16–27 hr (elderly)*	Yes	No	No	Renal	25 mg QD

* Half-life increases with renal insufficiency.

diomyopathy. Because experience with these compounds has been brief, little information is available on their pharmacology in elderly persons. However, a discussion of their properties may aid its safe use in older patients. Although many agents now have been introduced to inhibit the calcium channel, this discussion will be limited to verapamil and nifedipine. These agents produce a decrease in sinoatrial node activity, an increase in the atrioventricular node refractory period, an uncoupling of myocardial excitation-contraction (negative inotropy), decreased coronary vascular resistance (increased coronary flow), and decreased systemic vascular resistance (lowered blood pressure).[55,56] The negative inotropy is counter-balanced by a renal increase in cardiac contractility as a response to the peripheral vasodilation (afterload reduction) also caused by these agents. Pharmacologic differences between verapamil and nifedipine account for the variability of their clinical application; nifedipine has little electrophysiologic effect on the sinoatrial and atrioventricular nodes and is not useful in the treatment of supraventricular arrhythmias. Verapamil has less of a vasodilatory and afterload-reducing effect than nifedipine. Therefore, it causes more negative inotropy and is not as useful in patients with angina or congestive heart failure. Thus, verapamil is superior to nifedipine in the treatment of supraventricular arrhythmias, while nifedipine is better for the treatment of angina.[55,56]

Verapamil and nifedipine are well absorbed, highly protein bound, and metabolized in the liver. Plasma half-lives are between 3–8 hours. Data regarding the effects of aging on these properties are not available. Verapamil undergoes extensive first-pass metabolism in the liver and, thus, has a short half-life following oral administration.[57] Verapamil and nifedipine should be administered with caution in patients with extensive hepatic dysfunction. Nifedipine should be initiated with a low dosage in elderly persons (10 mg BID-QID) and may be increased, as tolerated, to a maximum of 40 mg QID. Oral verapamil should be initiated with 80 mg every 8–12 hours and increased gradually as tolerated. Intravenous verapamil is administered in doses of 0.075–0.15 mg/kg over a 2–3-minute period.

The side effects may be particularly troublesome in elderly persons. Verapamil may cause headaches, hypotension, flushing, dizziness, constipation, and nausea. High-grade heart block and congestive heart failure have been reported infrequently after the administration of verapamil; but are of concern in patients with pre-existing conduction disease or left ventricular dysfunction. Bradyarrhythmias and hypotension can be reversed by IV atropine sulfate, calcium gluconate, or norepinephrine. Verapamil is contraindicated in patients with moderate-to-advanced heart failure, sick sinus syndrome, second- or third-degree heart block, and hypotensive states. Verapamil may cause a non-cardiogenic pedal edema in about 25% of all patients, which is often a reason for its discontinuation. Adverse drug interactions of importance occur with other agents that affect inotropy and conduction, such as beta-blockers, disopyramide, and quinidine. Prior digitalization is not a contraindication except in the sick sinus syndrome or in cases of suspected digitalis toxicity when, verapamil is absolutely contraindicated.[58] The coadministration of digoxin and verapamil may lead to a decreased volume of distribution, reduced clearance, and increased half-life for digoxin, which suggests that the digoxin dose should be decreased (by about 50%) when initiating verapamil therapy.[59,60]

Nifedipine is likely to cause some symptoms and signs of vasodilation in all persons who receive it. These include dizziness, flushing, headaches, nausea and vomiting, diarrhea, palpitations, non-cardiogenic pedal edema, and paresthesias. These symptoms are of particular concern in elderly persons with pre-existing gait and central nervous system impairment. Severe hypotension may be a first-dose phenomenon or may appear as the drug dosage is increased, especially if there is concomitant beta-blocker therapy. The combined use of beta blockade and nifedipine usually is well tolerated.[61] However, an increased risk of congestive heart failure, conduction abnormalities, and symptomatic hypotension may follow, especially in patients with a pre-existing left ventricular failure, heart block, aortic stenosis, or low blood pressure.[62,63] There are rare reports of nifedipine-induced angina, infarction, and ventricular arrhythmias. Drug interactions include: 1) Imipramine, which may increase coronary vasospasm in patients on nifedipine via uncertain mechanisms; 2) Propranolol, with additive negative inotropy and conduction delay; and 3) Digoxin, whose serum level doubles after the administration of nifedipine.[60,64]

Indications for verapamil include the treatment of paraoxysmal supraventricular tachyarrhythmias,[65] conversion to sinus rhythm or slowing of the rate in atrial flutter, and rate control of atrial fibrillation. Verapamil may be used initially for its rapid effects in life-threatening supraventricular arrhythmias while awaiting the slower effect of digoxin, or it may be substituted for digoxin if adequate rate control cannot be achieved without resorting to potentially toxic doses. Digoxin and verapamil may be ad-ministered together in cases of chronic atrial fibrillation for improved rate control, or when heart failure and supraventricular arrhythmia coexist; but, the drug interaction noted above must be kept in mind.[55] Verapamil has also been used in the treatment of hypertrophic cardiomyopathy, both as a replacement for, and in combination with, beta-blocking drugs.[66]

Nifedipine and verapamil are useful in the treatment of coronary spasm, chronic stable angina, and unstable angina.[46,56,58,61,67] They may be used alone or in combination with nitrate and beta-blocking agents, but most authors recommend them only after failure of more traditional modes of therapy. Combination therapy carries a higher risk of congestive heart failure, conduction abnormalities, arrhythmias, and hypotension. Potential future applications for the calcium channel blockers include hypertension, afterload reduction in mild heart failure, pulmonary hypertension, and myocardial preservation after a myocardial infarction.[55,56]

Until more information is available on the use of these agents in elderly persons, it is prudent to begin with lowered doses and to observe closely for drug interactions and toxicities, which may prove to be life-threatening in the older population.

Vasodilators

Nitroglycerin is a vasodilator which exerts its strongest effect on the venous capacitance system at nitrate-specific receptors in the vascular smooth-muscle wall.[68] Nitrates decrease myocardial oxygen demand by causing venous pooling followed by a decreased ventricular volume and distention. An afterload-reducing effect also may contribute to decreased myocardial work, but reflex tachycardia may offset this action. Nitrates also increase coronary oxygen supply by redistributing blood flow along collateral vessels, and from epicardial to endocardial regions.[68] Sublingually administered nitrates are rapidly absorbed, with maximal effects after 3–15 minutes and little residual activity after 30 minutes. There is a considerable variation in nitrate sensitivity among individuals, but the pharmacokinetic factors responsible for these differences are not well understood. Nitrates are rapidly metabolized in the liver to inactive metabolites. Oral administration requires higher doses because of a first-pass effect. Oral agents other than isosorbide dinitrate are of unproven value. Longer-acting synthetic nitrates and topical preparations are also available (see Table 39-4).[70]

The toxic side effects of nitrate therapy include transient headaches, orthostatic hypotension with dizziness, flushing and palpitations, occasional nausea, and methemoglobinemia with prolonged high dosage. Adverse drug interactions may be expected when using other hypotensive agents, which include calcium channel antagonists, beta-blockers, vasodilators, and diuretics.

Indications for the use of nitrates are chronic stable angina, unstable angina (when IV nitroglycerin may prove to be beneficial), prophylaxis of exercise-induced angina, preload reduction in patients with left ventricular failure, and variant angina (coronary spasm). Their use in association with an acute myocardial infarction is controversial. The response of chest pain to nitrate therapy often is taken as evidence that the pain is cardiac in origin; however, nitrates also can relieve the pain of an esophageal spasm and renal or biliary colic. Partial hemodynamic tolerance may develop after the prolonged use of high-dose nitroglycerin therapy.[70] Nitrate dependence has been reported in munitions workers who are withdrawn from exposure to nitroglycerin; therefore, an abrupt discontinuation of therapy is not recommended.[68] Contraindications for the use of nitroglycerin include the angina of obstructive hypertrophic cardiomyopathy, severe anemia, hypoxia, and significant hypotension.[69,71]

Elderly patients should be advised to keep nitroglycerin in air-tight, amber glass containers, preferably in a cool place. Old pills should be replaced yearly. Should light-headedness follow therapy, patients should be instructed to lie down and elevate their legs. They should be warned of other likely side effects. Many older patients are afraid of addiction with nitrate therapy and must be educated about the need to use it with every episode of chest pain and before activities that usually precipitate angina.

The uses of prazosin, hydralazine, and nitroprusside in the treatment of hypertension and congestive heart failure are limited in elderly persons because of the risk of hypotension and other side effects. Prazosin is used in the treatment of high blood pressure and left ventricular failure as a pre- and afterload-reducing agent. Its mechanism of action is competitive blockade of the vascular, postsynaptic α-1-adrenergic receptor.[72] Prazosin is metabolized in the liver; in the presence of severe heart failure or hepatic dysfunction, its half-life may be prolonged. Increases in plasma renin activity may lead to significant fluid retention and edema, thus requiring diuretic therapy and leading to an increased risk of symptomatic hypotension.[72,73] Other side effects that are seen with prazosin include headache, fatigue, dry mouth, nausea, urinary incontinence (secondary to alpha-adrenergic blockade), polyarthralgias, rash, and depression.[73] A first-dose effect has been reported that leads to transient faintness, dizziness, palpitations, and (rarely) syncope. It is aggravated by pre-existing salt depletion or other hypotensive medications.[73] Patients should be advised to take their first dose at night in bed to protect against falls. Tolerance to its vasodilating effects may develop with chronic administration.[72] The drug should be tapered be-

TABLE 39-4   Nitrates

Preparation	Starting Dose in the Elderly	Dosage Schedule
Nitrolglycerin, sublingual tablets	0.15–0.3 mg	PRN
Nitroglycerin paste	0.5 inch	Q6h
Nitroglycerin patches	10 cm²*	Q24h
Isosorbide dinitate, oral tablets	10 mg	Q4–6h
Isosorbide dinitate, sublingual tablets	2.5 mg	Q3–6h

* 10 cm² = 5 mg/24 hr.

fore withdrawal.[72] The recommended starting dose in elderly persons is 1 mg at bedtime, followed by a gradual increase as tolerated.

Hydralazine is used to treat hypertension and as an afterload-reducing agent in congestive heart failure. It acts via direct arteriolar dilatation, and it also has a reflex positive inotropic effect. Reflex tachycardia may not be seen in patients with congestive heart failure, although it usually is observed in normal persons who are given hydralazine. Hydralazine is metabolized in the liver and excreted in the urine; the dose should be reduced in patients with significant renal or hepatic insufficiency.[74] Hydralazine often is discontinued by patients because of intolerable side effects, which include hypotension, anorexia, nausea and vomiting, drug fever, lupus syndrome, and tachycardia-induced angina.[75] Determination of hepatic acetylator status helps to predict patients who are at high risk for developing the lupus syndrome; patients who are slow acetylators and those treated with more than 200 mg/day of hydralazine are the most susceptible.[74] A drug-specific tolerance to hydralazine may develop and necessitates frequent re-evaluation of a patient on vasodilator therapy whose clinical condition does not improve or worsens.[76] As with other vasodilators, hydralazine must be tapered before it is discontinued. Drug initiation should be conservative in elderly persons, beginning with 10 mg orally BID and increasing the frequency and dosage gradually as tolerated.

Sodium nitroprusside has balanced pre- and afterload-reducing effects via direct vascular smooth-muscle relaxation. It has a rapid onset and offset of action and is used intravenously in monitored settings for the treatment of hypertensive crises, severe left ventricular failure, and dissecting aortic aneurysm. Its use in treating acute myocardial infarction to decrease mortality is controversial.[77,78] Nitroprusside decomposes non-enzymatically in the blood to cyanide, which converts to thiocyanate, and is excreted in the urine.[74]

Cyanide or thiocyanate toxicity limits both the duration of therapy and the dosage of nitroprusside to approximately 3 μg/kg/minute for less than 72 hours. The increasing use of IV nitroglycerin has diminished the need for toxic doses or duration of sodium nitroprusside therapy. Cyanide toxicity is heralded by a metabolic acidosis and tachyphylaxis, and thiocyanate toxicity causes confusion, hyper-reflexia, and convulsions. Renal failure increases the risk of thiocyanate accumulation; therefore, toxicity is likely to occur more frequently in elderly persons.[74] Treatment requires stopping the drug. The use of hydroxycobalamin, sodium thiosulfate, sodium nitrite, and hemodialysis, may be necessary as well.[74,79,80] Other side effects include increased perfusion of non-ventilated lung with a worsening $\dot{V}/\dot{Q}$ mismatching and hypoxia,[79] an inhibition of platelet aggregation, and thrombocytopenia.[79] Overtreatment may result in severe hypotension and cardiac ischemia.[74] The solution must be shielded from light. Nitroprusside should be tapered before its discontinuation. Its rapid disappearance from the plasma after stopping the infusion renders it a relatively safe vasodilator for use in elderly persons. Infusion should begin at low doses, approximately 0.1 μg/kg/minute, and should be increased as tolerated.

Antiarrhythmic Therapy

The use of antiarrhythmic drug therapy in elderly persons is a complex and confusing process not only because the indications for their use are seldom clear, but because of the significant risk that they pose of life-threatening toxicity. Asymptomatic elderly persons have a high incidence of complex supraventricular and ventricular arrhythmias on ambulatory monitoring. The value of antiarrhythmic drugs in preventing sudden death in these patients has not been established.[81] This casts doubt on the wisdom of treating a symptomatic elderly patient despite documented ectopy, unless a clear temporal relation exists between the symptom and the dysrhythmia.[81] There is increasing evidence that standard antiarrhythmic drugs can create malignant arrhythmias and increase mortality in patients who are receiving them.[82,83] Their use should be avoided until it is clear that antiarrhythmic agents are essential for patient safety. Characterization of the underlying cardiac disease and identification of reversible factors should be undertaken before committing a patient to long-term therapy with an antiarrhythmic agent.

Lidocaine

Lidocaine is the standard parenteral agent employed for suppression or prophylaxis of ventricular arrhythmias in association with an acute myocardial infarction, cardiac surgery, and acute illness.[84] Lidocaine decreases the rate of spontaneous depolarization of pacemaker tissues and the duration of the action potential, but does not effect the effective refractory period of the Purkinje cell. This renders the fiber inexcitable for a greater fraction of the depolarization-repolarization cycle. The fibrillation threshold is increased by lidocaine, and the conduction velocity in Purkinje fibers is decreased slightly.[85] These effects are presumed to suppress both reentrant arrhythmias and arrhythmias that are caused by increased automaticity.[85] The pharmacokinetics of lidocaine are altered significantly with age. Lidocaine is metabolized in the liver and its clearance is influenced by the rate of hepatic blood flow. A constant infusion of lidocaine will take about 6 hours (three 2-hour half-lives) to attain 90% of its steady-state concentration in healthy young adult subjects. Thus, lidocaine is usually initiated in bolus form to achieve steady-state levels rapidly, followed by a maintenance infusion designed to keep the blood levels in the therapeutic range. The half-life of lidocaine is prolonged in normal elderly subjects, while the volume of distribution is increased and total clearance is unchanged.[86]

In contrast, older patients with heart failure, hypovolemia, or hepatic disease have a reduced clearance with a prolonged half-life of the drug. Patients with heart failure or hypovolemia and normal liver function also have a decreased volume of distribution for lidocaine, with a resultant longer half-life and decreased clearance. These changes probably account for the increased incidence of adverse reactions to lidocaine that are seen in elderly persons.[87,88] Renal insufficiency does not appear to influence lidocaine pharmacokinetics,[88] although toxic metabolites may accumulate in ESRD.[89] Loading doses should be decreased by 50% for patients with heart failure or liver dysfunction (with greater reductions in those who have both), and smaller maintenance infusions on the order of 0.5–1.0 mg/minute instead of the usual 2.0–4.0-mg/minute infusion rate should be used. Adjustments should be made for weight with approximate total loading doses of 1.0–1.5 mg/kg. The bolus may be safer if administered in divided doses over 30–60 minutes, which avoids transiently toxic blood levels.[90] The bolus must be administered slowly (over several minutes) to avoid an immediate toxic reaction and to allow time for dilution and distribution of the drug.[85,87,88] If arrhythmias develop during a constant infusion, an increase in the maintenance dose must be accompanied by an additional small bolus to achieve the new desired steady state. Patients with a heart or liver disease take longer to reach a steady-state plateau phase, and late-onset toxicity is common in this population.

The assessment of serum blood levels, where available, may assist in monitoring patients who require lidocaine therapy. The length of time that is required to reach steady state in patients with heart failure or hepatic dysfunction must be kept in mind when evaluating these levels. For instance, a therapeutic level that is obtained 6 hours after beginning an infusion may progress to a toxic range 24 hours later, even though no change in the infusion rate has occurred.

Toxic reactions include central nervous system disturbances such as respiratory depression, somnolence, seizure, agitation, confusion, dizziness, tremor, visual changes, tinnitus, and nausea. Cardiovascular complications occur less frequently and include heart block, arrhythmia, hypotension, and cardiac arrest.[87] Toxicity is more common among patients with an acute myocardial infarction, congestive heart failure, and low body weight.[87] Age is correlated with an increased risk of toxicity, which probably is due to an increased incidence of cardiac disease and low body weight in this group.[87] There is no evidence of an intrinsic increase in sensitivity to lidocaine in elderly persons.[86]

The use of prophylactic lidocaine in suspected acute myocardial infarction is a controversial issue. Many trials have been conducted to examine this question, and no definitive evidence of benefit has been demonstrated to date.[85,89,91] Arguments in favor of its use suggest that 20–80% of all patients with primary ventricular fibrillation (unassociated with heart failure or cardiogenic shock) have no warning arrhythmia, and that about two thirds of all deaths thought to be due to ventricular fibrillation occur during the first hour after the onset of symptoms, with decreasing frequency over the ensuing 24 hours. Deaths following a myocardial infarction usually are due to mechanical difficulties such as a pump failure and cardiac rupture.[92] Even if a warning arrhythmia does occur in the monitored setting, about 50% are missed.

Opponents of the prophylactic use of lidocaine in a suspected myocardial infarction claim that primary ventricular fibrillation is not the major cause of mortality in coronary care units (CCU) and it can be effectively treated in a monitored situation with electrical cardioversion; also, that the period during which lidocaine is likely to be most effective usually occurs before admission to a CCU, and the risk of the drug may be greater than the benefit.

There is little controversy in most clinical settings over the use of lidocaine in patients with a suspected myocardial infarction who have any ventricular ectopy.[85,89,91] In view of the uncertain evidence in support of lidocaine as a prophylactic agent and the high risk of toxicity in elderly patients with a cardiac dysfunction, extreme care must be exercised in the use of this drug in the geriatric population. At present, most authors support its cautious use in patients with a suspected myocardial infarction.

Quinidine

Quinidine has direct depressant effects on excitability, conduction, and contractility in the heart, as well as indirect anticholinergic activity. This causes an increase in the effective refractory period throughout the heart, with an increased ratio of the effective refractory period to the action potential duration. The anticholinergic effects of the drug usually overcome the increase in the refractory period in the atrioventricular node, leading to an increase in nodal conduction.[93] The ECG reflects the effects of quinidine with an increase in the PR-interval, a widening of the QRS complex, and prolongation of the QT-interval. Quinidine is well absorbed and is largely bound to plasma proteins. It is about 60–85% metabolized by the liver, with renal elimination accounting for about 15–

40% of all total clearance. It usually is given in oral dosage forms. Significant pharmacokinetic changes in quinidine handling have been observed in elderly persons, although there is wide individual variation. Both the hepatic biotransformation and renal excretion of quinidine decrease with aging, which leads to a prolonged half-life (10 hours in an elderly person as opposed to 7 hours in younger adults) and a decreased total clearance.[94] Patients with hepatic dysfunction also have a significantly prolonged half-life. Patients with heart failure have been observed to have both a decreased volume of distribution and clearance of quinidine.[95] Patients with low serum proteins have a higher free fraction of the drug, and thus require lower serum levels for therapeutic efficacy.[95] Quinidine metabolites are active and probably contribute to both its therapeutic efficacy and toxicity. Drug interactions of particular concern include increased serum levels of digoxin with the coadministration of quinidine, hepatic enzymatic induction by drugs such as phenobarbital and phenytoin (necessitating an increased quinidine dosage), and a questionable decrease in quinidine clearance with the coadministration of propranolol.[95] Quinidine may suppress the synthesis of vitamin K-dependent clotting factors, and the coadministration of anticoagulants may lead to severe hypoprothrombinemia.[93] The toxic side effects of quinidine administration include a depression of cardiac conduction with an increased risk of ventricular arrhythmias, hypotension, reduced inotropy, "quinidine syncope," cinchonism (tinnitus, vertigo, and blurred vision), nausea, vomiting, diarrhea, thrombocytopenia, hemolytic anemia, and rash.[84,92,93,96] A periodic hematologic evaluation is recommended in patients on long-term quinidine therapy.

Indications for quinidine include the treatment of ventricular ectopy, conversion of atrial fibrillation or flutter to sinus rhythm (after pretreatment with digoxin to prevent an increase in conduction across the atrioventricular node), and the maintenance of sinus rhythm after pharmacologic or electrical cardioversion.[92,93,96] Quinidine should be avoided in patients with a pre-existing heart block, sick sinus syndrome, and prolongation of the QT-interval.[94] Doses should be initiated at lower levels in elderly persons (200 mg every 8–12 hours). Patients should be closely monitored both clinically and with serum quinidine levels, recalling that lower serum levels are therapeutics in patients with decreased protein binding.

Procainamide

Procainamide has electrophysiologic properties that are similar to those of quinidine, but it does not prolong the QT-interval to the same extent. It may be used both orally and intravenously.[84] Orally administered procainamide is well absorbed, and it is about 15% protein-bound with a half-life in healthy adults of 3.5 hours. The drug is metabolized in the liver to N-acetyl procainamide (NAPA), which is an active metabolite. Both the parent compound and the metabolite are excreted in the kidneys. Genetic factors determine a person's rate of acetylation, which can be measured and is a predictor of toxicity.

The measurement of the plasma concentration includes procainamide and NAPA, and a combined blood level of more than 16–20 μg/ml is associated with adverse reactions. Patients with renal insufficiency or congestive heart failure have a decreased volume of distribution and prolonged half-lives of both the parent compound and its metabolite.[93] Because of a decreased Ccr and diminished tubular secretion of this drug with age, a progressive age-related rise in steady-state serum levels of procainamide and NAPA is observed with any given dose of procainamide.[97] Thus, the dose must be decreased for age, renal dysfunction, and congestive heart failure. The pharmacokinetics of NAPA differ from procainamide as follows: It is well absorbed, has a lower volume of distribution than the parent compound, and is largely (80%) excreted unchanged by the kidneys. Its clearance by the kidneys also declines with age, but not as dramatically as procainamide. The half-life of NAPA is significantly longer than that of procainamide and ranges from 6–9 hours in young adults. It is longer in persons with renal insufficiency and progressively increases with normal aging.[97,98]

Adverse reactions to procainamide include a slowing of cardiac conduction, hypotension, negative inotropy, arrhythmia (especially increased ventricular rate in an atrial fibrillation or flutter), anorexia, nausea, vomiting, diarrhea, skin rash, and the lupus syndrome. Approximately 50% of patients on procainamide therapy will develop antinuclear antibodies, and at least 20% will develop the lupus syndrome. Slow acetylators are at particularly high risk; but, given a long-enough course of therapy, rapid acetylators are also susceptible. Drug-induced lupus differs from the idiopathic form in that neither renal nor central nervous system manifestations are described as part of the syndrome. It is characterized by fever, arthritis or arthralgia, myalgia, pleuritis, pleural effusion, pericarditis, Coomb's positive anemia, leukopenia, and rash.[99] The treatment involves discontinuation of procainamide. Although its use is controversial, NAPA induces the lupus syndrome only rarely, and may be used therapeutically in patients with a procainamide-induced lupus syndrome.[101]

The indications for procainamide are similar to those listed above for quinidine. Oral administration at 3–4-hour intervals may be necessary because of the short half-life of procainamide. Sustained-release preparations may be helpful for patients in whom compliance with a 3–4 hourly regimen is poor. Older patients with decreased renal function or congestive heart failure and a prolonged procainamide half-life may sustain therapeutic concentrations for longer periods of time—up to 6–12 hours with Ccr values between 10–50 cc/minute and 8–24 hours with Ccr values less than 10 cc/minute.[101] Plasma levels should be obtained to assist in choosing the optimal compound and dosing interval. In an elderly patient with a Ccr value greater than 30 cc/minute, procainamide should be initiated at about 250 mg orally every 6 hours. The dosing interval should be lengthened in cases of renal insufficiency. Serum levels are crucial for a safe administration of the drug, as considerable individual variation in metabolism exists. Parenteral therapy must be given slowly (no more than 100 mg every 5 minutes), with blood pressure and electrocardiographic monitoring, until toxicity, control of the arrhythmia is reached, or a 1-gram dose has been given.[93]

Because of its narrow therapeutic index, procainamide must be used with great caution in elderly persons. The dosage will depend on the acetylator status, renal function, and type of preparation used. Close monitoring for therapeutic end-points and toxicity, and use of plasma levels is essential in this age group.

Disopyramide

Disopyramide has electrophysiologic properties and indications for use that are similar to those of quinidine and procainamide. Its prominent vagolytic action also may contribute to its efficacy as an antiarrhythmic agent.[94] Disopyramide is well absorbed and has a half-life of about 7 hours in normal adults. Approximately 50% of the parent compound is metabolized by the liver and the remainder is excreted unchanged by the kidneys. Renal insufficiency and congestive heart failure lead to smaller volume of distribution and an increased half-life; smaller doses should be used in these clinical situations.[102] The decreasing Ccr that is seen with age would suggest that smaller dosages should also be employed in elderly persons.

The side effects of disopyramide have significantly limited its clinical use and are largely related to its anticholinergic and myocardial depressant properties. The side effects include urinary retention, dry mouth, constipation, blurred vision, worsening of glaucoma, nausea, vomiting, diarrhea, fatigue, headache, and an altered mental status. Fasting hypoglycemia via uncertain mechanisms also has been reported.[102] A prolonged QT-interval and malignant ventricular arrhythmias have been reported with disopyramide, as well as with quinidine and procainamide.[102] Disopyramide exerts a profound negative inotropic effect on the heart, which leads to a recurring congestive heart failure in about 50% of patients with a previous history of left ventricular dysfunction; it also precipitates new heart failure in approximately 5% of patients without such a history.[102–104] A previous history of congestive heart failure, thus, is a contraindication to the use of disopyramide.

Adverse drug interactions occur with procainamide, lidocaine, and phenytoin, which may cause severe conduction abnormalities and arrhythmias when used in combination with disopyramide.[105] Potassium has been reported to be synergistic with disopyramide, causing profound hypotension and conduction abnormalities.[106] The coadministration of propranolol causes additive negative inotropy,[20] and warfarin anticoagulants are potentiated by disopyramide.[102] Its use is contraindicated in the sick sinus syndrome and in advanced heart block. Disopyramide therapy should be initiated with 100 mg every 6 hours in elderly persons. The dosing interval should be lengthened in cases of renal insufficiency. Drug levels are a helpful guide to therapy.

The elderly population, with its high incidence rate of benign prostatic hypertrophy, constipation, glaucoma, susceptibility to central nervous system drug effects, and high frequency of pre-existing cardiac disease, is at a prohibitively high risk from this drug.

References

1. Whiting B, Lawrence JR, Sumner DJ: Digoxin pharmacokinetics in the elderly, in Crooks J, Stevenson IH (eds): *Drugs and the Elderly*. Chap 9, pp 89–101.
2. Smith TW: Digitalis: Ions, inotropy and toxicity, editorial. *N Engl J Med* 299:545–546, 1978.
3. Opie LH: Digitalis and sympathomimetic stimulants. *Lancet* 1:912–918, 1980.
4. Bresnahan JF, Vlietstra RE: Digitalis glycosides. *Mayo Clin Proc* 54:675–684, 1979.
5. Gerson CD, Lowe EH, Lindenbaum J: Bioavailability of digoxin tablets in patients with gastrointestinal dysfunction. *Am J Med* 69:43–49, 1980.
6. Lindenbaum J, Rund DG, Butler VP, et al: Inactivation of digoxin by gut flora: Reversal by antibiotic therapy. *N Engl J Med* 305:789–794, 1981.
7. Aronson JK: Clinical pharmacokinetics of digoxin 1980. *Clin Pharmacokin* 5:L137–L149, 1980.
8. Cusack B, Kelly J, O'Malley K, et al: Digoxin in the elderly: Pharmacokinetic consequences of old age. *Clin Pharmacol Ther* 25:772–776, 1979.
9. Stults BM: Digoxin use in the elderly. *J Am Geriatr Soc* 30:158–164, 1982.
10. Ewy GA, Kapadia GG, Yao L, et al: Digoxin metabolism in the elderly. *Circulation* 34:449–453, 1969.
11. Johnston GD, Kelley JG, McDevitt DG: Do patients take digoxin? *Br Heart J* 40:1–7, 1978.
12. Johnston GD, Harper DWG, McDevitt DG: Can digoxin prescribing be improved? *Eur J Clin Pharmacol* 16:229–235, 1979.

13. Johnston GD: Digoxin dose precision: Prescribing aids or intuition. *Drugs* 20:494, 1980.

14. Sloman J, Manolas EL: Cardiovascular disease, in Avery G (ed): *Drug Treatment*. Sydney and New York, Adis Press, 1980, chap 17, pp 554–637.

15. Howard JB, Strong KE, Facnha SR, et al: Medication procedures in a nursing home: Abuse of PRN orders. *J Am Geriatr Soc* 25:83–84, 1977.

16. Vestal RE: Drug use in the elderly: A review of problems and special considerations. *Drugs* 16:358–382, 1978.

17. Herrmann GR: Digitoxicity in the aged. *Geriatrics* 21:108–122, 1966.

18. Dall JLC: Digitalis intoxication in elderly patients. *Lancet* 1:194–195, 1965.

19. Green LH, Smith TW: The use of digitalis in patients with pulmonary disease. *Ann Int Med* 87:456–465, 1977.

20. Rahimtoola SH, Bunnar RM: Digitalis in acute myocardial infarction. Help or hazard? *Ann Int Med* 82:234–240, 1975.

21. Reicansky I, et al: The effect of intravenous digoxin on the occurrence of ventricular tachyarrhythmias in acute myocardial infarction in man. *Am Heart J* 91:705–711, 1976.

22. Leahey EB: Digoxin-Quinidine interaction: Current status, editorial. *Ann Int Med* 93:775–776, 1980.

23. Leahey EB, Reiffel JA, Giardina EGV, et al: Effect of quinidine and other oral antiarrhythmic drugs on serum digoxin. *Ann Int Med* 92:605–608, 1980.

24. Belz GG, et al: Digoxin plasma concentration and nifedipine. *Lancet* 1:844–845, 1981.

25. Martin DC, Mead K: Reducing medication errors in a geriatric population. *J Am Geriatr Soc* 30:258–260, 1982.

26. Selzer A: Digitalis in cardiac failure: Do the benefits justify the risks? *Arch Int Med* 141:18–20, 1981.

27. O'Malley K, Judge TG, Crooks J: Geriatric clinical pharmacology and therapeutics, in Avery G (ed): *Drug Treatment*. Sydney and New York, Adis Press, 1980, chap 5, pp 158–181.

28. McHaffie D, et al: The clinical use of digoxin in patients with heart failure and sinus rhythm. *Q J Med* 47:401–419, 1978.

29. Arnold SB, Byrd RC, Meister W, et al: Long term digitalis therapy improved left ventricular function in heart failure. *N Engl J Med* 303:1443–1448, 1980.

30. Lee DCS, et al: Heart failure in out-patients: A randomized trial of digoxin versus placebo. *N Engl J Med* 306:699–705, 1982.

31. Dall JLC: Maintenance digoxin in elderly patients. *Br Med J* 2:705–706, 1970.

32. Taggart AJ, McDevitt DG: Digitalis: Its place in modern therapy. *Drugs* 20:398–404, 1980.

33. Johnston DG, McDevitt DG: Is maintenance digoxin necessary in patients with sinus rhythm? *Lancet* 1:567–570, 1979.

34. Doherty JE: How and when to use the digitalis serum level. *JAMA* 239:2594–2596, 1978.

35. Melmon KL, Morelli HF: *Clinical Pharmacology*. Macmillan Co. 8 1972, chap 3.

36. Dirks JH: Mechanisms of action and clinical uses of diuretics. *Hosp Pract,* Sept 1979, pp 99–110.

37. Noble RJ, Rothbaum DA (eds): *Geriatric Cardiology*. Philadelphia, FA Davis, 1981, pp 195–210.

38. Greenblatt DJ, Duhme DW, Allen MD, et al: Clinical toxicity of furosemide in hospitalized patients. *Am Heart J* 94:6–13, 1977.

39. Laiwah ACY, Mactier RA: Antagonistic effect of non-steroidal anti-inflammatory drugs on furosemide-induced diuresis in cardiac failure. *Br Med J* 283:714, 1981.

40. Atallah AA: Interaction of prostaglandins with diuretics. *Prostaglandins* 18:369–372, 1979.

41. Opie LH: Drugs and the Heart. *Lancet* 1:693–698, 1980.

42. Shand DG: Propranolol. *N Engl J Med* 293:280–285, 1975.

43. Vestal RE, Wood AJJ, Branch RA, et al: Effects of age and cigarette smoking on propranolol disposition. *Clin Pharmacol Ther* 26(suppl 1):8–15, 1979.

44. Greenblatt DJ, Koch-Weser J: Adverse reactions to propranolol in hospitalized patients: A report from the Boston Collaborative Drug Surveillance Program. *Am Heart J* 86:478–484, 1973.

45. Fishman WH: Beta-adrenoceptor antagonists: New drugs and new indications. *N Engl J Med* 305:500–506, 1981.

46. Fishman WH: Atenolol and timolol, two new systemic beta-antagonists. *N Engl J Med* 306:1456–1462, 1982.

47. Castleden CM, George CF: The effect of aging on the hepatic clearance of propranolol. *Br J Clin Pharmacol* 7:49–54, 1979.

48. Wilkinson GR: Influence of liver in pharmacokinetic, in Evans W, Schentag JJ, Jusko W (eds): *Applied Pharmacokinetics: Principles of Therapeutic Drug Monitoring*. San Francisco, Applied Therapeutics, Inc, 1980, pp 57–59.

49. Koch-Weser J: Metoprolol. *N Engl J Med* 301:698–703, 1979.

50. Conolly ME, Kersting F, Dollery CT: The clini-

cal pharmacology of beta-adrenoceptor blocking drugs. *Prog CV Dis* 19:203–234, 1976.

51. The Norwegian Multicentre Study Group: Timolol induced reduction in mortality and reinfarction in patients surviving acute MI. *N Engl J Med* 304:800–807, 1981.

52. Traub YM, Rabinov M, Rosenfeld JB, et al: Elevation of serum potassium during beta-blockade: Absence of relationship to the renin-aldosterone system. *Clini Pharmacol Ther* 28:765–768, 1980.

53. Rosa RM, Silva P, Young JB, et al: Adrenergic modulation of extra-renal potassium disposal. *N Engl J Med* 302:431–434, 1980.

54. Bia MJ, DeFronzo RA: Extra-renal potassium homeostasis, editorial. *Am J Physiol* 240:257–268, 1981.

55. Deedwania K: Calcium channel blockers. *West J Med* 137:24–31, 1982.

56. Zelis RF: Calcium entry blockers in cardiologic therapy. *Hosp Pract* 1981, pp 49–56.

57. Ellrodt G, Chew CYC, Singh BN: Therapeutic implications of slow channel blockade in circulatory disorders. *Circulation* 62:669–679, 1980.

58. Opie LH: Calcium antagonists. *Lancet* 1980, pp 806–810.

59. Pederson KE, et al: Digoxin-verapamil interaction. *Clin Pharmacol Ther* 30:311–316, 1981.

60. Hansten PD: Digoxin and calcium antagonists. *Drug Inter News* 1:46, 1981.

61. Zelis R: Calcium channel blocker therapy for unstable angina pectoris, editorial. *N Engl J Med* 306:926–928, 1982.

62. Robson RH, Vishwanath MC: Nifedipine and beta-blockade as a cause of heart failure. *Br Med J* 284:104, 1982.

63. Gillmer DJ, Kark P: Pulmonary edema precipitated by nifedipine. *Br Med J* 284:1420–1421, 1980.

64. Belz GG, et al: Digoxin plasma concentrations and nifedipine. *Lancet* 1:844–845, 1981.

65. Mauritson DR, Winniford MD, Walker WS, et al: Oral verapamil for paroxysmal supraventricular tachyarrhythmia. *Ann Int Med* 96:409–412, 1982.

66. Rosing DR, Epstein SE: Verapamil in the treatment of hypertrophic cardiomyopathy, editorial. *Ann Int Med* 96:670–672, 1982.

67. Gerstenblith G, Ouyang P, Achuff SC, et al: Nifedipine in unstable angina. *N Engl J Med* 306:926–928, 1982.

68. Opie LH: Nitrates. *Lancet* 1:750–753, 1980.

69. Abrams J: Nitroglycerin and long-acting nitrates. *N Engl J Med* 65:53–62, 1978.

70. Aronow WS: Clinical uses of nitrates. *Mod Concep Cardiovasc Dis* 48:47–52, 1979.

71. Warren SE, Francis GS: Nitroglycerin and nitrate esters. *Am J Med* 65:53–62, 1978.

72. Colucci WS: Alpha-adrenergic receptor blockade with prazosin. *Ann Int Med* 97:67–77, 1982.

73. Graham RM, Pettinger WA: Prazosin. *N Engl J Med* 300:232–236, 1979.

74. Opie LH: Vasodilating drugs. *Lancet* 1:966–972, 1980.

75. Walsh WF, Greenberg BH: Results of long-term vasodilator therapy in patients with congestive heart failure. *Circulation* 64:499–505, 1981.

76. Packer M, Meller J, Medina N, et al: Hemodynamic characterization of tolerance to long-term hydralazine therapy in severe chronic heart failure. *N Engl J Med* 306:58–62, 1982.

77. Durrer JD, Lie KI, vanCapelle FJL, et al: Effect of sodium nitroprusside on mortality rate in acute myocardial infarction complicated by left ventricular failure. *N Engl J Med* 306:1129–1135, 1982.

78. Cohn JH, Franciosa JA, Francis GS, et al: Effect of short-term infusion of sodium nitroprusside on mortality rate in acute myocardial infarction complicated by left ventricular failure. *N Engl J Med* 306:1129–1135, 1982.

79. Cohn JN, Buirke LP: Nitroprusside. *Ann Int Med* 91:752–757, 1979.

80. Posner MA, Rodkey FL, Tobey RE: Nitroprusside-induced cyanide poisoning. *Anesthesiology* 44:330–335, 1976.

81. Glasser SP, Clark PI, Applebaum JH: Occurrence of frequent complex arrhythmias detected by ambulatory monitoring. *Chest* 75:565–568, 1979.

82. Velebit V, Podrid P, et al: Aggravation and provocation of ventricular arrhythmias by anti-arrhythmic drugs. *Circulation* 65:886–894, 1982.

83. Strasberg B, Sclaroosky S, Srdberg A, et al: Procainamide-induced polymorphous ventricular tachycardia. *Am J Cardiol* 47:1309–1314, 1981.

84. Opie LH: Antiarrhythmic agents. *Lancet* 1:861–868, 1980.

85. Collinsworth K: Clinical pharmacology of lidocaine as an antiarrhythmic drug. *West J Med* 124:36–43, 1976.

86. Nation RL, Triggs EJ, Selig M: Lidocaine Kinetics in cardiac patients, and elderly subjects. *Br J Clin Pharmacol* 4:439–448, 1977.

87. Pfeifer JH, Greenblatt DJ, Koch-Weser J: Clinical use and toxicity of intravenous lidocaine: A report from the Boston Collaborative Drug Surveillance Program. *Am Heart J* 92:168–173, 1976.

88. Thomson PD, Melmon KL, Richardson JA, et al: Lidocaine pharmacokinetics in advanced heart failure, liver disease and renal failure in humans. *Ann Int Med* 78:499–508, 1973.

89. Harrison DC, Berte LE: Should prophylactic antiarrhythmic drug therapy be used in acute myocardial infarction? *JAMA* 247:2019–2031, 1982.

90. Greenblatt DJ, et al: Pharmacokinetic approach to the clinical use of lidocaine intravenously. *JAMA* 236:273–277, 1976.

91. Noneman JW, Rogers JF: Lidocaine prophylaxis in acute myocardial infarction. *Medicine* 57:501–515, 1978.

92. Hillestad L, Bjerkelund C, Dale J, et al: Quinidine in maintenance of sinus rhythm after electroconversion of chronic atrial fibrillation. *Br Heart J* 33:418–421, 1971.

93. Federman J, Vlietstra RE: Antiarrhythmic drug therapy. *Mayo Clin Proc* 54:531–542, 1979.

94. Ochs JR, Greenblatt DJ, Woo E, et al: Reduced quinidine clearance in elderly persons. *Am J Cardiol* 42:481–485, 1978.

95. Ochs JR, Greenblatt DJ, Woo E: Clinical pharmacokinetics of quinidine. *Clin Pharm* 5:150–168, 1980.

96. Sodermark T, Edhag O, Sjogren A, et al: Effect of quinidine on maintaining sinus rhythm after conversion of atrial fibrillation or flutter. *Br Heart J* 37:486–492, 1975.

97. Reidenberg MM, Camacho M, Kluger J, et al: Aging and renal clearance of procainamide and acetylprocainamide. *Clin Pharmacol Ther* 28:732–735, 1980.

98. Galeazzi RL, Omar-Amberg C, Karlaganis G: N-acetylprocainamide kinetics in the elderly. *Clin Pharmacol Ther* 29:440–446, 1981.

99. Dubois EL: Procainamide-induction of a systemic lupus erythematosus-like picture. *Medicine* 48:217–218, 1969.

100. Kluger J, Drayer D, Reidenberg MM, et al: Acetylprocainamide therapy in patients with previous procainamide induced lupus syndrome. *Ann Int Med* 95:18–23, 1981.

101. Bennett WM, Muther RS, Parker RA, et al: Drug therapy in renal failure: Dosing guidelines for adults. *Ann Int Med* 93:(part I)62–89, (part 2)286–325, 1980.

102. Morady F, Scheinman MM, Desai J: Disopyramide. *Ann Int Med* 96:337–343, 1982.

103. Podrid PJ, Schoenberger A, Lown B: Congestive heart failure caused by oral disopyramide. *N Engl J Med* 302:614–616, 1980.

104. Leach AJ, Brown JE, Armstrong PW: Cardiac depression by intravenous disopyramide in patients with left ventricular dysfunction. *Am J Med* 68:839–844, 1980.

105. Ellrodt G, Singh B: Adverse effects of disopyramide: Toxic interactions with other antiarrhythmic agents. *Heart and Lung* 9:469–474, 1980.

106. Maddux BD, Whiting RB: Toxic synergism of disopyramide and hyperkalemia. *Chest* 78:654–656, 1980.

Chapter 40

Psychotherapeutic Drugs

Jane E. Stilwell, M.D.

Psychotherapeutic agents are so commonly used by the geriatric population that clinicians must become proficient in their use and be alert to potential risks. The anxiolytic sedatives, antidepressants, and antipsychotics may cause a significant morbidity and mortality not only by their own pharmacologic actions, but by complex interactions with other drugs and with natural aging processes. Clinicians should be aware of the general prescribing principles and the specific characteristics of the drugs that their patients use. By astute and judicious management of psychotherapeutic agents, elderly persons will benefit and avoid unnecessary ill effects.

Psychotherapeutic drugs are the second most commonly prescribed category of drugs for elderly persons. In one survey, 32% of all people 60–70 years of age had used a psychotropic drug within the previous year.[1] United States government studies have shown that 75% of all nursing home residents receive at least one of these agents,[2] and in 12 Veterans Administration hospitals, 70% of all elderly patients received at least one drug.[3] Paralleling the widespead use of psychotherapeutic drugs is a disproportionate incidence rate of adverse drug reactions.[4–7] In the over-70 age group, the incidence rate of adverse reactions is two-to-four times greater than in people younger than 40 years of age.[7,8] In Sydney, Australia, 16% of all admissions to one psychogeriatric unit were directly attributed to the ill effects of these drugs.[9]

Toxicity

The decrease in the functional reserve capacity of organ systems in older people results in an altered metabolism and clearance of drugs that lead to elevated plasma drug levels with customary therapeutic doses. Since the anxiolytic sedatives, antidepressants, and antipsychotics have direct central nervous system effects, their use in patients with a decreased cerebral reserve capacity may cause confusion and sedation; the consequences of both are falls, fractures, and further isolation in sensory-impaired individuals. Some of these drugs have cardiovascular effects and may cause a clinically significant cardiotoxicity in patients with an impaired myocardium or conduction system. A common and potentially serious side effect in elderly persons is orthostatic hypotension, which may be associated not only with falls and fractures, but also with arrhythmias, myocardial infarction, and cerebrovascular injury. Finally, elderly persons are especially sensitive to the anticholinergic effects of many psychotropic medications. A decreased functional reserve allows a bothersome side effect to become a clinically significant toxicity. Therefore, these drugs must be monitored carefully for toxic effects that often occur with lower dosages in elderly patients with a compromised functional reserve.

General Principles

There are some useful principles that should be applied when prescribing these drugs for an elderly patient:

1. Establish an accurate diagnosis, a clear indication for therapy, and a specific therapeutic goal;
2. Search for behavioral manifestations of somatic illnesses. Congestive heart failure, cerebrovascular insufficiency, chronic renal failure, and visual or hearing impairments may be present and associated with abnormal behavior;
3. Adjust the initial dose according to the expected pharmacokinetic changes in an elderly patient. Starting doses are often one third to one half of the doses for the general population;
4. Titrate the maintenance dose to the individual patient. Careful, frequent evaluation of both therapeutic and toxic effects will ensure maximum efficacy;
5. Observe a patient closely for toxic effects that may be both subtle and complex;
6. Search for potential drug interactions with other prescription and over-the-counter drugs;
7. Simplify the therapeutic regimen to promote compliance and to minimize toxicity;
8. Become familiar with a few drugs in each class and learn to use them properly and effectively;
9. Explore other modalities of therapy that will augment medication; and
10. Recognize the potential for abuse by physicians, patients, and care-givers.

The Anxiolytic Sedatives

Benzodiazepines

All benzodiazepines that currently are in clinical use are effective for the treatment of anxiety, tension, and insomnia without affecting perceptual or cognitive processes.[10] All exhibit some anticonvulsant activity and varying degrees of skeletal muscle relaxation. They have a lower incidence rate of drug interactions and side effects than other anxiolytic sedatives and are commonly used for that reason. Since there are no well-controlled, long-term trials that compare the efficacy of various benzodiazepines as hypnotics,[11,12] the choice of a benzodiazepine for use in elderly persons is commonly based on the potential for unwanted side effects. Toxic effects stem from both an apparent increase in sensitivity of elderly people to central nervous system effects and alterations in pharmacokinetics that may hamper drug elimination. Ordinarily, the benzodiazepines that rely on hepatic oxidative metabolism (diazepam, flurazepam, nitrazepam, and chlordiazepoxide) show an appreciable increase in their elimination half-life and show higher plasma levels of both the parent compounds and active metabolites. The consequences are lethargy, excessive sedation, confusion, orthostatic hypotension, and ataxia. Conversely, benzodiazepines that are metabolized by conjugation with glucuronic acid (temazepam, oxazepam, and lorazepam) do not show significant metabolic changes with age[12] and generally are considered safer for use in elderly persons. All benzodiazepines, however, share with the barbiturates the risk of causing a nightly reliance on drugs for sleep.[13] In addition, all are capable of producing paradoxic behavioral reactions that are characterized by increased agitation, aggressiveness, and confusion.[14] Studies concerning the effects of benzodiazepines on the sleep apnea syndrome are not available; therefore, these drugs should be used with caution in older patients in whom this syndrome is recognized.

Chlordiazepoxide

The prototype benzodiazepine, chlordiazepoxide, has significantly altered kinetics in elderly persons. The rate of gastrointestinal absorption following the administration is increased from less than 1 hour in young subjects to 3.3 hours in elderly subjects.[15] The elimination half-life is similarly prolonged to nearly double that found in young subjects after oral administration and eight to nine times that found after intravenous (IV) administration.[16] The total drug clearance, which is responsible for drug accumulation in chronic dosing, is reduced by 40%.[15,16] The fixed-dose administration of chlordiazepoxide may result in a slow accumulation of the drug to inappropriately high levels in elderly persons[16] and may lead to a substantial increase in central nervous system effects.[1]

Diazepam

Diazepam, which is the most extensively prescribed anxiolytic sedative, has been shown in controlled studies to alleviate anxiety in elderly patients,[10] to improve sleep, and to control hyperactivity and anxiety in geriatric patients with an organic brain syndrome.[17] Altered pharmacokinetics in older patients lead to higher and long-lasting plasma levels with attendant central nervous system side effects. Absorption of diazepam is slowed with lower peak concentrations.[13] The hepatic oxidative metabolism changes diazepam to three active metabolites that have a prolonged half-life of 20–200 hours and that may require 2–3 weeks to achieve steady-state plasma levels.[13] The elimination half-life of diazepam increases significantly with age, and the increase is greater among females.[18] The controversy about the effect of age on total drug clearance remains unresolved,[13,18,19] but it appears that it decreases.[18] The accumulation of high plasma drug levels with the chronic administration of diazepam may cause a long-lasting impairment of central nervous system function after the drug is withdrawn. Benzodiazepines with less complicated metabolic rates and shorter half-lives should be considered before chronic diazepam therapy is instituted.

Flurazepam

Flurazepam has become the most commonly prescribed hypnotic for hospitalized medical patients in the United States and Canada.[20] It is 80% absorbed after oral administration[13] and is metabolized in the liver to an active metabolite whose half-life is 47–100 hours.[13] This long-lasting metabolite is responsible for the persistent sedative effects of flurazepam.[13] Of all patients over 70 years of age, 39% experience side effects following the customary 30 mg-dose given to young adults. Adverse reactions are reduced

to less than 2% when patients receive a dose that is less than 15 mg.[20] These findings suggest that low-dose flurazepam may be an acceptable choice of a hypnotic drug in elderly persons if a surveillance for cumulative drug effects is made during chronic administration. However, even a low dose may produce deleterious effects in a frail elderly person with mental impairment.

Oxazepam

Oxazepam may be particularly suited for use in elderly persons.[10] Of 17 double-blind, placebo-controlled studies, 14 have shown oxazepam to be effective for the treatment of anxiety.[21] It is well tolerated and effective in the treatment of anxiety with or without depression,[22,23] and it is effective against irritability, insomnia, and agitation in geriatric patients.[24] Oxazepam is an hydroxylated metabolite of diazepam, but it has no active metabolites of its own. Its half-life of 7–10 hours is shorter than that of chlordiazepoxide, diazepam, and flurazepam,[23] and it shows no age-related changes.[25] Its major route of elimination is conjugation, which shows no appreciable decline with age. The side effects of an altered central nervous system function appear to be less frequently encountered with oxazepam than with chlordiazepoxide.[26]

Temazepam

Temazepam, which is a derivative of diazepam via hydroxylation, has a short half-life and no active metabolites. It reaches peak plasma concentrations in 3 hours, so it may be useful for sleep disorders that are characterized by difficulty in falling asleep.[11] Between 80–90% is excreted in the urine as the glucuronide conjugate, and its clearance is not affected by age.[11,27] It accumulates less than flurazepam or diazepam and may be particularly suitable for use in elderly persons.[10] However, it is more likely to cause rebound insomnia.

Lorazepam

Lorazepam is safe and effective for inducing sleep in elderly persons.[28] It is 10-fold more potent than its parent compound, oxazepam,[10] but it similarly has no active metabolites. Its short half-life of 16 hours is not significantly different in elderly persons.[13] It reaches peak plasma concentrations 2 hours after oral administration and is the most potent benzodiazepine in producing amnesia.[10] Drowsiness and daytime somnolence in elderly persons are more frequently associated with larger doses (2 mg/night).[28]

Nitrazepam

Nitrazepam probably is unsuited for use in elderly persons.[29] Its chronic use may result in considerable confusion, ataxia, and drowsiness. The kinetics of nitrazepam do not differ significantly in elderly persons, but an evaluation of performance following nitrazepam shows a significant impairment in elderly subjects.[30] Because kinetics are unchanged, the cerebral symptoms suggest an increase in central nervous system sensitivity to the drug.

Barbiturates

Barbiturates are effective soporifics; but, in elderly persons, they are especially prone to cause paradoxical agitation, aggressive behavior with confusion, and delirium.[10,31] In addition, they can cause central hypoventilation, which may compound dangers of sleep apnea or pneumonia. Their potential for habituation and addiction, cumulative action, and severe and often fatal effects following an overdose make them particularly unsuited for use in elderly persons.[31]

Tricyclic Antidepressants

Mechanism of Action

The tricyclic antidepressants share a common three-ring structure that is similar to the phenothiazine nucleus. Their differing pharmacologic properties are determined by side-chain substitutions of either secondary or tertiary amine groups. Although the mechanism of action is not established precisely, all tricyclic antidepressants inhibit the reuptake of the central nervous system neurotransmitters, norepinephrine and serotonin. This potentiates synaptic transmission and reverses the depletion of neurotransmitters which is associated with an

endogenous depression. The tertiary amine tricyclics, amitriptyline, doxepin, and imipramine, all inhibit the reuptake of serotonin; the secondary amine compounds, nortriptyline, protriptyline, and desipramine, inhibit the reuptake of norepinephrine.[32,33]

Pharmacology

Antidepressant Activity
Despite the controversy that surrounds their mechanism of action, tricyclic antidepressants have proven to be efficacious against depression in elderly persons.[10,34–37] There are six tricyclic antidepressants that are commonly prescribed in this country. Controlled comparative trials have usually demonstrated a generally equivalent efficacy.[38] Therefore, the choice of a specific drug often is made on the basis of side effects that are secondary to the antidepressant activity. Elderly persons are especially sensitive to these diverse actions; often, the tolerance of a tricyclic is determined by a patient's acceptance of these effects.

Anticholinergic Activity
All tricyclic antidepressants exert both central and peripheral anticholinergic activities, which do not contribute significantly to the antidepressant activity.[36] The six common tricyclics have varying degrees of anticholinergic activity (see Table 40-1). In general, tertiary amines are more anticholinergic than secondary amines.

Antihistamine Activity
Antihistamine activity with a blocking of H-1 and H-2 receptors is shared by all tricyclic antidepressants. It does not necessarily parallel anticholinergic activity.[36] The antihistamine activity of doxepin is greater than that of amitriptyline, while desipramine has the least.[39] This pharmacologic effect probably is responsible for the sedative properties of the tricyclics (see Table 40-1). Again, tertiary amines generally are more sedating than secondary amines. In clinical practice, the choice of a specific tricyclic agent often is based on the degree of sedation that is desired.[38] Antihistaminic effects on the central nervous system may be responsible for the weight gain that often occurs during tricyclic therapy. Caloric intake must be monitored if weight gain is undesirable.

TABLE 40-1   Side Effects of Antidepressants

	Anticholinergic Effects	Sedative Effects
High	Amitriptyline Doxepin Imipramine	Doxepin Amitriptyline
Moderate	Protriptyline Nortriptyline Amoxapine Maprotilline	Maprotilline Imipramine Nortriptyline
Low	Desipramine Trazodone	Amoxapine Trazodone Protriptyline Desipramine

Alpha-Adrenergic Blockade

Finally, tricyclic antidepressants exert both a central and peripheral alpha-adrenergic blockade that are responsible for orthostatic hypotension and for their interference with centrally acting antihypertensive medications.

Pharmacokinetics

The tricyclic antidepressants are administered orally and show a rapid gastrointestinal absorption. They undergo extensive first-pass hepatic extraction and metabolism. Tertiary amines are metabolized by microsomal enzymes to secondary amines. These generally are conjugated with glucuronic acid and are excreted in the urine. The tricyclics have large volumes of distribution because of their high lipid solubility. Only some kinetic parameters have been demonstrated in elderly persons. The half-lives of amitriptyline and imipramine are significantly prolonged. Similarly, elderly patients who are treated with equal doses of these two drugs develop higher steady-state plasma concentrations of parent compounds and active metabolites than younger patients.[25,36,40] Despite higher plasma levels, attaining a steady-state equilibrium may be considerably prolonged; the customary expectation of a 3-week onset of antidepressant activity may be optimistic in the geriatric population.[40] These data suggest that elderly persons should be treated with lower doses of antidepressants; indeed, one third to one half of the usual adult dose is administered initially. The return of a normal sleep pattern occurs rapidly, followed by an improvement of

nervousness, somatic complaints, appetite, and psychomotor retardation. Full antidepressant activity may not be evident for 3–6 weeks,[38] although an earlier response sometimes is observed in elderly persons.

Toxic Effects

Anticholinergic Effects

The extension of common anticholinergic side effects into clinically significant problems is a frequent occurrence. Urinary retention, constipation and fecal impaction, decreased visual accommodation, and a precipitation of acute glaucoma occur more frequently in elderly than younger patients.[4,35] Acute central anticholinergic effects can precipitate sedation, confusion, and even a florid toxic delirium.[36,37,41] Tolerance to adverse effects usually develops and can be aided by reducing the total dose or delivering it in a divided fashion. When adverse effects are intolerable, changing the therapy to a tricyclic agent with a milder anticholinergic acitivity often is successful.

Cardiotoxicity

Cardiotoxic effects are manifestations of a direct action on the cardiovascular system. Tricyclic antidepressants have quinidine-like effects on the myocardium[42] and may decrease cardiac conduction[43] while increasing cardiac repolarization. They also have direct anticholinergic effects and exert an adrenergic stimulation, while producing a peripheral alpha-adrenergic blockade.

The most common and serious cardiovascular effect is orthostatic hypotension, which is caused by this blockade of peripheral alpha-adrenergic receptors.[33] Of all young patients without a cardiovascular disease, 25% experience orthostatic hypotension when treated with imipramine. Elderly patients with a cardiovascular disease experience it three times more frequently.[44,45] Consequent falls and fractures, cardiac arrhythmias, and cerebrovascular accidents can result in a serious morbidity and mortality.[35] All tricyclics can cause orthostatic hypotension,[46] but the available literature is sparse regarding the frequency of hypotension that is caused by amitriptyline, doxepin, or desipramine in elderly persons. Nortriptyline may have significantly less of a hypotensive effect[44] and may be particularly useful in elderly persons.

Tricyclic antidepressants have significant effects on cardiac conduction with both therapeutic and toxic levels. Electrocardiographic alterations are common during therapy and include a prolongation of the PR- and QT-intervals and of QRS duration.[4,47] In patients with an existing bundle-branch block, a clinically significant AV or HV block may be precipitated. In addition, the quinidine-like action of tricyclics may exacerbate the sick sinus syndrome.[44] Imipramine has quinidine-like effects against a ventricular ectopy with therapeutic levels, but information regarding this action in other tricyclics is not known.[44,48] Toxic levels of tricyclics can be associated with a sinus tachycardia, supraventricular tachyarrhythmias, conduction defects, atrioventricular block, bundle-branch block, and with ventricular tachycardia or fibrillation.[49] In patients with normal left ventricular function, there is no evidence for its impairment with tricyclic use; but, the evidence is inconclusive in patients with left ventricular dysfunction.[44,50] A recent myocardial infarction is often regarded as an absolute contraindication to tricyclic therapy, but an intraventricular conduction delay is not.[37] There is little conclusive evidence that doxepin is less cardiotoxic with therapeutic levels than other tricyclics.[25] The simultaneous treatment with tricyclics and phenothiazines increases the risk of cardiotoxicity and should be undertaken with caution.[49]

Non-Tricyclic Antidepressants

Maprotiline

Maprotiline is a tetracyclic compound that inhibits the reuptake of norepinephrine but has no effect on serotonin. While it has demonstrated a significant antidepressant activity, it appears to offer little advantage over the tricyclics. Its adverse effects are similar, and there is no convincing evidence that its onset of action is shorter.[50,51]

Trazodone

Trazodone is structurally unrelated to either the tricyclic or tetracyclic compounds. It inhibits the reuptake of serotonin, but the relationship of this activity to its antidepressant effect is unknown. Its antidepressant activity equals that of the tricyclics, and it has demonstrated efficacy and safety in the geriatric population.[52-54] Trazodone has little, if any, anticholinergic effect, but its potential to induce dizziness and orthostatic hypotension equals that of the tricyclics. It has little apparent cardiotoxicity. Trazodone may make an important contribution to antidepressant medications for elderly persons, but further clinical experience is necessary to assess its usefulness.

Amoxapine

Amoxapine has significant antidepressant activity, but it offers no clear advantage over other tricyclics. In addition, its phenothiazine-like structure may confer clinically important extrapyramidal system activity.[55]

Monoamine Oxidase (MAO) Inhibitors

Monoamine oxidase (MAO) inhibitors were among the first antidepressants to be developed. While they are effacacious, their potential for important interactions with foods and other drugs and their precipitation of hypertensive episodes makes them less often suitable for the geriatric population.[36] Their use should be reserved for patients who have a history of previous response to them, a history of non-response to tricyclics, and who are able to attend to the details of dietary restrictions that are imposed by their use.[10,56]

Antipsychotic Medication

Antipsychotic medications have an important use in the treatment of geriatric patients for whom they are most frequently prescribed for symptoms that are associated with dementia. The antipsychotics comprise three groups of compounds with similar efficacy and pharmacology. The choice of a specific antipsychotic often is based on attempts to avoid side effects, rather than a clear superiority of one drug over another. The therapeutic and toxic effects of neuroleptic drugs often are exaggerated in elderly persons, so close supervision must accompany their use.

Classification

There are three major classes of antipsychotic drugs. The phenothiazines are three-ring compounds that are structurally and pharmacologically similar to tricyclic antidepressants. Phenothiazines with piperidine side chains are equal in antipsychotic potency, but they have more anticholinergic effects. Therefore, they cause extrapyramidal effects less frequently. By contrast, piperazine phenothiazines are more potent than chlorpromazine in inducing antipsychotic and extrapyramidal effects, but they are less anticholinergic. Thioxanthenes possess a similar three-ring structure. Individual thioxanthenes have less of an antipsychotic potency than homologous phenothiazines. The third class of antipsychotics, the butyrophenones, are structurally unlike the other classes. They most closely resemble the piperidine phenothiazines in structure and share a similar pharmacologic activity. In general, they possess less sedative and anticholinergic activity than aliphatic or piperidine phenothiazines, but they retain considerable potential for inducing extrapyramidal side effects.

Since comparative studies have not shown important qualitative differences in the antipsychotic effects of these drugs, and since no drug is without a potential for causing side effects,[57] a clinician should become familiar with, and master the use of, one or two drugs in each class.

Pharmacology

Antipsychotic Activity

The fundamental pharmacologic action of the phenothiazines is the blockade of dopaminergic receptors, which accounts for both therapeutic and toxic effects. The therapeutic effects include emotional calming, psychomotor slowing, and promotion of an indifference of affect.[57] They have significant effects on thought disturbances which accompany paranoid states delusions, and agitation. In the geriatric population, their efficacy has been demonstrated[58–60] in controlling symptoms that are associated with delirium and dementia, which may include restlessness, agitation, hostility, hallucinations and delusions, paranoid ideation, emotional outbursts, and lability of affect.[61]

Alpha-Adrenergic Blockade

The antipsychotics cause varying degrees of alpha-adrenergic blockade, which can result in orthostatic hypotension and sedation. Elderly persons are particularly sensitive to these effects[62] and may experience adverse consequences as a result.

Anticholinergic Activity

The neuroleptic drugs also possess an anticholinergic activity that usually causes visual blurring with therapeutic doses (see Table 40-2). They may cause dry mouth, urinary incontinence, and constipation, which may limit compliance.

Pharmacokinetics

Because of the increased sensitivity to the effect of the antipsychotics, one third to one half of the customary dose is prescribed for elderly persons. Sedative and anticholinergic activities appear within a few days, while neuroleptic effects may not be apparent for 1–3 weeks. Since steady-state plasma levels are reached in 5–8 days, increases in dosages at less than weekly intervals may lead to overmedication. Their in-

TABLE 40-2   Side Effects of Antipsychotic Agents

	Sedative Effects	Extrapyramidal Effects
High	Chlorpromazine Thioridazine	Haloperidol Thiothixene Trifluoperazine
Moderate	Acetophenazine Trifluoperazine	Chlorpromazine Acetophenazine Thiothixene
Low	Haloperidol	Thioridazine

herently long half-life makes a single daily dose practical, and night-time administration capitalizes on the sedative effects. Divided daily doses sometimes are used to minimize anticholinergic effects. A tolerance to the sedative and anticholinergic effects usually develops as therapy is continued.[57]

Toxic Effects

Anticholinergic Toxicity
(See pages 614–616)

Cardiotoxicity
Cardiotoxicity is a result of peripheral vasodilation, direct myocardial depression, and quinidine-like actions of the phenothiazines. Electrocardiographic changes are relatively common and include a prolongation of the PR-, QRS-, and QT-intervals, ST-segment depression, and T-wave notching, flattening, and inversion. With an impaired conduction system or with higher drug levels, atrioventricular conduction abnormalities, ventricular ectopy, and ventricular tachycardia of fibrillation may occur.[63] Cardiotoxicity is most common with piperidine phenothiazines (thioridazine and mesoridazine).[57]

Extrapyramidal Effects
The extrapyramidal effects of antipsychotics are particularly troubling (see Table 40-2). The extrapyramidal effects probably result from a depletion of dopamine by the phenothiazines, which leads to cholinergic overactivity. Typical antiparkinsonism medications often are effective against these side effects, probably by restoring the feedback inhibition.[64] Pheno-

thiazines (piperidines) that have the most anticholinergic activity are least likely to produce extrapyramidal effects. The butyrophenones, piperazine phenothiazines, and thioxanthenes have less anticholinergic activity and, therefore, more extrapyramidal side effects that are associated with their use (see Table 40-2).[57,58,60,64]

The manifestations of extrapyramidal effects include parkinsonian symptoms, acute dystonic reactions, akathisia, and tardive dyskinesia. Acute dystonic reactions are relatively rare in the geriatric population, but the other three types occur frequently.[65] Antipsychotic drug-induced parkinsonism is indistinguishable from the idiopathic type and is characterized by a shuffling gait, pill-rolling tremor, rigidity, and poverty of movement. It occurs at any time during therapy and usually is dose-related. It generally responds to a reduction in medication or an addition of anticholinergic medication. The use of L-Dopa is contraindicated because it vitiates the action of the antipsychotic medication, which is intended to block dopamine action.

Akathisia is a motor disturbance that is characterized by a subjective desire to be in constant motion.[57] It is not as common as parkinsonism in elderly persons, but it may be misinterpreted as an increased agitation and treated by increasing the antipsychotic agent.[62,66] There is an unpredictable responsiveness to anticholinergics, and proper treatment is the dose reduction of the neuroleptic.

Tardive dyskinesia has its highest incidence rate in elderly persons and is characterized by stereotypic movements of the eyes, lips, jaw, and tongue. It may be accompanied by dyskinesias of the trunk and upper extremities or by choreiform movements. Anticholinergics are ineffective, and the dyskinesia may worsen on reducing the antipsychotic agent.[67-69] Tardive dyskinesias are more frequent after prolonged treatment; since they are often irreversible after discontinuing the neuroleptic, early clues to their presence must be sought.

Other Toxicity

Other adverse effects include agranulocytosis and leukopenia, cholestatic jaundice, and dermatologic abnormalities that include urticaria, dermatitis, and photosensitivity. Phenothiazines may lower the seizure threshold and should be used with caution in patients with seizure disorders.

References

1. Parry JH, Balter MB, Mellinger GD, et al: National patterns of psychotherapeutic drug use. *Arch Gen Psychiatry* 28:269–283, 1973.
2. Special Committee on Aging, U.S. Senate: *Nursing Home Care in the U.S., Failure in Public Policy.* Washington, DC, United States Government Printing Office, 1974.
3. Prien F: A survey of psychoactive drug use in the aged at Veterans Administration Hospitals, in Gershon A and Raskin A (eds): *Aging.* New York, Raven Press, 1975, vol 2, pp 143–153.
4. Ouslander G: Drug therapy in the elderly. *Ann Int Med* 95:711–722, 1981.
5. Nithman CJ, Parkhurst YE, Sommers EB: Physician's prescribing habits. *JAMA* 217:585–587, 1971.
6. Peterson DM, Thomas CW: Acute drug reaction among the elderly. *J Gerontol* 30:552–556, 1976.
7. Blaschke TF, Cohen SN, Tatro DS: Drug-Drug interactions and aging, in Jarvik LF, Greenblatt DS (eds): *Clinical Pharmacology and the Aged Patient.* New York, Raven Press, 1981, pp 11–26.
8. Seidl LG: Studies on epidemiology of adverse drug reactions. *Bull Johns Hopkins Hosp* 119:299–315, 1966.
9. deGroot MHL: The clinical use of psychotherapeutic drugs in the elderly. *Drugs* 8:132–138, 1974.
10. Ban T: *Psychopharmacology for the aged.* New York, Karger, 1980.
11. *Medical Letter:* Temazepam. 24:16, 1982.
12. Conrad KA: Antianxiety agents and hypnotics, in Conrad KA, Bressler R (eds): *Drug Therapy for the Elderly.* St. Louis, The CV Mosby Co, 1982, pp 262–276.
13. Ban TA: Psychopathology, psychopharmacology and the organic brain syndrome. *Psychosomatics* 17:131–137, 1976.
14. Shader RI, et al: Absorption and disposition of chlordiazepoxide in young and elderly male volunteers. *J Clin Pharmacol* 17:709–718, 1977.
15. Roberts RK, Wilkinson GR, Branch RA, et al: Effect of age and parenchymal liver disease on the disposition and elimination of chlordiazepoxide (librium). *Gastroenterology* 75:479–485, 1978.
16. Cromwell HA: Management of anxiety/depression in geriatric patients. *Med Times* 101:47–53, 1973.
17. Greenblatt DJ: Diazepam disposition determinants. *Clin Pharmacol Therap* 27:301–312, 1980.
18. Klotz U, Avant GR, Hoyumpa A, et al: The effects of age and liver disease on the disposition and elimination of diazepam in adult man. *J Clin Invest* 55:347–359, 1975.
19. Greenblatt DJ, Allen MD, Shader RI: Toxicity in high dose flurazepam in the elderly. *Clin Pharmacol Therap* 21:335–361, 1977.
20. Blackwell B: A critical review of oxazepam: Efficacy and specificity. *Dis Nerv Syst* 36(suppl):17–22, 1975.
21. Merlis S, Koepke HH: The use of oxazepam in elderly patients. *Dis Nerv Syst* 36(suppl):27–29, 1975.
22. Ayd FJ: Oxazepam: An overview. *Dis Nerv Syst* 36(suppl):14–16, 1975.
23. Beber CR: Management of behavior in the institutionalized aged. *Dis Nerv Syst* 26:591–595, 1965.
24. Hicks R, Dysken MW, Davis JM, et al: The pharmacokinetics of psychotropic medication in the elderly: A review. *J Clin Psychiatry* 42:374–385, 1981.
25. Chesrow EJ, Kaplitz SE, Vetra H, et al: Blind study of oxazepam in the management of geriatric patients with behavioral problems. *Clin Med* 72:1001–1005, 1965.
26. Divol M: Effect of age and gender on disposition of temazepam. *J Pharm Sci* 70:104, 1981.
27. Baren DA, Resnick O: Lorazepam versus glutethimide as a sleep-inducing agent for the geriatric patient. *J Am Geriatr Soc* 21:507–511, 1973.
28. Evans IG, Jarvis EH: Nitrazepam and the elderly. *Br Med J* 4:487, 1972.
29. Dawson-Butterworth K: The chemopsychotherapeutics of geriatric sedation. *J Am Geriatr Soc* 18:97–114, 1970.

30. Castleden CM, George CF, Marcer D, et al: Increased sensitivity to nitrazepam in old age. *Br Med J* 1:10–12, 1977.

31. Mass W: Biogenic amines and depression. *Arch Gen Psychiatry* 32:1357–1361, 1975.

32. Rosenbaum AH, Maruta T, Richelson E: Drugs that alter mood: Tricyclic agents and monoamine oxidase inhibitors. *Mayo Clin Proc* 54:335–344, 1979.

33. Barnes R, Veith RC, Raskind MA: Depression in older persons: Diagnosis and management. *West J Med* 135:463–468, 1981.

34. Jarvik LF, Kakkar PR: Aging and response to antidepressants, in Jarvik LF (ed): *Clinical Pharmacology and the Aged Patient*. New York, Raven Press, 1981, pp 49–77.

35. Bressler R: Antidepressant agents, in Conrad KA, Bressler R (eds): *Drug Therapy for the Elderly*. St. Louis, The CV Mosby Co, 1982, pp 295–315.

36. Hollister LE: Treatment of depression with drugs. *Ann Int Med* 89:78–84, 1978.

37. Hollister LE: Tricyclic antidepressants. *N Engl J Med* 299:1106–1109 and 1168–1172, 1978.

38. Richelson E: Tricyclic antidepressants and histamine H_1 receptors. *Mayo Clin Proc* 54:669–674, 1979.

39. Nies A, Robinson DS, Friedman MJ: Relationship between age and tricylic antidepressant plasma levels. *Am J Psychiatry* 134:790–793, 1977.

40. Davies RK, Tucker GJ, Harrow M, et al: Confusional episodes and antidepressant medication. *Am J Psychiatry* 128:95–99, 1971.

41. Vohra J, Burrows G, Hunt D, et al: The effect of toxic and therapeutic doses of tricylic antidepressant drugs on intracardiac conduction. *Eur J Cardiol* 3:219–227, 1975.

42. Williams RB, Sherteri C: Cardiac complications of tricylic antidepressant therapy. *Ann Int Med* 74:395–398, 1971.

43. Glassman AH, Bigger JT: Cardiovascular effects of therapeutic doses of tricyclic antidepressants. *Arch Gen Psychiatry* 38:815–820, 1981.

44. Hayes JR: Incidence of orthostatic hypotension in patients with primary affective disorder treated with tricylic antidepressants. *Mayo Clin Proc* 52:509–512, 1977.

45. Ouslander JG: Drug prescribing for the elderly. *West J Med* 135:455–462, 1981.

46. Kantor SJ, Glassman AH, Bigger JT, et al: The cardiac effects of therapeutic plasma concentration of imipramine. *Am J Psychiatry* 135:534–538, 1978.

47. Giardina EG, Bigger JT, Glassman AH, et al: The electrocardiographic and antiarrhythmic effects of imipramine hydrochloride at therapeutic plasma concentrations. *Circulation* 60:1045–1052, 1979.

48. Benowitz NL, Rosenberg J, Becker CE: Cardiopulmonary catastrophes in drug overdosed patients. *Med Clin North Am* 63:267–296, 1979.

49. Veith RC: Cardiovascular effects of tricylic antidepressants in depressed patients with chronic heart disease. *N Engl J Med* 306:954–959, 1982.

50. Medical Letter. Maprotiline (Ludiomil): Another antidepressant. 14:585–590, 1981.

51. Stimmel GL: Maprotiline. *Drug Intell Clin Pharm* 14:585–590, 1980.

52. *Medical Letter*. Trazodone (Desyrel): A new non-tricyclic antidepressant. 24:47–48, 1982.

53. Rawls WN: Trazodone. *Drug Intell Clin Pharm* 16:7–13, 1982.

54. Gerner R, Estabrook KW, Steuer J, et al: Treatment of geriatric depression with trazodone, imipramine and placebo: A double blind study. *J Clin Psychiatry* 41:216–220, 1980.

55. *Medical Letter:* Amoxapine (Ascendin)—A new antidepressant. 23:39–40, 1981.

56. Lamy PP: *Prescribing for the Elderly*. Littleton, Massachusetts, PSG Publishing Co, 1982.

57. Bressler R: Neuroleptic agents, in Conrad KA, Bressler R (eds): *Drug Therapy for the Elderly*. The CV Mosby Co, 1982, pp 277–294.

58. Branchey MH, Lee JH, Amin R, et al: High and low potency neuroleptics in elderly psychiatric patients. *JAMA* 239:1860–1862, 1978.

59. Rudy WJ: An internist's observations on thioridazine in the very elderly. *J Am Geriatr Soc* 15:587–592, 1967.

60. Tsuang MM, Lu LM, Stotsky BA, et al: Haloperidol versus thoridazine for hospitalized psychogeriatric patients: Double blind study. *J Am Geriatr Soc* 19:593–600, 1971.

61. Charaton FT, Sherman FT, Libow LS: Geriatric psychiatry, in Libow LS, Sherman FT (eds): *The Core of Geriatric Medicine*. St. Louis, The CV Mosby Co, 1981, pp 59–84.

62. Hollister LE: Psychotherapeutic dugs, in Levenson A (ed): *Neuropsychiatric Side Effects of Drugs—The Elderly*. Aging. New York, Raven Press, 1979, vol 9, pp 79–88.

63. Fowler NO, McCall D, Chou TC, et al: Electrocardiographic changes and cardiac arrhythmias in patients receiving psychotropic drugs. *Am J Cardiol* 37:223–230, 1976.

64. Inversen LL: Dopamine receptors in the brain. *Science* 188:1084–1089, 1975.

65. Ayd FJ: A survey of drug-induced extrapyramidal reactions. *JAMA* 175:102–108, 1961.

66. Appleton WS: Psychoactive drugs: A usage guide. *Dis Nerv Syst* 32:607–616, 1971.

67. Fann WE, Davis JM, Janowsky DS: The prevalence of tardive dyskinesias in mental hospital patients. *Dis Nerv Syst* 331:182–186, 1972.

68. Siede H, Miller HF: Choreiform movements as side effects of phenothiazide medication in geriatric patients. *J Am Geriatr Soc* 15:517–522, 1967.

69. Greenblatt DL: Phenothiazine induced dyskinesia in nursing home patients. *J Am Geriatr Soc* 16:27–34, 1968.

CHAPTER 41

Pulmonary, Anti-Inflammatory, and Anti-Coagulant Medications

MICHAEL MYERS, R.PH.
JOHN R. WALSH, M.D.

Pulmonary Medications

Beta-Adrenergic Agents

Beta-adrenergic agonists are commonly prescribed for the treatment of airway disorders in elderly persons. Information from the few studies available suggests that the activity of beta agonists declines with age. The dose of isoproterenol that is required to raise the resting heart rate by 25 beats per minute increases with age,[1] which suggests a diminished responsiveness of beta adrenoceptors in elderly persons. If cardiovascular beta receptors undergo age-related changes, it is possible that pulmonary beta receptors also decrease in quantity or sensitivity. Variable responses were observed to inhaled salbutamol, known as albuterol in the United States, and to ipratropium in 29 asthmatic patients.[2] Albuterol was the most effective brochodilator in the majority of the patients studied. Of 15 patient characteristics, including the type of asthma, smoking history, concurrent medications, and pulmonary function results, age was the only significant discriminatory factor in achieving a maximal response to albuterol. All patients having a maximal response to albuterol were less than 40 years of age, which again shows a decreased response to beta-adrenergic agonists with increasing age.[1] The anticholinergic agent, ipratropium, produced less bronchodilation than albuterol in younger patients; however, the magnitude of the response was consistent with increasing age and equaled or exceeded the response to albu-

terol in some older patients. These studies have important implications for the treatment of elderly patients who require bronchodilators. In some patients, bronchodilators with different mechanisms of action may be needed in addition to, or in place of, the beta-adrenergic agents.

Theophylline

Theophylline and its salts constitute a major treatment regimen for bronchospastic diseases. Theophylline acts by inhibiting the enzyme phosphodiesterase, which converts cyclic adenosine monophosphate (cAMP) into an inactive form. Thus, cellular levels of cAMP are increased by theophylline. A wide variety of pharmacologic responses are produced by theophylline, which include central nervous system stimulation, cardiac stimulation, dilatation of coronary, pulmonary, and general systemic vessels, skeletal muscle stimulation, and diuresis. The clinical use of theophylline is primarily as a brochodilator due to its ability to relax smooth muscle.

Theophylline and its salts are well absorbed from the gastrointestinal tract. Peak levels from liquid or uncoated tablets are reached after approximately 1 hour. When taken with food, theophylline absorption may be delayed, but it is still complete. Rectal absorption from suppositories is erratic and incomplete, while rectal solutions of theophylline have an absorption similar to the oral route and are the preferred rectal method of administration.[3] The extremely alkaline pH (>9.5) level of aminophylline makes an intramuscular injection painful and delays absorption from the injection site.

Following absorption, theophylline is distributed throughout most body tissues, except fat. The volume of distribution averages 0.45 liters/kg and is unaffected by most factors that affect theophylline clearance.

Approximately 90% of theophylline is metabolized in the liver by oxidation and 1-demethylation.[3] The average elimination half-life for theophylline in adults is approximately 7–8 hours; however, this value may vary widely. Many factors will alter the theophylline clearance and elimination half-life in a given individual.

Cigarette smoking can have a marked effect on theophylline clearance. Substances in cigarette smoke induce hepatic enzymes that metabolize theophylline, which results in an increased theophylline clearance and decreased elimination half-life.[4] The theophylline half-life in young adult smokers averaged 4.3 and 4.1 hours in two studies.[3] The effect that smoking has on theophylline clearance in elderly persons is less clear-cut. Elderly persons are less responsive to the enzyme-inducing effects of smoking[5]; however, two studies have shown an increased theophylline clearance in elderly smokers.[6,7]

Diseases such as congestive heart failure, hepatic cirrhosis, and severe airway obstruction all are associated with a decreased theophylline clearance. Theophylline elimination half-lives of 3.1–82 hours have been reported in patients with acute pulmonary edema and 10.4–56 hours in cirrhotic patients.[3]

Aging also appears to affect theophylline clearance, but conflicting data exists. No age-related differences in theophylline pharmacokinetics were found in three studies.[6–9] However, when the values for unbound theophylline were compared, the apparent volume of distribution and plasma clearance were reduced in elderly persons by 37% and 30%, respectively. In addition, the unbound theophylline level was significantly higher in elderly persons. A study of the excretion of theophylline metabolites showed that the elderly age group had a 37% decrease in clearance by N-1-demethylation and a 20% decrease in clearance by oxidative pathways.[8] These data suggest that the hepatic

metabolism of theophylline is decreased in elderly persons.

Drug interactions also can alter theophylline pharmacokinetics. Both cimetidine and erythromycin inhibit the hepatic metabolism of theophylline and lead to higher serum theophylline levels.[10,11] Influenza vaccination also appears to decrease the theophylline elimination rate with half-lives increasing by an average of 122% after vaccination.[12] These interactions can lead to serious theophylline toxicity and require close monitoring.

Theophylline exemplifies a drug with a narrow therapeutic index by producing toxicity at blood levels close to those that are needed for a therapeutic effect. As might be predicted from the variety of organ systems affected by theophylline, the manifestations of theophylline toxicity are diverse. Toxicity is closely related to the theophylline serum concentration. Most adverse reactions occur at levels greater than 20 μg/ml, although they may occur at lower levels in some patients. Tachycardia, nausea, vomiting, headache, irritability, and insomnia generally occur at the lower end of the toxic range. Higher levels have resulted in seizures, brain damage, cardiac arrhythmias, and death. Rapid intravenous (IV) administration, especially through a central venous catheter can expose the heart to extremely high concentrations and can lead to cardiac arrhythmias and death. It is important to note that the relationship between the theophylline serum level and the toxic symptoms is not absolute. Some patients have developed seizures without experiencing previous minor symptoms.[13] Obviously, administering doses of theophylline based on the development of a minor toxicity as a therapeutic end-point is irrational and risky. Only the use of plasma theophylline measurements can give a physician an accurate assessment of a patient's theophylline pharmacokinetics and determine if the serum level is within the safe range.

A number of dosage nomograms or guidelines for theophylline have been published to aid in determining a maintenance dose.[14–17] A continuous IV infusion of aminophylline is recommended to provide a constant serum level and to make the interpretation of serum levels easier. For elderly patients, an initial maintenance infusion rate of 0.3–0.6 mg/kg/hour is suggested. If diseases such as congestive heart failure or liver disease are present or a patient is taking drugs such as cimetidine or erythromycin, the maintenance dose should be reduced even further to a range of 0.2–0.4 mg/kg/hour. If a patient has been taking sustained-release theophylline preparations before starting IV aminophylline therapy, the maintenance dose should be lowered for the first 12–24 hours, since the oral theophylline will continue to be absorbed. Theophylline serum level measurements should be used to adjust the dosage to provide serum levels between 10–20 μg/ml. At this point, two approaches are available for monitoring serum levels. The first approach is to wait until a steady state has been achieved and to draw a single serum level. A patient's theophylline clearance can be calculated and used to make any dosage adjustment.[3] The drawback to this method is that a steady state will not be reached until 4–5 half-lives, which may be 24 hours (or longer if a patient has a prolonged elimination half-life). A second option is the use of two serum levels before achieving a steady state to estimate the theophylline clearance rate.[18,19] This method can estimate the theophylline clearance and the eventual steady-state serum level as soon as 6 hours after initiating therapy. Unfortunately, this method will not work for patients who have recently taken sustained-release theophylline preparations.

When starting oral therapy, the same guidelines may be used; however, the dose must be adjusted for theophylline content. In addition to anhydrous theophylline, a wide variety of theophylline salts are used to formulate oral theophylline products. The theophylline content of these commonly used products is listed in Table 41-1. Aminophylline contains 80% theophylline; therefore, the suggested aminophylline dose of 0.4–0.6 mg/kg/hour converts to 0.32–0.48 mg/kg/hour of anhydrous theophylline or 0.5–0.75 mg/kg/hour of oxtriphylline. These doses should be based on the lean body weight in obese patients.

The dosage interval is determined by the theophylline elimination half-life and the type of preparation that is chosen. Patients with short theophylline elimination half-lives must take the drug more often to avoid large fluctuations between peak serum levels and trough serum levels, while patients with longer half-lives can take it less often. The product formulation also affects the dosing interval, since sustained-release preparations can be given less often than the regular tablets or liquid preparations. Most sustained-release products will maintain therapeutic serum levels for 8–12 hours. Few geriatric patients should ever need to take a sustained-release product more often than every 8 hours.

Once the dosage form and formulation have been chosen, the dose can be determined by:

$$\text{DOSE} = (\text{mg/hour of theophylline/}F) \times \text{Dosing interval}$$

Where F = the percentage of theophylline/100 and the dosing interval is in hours. When converting from a continuous aminophylline infusion to a sustained-release anhydrous theophylline product, such as Theodur, the dose to be given every 12 hours can be quickly estimated by multiplying the hourly dose of aminophylline by 10.[20] For example, a patient who is receiving 40 mg/hour of aminophylline should achieve comparable serum levels when given 400 mg of Theodur every 12 hours.

Patients who have difficulty in swallowing or who are receiving oral therapy via a nasogastric tube will not tolerate sustained-release products. It is important to educate a patient's family or the nursing staff to not crush sustained-released products, as this may cause alternating excessive and subtherapeutic serum levels.

TABLE 41-1 Theophylline Content of Common Theophylline Salts

Drug	Theophylline (%)	Example Product
Anhydrous theophylline	100	Theodur, Theolair
Aminophylline	80	Aminodur
Theophylline monoethanolamine	75	Fleet's theophylline
Oxtriphylline	64	Choledyl
Theophylline calcium salicylate	48	Quadrinal

Some patients will be able to take the pellets from a sustained-release capsule, such as Slophyllin gyrocaps or Theodur Sprinkles, mixed with food; however, many patients will need a liquid preparation. When changing from a solid dosage form to a liquid theophylline product, it is important to make certain that the salt form is the same (and make the appropriate dosage adjustment if it is not) and that the dosing interval is appropriate to the new formulation. Finally, many liquid preparations, such as Elixophyllin, are elixers that contain significant amounts of ethanol. Possible contraindications to ethanol should be reviewed and a non-alcoholic product chosen if necessary.

Antiarthritic Drugs

Aspirin

Aspirin, which is a widely used drug for elderly persons, is customarily used in large doses for the treatment of arthritis and in low doses for its antiplatelet activity in preventing transient ischemic attacks (TIAs). The adverse effects of aspirin may produce serious problems in elderly persons. Aspirin, even in small doses, may prolong bleeding time and cause gastric erosions with bleeding. In addition, low doses of aspirin modifies platelet aggregation, thereby interfering with thrombus formation. Aspirin abolishes both platelet and endothelial cyclo-oxygenase (Fig. 41-1) by irreversible acetylation in doses as low as 160 mg, orally. The resulting inhibition of endoperoxides and thromboxane A_2 synthesis[21] interferes with platelet aggregation and subsequently prolongs bleeding time. The effect lasts as long as the platelet survives (9–13 days). Prostacyclin that is produced by blood vessel walls is a strong vasodilator and an inhibiter of platelet aggregation. Aspirin inhibits prostacyclin formation, but at a higher dose than that needed to suppress thromboxane A_2. The platelet cyclo-oxygenase appears to be more sensitive to aspirin inhibition than the enzyme from the vessel wall, and cyclo-oxygenase in vessel walls recovers from the inhibitory effect of aspirin within 24 hours. For its antiplatelet effect, one tablet of aspirin (320 mg) usually is given once daily. This is a greater dose than needed, but it is an easy regimen to adhere to.

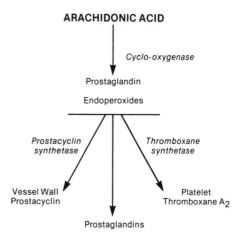

FIGURE 41-1 Prostaglandin synthesis. Aspirin irreversibly inhibits cyclo-oxygenase by acetylation.

Aspirin is considered to be the treatment of choice for arthritis. An anti-inflammatory effect requires doses that are high enough to yield serum salicylate levels in the range of 20–30 mg/dl. This effect is achieved in young adults by administering 12–16 (320 mg) tablets per day divided into four doses. Therapy in elderly patients, however, should be initiated at a lower dose; approximately two 320-mg tablets four times per day with meals and with a snack at bedtime. Upward adjustments in increments of one to two tablets per day are prescribed until a patient has obtained symptomatic relief or develops toxicity. Tinnitus, which is a common complaint of younger patients who have serum levels greater than 30 mg/dl, often does not develop in elderly persons because of a sensorineural hearing loss. Therefore, salicylate serum levels should be used as a more reliable method of monitoring aspirin therapy in older persons. Enteric-coated aspirin has less of a risk of gastrointestinal erosion and bleeding compared to ordinary aspirin, and it may be used in patients who are unable to tolerate regular aspirin.

Non-Steroidal Anti-Inflammatory Drugs (NSAIDs)

These are a heterogenous group of drugs possessing similar pharmacologic effects that include significant analgesic, antipyretic, and anti-inflammatory properties. These drugs include the following:

1. Propionic acid derivatives (ibuprofen, fenoprofen, naproxen);
2. Indoleacetic acid derivatives (indomethacin, sulindac, tolmetin); and
3. Fenamates (meclofenamate).

Adverse reactions are similar to those of salicylates, but some are unique to this group of drugs. Gastrointestinal side effects with dyspepsia, nausea, diarrhea, ulcers, and hemorrhage may occur. These agents should not be used in patients with known active peptic ulcer disease. Central nervous system symptoms of somnolence, dizziness, tinnitus, tremor, and confusion usually are mild, but if bothersome, then the drug should be discontinued. Fluid and sodium retention are found with all NSAIDs. Edema may be more overt in elderly patients with congestive heart failure or with lowered renal reserve. NSAIDs can decrease the glomerular filtration rate (GFR), and produce volume retention that is resistant to diuretics,[22] hyponatremia due to an increased renal sensitivity to an antidiuretic hormone (ADH),[23] hyporeninemic hypoaldosteronism with hyperkalemia,[24] aggravation of pre-existing hypertension, and resistance to antihypertensive drugs.[25] The NSAIDs can cause a deterioration of renal function through several mechanisms. Prostaglandins regulate renal blood flow, by means of vasodilatation or vasoconstriction, via enhancing sodium and water excretion and renin secretion. The NSAIDs act by inhibiting renal prostaglandin synthesis[26,27] through interfering with the enzyme cyclo-oxygenase, which increases vasoconstriction, and decreases renal blood flow and the GFR. The NSAIDs also cause nephrotoxicity that is unrelated to prostaglandins, thus producing allergic interstitial nephritis or chronic interstitial nephritis with papillary necrosis. Functional renal insufficiency without proteinuria is the most common adverse nephrotoxic effect that involves, perhaps, 10–20% of all elderly patients. Prerenal azotemia and acute renal failure may result.[28] Massive proteinuria and a nephrotic syndrome has been reported after the administration of fenoprofen, naproxen, and indomethacin.[29–31] All NSAIDs inhibit platelet aggregation through an inhibition of prostaglandin synthesis, leading to increased bleeding time, and the potential to cause bleeding problems in patients with hematologic disorders. Contrary to the effect of aspirin, the inhibition of platelet aggregation with ibuprofen is short-lived; it lasts only while the drug is present (approximately 24 hours).

A cognitive dysfunction manifested by memory loss, inability to concentrate, confusion, and personality change has been reported in patients over 65 years of age who have received either naproxen or ibuprofen.[32]

Cimetidine

Cimetidine is a histamine H-2-receptor antagonist that is used primarily to decrease gastric acid secretion. Although widely used, it is not an entirely benign drug in elderly persons. About 75% of cimetidine is excreted unchanged in the urine and 19% is converted to the sulfoxide metabolite in the liver. Cimetidine has an increased half-life in elderly patients due to the age-related renal changes that diminish the excretion of the drug and, consequently, increases blood levels of cimetidine.[33,34] The administration of a full dose of cimetidine to elderly patients frequently will provoke a confusional state. Patients with an impaired renal function are predisposed to cimetidine-associated central nervous system symptoms that include confusion, delirium, drowsiness, dizziness, slurred speech, agitation, and hallucinations.[35,36] Mental status changes usually occur within 48 hours after the initial dose.[36] Symptoms appear to be dose-related and subside after discontinuing the drug, decreasing the dose, or lengthening the dosing interval. In most patients, mental symptoms improve in 24–48 hours after lowering the dose or stopping the drug.

The usual dose regimen for cimetidine is 300 mg every 6 hours in patients with normal renal function. Lower doses are indicated for patients with renal impairment (see Table 41-2). The half-life of the drug almost doubles as the creatinine clearance (Ccr) is reduced below 50 ml/minute, from 1.5 hours in normal persons to 2.89 hours in persons with moderate renal failure.[33] A Ccr value below this level is usual in elderly people who are considered to have a "normal" renal function.

Mental disturbances have been reported in patients with associated renal and liver im-

TABLE 41-2 Dose of Cimetidine with Renal Impairment

Renal Function	Creatinine Clearance (ml/min)	Regimen
Normal	100	300 mg q6h
Mild renal failure	50–100	300 mg q6h
Moderate renal failure	20–50	300 mg q8h
Severe renal failure	0–20	300 mg q12h

pairment.[36] An impaired hepatic function is another predisposing factor for cimetidine-induced mental problems. A clinician should always consider the possibility of a cimetidine-induced mental change in any patient with renal or hepatic impairment who is confused. Furthermore, initiating cimetidine therapy in older patients always should be done with lower dosage levels to avoid this problem.

Several clinically significant drug interactions have been reported with cimetidine. Cimetidine inhibits hepatic microsomal drug metabolism, which reduces the clearance of warfarin,[37] phenytoin,[38] theophylline,[11,39,40] diazepam,[41] and chlordiazepoxide[42] from the body. Propranolol clearance is reduced by cimetidine via an inhibition of hepatic enzymes and a reduction of hepatic blood flow.[43] The consequence of the interaction of cimetidine with each of these drugs is to increase the blood level and activity of the drug. Because these drugs frequently are used in elderly persons and have narrow therapeutic indexes, concurrent administration with cimetidine may cause adverse effects.

Useful guidelines for the use of cimetidine in elderly persons are (modified from Jenike)[44]:

1. Use a lower dosage, because of a decreased renal clearance of cimetidine in elderly persons.
2. Be alert for neuropsychiatric changes:
   a. If an elderly patient becomes confused, stop cimetidine;
   b. Consider a trial of physostigmine if clinically indicated.
3. Decrease dosages of other drugs that are known to be potentiated by cimetidine (especially phenytoin, diazepam, chlordiazepoxide, warfarin, and theophylline). Observe phenytoin blood levels and prothrombin

time closely when cimetidine is added to the regimen.
4. Oxazepam or lorazepam are unaffected by cimetidine and are preferable if a benzodiazepine is indicated.
5. Lower doses of cimetidine are indicated for patients with renal failure.

Warfarin Anticoagulation Therapy

Warfarin, which is a coumarin derivative, produces its anticoagulant effect by interfering with clotting factors II, VII, IX, and X (Vitamin K-dependent coagulation factors) in the liver. Vitamin K is a cofactor for the carboxylation of glutamic acid residues of these factors. Oral anticoagulants interfere with the carboxylation that is essential for calcium binding, thereby producing biologically inactive factors. The onset of anticoagulation with warfarin is delayed until pre-existing Vitamin K-dependent factors are cleared from the circulation. The activity of factor VII (whose half-life is approximately 5 hours, falls rapidly after initiating warfarin therapy), whereas factors II, IX, and X (the most important factors for antithrombotic effect) fall slowly over 3–4 days. The early decrease in factor VII produces a prolongation of the prothrombin time, but there actually is little antithrombotic effect. A decrease in the levels of factors II, IX, and X occur at similar rates whether a large loading dose or smaller therapeutic doses are given.

For early anticoagulation, it is standard practice to give an IV bolus of heparin followed by continuous infusion for 7–10 days. Oral anticoagulation with warfarin is started on the fifth day, thus overlapping with heparin therapy for at least 3 days to insure good antithrombotic effect. Another reason for overlapping warfarin with heparin therapy is to provide anticoagulant coverage during a time that antithrombin III levels may be low following heparin therapy.

Warfarin is well absorbed from the gastrointestinal tract. It is extensively bound to albumin (98%), although there is a great interindividual variation in the bound and free fractions of warfarin that is caused by a diminished serum albumin or displacement from protein-binding sites by other drugs that may produce a considerable increase in the prothrombin time. Patients over 70 years of age often show an excessive anticoagulant effect.[45,46] Elderly patients appear to be more sensitive to the anticoagulation effect of warfarin and frequently require lower doses to produce comparable degrees of anticoagulation compared to younger adults.[47] Therefore, they have a greater risk of bleeding. The cause of this age-related sensitivity to warfarin is unclear. Diminished serum albumin concentrations that sometimes are found in older patients may cause a diminished protein binding to partly explain this sensitivity.

Pharmacokinetics are unchanged in elderly persons.[45,48] At the same plasma warfarin concentrations, there is a greater inhibition of Vitamin K-dependent-clotting factor synthesis in elderly persons.[45] Yet, plasma half-life (20–40 hours), volume of distribution, plasma clearance, and plasma protein binding are similar to younger adults.[45,48]

While it has been traditional to continue oral anticoagulants for a period of 3–6 months, there still is uncertainty about the duration of therapy following a major thromboembolic event. The evidence indicates that such patients are at high risk for a recurrence for 3 months,[49,50] but recurrences are encountered frequently enough up to 6 months to warrant continuation of anticoagulation.[50,51] It still is a reasonable assumption that high-risk patients with coexisting congestive heart failure, venous insufficiency of the lower extremities, or who are undergoing prolonged immobilization, should receive anticoagulant drugs for longer periods of time. Conversely, elderly patients with only a calf-vein thrombosis may be given warfarin therapy for a minimum of 6 weeks.[51] Subcutaneous heparin given every 12 hours in a dose that is adjusted to prolong the midinterval partial thromboplastin time to 1.5 times the control value is as effective as warfarin in preventing a thromboembolism.[50] Heparin therapy, however, is more expensive, requires parenteral administration, and may uncommonly produce thrombocytopenia and osteoporosis as a side effect.

The therapeutic goal of warfarin therapy is to maintain the prothrombin time at 2–2.5 times that of normal, although it is known that a thrombosis occurs less frequently in more intensely treated patients. However, the frequency of bleeding is noted to be considerably higher with prothrombin times that are greater

TABLE 41-3 Drugs That Interact with Oral Anticoagulants

Increased Anticoagulant Effect		Decreased Anticoagulant Effect	
Drug	Mechanism	Drug	Mechanism
Nortryptyline	Increased absorption	Cholestyramine	Decreased absorption
Allopurinol Cimetidine Disulfiram Acute alcoholism	Decreased metabolism	Barbiturates Chronic alcoholism	Increased metabolism Increased metabolism
Sulfonamides Phenylbutazone Salicylates > 3 g/day	Displacement from protein-binding sites		
Antibiotics	Displacement from protein-binding sites, Vitamin K synthesis inhibition by bacteria		

than 2.5 times the control levels. There is an increased risk of bleeding, especially in elderly females, patients with liver disease, and older persons with a Vitamin K deficiency. High-risk patients who have undergone recent surgery or trauma may have major bleeding episodes, even when coagulation levels are within therapeutic ranges. With a prothrombin time in the therapeutic range, a clinician should always consider an underlying disease as a cause for bleeding, particularly if either gastrointestinal or urinary tract bleeding occurs. Conversely, if the prothrombin time is remarkably prolonged, bleeding can occur in the absence of a local lesion. Patients with hypertension or a recent cerebral infarction are at an increased risk for a central nervous system hemorrhage. A subdural hematoma is a common complication in patients on long-term anticoagulant therapy.

Older persons who are receiving several drugs are at greater risk for drug interactions that may lead to enhanced or diminished effects of warfarin (*see* Table 41-3).

References

1. Vestal RE, Wood AJJ, Shand DG: Reduced B-adrenoceptor sensitivity in the elderly. *Clin Pharmacol Ther* 26:181–186, 1979.
2. Ullah MI, Newman GB, Saunders KB: Influence of age on response to ipratropium and salbutamol in asthma. *Thorax* 36:523–529, 1981.
3. Hendeles L, Weinberger M, Johnson G: Theophylline, in Evans W, Schentag JJ, Jusko W (eds): *Applied Pharmacokinetics: Principles of Therapeutic Drug Monitoring.* San Francisco, Applied Therapeutics, Inc, 1980, pp 95–138.
4. Ogilvie RI: Smoking and theophylline dose schedules. *Ann Int Med* 88:263–264, 1978.
5. Vestal RE, Wood AJJ: Influence of age and smoking on drug kinetics in man. *Clin Pharmacokinet* 5:309–319, 1980.
6. Bauer LA, Blouin RA: Influence of age on theophylline clearance in patients with chronic obstructive pulmonary disease. *Clin Pharmacokinet* 6:469–474, 1981.
7. Cusack B, Kelly JG, Lavan J, et al: Theophylline kinetics in relation to age: The importance of smoking. *Br J Clin Pharmacol* 10:109–114, 1980.
8. Antal EJ, Kramer PA, Merick SA, et al: Theophylline pharmacokinetics in advanced age. *Br J Clin Pharmacol* 12:637–645, 1981.
9. Talseth T, Boye NP, Kongerud J, et al: Aging, cigarette smoking and oral theophylline requirement. *Eur J Clin Pharmacol* 21:33–37, 1981.
10. May DC, Jarboe CH, Ellenburg DT, et al: The effects of erythromycin on theophylline elimination in normal males. *J Clin Pharmacol* 8:263–264, 1982.
11. Reitberg DP, Bernhard H, Schentag JJ: Alteration of theophylline clearance and half-life by cimetidine in normal volunteers. *Ann Int Med* 95:582–585, 1981.
12. Renton KW, Gray JD, Hall RI: Decreased elimination of theophylline after influenza vaccination. *CMA Journal* 123:288–290, 1980.
13. Zwillich CW, Sutton FD, Neff TA, et al: Theophylline–induced seizures in adults. *Ann Int Med* 82:784–787, 1975.
14. Talseth T, Kornstad S, Boye NP, et al: Individualization of oral theophylline dosage in elderly patients. *Acta Med Scand* 210:489–492, 1981.
15. Anonymous: IV dosage guidelines for theophylline products. *FDA Drug Bull* 10:4–6, 1980.
16. Jusko WJ, Koup JR, Vance JW, et al: Intravenous theophylline therapy: Nomogram guidelines. *Ann Int Med* 86:400–404, 1977.
17. Powell JR, Jackson JE: Counterpoint discussion: Theophylline, in Evans W, Schentag JJ, Jusko W (eds): *Applied Pharmacokinetics: Principles of Therapeutic Drug Monitoring.* San Francisco, Applied Therapeutics, Inc, 1980, pp 139–166.
18. Anderson G, Koup J, Slaughter R, et al: Evaluation of two methods for estimating theophylline clearance prior to achieving steady state. *Ther Drug Mon* 18:473–477, 1981.
19. Vozeth S, Kewitz G, Wenk M, et al: Rapid prediction of steady-state serum theophylline concentration in patients treated with intravenous aminophylline. *Eur J Clin Pharmacol* 18:473–477, 1980.
20. Wightkin WT, Buchhammer CR: A simple method for intravenous-to-oral theophylline dose conversion. *Clin Pharm* 1:300–301, 1982.
21. Moncada S, Vane JR: Arachidonic acid metabolites and the interactions between platelets and blood-vessel walls. *N Engl J Med* 300:1142–1147, 1979.
22. Smith DE, Brater DC, Lin ET, et al: Attenuation of Furosemides' diuretic effect by indomethacin: Pharmacokinetic evaluation. *J Pharmacokinet Reopharm* 7:265–274, 1979.
23. Gross PA, Schrier RW, Anderson RJ: Prostaglandins and water metabolism: A review with emphasis on *in vivo* studies. *Kidney Int* 19:839–850, 1981.
24. Tan SY, Shapiro R, Franco R, et al: Indometha-

cin-induced prostaglandin inhibition with hyperkalemia: A reversible cause of hyporenimic hypoaldosteronism. *Ann Int Med* 90:783–785, 1979.

25. Romero JC, Beierwalter WH: Renal prostaglandins in hypertension. *Min Electrol Metab* 6:90–104, 1981.

26. Kimberley RP, Bowden RE, Keiser HR, et al: Reduction of renal function by newer nonsteroidal anti-inflammatory drugs. *Am J Med* 64:804–807, 1978.

27. McCarthy JT, Tones VE, Romero JC, et al: Acute intrinsic renal failure induced by indomethacin: Role of prostaglandin synthetase inhibition. *Mayo Clin Proc* 57:289–296, 1982.

28. Torres VE: Present and future of the nonsteroidal anti-inflammatory drugs in nephrology. *Mayo Clin Proc* 57:389–393, 1982.

29. Finkelstein A, Fraley DS, Stachura I, et al: Fenoprofen nephropathy: Lipoid nephrosis and interstitial nephritis. *Am J Med* 72:81–87, 1982.

30. Brezin JH, Katz SM, Schwartz AB, et al: Reversible renal failure and nephrotic syndrome associated with non-steroidal anti-inflammatory drugs. *N Engl J Med* 301:1271–1273, 1980.

31. Brandsetter RD, Mar DD: Reversible oliguric renal failure associated with ibuprofen treatment. *Br Med J* 2:1194–1195, 1978.

32. Goodwin JS, Regan M: Cognitive dysfunction associated with naproxen and ibuprofen in the elderly. *Arth Rheum* 25:1013–1014, 1982.

33. Ma KW, Brown DC, Masler DS, et al: Effects of renal failure on blood levels of cimetidine. *Gastroenterology* 74:473–476, 1978.

34. Drayer DE, Romankiewiaz J, Lorenzo B, et al: Age and renal clearance of cimetidine. *Clin Pharmacol Ther* 31:45–50, 1982.

35. McGuigan JE: A consideration of the adverse effects of cimetidine. *Gastroenterology* 80:181–192, 1981.

36. Schentag JJ, Cena FB, Calleri G, et al: Pharmacokinetic and clinical studies in patients with cimetidine-associated mental confusion. *Lancet* 1:177–181, 1979.

37. Silver BA, Bell WR: Cimetidine potentiation of the hypoprothrombinemic effect of warfarin. *Ann Int Med* 90:348–349, 1979.

38. Hetzel DJ: Cimetidine-phenytoin interaction. *Br Med J* 282:1512, 1981.

39. Roberts RK, Grice J, Wood L, et al: Cimetidine impairs the elimination of theophylline and antipyrine. *Gastroenterology* 81:19–21, 1981.

40. Weinberger MM, Smith G, Milavetz G, et al: Decreased theophylline clearance due to cimetidine. *N Engl J Med* 304:672, 1981.

41. Klotz U, Reimann I: Delayed clearance of diazepam due to cimetidine. *N Engl J Med* 302:1012–1014, 1980.

42. Desmond PV, Patwardhan RV, Schenker S, et al: Cimetidine impairs elimination of chlordiazepoxide (librium) in man. *Ann Int Med* 93:266–268, 1980.

43. Feely J, Wilkinson GR, Wood AJ: Reduction of liver blood flow and propranolol metabolism by cimetidine. *Ann Int Med* 93:266–268, 1980.

44. Jenike MA: Cimetidine in elderly patients. Review of uses and risks. *J Am Geriatr Soc* 30:170–173, 1982.

45. Shepherd AMM, Hewick DS, Morland TA, et al: Age as a determinant of sensitivity to warfarin. *Br J Clin Pharmacol* 4:315–320, 1977.

46. O'Malley K, Stevenson IH, Ward CA, et al: Determinants of anticoagulant control in patients receiving warfarin. *Br J Clin Pharmacol* 4:309–314, 1977.

47. Routledge PA, Chapman PA, Davies DM, et al: Factors affecting warfarin requirements. *Eur J Clin Pharmacol* 15:319–322, 1979.

48. Hotraphinyo K, Triggs EJ, Maybloom B, et al: Warfarin sodium: Steady state plasma levels and patient age. *Clin Exp Pharmacol Physiol* 5:143–149, 1978.

49. Coon WW, Willus PW III: Recurrence of venous thromboembolism. *Surgery* 73:823–827, 1973.

50. Hull R, Delmore T, Carter C, et al: Adjusted subcutaneous heparin versus warfarin sodium in the long term treatment of venous thrombosis. *N Engl J Med* 306:189–194, 1982.

51. Hull RB, Delmoret L, Genton E, et al: Warfarin sodium versus low dose heparin in the long-term treatment of venous thrombosis. *N Engl J Med* 301:855–858, 1979.

Index

All page numbers in italic refer to Volume II.